Introduction		iv
Unit 1	**Equal opportunities and clients' rights**	1
	1.1 Promoting equality in care practice	2
	1.2 Legislation, policies and codes of practice for promoting equality	4
	1.3 How care organisations promote equality	6
	1.4 The effects of discriminatory practices on individuals	8
	1.5 Organisations that challenge discrimination	10
	OHTs	13
	Activities	26
Unit 2	**Communicating in health and social care**	33
	2.1 Types of interaction	34
	2.2 Effective communication	36
	2.3 Communication skills in groups	38
	2.4 Evaluating communication skills	41
	2.5 Maintaining client confidentiality	42
	OHTs	48
	Activities	58
Unit 3	**Physical aspects of health**	67
	3.1 Physiology and anatomy	68
	3.2 Homeostasis	70
	3.3 Physiological measurements of individuals in care settings	70
	3.4 Safe practice	72
	3.5 Analysis and accuracy of results	72
	OHTs	77
	Activities	83
Unit 4	**Factors affecting human development and growth**	97
	4.1 Human development	97
	4.2 Development of skills and abilities	97
	4.3 Factors affecting development	99
	4.4 Theories of human development	102
	OHTs	105
	Activities	121
Unit 5	**Health, social care and early years services**	130
	5.1 Origins and development of services	130
	5.2 National and local provision of services	131
	5.3 Informal carers	132
	5.4 The funding of services	133
	5.5 The effects of government policies on services	134
	5.6 Access to services	134
	OHTs	137
	Activities	160
Unit 6	**Research perspectives in health and social care**	172
	6.1 The purpose of research in health and social care	172
	6.2 Research methods	174
	6.3 Planning research, methods of analysis and validation	174
	6.4 Presenting research	175
	6.5 Ethical issues	176
	OHTs	179
	Activities	206

INTRODUCTION

THE AIMS OF THE TUTOR RESOURCE FILE

This file will provide a useful resource to complement the AVCE textbook. Like the textbook, the file is designed in six chapters which cover the compulsory units of the Curriculum 2000 National Standards. These six compulsory units form the core of the different vocational A-level awards that are offered by all awarding bodies. The file aims to complement the textbook by:

- providing additional advice and information relevant to the national standards
- providing advice and guidance on the organisation of the learning experience for students
- providing a range of practical activities which can be adapted to suit the needs of different learners
- providing a range of handouts and/or overhead transparencies which may assist students to engage with the learning process during each unit.

The file aims to provide a resource for teachers, but it is not intended to be a definitive open learning manual. Teaching activities and exercises within this pack will need to be adapted if the needs of individual students, as well as the needs of different groups of students across the country, are to be met.

THE AVCE IN HEALTH AND SOCIAL CARE

The AVCE replaces the Advanced GNVQ which preceded it. Like the GNVQ, this new qualification enables students to explore the health and social care sector. The AVCE also enables students to gain a qualification at level 3 of the National Qualifications Framework that will assist progression to a career in health or care work.

The AVCE is designed to offer a greater range of flexibility than the GNVQ. Students may take a three-unit part award, a six-unit single award, or a twelve-unit full award. In this way students may explore the health and social care sector and career opportunities that may exist within this sector, without losing the flexibility to explore other academic or occupational qualifications.

One-third of the AVCE is externally assessed, including both compulsory and optional units. Both Units 1 and 4 are currently externally assessed. It is likely that there will be several rounds of testing before tests settle into a predictable and reliable format. Initially, past tests may not provide reliable guidance for students as to what they may expect. In time, past tests are likely to provide a sound guide for revision.

THE STRUCTURE OF THE AVCE

Students must complete all six of the compulsory units if they take the full twelve-unit award. The single award may consist of four compulsory units and two optional units. The part award consists of three compulsory units. Each awarding body will have their own list of optional units. The six compulsory units are:

Unit 1 Equal opportunities and clients' rights

Unit 2 Communicating in health and social care

Unit 3 Physical aspects of health

Unit 4 Factors affecting human growth and development

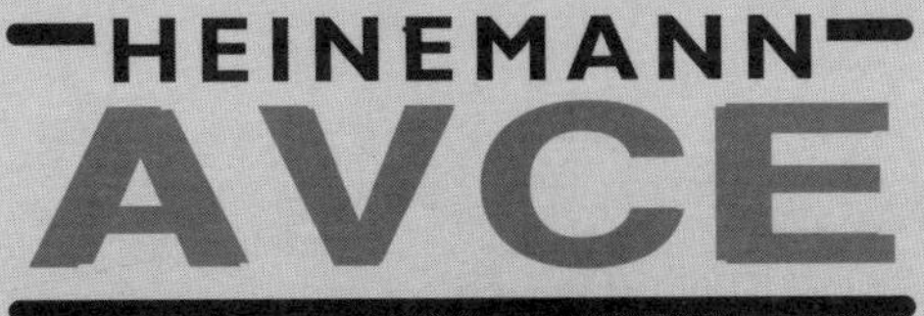

ADVANCED

Health and Social Care

Editor: Neil Moonie

TUTOR'S FILE

Heinemann Educational Publishers
Halley Court, Jordan Hill, Oxford, OX2 8EJ
a division of Reed Educational & Professional Publishing Ltd
Heinemann is a registered trademark of Reed Educational & Professional Publishing Ltd

OXFORD MELBOURNE AUCKLAND
JOHANNESBURG BLANTYRE GABORONE
IBADAN PORTSMOUTH NH (USA) CHICAGO

First published 2001

04 03 02 01
10 9 8 7 6 5 4 3 2 1

A catalogue record for this book is available from the British Library
on request

ISBN 0 435 45590 7

Typeset by TechType, Abingdon, Oxon
Printed in Great Britain by Thomson Litho Ltd, Scotland

Tel: 01865 888058 www.heinemann.co.uk

Unit 5 Health, social care and early years services

Unit 6 Research perspectives in health and social care

USING THE TEXTBOOK TO SUPPORT STUDENT LEARNING

Knowledge

This file has been designed to be used in conjunction with the student textbook. The textbook contains the essential knowledge needed for successful performance to national standards. The textbook has also been designed to stimulate reflective thinking and to assist students to develop a depth of understanding as they learn to apply new concepts to their experience.

Assessment and tests

The textbook has also been designed to offer guidance on meeting the requirements of the assessment evidence grids. Each chapter of the textbook contains a test to assist reflection or to help prepare students for external assessment.

This tutor resource file provides extensive additional advice on supporting learners to meet the demands of assessment.

The tutor resource file also builds on the content of the textbook. Activities are often linked to sections of the textbook and page numbers in the textbook are often referred to.

Differentiation

The tutor resource file has been designed to provide a range of different types of learning activity and stimulus material. For each unit there are visual diagrams or representations which may assist learners who prefer to visualise ideas. Each unit contains activities which may appeal to those learners who need to engage in practical tasks in order to make sense of new ideas. Many tasks involve discussion and this may appeal to the developing social skills of health and social care students. Grids and tables have been designed to offer a structure to those students who need to anchor ideas in a simple framework.

Although there is diversity in the range of material provided, it is likely that teachers will need to make adaptations in the way activities or materials are employed in order to meet the specific needs of their own groups. Some activities might be adapted to provide learning checks within the classroom. Some OHTs might be better used as handouts with some groups. Some handouts might be adapted to be given out in stages during a lesson. Some exercises and activities should be linked with placements or visits to health and social care settings.

UNIT 1 – EQUAL OPPORTUNITIES AND CLIENTS' RIGHTS

OVERVIEW

This unit will provide students with the intellectual underpinning to good practice in health and social care. It gets to the core of the knowledge required to deliver care in a manner that is empowering to clients and respectful of their dignity and rights. By the time they complete this unit, students should have an awareness of the moral, statutory and administrative background to client rights, and the obligations these rights place on care workers in their everyday work with clients. They should understand the negative psychological, social and economic consequences of discrimination on people generally, and the effect on clients of poor practice in care work. This should be balanced with an awareness of how informed and thoughtful practice enhances the quality of clients' lives

Students should be beginning to appreciate the complexity of the care environment, and how rights and obligations of clients and workers may conflict. They should be aware of the moral as well as the practical dimensions of choices that have to be made in caring environments. They should understand the processes and mechanisms that exist to help care workers in their everyday work, and also those that will assist them to deal with more complex issues.

It will give them an understanding of the relevant issues and the statutory restraints within which care organisations operate. They should begin to understand the circumstances in which clients' rights and choices may be overruled, and should have a basic understanding of the sources of guidance and means of redress available to people who think their rights have been infringed.

This knowledge should not be compartmentalised. Students should be encouraged to make links between the different areas of the unit to promote their understanding, self-awareness and ability to apply the knowledge to real life situations. Students will be aided in this by inputs from practicing professionals and by extensive use of live material from the professional and general press. The unit covers a dynamic and fast-changing area of knowledge. By their nature, textbooks quickly become out of date and need to be supplemented by additional sources of information such as the press and the Internet. Reports about changes in the law, court judgements and tribunal findings are frequently published in the broadsheet press, and it does not take long to build up a library of cuttings suitable for use as teaching material.

This unit is organised into five sections that are numbered for ease of reference:

1.1 Promoting equality in care practice
1.2 Legislation, policies and codes of practice for promoting equality
1.3 How care organisations promote equality
1.4 The effects of discriminatory practices on individuals
1.5 Organisations that challenge discrimination

Aims and objectives

This unit covers:

- promoting equalities in care practice
- the use of the legal framework and policies for promoting equality in care work
- the effects of discriminatory practices on individuals
- the promotion of individuals' rights in health, social care and early years settings
- the sources of support and guidance for clients and care workers in promoting equal rights.

Students should be able to:

- explain how ethical issues can arise when balancing the rights of clients with the rights of others
- make judgements regarding interventions or disclosures to safeguard the rights of clients
- identify the boundaries that apply in clients' rights, including when the clients' wishes can be overruled
- explain how policies to promote clients' rights are interpreted and used in practice
- identify how levels of resourcing may influence the effectiveness of policies promoting clients' rights
- explain the key principles of current legislation to promote equality
- explain why users of care services may be particularly vulnerable to infringement of

their rights and the applications of current laws
- identify differences between the key principles of rights legislation in England, Wales, Scotland and Northern Ireland
- explain whether relevant charter standards are being achieved by examining policies and procedures in place in care settings
- identify how individuals' rights are promoted and monitored in daily practice within care settings
- explain the different ways in which discriminatory practice can affect clients' well-being
- identify the ways in which non-oppressive practice can enhance clients' self-esteem and self-worth.

TEACHING NOTES

1.1 Promoting equality in care practice

The starting point for this unit must be an understanding that there are such things as human rights, and where they come from. It is necessary to look at various documents which convey rights, such as the UN and Council of Europe Declarations, and European Union law. Students should be assisted to arrive at a consensus of basic human rights, and an understanding that granting a right to one person imposes an obligation on another. This means that rights are not always achieved in the absence of conflict. Material which would help with this includes the history of the emancipation of slaves, the struggle of women to obtain the vote and achieve equal rights in the workplace, the campaign for gay rights and the current conflict over the abolition of Section 28, and the political controversy surrounding the passing of the Human Rights Act.

Students should be encouraged to discuss issues such as: Should human beings have rights that are different from other animals and if so, why? Are rights separable from responsibilities, and can you have one without the other? Do different people have different rights, and what makes the difference? When, and to what extent, can people's rights be taken away from them? The 2 October 2000 saw the implementation of the Human Rights Act 1998, and so there is now a clear statement in UK legislation as to what human rights are.

This discussion should inevitably lead to a consideration of ethical issues. This is a particularly difficult area for students, and it may help them if they are given a very brief introduction to two different ethical systems. They could, for instance, be introduced to an absolute system of ethics, such as the Ten Commandments, and be encouraged to compare that with a utilitarian ethical system. If they have a broad understanding of different ethical positions, they should be able to identify the pitfalls of each, and recognise where different ethical systems conflict, for instance in arguments about contraception, abortion and euthanasia. When asked about ethical issues in tests, the great majority of candidates struggle to identify or explain them. They will often settle on issues of practicality and efficiency, and fail to see the underlying ethical problem. They need practice with case studies to enable them to analyse problems and extract the moral dimension.

It is important that they have practice in analysing a variety of situations to appreciate how different rights of an individual (independence/protection) and the rights of two people (choice of one person/risk to others) may conflict. Students also need to explore situations where the obligations of care workers may conflict (respecting choice/maintaining confidentiality or duty to the client/duty to employers or society). Students must understand that situations where scarcity of resources results in rationing may have an ethical dimension.

Activity 1.1.1 provides students with an ethical dilemma for them to discuss and to reach some solution. The dilemma is set out in **OHT** 1.1.3, and there is supporting material in **OHT** 1.1.1, which provides an outline of the nature of ethical dilemmas, and **OHT** 1.1.2, which outlines human rights stated in the European Convention of Human Rights. The activity can be used to cover any situation in the news to enable the use of current stories as support material.

The issues which should arise and be explored are:

- Conflicts between the rights of the parents and the state to determine who should make decisions on behalf of children.

- Conflicts between utilitarian and absolute value systems.
- Conflicts between the rights of life of both twins.
- The relevance of resource issues.
- The relevance of disability issues.

The aims of this activity are to:

- assist students to understand that ethical problems do not have straightforward solutions
- enable students to name some of the basic principles involved in ethical decision making
- prepare students, through practical work, in using principles of consistency and quality of outcome when analysing ethical dilemmas.

It is important that students have a basic understanding of issues of competence and consent. When tested, candidates often appear to believe that things can be done to people, regardless of consent, providing it is in their interests. Students must have some idea of the notion of consent, especially in relation to children, older people and people with mental disorders, and they also need to know about competence and the capacity to make decisions. They must understand the interrelationship between competence and consent, and that there has to be a statutory basis for compulsory action. An issue of competence, which many students would see as being relevant to them, would be the Gillick judgement, and what has flowed from that in terms of young people being able to consent to medical procedures. Students sometimes give the impression in tests that some groups, particularly older people, have

Notes on Activity 1.1.1

1 Students should be introduced to theories of ethics such as utilitarianism and the consistency principle (see pages 10–17 in the advanced textbook).

2 Details of the ethical problem to be analysed should be discussed with the whole student group.

3 Students might work in groups of two or three in order to make a list of the practical issues involved in the dilemma.

4 Students should also name the values and beliefs that will influence decisions. These values might include:

- The care value base and empowerment.
- Cultural and religious beliefs.
- Fairness and consistency.
- The likely consequences of any ethical decision judged in relationship to the creation of 'the greater good of humanity'.

5 Each group should identify a solution to the problem and explain how this solution links with the values listed above. Students could record their decision and then check the decision against the principles listed above.

6 The tutor should take feedback from the student group (see options below).

7 In taking a whole group feedback it will be important to emphasise that there is no simple right or wrong answer to the question and that it is the quality of analysis and thinking which is important in relation to the assessment of this unit.

Options

1 Students might be asked to write their solution on a sheet of paper and write down how their answer relates to the ethical principles before handing their work in. Answers might be pinned on a suitable board or wall space as a focus for feedback, as an alternative to taking oral feedback.

2 Students might be able to role-play a debate between different views as if they were simulating a court hearing or a case conference.

fewer rights than others, and that their wishes can be overruled if they are inconvenient or incompatible with what others see as their interests.

At this point, there is a need to introduce the legislation which allows compulsory action – Mental Health Act 1983, National Assistance Act 1948, and the Crime and Disorder Act 1998. Candidates do not need a detailed knowledge of the legislation, but do need to have a broad grasp of the situations which justify overriding the wishes of clients, i.e. when the client's interests, or the interests of others, require it. They also need to know in general terms which professionals have duties under the legislation, and what those duties are.

A number of sources of information are available to tutors, for instance *Community Care* magazine has a Practice section most weeks which analyses a situation of risk, presents arguments for and against, and provides case notes and an independent professional comment. This material will be invaluable, either given in its original form to students to help them understand the nature of ethical issues which arise in social care work, or adapted to use as case material in exercises. Within a short time it is possible to build up a library of situations – children at risk, older people and mental health – which will give a wide range of material for students to work with, and which will also give an insight into the workings of the relevant legislation.

OHTs 1.1.4, 1.1.5, 1.1.6 may be helpful in supporting the teaching on valuing diversity, the application of utilitarian principles and the logical theory of ethics.

1.2 Legislation, policies and codes of practice for promoting equality

Having introduced the subject of the law relating to overruling clients' wishes, the unit then moves on to the main body of legislation which provides client rights and promotes equality. The list in the unit is not exhaustive, and could not be as there are constant changes in legislation and the unit would already be out of date if it attempted to provide a prescriptive list. This causes problems for tutors, because textbooks become similarly outdated very quickly, and it appears to be a problem with test candidates, particularly in the area of disability, that when asked questions they tend to produce outdated answers from superseded legislation. The latest editions of general guides to the law – the *Liberty Guide to Your Rights* and the *Which? Guide to Employment* are at an appropriate level – will provide most information required about the legislation, and also include interesting case material. These, together with keeping a cuttings file from a broadsheet newspaper, should be sufficient to provide the knowledge required.

The obvious legislation to start with is that providing protection to particular groups: the Disability Discrimination Act 1995, the Race Relations Act 1976, the Sex Discrimination Act 1986 and the Equal Pay Act 1970. Much of this legislation is concerned with employment (the Equal Pay Act exclusively so) so the intention must be that these aspects will be tested, as they have been in the past. Students will need to know the outline of the legislation: the group it applies to, the contexts (i.e. employment, services, education, etc.) it applies to, and its scope (direct and indirect discrimination, harassment, etc.). Students also need to know the means of redress for people who think their rights have been infringed (employment tribunals, county courts) and, looking forward to the resources at the end of these notes, the bodies set up to exercise functions under the legislation. Candidates for testing are often very weak on stating the functions of bodies such as the Equal Opportunities Commission, the Commission for Racial Equality and the Disability Rights Commission. They will frequently give vague generalisations like 'make sure people get their rights' or 'stop discrimination' which do not convey the impression that they have any real knowledge. These bodies all have web sites where current information about their roles, responsibilities and activities can be found (see web sites on page 11).

There is a requirement to understand how the law differs in Northern Ireland. Students in England and Wales should have a cursory knowledge of the Fair Employment Act, and an understanding that, unlike the UK, Northern Ireland has primary legislation which makes discrimination on the basis of religion illegal in itself. The situation in Northern Ireland has also been changed recently by the Northern Ireland Act 1998, which merged the separate equality bodies – the CRE (NI), the EOC (NI), the Fair Employment Commission and the Disability Council – to form the Equality Commission. The Equality Commission will work alongside the Northern Ireland Human Rights Commission.

Students should be aware of the two distinct strands of European influence on domestic law, firstly through the EU which has profoundly influenced the law in relation to women's employment rights, and secondly through the Council of Europe's Convention on Human Rights. This, for instance, has provided protection against discrimination on the basis of sexuality, which was otherwise absent from domestic legislation. This knowledge will also be important later in the unit when the Council of Europe's Convention on Human Rights is explicitly mentioned. If the European dimension is not covered within the context of domestic legislation, it may be difficult to integrate later.

The law relating to discrimination has little direct impact on clients in that it is unlikely that they would use it to enforce their rights. It is important that students know about it because it does set the context in which services are provided and informs the standards of service providers. An area that tutors need to be particularly aware of is the implementation of the Human Rights Act in October 2000. This will incorporate the European Convention on Human Rights into domestic law, which will have a profound effect, not only clients' rights, but also on the way that clients can enforce them through the courts.

Discrimination is a very difficult concept for some students to use effectively. Sometimes the word is used to cover any unpleasant experience or any perceived form of injustice. It will be important to guide students to understand how the concept of discrimination should be used in care work.

Activity 1.2.1 aims to enable students to employ the concept of discrimination appropriately.

Students should be introduced to the concept of discrimination as treating some groups of people less well than others. Discrimination often involves making assumptions such as all gender, ethnic, religious and age groups should have the same needs. The idea that it is fair to 'treat everybody the same' should be challenged.

Students might be asked to identify the correct use of the term 'discrimination' in multiple choice activities such as those in Activity 1.2.1.

Options to Activity 1.2.1

Students might work in small groups to discuss their answers to the problem. Alternatively, they might be asked to work individually in order to explore their own understanding of the concept of discrimination.

It might be important to explore the reasons why we would not obviously use the concept of discrimination to classify many of the situations in the activity. Students might work in small groups in order to offer an explanation of why certain situations do not involve discrimination. Alternatively, a full explanation might be discussed with the whole student group.

It will also be important to discuss how far the law provides protection for people who experience discrimination. Students should recognise that the law provides redress for only a limited range of discriminatory situations.

The points that follow are a discussion of the issues.

Discussion of Activity 1.2.1

1 Unpleasant situations and pain do not necessarily indicate discrimination. Zoe's dentist is behaving appropriately and in her best interests.

2 Treating people differently does not necessarily indicate discrimination. The nurse is probably behaving appropriately in treating Ahmed differently because he is diabetic. The use of scissors may be less safe in his case – he was not refused a service but simply told he would need a different service.

3 Being short of money is not necessarily an issue of discrimination. There might be many reasons why Ola's parents cannot afford a new computer. Discrimination could be a reason and an interesting debate could take place to identify possibilities. However, there is no direct information to identify Ola's disadvantage as an act of discrimination.

4 Michelle has been discriminated against because she is a member of a religious group. She has been treated less well than people who belong to other groups. Michelle may have been very flexible outside of her commitment – not to work on Sundays. Her potential employers have made assumptions which discriminate against people who hold her beliefs. Michelle may have difficulty in using the law to protect herself in this situation though.

5 Having to do things differently does not necessarily indicate discrimination. Andreas does have access to facilities even though he may prefer to work on the ground floor. Once again there are issues to debate, but having to move floors does not necessarily prove discrimination.

The previous section of the unit raises issues of confidentiality and access to services under 'promoting equality', so there is clearly a need to look at legislation concerned with other client rights. Tutors should be aware of the new Data Protection Act, which not only supersedes the old Data Protection Act, but also the Access to Personal Files Act and the Access to Health Records Act. Students need to be aware of those parts of the Act relating to the collection, storage and use of information, and the way in which these provisions support clients' rights to confidentiality. They need to be able to link this information back to the previous section of the unit to establish when it is justifiable to breach confidentiality. Tutors can obtain information from the office of the Data Protection Commissioner, who also has a web site (www.dataprotection.gov.uk).

Students should be aware of those parts of general legislation – NHS and Community Care Act, Children Act, etc. – which give clients rights, e.g. to an assessment of need. Students should know that this is an area of legislation with a direct bearing on client rights. This leads naturally into the area of charters, the rights they give clients and the means of redress built into them. Students should be familiar with the rights and standards of the charters. They are often unable to differentiate between rights and standards when asked in tests, and some make up desirable rights that do not appear in the charters, but which actually originate in the relevant legislation. They should have no difficulty in obtaining copies of the Patient's Charter from local hospitals or primary health care practices, and copies of the Community Care Charter should be available from local social services offices. Students need not only an appreciation of the contents of the charters, but also of their practical application in care settings. Input from a current practitioner would be valuable here.

Once students have a clear concept of what discrimination is they might be asked to explore newspapers or magazines in order to find a story which exemplifies the idea of discrimination, as in **Activity** 1.2.2.

The objective is to extend students' understanding of the concept of discrimination, in relation to current events.

1.3 How care organisations promote equality

Since the charters are fundamental to an understanding of client rights in the area of service provision, students should now be ready to develop an understanding of the way in which care organisations promote equality. It is clearly the intention that the section should go beyond this title, and encompass the wider issue of client rights.

Students must develop an understanding of the interrelationship of the organisational factors which promote client rights. This may be best achieved by looking at a number of areas: how organisations set standards; how they ensure the quality of staff; how they ensure that these standards are transmitted and promoted to staff, so that they become part of the culture and practice or the organisation.

Students will by now have an understanding of the legislative and other government-imposed obligations on organisations to promote client rights. They also need to have a clear understanding of the care value base, and how this combines with legislation and charters to inform the policies of care organisations. Students should have no difficulty in obtaining information from health and social care organisations outlining the services they provide, the standards clients should expect, and the systems of redress in place if the standards are not met. Students need practice at implementing the care value base through the consideration of case studies, to ensure that they fully understand its importance in everyday care work, and are able to apply it correctly to everyday working situations.

They need to understand the role of staff selection, the qualifications and personal qualities employers look for to ensure that they recruit staff of the appropriate quality to provide high-calibre services. To fully understand this they will require an appreciation of the ethical dimensions of academic and professional qualifications. They also need to understand how employers develop the skills of staff through in-service training, supervision and management. This area will link back to earlier work done with the Race Relations and Sex Discrimination Acts, and promote student understanding of the exemptions provided in the Acts for genuine occupational qualifications.

The way in which organisations promote the culture of respect for clients' rights is central to the promotion of those rights. Students will by now understand the statutory requirements on organisations, and other requirements imposed by the care value base. They next need to investigate how these are translated into the culture of organisations, through mission statements, service principles, etc. Most large organisations, such as social services departments, health trusts and primary care groups, will publish these and so they should be generally available to students.

The next layer is that of employment contracts and practice directives and manuals which organisations use to communicate expected standards of conduct to their staff. These will not be generally available to students unless they are in employment, and so this is another area where the input of current practitioners would be valuable. In addition to this, employers will circulate a plethora of information from, for instance, codes of practice associated with legislation, government directives, etc. which indicate standards expected. Local authorities currently also have regulatory powers over private providers through their inspection function, and students should be aware of these. Tutors do need to bear in mind that inspection arrangements will shortly change with the implementation of the Care Standards Act.

Students also need to understand that there are outside influences other than training that impact on the conduct of care workers and protect and promote client rights, such as the codes of conduct of professional organisations. Students need to be able to integrate this knowledge and develop an understanding of how these influences interrelate to create a climate which is respectful of clients' rights.

An approach to help students do this would be to consider a number of situations which could arise in the workplace in a hierarchy of difficulty, and discuss with the students how they could be resolved – in discussion with colleagues, by reference to procedures, in supervision with a manager, in consultation with a professional body, or by reference to the courts. This again links back to the area of ethical issues, and consideration of how the most difficult of these are resolved by the courts will reinforce students' understanding.

Tutors should watch for other changes as a result of the forthcoming Care Standards Act.

This is a major piece of legislation which will impact on many aspects of this unit. Not only will it establish a new regulatory body for social care and private and voluntary health care service, but will set up independent councils to register social care workers. This means that for the first time many care workers will be subject to the code of conduct and associated disciplinary procedures of a regulatory body. This has considerable implications for the promotion of clients' rights. The advantage of this for tutors is that the implementation will generate a volume of excellent teaching material in the professional press.

The aim of **Activity 1.3.1** is to enable students to understand how client rights are promoted within care environments through all of the influences operating on the worker. **OHT 1.3.1** and **OHT 1.3.2** will help in preparing students for the activity. The activity involves students obtaining and reading through codes of practice and identifying how far these codes promote clients' rights, promote the valuing of diversity and the maintenance of confidentiality.

The objective of **Activity 1.3.2** is to enable students to investigate how client rights are promoted within care environments through the totality of influences operating on the worker. Two OHTs are provided. **OHT 1.3.3** provides a diagrammatic representation of the influences on a worker, and **OHT 1.3.4** provides a more detailed list of what might constitute those influences.

The aim is to enable students to integrate interpersonal skills and research approaches to the study of care organisations.

This activity would work as a question and answer session with an invited care professional. Alternatively, it could be used to design a questionnaire which students could take out into the community to use as the basis to interview a range of social care workers. The advantage of the second approach would be that the students *could* return to class and evaluate differential responses from workers operating with differing levels of autonomy and responsibility.

The object is to reinforce learning and enable students to investigate how a culture promoting equal opportunities and client rights is promoted in the workplace.

Notes to Activity 1.3.2

1 Students should be introduced to some basic theory about asking open questions and the need to prepare questions in advance of a meeting. This work might be linked to work for Unit 2, or Unit 6.

2 Students might work in pairs or groups in order to prepare questions which might form part of a questionnaire or which the group might ask a visiting practitioner.

3 In order to explore ways in which organisations promote equality students should consider questions about:

- Training
- Organisational policies and procedures
- Advocacy
- Codes of practice
- Charters
- The impact of legislation on policies at work.

4 The tutor should check suggested questionnaires or prepared questions before the student uses them in practice.

5 Students should record the responses they obtain from a questionnaire or from the visiting practitioner and should use these responses to write a report on how a specific organisation sets about promoting equality in practice.

1.4 The effects of discriminatory practices on individuals

Students should now have a good understanding of what constitutes good practice and how it is maintained. The unit now deals with the effects of discriminatory practice on individuals. This provides students with opportunities to look at the real world, and to understand that despite legislation and good intentions, discrimination still exists in society, and it has negative effects on individuals.

Students must have an understanding of the bases and roots of individual discrimination and be encouraged to examine their own attitudes. Concepts such as labelling and stereotyping, direct and indirect discrimination, overt and covert discrimination, victimisation and harassment should be familiar to them. Students typically find it easier to identify examples of these than to explain what they are. They must be able to appreciate that discrimination comes in many guises, some of them apparently positive.

They need to understand the psychological effects of discrimination on the individual, though this must be taught in a way that is not patronising towards groups discriminated against. Whilst students must understand that discrimination has negative consequences, they should understand that there is not a simple relationship between discrimination and self-esteem. Those subject to discrimination should not be presented as mere passive recipients. Students should be able to produce a sophisticated analysis of the relationship between self-esteem and life chances.

Students must understand how individual discrimination builds into institutional and structural discrimination, and that this has widespread and pernicious effects on the health and the social and economic status of individuals. There is a lot of material surrounding the Stephen Lawrence enquiry which would be useful in examining these issues.

Areas for investigation and discussion could include differential treatment of people from different racial groups within the health and criminal justice systems, failure of social care organisations to provide services to minority groups, and continuing differentials in the employment and pay of men and women.

With this grounding, students should now be able to revisit the care value base and through the use of case studies analyse the positive effects on clients of non-oppressive practice. In tests, students often appear to find it easier to give the negative effects of poor practice than the positive effects of good practice, and sometimes appear to lack understanding of the practical purpose of the care value base.

The impact of discrimination on individuals will not be easy for many students to understand. Nearly all students will have experienced put-downs, verbal abuse and tensions with people. Some students may be tempted to assume that whilst 'sticks and stones may break my bones – words can never hurt me'! It will be important that students can understand that persistent discrimination by people who have power can lead to a poor self-concept and low self-efficacy. When this happens, words and the non-verbal communication of others may have far more wide-ranging effects than the sticks and stones of the old saying above.

One way of attempting to help students understand the role of power and vulnerability in influencing people, might be to appeal to their powers of imagination.

Activity 1.4.1 asks students to imagine an unpleasant situation and list the problems that they imagine they might face in such circumstances. **OHT** 1.4.1 and **OHT** 1.4.2 provide support for preparing students for this activity.

Options to Activity 1.4.1

This script could be used as part of a whole group exercise employing whole group discussion or students might be asked to write out a list and go on to give their responses in writing to Task 2. The story could be supplied as a simple written script or it could be developed into a full emotive story that students listen to.

However the story is used it will be important to follow it up with discussion of the concept of vulnerability. A single abusive comment or abusive joke may not affect an individual who has a strong sense of his or her own self-worth. When people are powerless – such as young children, hospital patients, people with learning difficulty, or older people in care – discriminatory behaviour may cause far more damage.

Students might move on to imagine a child, or a vulnerable adult in a care situation where their rights are not respected. **OHT** 1.4.2 could be used as a stimulus for a piece of written work where the student explains the impact that discrimination could have on a vulnerable person.

1.5 Organisations that challenge discrimination

Much of this section will involve revisiting and elaborating on work done earlier in the unit. Students should have an appreciation of the role of the Equal Opportunities Commission and the Commission for Racial Equality. The Disability Rights Commission must be added to this list, in the place of the National Disability Council, which no longer exists. Students should have a clear view of the roles and responsibilities of these organisations, something they are often unable to demonstrate in tests. The activities of the Disability Rights Commission are currently being reported in the specialist press as it is a new body testing the boundaries of its responsibilities, currently establishing, for instance, that mental health as well as physical impairments fall within its remit.

It is not clear what the role of the Health Education Council is in challenging discrimination and acting on behalf of, and supporting, individuals.

The earlier work done on the role of Europe in informing domestic legislation will also contribute towards the students' understanding of the European Commission of Human Rights, and the Commission's role as the gateway to the European Court of Human Rights. Students need to have a basic understanding of the roles of these organisations in the promotion of individual's rights, and some understanding of the major impact that judgements have had on the UK. They need to understand that these organisations have provided protection for groups (e.g. gay people) who are not covered by domestic legislation. Tutors must be aware that this is a fast-moving area and that the implementation of the Human Rights Act will mean that groups and individuals who would previously have had to go to Europe for redress will now be able to obtain it in the domestic courts. It remains to be seen what effect this will have.

According to Thompson (1997) discrimination can work on three different levels (see **OHT 1.5.1**). There is the personal and psychological level, there is the cultural and conformity to norms level, and there is the structural and social forces level. Organisations that challenge discrimination will need to work on each of the three levels.

Students might undertake an Internet search in order to explore the degree to which material available on an organisation's web site indicates that the organisation is addressing each of these three levels.

Activity 1.5.1 aims to enable students to use Thompson's theory of levels of discrimination in order to analyse the effectiveness of organisations that challenge discrimination.

Notes to Activity 1.5.1

1 Students should discuss examples of discrimination at each of the three levels. They should then list ways in which an organisation might attempt to challenge discrimination at each level.

   On a personal level, organisations might offer training, codes of conduct, procedures, and careful use of language so as to challenge discrimination. On a cultural level, organisations may be attempting to change public assumptions through advertising and through promoting their own image as an effective centre for challenging discrimination. On the structural level, organisations might lobby public opinion and politicians for changes in policy or laws which may challenge discrimination.

2 Students should select an organisation's web site and evaluate how far the information on the site suggests that the organisation is challenging discrimination on each of the three levels. (For web sites, see page 11.)

3 Students might print pages which provide evidence of ways in which the organisation challenges discrimination.

4 Students should prepare written notes to support an oral presentation to their group or to the whole class. This presentation should provide examples of evidence that a particular organisation is challenging discrimination. Students should also evaluate the degree to which the organisation is likely to be successful on each of the three levels.

➡

5 Students might progress to providing a full report of their findings following feedback from their oral presentation. This work might also contribute to the completion of portfolio work for key skills in communication.

Options

Students might work in small groups and select key web sites amongst themselves – reporting back to each other. Alternatively, students might choose a web site within the class group, and present back to the whole class. Another option might be to select key web sites, such as the Commission for Racial Equality or the Equal Opportunities Commission, and ask small groups of students to research a web site between themselves. This last option may be less effective for meeting key skills criteria, but some groups may find it easier to manage this option.

ASSESSMENT SUMMARY

Grade E

To achieve **grade E** the work investigating one health, social care or early years setting must show:

- A clear description of the possible effects of discrimination on the well-being of clients in the chosen setting.
- An explanation of the ways in which legislation, policies and codes of practice are used in the setting to promote clients' rights and confidentiality.
- An identification of the way clients' rights may be respected and promoted within the chosen setting.
- An explanation of the principle of non-discriminatory practice in relation to the setting.

Grade C

To achieve a **grade C** the work must show:

- Analysis of how the organisation supports workers in promoting clients' rights and an evaluation of the effectiveness of the support.
- A clear explanation of why users of the care service may be particularly vulnerable to infringement of their rights.
- Analysis of the benefits to clients of any day-to-day practice or procedures in place in the setting as a result of a code of practice or charter of rights.

Grade A

To achieve a **grade A** the work must show:

- An evaluation of the effectiveness of equal opportunities legislation in influencing care workers' attitudes and behaviour.
- Use of sources of information and support from the chosen setting, and explaining with examples the ways in which carers can improve practice in promoting equal opportunities and clients' rights.

NOTE

This unit is already out of date in some respects, and tutors may be concerned whether they should teach to the unit or to the current situation. It is arguable that if this qualification is to be of any vocational use, there is little point in teaching history. The realities may be changing faster than tests can be prepared, but if students do possess the most up-to-date knowledge possible, it is inconceivable that this would not be credited in tests.

RESOURCES

Useful web sites include:

Ombudsman schemes in the UK
www.bioa.org.uk

Commission for Racial Equality
www.cre.gov.uk

Data Protection Commissioner
www.dataprotection.gov.uk

Disability Rights Commission
www.drc-gb.org.uk

Equality Commission for Northern Ireland
www.cre.gov.uk

Equal Opportunities Commission
www.eoc.org.uk

Northern Ireland Human Rights Commission
www.nihrc.org.uk

Local Government Ombudsman
www.open.gov.uk

Official Solicitor to the Supreme Court
www.offsol.demon.co.uk

Parliamentary and Health Service Ombudsman
www.ombudsman.org.uk

Many voluntary organisations also have web sites, which students will easily be able to access by typing the name of the organisation into a search engine.

Note: Useful archived press stories and other material is available at:
www.community.care.co.uk

OHTs

The OHTs to help deliver this unit are:

1.1.1 Promoting equality
1.1.2 The European Convention on Human Rights
1.1.3 Ethical dilemma
1.1.4 Valuing diversity
1.1.5 The application of utilitarian principles
1.1.6 Alternative logical theory of ethics
1.3.1 The care value base: Foster people's equality, diversity and rights
1.3.2 Anti-discrimination influences on client care
1.3.3 Outline of influences on care workers
1.3.4 Details of influences on care workers
1.4.1 How discrimination may block human needs and change people
1.4.2 Outcomes of discrimination
1.5.1 Different levels of discrimination

ACTIVITIES

The activities are designed to promote learning and understanding and develop logical thinking and a rational approach to studies.

1.1.1 An ethical problem
1.2.1 Clarifying the concept of discrimination
1.2.2 Creating a group scrapbook
1.3.1 Comparing codes of practice with the care value base
1.3.2 Investigating how client rights are promoted in care environments
1.4.1 The effect of discrimination
1.5.1 Levels of discrimination

Ethical Issues

- One person's rights vs the rights of others
- Two conflicting rights of a person
- Two conflicting obligations of a care worker
- Conflicting philosophical positions
- Conflicting cultural values
- Rationing services

OHT 1.1.2 THE EUROPEAN CONVENTION ON HUMAN RIGHTS

Outline of Human Rights

As incorporated into British Law (not Article 1)

Article 2	Protection of life
Article 3	Freedom from inhuman treatment
Article 4	Freedom from slavery, servitude or forced or compulsory labour
Article 5	Right to liberty and security of person
Article 6	Right to a fair and public hearing
Article 7	Freedom from retrospective effects of penal legislation
Article 8	Right to respect for privacy
Article 9	Freedom of thought, conscience and religion
Article 10	Freedom of expression
Article 11	Freedom of association and assembly
Article 12	Right to marry and found a family
Article 13	Right to an effective remedy before a national authority
Article 14	Prohibition of discrimination on the grounds of: Sex, race, colour, language, religion, political or other opinion, national or social origin, association with a national minority, property, birth or other status.

OHT 1.1.3 ETHICAL DILEMMA

This ethical dilemma is to be used for Activity 1.1.1.

- Conjoined twins have been born in a British hospital.
- One twin has no functioning heart or lungs and only a primitive brain.
- If the twins are separated, the weaker twin will die.
- If the twins are separated, the stronger twin has a good chance of survival, but may have serious physical impairments.
- If the twins are not separated, both will die.
- Doctors want to separate the twins.
- The parents are deeply religious and oppose the operation.
- The parents come from a remote community where there are few specialised facilities for children with special needs.
- The doctors have applied to the court for permission to perform the operation to separate the twins.

OHT 1.1.4 VALUING DIVERSITY

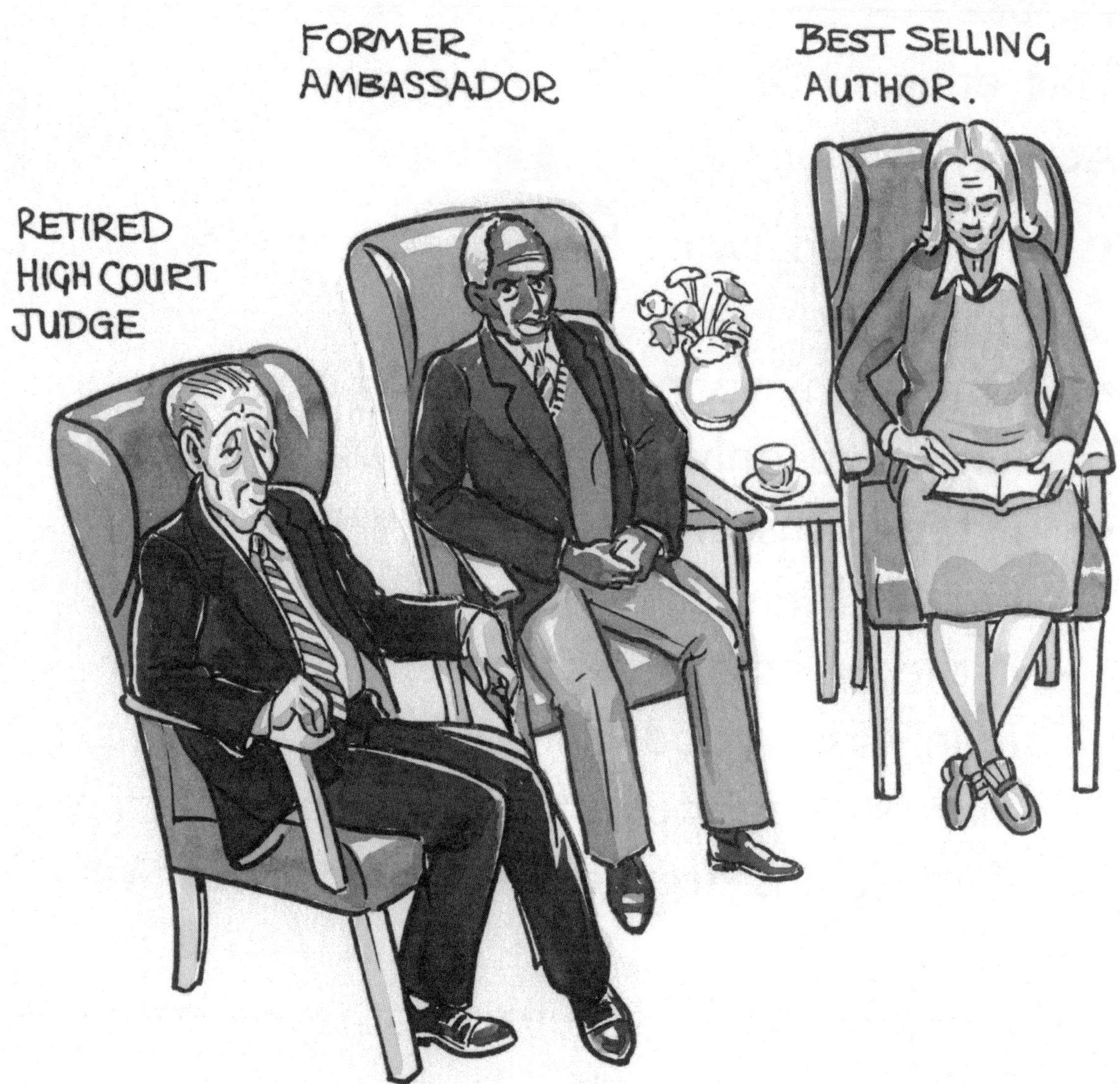
FORMER AMBASSADOR
BEST SELLING AUTHOR.
RETIRED HIGH COURT JUDGE

OHT 1.1.5 THE APPLICATION OF UTILITARIAN PRINCIPLES

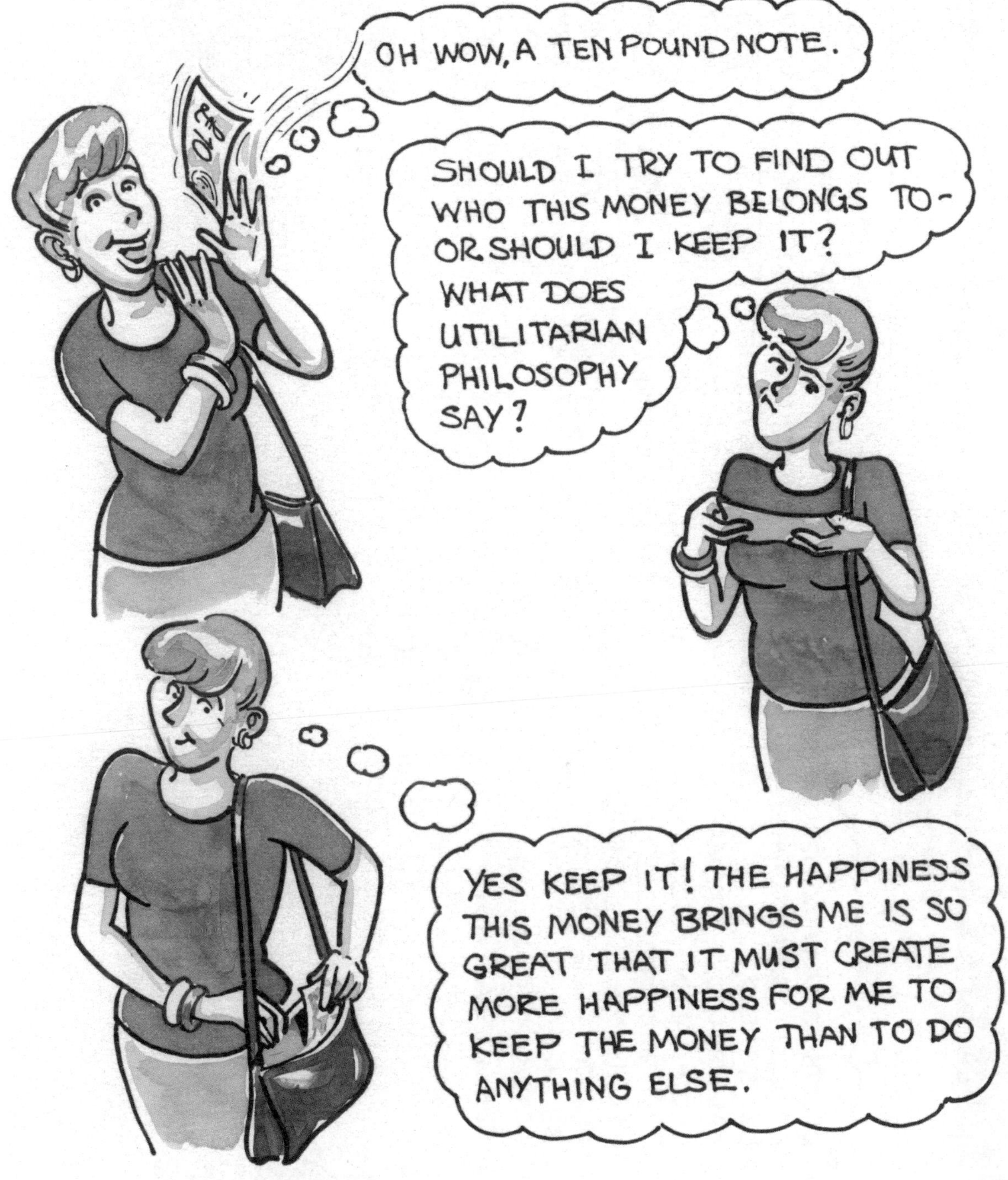

OH WOW, A TEN POUND NOTE.
SHOULD I TRY TO FIND OUT WHO THIS MONEY BELONGS TO - OR SHOULD I KEEP IT? WHAT DOES UTILITARIAN PHILOSOPHY SAY?
YES KEEP IT! THE HAPPINESS THIS MONEY BRINGS ME IS SO GREAT THAT IT MUST CREATE MORE HAPPINESS FOR ME TO KEEP THE MONEY THAN TO DO ANYTHING ELSE.

OHT 1.1.6 ALTERNATIVE LOGICAL THEORY OF ETHICS

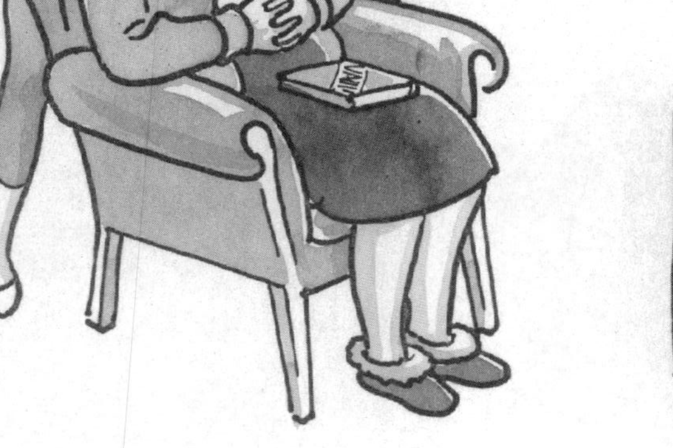
DOROTHY IS WATCHING HER FAVOURITE T.V. PROGRAMME BUT WE NEED TO GET THE BATH ROTA DONE. OK, ACT UTILITARIANISM- LET'S SEE, TWO OF US WOULD BE VERY HAPPY IF WE DRAGGED HER OFF- SHE WOULDN'T BE HAPPY. OK, TWO AGAINST ONE, WE WIN- SHE GETS A BATH!

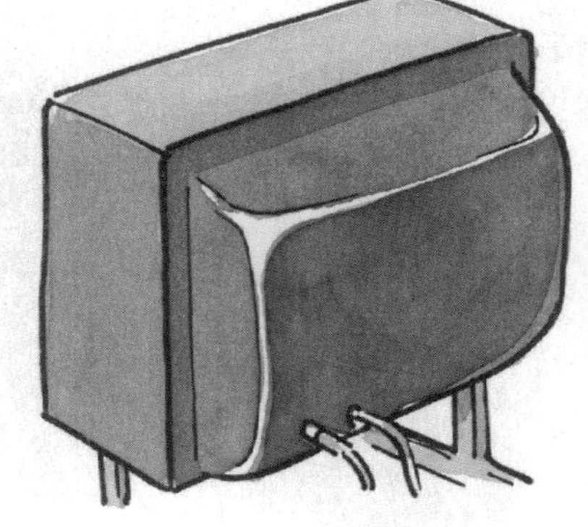

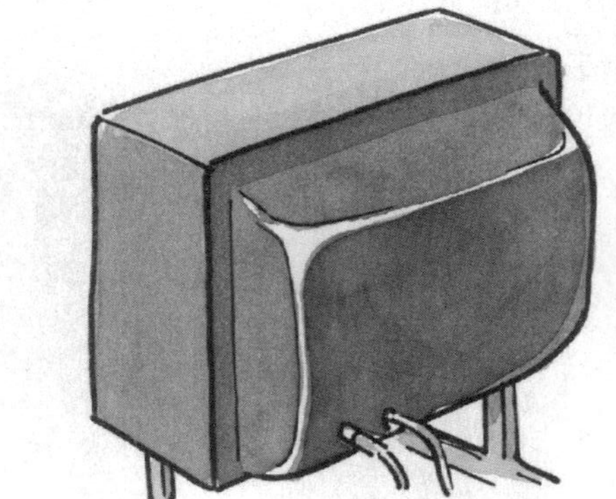
BUT THE CARE VALUE BASE SAYS I HAVE A RIGHT TO DIGNITY, RESPECT AND CHOICE-THESE RIGHTS ARE JUSTIFIED IN TERMS OF SOCIETY'S VALUE AND QUALITY CARE - THIS IS WHERE THE PRINCIPLE OF UTILITARIAN DECISION-MAKING COMES IN- NOT IN JUSTIFYING INDIVIDUAL ACTIONS.
VALUES

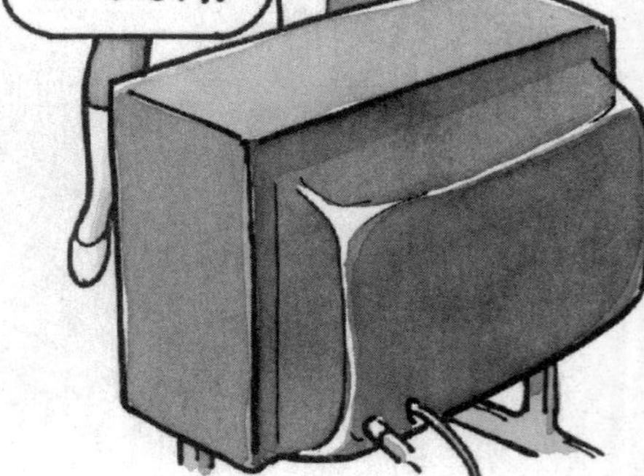
OK, DOROTHY WINS, WE HAVE TO ACT IN TERMS OF THE VALUE BASE - THE VALUE BASE MIGHT BE JUSTIFIED IN TERMS OF THE GREATEST HAPPINESS FOR PEOPLE IN SOCIETY.

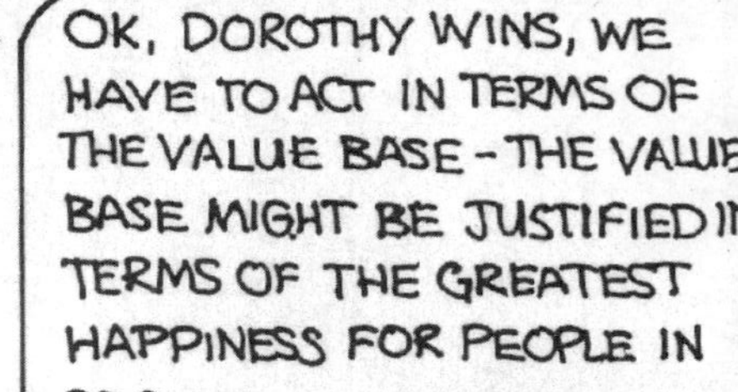

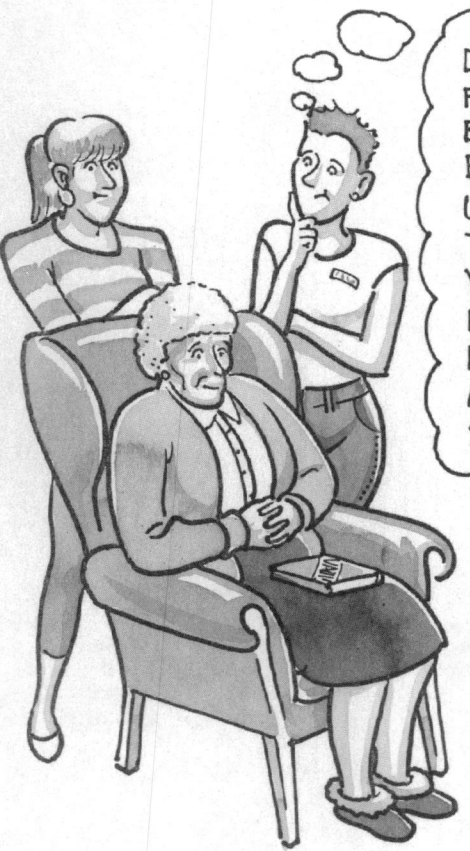

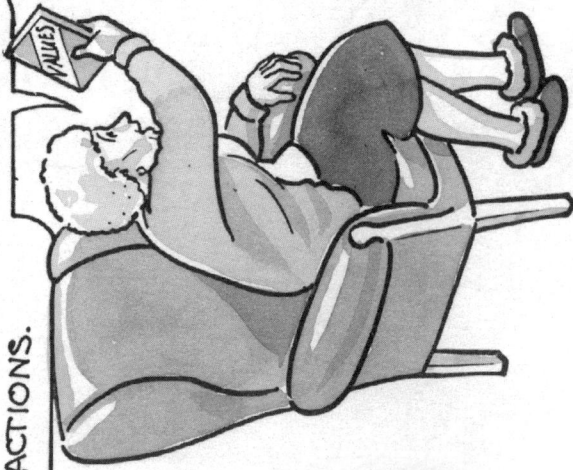

OHT 1.3.1 THE CARE VALUE BASE

Foster people's rights and responsibilities

- Rights: The right to be different
  Freedom from discrimination
  Confidentiality
  Choice
  Dignity
  Effective communication
  Safety and security
- Advocacy
- Effective relationships
- Role boundaries
- Needs and resources
- Challenging when other's rights are not met

Foster equality and diversity of people

- Understand assumptions and oppressions such as those which surround gender, race, age, sexuality, disability, class.
- Understand prejudice, stereotyping and labelling and their effects.
- Understand own beliefs, assumptions and prejudice.
- The benefits of diversity.

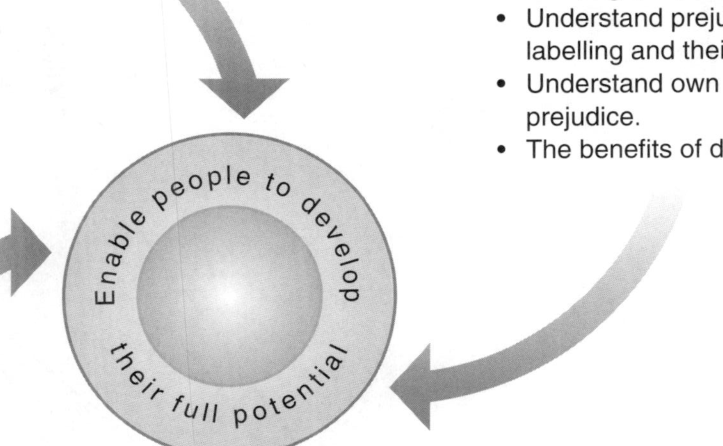
Enable people to develop their full potential

Maintain the confidentiality of information

The legal framework: Data Protection Acts, 1984 and 1998,Access to Personal Files Act 1987

- The security of recording systems
- The need and right 'to know'
- Confidentiality can value and protect a client
- Policies, procedures and guidelines
- Boundaries and tensions in maintaining confidentiality.

OHT 1.3.2 ANTI-DISCRIMINATION INFLUENCES ON CLIENT CARE

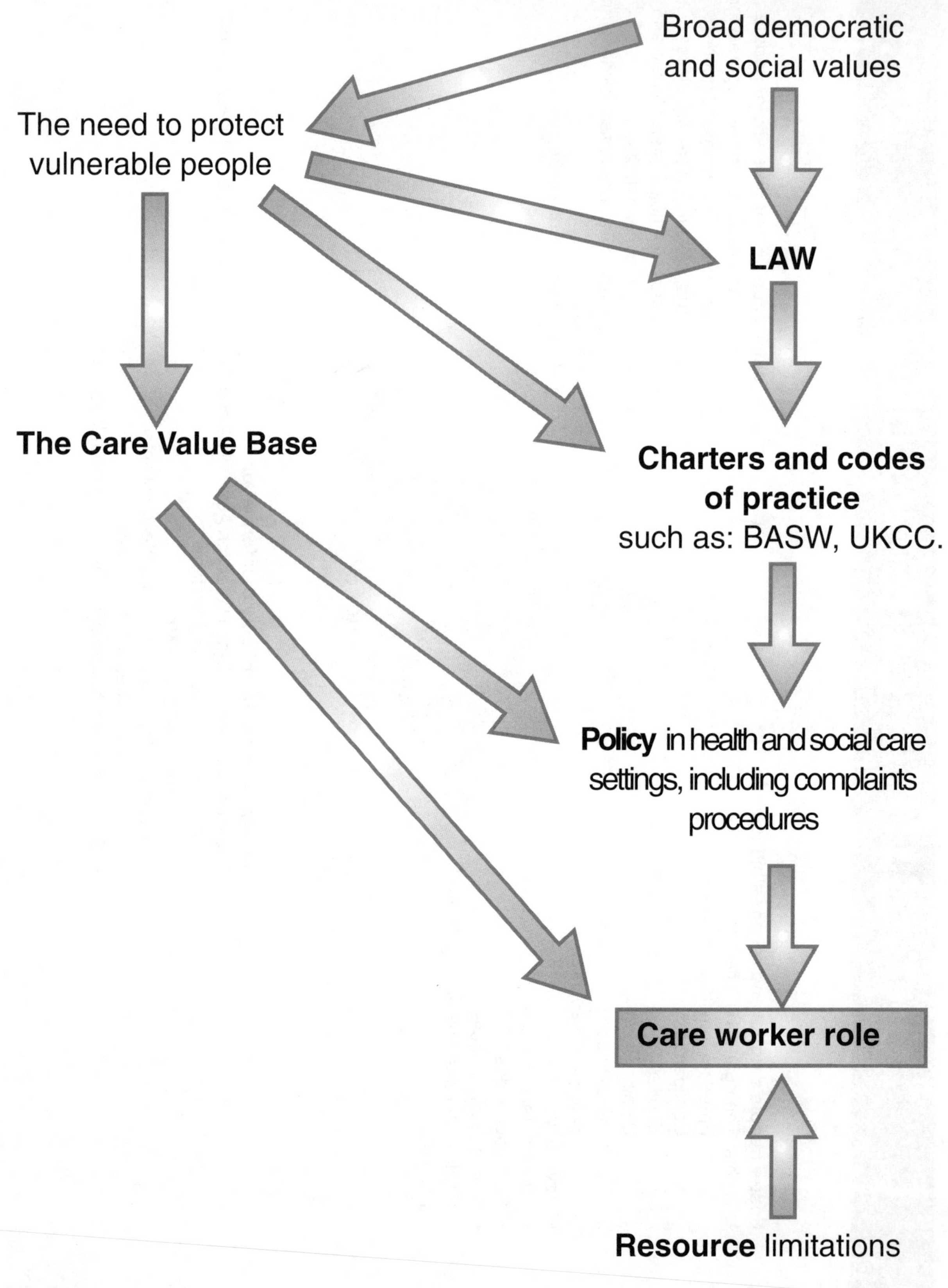

Broad democratic and social values
The need to protect vulnerable people
LAW
The Care Value Base
Charters and codes of practice such as: BASW, UKCC.
Policy in health and social care settings, including complaints procedures
Care worker role
Resource limitations

OHT 1.3.3 OUTLINE OF INFLUENCES ON CARE WORKERS

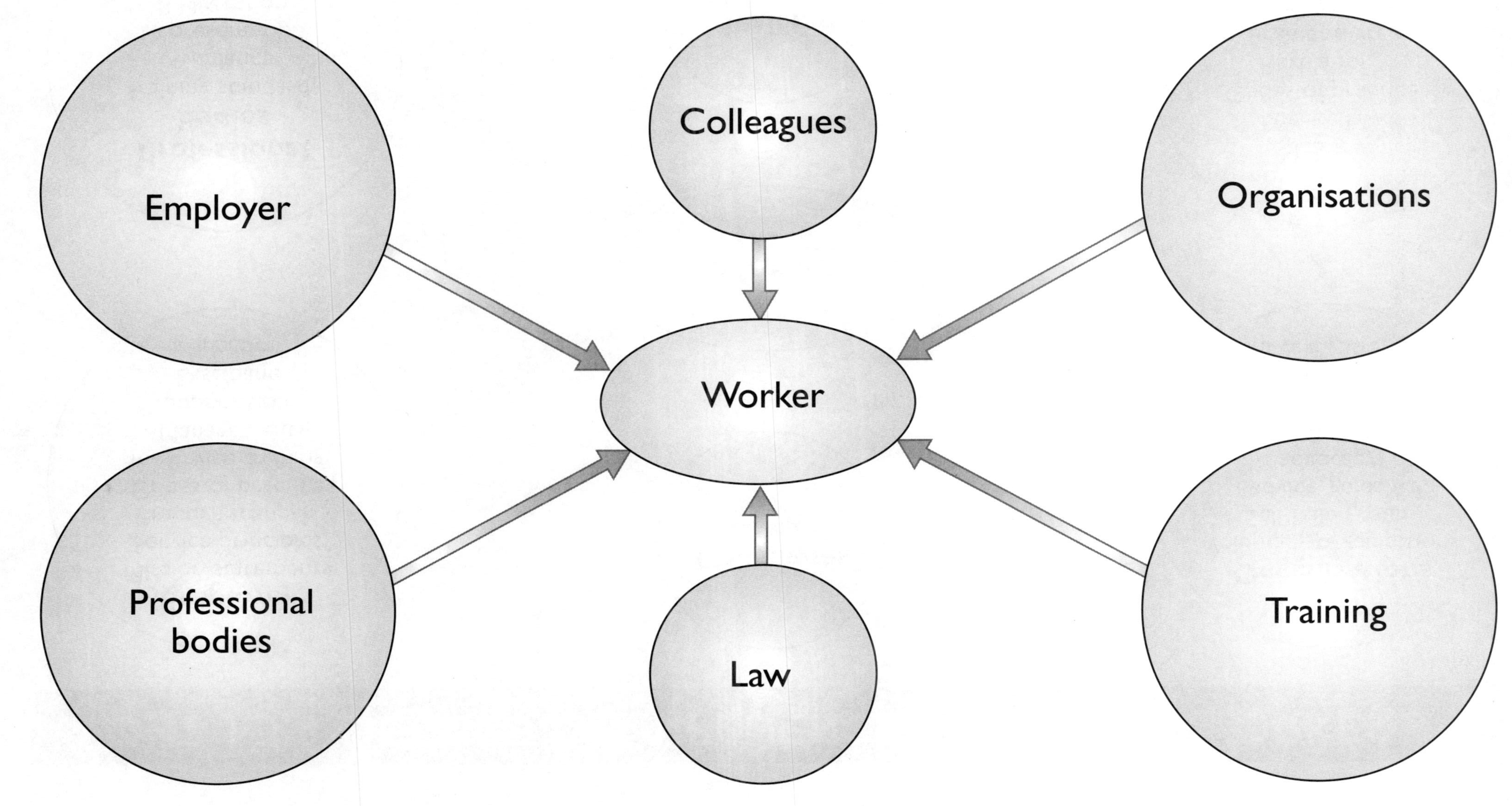
Employer
Colleagues
Organisations
Worker
Professional bodies
Law
Training

OHT 1.3.4 DETAILS OF INFLUENCES ON CARE WORKERS

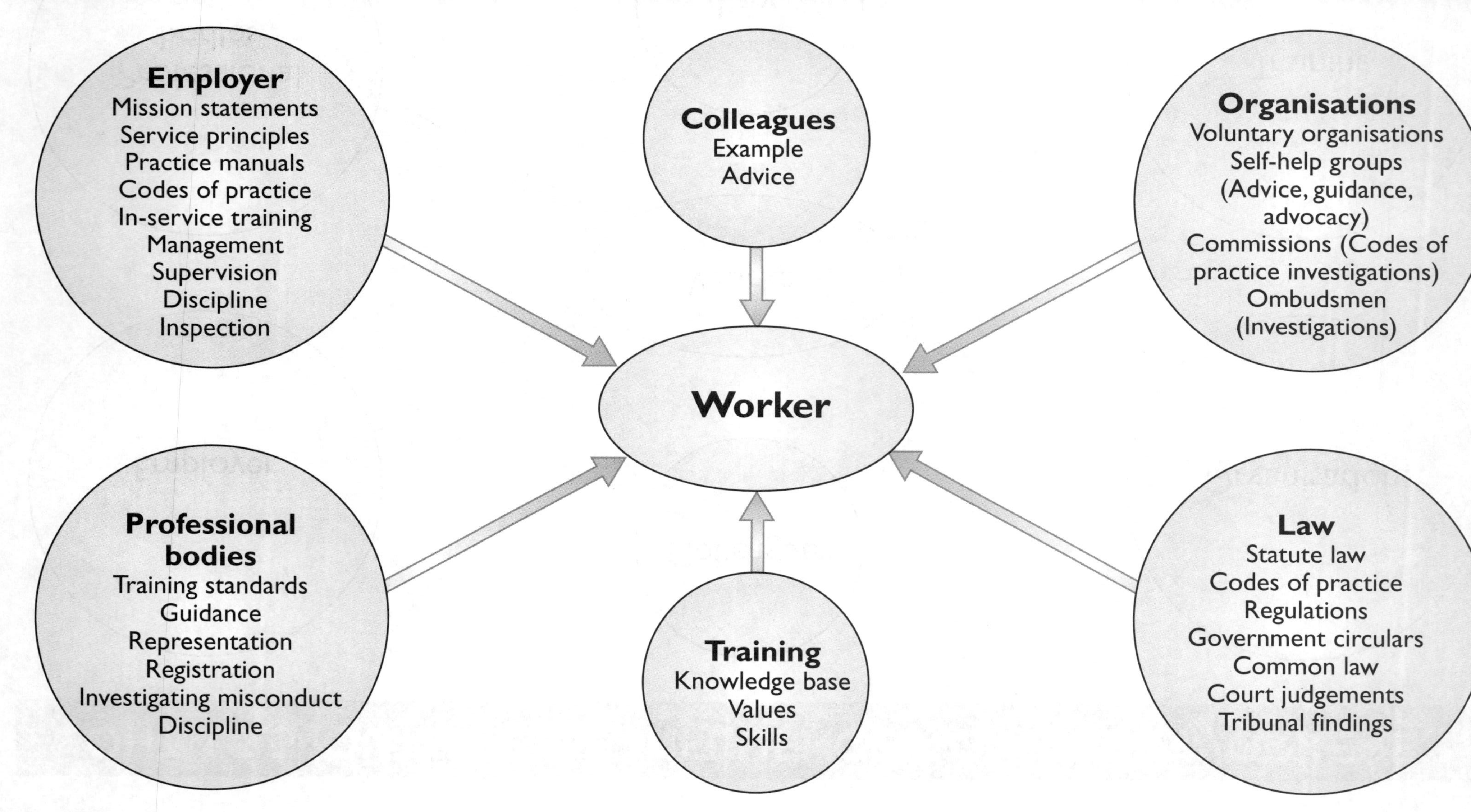
Employer
Mission statements
Service principles
Practice manuals
Codes of practice
In-service training
Management
Supervision
Discipline
Inspection
Colleagues
Example
Advice
Organisations
Voluntary organisations
Self-help groups
(Advice, guidance, advocacy)
Commissions (Codes of practice investigations)
Ombudsmen
(Investigations)
Worker
Professional bodies
Training standards
Guidance
Representation
Registration
Investigating misconduct
Discipline
Training
Knowledge base
Values
Skills
Law
Statute law
Codes of practice
Regulations
Government circulars
Common law
Court judgements
Tribunal findings

OHT 1.4.1 HOW DISCRIMINATION MAY BLOCK HUMAN NEEDS AND CHANGE PEOPLE

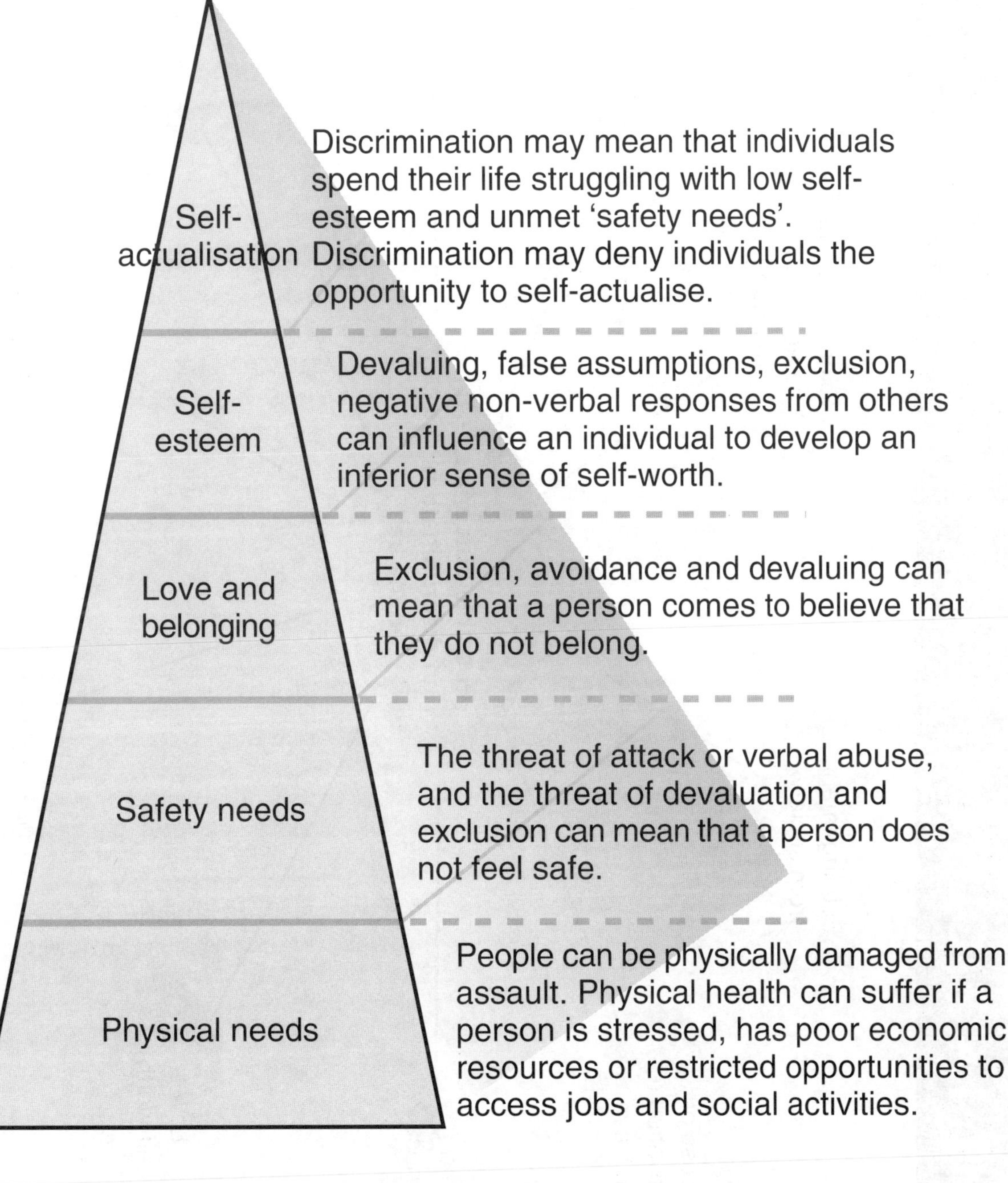
Self-actualisation
Discrimination may mean that individuals spend their life struggling with low self-esteem and unmet 'safety needs'. Discrimination may deny individuals the opportunity to self-actualise.
Self-esteem
Devaluing, false assumptions, exclusion, negative non-verbal responses from others can influence an individual to develop an inferior sense of self-worth.
Love and belonging
Exclusion, avoidance and devaluing can mean that a person comes to believe that they do not belong.
Safety needs
The threat of attack or verbal abuse, and the threat of devaluation and exclusion can mean that a person does not feel safe.
Physical needs
People can be physically damaged from assault. Physical health can suffer if a person is stressed, has poor economic resources or restricted opportunities to access jobs and social activities.

OHT 1.4.2 OUTCOMES OF DISCRIMINATION

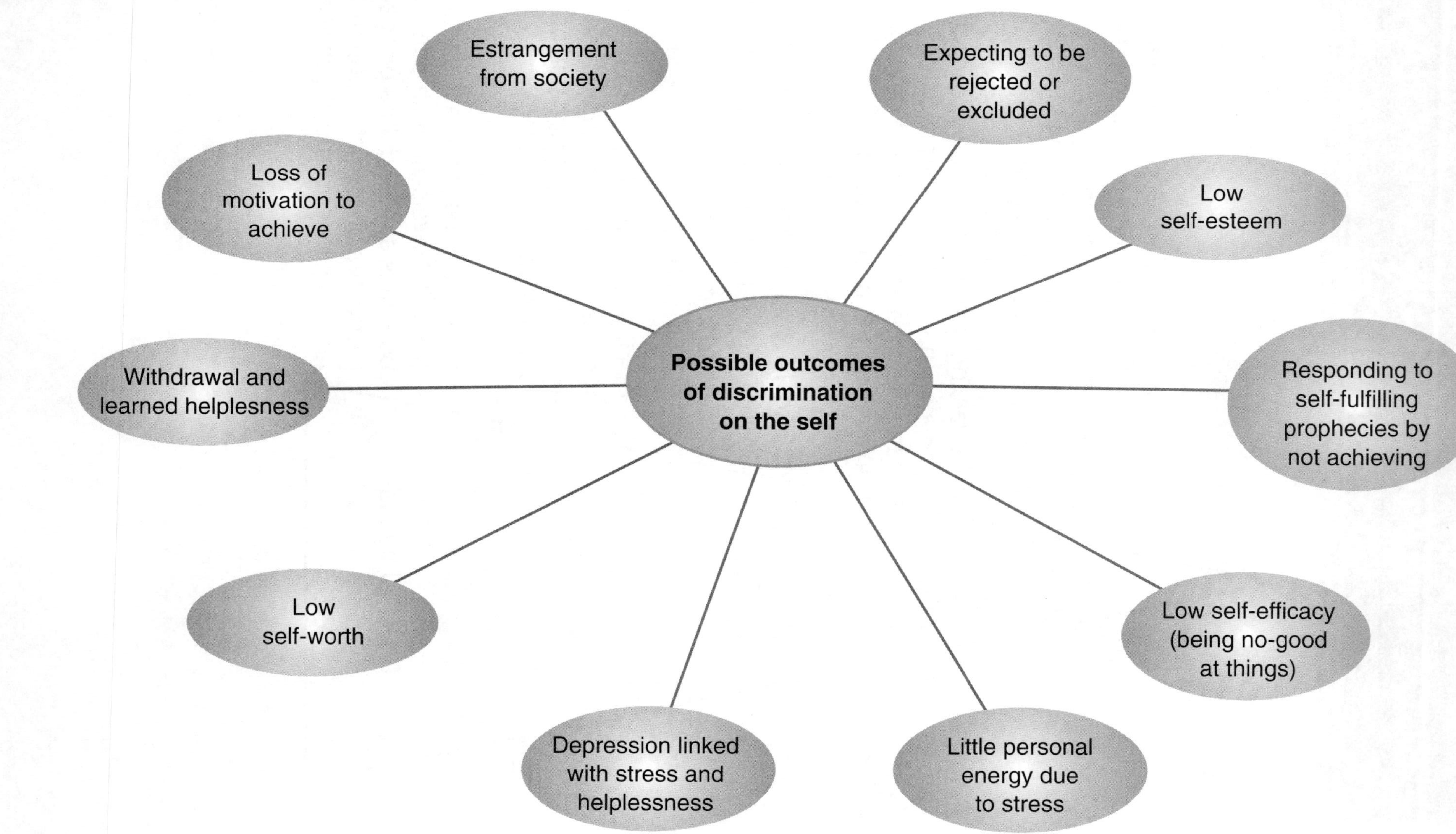
Possible outcomes of discrimination on the self
Estrangement from society
Expecting to be rejected or excluded
Low self-esteem
Responding to self-fulfilling prophecies by not achieving
Low self-efficacy (being no-good at things)
Little personal energy due to stress
Depression linked with stress and helplessness
Low self-worth
Withdrawal and learned helplesness
Loss of motivation to achieve

OHT 1.5.1 DIFFERENT LEVELS OF DISCRIMINATION

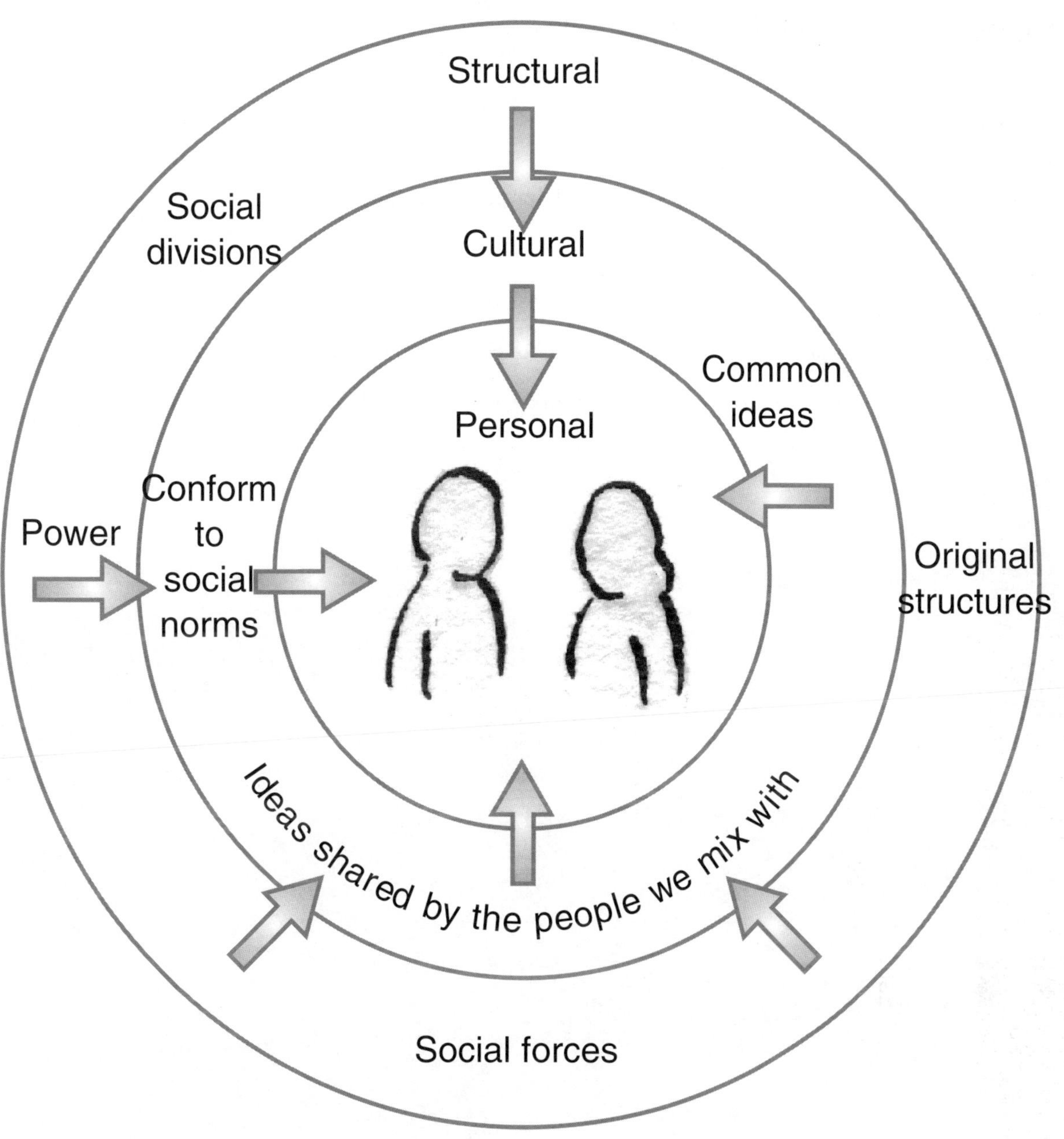

Structural
Social divisions
Cultural
Common ideas
Personal
Conform to social norms
Power
Original structures
Ideas shared by the people we mix with
Social forces

ACTIVITY 1.1.1 AN ETHICAL PROBLEM

This activity involves discussing the ethical dilemmas raised by the case in OHT 1.1.3 and attempting to find a solution to that problem.

You may work in groups of two or three.

TASKS

1 Make a list of the practical issues involved in the dilemma.

2 List the values and beliefs that will influence decisions.

3 Identify a solution to the problem and explain how this is linked to the values you have listed.

4 Prepare your case according to the format chosen by the tutor.

5 Prepare a written summary of the arguments employed on both sides of the dilemma.

ACTIVITY 1.2.1 CLARIFYING THE CONCEPT OF DISCRIMINATION

TASK 1

Read the details below and identify which person is likely to have been discriminated against.

1 Zoe went to the dentist with a painful abscess. The dentist prescribed antibiotics and said that Zoe would have to wait for a week before he could operate. Zoe is still in pain.

2 Ahmed is diabetic and is in hospital being treated for a heart condition. A nurse provided manicure services to other patients on the ward but refused to cut Ahmed's nails saying that he would need specialist attention because of his diabetes.

3 Ola's parents cannot afford to buy her a computer with Internet access, yet all her friends at school have good computer systems at home.

4 Michelle went for a job interview where she explained that her religious views prevented her from working on Sundays. She was not appointed and was told that she was not sufficiently flexible in her attitude to being available for work.

5 Andreas is a wheelchair user working on the first floor of a building. Andreas has to use the lift in order to access the disabled toilet on the ground floor of his work setting. His able colleagues can access a toilet on the first floor.

TASK 2

a As a group discuss why you think the person you have chosen was discriminated against and why the others were not.

b Discuss how the person discriminated against could be protected by the law and could seek compensation under the law.

ACTIVITY 1.2.2 CREATING A GROUP SCRAPBOOK

TASKS

1 Working in groups or a whole class, compile a scrapbook of stories which exemplify discrimination. Each student should explore newspapers or magazines over a two-week period in order to identify a story which suggests that some type of discrimination has taken place.

2 Write a brief statement explaining why discrimination is an issue in the story. Make sure you identify what kind of discrimination has taken place, e.g. sexism, racism, ageism, etc.

3 Comment on how far the law provides a remedy for people who have been discriminated against in the context of the story.

4 Attach your stories and statements to large sheets of sugar paper which could be used to create a general resource book or used for display purposes.

ACTIVITY 1.3.1 COMPARING CODES OF PRACTICE WITH THE CARE VALUE BASE

TASKS

1 Obtain a code of practice or a policy document from the Internet, or a service or setting you have visited or worked in.

2 Working in pairs, evaluate how far these documents include content on clients' rights, valuing diversity, combating discrimination, and maintaining confidentiality.

3 Write your own individual report on a code or document which records details of links between the care value base and the code.

4 Consider the likely impact of resource limitations on the implementation of codes and policies and offer a brief evaluation of the usefulness of the code or policy which you have reviewed.

ACTIVITY 1.3.2 INVESTIGATING HOW CLIENT RIGHTS ARE PROMOTED IN CARE ENVIRONMENTS

For this activity you may work in pairs or in a group.

TASKS

1 Design a questionnaire to use to investigate how the range of influences which promote client rights and equal opportunities impact on a care worker.

2 Interview care workers in an organisation, using the questionnaire to record their responses to the questions.

3 Write a report on how a specific organisation sets about promoting equality in practice.

ACTIVITY 1.4.1 THE EFFECT OF DISCRIMINATION

Read the case study below and do the tasks that follow.

Imagine you went on holiday with friends to a distant place that you had never been to before. The people in this place do not speak any languages that you know and they have an entirely different culture, beliefs and values from those you are familiar with. You share little in common with the people in this country except that you are a tourist and these people are welcoming and friendly towards tourists.

Towards the end of your holiday you become ill and you are taken to hospital many miles away from the resort you were staying in. Your friends all have to return home, and you are left in a hospital without anybody you know or anyone you can talk with. You have little money and do not understand what is expected of you in the hospital. You are weak, you are in pain and you feel vulnerable. Staff in the hospital cannot communicate with you and you might worry that they do not really like you or care about you.

TASKS

1 Make a list of the emotions that you would feel in this situation.

Assuming that it is not possible for you to go home and not possible for your friends and relatives to fly out to be with you, make a list of all the opportunities that you would hope care staff would provide. Also list the ways in which you hope care staff would treat you. In other words, make a list of the kind of care you hope you would receive.

2 Now imagine that none of the things on your list were provided. The staff treat you roughly and do not respect you. You would long to leave. Now imagine that you were told you would be ill for the next 10 years and you could not go home. What would be the long-term consequences for you?

ACTIVITY 1.5.1 LEVELS OF DISCRIMINATION

TASKS

1 Discuss together examples of Thompson's levels of discrimination.

2 List ways in which an organisation might attempt to challenge discrimination at each level.

3 Select an organisation's web site and evaluate how far the information on the site suggests that the organisation is challenging discrimination on each of the three levels.

4 Print out pages which provide evidence of ways in which the organisation challenges discrimination.

5 Prepare written notes to support an oral presentation to your groups or to the whole class. Include an evaluation of the degree to which you think the organisation is likely to be successful on each of the three levels of discrimination.

UNIT 2 – COMMUNICATING IN HEALTH AND SOCIAL CARE

OVERVIEW

In this unit students will need to concentrate on developing an understanding of effective communication skills in both individual and group situations. The grade awarded for this unit will depend on students' ability to evaluate their own and others' communication skills. Whilst these topics will form the bulk of the students assessed work it is important that students understand the importance of maintaining confidentiality. Students also need to be aware of the varied range of communication skills needed in different care roles.

This unit will require a range of practical exercises in order to build an understanding of the skills involved. Students will also need to access care settings in order to observe individual and group communication in practice. Students will also need to be involved in practical communication work with staff and service users in order to record, develop and evaluate their own skills.

The unit contains five defined areas which are numbered for ease of referencing in this file:

2.1 Types of interaction
2.2 Effective communication
2.3 Communication skills in groups
2.4 Evaluating communication skills
2.5 Maintaining client confidentiality

Aims and objectives

The unit covers:

- effective communication skills relevant to care settings
- types of interaction involved in care settings
- valuing individuals through communication
- factors that inhibit interaction and their potential impact on an individual's health and well-being
- methods used to evaluate interactions.

Students should be able to:

- identify different types of interactions
- explain different purposes of interactions
- interact in formal and informal situations
- interact in one-to-one situations
- interact in group situations.
- build a professional relationship with clients
- explain how different factors may affect interaction
- minimise communication barriers
- explain the differences between one-to-one and group interactions
- analyse one-to-one and group interactions
- explain the theories behind group interaction
- evaluate own effectiveness in one-to-one and group interactions
- demonstrate an openness to feedback from others
- promote clients' rights and confidentiality during interactions with other carers and clients during conversations or by written records
- explain how the recording and storage of client information is protected by Acts of Parliament
- identify potential dilemmas associated with maintaining confidentiality.

Assessment

Students are required to produce a report which identifies and preferably evaluates the communication skills employed in a care setting. In addition to this report students must also produce records which demonstrate effective personal communication skills in a one-to-one and a group interaction with clients.

Evidence for assessment might be partly provided by records of communication activity. Students might be encouraged to maintain a **log book** which will help them to identify, and later to evaluate, the quality of communication within a care setting. Students will also need help to identify how communication is working in practical settings. One way of trying to help students is to provide them with key concepts laid out in **grids.** These grids can then be used to identify and analyse interactions which they have seen. A range of grids are provided in this file.

TEACHING NOTES

Because this unit requires many practical exercises and much discussion of individual behaviour it may be important to establish the ground rules or values of caring behaviour before practical exercises begin. Students should be aware of the care value base and of the importance of offering positive feedback to other students. It is important that students recognise the importance of contributing to others' self-esteem rather than threatening their self-esteem or self-concept. Students should also be aware of the importance of maintaining confidentiality in relation to the practice which they observe.

2.1 Types of interaction

It may be useful to provide some overview of the types of interaction that students may experience in health and social care settings. The value of descriptive information is likely to be limited and students are most likely to develop an understanding of interaction through practical experiences. Students should be encouraged to maintain a log book during their placement experience or at least to maintain records of visits to care settings which they have made. Log book records should be reviewed during tutorial or small group discussions with students.

Designing a log book

Students will need a great deal of advice and guidance in order to design an effective placement log book. The log book should not be a diary of activities. Students should be invited to make records of one-to-one conversations and group discussions which they have joined in.

One way of encouraging effective recording might be to ask students to record the detail of conversation and group discussion using the headings set out below. Students might then be invited to use a separate set of headings in order to evaluate what happened. The log book might be based on a notebook where the left-hand page is used to record details of conversations and the right-hand page used to evaluate those details.

Describing what happened during communication

- Describe the background to the conversation or discussion (what had happened immediately before you began talking).
- Who was involved in the discussion? (Be careful to maintain confidentiality by not using clients' real names.)
- Record details of the most important things that were said and the responses that other people made.
- Record details of non-verbal behaviour such as tone of voice, eye-contact and gestures.
- When describing a conversation try to record objective factual details. Record some of the phrases that people actually said and describe their facial expression and other precise details of non-verbal behaviour. Be careful not to interpret behaviour by making judgements such as: 'The client was angry', or 'We got on very well together'. The description of communication should give as much factual information as possible, so that other people can come to their own conclusions about the conversation.
- Record how other people were affected by the communication that took place. Was there evidence that clients might have felt supported or helped? Did your communication have the effects that you expected?

Analysing log book records

If a conversation or discussion has been clearly described it will be possible to analyse and evaluate its effectiveness using some of the questions below.

- Was an effective communication cycle developed during communication? (See page 88 of the textbook.)
- How effective were your own listening skills? (See pages 88 and 89.)
- How did any questions that you may have asked influence the communication? (See pages 90–91.)
- How did cultural differences influence the communication? (See pages 84 and 85.)
- How did your own non-verbal behaviour influence the communication? (See pages 77–80.)
- Were you able to be supportive towards others during the communication? (See pages 80–83.)
- Were there any barriers or blocks to communication? (See pages 96–98.)
- What did you learn from other people's non-verbal reactions to your behaviour?
- What aspects of communication practice could be improved in future?

Formal and informal interaction might be discussed in the context of class teaching designed to introduce the concepts of verbal and non-verbal communication. The teaching for this section of the standards might be comfortably integrated with teaching for the section on effective communication.

At the start of the unit it may be worth introducing students to the importance of communication work by using an 'ice breaker' exercise.

Activity 2.1.1 is designed to explore the barriers created by restricting communication to verbal explanation.

Explain the task to the students. Then ask them to organise themselves in pairs sitting back to back with each other. Provide one student with a blank sheet of paper and the other student with one of the two diagrams provided as handouts (see **Activity 2.1.1**). The student with the diagram may not show the diagram to their partner. The student with the diagram has a maximum of five minutes to explain the diagram orally to their partner who will attempt to draw what is being explained. The student with the diagram may not look at their partner's drawing during the exercise. All communication is to be restricted to oral communication with no feedback or visual contact between the two members. It may be helpful to give different students a different diagram to ensure that the students who are drawing cannot be sure of the nature of the diagram that their partner has, should they be in a position to hear instructions or see the results of other students' work.

Each pair of students will then swap roles and repeat the exercise with a different diagram.

At the end of the exercise take feedback from the whole group. Emphasise the importance of clear verbal feedback and of being able to use non-verbal behaviour and visual information when trying to communicate.

Introduce the notion of barriers to communication and the role in building skills of overcoming barriers to communication.

Activity 2.1.2 might help students to map the kind of interactions which they may come across in a care setting. The purpose of this exercise is to explore the expectations and roles which care staff may take on.

Students should be introduced to the idea of making pattern notes. They should then be asked to talk to 4 or 5 different members of staff in a *given care setting*. They should ask staff to describe the range of people that they have to work for – or with – such as managers, clients, relatives and colleagues. Students should then ask what expectations other people have of their role. Students might probe whether different people have different expectations of members of staff. If there are varied expectations a final follow up question might be to ask staff how they have to alter their communications skills in order to meet the different expectations of people. The range of people that staff in the care setting have to work with could then be drawn into a pattern diagram such as the one below:

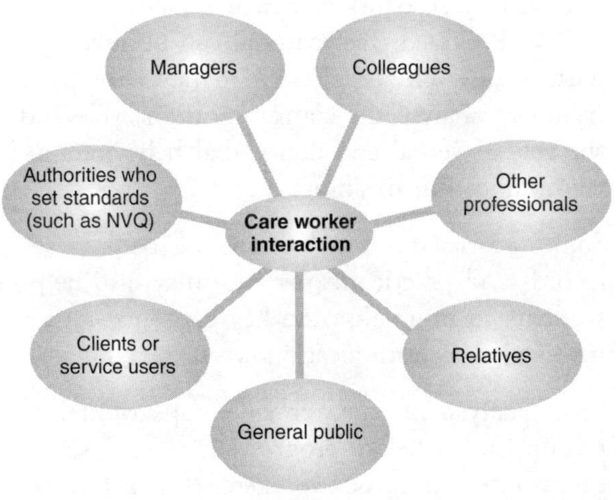
Managers
Colleagues
Authorities who set standards (such as NVQ)
Care worker interaction
Other professionals
Clients or service users
Relatives
General public

Notes on Activity 2.1.1:

- Arrange students into pairs sitting back to back.
- Explain the nature of the exercise.
- Give out plain paper to students who will draw their version of the oral description.
- Give out diagrams to the instructors.
- Allow five minutes for communication to take place.
- Allow students to swap roles and repeat the exercise with a different diagram.
- Stop the exercise and ask students to form one group. Take feedback from the whole group. Emphasise the importance of clear verbal feedback and of being able to use non-verbal behaviour and visual information when trying to communicate.
- Introduce the notion of barriers to communication and the role of Unit 2 in building skills of overcoming barriers to communication.

Different types of communication to meet different kinds of need could be discussed either in a classroom setting or individually in a tutorial following a review of log book notes. **OHTs** 2.1.1, 2.1.2, 2.1.3 could be used to stimulate a class discussion on the nature of communication.

2.2 Effective communication

Students will need to be able to analyse communication using the concepts set out in the grid activities in this file. Teaching for this section should be experiential, involving a range of practical exercises where students are required to analyse their own and others' performances.

It will be important to develop a range of video-taped material which can be used to illustrate the concepts involved in verbal and non-verbal communication. There are some commercially produced videos which illustrate communication in care and nursing settings. There are also a range of commercially available video tapes which illustrate basic counselling skills. It might also be interesting to analyse episodes of communication between fictitious characters. Many 'soaps' are avidly followed by students who will undertake the AVCE. Provided this material can be used within copyright restrictions it may be worth trying to analyse the communication cycle and the role of verbal and non-verbal behaviour in communicating meaning.

Some tutorial discussion of the log book records and practical experience may also help students to internalise the key concepts involved in communication work.

Some analysis of taped or video-tape work is recommended before progressing to analyse group interaction. Group exercises will form the basis for experiental learning and this section might be partly integrated with the learning experiences required to analyse communications skills in groups.

Students will need guidance in order to make effective notes on their own communication. It may be important to encourage students to analyse verbal and non-verbal behaviour as set out in the textbook. One idea for doing this might be to use video material and ask students to discuss the quality of verbal and non-verbal interaction in relation to a specific character. Videos need not necessarily relate to care settings and it might be better not to use professional counselling tapes. Any acted material which can be used within copyright guidelines may be appropriate for drawing students' attention to verbal and non-verbal components of communication.

Activity 2.2.1 aims to develop the ability to analyse verbal and non-verbal communication. Students should be asked to watch a short sequence of communication between two characters. This sequence might be appropriately only five minutes in length. Students might then use the grid in the activity to analyse what they have seen. They might initially rate the behaviour they have seen and then share their thoughts either with a partner or in small group discussion.

By integrating these tasks into learning experiences students will be able to analyse the verbal and non-verbal behaviour in terms of the concepts and categories set out in the tables.

Notes on Activity 2.2.1:

- It will be important to explain and provide examples of each skill area before students can use the grid. It may be worth checking that students understand ideas such as reflection and prompts before using the grids in an exercise.
- Students might be asked to make brief notes while they watch a short video or other interaction. Taking notes may help students to remember incidents that may influence their final rating.
- Students might rate the skill areas that they have seen individually at the conclusion of the observation.
- Pair work or small group discussion may help students to clarify their ideas and develop their ability to analyse communication.
- Whole group discussion may provide a learning check with respect to a student's ability to analyse communication.

The grids might provide a focus for helping students to reflect on their own communications skills within placements. Grids for verbal and non-verbal behaviour might provide a focus for activity within the 'Improve own Learning and Performance' and 'Working with Others' additional key skills units.

The grids can be used to explore behaviour within classroom settings or within other small group activities. The key value of using the grids is to help students develop skills of analysis as applied to real-life behaviour.

Assertiveness

Assertiveness is often confused with aggressive behaviour. Some people interpret assertiveness to mean 'sticking up for yourself' at the expense of others. Assertiveness is quite a difficult concept to understand. The natural tendency in many people is to 'fight or run' when they encounter difficulty in their relationships with others. Assertiveness should be presented as an alternative to being defeated or defeating others. It might be explained as attempting to achieve a 'win/win' situation rather than a 'you lose/I win' situation.

The following activity explains how a 20-minute game might be played. This game may encourage students to reflect on the advantages of assertive strategies in life.

The aim is to encourage an understanding of the win/win theory of interpersonal interaction, and the objective is to enable students to discuss assertiveness in the context of win/win philosophy.

Notes on the assertiveness activity:

- Explain the procedures and rules for the game.
- Get the class group to form into groups of three with a score keeper and two opponents.
- Check that the groups understand the nature of the game.
- Ask the score keeper to make a list from 1 to 20 with two columns to record the score for each opponent.
- Start the game.
- Allow people to change over with the score keeper after the first game has been completed (the score keeper might play the winner of the game).
- Discuss the strategies involved in being successful at the game.
- Discuss links between successful strategies and assertive strategies within the context of care work and employment.
- Explore specific skills used in assertiveness in relation to the win/win theory that emerges from this exercise. **OHT 2.2.1** may assist with this discussion.

Activity – on assertiveness

Students will need two small pieces of card or paper, together with a sheet of paper on which they can record the results of the exercise. Students will write 'Yes' on one card and 'No' on the other. They then hold both cards behind their back so their opponent cannot see them. Ideally this game should be played in groups of three, where one person acts as referee and score keeper and the other two are opponents. The referee announces 'Go' and both opponents simultaneously produce one card from behind their back. If there is hesitation on behalf of one player the round is declared void. The game should be played for perhaps 20 rounds. The scoring system for the game is set out below:

- Whenever a player produces a 'No' card they will receive one point.
- If both players produce a 'Yes' card then they both receive two points.
- If one player produces a 'Yes' card but the other produces a 'No' card then the 'Yes' scores a zero and the 'No' scores the usual one point.

The object of the game is to try to beat your opponent's score and to score more than other people in the same class. No negotiation or discussion of strategies is permitted during the game. An alternative rule is that people may break any agreements they have made with respect to the cards that they will show.

This game involves a conflict between the desire to maximise one's score and the need to beat your opponent. Producing a 'No' card is a safe strategy, but this strategy will result in a low score which will almost certainly fail to beat other people in the class group. If both players produce 'Yes' cards, then they will maximise their score. However, it is difficult to be sure that you can trust your opponent. The students who score highest in this game will be students who establish a co-operative arrangement as they play it. But negotiation to co-operate is not permitted in the rules of the game.

The outcome from a group of people who play this game should be a discussion of strategies for co-operation or 'going it alone'. The strategies involved in the game may be seen as a metaphor for aggressive or co-operative behaviour in real life. Businesses that co-operate often achieve higher profits than businesses which undertake ruthless competition against each other. Biologists argue that species that co-operate amongst themselves are often more successful than species where individuals compete with each other. In a social context co-operation involving assertive strategies may often prove to be more successful than competitive strategies aimed at defeating an opponent.

It is recommended that this game might lead to a discussion of the value of using assertive strategies within employment situations.

2.3 Communication skills in groups

It may be useful to introduce this section with a discussion on the nature of groups. Pages 103–104 in the textbook offer an explanation of how groups form and how the term 'Group' might be used in health and care settings. Students might be asked to reflect on their own group behaviour and how they may have come to identify themselves as a group. Tuckman's four stages of group development provides a useful theory for explaining the importance of norms and value systems in enabling individuals to identify with a wider group. (See **OHT** 2.3.1.) Students might be asked to identify the values which enable then to identify with a feeling of group belonging. Some discussion of team work within care settings may also be appropriate at this stage. It will be important for students to understand that groups form around systems of values and norms and that values are central to the caring task. Students might identify the task of establishing ground rules of behaviour as linked to Tuckman's stages of group development. They might be invited to consider the parallels between becoming a member of the student group and a member of a team within a work setting.

Following an introduction to the importance of value systems in groups, students may progress to exploring communication patterns and group task and maintenance behaviours. At this point students will need to undertake some practical group activities in order to understand the key concepts involved. Some potential activities are described in this file.

These activities might integrate with work for the previous section.

As well as learning to analyse one-to-one communication in terms of verbal and non-verbal skills students will need to be able to analyse group communication. Students will also need to be able to provide evidence of their own effective group interaction. It will be important to encourage students to undertake activities where they analyse group behaviour. A possible profile which may be useful for analysing group behaviour is that in **OHT** 2.3.2.

Analysis of group behaviour – participation patterns

An important aspect of group interaction is the extent to which individuals participate in a group discussion. Pages 108 and 109 of the textbook explain how to observe and record participation patterns (see also **OHTs** 2.3.3 and 2.3.4.)

Activity 2.3.1, which involves playing the game of noughts and crosses, can be used by students to record patterns of interaction. The aim is to provide a setting for students to analyse and record participation patterns. The activity will enable the students to map individual patterns within a group.

The game is played by two players, each taking it in turns to place an X or a 0 in one section of the noughts and crosses grid. Whoever makes a line first is the winner.

Ask the students to form groups of between six and eight members. Then ask the group to try to work out a strategy, using the grids to practise on, whereby they can ensure that their group can never lose at this game, without altering the fundamental rules of the game and without deliberately cheating.

The answer is quite simple. Players have to try to block their opponent rather than try to win the game. Most people will not be fully aware of this strategy however, and will need to practise the game in order to satisfy themselves that there is a strategy for not losing. Some students become confused and assume that they have to try to win the game – however there is no strategy within the rules which can ensure this!

The key point in using this game is that groups will find many different ways of working. Some groups will work as one whole group, but most of the interaction may take place between a few people. Some groups will split into a number of sub-groups, and interaction patterns can be mapped to show which groups are which.

Notes on Activity 2.3.1:

- Explain methods used for mapping group participation patterns. Issue students with a series of circles drawn on a sheet of paper which they can use to represent groups that they will observe.
- Explain that students might like to use numbers or real names in order to record participation within a group.
- Split the class group into observers and participants for the game. This activity can be undertaken as a 'fish bowl' exercise.
- Explain the noughts and crosses game.
- Check that the observers have numbered or named the participants in the exercise.
- Begin the activity.
- Take feedback on the outcome of the game.
- Take group feedback from the observers on the participation patterns which they have seen.
- Alternatively, the observers may discuss the participation patterns they have recorded with members of the group or with each other before group feedback is taken.
- Summarise the importance of mapping group participation in class discussion.

Group communication – analysing behaviour during an ethical debate

It is important that students can reflect not only on the content of what they say but also on the nature of interaction within groups that they belong to. Students will need to practise using profiling systems in order to develop analytic skills in monitoring group behaviour. The profile in OHT 2.3.2 might be used in a fish bowl exercise in order to assist students to analyse task and maintenance behaviour within groups.

Activity – monitoring an ethical debate

For this activity students might be asked to form groups of about 10. Each group of 10 might be subdivided into five members who will hold a debate and five members who will act as observers. The observers will complete a group profile on the behaviour which they observe.

The aim of the activity is to enable students to identify and understand how task and maintenance behaviours influence group processes.

The objectives are to enable students to:

- identify examples of group maintenance behaviour and examples of group task behaviour.
- Evaluate their own contributions in relation to task and maintenance behaviour.
- Identify behaviour which maintains group interaction, keeps a group on task, or blocks group behaviour within practice or placement settings.

See notes on page 40.

When to introduce fish bowl observation

The method of observing described above is called the fish bowl method – it is explained on page 112 of the textbook. The people on the inside, that is, those holding the debate, might feel like goldfish in a bowl. The people on the outside are studying their behaviour. If students have never practised the goldfish bowl method before, they may need to undertake a more simple exercise than an ethical debate as their first introduction to this method. The noughts and crosses game in Activity 2.3.1 might provide a good starting point for introducing the fish bowl method.

Unit 2 might be taught alongside Unit 1, in which case it would be highly appropriate to link the activities for Unit 1 to group observation. If Unit 2 is taught together with Unit 1 then the fish bowl method might provide a useful method of revision for the Unit 1 test. Alternatively, fish bowls might be used in relationship to any area of teaching where students might be expected to have an opinion.

Notes on monitoring ethical debate activity:

- Only introduce a serious debate with student groups who have established appropriate supportive norms and ground rules.
- Select a suitable topic in relation to what is known about the needs and the abilities of the student group.
- Check that all students are sufficiently confident to cope with being observed.
- Check the topic with the student group for appropriateness.
- Check that students have successfully undertaken fish bowl observation before undertaking a serious debate.
- Organise the group into observers and participants, perhaps five observers and five participants in each fish bowl sub-group, i.e. a group of 20 students might be split into two sets of observers and participants.
- Ensure that observers have copies of the group observation grid (see OHT 2.3.2) and that they are clear what the different categories mean.
- Set a time limit for the discussion, say 10 minutes.
- Confirm the time interval for recording behaviour on the grid and check that students have a method for identifying when to move columns. It may be appropriate for the tutor to announce minute-by-minute column changes by pointing to a clock. Verbal announcement may disrupt the group discussion.
- Stop the discussion and debrief the participants about he content of their debate.
- Observers may discuss the content of their observations whilst participants debrief.
- Ask for feedback from the observers to clarify the task and maintenance behaviour observed. Summarise observations in a supportive way.
- Ask participants to change places with observers so that all students have had a chance to observe a group.
- Repeat the feedback procedures.
- Ask students to identify how they might use their observational skills in a real care setting.

Possible topics for discussion

The fish bowl method provides an opportunity to analyse any discussion. Choice of topic will need to be carefully judged in relation to the abilities, sensitivities and maturity of the student group. A simple topic might be to ask students to discuss their beliefs about animal rights – some people may be vegetarian, others may believe that eating meat is ethically justified. Such an area of debate may create an interesting discussion which can be analysed using the observation grid (see OHT 2.3.2). It will be important to consider the nature of individual belief systems before introducing such a topic however, as it is possible that an individual could be isolated or discriminated against by other group members during the debate. Provided that student groups have established supportive norms of personal working it might be possible for them to undertake a mature discussion of ethical issues. The topics in **OHT 2.3.5** represent further ideas that might be appropriate for discussion in some circumstances.

Developing listening skills

Many students will have difficulty in understanding the difference between hearing the words that people say and active or reflective listening. It may be important to introduce students to video material which explains the way that counsellors listen to and encourage their clients to talk. As well as demonstrating the skill of listening it may be important to encourage students to practise listening and so offer feedback and guidance on the development of students' skills. It may also be worth encouraging students to understand the difference between offering advice and trying to help a person by listening to their views. Many students may believe that they should give people advice as part of their caring role. Students may understand the importance of listening if they perceive it as an alternative to giving advice.

Activity – listening skills

You could set up an activity to help students to develop listening skills and so be able to analyse the effectiveness of listening skills in care contexts. This could involve observing demonstrations and undertaking practical work, after which students will be able to employ basic listening skills and recognise effective listening skills in others. Students will be able to avoid offering inappropriate advice in care contexts.

The activity might involve students explaining a personal hobby or activity to a partner. This conversation might be tape-recorded or video-recorded. The skills of the listener should be analysed as well as the communication skills of the speaker. This activity might also contribute towards communication key skills.

When students are familiar with recording conversational work they might undertake a role-play exercise. Students might compile their own list of day-to-day problems or might be offered a scenario to act out. One student should attempt to display listening skills whilst the other student relates a problem, such as being short of money or worried about the health of a pet. The outcome of the tape-recorded conversation might be analysed in terms of the student's ability to avoid giving advice and to use effective listening skills instead.

Notes on listening skills activity:

- Students should observe demonstrations of effective listening skills either via real-life demonstration or through watching video material.
- Students should undertake a range of simple conversational activities which they may tape-record and analyse in terms of listening skills.
- Observation of student activity and resulting class discussion should indicate that students have sufficient understanding of listening skills to make role-playing effective.
- Students undertake role-plays in pairs without being observed by others.
- Students evaluate their own performance before discussing their performance in a wider class context.

Students will need a degree of privacy and a relatively quiet setting if they are to work effectively and tape-record conversations.

2.4 Evaluating communication skills

This section might be taught separately from the main focus on effective communication. Teaching might integrate work for this section with teaching for the additional key skill of 'Improving Own Learning and Performance'. Students might be set specific tasks which ask them to reflect on practice such as the evaluating communication skills activities in this file. Students might also use the rating scale set out in Table 2.3 on page 116 of the textbook (reproduced in this file as **OHT** 2.4.1). Lesson plans might be designed to focus work on the assessment requirements as set out at the end of these teaching notes.

One of the most successful ways of assisting students to understand evaluation might be to encourage them to develop peer assessment skills. Students will need to have established supportive values and norms within the group, and tutors will need to be confident that ground rules will be adhered to before peer assessment can be used. Students will probably need to have covered most of the theory required for this unit and perhaps for Unit 1, before they will be ready to engage in peer assessment. Students might work in groups of two or three in order to rate the quality of acted communication portrayed in video clips. Students might subsequently build on this experience by rating one another's performance on short acted examples of communication work. If students make presentations to their group these presentations could be rated using a grid – such as OHT 2.4.1 – and peer assessment. The skill of self-assessment might develop from experience of peer assessment work. Once students have developed the idea of self-assessment using rating scales, they may be able to use theories such as the 'Kolb learning cycle' (See **OHT** 4.4.2 and page 114 of the textbook) in order to explain their practice. This theory is likely to be too abstract to assist students from the outset of the unit however.

Students will undertake many practical activities within the classroom to assist them in understanding and evaluating their own and others' communication. Preparation for the assessment will require students to evaluate their own skills in two different care settings. As part of the formative assessment work that they need to do students might evaluate barriers to communication that they perceive in a care setting.

Activity 2.4.1 will assist them in identifying issues for their report. **Note**: This activity might be used as preparation for the formal unit assessment.

In the activity students should be asked to keep a log book and to record their thoughts and observations in relation to conversation and group activities that they have observed. Students might be asked to write up a brief description of a conversation or group session which they observed. They might then rate the conversation in relationship to barriers. The written description and rating might form the basis of a tutorial discussion with each student.

In discussion the student might explore the reasons for the quality of communication that they have observed. The student might also discuss improvements which they may be able to make or suggest in order to reduce barriers. A final piece of written work might be to write up suggestions for improving communication in preparation for the assessment.

The aim of the activity is to encourage students to employ the concept of barriers when evaluating the quality of communication in care settings.

The objective is for the student to be able to identify barriers to communication and understanding within care settings and propose methods for improving communication.

2.5 Maintaining client confidentiality

Once again this section of the standards might be taught separately from the bulk of the teaching on effective communication. This section could be integrated with teaching for Unit 1. A thorough analysis of the issues involved in maintaining client confidentiality might be covered in the context of the value base and for the ethical dilemmas as specified within the standards for Unit 1. Information on the Data Protection Acts and other relevant legislation might be provided in the context of Unit 1.

The assessment for Unit 2 requires that students should give an explanation of the way in which client confidentiality can be maintained. It may be useful to consider confidentiality under the following headings:

- Client's rights with respect to confidentiality.
- Agency policies on confidentiality.
- The storage and transmission of confidential documents.
- Access to confidential documents.
- Maintaining confidentiality in conversations.
- Understanding the boundaries to confidentiality.

Client's rights

Students should make outline notes on the rights which people have under the Data Protection Act 1998. These rights will influence agencies' policies on confidentiality.

Notes on Activity 2.4.1:

- Ensure that students are maintaining notes of individual and group communication activities in their log books.
- Set students the task of writing a short description of a specific individual or group interaction.
- Advise students of tutorial arrangements to discuss their description and hand out copies of the barriers to communication grid that accompanies this activity. Ask students to rate their description using this grid.
- Organise a brief discussion between pairs of students so that they can collect their thoughts about rating their observations.
- Undertake tutorial discussion with students to assist them in developing evaluation skills. Clarify plans for a written evaluation of the observed conversations based on their ratings using the grid.
- Mark the formal written work which results from this activity as a foundation for formal assessment work.

Agency policy

Students should be encouraged to obtain copies of policy documents from placements or settings which they visit. These policy documents should outline procedures for maintaining confidentiality and may well provide the central focus for the student's notes on confidentiality.

The storage and transmission of confidential documents

Students should make notes on policy and procedures within the care settings which they visit with respect to the storage and transmission of confidential documents. It may be appropriate for students to interview senior staff in order to establish the degree of security which surrounds confidential documents. Students might make a short list of documents which are confidential in one column in their notebook and arrangements to protect the security of documents might be recorded in another column of their notes. Details relevant to the storage of manual and electronic records may be found on page 120 of the textbook.

Access to confidential documents

Students should note which staff have access to confidential documents, fax reports, electronic information and oral information relevant to the personal welfare of clients. They will be able to note that their own access is restricted.

Maintaining confidentiality in conversations

Students should have undertaken discussions, both within the classroom and during placements or visits, which explore the importance of maintaining confidentiality. Students should be able to identify in their notes the possible negative consequences of breaking confidentiality. The importance of maintaining confidentiality should be reflected in student records which demonstrate effective communication skills for the assessment.

Understanding the boundaries to confidentiality

It will be important to discuss this issue if students are to receive a high grade for Unit 2 work. The concept of boundaries is abstract and not easy to understand. It may be important to undertake some problem-solving work with students to help them to build an understanding of how care staff make appropriate judgements with respect to confidentiality.

Exploration of log book recordings, tutorial discussion and practice supervision might concentrate on understanding the boundaries involved in maintaining confidentiality. Some class problem-solving activity should be organised using brief case study outlines to help students to analyse the issues involved in making decisions about confidentiality.

Students might be asked to undertake a practical research project. They could design a series of questions, which they might ask staff within a placement setting. The design of an interview would provide a way of teaching the theory of funnelling as described on page 91 of the textbook. Students could ask straightforward questions about the security of information within a centre. These might concern specific issues such as who has access to incoming fax data, the security of filing cabinets, and the possibility of confidential conversations being overheard. Alternatively, students might undertake a more in-depth style interview and interview staff about situations where the boundaries of confidentiality have been an issue of practical importance for them. Students might make a checklist or even a rating scale of issues relevant to the maintenance of confidentiality in a work setting. It might be important for tutors to check students' proposed questionnaires or interview schedules before they are used in practice.

The aim of the boundaries to confidentiality activity that follows is to enable students to understand how to apply the concept of boundaries in relation to decisions about maintaining confidentiality.

The objectives are for the students to be able to evaluate the implications of breaking confidentiality or maintaining confidentiality in difficult situations.

Activity – boundaries to confidentiality

Students should be asked to discuss the conditions under which information told to them in confidence might be passed on to others. If possible, it might be useful to introduce students to the issues by outlining a real story; perhaps a story about a client who neglected themselves but did not want other people to know about this. Students should be invited to consider the principles which guide decision-making, perhaps constructing their own list.

Principles for guiding decisions include:

- Assessing the level of risk involved.
- The likely consequences of maintaining or breaking confidentiality.
- The consequences of maintaining or breaking confidentiality for the staff member as well as the client and their friends and relatives.
- The need to be fair and consistent.
- Clients' rights and responsibilities, including the right to make their own decisions.

Once students have a list of the principles which guide decision-making they might use it as a checklist to record their thoughts as they discuss a series of scenarios.

Further notes

Ground rules

An exercise on ground rules might be designed to build on work undertaken for Unit 1. A class or group of students might undertake a discussion exercise in order to list ground rules for debating and analysing others' communication skills. Alternatively, guidance on working within a caring value base might be given before students set out on visits or placements. It may be important to emphasise the role of values before any placement or practical activities begin.

Placements

Teaching this unit might capture the imagination of students who can see the relevance of classroom activities to their own social skills and impact on others. Students may need to link classroom teaching with practical experience in order to be motivated to achieve. It is recommended that students undertake visits or placements in order to focus their work for this unit.

ASSESSMENT SUMMARY

Unit 2 is a very practical unit. Students will base their work on placements or visits to care settings. Preparation will therefore have to begin at the outset of the unit. By the conclusion of the unit students must **report on the use of communication skills**

Notes on boundaries to confidentiality activity:

- Introduce the topic of confidentiality with reference to a real story.
- Establish a list of criteria for making decisions about confidentiality.
- Present a range of short stories or scenarios which illustrate the problems that can occur with confidentiality – there is a brief list on page 119 of the textbook. Other situations might include:
  - A person who has a serious illness but who does not want their relatives to know.
  - A client who appears to be very ill but does not want their doctor to know about their illness.
  - A client who would like to give you an expensive gift and asks you to keep this confidential to stop your employer from interfering.
  - A client who claims that they are being abused by another member of staff but who does not want you to disclose this information because they are afraid of retaliation.
- Ask students to discuss each story in relation to the criteria for decision-making. Take discussion after the first situation has been evaluated.
- Take general class feedback on the use of principles to help make ethical decisions.
- Emphasise the importance of discussing confidentiality principles with others and explain that care work cannot be based simply on following rules.
- Evaluate the discussion on confidentiality in relation to the needs of the assessment.

within a health, social care or early years setting. Students must also produce records of their **own effective communication skills** in:

- A one-to-one interaction
- A group interaction.

The client groups must be different for each interaction.

In order to undertake these tasks students will need to develop skills in recording details of communication. It is unlikely that students will be able to video or audio-tape real communication in care settings as such recordings might breach clients' rights to confidentiality. Students will therefore have the very difficult task of reconstructing details of conversations after they have occurred. Students will not be able to write useful accounts of conversations unless they understand a range of useful concepts which will enable them to analyse verbal and non-verbal communication. They are likely to need a great deal of support with recording details of communications. The following approaches may be needed if students are to gather the basic material they need in order to complete the assessment.

- Practice in analysing communication using the grids supplied in the textbook and in this file. Students might be introduced to activities, such as Activity 2.4.1, so that they become used to using grids to help them interpret their own practical experiences.
- Guidance on maintaining log book records of their own and others' conversations whilst on visits or placements. Students might be asked to use grids or simply to record conversations noting verbal and non-verbal categories of communication.
- Regular tutorial review of log book records to provide appropriate feedback in order to assist students to improve their recording techniques.
- Class activities such as the 'fish bowl' activity in Section 2.3 of this file (monitoring ethical debate) to help students employ grids to analyse group communication.
- Class discussion and presentations where students present details of their practical experience analysed in terms of the concepts taught in this unit.

Only after students have become familiar with recording and analysing individual and group communication will it be appropriate to undertake the formal assessment required for Unit 2.

Grade E

To achieve a **grade E** the work must show:

- Examination of communication skills in a health, social care or early years setting.
- Records of effective communication skills in one-to-one and group interactions using different client groups.
- A review of the communication skills demonstrated in the interactions.
- A clear explanation of the factors that influenced the interactions and how potential barriers to communication were avoided.
- An explanation of how effective communication by carers in the chosen setting contributes to valuing people as individuals.
- An explanation of how client confidentiality can be maintained.

Grade C

To achieve a **grade C** the work must show:

- A review of the effectiveness of the interactions and how improvements could be made.
- An analysis of the implications of inappropriate communication on the health and well-being of clients from the chosen setting.

Grade A

To achieve a **grade A** the work must show:

- A critical evaluation of personal use of communication skills.
- A realistic action plan for improvement of skills in one-to-one and group interactions.
- An evaluation of the extent to which appropriate communication skills are used in the chosen setting and realistic recommendations for improvement in interactions.

ASSESSMENT GUIDELINES

The guidance set out below might be used as an initial outline to assist students with the completion of the assessment work for this unit. These guidelines are aimed at helping students to attain an A grade. Work which does not follow all of these headings might achieve a lower grade.

Communication skills in a one-to-one interaction

1 **Explain the context in which the interaction took place.** Students should give details of:

- Where the interaction happened – what was the setting like? Give details of the size of the room layout, of seating, and so on.
- Who was involved in the interaction as well as yourself. Describe the roles of people rather than their real names.
- What had happened leading up to the interaction. Explain the events which happened before the interaction.

2 **Describe the verbal and non-verbal details of the interaction.** Students should provide an objective statement which describes the detail of the interaction. They might use the grid in Table 2.3 (page 116 of textbook), reproduced as OHT 2.4.1, to provide headings which could be used to explain what happened. The section should not seek to interpret or explain the events but just to describe what was heard and seen.

3 **Identify potential barriers to communication.** Students should explain any potential barriers which may have existed and what actions they took to avoid barriers to communication.

4 **Provide a critical evaluation of the use of interaction skills.** Students should interpret and evaluate the interaction and evaluate their own effectiveness at this point. It may be important to provide a clear evaluation which is separate from the detail of the interaction.

5 **Provide a realistic action plan for improving one-to-one communication skills.** Students need to explain how they might improve their one-to-one interaction skills. They can use the action plan guidance in the textbook (pages 111–114) to help.

Communication skills in a group interaction

1 **Explain the context in which the interaction took place.** The student should give details of the following:

- The setting that the group meeting took place in. Explain and/or draw the layout of the group. Describe any seating pattern.
- Who the group members were; describe their roles rather than their real names.
- Any events which led to the group meeting. Give a brief account of any previous meetings of this group. Describe any function or purpose which members may have had for the group.

2 **Describe the interaction patterns observed in the group and provide a detailed description of individual behaviour relevant to group functioning.** The student might like to use the grid set out in OHT 2.3.2 (Figure 2.25 on page 111 of textbook) to monitor individual behaviour among group members. They might also like to draw and/or describe the participation patterns they observed. They should explore the extent to which group **maintenance** and **task** behaviours were observed. Some non-verbal communication may need to be described, but details of verbal and non-verbal analysis may be more limited than in the individual interaction.

3 **Identify potential barriers which might block group communication or group processes.** The student should describe any emotional, environmental, behavioural, listening, language or skills-based barriers which might interfere with group communication or with the successful working of the group.

4 **Provide a critical evaluation of your own interaction skills within the group.** The student should evaluate the effectiveness of the group in achieving its aims or at least working within a value system. The student should also evaluate the effectiveness of their own communication within the group. It may be important to provide an evaluation which is separate from the detail of the group observation.

5 **Provide a realistic action plan for improving your group communication skills.** The student needs to explain how they might improve their group communication skills. Use the action plan guidance in the textbook (pages 111–114) to help.

Report examining communication skills within a health, social care or early years setting

1 **The student should provide an explanation of how effective communication can contribute to valuing people.**

- This explanation might draw on the theory as set out in OHT 2.1.1 (Figure 2.1 on page 74 of the textbook).
- The student should also draw on the theory of emotional work in care as set out on page 80 of the textbook.
- The student should also draw on the theory of valuing differences between people as set out on page 84 of the textbook and the theory of empowerment as set out on page 94.

2 **The student should provide an evaluation of the extent to which appropriate communications skills are demonstrated in a chosen care setting.** This evaluation might be based on the theory explained in Section 2.1 above. The student should evaluate how well communication is working within a setting they have been on placement in or which they have visited. They should explain to what extent communication fits the theory of meeting different levels of human need. The student should also explain how inappropriate communication might damage the well-being of clients.

3 **Make realistic recommendations for improving interactions in care settings.** The student should offer a range of detailed ideas for improving communication in a setting that they have worked in.

4 **Provide an overview of ways in which client confidentiality can be maintained.** Use Section 2.5 on pages 117–120 of the textbook to help structure a set of ideas which will ensure that client confidentiality is maintained in relation to the care setting described previously.

OHTs

The OHTs to help tutors to deliver this unit are as follows:

2.1.1 Communication related to Maslow's levels of need
2.1.2 Informal interaction in care
2.1.3 Examples of formal interaction
2.2.1 Some differences between aggressive, assertive and submissive behaviour
2.3.1 Tuckman's 4 stages of group formation
2.3.2 A profile to monitor group behaviour
2.3.3 Two patterns of participation
2.3.4 Group participation
2.3.5 Ethical dilemmas
2.4.1 Analysing communication

ACTIVITIES

The activities are designed to promote learning and understanding, provide consolidation and develop logical thinking.

2.1.1 Exploring the importance of communication
2.1.2 Exploring the role of staff in a care setting
2.2.1 Effective communication
2.3.1 Noughts and crosses
2.4.1 Evaluating barriers to communication

OHT 2.1.1 COMMUNICATION RELATED TO MASLOW'S LEVELS OF NEED

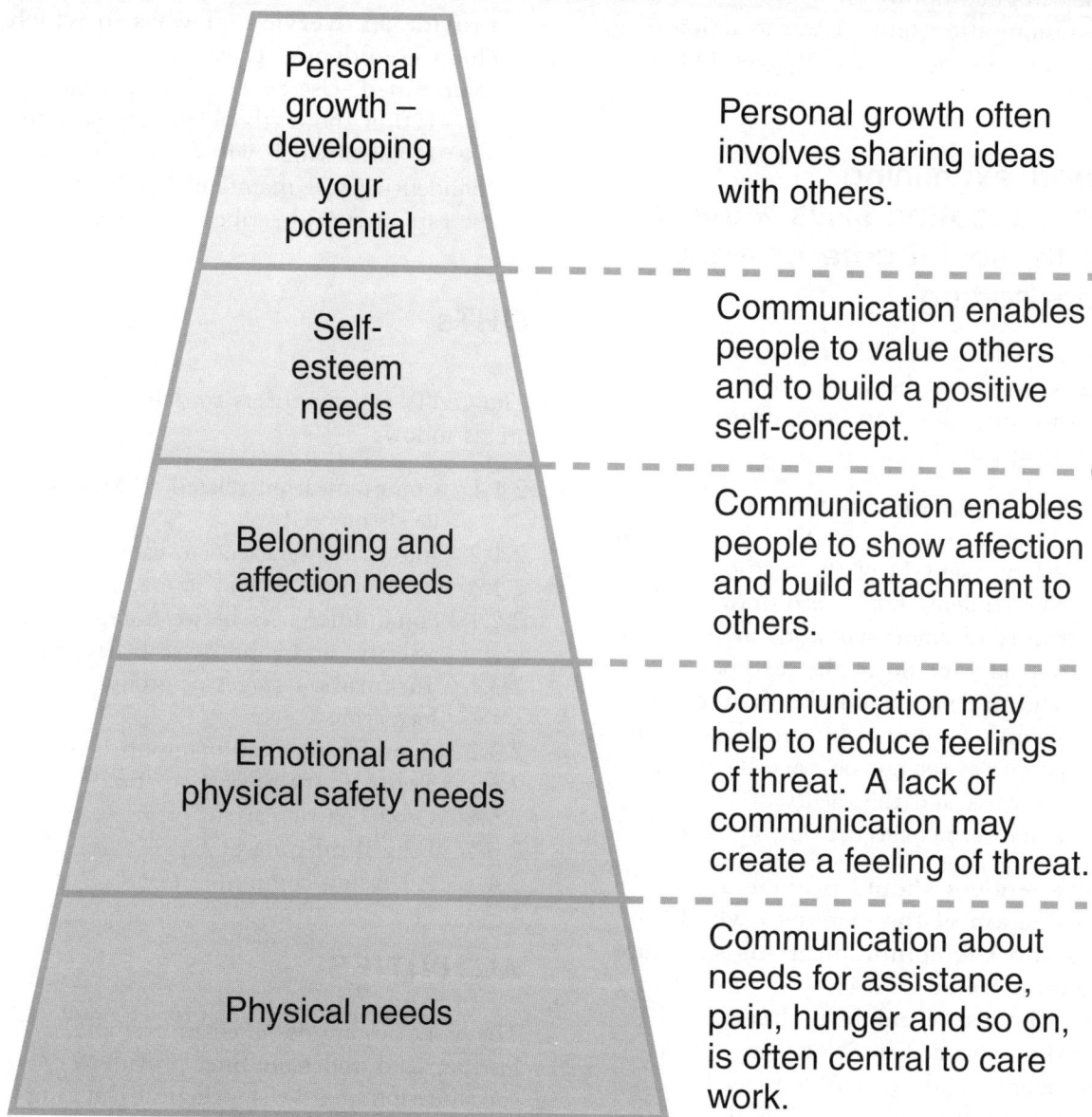

Level of need	Role of communication
Personal growth – developing your potential	Personal growth often involves sharing ideas with others.
Self-esteem needs	Communication enables people to value others and to build a positive self-concept.
Belonging and affection needs	Communication enables people to show affection and build attachment to others.
Emotional and physical safety needs	Communication may help to reduce feelings of threat. A lack of communication may create a feeling of threat.
Physical needs	Communication about needs for assistance, pain, hunger and so on, is often central to care work.

OHT 2.1.2 INFORMAL INTERACTION IN CARE

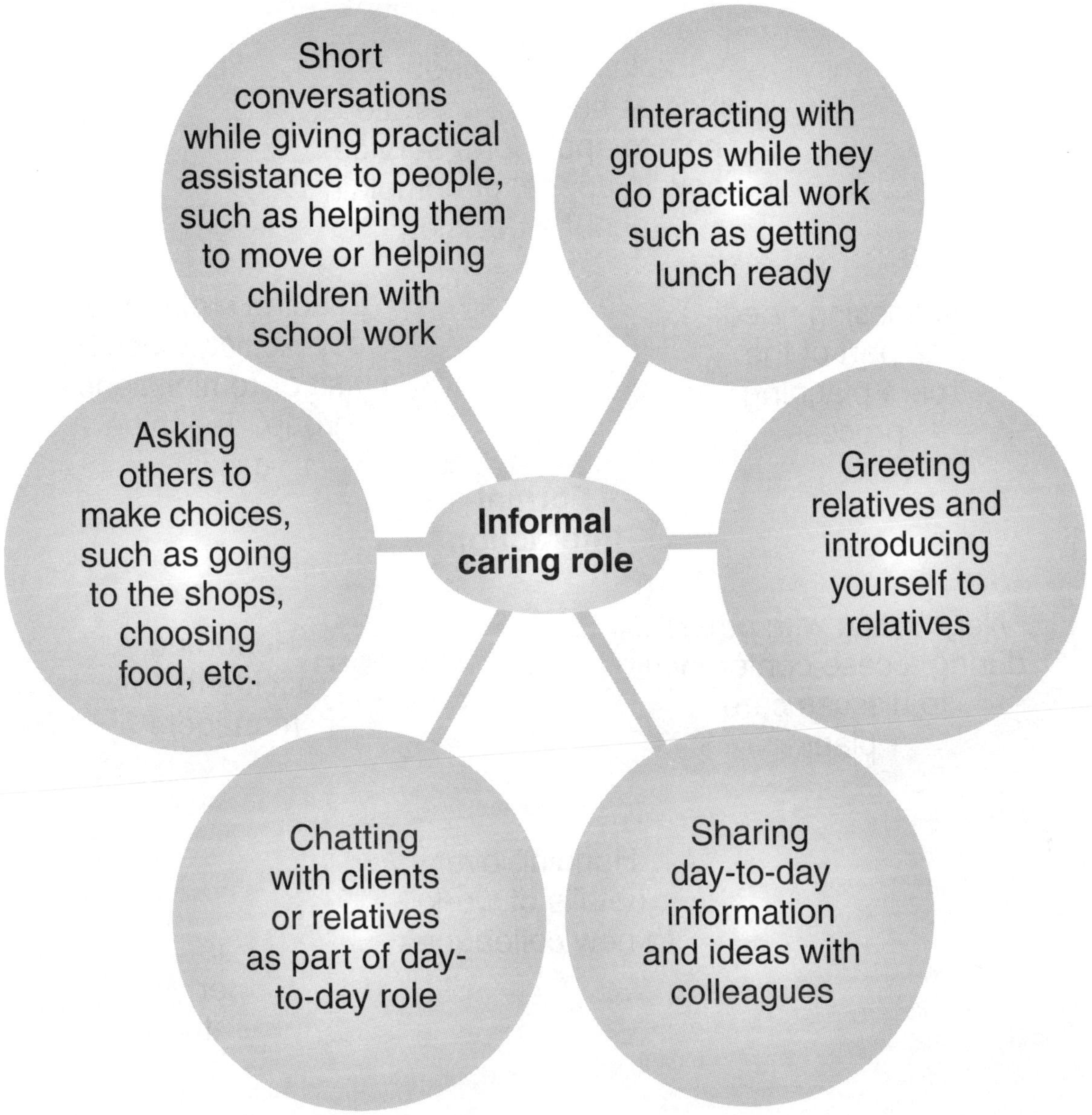

Informal caring role

- Short conversations while giving practical assistance to people, such as helping them to move or helping children with school work
- Interacting with groups while they do practical work such as getting lunch ready
- Greeting relatives and introducing yourself to relatives
- Sharing day-to-day information and ideas with colleagues
- Chatting with clients or relatives as part of day-to-day role
- Asking others to make choices, such as going to the shops, choosing food, etc.

OHT 2.1.3 EXAMPLES OF FORMAL INTERACTION

Formal interaction

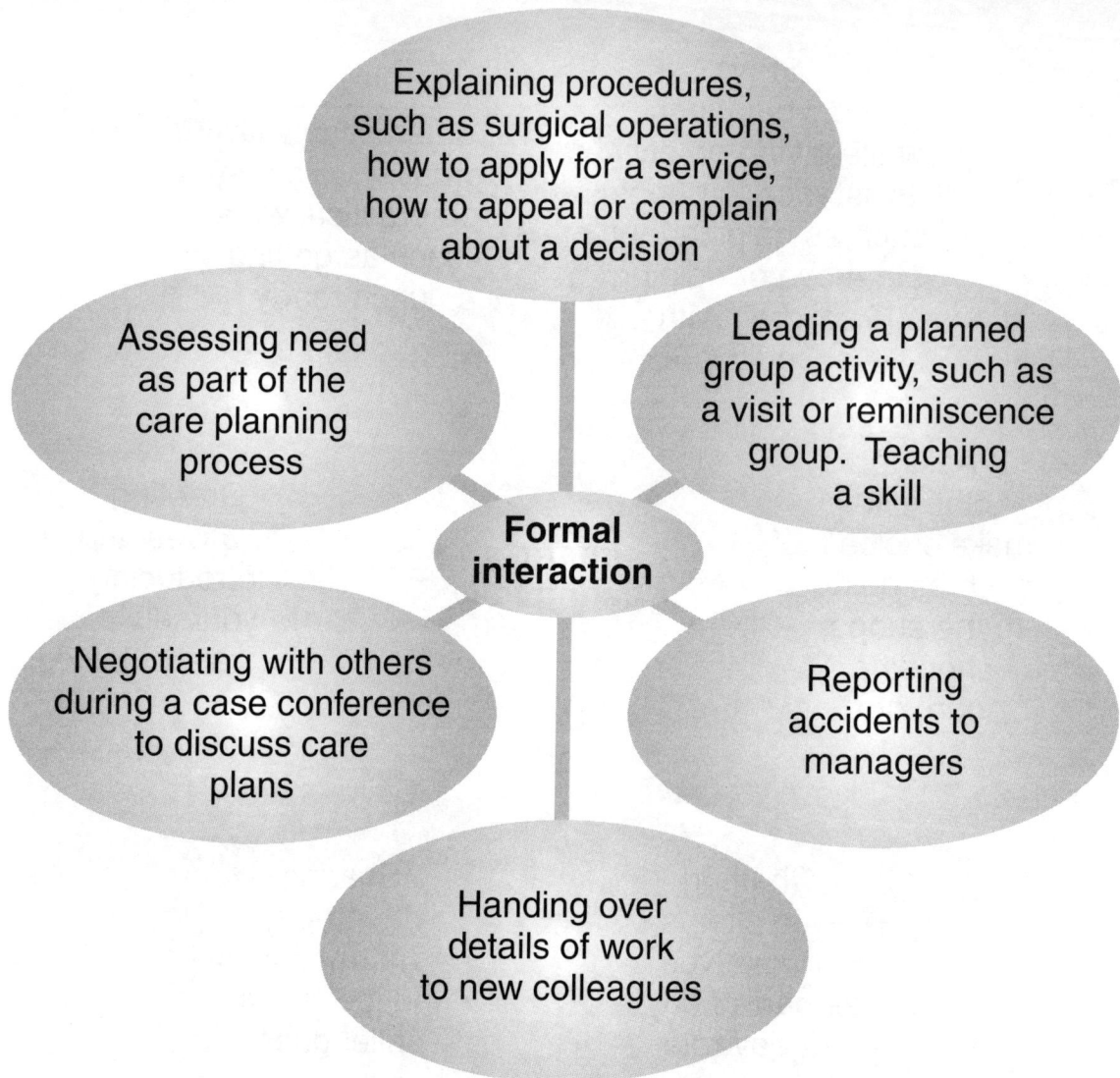

- Explaining procedures, such as surgical operations, how to apply for a service, how to appeal or complain about a decision
- Leading a planned group activity, such as a visit or reminiscence group. Teaching a skill
- Reporting accidents to managers
- Handing over details of work to new colleagues
- Negotiating with others during a case conference to discuss care plans
- Assessing need as part of the care planning process

OHT 2.2.1 SOME DIFFERENCES BETWEEN AGGRESSIVE, ASSERTIVE AND SUBMISSIVE BEHAVIOUR

Aggressive behaviour	**Assertive behaviour**	**Submissive behaviour**
Main emotion: anger	*Main emotion*: staying in control of own actions	*Main emotion*: fear
Wanting your own way Making demands Not listening to others 'Putting other people down' Trying to win Shouting or talking very loudly	Negotiating with others Trying to solve problems Aiming that no one has to lose Listening to others Showing respect for others Keeping a clear, calm voice	Letting others win Agreeing with others Not putting your views across Looking afraid Speaking quietly or not speaking at all
Threatening non-verbal behaviour including: fixed eye contact, tense muscles, waving or folding hands and arms, looking angry	**Normal non-verbal behaviour** including: varied eye contact, relaxed face muscles, looking 'in control', keeping hands and arms at your side	**Submissive non-verbal behaviour** including: looking down, not looking at others, looking frightened, tense muscles

OHT 2.3.1 TUCKMAN'S 4 STAGES OF GROUP FORMATION

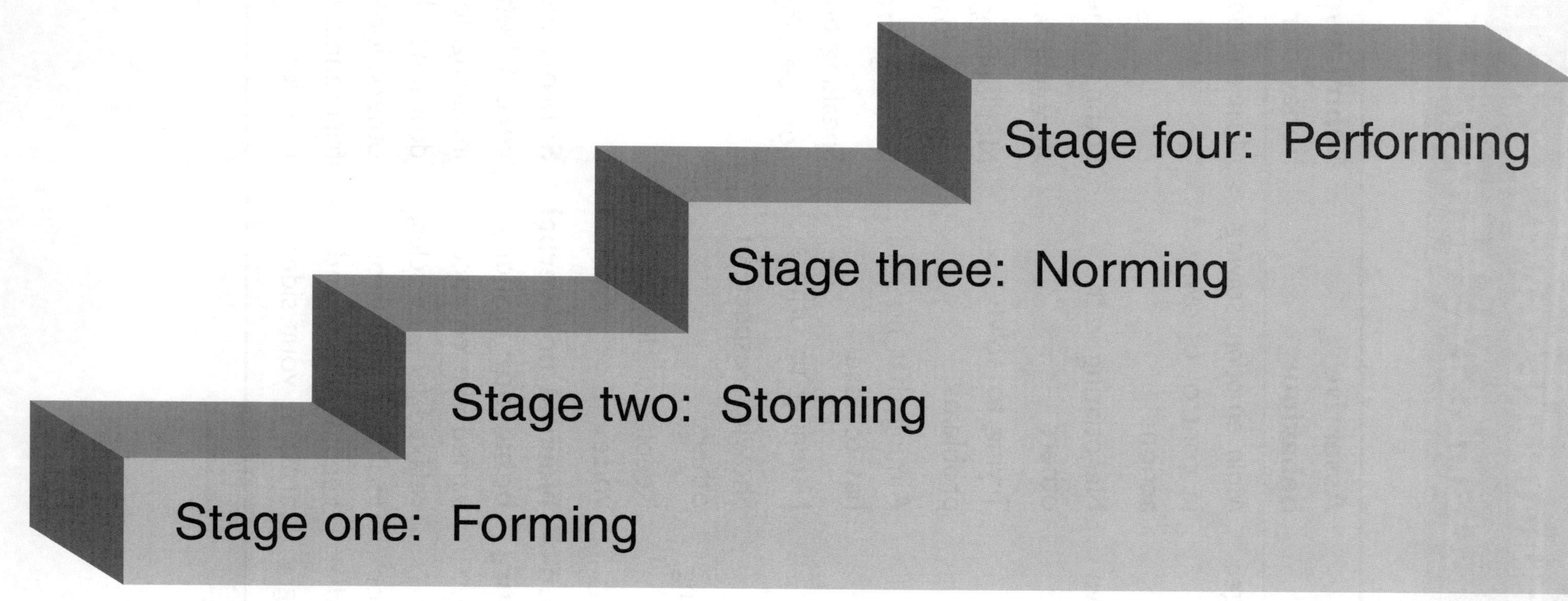
Stage four: Performing
Stage three: Norming
Stage two: Storming
Stage one: Forming

OHT 2.3.2 A PROFILE TO MONITOR GROUP BEHAVIOUR

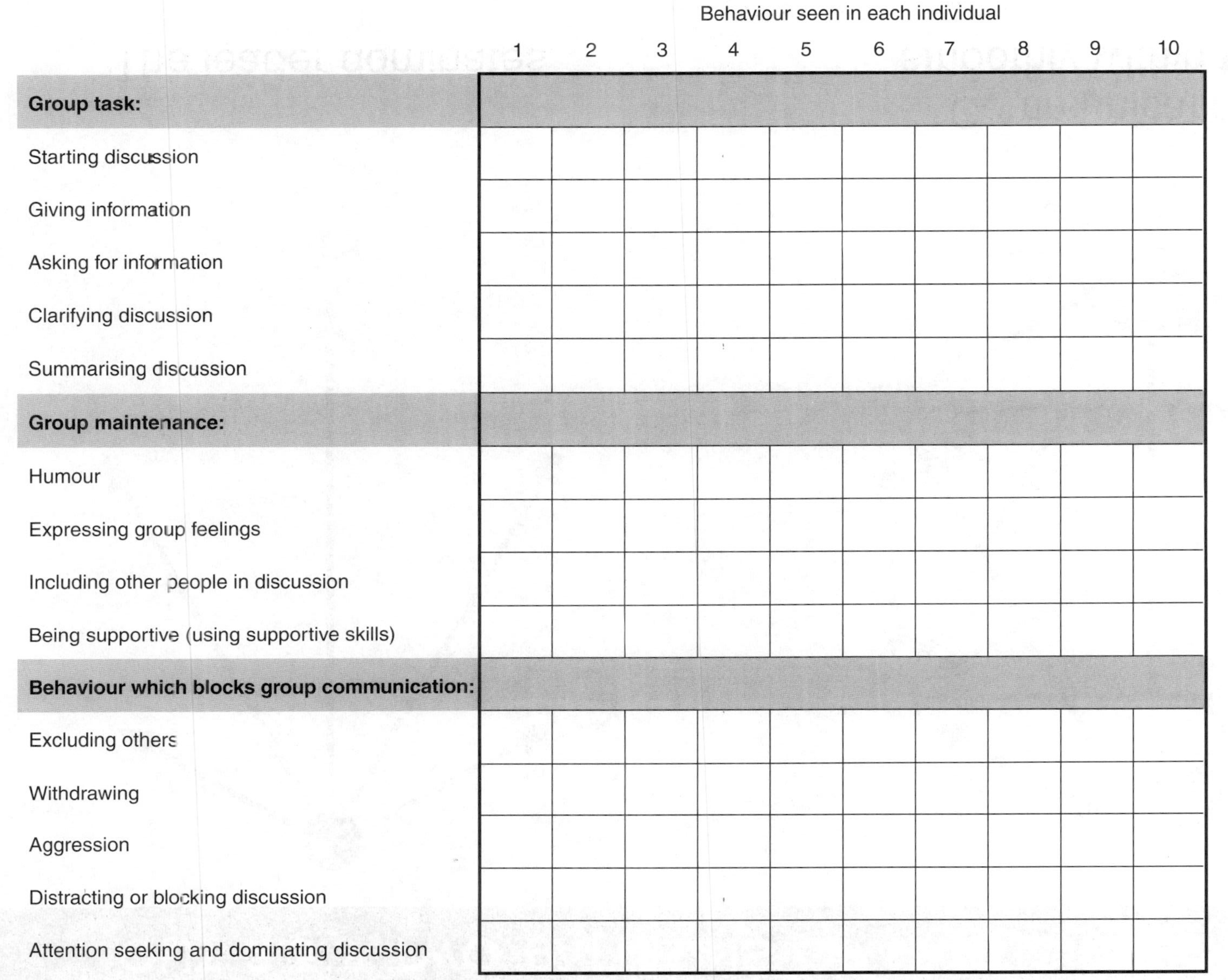

	Behaviour seen in each individual									
	1	2	3	4	5	6	7	8	9	10
Group task:										
Starting discussion										
Giving information										
Asking for information										
Clarifying discussion										
Summarising discussion										
Group maintenance:										
Humour										
Expressing group feelings										
Including other people in discussion										
Being supportive (using supportive skills)										
Behaviour which blocks group communication:										
Excluding others										
Withdrawing										
Aggression										
Distracting or blocking discussion										
Attention seeking and dominating discussion										

OHT 2.3.3 TWO PATTERNS OF PARTICIPATION

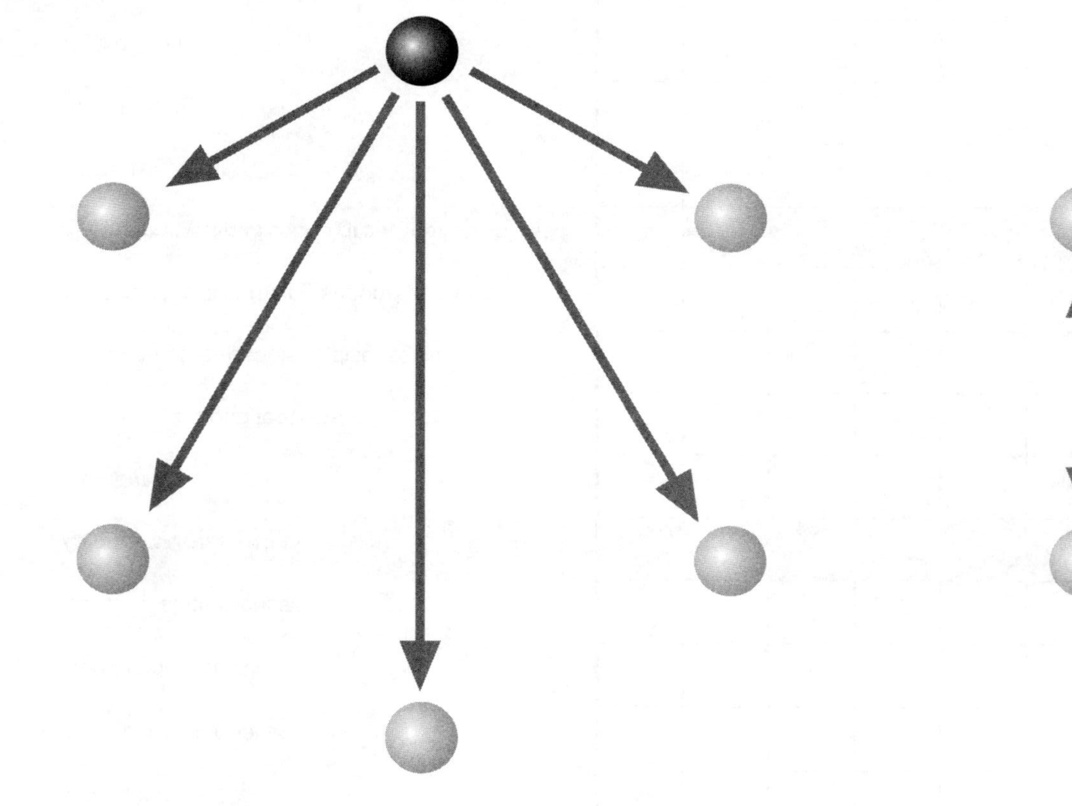

The leader dominates

Communication runs smoothly within the group

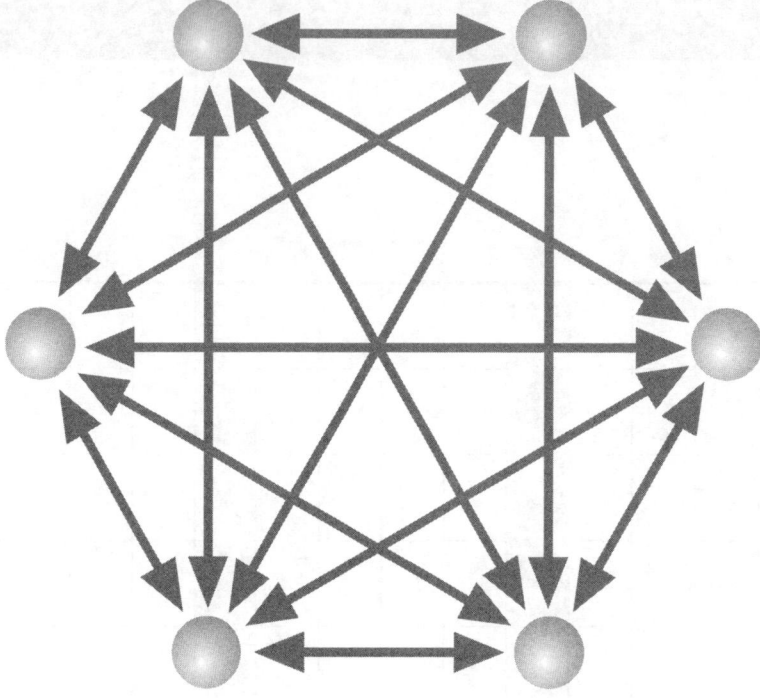

OHT 2.3.4 GROUP PARTICIPATION

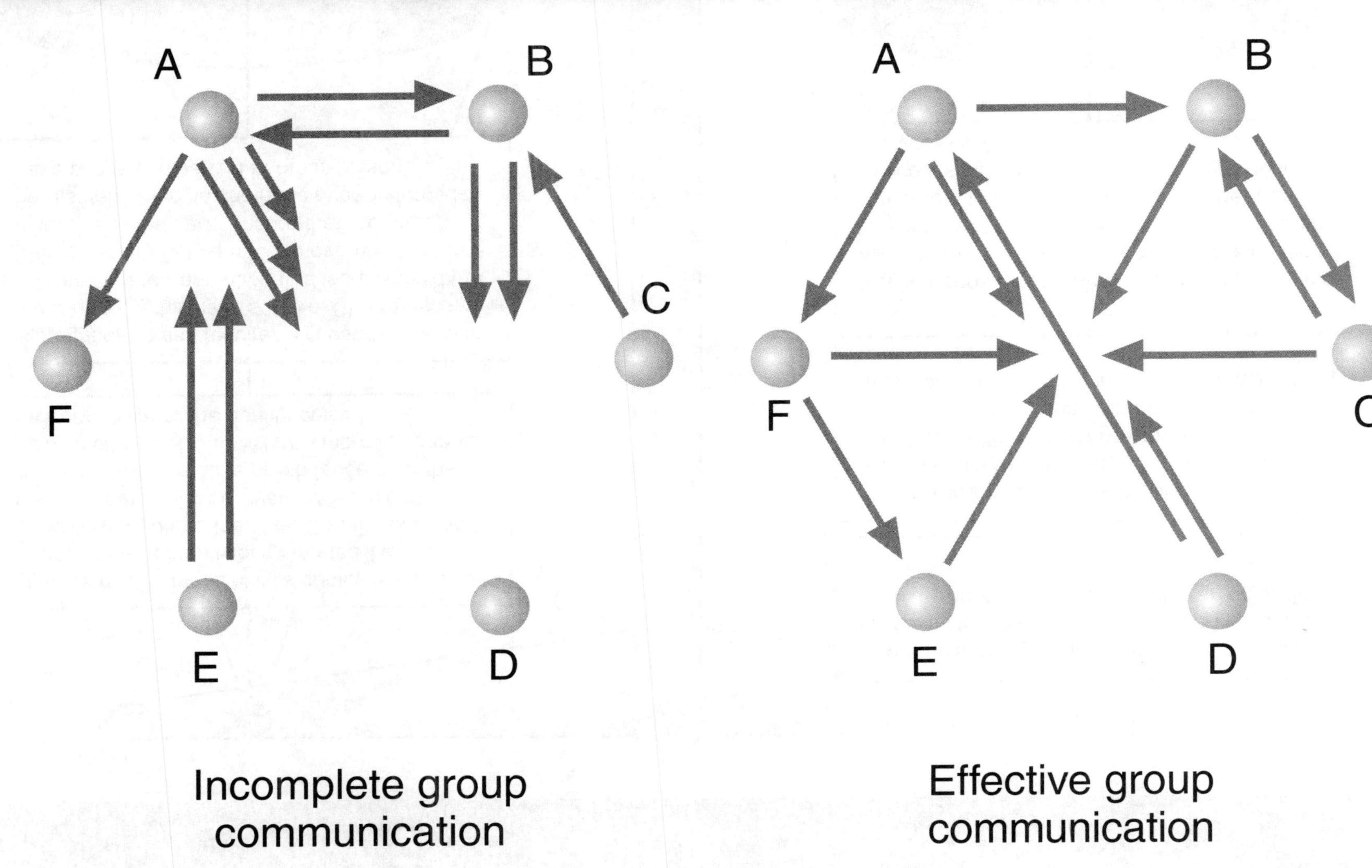
A
B
C
D
E
F
Incomplete group communication
A
B
C
D
E
F
Effective group communication

OHT 2.3.5 ETHICAL DILEMMAS

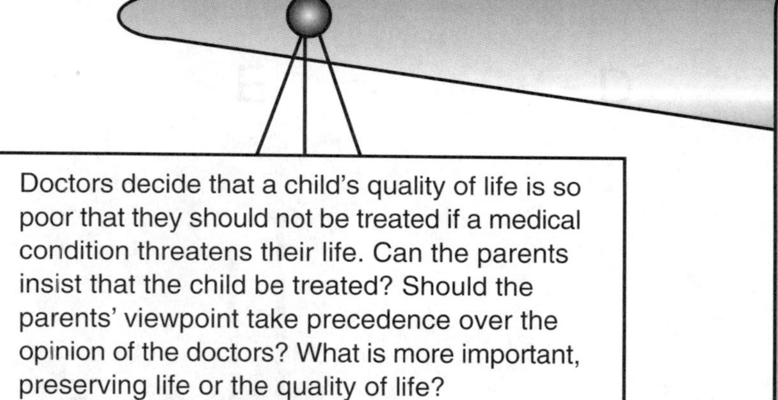

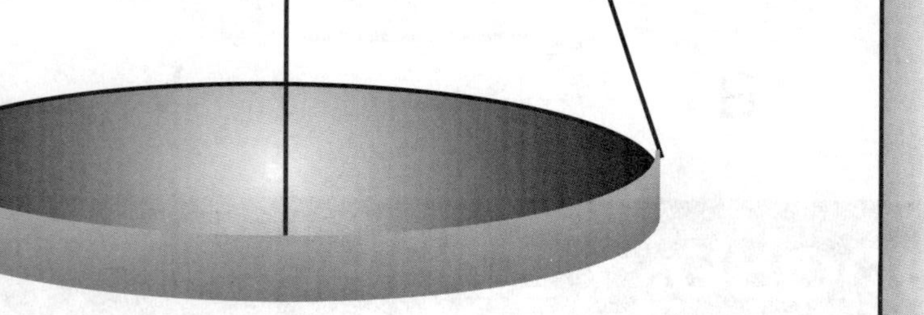

Doctors decide that a child's quality of life is so poor that they should not be treated if a medical condition threatens their life. Can the parents insist that the child be treated? Should the parents' viewpoint take precedence over the opinion of the doctors? What is more important, preserving life or the quality of life?

A pregnant woman requires a caesarean section if her unborn child is to survive. She refuses, without an apparent rational reason. Should the Mental Health Act be used to override the woman's wishes and ensure that the child is born safely? Should someone ever be forced to have surgery to benefit another person?

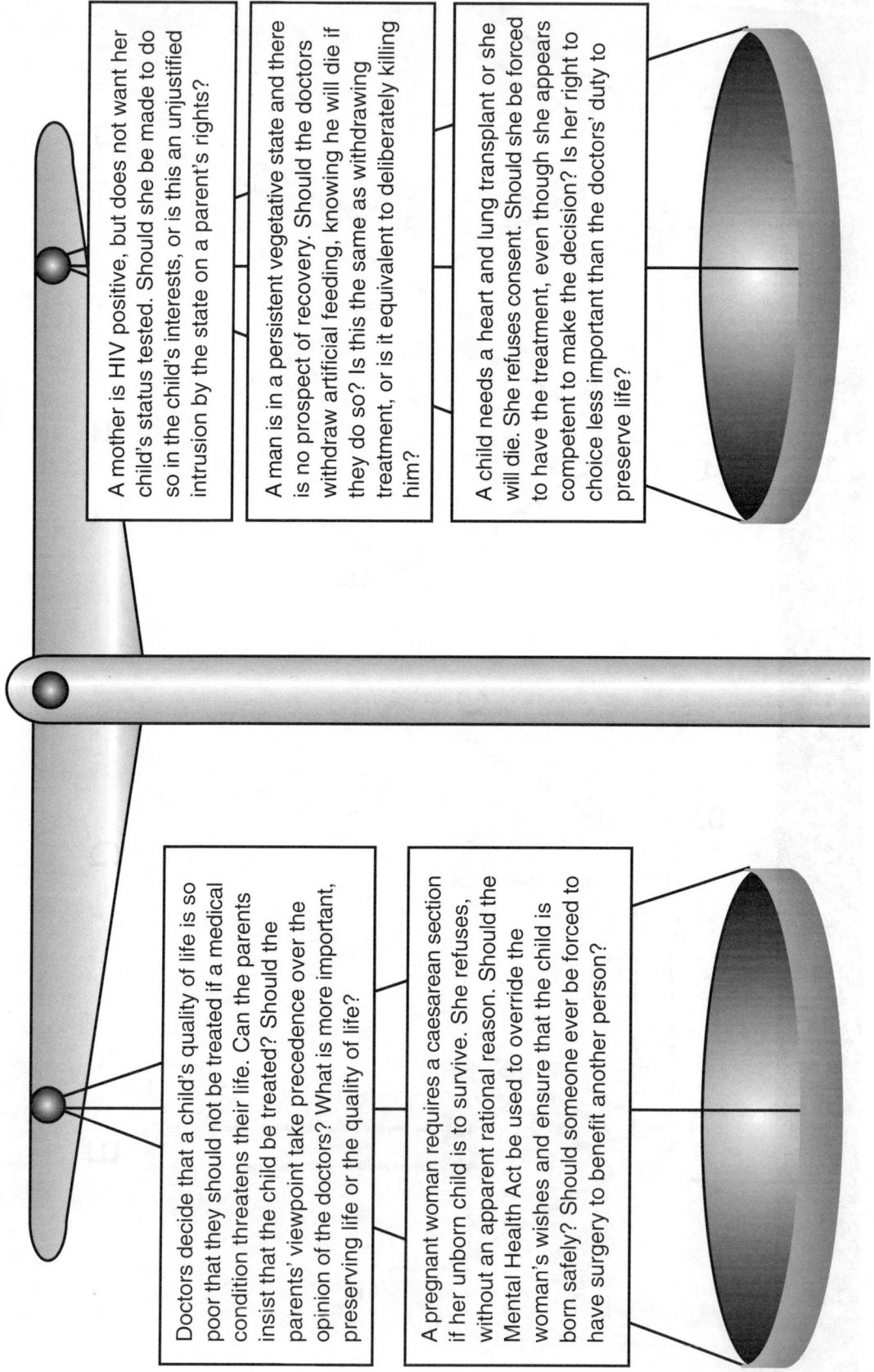

A mother is HIV positive, but does not want her child's status tested. Should she be made to do so in the child's interests, or is this an unjustified intrusion by the state on a parent's rights?

A man is in a persistent vegetative state and there is no prospect of recovery. Should the doctors withdraw artificial feeding, knowing he will die if they do so? Is this the same as withdrawing treatment, or is it equivalent to deliberately killing him?

A child needs a heart and lung transplant or she will die. She refuses consent. Should she be forced to have the treatment, even though she appears competent to make the decision? Is her right to choice less important than the doctors' duty to preserve life?

OHT 2.4.1 ANALYSING COMMUNICATION

	Rating scale Mark 1, 2, 3, 4 or 5	Evidence seen
Non-verbal communication Eye contact Facial expression Angle of head Tone of voice Position of hands and arms Gestures Posture Muscle tension Touch Proximity Dress and appearance		
Verbal communication: listening skills Encouragement Reflection Use of prompts Conversational skills Questioning Use of silence Clarity Pace of conversation Turn taking		
Creating emotional safety Understanding Warmth Sincerity Appropriate responsiveness and calmness		
Attention to values Rapport Respect for diversity in others Appropriate choice of language Understanding the influence of culture and gender on communication		
The quality of the environment for communication Physical barriers to communication Privacy Maintaining confidentiality		

ACTIVITY 2.1.1 EXPLORING THE IMPORTANCE OF COMMUNICATION

This activity enables you to understand the importance of non-verbal and visual clues when communicating.

In doing it you will be able to explain the importance of context and visual information when you attempt to communicate.

The diagrams on the following pages will be needed for this activity.

How to do the activity

1 Organise yourselves into pairs sitting back to back with each other.

2 One of you will be given a blank sheet of paper and the other a diagram. The one with the diagram must not show it to their partner.

3 The one with the diagram has to explain it orally to their partner. They have 5 minutes to do this. The one with the blank sheet of paper has to try to draw the diagram that is being explained to them.

4 You will then swap roles and repeat the activity using a different diagram.

5 After you have completed the activity you will give feedback to the class on what you learned.

ACTIVITY 2.1.1 (CONTINUED) HANDOUT 1

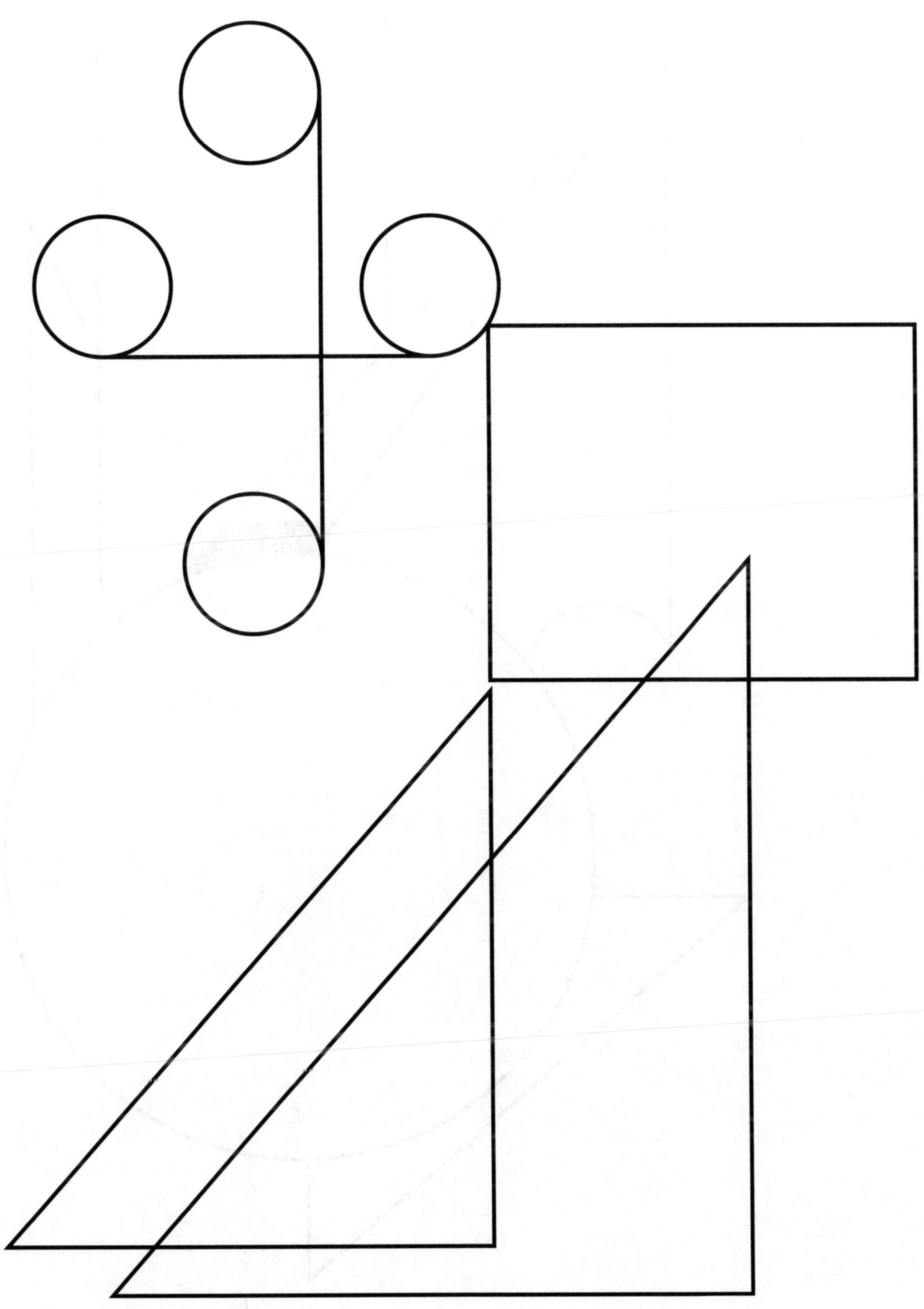

ACTIVITY 2.1.1 (CONTINUED) HANDOUT 2

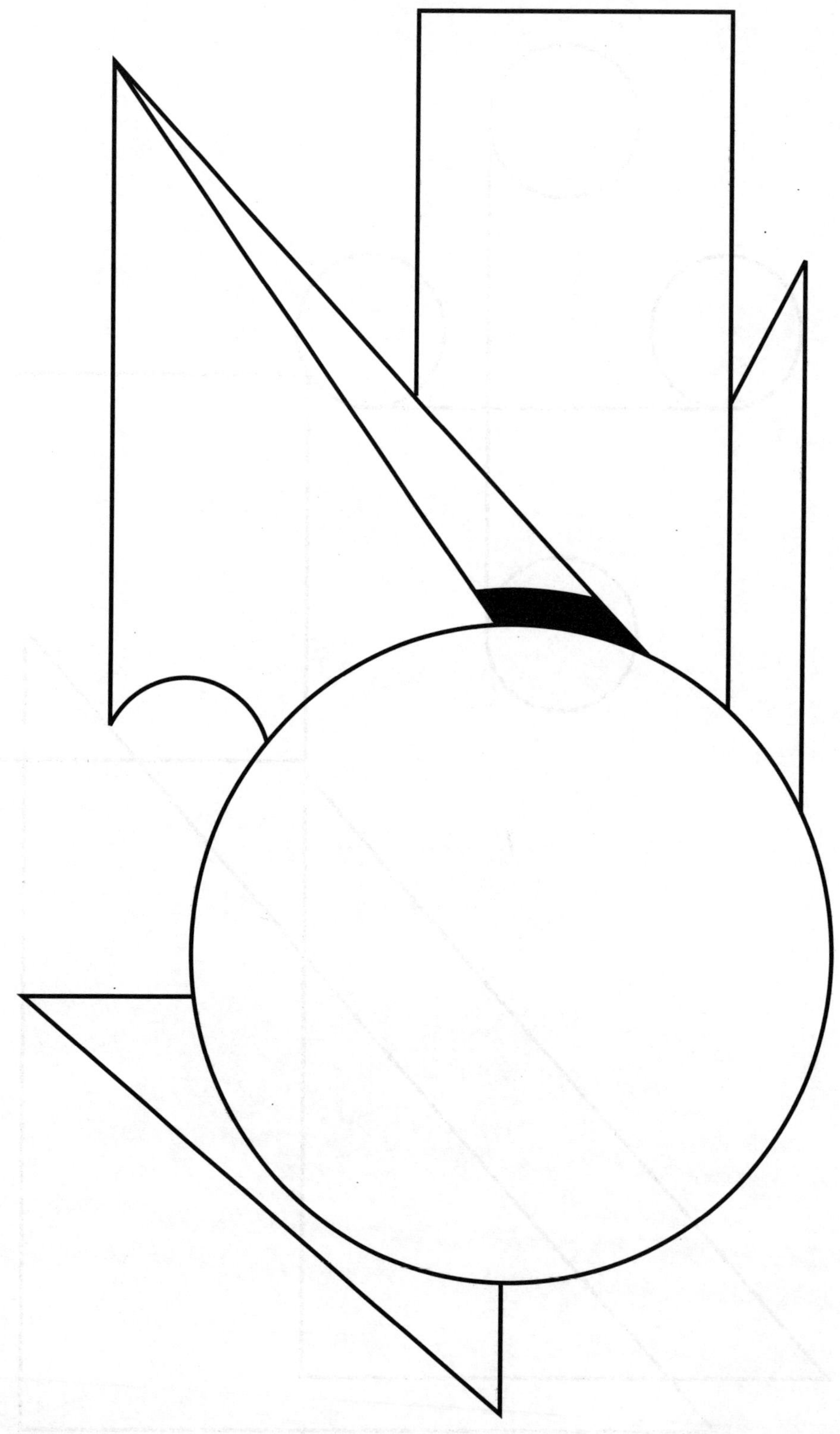

ACTIVITY 2.1.2 EXPLORING THE ROLE OF STAFF IN A CARE SETTING

This activity will help students map the kind of interaction they may come across in a care setting.

TASK 1

Talk to 4 or 5 different members of staff in a given care setting and ask them the following:

- To describe a range of people that they have to work for or with (e.g. manager, clients, relatives, colleagues).
- What expectations they have of their role.
- Whether different people have different expectations of members of staff.
- How they have to alter their communication skills to meet the different expectations of people.

TASK 2

Draw a pattern diagram of the range of people that staff in a care setting have to work with – the diagram below is an example.

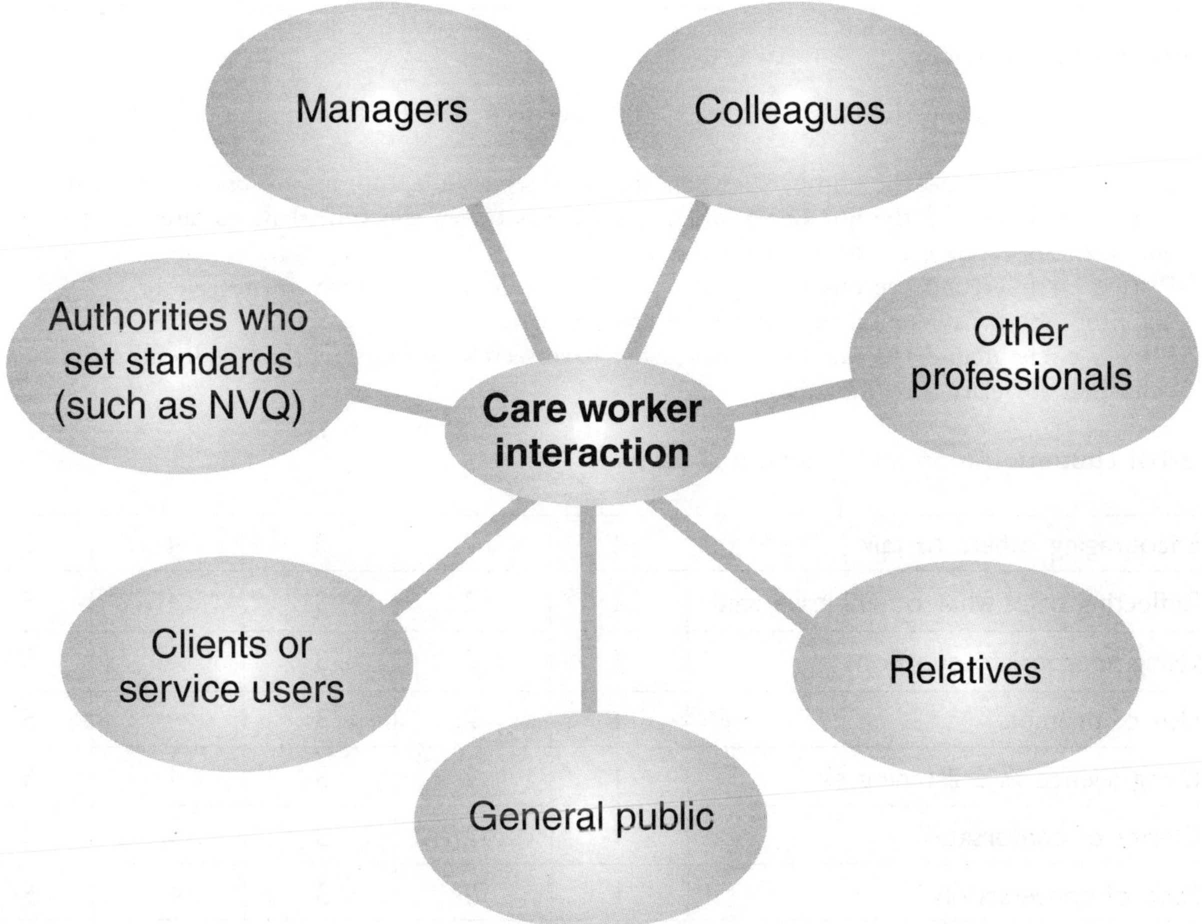
Managers
Colleagues
Authorities who set standards (such as NVQ)
Other professionals
Care worker interaction
Clients or service users
Relatives
General public

ACTIVITY 2.2.1 EFFECTIVE COMMUNICATION

This activity aims to develop the ability to analyse verbal and non-verbal communication.

Non-verbal communication

Eye contact	1	2	3	4	5
Facial expression	1	2	3	4	5
Angle of head	1	2	3	4	5
Tone of voice	1	2	3	4	5
Position of hands and arms	1	2	3	4	5
Gestures	1	2	3	4	5
Posture	1	2	3	4	5
Muscle tension	1	2	3	4	5
Touch	1	2	3	4	5
Proximity	1	2	3	4	5

How to rate behaviour:

- Place a circle around the number 1 when you have seen very effective and appropriate use of a skill.
- Place a circle around the number 2 when you have seen some appropriate use of the skill.
- Place a circle around the number 3 when you have not seen the skill demonstrated or if it does not seem appropriate to comment on the area.
- Place a circle around the number 4 when you have seen some slightly ineffective or inappropriate behaviour in relation to the area.
- Place a circle around the number 5 when you have seen very inappropriate or ineffective behaviour in relation to the area.

Verbal communication and listening skills

Encouraging others to talk	1	2	3	4	5
Reflecting back what others have said	1	2	3	4	5
Using appropriate questions	1	2	3	4	5
Use of prompts	1	2	3	4	5
Using silence as a listening skill	1	2	3	4	5
Clarity of conversation	1	2	3	4	5
Pace of conversation	1	2	3	4	5
Turn taking	1	2	3	4	5

How to rate behaviour:
Use the same rating instructions used for non-verbal communication above.

ACTIVITY 2.3.1 NOUGHTS AND CROSSES

To do this activity you should form into groups of 6–8 members for the game of noughts and crosses. Each group will be divided into observers and participaants. The observers will record in circles on a sheet of paper the pattern of the other members' participation in the game. Your aim is to work out a strategy which makes it impossible to lose playing the game of noughts and crosses; that is, without changing the rules of the game or cheating.

TASK 1

Play the game using the noughts and crosses grids on the following page.

TASK 2

As a group try to work out a strategy, using the grids on the following page to practise on, by which you, as a group, can never lose at the game.

TASK 3

The observers will feedback to the tutor the participation patterns they have recorded, or will discuss these patterns with members of the group before giving feedback.

ACTIVITY 2.3.1 (CONTINUED) HANDOUT – NOUGHTS AND CROSSES GRIDS

ACTIVITY 2.4.1 EVALUATING BARRIERS TO COMMUNICATION

This activity will help you identify issues for your assessment report. You can use the grid on the following page to help in identifying the barriers to communication and the issues involved.

TASKS

1. Keep a log book in which to record your thoughts and observations of conversations and group activities you have observed.
2. Write a brief description of a conversation or group session you have observed.
3. Using the grid, rate the conversation in relation to the barriers.
4. Explore the reasons for the quality of the communication you observed.
5. Think of any improvements you would suggest to reduce the barriers to communication.
6. Write up any suggestions you have to make for improvements to communication.

ACTIVITY 2.4.1 (CONTINUED) HANDOUT – BARRIERS TO COMMUNICATION GRID

Rating scale:
1 Good – there is no barrier
2 Quite good – few barriers
3 Not possible to decide or not applicable
4 Poor – barriers identified
5 Very poor – major barriers to communication

Barriers	**Rating scale**				
In the environment					
Lighting	1	2	3	4	5
Noise levels	1	2	3	4	5
Opportunity to communicate	1	2	3	4	5
Language differences					
Carers' skills with different languages	1	2	3	4	5
Carers' skills with non-verbal communication	1	2	3	4	5
Availability of translators or interpreters	1	2	3	4	5
Assumptions and/or stereotypes	1	2	3	4	5
Emotional barriers					
Stress levels and tiredness	1	2	3	4	5
Carers stressed by the emotional needs of clients	1	2	3	4	5
Cultural barriers					
Inappropriate assumptions made about others	1	2	3	4	5
Labelling or stereotyping present	1	2	3	4	5
Interpersonal skills					
Degree of supportive non-verbal behaviour	1	2	3	4	5
Degree of supportive verbal behaviour	1	2	3	4	5
Appropriate use of listening skills	1	2	3	4	5
Appropriate use of assertive skills	1	2	3	4	5
Appropriate maintenance of confidentiality	1	2	3	4	5

UNIT 3 – PHYSICAL ASPECTS OF HEALTH

OVERVIEW

In this unit students are introduced to the human physiology of six major organ systems in the human body and how these are dependent on each other so that the whole body can function as a co-ordinated whole.

Each body system has a self-regulatory or homeostatic control mechanism to maintain vital body features within a fairly narrow range, and students will learn about these.

Your class group will need to carry out practical work by taking external physiological measurements, preferably from real clients, and learn how to use the equipment safely to produce accurate results. They will use analytical skills in the interpretation of their results.

The unit is divided in the textbook into five sections and the teaching notes in this file are similarly sub-divided. The sections are:

3.1 Physiology and anatomy
3.2 Homeostasis
3.3 Physiological measurements of individuals in care settings
3.4 Safe practice
3.5 Analysis and accuracy of results

Each section will include references to overhead transparencies and activities relevant to that section.

Aims and objectives

The aims of this unit are to:

- identify the structures relating to functions of specified human body systems
- recognise the ways in which these body systems relate to each other
- identify the homeostatic processes regulating vital physiological factors relating to the body systems
- explain how routine physiological measurements are obtained and how results of monitoring are interpreted
- apply science in a care context.

Students should be able to:

- explain the gross structure and function of the respiratory, cardio-vascular, digestive, renal, nervous and endocrine systems
- describe the relationships between these systems
- describe the homeostatic processes operating in specified body systems to control blood glucose levels, body temperature, heart rate, respiratory rate and water content
- use physiological measuring equipment under supervision to take and record measurements from individuals
- interpret results of physiological measurements including deviations from expected results
- describe ethical issues which may arise from taking physiological measurements
- identify potential health and safety risks associated with physiological measurements and the ways of minimising these risks
- describe possible sources of error associated with physiological monitoring and the ways of reducing these errors
- analyse results accurately and in an appropriate scientific manner.

Assessment

The unit is assessed through portfolio work and extra depth, breadth, originality and independence will all count towards higher grade achievement.

For the assessment, students will make routine physiological measurements involving at least three body systems. They will be expected to know the normal ranges for these measurements and be able to explain any deviations from the expected range. After choosing the three systems, they will describe their gross structure and function and explain how the homeostatic mechanisms control the factors they have measured.

While using equipment to monitor the chosen physiological factors, students will both use and describe safe practice in using equipment and comment on any potential health and safety risks and ways to reduce these.

In addition grade C students will review their methods of monitoring and identify possible sources of error. They will use their data to demonstrate how the systems are working together and explain how a failure of homeostatic control can produce data outside the expected range.

Grade A students will be able to suggest and justify ways to improve the accuracy of the results. They will be able to harness complex analytical skills in interpreting their data to demonstrate the inter-relationships of the body systems which bring about homeostasis. For further details on how to organise the unit assessment see textbook.

TEACHING NOTES

3.1 Physiology and anatomy

Most tutors will begin this section with either the cardio-vascular system or the respiratory system. The former is perhaps the most popular, but the latter makes a logical approach to dealing with the cardio-vascular as the second system. Sadly, even students who have achieved GCSEs in Biology or Human Biology still believe that respiration is breathing!

The respiratory system

It is useful then to begin with the process of respiration as a cellular activity and to introduce the systems as a means of delivering the raw materials to the cells for the purpose of respiration without which nothing can function. At the same time, mention can be made of anaerobic respiration as an emergency measure in the absence of a sufficient supply of oxygen.

The respiratory system can then be introduced as the physical way in which oxygen is delivered to the cells and the waste products of carbon dioxide and water are removed. You can then revise this for reinforcement when you come to the cardio-vascular system.

It is useful then to break up this 'delivery' process into breathing, gaseous exchange and carriage of gases by the blood. Students should understand the scientific concept underlying the pressure/volume relationship that is fundamental to inhalation and exhalation and to the pull of surface tension that allows the lungs to follow in the wake of the chest wall. This will enable them to understand emergencies and treatments for conditions such as a collapsed lung or chest wounds.

(See **OHT** 3.1.1).

If this is followed by lung volume measurement, using either spirometer or simple tubing and calibrated container, try to let students see some animal lungs and appreciate the spongy nature and smooth texture of the external surface. Trying to squeeze all the air out of a piece of lung tissue (unsuccessfully, as it still floats in water) emphasises that fresh lung tissue always contains some air (residual air).

A circus of practical activities can be very successful in sustaining interest, as each one takes only a short time to do. It is better to devote a session to participating in all the activities than losing time with individual practical tasks.

This is also a good place to explain diffusion and osmosis; very few school-leavers appreciate that osmosis is a special case of diffusion concerned only with water and selectively permeable membranes which they rarely equate with cell membranes. If you have ex-Intermediate students or mature students in your group you will certainly have to spend some time investigating diffusion as well. All too often in the past with GNVQ curricula in health and social care there was a lack of interesting and reinforcing practical work, so you should endeavour to re-introduce laboratory sessions.

Getting students used to practical work will increase confidence for their own assessment and may improve manual dexterity.

Many tutors will show students how to measure lung volumes, breathing rates and utilisation of oxygen by using a spirometer. There are many different models of biological spirometer, some old and some more modern. It must be emphasised that students should have sheets showing the standard operating procedure for the particular spirometer, as well as having the spirometer demonstrated beforehand and being supervised during its use.

This will inevitably take a considerable time and students clearly cannot transport a spirometer into a care setting to use with a client. Neither can they transport calibrated containers, water troughs and rubber tubing with them. Being practical, it may be more profitable for the tutor to demonstrate using a spirometer so that students fully understand its use, but allow them to measure lung volumes on each other with calibrated containers, etc. This is a relatively safe procedure, if somewhat inaccurate, although they may get a little wet! Measuring lung volumes in a care setting is therefore going to be impractical for most students. They can, however, with permission, make peak flow readings and take breathing rates. It might be possible for some students to visit a physiological measurement unit in a hospital or have a guest speaker with a portable medical spirometer.

Activity 3.1.1 is designed to be trouble-free for the tutor so simple laboratory equipment is used to determine the vital capacity and tidal volume. You might wish students to compare the accuracy of reading from the equipment with spirometer readings. However, using a spirometer individually will involve close supervision and considerable time.

The aim of this activity is for students to learn how to take peak flow readings and to measure vital capacity, and to determine whether there is a correlation between the two physiological measurements. Label each group with a letter and instruct the students to number themselves within the group; this is to ensure some confidentiality in the whole group (e.g. Morag Smith may be represented by B4).

Students will be able to achieve key skills in number, problem-solving and working with others in this activity.

Students should also be able to analyse and interpret a spirometer reading.

Activity 3.1.2 is designed to test a student's learning and understanding of the anatomy and physiology of the respiratory system.

The cardio-vascular system

The cardio-vascular system is fairly straightforward. This should of course include an outline of the structure and functions of blood as well as the heart and circulation. See **Activity** 3.1.3 and **OHTs** 3.1.2 and 3.1.3.

A brief mention should be made about the lymphatic system, as students will find it difficult to fully comprehend the absorption of fats and oedema if it is omitted.

Many students appreciate the chance to dissect a sheep's heart, but this should be voluntary, as it can be very distasteful to vegetarians, animal lovers or those of a squeamish disposition. It is useful to have overhead transparencies on a screen during this procedure, as it is easier to look up at a screen to identify a structure than thumb through several pages of instructions.

The digestive system

This is the next logical step. Although students should understand the way in which enzymes work, and their sensitivities, it seems inappropriate to spend much time on specific enzyme names and actions other than the most common. (See **Activity** 3.1.4.) It will be more profitable to explain that complex macromolecules in food must be broken down before they can be absorbed through the wall of the gut lining into the bloodstream. There is also no real monitoring of the digestive system, as you will not wish your students to be examining vomit or faeces, that is, from a safety point of view.

This is unlikely to be a system that students will utilise in their assessment and the unit does not involve nutrition. A diffuse link could be made between the cardio-vascular and respiratory systems and mealtimes. In other words, students could routinely monitor these two systems before, during and after meals, although the results may be not too different.

The renal system

The renal system has similarities to the digestive system. Although students could test urine, you are unlikely to wish them to be involved in examining body fluids. Some students may have part-time work in care settings and may already be involved in testing urine as part of their daily routine. There would be no reason why this should not be used in that particular case. There is, however, sound educational reasons for delivering a broad outline of the renal system, including the functions of a nephron. (See **Activity** 3.1.5.) A student will need to appreciate the links between renal function and blood pressure, and that hypertension can be both a cause and effect of renal failure. This will be particularly useful if students intend to add Unit 13, 'Physiological disorders', to their curriculum.

The nervous system

The nervous system will also be delivered in a broad outline as students will need a basic understanding to fully comprehend homeostatic control through receptors, effectors and central control. (See Activities 3.1.5, 3.1.7, 3.1.9.)

Students need to have learned the basic facts about this system or read pages 159–163 of the textbook before attempting **Activity 3.1.7**.

The nervous system assists with communication and co-ordination inside and outside the body. It is composed of special excitable cells called neurones and supporting cells. Neurones are organised into particular areas.

Down the main axis of the body lies the central nervous system and branching out from this are the peripheral nerves.

One neurone communicates with another by the passage of nervous impulses that are waves of minute electrical activity. There is a minute space between the endings of one neurone as it impinges on the next and this is called a synapse.

Skin can be considered here as an organ of the nervous system as it clearly plays a vital part in the regulation of body temperature. (See **Activity 3.1.6.**) Students should learn about the structure of skin and it's sensitivity (see **OHT** 3.1.4).

The endocrine system

For the endocrine system, students will need to learn the positions of the major endocrine glands, their hormones and principal actions. Although at first sight it would seem that there is no routine monitoring here either, students could link the release of adrenaline during exertion with the cardio-vascular system and the respiratory system. There is also ADH secretion and temperature regulation (see **Activities** 3.1.8 and 3.1.9).

Reviewing all the anatomy and physiology of these body systems, the trios most likely to provide suitable material for assessment are:

- Cardio-vascular system
  Respiratory system
  Endocrine system
  (Resting and exercise)
- Nervous system (skin)
  Cardio-vascular system
  Endocrine/renal systems
  (Temperature regulation)
- Cardio-vascular system
  Respiratory system
  Digestive system
  (Around mealtimes)
- Cardio-vascular system
  Renal system
  Endocrine system
  (Water regulation and blood pressure)

3.2 Homeostasis

After providing a definition and explanation of the concept of homeostasis, it is often useful to deviate to a control system the students are likely to be familiar with, and an oven thermostat is a popular example. This example illustrates the need for a central control, and receptors and effectors with connecting links to form the control system. Returning to the body systems, the analogy can be transferred to human physiology. See page 168 of the textbook.

Each homeostatic control system can then be studied in turn:

- Blood glucose level (Activity 3.1.8)
- Body temperature (Activity 3.1.6)
- Heart rate (Activity 3.1.2)
- Respiratory rate (Activity 3.1.2)
- Water regulation (Activity 3.1.5)

The textbook provides full details of these control systems, see pages 168–175.

3.3 Physiological measurements of individuals in care settings

It is most likely to prove difficult for tutors to arrange for students to take these physiological measurements in care settings. This is because of the increasing pressure to obtain care work placements and the ground rules established between care placements and educational establishments regarding the tasks untrained voluntary helpers can be permitted to carry out.

Many work experience placements are in schools, nurseries, clinics and residential homes and many of these clients will not require routine monitoring. To do so for the purposes of students' work records may be considered unethical. You should discuss this with your students and include invasion of privacy as an issue. If you are fortunate enough to obtain work placements in a hospital environment, then life can still be difficult for you. Such establishments tend to be extremely wary of possible litigation and very reluctant to allow students to carry out tasks involving client care, whether or not the task is non-invasive.

There are various steps you can take to find opportunities for your students to do routine monitoring.

- Discover how many of your students work in real care establishments as part-time care assistants. These students are more likely to be able to ask and receive permission for their own routine monitoring. They are also likely to have suitable equipment available and already know the health and safety practice that runs alongside equipment use. However, you must clearly establish this, rather than assume it.
- Find out how many of your students have a friend or relative cared for by professionals but living in their own home environments.

  They are also more likely to ask for and get permission from people they know who are anxious to help them. You will need to investigate availability of equipment and ensure safe practice.

- You might wish to distribute an internal e-mail or memo asking if any staff in your organisation would be willing to assist by volunteering to be routinely monitored by your students. You could also ask the same or other students in other groups, and of course your own group. You might get an improved response if you identify a few conditions such as asthma, diabetes, hypertension, etc. to assist would-be participants decide whether they are suitable and willing.
- You might like to write to or visit placements that have benefited from helpful students in the past, or who in the past have been very co-operative with your establishment.
- The final resort is to allow students to take measurements from each other. This is not recommended as they are unlikely to be well-motivated and are unlikely to take any measurements outside the expected ranges.

Students should have the support of either you or a professional when taking measurements. If students do take measurements of people with serious health care needs, it will be vital that the students understand the risk of emotional threat which taking measurements can produce. Students will need to maintain sensitive communication with real patients and maintain confidentiality.

The next step is for each student to agree the nature of the measurements and the time-scale and intervals for the monitoring.

It will save you time if you ask each student to write a summary of their proposed investigations and submit it to you by a set deadline. Students will also need access to expected ranges of data and be able to research care magazines and other published data.

Students should be able to measure pulse rates (manually and electronically), body temperature, blood pressure, respiratory rates, and peak flow at different times of the day and during/after different activities. They also need to know how these measurements will vary with emotion and age. They will need to use different types of equipment and be aware of the expected range of each measurement. You are not likely to have many pieces of modern equipment and you might need to plan a circus of activities so that a group of students learn how to use each type of equipment before moving on to the next task. This will take a few sessions depending on the size of your group.

Once again, it is sensible to review the ethics of taking physiological measurements from people and maintaining confidentiality of results while students are learning how to investigate a physiological function.

Students should be told what to do if they find any measurement outside the expected range for a member of their class group. You will not wish to have an 'abnormal' reading shouted out in a class session, as this could cause the person being measured to become anxious and embarrassed. Quiet reflection and individual counselling will need to follow after you have double-checked the reading for yourself. You may find it necessary to advise a class member to see his or her medical advisor. Forewarned is forearmed and if the group is told this at the beginning of the session, then they will be prepared.

It is not so unusual to find a higher than normal pulse rate or blood pressure during a class session and you can present it as a bonus that they, the students, are checking their own health at the same time. Some students may know that they have a fast pulse or high/low blood pressure and it is a good idea to check on this too. Many young people have blood pressure readings in the 90/60 mm.Hg range, and this is quite normal.

You are also advised to obtain the manufacturer's instructions for equipment that will be in use and to have several photocopies of these available in the classroom for student use. This is particularly useful for spirometers as there are so many different types in circulation.

Spirometers should only be used in the presence of a qualified member of staff.

Students will need to understand the various reasons for monitoring individuals and how measurements relate to the subsequent care of a client. For example, a client with a high blood pressure may need to be prescribed diuretics to reduce the amount of water in the bloodstream, or a client with a high body temperature may need cooling with a fan or tepid sponging.

3.4 Safe practice

You will find the safe practice for using different equipment incorporated in the details of each method of use, and it is probably best delivered in that way, along with the accuracy of equipment. This is to avoid fragmentation of information. Students will also need to know how to reduce risks applied to the use of equipment.

You will find that there are some generic hazards and risks that occur when using any piece of electrical equipment and specific hazards and risks that apply to one piece of equipment. It is better to teach the generic risks first.

Students should also be aware of the legislation that applies to the workplace, such as HASAW, COSHH and RIDDOR. These are all documented in the student textbook, see pages 191–193, and **OHTs** 3.4.1 and 3.4.2.

You will need to deliver all the health and safety topics before students handle any equipment. Standard operating procedures and manufacturers' instructions should be readily available for students to access.

When students are in a workplace, either as volunteers or employees, they should be aware of the responsibilities of employers to provide proper training before anyone uses a piece of equipment. They should, as responsible adults, know the value of reading all manufacturers' instructions before using any equipment even if they have previous knowledge of similar models. This applies not only to care equipment.

3.5 Analysis and accuracy of results

In the case of some of the latest equipment used for making measurements, you may not know the limits of accuracy to be able to assist your students. Manufacturers' instructions if compiled correctly should contain this information. It would be wise to instruct a technician to check the availability of this information before the unit is delivered. Most manufacturers are anxious to assist their customers and will be co-operative in sending a replacement photocopy if the original information has been lost.

Calculating and detecting errors

You will need to show students how to calculate possible errors in their measurements and to be aware of 'calculator' errors. For example, if a student is reading a scale that shows small one degree calibration marks, the nearest estimation between two marks that they can read is probably 0.5 degree. However, if they are using this in a calculation with the use of a calculator the answer may be shown to several decimal places. This degree of accuracy is nonsense if the apparatus is much less sensitive; many students find it very difficult to appreciate this. An answer to a calculation should not contain more significant figures than the least number of significant figures used among the given measurements. There is no requirement to deliver calculations of statistical error within the unit, however on rare occasions a student transferring to a health and social care pathway may have previous learning, so and he or she should be encouraged to deploy these techniques.

The unit requires a logical common sense approach to the detection of possible errors given the limitations of equipment as described above or the monitoring process. Examples of the latter may be found in counting an arterio-sclerotic pulse, an erratic or unusually fast pulse rate.

Students need to use common sense in determining how to reduce such errors, for example using a pulse meter for a faster pulse rate or using another piece of equipment that measures in smaller intervals. Gaining more experience in monitoring by measuring at shorter intervals will increase expertise and reduce errors.

Plotting graphs

You are advised to give students practice in plotting graphs as many will not yet be expert in this. Common mistakes or incompetences are:

- Reversing the axes so that the graph is upside down.
- Not being able to calculate the best scales for producing a graph that maximises the space available.
- Not having regular intervals marked on the scales.
- Not realising that graph scales do not have to commence at zero.
- Errors in the actual plotting of points.
- Being unaware of the convention in joining plots with straight lines or freehand curves.
- Having little or no practice in plotting or reading graphs with more than one vertical scale.
- Being unable to extrapolate graphs where relevant.
- Omitting graph titles and axis labels, including the units used in measurement.
- Constructing graph lines with ballpoint so that errors cannot be rectified.
- Being unable to read a graph to find other values.
- Being unable to describe the trends in a graph.
- Not appreciating how the use of different scales changes the appearance of a graph.

Some students will also be unable to use fractions and decimals competently, particularly the former. There is little everyday use in the handling of fractions, so young people quickly forget how to deal with them. They may also require practice in constructing histograms and bar charts; very few students appreciate the difference between the two. The student textbook deals with graphical displays and provides opportunities for practice, see pages 195–201.

As many students are not competent in handling graphs, so they will be unaware how to calculate rates of change in a graph. Some will not appreciate that the steepness of the slope of a graph indicates a faster rate of change, so you will need to emphasise this and demonstrate the calculation of rate of change, see pages 198–199 of the textbook.

Although not specifically required for the unit assessment, your students should be aware of some common formulae in use in the caring field and everyday life. They should be able to demonstrate to you that they can use a formula to calculate electrolyte concentrations. Clear explanations of these are provided in the textbook, and some examples and questions are provided for practice, see pages 189–191 and page 201.

ASSESSMENT SUMMARY

We have covered some of the material within the teaching notes, particularly the routine measurements involving three human body systems and some of the problems encountered in meeting the requirements from non-invasive techniques. However, the unit text may have scope for eliminating some of these difficulties. Students are only required to produce information about routine measurements, not to necessarily carry out all the monitoring themselves. Clearly, the assessment should contain some monitoring carried out by students, but not necessarily for all three systems. This does create another ethical issue, as students will need access to some recorded information about clients having medical conditions such as diabetes or renal failure.

This does give your students more scope to be innovative and original, provided they can get permission to access this type of information. Certainly this provides material for obtaining monitoring values outside the expected range and being able to link the physiological factors to the homeostatic function in a more precise way. Students would still have to investigate the safe use of equipment, potential health and safety risks and their methods of reduction, and this will involve considerable research on their behalf.

Do not allow your students to produce a wholly theoretical study or they will lose out on valuable experience of dealing with real clients. Motivation decreases as they delve further than necessary into advanced medical reference texts and re-write material that they do not understand. The unit intention is essentially practice-based, and you should ensure that your students understand this.

It might be wiser to delay mentioning that recorded data can be used until you have rough plans of their assessments to hand and can see the direction in which they are travelling. When there is an obstacle to monitoring, the use of recorded data can be introduced, provided the student is aware of the safe use of data, the health and safety risks, etc. that will still be required.

Presumably a student who produces a completely theoretical assessment cannot achieve a higher grade, as grade C specification includes a review of the students' monitoring methods. This would not be possible if someone else had recorded all the data.

Grade E

To achieve **grade E** the work must show the results of monitoring the physiological status of individuals to demonstrate an understanding of human body systems.

- Recordings of routine measurements of at least three body systems with recognition and explanation of any deviations from the normal expected range of values.
- Safe use of equipment to monitor physiological status.
- Description of potential health and safety risks when monitoring and their methods of reduction.
- Explanation of the gross structure and function of the body systems involved in the monitoring and their inter-relationships.
- Description of the homeostatic mechanisms appropriate to the body systems used in the monitoring.

Grade C

To achieve **grade C** the work must show:

- Review of methods used in monitoring to identify possible sources of error.
- How and why homeostatic dysfunction can produce abnormal data.
- How the data collected demonstrates the inter-relationships of body systems for effective function.

A student must show that they have done the following:

- They have carried out *some* routine non-invasive measurements that are clearly tabulated and explained.
- They have included measurements from at least three body systems that reach conclusions about the physiological status of the individual. 'Physiological status' is open to interpretation, as there is no supplied definition. It might mean that an individual suffers from moderately severe diabetes mellitus that is well controlled by insulin or that an individual has periodic attacks of asthma when exposed to certain allergens or respiratory infection but is fit and well between attacks. You should make clear to your students that they must make a specific statement concerning the individual's physiological health and place this under a clear heading of 'Physiological status' so that it can be easily identified by the assessor and verifiers.
- Analysed and interpreted (and this will produce the physiological status statement) collected data by the most appropriate means, usually graphical displays. This must include identifying and explaining any deviations from the expected range of values that must be included.
- Provided brief descriptions of the equipment used in the monitoring of the

three systems and how it is used safely.
- Provided descriptions of any potential health and safety risk that might be encountered during the monitoring and explained how these are reduced or minimised.
- Explained the gross structure and functions of the three systems and how they relate to one another.
- Provided descriptions or charts showing how homeostatic mechanisms control the physiological factors they have monitored, *referring to the data they have collected or obtained.* You would expect a minimum of two control systems to be described, and in many cases three.

Grade C students need to show careful planning and carrying out of tasks in their work, which should contain appropriate scientific terminology.

They must reflect on their own monitoring and identify possible sources of error, practically about a minimum of three. Make sure that your students put these extra requirements under appropriate headings so that inspection of the work shows the evidence clearly. Following this, they should be able to demonstrate, preferably numerically, the effect of the errors on their results.

At this grade, students must use the data they have collected to show how the systems are working together to bring about homeostasis. For instance, they might show how the levels of blood glucose return after a meal has been digested and absorbed as a result of the circulatory and endocrine systems working together with the digestive system.

When homeostatic control is not working properly, the rates or levels of physiological factors cannot be maintained within the expected range and may spiral out of control. Using secondary source data, students need to show how abnormal data can be produced and explain why this happens.

Grade A

A student working at **grade A** will produce a portfolio of evidence that shows depth and breadth of understanding, increased analytical skills and evaluation. He or she can work well on their own and display critical understanding. Many students fear that if they are critical of work they will lose credit, so you will need to explain the advantages of a broad, independent, critical approach.

After reviewing their work to identify possible sources of error at grade C, students need to suggest with a reasoned explanation, how they could have improved on the ways in which they collected their physiological data.

In addition, they will have to show a comprehensive interpretation and analysis of their data to show how the body systems work together to bring about homeostasis. This involves displaying relevant work of a detailed nature with graphical displays and full interpretation and analysis that constantly refers back to homeostatic control systems.

Students working at this level should be able to relate abnormal data and failure of homeostasis to the potential care of the individual client. For example, a client with diabetes mellitus will have to be observed carefully for signs of impending coma or hypoglycaemia. Body temperature regulation will be an important factor in predicting potential infection and blood glucose and glycosuria will be monitored regularly.

OHTs

Some useful overhead transparencies are included to facilitate delivery. These are:

3.1.1 Vertical section through the thorax
3.1.2 Vertical section of the heart
3.1.3 Blood circulation
3.1.4 Vertical section through the skin
3.4.1 Health and safety in the workplace
3.4.2 Responsibilities of employers using hazardous substances in the workplace

ACTIVITIES

The activities are designed to promote learning and understanding, provide consolidation and develop logical thinking and a rational approach to studies. In many exercises there is the potential to achieve key skills.

3.1.1 Comparing peak flow readings with lung volumes
3.1.2 Respiratory system
3.1.3 Exercise on blood circulation
3.1.4 The digestive system
3.1.5 Water and renal function
3.1.6 Monitoring some routine measurements
3.1.7 The nervous system
3.1.8 Blood glucose levels
3.1.9 Endocrine physiology

OHT 3.1.1 VERTICAL SECTION THROUGH THE THORAX

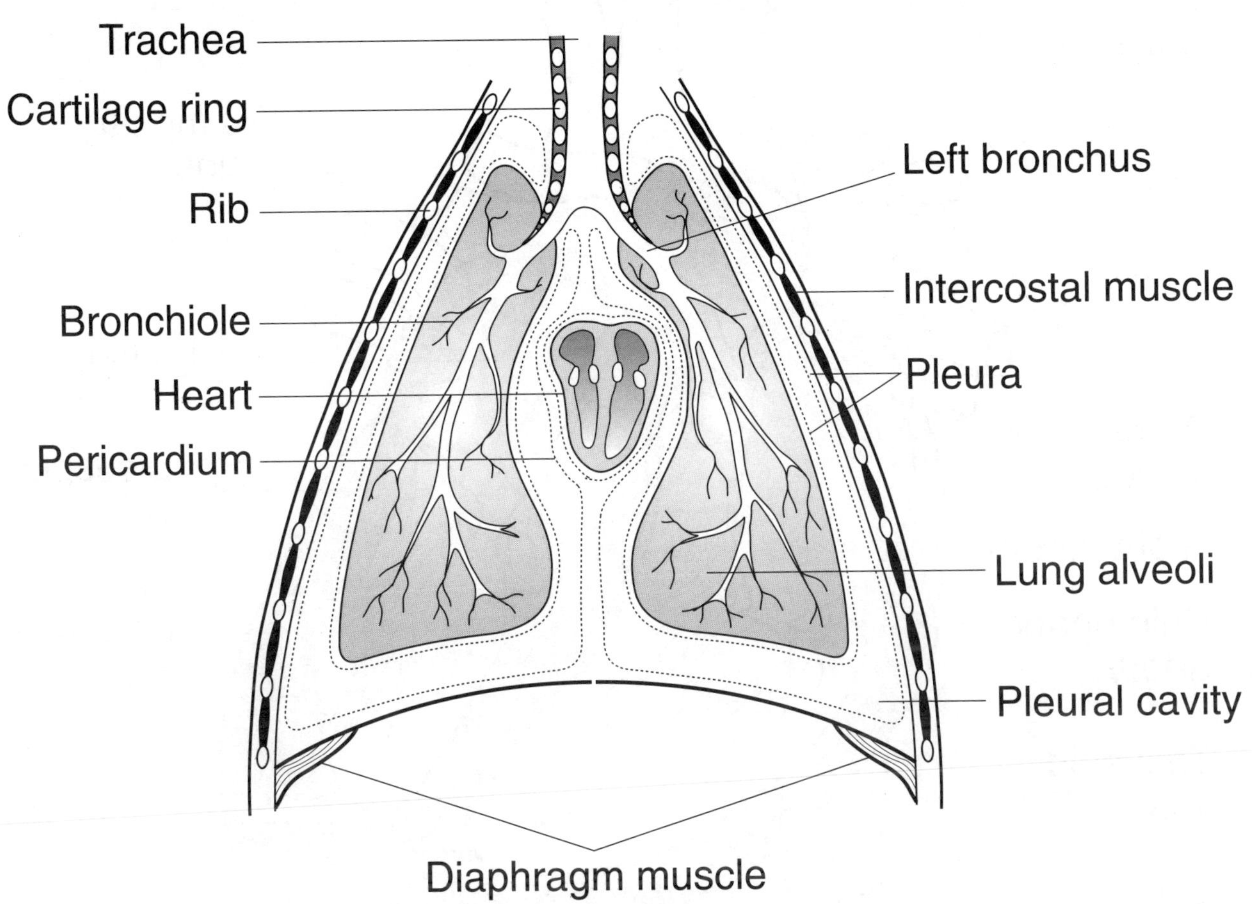
Trachea
Cartilage ring
Rib
Bronchiole
Heart
Pericardium
Left bronchus
Intercostal muscle
Pleura
Lung alveoli
Pleural cavity
Diaphragm muscle

OHT 3.1.2 VERTICAL SECTION OF HEART

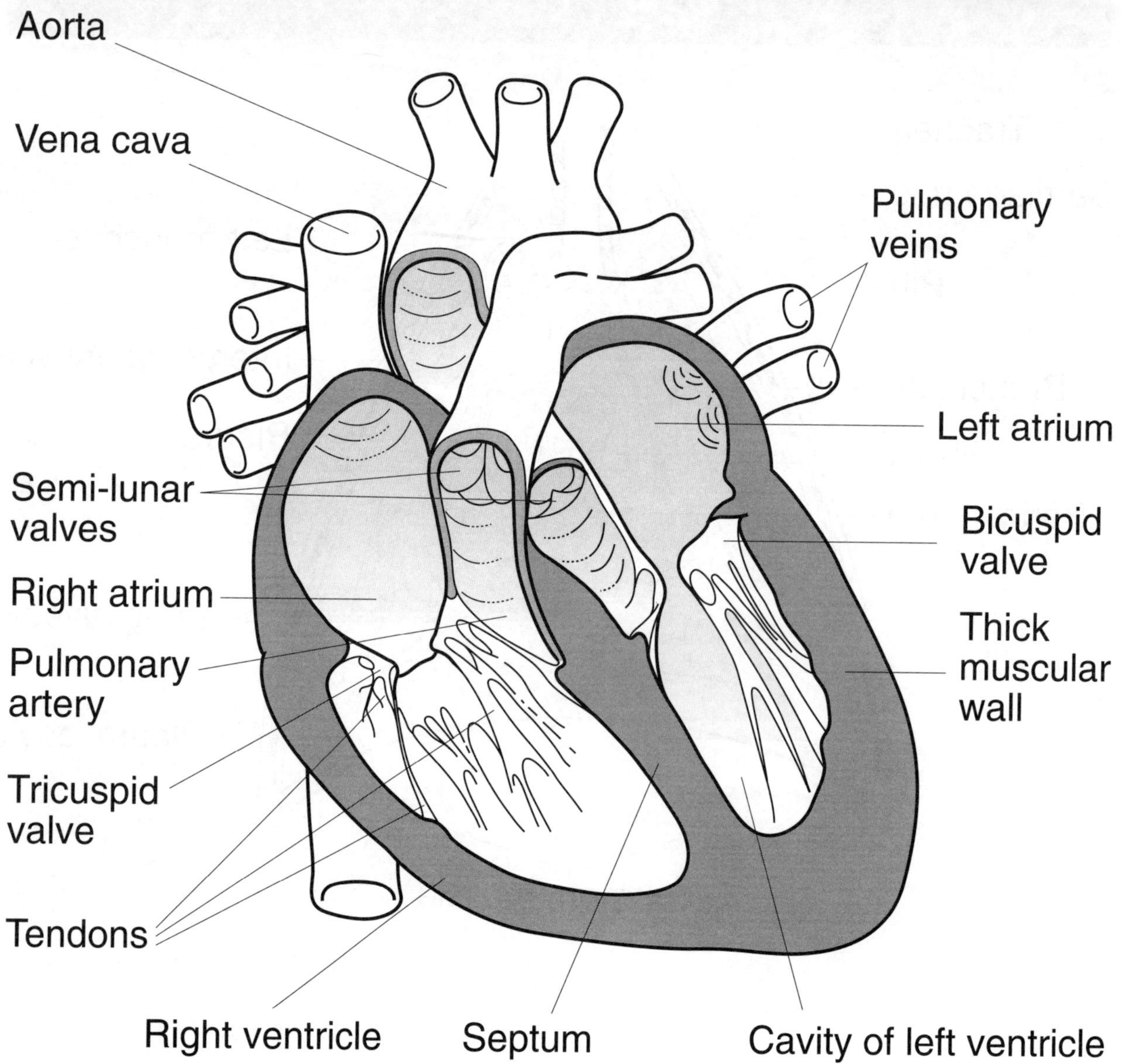
Aorta
Vena cava
Pulmonary veins
Left atrium
Semi-lunar valves
Bicuspid valve
Right atrium
Thick muscular wall
Pulmonary artery
Tricuspid valve
Tendons
Right ventricle
Septum
Cavity of left ventricle

OHT 3.1.3 BLOOD CIRCULATION

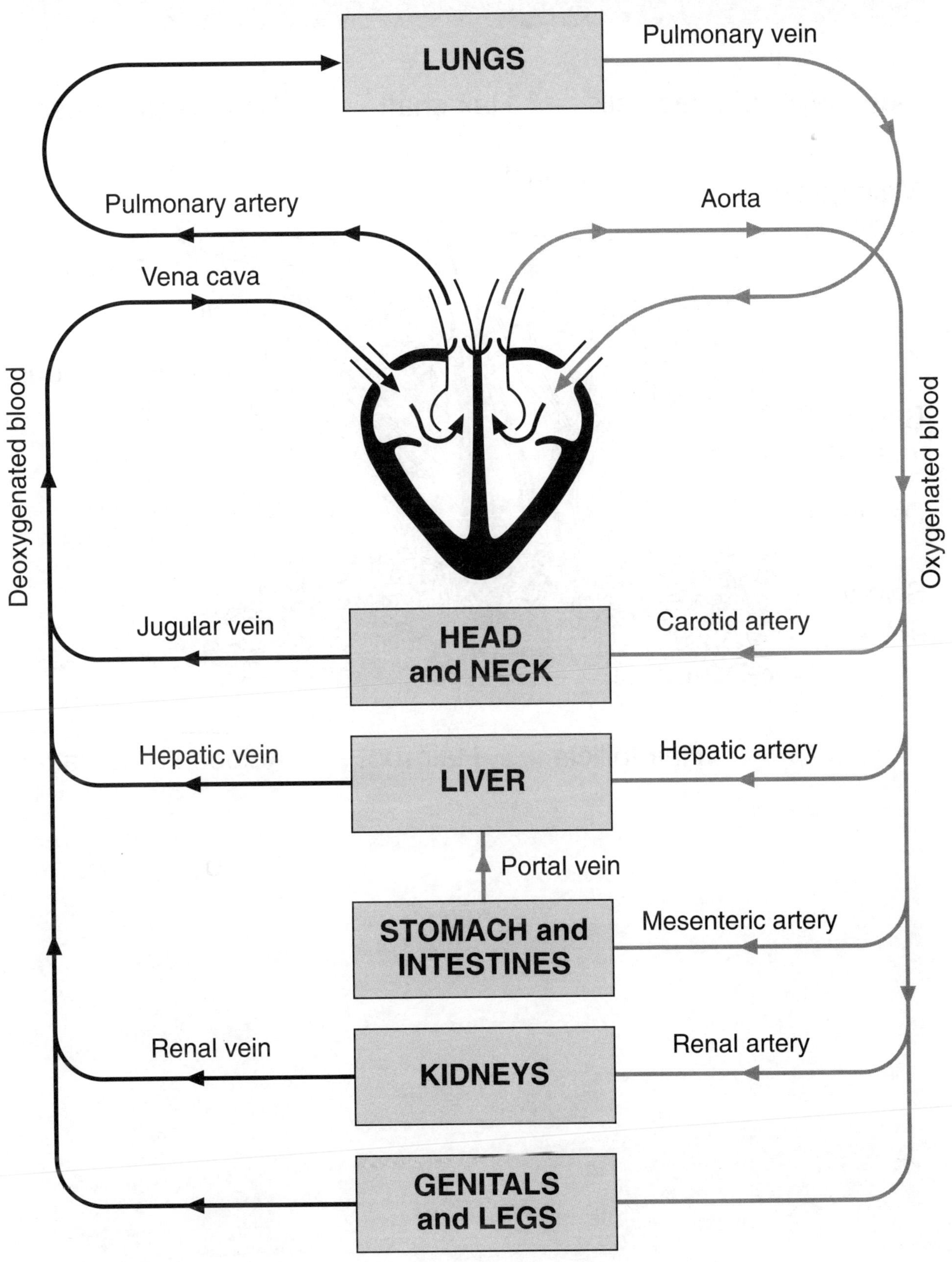
LUNGS
Pulmonary vein
Pulmonary artery
Aorta
Vena cava
Deoxygenated blood
Oxygenated blood
HEAD and NECK
Jugular vein
Carotid artery
LIVER
Hepatic vein
Hepatic artery
Portal vein
STOMACH and INTESTINES
Mesenteric artery
KIDNEYS
Renal vein
Renal artery
GENITALS and LEGS

OHT 3.1.4 VERTICAL SECTION THROUGH SKIN

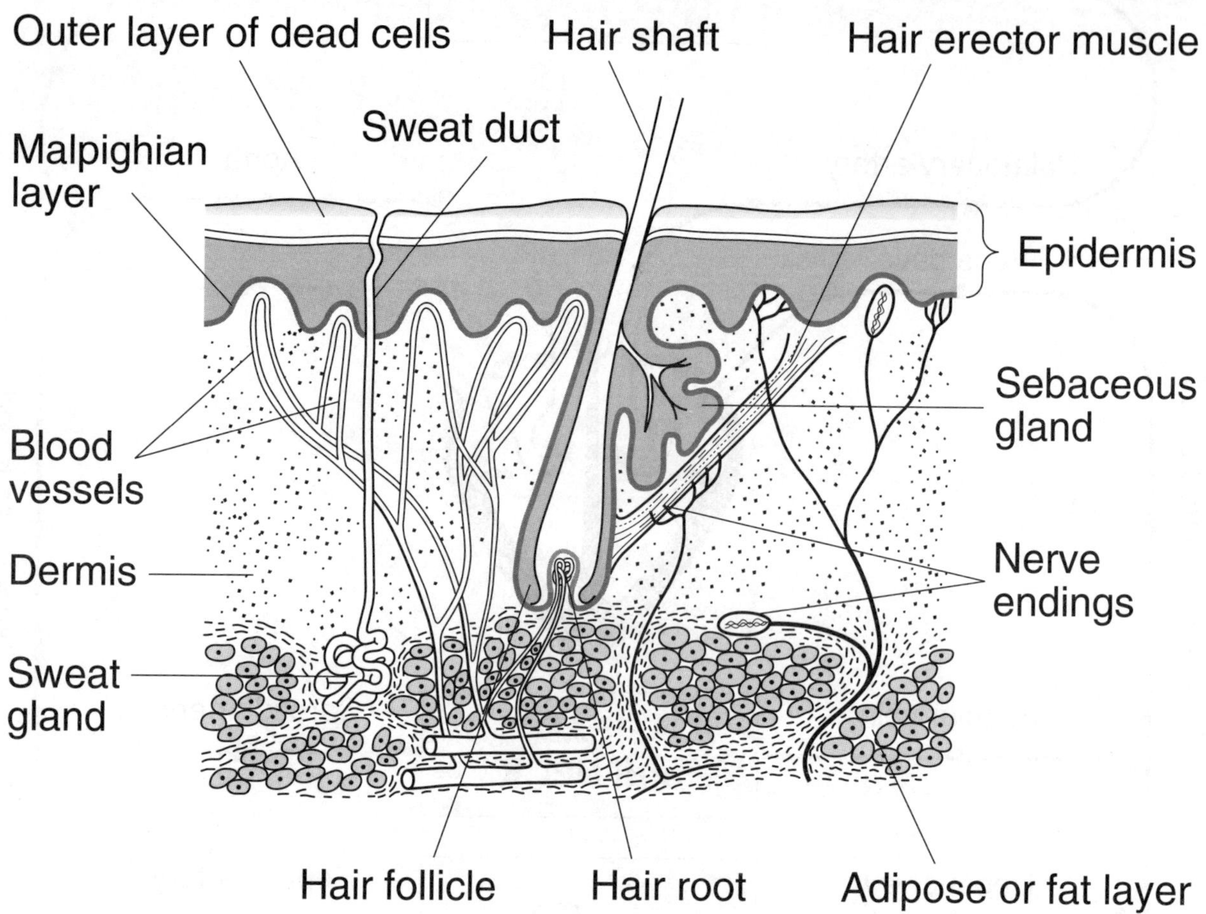

Outer layer of dead cells
Hair shaft
Hair erector muscle
Malpighian layer
Sweat duct
Epidermis
Sebaceous gland
Blood vessels
Dermis
Nerve endings
Sweat gland
Hair follicle
Hair root
Adipose or fat layer

OHT 3.4.1 HEALTH AND SAFETY IN THE WORKPLACE

This is summarised from the Health and Safety at Work Act 1974.

You should know:

- How to do a job safely and not put yourself or others at risk.
- The risks identified with your job that may affect you.
- What has been done to protect you from the risks.
- How to use the protective measures.
- How to take reasonable care of yourself and others who may be affected by your job.
- Not to undertake jobs or use equipment unless trained to do so.
- To let the manager or other appropriate person know if you have seen any occurrence or near miss that could place yourself or others at risk.
- What to do in an emergency.
- How to get first aid.
- You must co-operate with your employers on health and safety matters.
- About the Health and Safety at Work Act 1974 and the amendments to the act.
- The contents of your health and safety policy.
- That you are entitled to proper safety training.
- That your employer should supply protective clothing and equipment.

OHT 3.4.2 RESPONSIBILITIES OF EMPLOYERS USING HAZARDOUS SUBSTANCES IN THE WORKPLACE

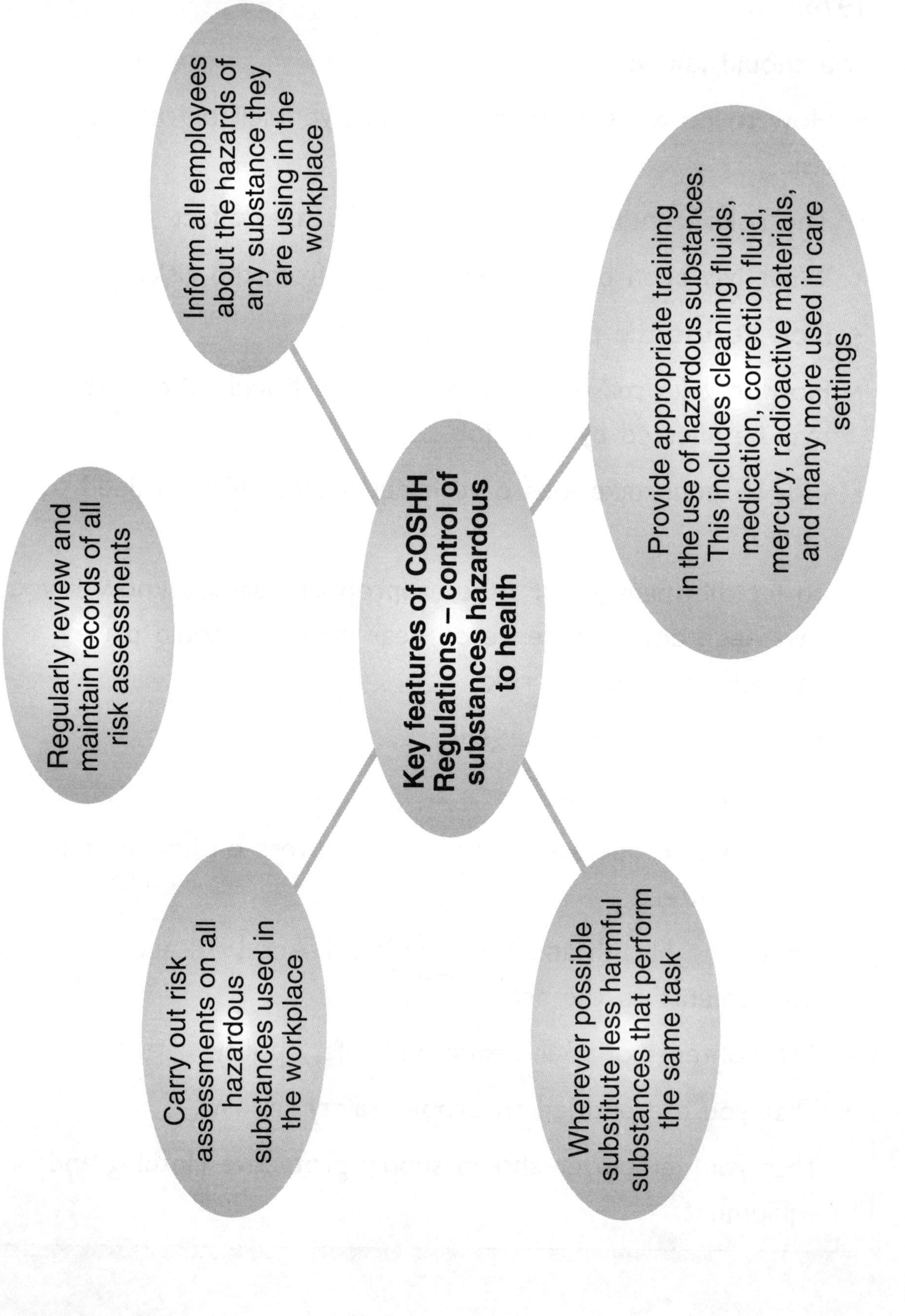

Key features of COSHH Regulations – control of substances hazardous to health

- Inform all employees about the hazards of any substance they are using in the workplace
- Provide appropriate training in the use of hazardous substances. This includes cleaning fluids, medication, correction fluid, mercury, radioactive materials, and many more used in care settings
- Wherever possible substitute less harmful substances that perform the same task
- Carry out risk assessments on all hazardous substances used in the workplace
- Regularly review and maintain records of all risk assessments

ACTIVITY 3.1.1 COMPARING PEAK FLOW READINGS WITH LUNG VOLUMES

In this activity you will learn how to take peak flow readings and to measure vital capacity, and to determine whether there is a correlation between the measurements.

You will work in groups of five. Each group is provided with the following laboratory equipment:

- Calibrated container of at least 5 dm^3 capacity
- Rubber tubing
- Clean water and antiseptic wipes
- Trough or bucket
- Peak flow meter
- Disposable mouthpieces or warm soapy water.

TASKS

1 Set up the first four items above so that you can measure each individual's vital capacity and tidal volume. If you are uncertain how to do this read through the 'Try it out' on page 140 in the textbook.

Make sure that you carefully clean the outside of the rubber tubing with water and antiseptic wipes in between measuring each person.

2 You should then measure the peak flow for each individual. Each person should take a deep breath, blow as hard as they can through the mouthpiece and you record the reading on the scale.

Make a table to record your readings for each group member on a flip chart sheet. Do not give your group members' names; use your group letter and number each individual, e.g. B5. Display the flip chart sheet on the wall of the room.

3 Copy at least three more sheets of results, making 20 sets, or the whole group if less than 20 members.

4 Plot a graph of vital capacity against peak flow for the set of figures and determine whether there is any correlation between the two physiological measurements. See pages 199–200 in the textbook for information on correlation.

5 Using your own group members' results, work out the fraction from the formula:

Tidal volume in cm^3 divided by vital capacity in cm^3.

You will have to convert the result of vital capacity into cm^3. What is the range for your group for this fraction? Compare it with results from other groups.

6 Viewing the results from the whole set, are any of the results for peak flow or vital capacity outside the range you would expect? Suggest explanations for these results.

7 Suggest why peak flow monitoring in clients might take place.

8 What safety precautions are necessary during peak flow monitoring? How would you reduce these to a minimum?

9 Comment on the accuracy of:

a Measuring peak flow.
b Measuring vital capacity by the method you have used.

10 If you collected the air expelled in a vital capacity measurement and analysed the gaseous content, how would this differ in content from the air in the lung alveoli (known as alveolar air)? Explain the difference.

ACTIVITY 3.1.2 RESPIRATORY SYSTEM

This activity tests your learning and understanding of the anatomy and physiology of the respiratory system.

Hamid measured his tidal volume using a spirometer and found that it was 510 cm^3.

He had no means of measuring the dead air space that filled his trachea, bronchi and bronchioles, so he used a standard figure of 150 cm^3 for this. Dead air space does not reach the respiratory surfaces in the lungs so gaseous exchange cannot occur. He counted his breathing rate at rest four times and found that the mean respiratory rate was 16 breaths every minute.

TASKS

1 Calculate Hamid's pulmonary ventilation at rest.

2 Calculate Hamid's resting alveolar ventilation.

3 After chemical analysis Hamid's exhaled air contains 3.9% carbon dioxide. How much carbon dioxide was exhaled in one minute?

4 Hamid's alveolar air had a much higher carbon dioxide level at 5.9%. How much more carbon dioxide left the alveoli in one minute?

5 Account for the difference in carbon dioxide between the air leaving the lungs and what was actually exhaled.

6 Hamid is a keen underwater swimmer, using a snorkel to explore the sea bed in quiet, shallow coves. Until he studied the respiratory system, he had not understood why snorkels were not made longer or wider. Explain why.

7 Explain the homeostatic control of respiratory rate that adjusts the level of breathing to different demands of the body.

8 Hamid and his tutor used a spirometer to find his tidal volume at rest and during mild exercise. He collected a trace of the experiment. A copy of the trace is provided in the figure. Calculate the tidal volumes and oxygen utilisation at rest and during exercise.

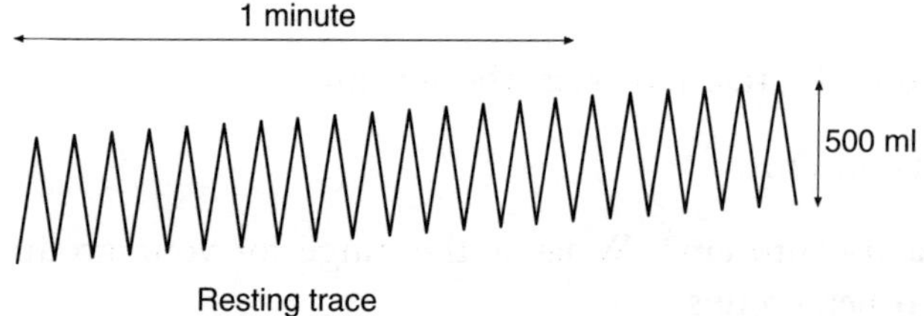
1 minute
500 ml
Resting trace

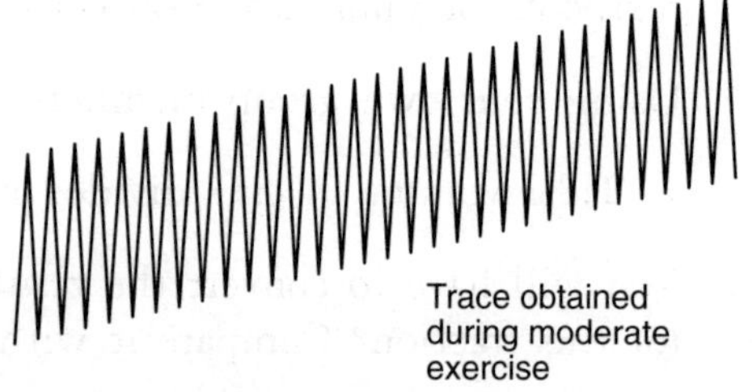
Trace obtained during moderate exercise

9 While on work experience, Hamid helps to care for an older man with bronchitis and emphysema. This condition is the result of chronic infection or irritation that has caused the walls of many alveoli to break down so that larger spaces have formed.

a What effect will this have on the man's blood oxygenation levels? Justify your answer.
b How will this affect his respiratory rate? Justify your answer.
c How will this affect his lifestyle?
d Suggest how the care given to this client might improve his respiratory health.

ACTIVITY 3.1.3 EXERCISE ON BLOOD CIRCULATION

The following table shows the distribution of blood to various organs at rest and during severe exercise. The figures represent the percentage of blood volume delivered from the heart.

At rest the cardiac output was 5 dm^3 per minute (5 dm^3 min-1), but this rose to 25 dm^3 min-1 during the exercise.

Organ	At rest (%)	During exercise (%)
Lungs	100	100
Heart muscle	5	5
Digestive organs and liver	25	5
Kidneys	20	3
Skin	5	1
Muscles	20	80
Brain	15	4
Bone marrow	4	1
Fat	6	1

TASKS

1 Draw two fully labelled bar charts to display these results graphically.

2 Explain why the distribution of blood is different in the two bar charts.

3 Which hormone is principally responsible for the change in the distribution of blood?

4 What is the blood volume passing through the following organs at rest and during exercise?

a The lungs

b The heart muscle

c The muscles.

5 What changes occur in the action of the heart to increase cardio-vascular output when the body undertakes exercise?

6 What happens to the production of urine during exercise? As urine is a product of blood filtration, calculating the blood flow through the kidneys at rest and during exercise will provide the answer.

7 Urine production at rest with 5 dm^3 min-1 cardiac output is 1 ml min-1. Calculate how much urine is produced during exercise with a cardiac output of 25 dm^3 min-1.

8 Calculate the blood flow through the skin at rest and during exercise. Comment on the result.

9 Describe the homeostatic control of heart rate.

10 How does the process of altering the blood supply to an organ actually happen?

11 Why is the percentage of blood passing through the lungs 100% in both columns of the table?

12 Explain what happens to blood pressure during exercise.

13 Describe the way in which muscle action assists in the return of blood to the heart.

14 Produce a fully labelled diagram of the heart in vertical section and show the direction of blood flow with arrows.

15 Describe the structures that ensure there is one-way flow of blood through the heart.

16 Describe the heart sounds heard through a stethoscope and explain how they are caused.

ACTIVITY 3.1.4 THE DIGESTIVE SYSTEM

TASKS

1 Label the diagram on the following page to show that you understand the structure of the alimentary canal.

2 Why is digestion of food necessary?

3 Where does ingestion take place?

4 Which organ acts as an endocrine gland and as an exocrine gland (this type of gland produces secretions that travel down a duct)?

5 Name the organ that forms bile and the structures involved in the passage of bile to its destination. Where is the destination of bile?

6 Which part of the alimentary canal contains villi? What is the function of villi and how are they specially adapted to perform their functions?

7 Describe the functions that the structures in the mouth carry out.

8 Which part of the alimentary canal contains acid juices? What is the purpose of the acid juices?

9 Some clients produce excess acid. Explain how this might affect their health and well-being.

10 Carbohydrate food is digested to form glucose and other monosaccharide sugars. Explain the fate of glucose when digestion is complete.

11 Which organ manufactures urea? What is the source of urea and why must it be continuously eliminated from the body in urine?

12 Many glands pour watery juices onto food as it passes down the alimentary canal. The body would rapidly become dehydrated if the water were allowed to leave the body in these large volumes. Describe how this water is moved from the alimentary canal back into the bloodstream.

13 When the alimentary canal is irritated or poisoned by toxins from microbes and some foods, the contents are rushed through the parts of the system by strong peristaltic muscular waves that often produce colicky pain. Explain the effect of this type of illness on the production of faeces.

14 Which parts of the alimentary canal as shown in the figure do not produce any enzymes to digest food?

15 Describe the characteristics of enzymes that carry out food digestion.

16 Explain the functions of all the secretions that enter the first part of the intestines.

17 Explain what is meant by a sphincter muscle and give the location of one sphincter muscle in the alimentary canal.

18 Some end-products of digestion pass into the lymphatic system. Explain where, how and why this happens.

19 List four functions of the liver.

20 Describe the digestion of a piece of dry wholemeal bread.

ACTIVITY 3.1.4 (CONTINUED) HANDOUT

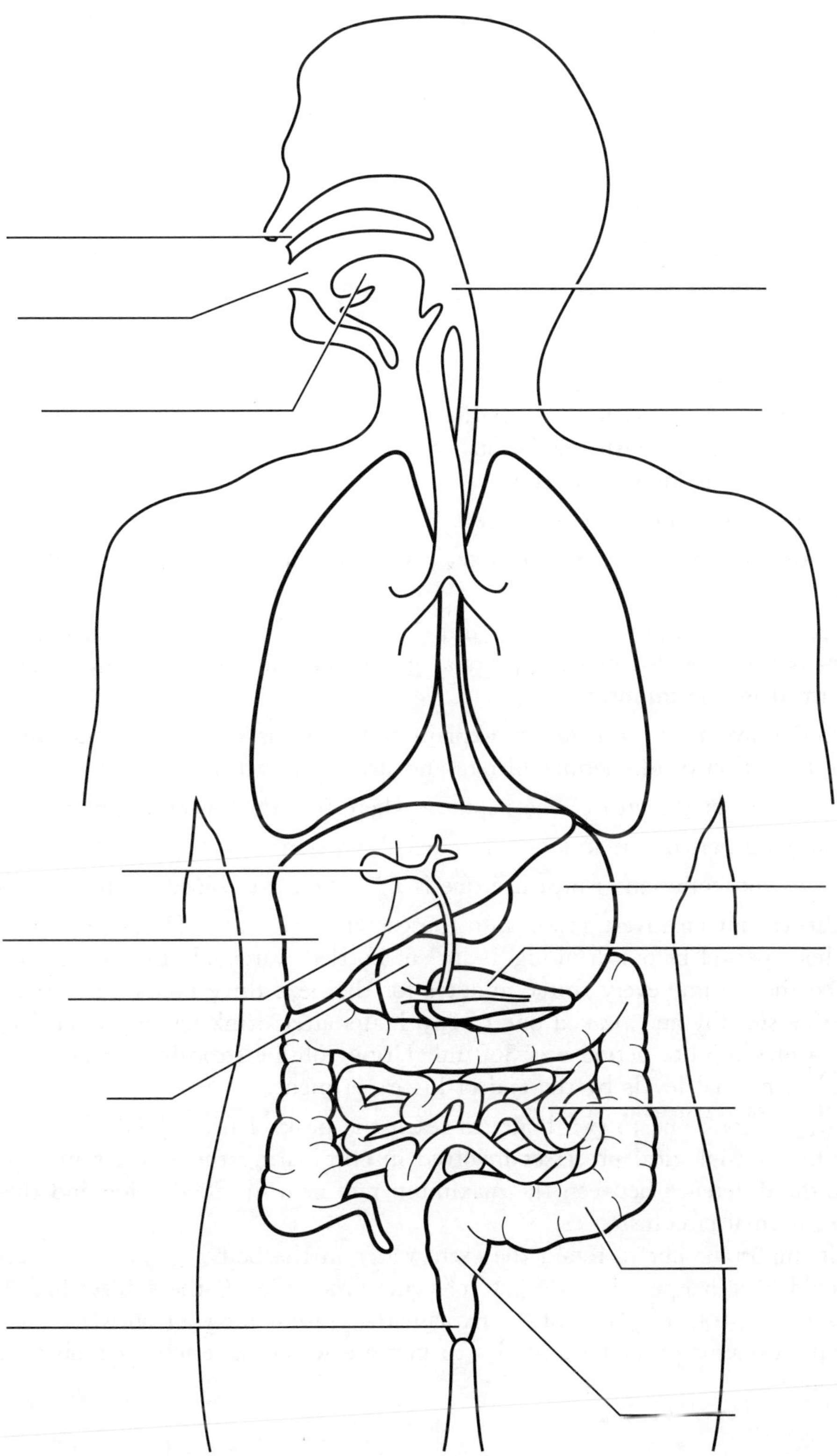

ACTIVITY 3.1.5 WATER AND RENAL FUNCTION

The diagram on the following page shows a microscopic renal nephron. Most of the surrounding capillary network has been omitted for clarity.

TASKS

1 Label the numbered parts in the diagram.

2 State which numbered part represents the area where:
- capillary blood pressure is high
- glomerular filtrate forms
- amino acids are absorbed
- a build up of sodium ions occurs
- water absorption occurs without regulation
- water absorption occurs with regulation
- glomerular filtrate is known as urine.

3 Explain how glomerular filtrate is produced.

4 Explain why plasma proteins found in blood plasma are not found in glomerular filtrate in any quantity.

5 A client has a cardiac output of 5.5 dm^3 min-1 and one quarter of this blood goes to his kidneys. Ten per cent of this blood appears as glomerular filtrate. How much glomerular filtrate is formed in one minute?

6 Urine production averages 1 ml min-1. Explain why there is such a difference in volume between the formation of glomerular filtrate and urine production.

7 Explain the purpose of the area of the nephron where sodium concentration rises considerably.

8 Which is the main part of the kidney for water absorption?

9 Explain why the concentration of urea in urine is 2% whereas in blood plasma it is only 0.02%.

10 A student carried out an investigation into the excretion of water. He emptied his bladder over a two-hour period before drinking 1 dm^3 of bottled water. He then collected his urine and measured the volume every thirty minutes for the next three hours. He found that urine production rose steadily and peaked one to two hours after drinking the water. The highest volume in a thirty-minute period was 360 ml. Urine volume steadily decreased after the peak and returned to normal levels by the end of his experiment.

a Explain why it took one to two hours to reach the peak of urine production.
b Describe the physiological processes involved in eliminating the excess water.
c Calculate the difference between the maximum rate of urine production and the average rate under normal circumstances.
d Why is it important not to retain the extra water in the body?
e What would have happened to the rate of urine production if the subject had drunk isotonic saline instead of plain water? Explain the reasons for your answer.
f Why would a doctor prescribe diuretics to increase water excretion for a client with hypertension?

ACTIVITY 3.1.5 (CONTINUED) HANDOUT

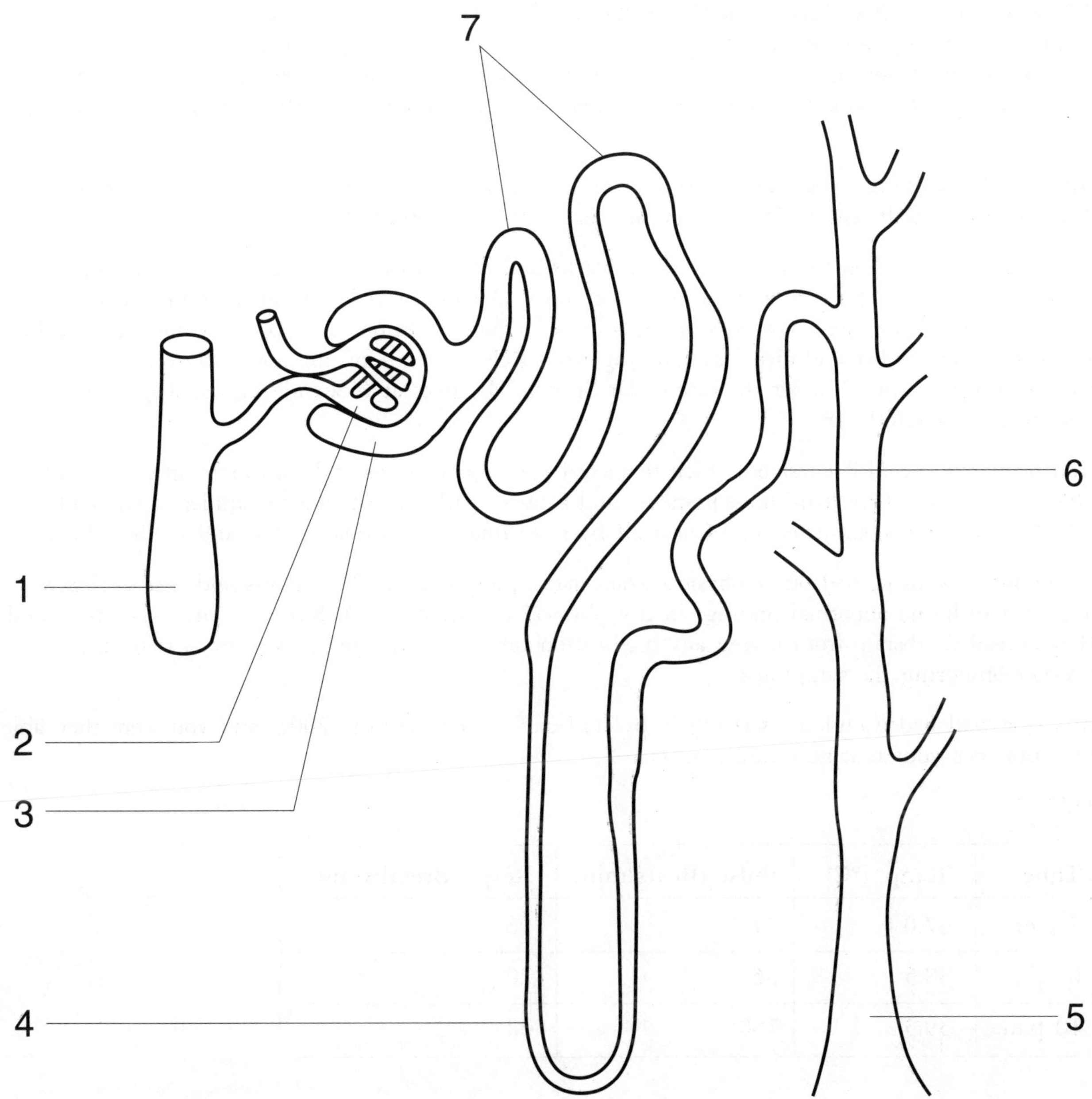
7
6
1
2
3
4
5

ACTIVITY 3.1.6 MONITORING SOME ROUTINE MEASUREMENTS

You are on work experience in Heinemann Hospital and have been assigned to Medical Unit 5, REPP Ward. You have become quite familiar with the routine work of the ward and have shadowed a health care assistant for three days. Prior to your visit, your tutor negotiated with the placement supervisor and it has been agreed that subject to satisfactory performance, you will be able to carry out routine measurements on a selected client for the last three days of your week's placement.

You will be working under the supervision of the client's named nurse and have been allocated to Mrs Idina Cornwall who is 52 years old and has just been admitted for observations.

Mrs Cornwall has been feeling ill for three weeks and complains of pyrexia (raised temperature), anorexia (depressed appetite) and fatigue. Her family doctor has referred her for observations and investigations. There are a few possible diagnoses for her condition, but no one knows the precise diagnosis. She has been admitted as suffering from PUO (pyrexia of unknown origin). Mrs Cornwall was admitted under the care of Dr Stretch, she lives at 6 Seaside Mews, Rugby, and her date of birth is 20.02.48.

You have a blank TPR chart on which to record your observations and measurements. You will be able to carry out three daily measurements and a nurse will perform the remainder of the daily schedule. The nurse admitted Mrs Cornwall by recording her personal details and medical history.

A younger doctor carried out a physical examination, and checked her details and history. There appeared to be no abnormal findings in the physical examination. Dr Stretch visited the client and they agreed to abstain from giving any medication until the investigations were carried out, to prevent obscuring the symptoms.

Mrs Cornwall had completed settling in by mid-day on 6 November 2000, and you were then able to commence your routine measurements.

DAY 1

Time	Temp. (°C)	Pulse (Beats/min)	Resp. (Breaths/min)
2 p.m.	37.0	71	16
6 p.m.	38.5	86	20
10 p.m.	39.3	100	22

Bowels opened 6 p.m., urine passed 4.30 and 10 p.m.

DAY 2

Time	Temp. (°C)	Pulse (Beats/min)	Resp. (Breaths/min)
2 a.m.	40.3	124	25
6 a.m.	38.0	95	21
10 a.m.	36.9	69	17
2 p.m.	37.0	72	17
6 p.m.	38.4	85	18
10 p.m.	40.0	101	21

Bowels opened 5 p.m., urine passed 8.00 a.m, 1.00 p.m., 5.30 p.m. and 10 p.m.

You notice a fan has appeared in the room and Mrs Cornwall explains that this was switched on after 10 p.m., and she was sponged down with tepid water around midnight.

DAY 3

Time	Temp. (°C)	Pulse (Beats/min)	Resp. (Breaths/min)
2 a.m.	40.1	120	23
6 a.m.	37.3	80	22
10 a.m.	36.8	70	16
2 p.m.	37.0	75	18
6 p.m.	38.8	118	24
10 p.m.	40.0	120	24

Bowels opened 6 p.m., urine passed 7.00 a.m., 1.30 p.m., 5.30 p.m. and 10 p.m.

The same care was given nightly when Mrs Cornwall's temperature rose, as on Day 2.

After your placement was completed you visited Mrs Cornwall one more time. She had been in hospital for three weeks and the doctors had found some anomalies from scans but nothing to account for her pyrexia. It seemed that the peaks of temperature were slowly decreasing and Mrs Cornwall was to visit as an outpatient for a year to keep up the observations. She was cheerful and happy to be going home although she had lost several kilograms in weight.

TASKS

1 Complete the TPR chart in full for Mrs Cornwall.

2 Interpret and analyse the chart by summarising the information displayed.

3 Describe precisely how you measured Mrs Cornwall's temperature, pulse and respiration.

4 Comment on the accuracy of the measurements, assuming that you had become competent in the first part of your placement.

5 Describe the potential health and safety risks associated with taking these measurements.

6 State how you would keep the health and safety risks to a minimum.

7 Relate the care Mrs Cornwall received to her routine measurements.

8 Describe the inter-relationships of the human body systems you have measured.

9 Describe the homeostatic mechanisms involved in regulating body temperature.

10 Use the data to show how the body systems work together to bring about homeostasis.

Mrs Cornwall was advised that she had suffered from a serious illness, even though the consultant did not know the precise nature of the diagnosis. As she improved over a period of six weeks there was no further action to investigate the illness, as laboratory investigations were costly and time-consuming. Discuss the ethics of this course of action.

Heinemann Hospital

T.P.R. CHART

4 HRLY.

SURNAME	UNIT No
FIRST NAME	SEX
ADDRESS	DATE OF BIRTH

CONSULTANT
WARD OR DEPT

DATE														
TIME	A.M.	P.M.	A.M.	P.M.	A.M.	P.M.	A.M.	P.M.	A.M.	P.M.	A.M.	P.M.	A.M.	P.M.
TIME. HR	2 6 10	2 6 10	2 6 10	2 6 10	2 6 10	2 6 10	2 6 10	2 6 10	2 6 10	2 6 10	2 6 10	2 6 10	2 6 10	2 6 10
BOWELS														
URINE														

TEMPERATURE

°C	°F
40.5	105.0
40.0	104.0
39.5	103.0
39.0	102.0
38.5	101.2
38.0	100.4
37.5	99.5
*37.0	98.6*
36.9	98.4
36.5	97.7
36.0	96.8
35.5	95.5

PULSE.

170
160
150
140
130
120
110
100
90
80
70
60
50
40
30

RESP'N.

20
10
0

*The figures 37.0 and 98.6 refer to the top of the thick line and the figures 36.9 and 98.4 refer to the bottom of the thick line.

ACTIVITY 3.1.7 THE NERVOUS SYSTEM

TASKS

1 Which parts of the nervous system make up the central nervous system?

2 Describe the events at a synapse when an impulse arrives.

3 What is the function of a synapse?

4 The correct biological term for an impulse is an action potential. What is a resting potential?

5 How can the central nervous system differentiate between strong stimuli and weak stimuli?

6 How does the central nervous system differentiate between an action potential arising from a light stimulus and one from a sound stimulus?

7 Another part of the nervous system is called the autonomic nervous system. It has two divisions called the sympathetic and the parasympathetic nervous systems. Differentiate between the basic functions of these two systems.

8 Give three differences in the way these two branches of the autonomic systems are organised.

9 Some actions of the nervous system are classed as voluntary actions because they are under a person's control or will, but others are reflex actions. What are the characteristic features of a reflex action?

10 The diagram on the following page shows a spinal reflex action called a knee jerk reaction. Doctors may test the knee jerk reflex of a client. What would be the purpose of testing such a reflex action?

11 Label the diagram fully.

12 Explain how the impulse travels from the receptor to the effector in this diagram.

13 Give one example of a cerebral reflex action that may also be used by medical practitioners in a clinical examination involving the nervous system.

14 Some reflex actions can be over-ridden by an individual's voluntary control. Give an example of a reflex occurring in an organ belonging to the renal system that is commonly controlled until a convenient time.

15 Some clients with neurological problems, such as stroke victims, often lose voluntary control of the organ belonging to the renal system and the reflex action becomes operative again. What term is used to describe this loss of control?

ACTIVITY 3.1.7 (CONTINUED) HANDOUT

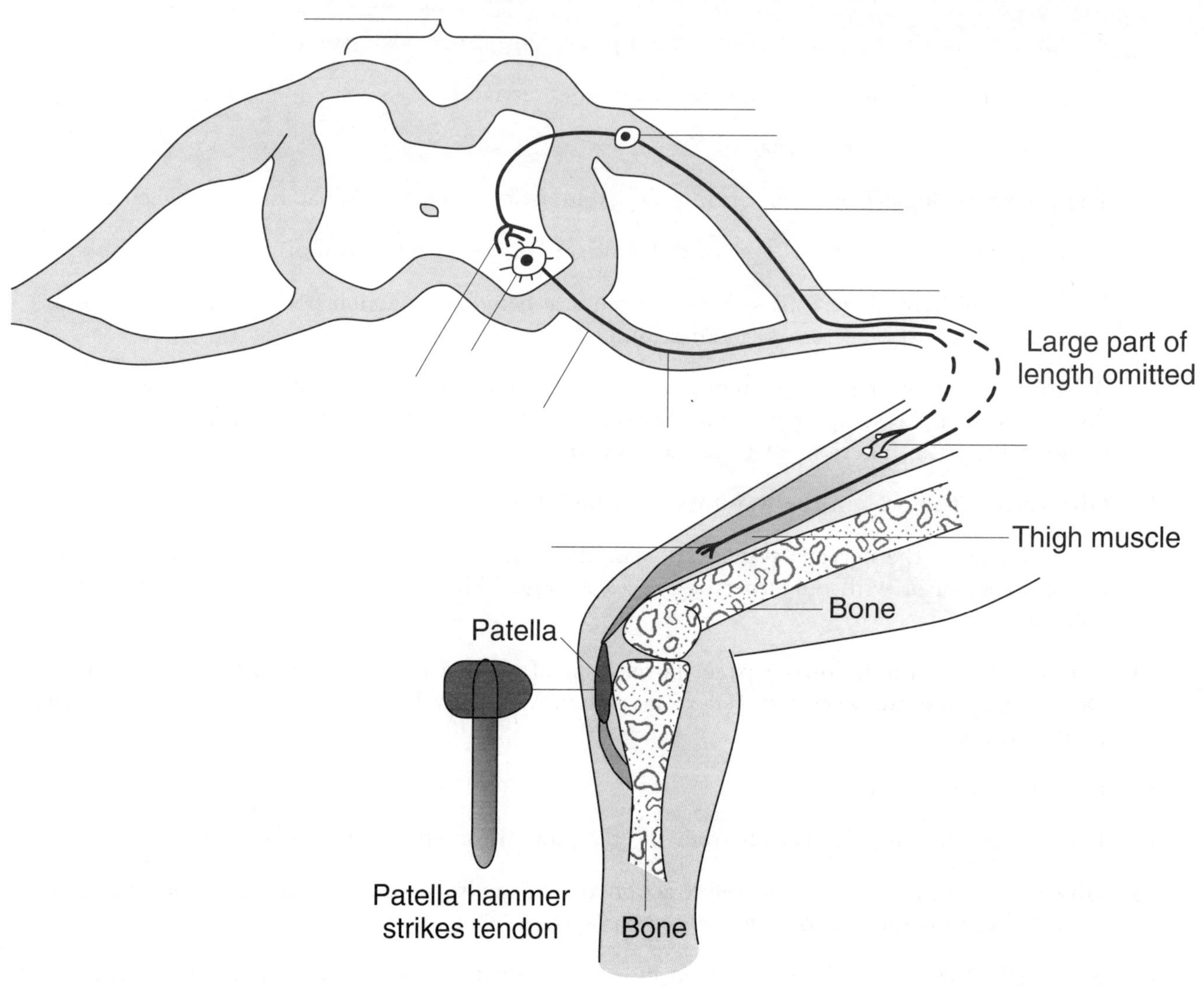
Large part of length omitted
Thigh muscle
Bone
Patella
Patella hammer strikes tendon
Bone

ACTIVITY 3.1.8 BLOOD GLUCOSE LEVELS

Mr Abbot, Mr Lu and Mr Costello had all been referred to the local hospital for a glucose tolerance test as they were suspected of having diabetes mellitus. Mr Abbot needed new glasses and his optician recommended that his blood glucose be tested first. Mr Lu always seemed to be thirsty and he had suffered several infections recently. Mr Costello kept falling asleep and his wife was so exasperated with him that she made him go to the surgery for an appointment with his family doctor.

They had all been asked to fast for twelve hours before attending the unit and told that they would have to be there for nearly three hours. At 9.00 a.m. they were all given 150 ml of water in which 50 g of glucose had been dissolved. At the same time they had their blood glucose tested – the fasting blood glucose.

Thereafter, all three men had their blood tested for glucose every thirty minutes for two and a half hours.

The following table represents their blood glucose levels from 9.00 a.m. until 11.30 a.m.

Time a.m.	Blood glucose mg 100 ml-1		
	Mr Abbot	Mr Lu	Mr Costello
9.00	65	110	200
9.30	130	165	275
10.00	150	230	335
10.30	120	145	300
11.00	80	125	290
11.30	65	100	280

TASKS

1. Plot a single graph to show the blood glucose levels of all three men over the period of the glucose tolerance test.
2. You should understand the expected range for blood glucose and be able to determine which man was not suffering from diabetes mellitus, which man had the condition in a mild form and which man was severely diabetic. Justify your choice.
3. The kidneys excrete glucose in the urine above 180 g 100 ml–1. A diabetic may excrete glucose in the urine. Which men would show a positive test for urinary glucose and for how long?
4. Why was it necessary for the men to fast before coming to the unit for the glucose tolerance test?
5. Why did the test last for two and a half hours?
6. Why was blood glucose tested every thirty minutes?
7. Describe the cause of diabetes mellitus.
8. Why is it important to diagnose this condition as soon as possible?
9. Describe the homeostatic control of blood glucose.
10. Describe the inter-relationships of body systems involved in the regulation of blood glucose.
11. Explain how and why the failure of blood glucose homeostasis leads to abnormal data.
12. Which man needs treatment as soon as possible? Explain the reasons for your answer.

ACTIVITY 3.1.9 ENDOCRINE PHYSIOLOGY

The diagram below shows the interaction between the brain, pituitary gland and the kidneys. The arrows indicate probable pathways of influence.

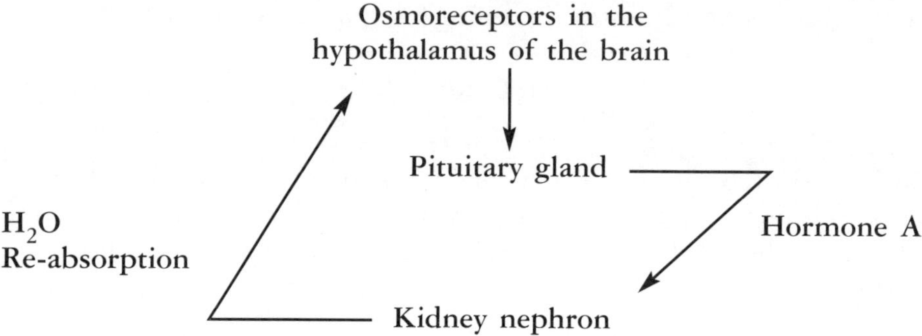

Osmoreceptors in the hypothalamus of the brain
Pituitary gland
H_2O Re-absorption
Hormone A
Kidney nephron

TASKS

1 What are osmoreceptors?
2 Which part of the pituitary gland is affected by their action?
3 Name hormone A.
4 Which part of the nephron does this hormone affect?
5 What is the effect of this hormone on the nephron that causes water re-absorption?
6 How does water re-absorption affect the osmoreceptors?
7 This process is an example of homeostasis. Where is the central control?
8 Where are the receptors?
9 Where are the effectors?
10 How do hormones reach their destinations?
11 Suggest the period of time for water levels to re-adjust by hormonal action.
12 Differentiate between an enzyme and a hormone.
13 Produce a table showing five named hormones, the endocrine glands that produce them, their target organs/cells and a summary of their actions.
14 Insulin is a hormone that is not controlled by the nervous system like many other hormones. What is the main stimulus for the outpouring of insulin?
15 Adrenaline is a hormone closely linked to one part of the nervous system. Name this part.
16 Under what conditions is adrenaline produced in quantity?
17 How does adrenaline affect:

- The heart
- The digestive system
- The skin
- The skeletal muscles
- The liver
- Blood pressure.

18 A client is performing a stressful job and is also having marital problems. He or she is at risk of heart disease. Explain how stress, linked to adrenaline production, may give rise to heart disease.
19 The chemical nature of hormones can be either protein-based or steroid-based. Name one example of each type.
20 The endocrine and nervous systems both assist in communication and co-ordination within the body. Give four major differences in the way these two systems function to effect communication and co-ordination.

UNIT 4 – FACTORS AFFECTING HUMAN GROWTH AND DEVELOPMENT

OVERVIEW

This unit provides the understanding that is fundamental to the appreciation of how human beings grow and develop. It explores traditional and modern viewpoints, so students will be able to consider all aspects and theories and gain a balanced perspective of human growth and development.

The unit consists of four sections which are numbered for ease of referencing in this file:

4.1 Human development
4.2 Development of skills and abilities
4.3 Factors affecting development
4.4 Theories of development

Assessment is by external assessment only.

Aims and objectives

The aims of this unit are to:

- consider human growth and development across the lifespan
- identify skills and abilities developed throughout the lifespan
- appreciate the range of factors that influences growth and development
- consider the different theories concerning development.

Students should be able to:

- explain the key factors relating to human development in infancy, early childhood, adolescence, early, middle and late adulthood
- describe the skills and abilities developed across the lifespan, including gross and fine motor skills, intellectual ability, emotional development, language skills and social skills
- understand the importance of different skills at different life stages and that development is a continuum with different rates at different times
- discuss the impact of genetic and environmental factors on development
- consider the effects of socio-economic factors on the development of different individuals
- discuss the effects of local and global environmental issues on the growth and development of individuals
- consider the inter-relationships of genetic, socio-economic and environmental factors on growth and development
- examine the different theories of development described by Gesell, Freud, Erikson, Skinner, Bandura, Vygotsky and Piaget.

TEACHING NOTES

After introducing the unit and the method of assessment, students should be informed that they will learn about the different life stages from infancy to adulthood and about the range of factors affecting that development. They should understand the difference between growth and development and consider why individuals develop in different ways and what the influences are that could have made an impact.

Students would also benefit from a short introduction to sociological and psychological aspects.

4.1 Human development and 4.2 Development of skills and abilities

Human growth and development is a complex issue and not easy to deliver to students. Pursuing a chronological approach means that the tutor is darting about between physical, social, emotional and intellectual aspects of development in a limited age range; as a result there is often a lack of continuity. On the other hand, dealing with all the physical aspects first, then the social, and so on, does not lead to a holistic view of growth and development in one individual.

On the whole, students probably learn better if the latter strategy is adopted and the unit has been written to follow that order. It is commonplace to stress early years development at the expense of other life stages. However, this is not a unit specialising in early years and it is important to reduce the information at this stage so that all life stages are considered equally.

The life stages of development stated in the unit are:

- Infancy (0–2years)
- Early childhood (2–8 years)
- Puberty and adolescence (9–18 years)
- Early adulthood (19–45 years)
- Middle adulthood (46–65 years)
- Later adulthood (65+years)

See **OHTs** 4.1.1, 4.1.2 and 4.1.3.

Infancy and early childhood

You might wish to start with an introductory video on pregnancy and birth. There are several available; try to choose one with a section on intra-uterine development because you are not really concerned with pregnancy other than as an influencing factor.

Starting with infancy and early childhood, it might be useful to find out how many of your students have their own children, siblings, nieces and nephews in those age groups. Ask them to bring in photographs and tell other students about their skills and abilities.

Some students might be able to arrange an observational visit to children. Students find it much easier to study with visual examples. You could divide the students into groups and ask each group to prepare an activity that will illustrate some aspect of physical or intellectual development. Warn students that children frequently will not perform to 'order', especially if a lot of people are in the room.

Some students with family babies or young children might be able to video some activities at home and show them in the group. Videos may already exist, so it is worthwhile exploring this. This type of activity needs careful planning so it is well to explore the resources of the group at the beginning of the unit. The students can spend the intervals between visits receiving more formal information and de-briefing the observations from the visits.

When the unit coincides with student work placements in child settings, a great deal of useful material can be obtained. There are useful child development videos obtainable from various sources if you have to resort to commercial products.

If you have an early years curriculum unit in your establishment then share resources or information with those staff. Otherwise surf the web! There are some useful videos on www.childhoodstudies.com on the UK web.

A series of visits to a nursery or pre-school playgroup can also provide a wealth of information. If you live in a town or city with several resources available, you could arrange a morning or afternoon visit and send two or three students to each one. Ensure that they have a precise agenda, otherwise the students will probably play with the children and not carry out the necessary observations. Two or three such visits would really reinforce their learning. You could divide up the visits into looking at physical, social and intellectual/language development and ask them to observe emotional aspects all the time.

When de-briefing students' observations emphasise the key features mentioned in the unit, such as cephalo-caudal development, midline to extremities and sequential development. They should also be encouraged to view each individual child developing at his or her own pace.

Puberty and adolescence

Moving on to the next phase of puberty and adolescence, you should find that most of your students remember the events of their own lives. It would be advantageous to ask them to read the sections in the student textbook first (see pages 222–223, 232–234, 242–243, 255).

Ask your students to write an anonymous piece about their own experience of this stage of their lives under the five headings of skills and abilities:

- Physical
- Intellectual
- Language
- Emotional
- Social

If they can word-process the piece it would preserve anonymity. This could present some difficulty if there is only one or two of one gender; it is far easier to do in a good gender mix or a single gender class.

You can then divide the class into groups of four or five and ask them to analyse the scripts and produce examples of each of the five aspects. Stress that the information is confidential and is not to be attributed to any one person. The students are young adults and should be able to carry out the task in a proper manner. You will not be able to trust their confidentiality in work experience if they cannot keep the confidence of their peers.

If you do not wish to build on your students' experience in this way, you could try using discussion groups, again using the five aspects. If you have a single gender group you will have to deliver the other gender in a lesson. In considering the personalities of your mixed gender group, you will have to decide whether to mix genders or keep them separate. There could be advantages and disadvantages either way.

Activity 4.1.1 and **Activity** 4.1.2 give students the opportunity to explore life events up to adolescence.

Middle age–later adulthood

Many student groups will not have adults beyond their thirties in the group and some will not have any mature students in the group at all. You will inevitably receive confidences regarding parents and grandparents when you come to middle and late adulthood. This can lead to difficulties, although you will not wish to stop students from contributing in class. You might try asking them to take a confidential approach by saying something like, 'I know someone who…' to prevent awkward moments, but many students will forget this in their eagerness to contribute an anecdote. Explaining how older people do not like personal details discussed in public might strike home! Immediately correct any student who forgets to observe confidentiality. Due to the age group of your class, you will receive many anecdotes from members of the class regarding the menopause of their female family members, so it is essential to maintain control over class time or you can find the session running out of time without achieving very much. It is useful to demonstrate this from the very beginning of the unit, allowing only a little time for relevant anecdotes and none for irrelevant ones. Do not be afraid to cut a story short if it is not leading towards useful learning. The class group will soon realise that you will not allow time-wasting

Developing skills and abilities

The unit is about people's development and if it is totally theoretical it will be boring for students. Relating theory to practice in their lives is really useful and will maintain interest, but take care. See **OHT** 4.2.1.

It is useful to extend an anecdote with questions such as:

- Why do you think that happened?
- What might have caused you, him or her to feel/act that way?
- How could things have been different?
- On reflection, would you, him or her act the same way again?
- Did anything else influence the way you, him or her felt/acted?

In this way, you will have either a natural lead in to the factors that influence development or be able to recall the example.

When considering skills and abilities of older people, the unit specification asks for a positive viewpoint and not just a lessening of skills and abilities of those people. A useful exercise for students to carry out is to produce a two-column chart, one for positive effects of ageing and one for negative effects. Make a rule that the two sides must be equal; in other words, they cannot put a negative effect without producing a positive one.

Another activity could be to research their local area and find out about all the clubs, societies, academic lectures, etc. available for the over-fifties. There is clearly more scope for this in larger villages and towns than in rural areas, however the students might be surprised how much activity is going on.

Students are also asked to consider the effects of accident or stroke on a person's skills and abilities, but again it is also encouraging to see how much can be accomplished even after a disabling event.

Activity 4.2.1 involves devising a questionnaire to discover the most stressful life events in people's lives, using the Holmes-Rahe scale. If you wish to test a large sample of questionnaires, you could merge the groups for analysis.

4.3 Factors affecting development

You might begin this section with some interesting discussion on the inter-relationships between genetic and environmental influences on development.

The textbook gives some fascinating examples on pages 280–284. A short introduction to cell biology, DNA, dominant and recessive alleles might be useful if students have little or no learning in the field of inheritance. Another simple example that many will have heard about is 'handedness' that is inherited genetically. In the past, when left-handedness had sinister overtones, parents would bind up a child's left hand and force them to use the right hand. Genetically, the child would have favoured the left hand but environmentally (through the parents) the child became right-handed. This might have had an effect on language development, co-ordination and dexterity. In turn, this might have affected job or career choice and subsequent socio-economic circumstances.

Activity 4.3.1 explores motor skills and **Activity 4.3.2** explores the development of language skills in early childhood. You might wish to divide your class group in half so that one group is researching motor skills and the other language skills. They could prepare a short talk on their experiences to share with other students.

Students might be able to think of more examples of the factors affecting development. They could examine the 'Nature versus Nurture' debate and actually have an end-of-term debate on this issue with Intermediate students invited to hear the arguments and vote at the end. This is often a good way to incorporate some of the communication key skills.

Students could explore their local environmental influences, such as access to health services, housing, education and pollution. Your local government and health authority reports and newspapers will prove invaluable resources to assist them. *The Health of the Nation* reports will provide a broad view of national concerns. (See **OHT 4.3.1** and **OHT 4.3.2**.)

It is important that students can link theory to case studies. One way of assisting them to make sense of case studies might be to encourage them to create characters based on their knowledge of life and the theory in Unit 4. A possible activity might be to design profile sheets which can be given to small groups of students. In **OHT 4.3.3** you will find a sheet which can be filled in for this purpose. Students might be asked to imagine a short life history based on the information they are given.

For example, **Activity 4.3.3** involves imagining how a person would have developed over 16 years of being subject to a range of influences.

The aim is to help students to relate theory to practice. The students' objective will be to assess the significance of theoretical information and use theory to predict human development.

Notes on Activity 4.3.3:

1 Use a task such as the time-line exercise (Activity 4.2.1) to encourage students to think about their own and others' development. The time-line exercise involves asking students to make a simple graph of their own memories of happiness since the age of five. Students may then share discussion of some of the factors which have influenced their own lives.

2 Explain the use of the profile set out in OHT 4.3.3 and ask students to briefly discuss how these factors might influence people.

3 Issue students with copies of the sheet in OHT 4.3.3. Each sheet could have the character's name at the top and then a profile of the influences on them.

4 Ask students to work in groups of two or three in order to imagine how the first 16 years of life might work out for a person given the pattern of influences described on the work card that they receive.

5 Ask students to write up an outline story based on their discussion of the influences.

6 Invite students to share the stories which they have created with each other.

7 Engage the whole class in discussion of the way in which genetic and environmental factors will influence human development.

This activity might be used as a revision exercise, or towards the end of teaching for Unit 4. Students will need a warm up exercise to engage them with thinking about human development before attempting to use profiles. They might be asked to work in groups of two or three. Each group might be given a profile sheet, each filled in with the details of a different person for each sheet. Each small group might then attempt to create a brief life story which would fit the information which they had been given. Stories could be shared between groups.

Using life stories

If students can record or invent life stories, the stories might be used as a basis for developing further links with theory. The overview on page 325 of the textbook and on **OHT 4.3.4** in this file might be used as a stimulus for asking students to conceptualise the way in which theory can be used to both interpret and influence life development.

Students could be asked to review their case study in terms of questions such as 'How might the character's development have been influenced if . . .'

- friends and relatives had reinforced good study habits (Skinner)
- the growing child had seen people around being praised for good work at school (Bandura)
- parents and teachers had helped the child to internalise their knowledge and skills (Vygotsky)
- the local school and community provided stimulating and effective opportunities to encourage learning (Piaget)
- parents had been sensitive to their potential impact on the environmental development of the child (Freud and Erikson).

Alternatively, students might be asked to explore the extent to which these theories might explain some of the environmental influences on the character's development.

In **Activity 4.3.4**, the students will prepare a talk for their peers. Each pair of students will prepare three questions on their work and hand them in to you. You will need to review the suitability of their questions and their answers and put them into a format suitable for informal assessment. On completion of the talks, you can present the quiz as an assessment tool and indicate the areas of weakness for each student. You will need to set a deadline for the questions so that you can prepare the quiz in plenty of time. If the class is large you might have two pairs working on, say, Piaget and Freud and divide up the work.

Students should be able to achieve communication and IT skills through this activity. They should be warned about the informal assessment, as they will be motivated to listen carefully.

If time is scarce and you do not wish to take the time for the talks, you can ask the students to prepare a maximum of two flip chart sheets with the information. Allow the students one session for reading and assimilation and deliver the quiz at the end. Leaving the sheets on display will assist reinforcement.

Social and economic factors which influence development

Understanding interaction

It will be useful for students to understand that current government policy on social exclusion is based on the idea that different levels of social factors interact. Both the Acheson report and 'Opportunity for All' documents show how different social and environmental factors may interact to affect the life chances of people. The unit should explore students' understanding of the concept of interaction. Two diagrams which will help explain the theory of interaction are in **OHTs 4.3.5** and **4.3.6**.

The interaction matrix

The interaction of multiple genetic and environmental factors is immensely, and possibly infinitely, complex. A simplified way of trying to understand interaction is set out in **OHT 4.3.7**. Nothing is completely fixed either by the environment or by genetics; both the environment and genetics interact to influence what happens.

How fixed is your future?

Ask yourself questions such as:

- What are my chances of living a long and healthy life?
- What are my chances of avoiding serious illnesses during my adult life?
- What are my chances of becoming a top athlete?

- What are my chances of achieving a high-paying career?
- What are my chances of achieving high academic qualifications?

OHT 4.3.7 provides an outline of how to find an answer to these sort of questions.

How different factors interact
Activities 4.3.5 and **4.3.6** aim to assist students to understand the ways in which social factors may interact to improve or reduce an individual's life chances. Students will be able to explain how a range of factors may interact to improve or reduce life chances.

Students should be introduced to information on low income, employment and unemployment, differences in housing, the risk of discrimination and problems with access to services. They will need to discuss and explore how this information relates to real life if they are to internalise their understanding in preparation for a test. Activity 4.3.5 may assist students to explore how factors may interact.

After receiving some initial guidance and information students should complete the table in Activity 4.3.5. Students might be presented with a case study, such as the case study of Stephen on page 326 and in **OHT 4.3.8** in this file, or they might be asked to research their own case study. This is intended to help individual students to focus their thoughts before moving on to discuss a case study using a further grid, in Activity 4.3.6.

Notes on Activity 4.3.5:
1 Provide students with background information and ideas.

2 Ask students to complete the grid giving examples of situations.

3 Discuss the outcomes of the activity with the whole group. Alternatively, students might discuss the outcomes in pairs.

Notes on Activity 4.3.6:
1 Ask students to complete the activity grid in relation to the supplied case study in OHT 4.3.8.

2 Using whole group discussion explore the idea of upward or downward spirals of development in relationship to the interaction of variables.

3 Ask students to produce an elaborated case study that describes the life story of two people with similar genetic inheritances, but who experience a different balance of life chances.

4.4 Theories of human development

In many ways this section of the standards may prove to be the most interesting but also the most challenging section to teach. Many students may assume that there should be one correct or right way to explain influences on human development. Some students may have difficulty coping with the idea of multiple interpretations, or theories of development.

One way of attempting to cope with abstract theory is to present it as a series of concrete sets of information associated with each theorist's name. In this way the theories of Freud, Erikson, Skinner, Bandura, Vygotsky and Piaget can be reduced to simple, easy to remember, ideas. (See **OHT 4.4.1**.) There are two major limitations to this strategy however:

1 Information overload. Some students will still have trouble making sense of the different theories and memorising sufficient information to use effectively under test conditions.

2 Teaching each theory as an independent range of facts and information will not assist students to develop the analytic skills and understanding which will be required for higher grades, under test conditions.

A more appropriate teaching strategy might be to mix a range of step-by-step information with some more holistic work aimed at enabling students to analyse life events in terms of theory. For example, it may be appropriate to outline theories such as Skinner's and Freud's and then introduce a brief case study and invite students to debate the rival interpretations that the different theorists would offer. A model for using this type of case study is set out on page 326 of the textbook and in OHT 4.3.8 of this file. Able students may be capable of relating theory directly to short case studies. Some students may need to be guided through case studies, such as Stephen's in OHT 4.3.8, before they understand the idea of using theory to analyse life events. Students might be invited to supply short stories describing an individual's behaviour, and they might then briefly discuss how the different theories would explain the stories. Alternatively, you may wish to provide interpretations from the different theoretical perspectives in order to model how theory can be used to interpret human behaviour.

Case studies will provide a basis for a whole group of small group work following the teaching of the various theories. Students should be encouraged to see the different theories as each supplying a section of the jigsaw that makes up the truth about influences on development. Each theory may have something to offer but perhaps no one author has completely explained how our biology and environment interact to create unique individuals. Students should be encouraged to debate and discuss ways in which the different theories can explain what has happened to an individual. Students should also be encouraged to understand the dangers of making assumptions about people based on a single theoretical interpretation.

Students might be invited to research information about the developmental theories in this section. They might for example research information in order to write a short paper as part of a group project. The group might present their conclusions on the interpretation of a case study using contributions from a range of individuals who have each researched a different theory. Initially, students might be invited to use A-level Psychology or Human Development textbooks. Many students will gain satisfaction from hunting information out from the World Wide Web. It may be important to caution students that much of this information is likely to be advanced and specialised. Some students may be put off if they cannot make sense of the material they have retrieved.

Tutorial discussion may provide a useful tool to sensitise students to the practical application of theory to care work. If some students are studying the additional key skill of 'Improving Own Learning and Performance', they may explore the development of their own problem-solving and reflective ability using the Kolb learning cycle as set out on page 114 of the textbook and in **OHT 4.4.2** in this file. It will be important to encourage students to use theories of development in the context of explaining life events.

Where students are sufficiently motivated it might be possible to revise theories of development using a 'Trivial Pursuit' type of quiz game. Each team can devise short descriptions of life events, or people's behaviour, and the opposing team can attempt to explain each story using one or more theories.

ASSESSMENT SUMMARY

Grade E

To achieve a **grade E** the work must show an understanding of human development based on a study of the human development of two individuals at different life stages (over eight years old and over nineteen years old) including:

- A clear description of the growth and development of two individuals at different life stages.
- The development of two major skill areas in each individual.
- A description of the range of factors that may have affected the development of the two individuals.
- A description of the four main theories of development and how they relate to individuals.

Grade C

To achieve a **grade C** the work must show:

- Contrast and comparison of the differences in development of the two individuals.
- An accurate explanation of the influence of the skill areas on the development of the two individuals.

- The use of appropriate theories to analyse the influence of the range of factors on development and the presentation of well-considered conclusions.

Grade A

To achieve a **grade A** the work must show:

- Coherently presented arguments based on a comprehensive analysis of the relative importance of the factors that affected the development of the individuals.
- An explanation of how the effect of the factors may be enhanced or minimised.
- A reflection of how the use of different theories might influence the interpretation of the development of a chosen individual.

OHTs

The OHTs to help tutors deliver this unit are as follows:

4.1.1 Life stages of human development

4.1.2 Differences in self-concept between different age groups

4.1.3 The Holmes-Rahe life event scale

4.2.1 Gardner's seven intelligences

4.3.1 Circles of influence

4.3.2 Death rates for men aged 20–64

4.3.3 Handout – A profile for creating characters

4.3.4 An overview of theories and theorists

4.3.5 Different levels of influence on development

4.3.6 Factors that can contribute to social exclusion

4.3.7 Interaction of genetic and environmental factors

4.3.8 How factors interact

4.4.1 Freudian mental mechanisms

4.4.2 Kolb's learning cycle

ACTIVITIES

The activities are designed to promote learning and understanding, provide consolidation and develop logical thinking and a rational approach to studies.

4.1.1 Growth profiles

4.1.2 Primary socialisation in your development

4.2.1 Testing the Holmes-Rahe scale

4.3.1 Motor skills in early childhood

4.3.2 Language skills in early childhood

4.3.3 Inventing a character

4.3.4 Exploring theories and theorists

4.3.5 Factors which can contribute to social exclusion

4.3.6 Assessing the life chances of two similar people born into different environments

OHT 4.1.1 LIFE STAGES OF HUMAN DEVELOPMENT

These are some examples of Havighurst's description of the stages of development in human life.

Infancy and early childhood

- Learning to take solid foods
- Learning to walk
- Learning to talk
- Learning bowel and bladder control
- Learning sex differences and sexual modesty

Middle childhood

- Learning physical skills necessary for ordinary games
- Learning to get along with peers
- Learning an appropriate masculine or feminine role
- Developing basic skills in reading, writing and calculating
- Developing concepts necessary for everyday living
- Developing conscience, morality and a scale of values

Adolescence

- Achieving new and more mature relations with peers of both sexes
- Achieving a masculine or feminine role
- Achieving one's physique and using the body effectively
- Achieving emotional independence of parents and other adults
- Preparing for marriage and family life
- Preparing for an economic career

OHT 4.1.1 (continued)

Early adulthood

- Selecting a mate
- Learning to live with a marriage partner
- Starting a family
- Rearing children
- Managing a home
- Getting started in an occupation

Middle age

- Assisting teenage children to become responsible and happy adults
- Reaching and maintaining satisfactory performance in one's occupational career
- Relating to one's spouse as a person
- Accepting and adjusting to the physiological changes of middle age
- Adjusting to ageing parents

Later maturity

- Adjusting to decreasing physical strength
- Adjusting to retirement and reduced income
- Adjusting to the death of one's spouse
- Establishing satisfactory physical living arrangements

OHT 4.1.2 DIFFERENCES IN SELF-CONCEPT BETWEEN DIFFERENT AGE GROUPS

Age	Expression of self-concept
Young children	Self-concept limited to a few descriptions, for example, boy or girl, size, some skills
Older children	Self-concept can be described in a range of 'factual categories', such as hair colour, name, details or address, etc.
Adolescents	Self-concept starts to be explained in terms of chosen beliefs, likes, dislikes, relationships with others
Adults	Many adults may be able to explain the quality of their lives and their personality in greater depth and detail than when they were adolescents
Older adults	Some older adults may have more self-knowledge than during early adult life. Some people may show 'wisdom' in the way they explain their self-concept

OHT 4.1.3 THE HOLMES-RAHE LIFE EVENT SCALE

Life event	Value
Death of partner	100
Divorce	73
Marital separation	65
Going to prison	63
Death of a close family member	63
Personal injury or illness	53
Marriage	50
Being dismissed at work	47
Marital reconciliation	45
Retirement	45
Change in health or family member	44
Pregnancy	40
Sexual difficulties	39
Gaining a new family member	39
Business or work adjustment	39
Change in financial state	38
Death of a close friend	37
Change to a different line of work	36
Change in number of arguments with partner	35
Mortgage larger than one year's net salary	31
Foreclosure of mortgage or loan	30
Change in responsibilities at work	29

Life event	Value
Son or daughter leaving home	29
Trouble with in-laws	29
Outstanding personal achievement	28
Partner begins or stops work	26
Begin or end school	26
Change in living conditions	25
Revision of personal habits	24
Trouble with boss	23
Change in work hours or conditions	20
Change in residence	20
Change in schools	20
Change in recreation	19
Change in religious activities	19
Change in social activities	18
Mortgage or loan less than one year's net salary	17
Change in sleeping habits	16
Change in number of family get-togethers	15
Change in eating habits	15
Holiday	13
Major festival, e.g. Christmas	12
Minor violations of the law	11

OHT 4.2.1 GARDNER'S SEVEN INTELLIGENCES

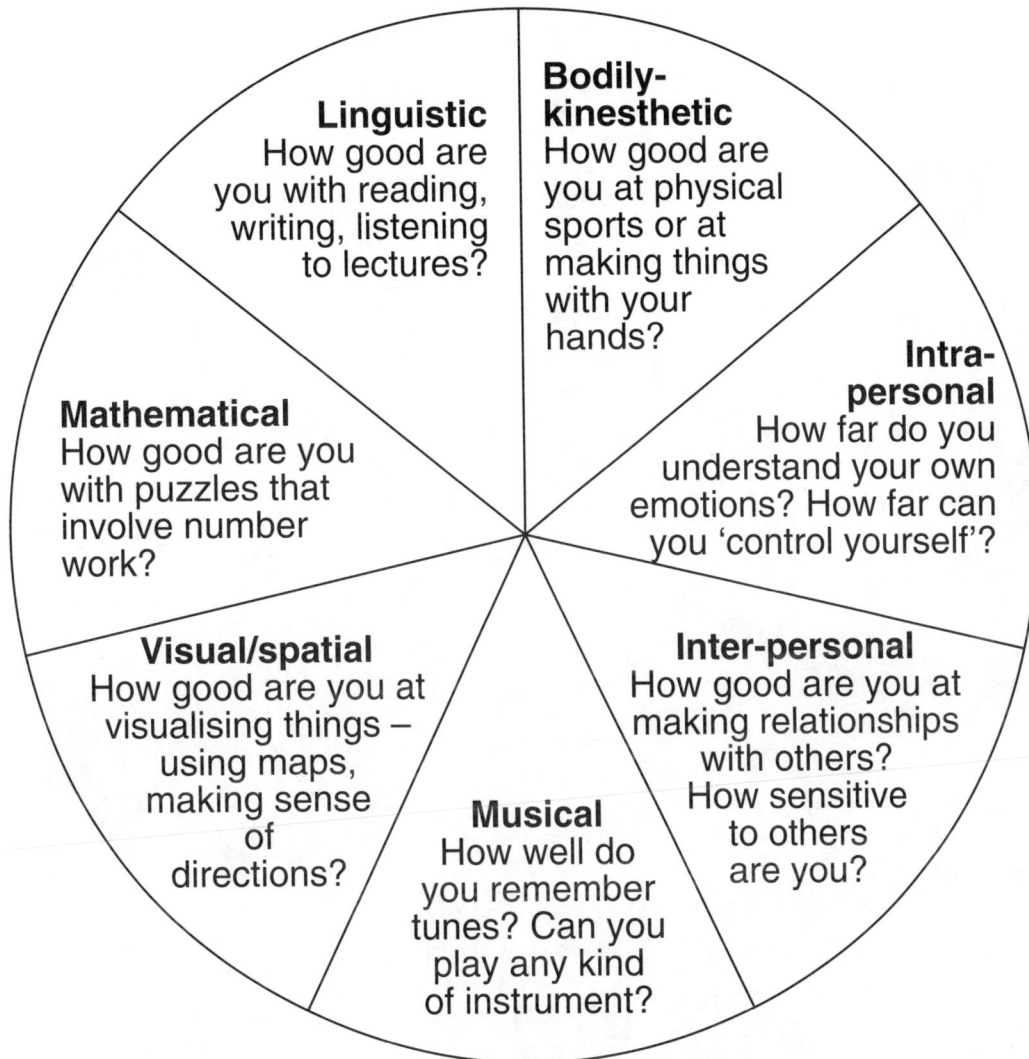

Linguistic
How good are you with reading, writing, listening to lectures?

Bodily-kinesthetic
How good are you at physical sports or at making things with your hands?

Intra-personal
How far do you understand your own emotions? How far can you 'control yourself'?

Inter-personal
How good are you at making relationships with others? How sensitive to others are you?

Musical
How well do you remember tunes? Can you play any kind of instrument?

Visual/spatial
How good are you at visualising things – using maps, making sense of directions?

Mathematical
How good are you with puzzles that involve number work?

OHT 4.3.1 CIRCLES OF INFLUENCE

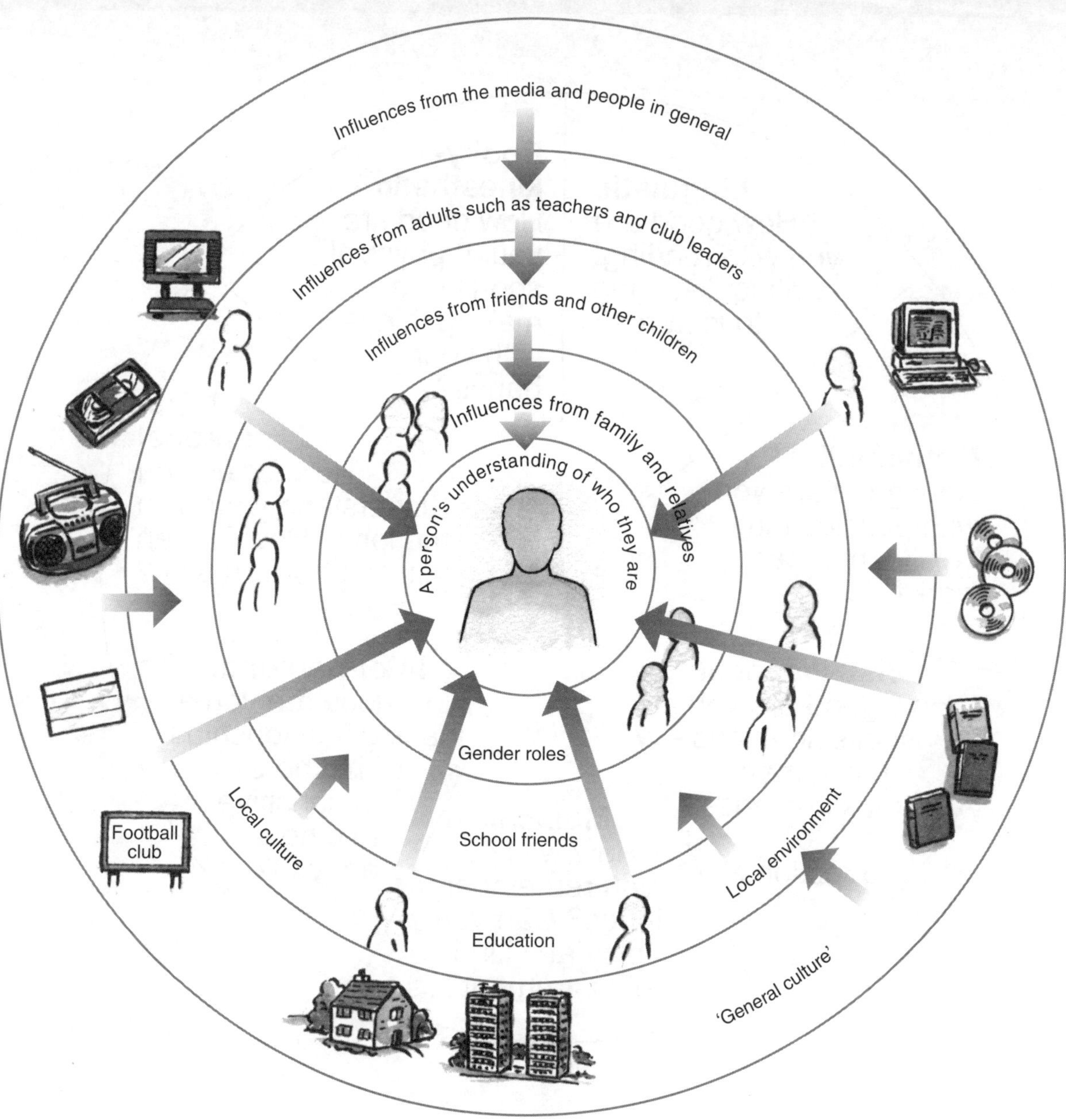
Influences from the media and people in general
Influences from adults such as teachers and club leaders
Influences from friends and other children
Influences from family and relatives
A person's understanding of who they are
Gender roles
School friends
Education
Local culture
Local environment
'General culture'
Football club

OHT 4.3.2 DEATH RATES FOR MEN AGED 20–64

All causes
rates per 100,000

Social class	*Year*		
	1970–72	1979–83	1991–93
I – Professional	500	373	280
II – Managerial & Technical	526	425	300
III(N) – Skilled (non-manual)	637	522	426
III(M) – Skilled (manual)	683	580	493
IV – Partly skilled	721	639	492
V – Unskilled	897	910	806
England and Wales	624	549	419

Lung cancer
rates per 100,000

Social class	*Year*		
	1970–72	1979–83	1991–93
I – Professional	41	26	17
II – Managerial & Technical	52	39	24
III(N) – Skilled (non-manual)	63	47	34
III(M) – Skilled (manual)	90	72	54
IV – Partly skilled	93	76	52
V – Unskilled	109	108	82
England and Wales	73	60	39

Coronary heart disease
rates per 100,000

Social class	*Year*		
	1970–72	1979–83	1991–93
I – Professional	195	144	81
II – Managerial & Technical	197	168	92
III(N) – Skilled (non-manual)	245	208	136
III(M) – Skilled (manual)	232	218	159
IV – Partly skilled	232	227	156
V – Unskilled	243	287	235
England and Wales	209	201	127

Stroke
rates per 100,000

Social class	*Year*		
	1970–72	1979–83	1991–93
I – Professional	35	20	14
II – Managerial & Technical	37	23	13
III(N) – Skilled (non-manual)	41	28	19
III(M) – Skilled (manual)	45	34	24
IV – Partly skilled	46	37	25
V – Unskilled	59	55	45
England and Wales	40	30	20

Accidents, poisoning, violence
rates per 100,000

Social class	*Year*		
	1970–72	1979–83	1991–93
I – Professional	23	17	13
II – Managerial & Technical	25	20	13
III(N) – Skilled (non-manual)	25	21	17
III(M) – Skilled (manual)	34	27	24
IV – Partly skilled	39	35	24
V – Unskilled	67	63	52
England and Wales	34	28	22

Suicide and undetermined injury
rates per 100,000

Social class	*Year*		
	1970–72	1979–83	1991–93
I – Professional	16	16	13
II – Managerial & Technical	13	15	14
III(N) – Skilled (non-manual)	17	18	20
III(M) – Skilled (manual)	12	16	21
IV – Partly skilled	18	23	23
V – Unskilled	32	44	47
England and Wales	15	20	22

OHT 4.3.3 HANDOUT – A PROFILE FOR CREATING CHARACTERS

This profile sheet can be used for Activity 4.3.3.

Name	
General physical constitution	Very healthy, healthy, liable to poor health ____________________ ____________________
Ability:	Give marks out of five for each ability, i.e. 1 2 3 4 5
Linguistic	☐
Mathematical	☐
Visual/spatial	☐
Musical	☐
Bodily-kinesthetic	☐
Intra-personal	☐
Inter-personal	☐
Social class and income of parents	Give a brief description of the social class, wealth and income of the parents (high, average or low) ____________________ ____________________
Housing	Describe the house or flat that the child grows up in. Rate housing as stress-free, restricting or stressful. ____________________ ____________________
Local community, including pollution, crime and stress	Outline any sources of pollution, crime or stress using three categories, such as serious air pollution, some air pollution, little air pollution; serious crime, some crime, little crime, etc. ____________________ ____________________
Family support	Relationships between family members may be warm and supportive, neutral, or rejecting. ____________________ ____________________
Quality of learning opportunities	Children might receive lots of encouragement from relatives friends and teachers, some encouragement or little encouragement. ____________________ ____________________

OHT 4.3.4 AN OVERVIEW OF THEORIES AND THEORISTS

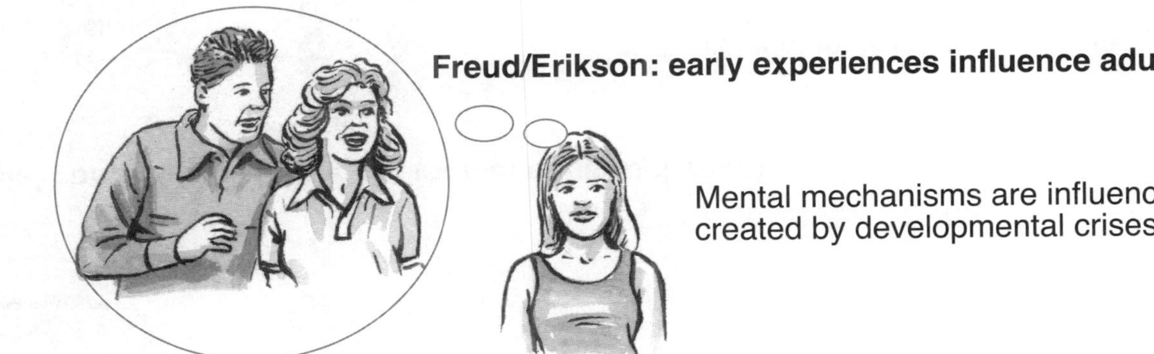

Freud/Erikson: early experiences influence adult life

Mental mechanisms are influenced and created by developmental crises

Piaget: children progress through stages of cognitive development

Child matures in stages
Adults may facilitate or help but children build their own systems of thinking

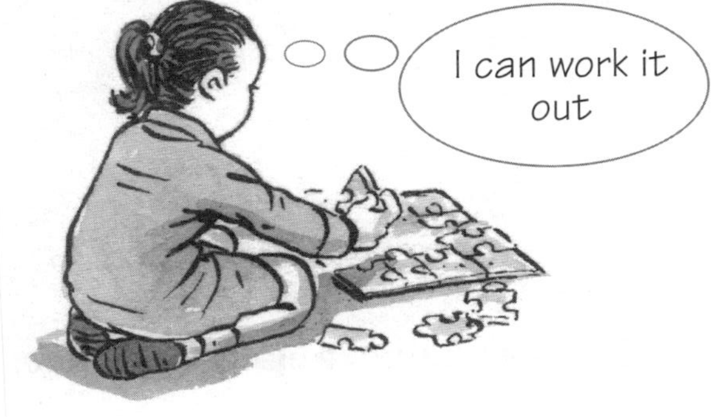
I can work it out

OHT 4.3.4 (continued)

Skinner and Bandura: children are conditioned to learn from their experiences

Reinforcement or punishment moulds our behaviour

Learning by imitation:Bandura

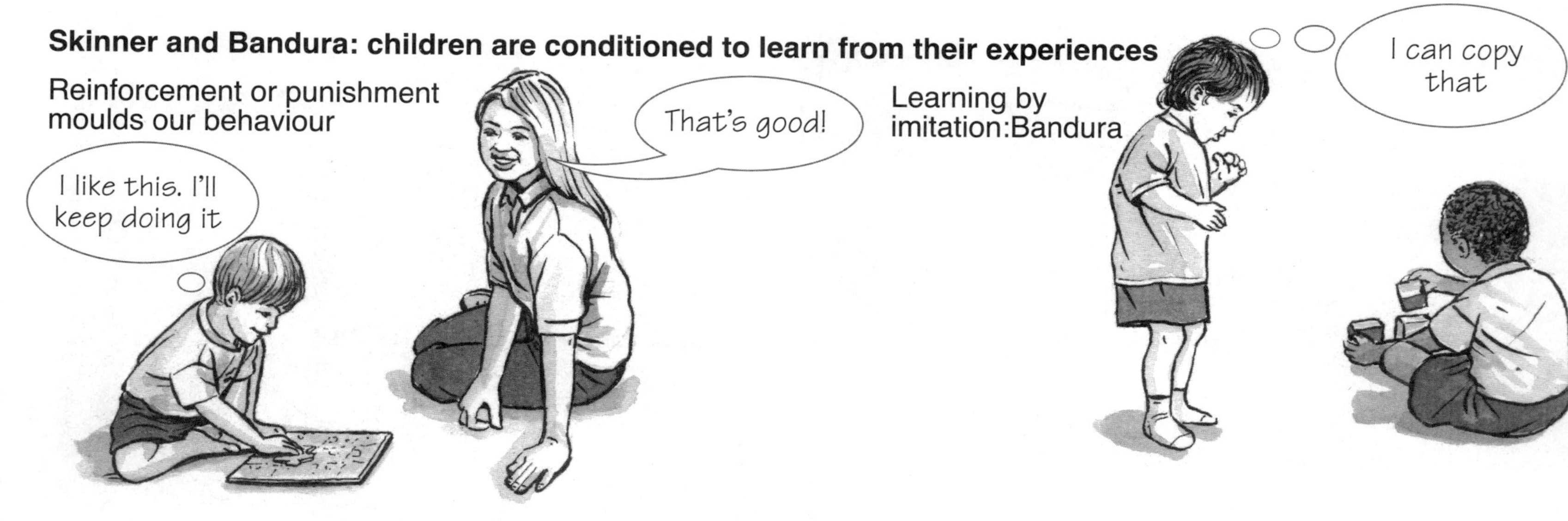

I like this. I'll keep doing it
That's good!
I can copy that

Vygotsky: social context is all important (social constructivism)

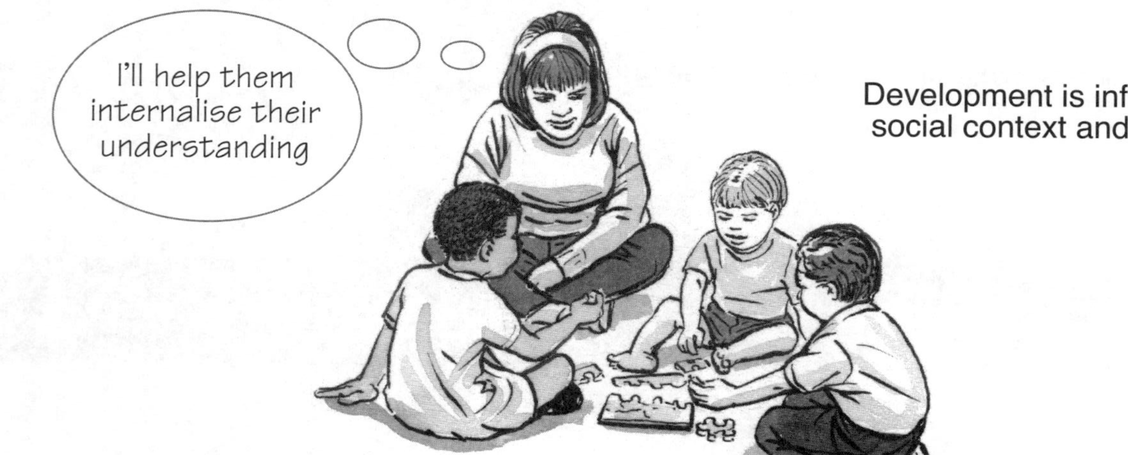

I'll help them internalise their understanding

Development is influenced by language, social context and adult guidance

OHT 4.3.5 DIFFERENT LEVELS OF INFLUENCE ON DEVELOPMENT

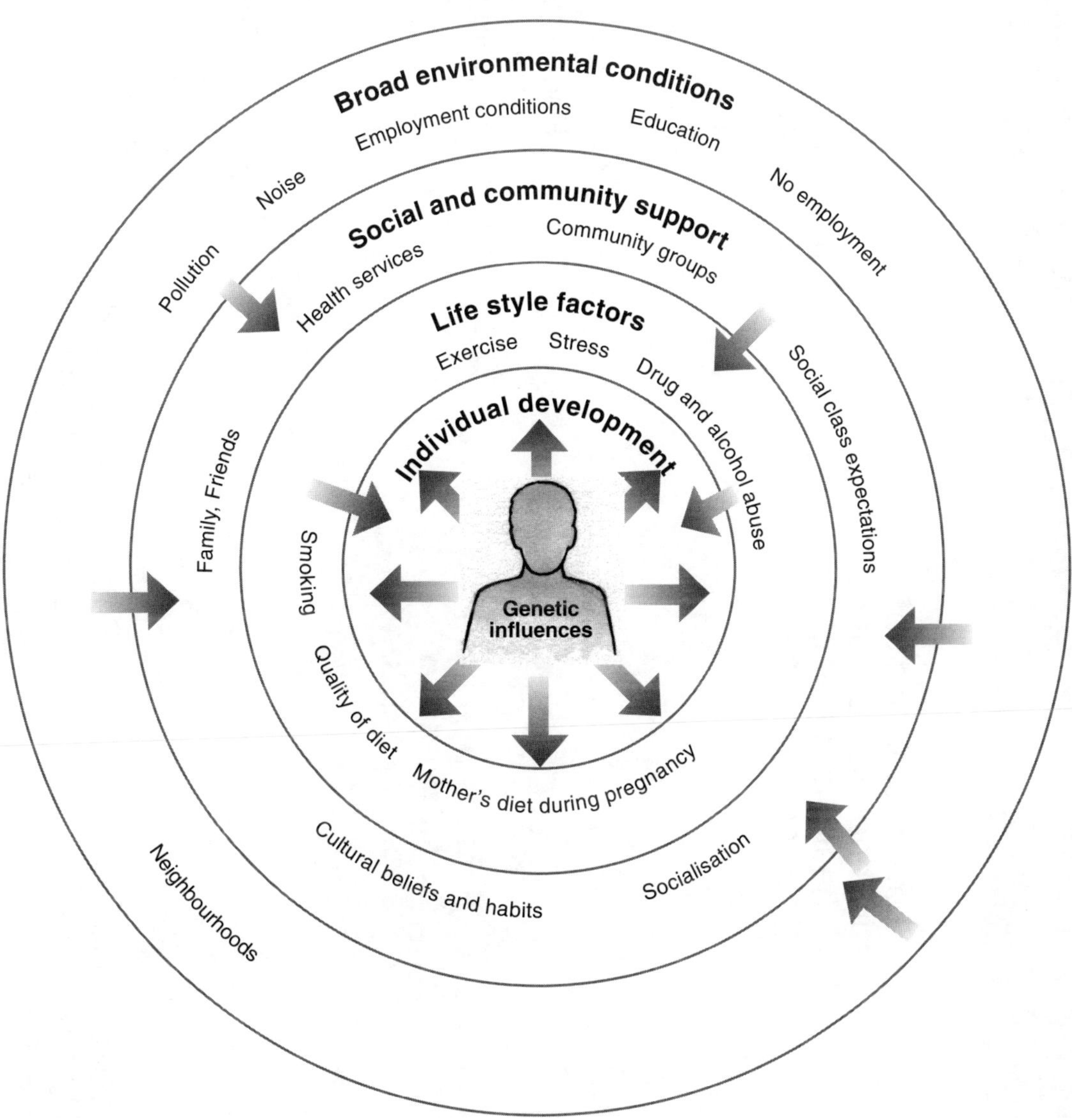

Broad environmental conditions
Employment conditions
Education
Noise
No employment
Pollution
Social and community support
Health services
Community groups
Life style factors
Exercise
Stress
Drug and alcohol abuse
Social class expectations
Individual development
Family, Friends
Smoking
Genetic influences
Quality of diet
Mother's diet during pregnancy
Cultural beliefs and habits
Socialisation
Neighbourhoods

OHT 4.3.6 FACTORS THAT CAN CONTRIBUTE TO SOCIAL EXCLUSION

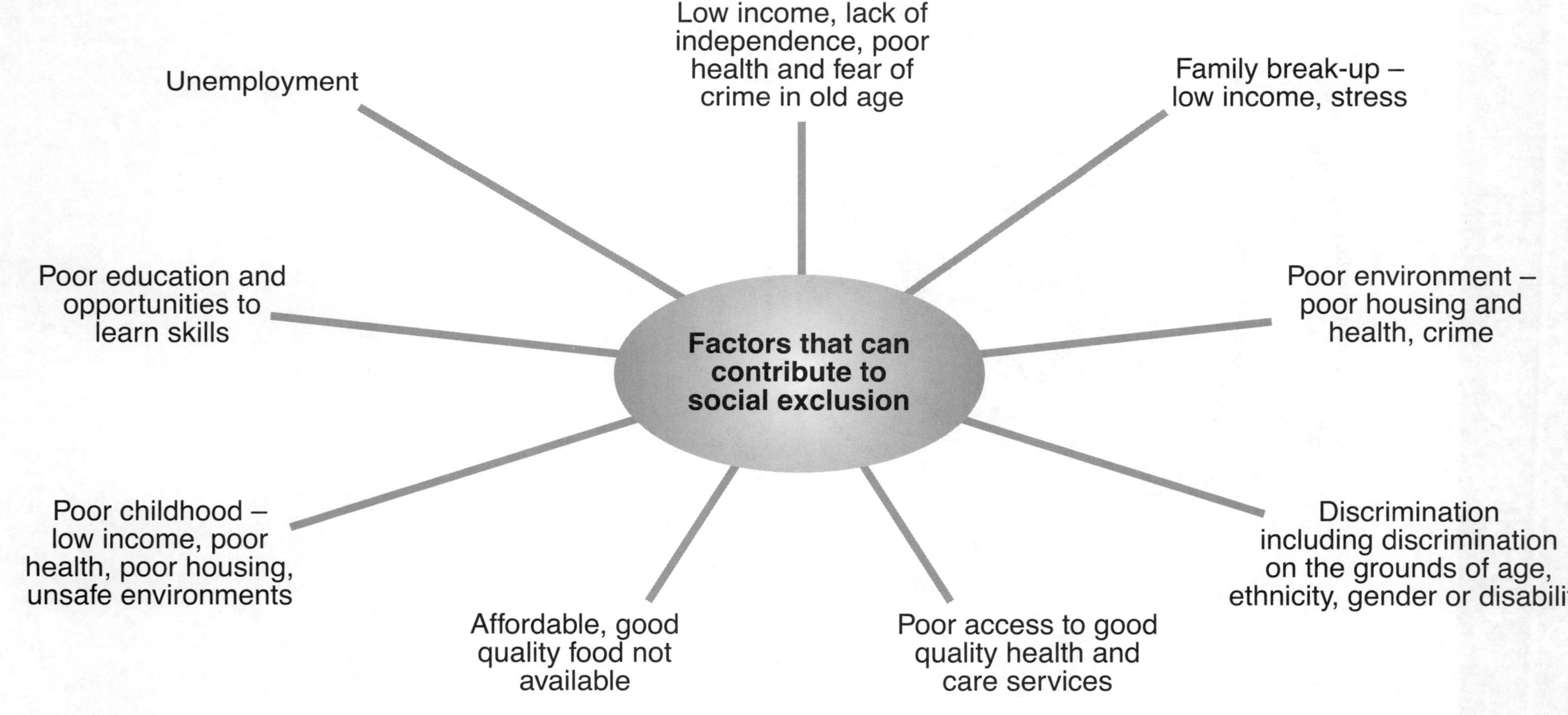

Factors that can contribute to social exclusion
Unemployment
Low income, lack of independence, poor health and fear of crime in old age
Family break-up – low income, stress
Poor education and opportunities to learn skills
Poor environment – poor housing and health, crime
Poor childhood – low income, poor health, poor housing, unsafe environments
Affordable, good quality food not available
Poor access to good quality health and care services
Discrimination including discrimination on the grounds of age, ethnicity, gender or disability

OHT 4.3.7 INTERACTION OF GENETIC AND ENVIRONMENTAL FACTORS

	Ideal environment	**Satisfactory environment**	**Poor environment**
Ideal genetic inheritance	You should do well. You have everything going for you.	You will probably do well.	How well you do may be down to chance.
Satisfactory genetic inheritance	You will probably do well.	How well you do may be down to chance.	You will probably do badly.
Poor genetic inheritance	How well you do may be down to chance.	You will probably do badly.	You have little chance. Everything is against you.

OHT 4.3.8 HOW FACTORS INTERACT

Case study: Stephen

Stephen is now 20 years old. Stephen appeared to enjoy a healthy and happy childhood but he never did very well at junior school. When Stephen was 12 years old his mother and father got divorced and his mother remarried. Stephen did not get on well with his new stepfather. Stephen stayed at school until he was 18 but never did very well in his exams. He went to work for a DIY store as his first job but found that he couldn't get on with the other staff. Stephen left his job because of arguments with his employers.

OHT 4.4.1 FREUDIAN MENTAL MECHANISMS

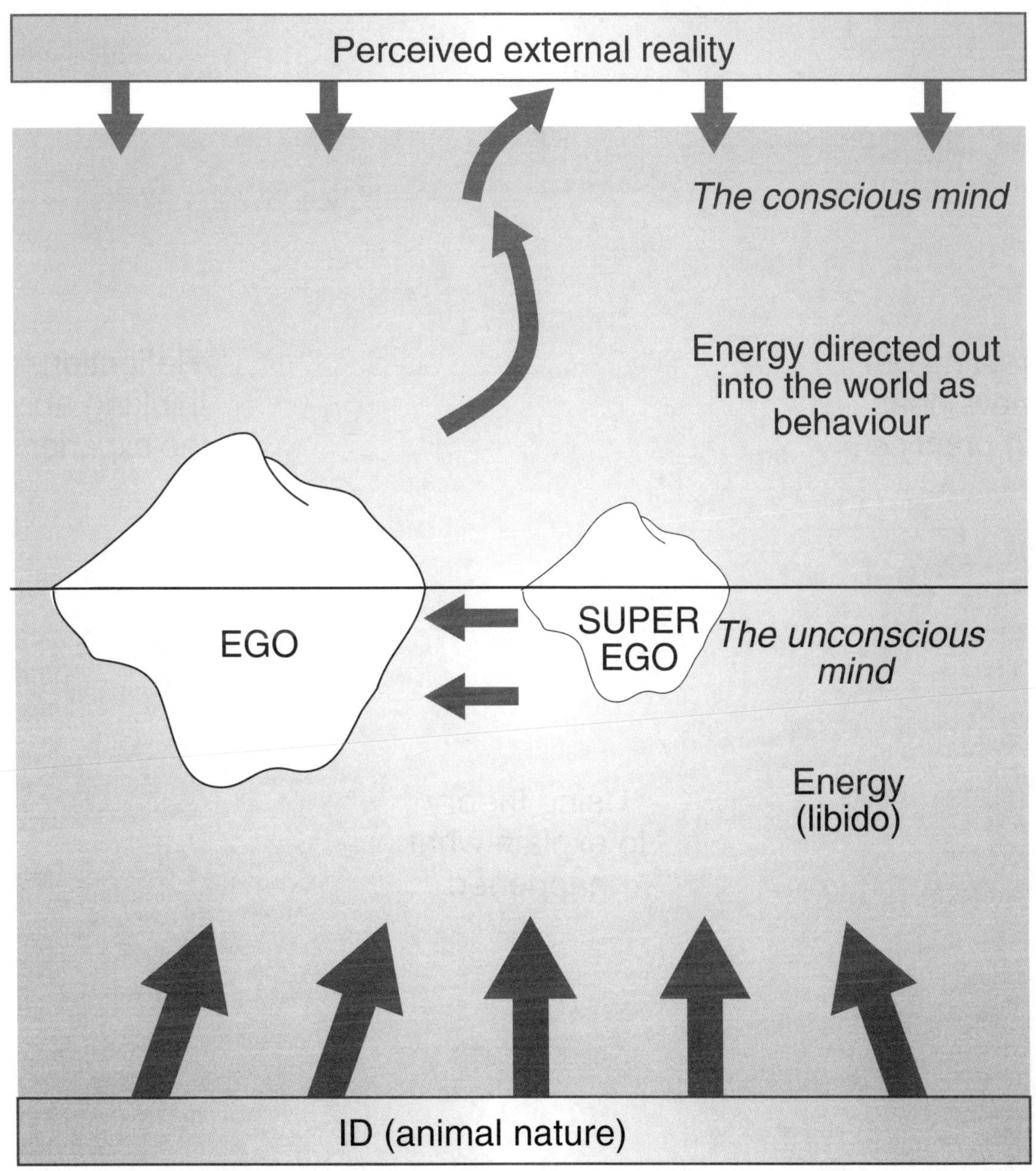
Perceived external reality
The conscious mind
Energy directed out into the world as behaviour
EGO
SUPER EGO
The unconscious mind
Energy (libido)
ID (animal nature)

OHT 4.4.2 KOLB'S LEARNING CYCLE

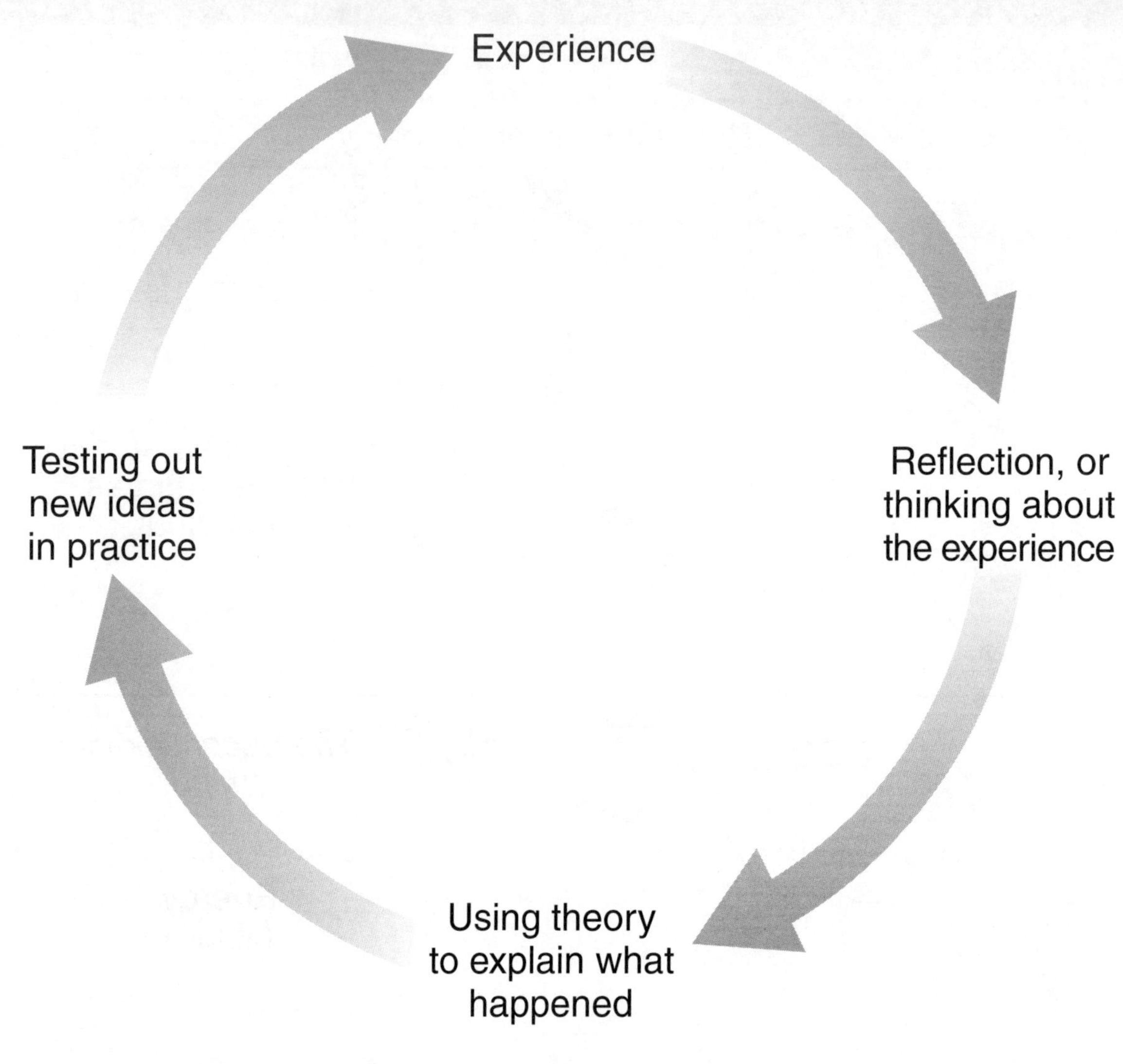
Experience
Reflection, or thinking about the experience
Using theory to explain what happened
Testing out new ideas in practice

ACTIVITY 4.1.1 GROWTH PROFILES

A group of researchers measured the body mass of a large number of young males and females of different ages. After calculating the mean body mass for each age group in years, they tabulated their results in the table:

Age in years	Males (Mean body mass in kg)	Females (Mean body mass in kg)
0	6	5.5
1	11	10
2	13	12
3	15.5	14
4	18	17
5	19.5	18
6	23	22
7	25	23
8	28	26
9	31	29
10	33	32
11	35	36
12	38	41
13	42	43
14	50	47
15	55	52
16	59	54
17	63	55
18	64	55

TASKS

1 Carefully plot a graph of these results with a title and labelled axes.

2 Describe the pattern of growth for males and females shown by your graph.

3 For how many years are males heavier than females?

4 State the age range when the increase in mass for males is the greatest.

5 How much extra mass do males put on in this period?

6 Place an X on your graph to represent the mean age for walking independently.

7 Represent the mean ages for the start of puberty in males and females by placing Y and Z on the correct graph lines.

8 Calculate the rate of change for males between the ages of 14 and 16.

9 Describe the changes that occur in girls during puberty.

10 Olympic female swimmers are often girls in the age range from 12 years to 15 years whereas male swimmers are usually from 19 to 25 years of age. Suggest a physical reason for this.

11 By how many kilograms are males heavier than females at the age of 18 or the end of adolescence?

12 Describe the changes in males during puberty.

ACTIVITY 4.1.2 PRIMARY SOCIALISATION IN YOUR DEVELOPMENT

Before you begin this activity, read pages 230–234 on socialisation in the textbook.

TASKS

1. Write down the norms of behaviour in your home upbringing in two sections:

   a up to the age of eight years
   b from nine years to eighteen, or the present day if you are younger than eighteen.

2. Who set those norms?
3. What do you think were the underlying reasons for those norms?
4. If you have brothers or sisters, were the norms the same for all children? If you do not have brothers or sisters, were they the same for any other relatives you have?
5. Thinking about your peers in the two age groups, did they have different norms of behaviour? Explain the differences.
6. How did these norms of behaviour influence your development?
7. How did different norms of behaviour affect other young people that you know?
8. When you have children of your own, which norms of behaviour from your own upbringing would you keep? Explain the reasons for your answer.
9. When you have children of your own, which norms of behaviour from your own upbringing would you reject? Explain the reasons for your answer.
10. Predict the consequences of your answer to question 9.
11. Join with two other class members and discuss the similarities and differences of your answers.
12. Review your answers in the light of your peer discussion and make changes if you wish.
13. Re-form your group and prepare a flip chart sheet of the major norms of behaviour in the two age ranges from all answers. Write in a non-personal way.
14. Display your poster in the classroom and compare with your experiences.

ACTIVITY 4.2.1 TESTING THE HOLMES-RAHE SCALE

Read pages 235–239 of the textbook until you are familiar with social and emotional development in early, middle and late adulthood.

TASKS

1 Devise a questionnaire involving the Holmes-Rahe scale of the most stressful life events – see OHT 4.1.3. Ensure that you mix up the categories so that they are in a different order to that in the scale. You are doing this to prevent your subjects from realising that this is a descending scale. Under each category place a scale numbered one to ten; your scale might look something like this:

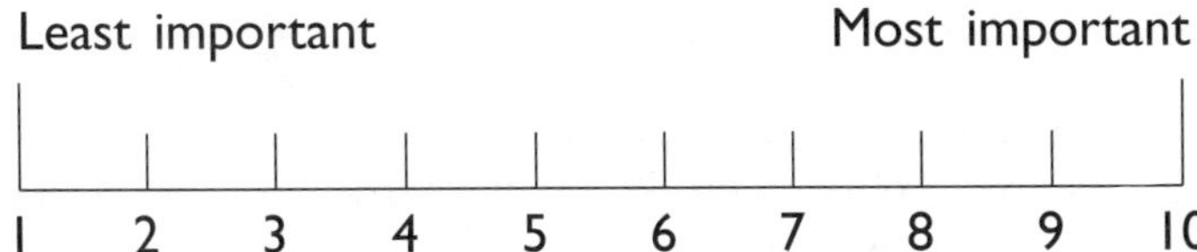
Least important
Most important
1 2 3 4 5 6 7 8 9 10

or you may prefer to work in tens up to a hundred.

2 Ask each person who receives the questionnaire to place a mark on the scale to represent his or her feelings about the degree of stress for that category. As an example, you or a member of your family receives a jail sentence. How stressful would that be to you? Mark the scale with a line.

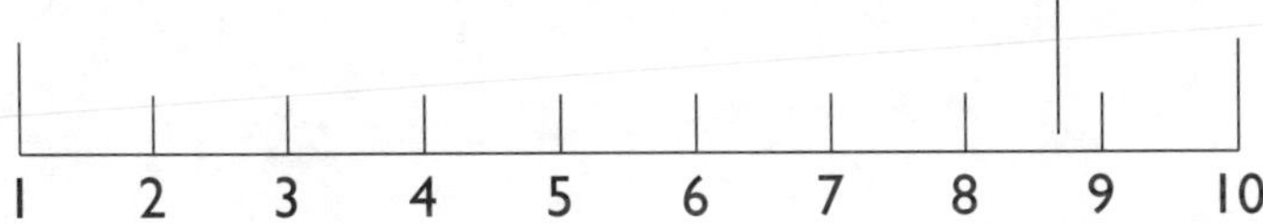
1 2 3 4 5 6 7 8 9 10

Make sure that you ask at least five people from each of the three sections of adulthood.

You might wish to add one or two categories of life events from OHT 4.1.1 as some may not be relevant to all sections of adulthood. For instance, a member of the group in late adulthood will not find pregnancy stressful! They might, however, find a change of residence very stressful. You will need to consider the relevance of your findings in accordance with the section of adulthood you are exploring. You might wish to ask people to mark only whole numbers to make evaluation easier. Do not forget to make the questionnaire confidential although you will need the recipient to state the age range they are in, and the gender might prove interesting. You can test people from any location with this questionnaire.

3 When you have the 15 replies, sort them into the relevant sections of adulthood and compare them within your sections.

Compare the results from the different sections with each other and then compare them with the standard Holmes-Rahe scale.

4 Write an analysis of your results and evaluate your method of operation.

Try to incorporate some statistical information from your results.

ACTIVITY 4.3.1 MOTOR SKILLS IN EARLY CHILDHOOD

Read pages 239–242 in the textbook before you begin this activity.

TASKS

1 Organise at least two visits to a playgroup or nursery in your locality. Explain what it is that you plan to do during your visit.

You will be observing gross and fine motor skills of babies and/or young children at different stages of development.

2 Prepare a chart to enable you to log your observations and the ages of the children concerned. You might find that it is more convenient to focus on three particular children of different ages in one session rather than attempt to observe all the children.

Focusing would enable you to encourage different play activities during your observation period. You can also talk to the care staff if there is any problem. For instance, if the weather is poor, the children are unlikely to play outside and you may not get the opportunity to observe a skill such as riding a tricycle.

3 When your observations are complete, write an account of your observations of gross and fine motor skills of the children, commenting on any child whose rate of development is faster or slower than the expected or average rate of development.

ACTIVITY 4.3.2 LANGUAGE SKILLS IN EARLY CHILDHOOD

Read pages 266–272 in the textbook on language skills in babies and young children.

TASKS

1 Organise at least two visits to a playgroup or nursery in your locality. Explain what it is that you plan to do during your visit.

You will be observing communication and the acquisition of language skills of babies and/or young children at different stages of development.

2 Prepare a chart to enable you to log your observations and the ages of the children concerned. You might find that it is more convenient to focus on three particular children of different ages in one session rather than attempt to observe all the children.

Focusing would enable you to encourage different play activities during your observation period to stimulate communication. You can also talk to the care staff if there is any problem. For instance, a few children will take a longer time to talk to a stranger.

3 When your observations are complete, write an account of your observations of communication and language skills of the children, commenting on any child whose rate of development is faster or slower than the expected or average rate of development.

ACTIVITY 4.3.3 INVENTING A CHARACTER

In groups of two or three you are going to imagine how a 16-year-old person has developed given the range of influences they have been subjected to in their life so far.

TASKS

Each group will be provided with a profile sheet (OHT 4.3.3) on a person which they will fill in. From this you have to construct a life history of the person.

1 Write up an outline story based on your discussion of the influences on the person in the profile sheet.

2 Share the story with the other groups.

3 As a class discuss the way in which genetic and environmental factors influence human development.

4 To make the link between theory and your story, review your story in terms of the question: 'How might the character's development been influenced if …

… friends and relatives had reinforced good study habits?' (Skinner)

… the growing child had seen people around being praised for good work at school?' (Bandura)

… parents and teachers had helped the person to internalise their knowledge and skills?' (Vygotsky)

… the local school and community provided stimulating and effective opportunities to encourage learning? (Piaget)

… parents had been sensitive to their potential impact on the emotional development of the child?' (Freud and Erikson)

ACTIVITY 4.3.4 EXPLORING THEORIES AND THEORISTS

TASKS

1 After you have read this unit in the textbook you will have become acquainted with different theorists and how their theories relate to human development.

Working in pairs and using material from other sources as well as the textbook, prepare a talk about one of the theorists in the list below. You may work in pairs, providing both of you participate in the talk. The talk should be at least five minutes long and no longer than ten minutes. You should not read your notes and may have two overhead transparencies for illustrative purposes. You should speak about the theorist and the context in which he or she worked and then give a summary of their major theories. Finally, you should give a personal opinion about the relevance and importance of his or her work in modern society.

Piaget	Erikson
Bandura	Gesell
Skinner	Vygotsky
Freud	

2 Prepare three questions and their answers on your work to give to your tutor. The questions should be relevant to the unit and not, for example, the dates of the theorist's lifetime!

ACTIVITY 4.3.5 FACTORS WHICH CAN CONTRIBUTE TO SOCIAL EXCLUSION

This activity aims to help you to understand the way in which social factors may interact to improve or reduce an individual's life changes.

TASK 1

Using the case study of Stephen in OHT 4.3.8, or one that you have researched yourself, complete the grid below.

Factor	Examples
Poor employment opportunities and unemployment	
Low income	
Family break-up	
Poor environment: poor housing, crime, etc.	
Poor access to good quality health and care services	
Poor educational opportunities	
Discrimination – including discrimination on grounds of age, ethnicity, gender or disability	
Affordable good quality food not available	
Poor health due to stressful living conditions	
Unsafe, polluted and stressful living environments	

(Adapted from *Opportunity for All* 1999)

TASK 2

As a group, or in pairs, discuss the outcomes from the information in the table.

ACTIVITY 4.3.6 ASSESSING THE LIFE CHANCES OF TWO SIMILAR PEOPLE BORN INTO DIFFERENT ENVIRONMENTS

This activity will enable you to assess the development of the lives of two people who are genetically similar but grow up in different environments.

TASK 1

Using the case study provided in OHT 4.3.8 complete the grid below.

Factors	How negative instances may restrict life chances	How positive instances may enhance life chances
Employment opportunities		
Income		
Family cohesion and support between family members		
The quality of housing and the degree of crime and stress locally		
Access to good quality health and care services		
Educational opportunities to learn skills and achieve qualifications		
Exposure to discrimination		
Quality of diet		
The impact of living conditions on health		
The degree of pollution and safety within the environment		

TASK 2

As a group explore the idea of upward or downward spirals of development in relation to the interaction of variables.

TASK 3

Produce a case study about two people with similar genetic inheritances who grow up in different environments and experience different chances in life.

UNIT 5 – HEALTH, SOCIAL CARE AND EARLY YEARS SERVICES

OVERVIEW

This unit is covered in six sections in the textbook. These are numbered for ease of referencing in the file.

5.1 Origins and development of services
5.2 National and local provision of services
5.3 Informal carers
5.4 The funding of services
5.5 The effects of government policies on services
5.6 Access to services

Aims and objectives

The unit covers:

- origins and development of health, social care and early years services
- national and local provision of services
- access to services
- funding of services
- organisation of services
- informal carers.

Students should be able to:

- explain how and why health, social care and early years services have developed and changed over time
- explain how demographic characteristics have influenced the development and delivery of services
- describe the management and function of services at national, regional and local levels in their country of the U.K.
- explain the impact of national strategic policies on local care organisations
- explain how local independent services are organised
- describe how access is gained to health, social care and early years services
- describe how these services may inter-relate
- identify barriers to access for some individuals and how access could be improved
- explain how services are funded
- identify differences in the methods of funding for different organisations
- describe how methods of funding could affect clients
- explain how government policies may affect the structure, development and delivery of health, social care and early years services
- identify how recent legislation, policies, reforms and proposals have affected the structure and funding of services
- describe the ways in which government policy may be influenced by the general public and clients
- describe the importance of support from informal carers
- identify the support needs of informal carers and assessment by statutory services
- explain the importance of the Carers Recognition Act 1995

TEACHING NOTES

5.1 Origins and development of services

This section provides the following:

- An historical background to the development of health and social care and early years services from the 1300s to the 1990s – including an explanation of how services are structured and an introduction to different approaches to health care. (See **OHT 5.1.1.**)
- An explanation of some of the main demographic influences on the provision of care.
- An introduction to the issue of 'inequalities' in the provision of health care.

When studying the historical development of the services, it is important the student understands why changes were introduced and understands the inter-relatedness of economic, political, technological and social attitudes that influenced these changes.

The first **Think it over** on page 348 of the textbook asks students to find out what influenced the deterioration of the industrial relationships between health care workers, the NHS management and the government in the 1970s.

The students' answers may include some of the following:

- Long working hours – especially for junior doctors.
- Poor pay and conditions of services – especially for nurses.

- The introduction of more senior administrators from outside the health service.
- The introduction of more management tiers within the health service – sometimes taking senior practitioners away from their primary caring role into management.
- Increasing changes within the health service.
- Maladministration within the health service.
- Health workers feeling that they were not valued by government.

Students should be encouraged to research newspaper articles from that period.

The second **Think it over** on page 348 encourages the student to think about private health care and how low income affects what health care may be available to people. Students should again be encouraged to look at newspapers and talk to people who have chosen to have private health care. Their answers may include some of the following:

- Swifter access to health care.
- Being able to determine themselves when to have treatment.
- Better accommodation in hospitals.
- More expensive treatment than that available on the NHS, e.g. special expensive drugs.
- More intensive treatment than is available on the NHS, e.g. intensive physiotherapy.
- Access to rehabilitation facilities, e.g. a recuperation period in a nursing home following an operation, or 24-hour nursing support.

On page 351 the **Think it over** requires the student to think about the role of women in our society. They should consider the way that women may contribute to the financial stability of the family; increased career opportunities; equal pay issues; how the use of contraception and the increased earning power of women has provided opportunities for variations in child caring patterns.

The **Think it over** on page 353 is used as an example of how lifestyles affect health. Students need to understand how lifestyles affect health, which in turn affects what health care services are required; how this affects the cost associated with health care and thus why governments need to introduce changes in the structure of health care services and campaigns aimed at developing healthier lifestyles. However, the student also needs to understand that health care provision is not the same all over the UK – and why this is. They should be aware that health care needs are different in different areas, and that the availability and the effectiveness of health care can vary from area to area. (See **OHTs** 5.1.2 and 5.1.4.)

Activity 5.1.1 provides students with a case study and questions for them to explore the services required to support Mrs Williamson. (See **OHT** 5.1.3.)

Students should also consider why health care in children is very important and that poor health care can result in long-term and social care needs.

Activity 5.1.2 is a case study, providing students with the opportunity to consider what could be done to improve a child's health.

The **Think it over** on page 356 introduces the notion that choices need to be made when accessing some treatments that could involve a risk associated with them. It may be useful to debate this with a group of students.

5.2 National and local provision of services

This section provides the following:

- An explanation of the structure of health and social care services and how this differs in England, Wales, Scotland and Northern Ireland. (See **OHTs** 5.2.1 and 5.2.2.)
- An explanation of how the NHS is structured at central government, regional and local levels. (See **OHTs** 5.2.3 and 5.2.4.)
- An explanation of how early years services are structured. (See **OHTs** 5.2.5 and 5.2.6.)
- An introduction to the role of independent organisations in the provision of health and social care.

Students should understand that health and social care are provided as a result of national strategies. It may be helpful for students to do some research into the different government departments and what they are responsible for. They can do this by additional reading or by accessing government department web sites.

In the past few years the structure of health and social care services have undergone many changes and these changes are continuing to occur, especially in relation to the way services are provided (See **OHTs 5.2.7** and **5.2.8**.). It is therefore essential that they understand the importance of the introduction of NHS Hospital Trusts, in respect of secondary services, and Primary Care Groups – and subsequently Primary Care Trusts – in respect of primary (or community) services (see pages 365 and 370 of the textbook). Students should be encouraged to find out about the Hospital Trusts and Primary Care Groups/Trusts in their own area. They may do this by looking at articles in local newspapers or by contacting the local health authority for information.

It is also important that students understand the changing role of the social services department from being a provider of care to an assessor of need and commissioner of care services. The **Think it over** on page 367 will begin to help them understand the extent of the assessing role that social services undertake. Each social services department publishes a community care plan detailing the services that they are responsible for and how these can be accessed. Students may obtain these from their local social services department. The **Try it out** on page 369 and the one on page 368 will help them understand the effects of these changes.

Early years services are delivered under three broad areas: health services, educational services and social services (see page 369). Students should understand what provisions are made under each of these services. Figures 5.18 and 5.19 on page 370 of the textbook and the OHT 5.2.5 in this file explain about these provisions for child health care.

Educational provision is detailed on pages 372–374. Students need to understand that although the overall provision of education is determined at a central government level, the way that it is provided at a local level can vary considerably.

Figure 5.23 on page 374 and **OHT 5.2.9** in this file shows how the provision of social care is structured at central government, regional and local levels.

Students should be aware that apart from nurseries, childminders and foster care, etc., care for children is also provided, indirectly, through the housing department and through the benefits system (see page 375).

The **Think it over** on page 376 asks students to think about the effects of poor communication between agencies who provide child care. Their answers may include:

- Children being abused – physical, emotional, sexual or financially.
- The death of a child.
- Children not receiving appropriate or timely health care treatment.
- Children not receiving education appropriate to their needs or ability.
- Children living in poverty and/or poor housing.

5.3 Informal carers

Students should have an understanding of the extent to which the needs of sick, disabled and elderly people are met by informal carers and that there are many 'young carers' as well as adult carers. They should also be aware of carers' needs that enable them to continue in the role of carer and how these needs will differ from person to person, depending on a whole range of variables, which will include the following:

- The particular needs of the person they are caring for.
- The age of the person they are caring for.
- Their own age.
- Their own physical and emotional abilities to care.
- Their cultural and religious background.
- Other personal commitments.
- Their financial situation.
- Where they live.

See pages 379 and 380 in the textbook.

Activity 5.3.1 explores the needs of informal carers through a case study and questions.

The **Think it over** on page 378 will encourage students to think about the role of women in society. Their answers may include the following:

- Females are often socialised into the caring role from childhood and therefore the caring role is often seen as being best carried out by women.

- Caring jobs have often been low paid.
- Jobs in the caring services are often part-time and give more flexibility for juggling other commitments.
- Caring jobs often have a low status.

In the past few years the contribution of young people in a caring role has become more acknowledged and their special needs are now being taken into account and considered more fully. The case study on page 382 of the textbook will begin to help students to consider the needs of young carers. **Activity 5.3.2**, which is a role-play, will help to extend their understanding of what it may feel like to be a young carer.

Information in this section will give students an understanding of the initiatives that the government has introduced in recognition of the vital role that individual informal carers play and of the support mechanisms that they have put in place to assist carers (see pages 381–384).

The final part of this section looks at the role of voluntary organisations, helplines and self-help groups, and the caring roles that they have and how they support informal carers. Answers to the **Think it over** box on page 385 may include:

General organisations

- Child Poverty Action Group
- Citizens Advice Bureaux National Association
- Disability Information Trust
- Family Rights Group
- Jewish Care
- Salvation Army
- Social Care Association
- SSAFA Forces Help

Specific organisations

- British Heart Foundation
- Cystic Fibrosis Trust
- Headway
- National AIDS Helpline
- National Council for One Parent Families
- Patient's Association
- Sickle Cell Society
- The Stroke Association

5.4 The funding of services

The funding of health and social care provision is very complex. Students need to understand where the money for these services is obtained from and then how it is allocated to the statutory health and social care services (see pages 386–389 in the textbook).

The funding of early years services is also complex, but Figure 5.25 on page 388 of the textbook (**OHT 5.4.1** in this file) gives an outline of these services, and Table 5.12 on page 389 shows the amount of government spending on education during the period 1988–1997.

Activity 5.4.1 involves finding out about some of the organisations involved in early years provision of services.

Students should be aware of the increasing demand on services; the higher expectations of people regarding the availability and quality of services; the increasing costs and therefore the importance of the use of voluntary and private service providers.

OHT 5.4.2 shows where voluntary organisations get their funds from.

Government initiatives encourage people to take an increasing personal responsibility for making provision so that in future they will be able to contribute towards the cost of their own care. The government is also keen to ensure that whatever monies they spend on services, they will get value for money and there will be a good quality of care.

A complex system of contracts and grant-giving has developed between the government and health and social care providers (see pages 390–392).

A new system of 'Direct Payments' is briefly described on page 392 of the textbook. The use of Direct Payment (or Voucher) Schemes is likely to increase and students should therefore be aware of this.

The final part of this section deals with welfare benefits and **OHT 5.4.3** has further information about some of the most widely available benefits and some brief case studies are provided in **Activity 5.4.2** which will help students to understand the criteria for claiming these. However, they should also understand that benefits are constantly changing, and how one benefit may affect the ability to claim another is a very specialised area of work. There are now a number of benefits officers and welfare rights agencies that provided advice and assistance in claiming benefits.

5.5 The effects of government policies on services

Services need to change and adapt according to the policies introduced by government. In the past twenty-five years the number of changes and the speed at which these have been introduced has become increasingly rapid (see Figures 5.29 and 5.30 on page 397 of the textbook). Students need to be aware of the legal framework within which services are developed and provided.

In order to understand the variations that occur they must understand the difference between mandatory legislation and permissive legislation, and the difference between the duties and powers that legislation creates (see pages 394–395). Legislation covers all areas of health and social care, from the protection of children, the provision of services for disabled people and older people, to the payment of benefits, the protection of people at work and the detention of people with a mental illness or those who have committed a criminal act. Three major pieces of legislation are described in this section:

- The Mental Health Act 1983 (see page 398).
- The Children Act 1989 (see page 399).
- The NHS and Community Care Act 1990 (see page 401).

All three Acts have resulted in major changes to the way that services are structured and provided.

In addition to legislation, the government issues guidelines and introduces 'strategies' regarding health and social care. Some of these are described on pages 395 and 396. One of the main initiatives at this time are the Health Improvement Targets, which were developed in response to the government's *Health of the Nation* strategy (see page 396 and **OHTs** 5.5.1 and 5.5.2). **Activity** 5.5.1 will assist students to think about how lifestyles can affect health and how changing to healthier lifestyles can help meet health improvement targets.

Government often commissions special reports before making changes, but there are also many ways in which the public may affect government policies. These include the opinion of voters, the views of pressure groups, the strength of lobbying groups and political campaigners. How these work are described on pages 402 and 403. In addition, **OHT** 5.5.3 provides some further information about how pressure groups can influence government policies.

The final part of this section describes the role of Community Health Councils in representing the interests of the public in health matters (see page 403).

5.6 Access to services

The final section deals with the issue of accessing services and the different ways that this can be done. Different services are accessed in different ways, however whichever way they are accessed, people first need to know what services exist. They may find out about the services themselves or they may be informed by someone else, who may be a professional or non-professional person (see pages 404 and 405). Having clear and accurate information regarding services and how they can be accessed is very important. **Activity** 5.6.1 will help students to think about how information is presented.

There are many reasons why someone may not be able to access services. These 'barriers' are briefly described on pages 405 and 406. **Activity** 5.6.2 will help the student think more about these barriers.

ASSESSMENT SUMMARY

Pass grade

To obtain a **pass** in this unit the student must prepare a **case study** which shows an investigation into one local health, social care or early years organisation. Examples of these might include a health clinic, a residential home for older people or a day nursery. The organisation may be set in the statutory, private or voluntary sector. The investigation may be based on a real or fictitious care setting.

The investigation must include the following:

- The functions and purpose of the organisation.

- Information about how the local organisation provides services – with reference to the function and purposes of the national framework, local demographic characteristics and government policies.
- How individuals gain access to the services of the organisation, and barriers they may encounter.
- Ways in which one national and/or local organisation is funded.
- Recent changes in legislation that have affected the organisation.

E grade

In order to obtain an **E grade** the student must show that they can:

- Explain clearly the functions and purpose of the organisation that they have chosen.
- Explain clearly how clients gain access to the service and identify any barriers which they may face in accessing the chosen service.
- Explain accurately and clearly how the service is organised and funded at national, regional and local level.
- Describe in detail the effects of any recent government reforms on the chosen organisation.

C grade

In order to obtain a **C grade** the student must, in addition to the above, show that they can:

- Analyse the impact of government policies on the way the organisation functions and is funded.
- Describe how the chosen organisation co-ordinates or interacts with at least one other service.
- Make realistic suggestions about how access to the service can be improved.
- Analyse the ways in which an aspect of the service has developed over a long period of time, as government policies have changed and new legislation has been introduced.

A grade

In order to obtain an **A grade** the student must complete both parts above and show that they can:

- Analyse ways in which the public or clients have influenced the practices of the organisation.
- Evaluate the ways in which the organisation monitors changes in government policy and may alter the service it provides accordingly.
- Analyse how the work of the organisation relates to the work of other organisations at either local, regional, or national level, and how inter-agency co-ordination is managed.

OHTS

The OHTs to help tutors deliver this unit are as follows:

5.1.1	Types of health care approach
5.1.2	Purchasers and providers in the NHS (1990s)
5.1.3	Mixed economy of care
5.1.4	Factors influencing population size (demographic changes)
5.2.1	The structure of health and social care in England and Wales
5.2.2	The structure of health and social care in Scotland and N. Ireland
5.2.3	Structure of the NHS (England) – late 1990s
5.2.4	Structure of social services
5.2.5	Child health care
5.2.6	Child health care services
5.2.7	The future structure of health and social care
5.2.8	Understanding new terminology in health and social care services
5.2.9	Provision of social services for children
5.4.1	Services for early years
5.4.2	Financing voluntary organisations
5.4.3	Welfare benefits
5.5.1	Health improvement programme targets
5.5.2	Healthier lifestyles
5.5.3	Child poverty, pressure groups and the government

ACTIVITIES

The activities are designed to promote learning and understanding, provide consolidation and develop logical thinking and a rational approach to studies.

5.1.1 Mixed economy of care
5.1.2 Improving child health care
5.3.1 The needs of informal carers
5.3.2 The needs of young carers
5.4.1 Services involved in early years provision
5.4.2 Welfare benefits
5.5.1 A healthier lifestyle
5.6.1 Accessing services
5.6.2 Case study: accessing services

OHT 5.1.1 TYPES OF HEALTH CARE APPROACH

Emergent	■ Health care viewed as item of personal consumption ■ Physician operates as solo entrepreneur ■ Professional associations powerful ■ Private ownership of facilities ■ Direct payments to physicians ■ Minimal role in health care from the state
Pluralistic	■ Health care viewed mainly as a consumer good ■ Physician operates as solo entrepreneur and in organised groups ■ Professional organisations very powerful ■ Private and public ownership of facilities ■ Payments for services direct and indirect ■ State's role in health care minimal and indirect
Insurance/social security	■ Health care as an insured/guaranteed consumer good or service ■ Physicians operate as solo entrepreneurs and as members of medical organisations ■ Professional organisations strong ■ Private and public ownership of facilities ■ Payment for services mostly indirect ■ State's role in health care central but indirect

OHT 5.1.1 (continued)

National Health Service	■ Health care as a state-supported service ■ Physicians operate as solo entrepreneurs and as members of medical organisations ■ Professional organisations fairly strong ■ Facilities mainly publicly owned ■ Payment for services indirect ■ State's role in health care central and direct
Socialised	■ Health care a state-provided public service ■ Physicians are state-employed ■ Professional organisations weak or non-existent ■ Facilities wholly publicly owned ■ Payments for services entirely indirect ■ State's role in health care is total

Source: Field (1989)

OHT 5.1.2 PURCHASERS AND PROVIDERS IN THE NHS

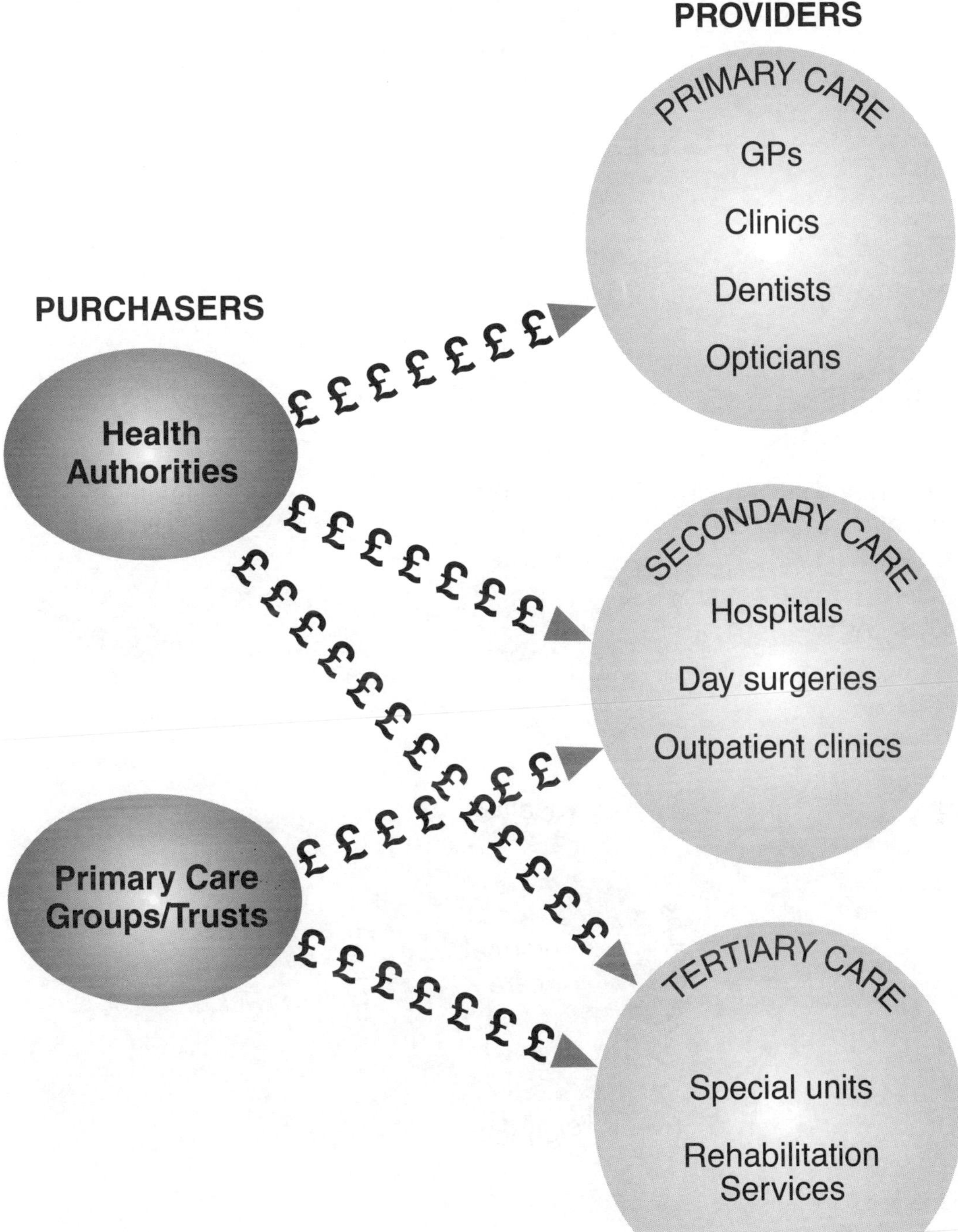

PROVIDERS
PRIMARY CARE
GPs
Clinics
Dentists
Opticians
PURCHASERS
Health Authorities
SECONDARY CARE
Hospitals
Day surgeries
Outpatient clinics
Primary Care Groups/Trusts
TERTIARY CARE
Special units
Rehabilitation Services

OHT 5.1.3 MIXED ECONOMY OF CARE

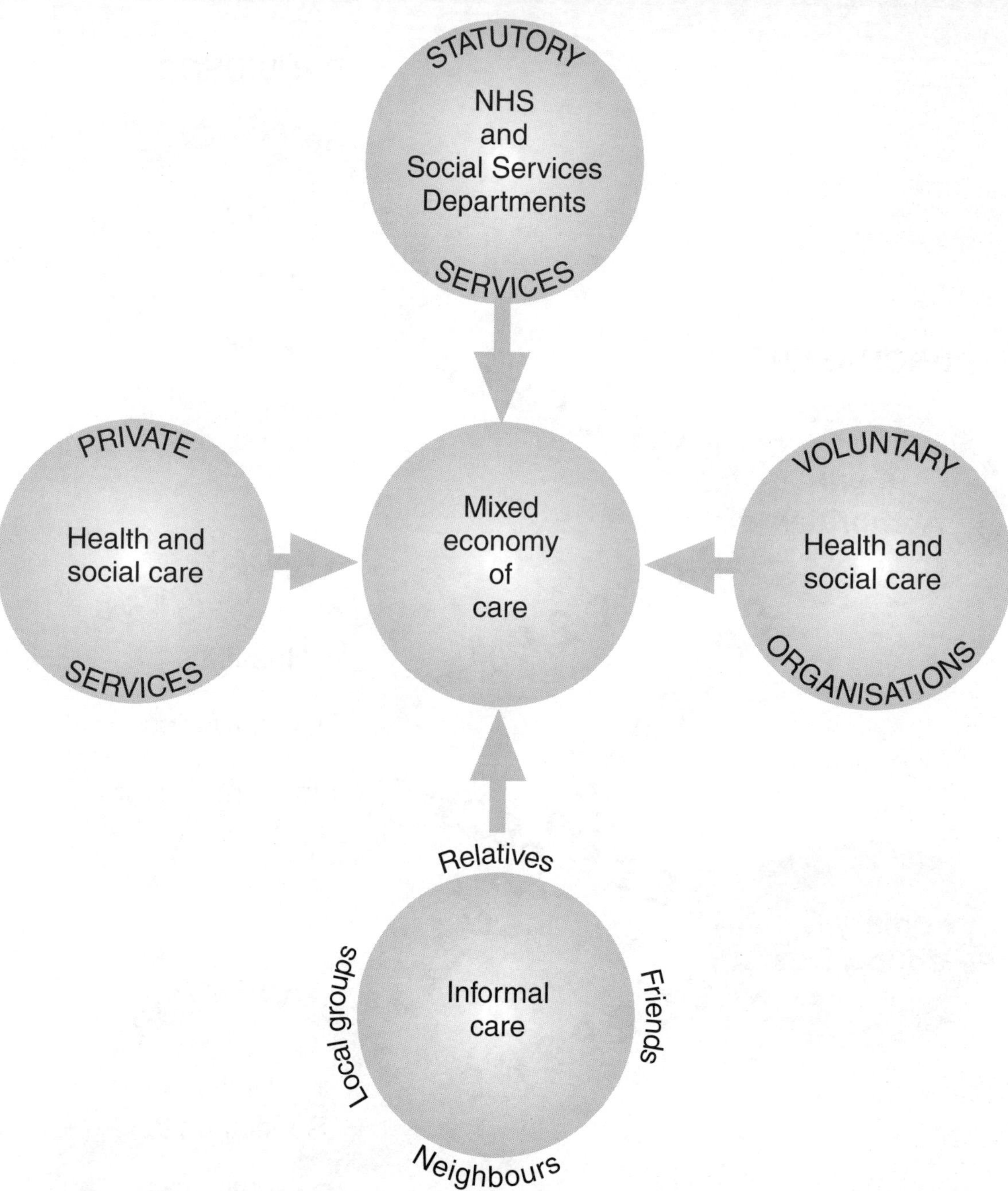

STATUTORY
NHS and Social Services Departments
SERVICES
PRIVATE
Health and social care
SERVICES
Mixed economy of care
VOLUNTARY
Health and social care
ORGANISATIONS
Relatives
Local groups
Informal care
Friends
Neighbours

OHT 5.1.4 FACTORS INFLUENCING POPULATION SIZE (DEMOGRAPHIC CHANGES)

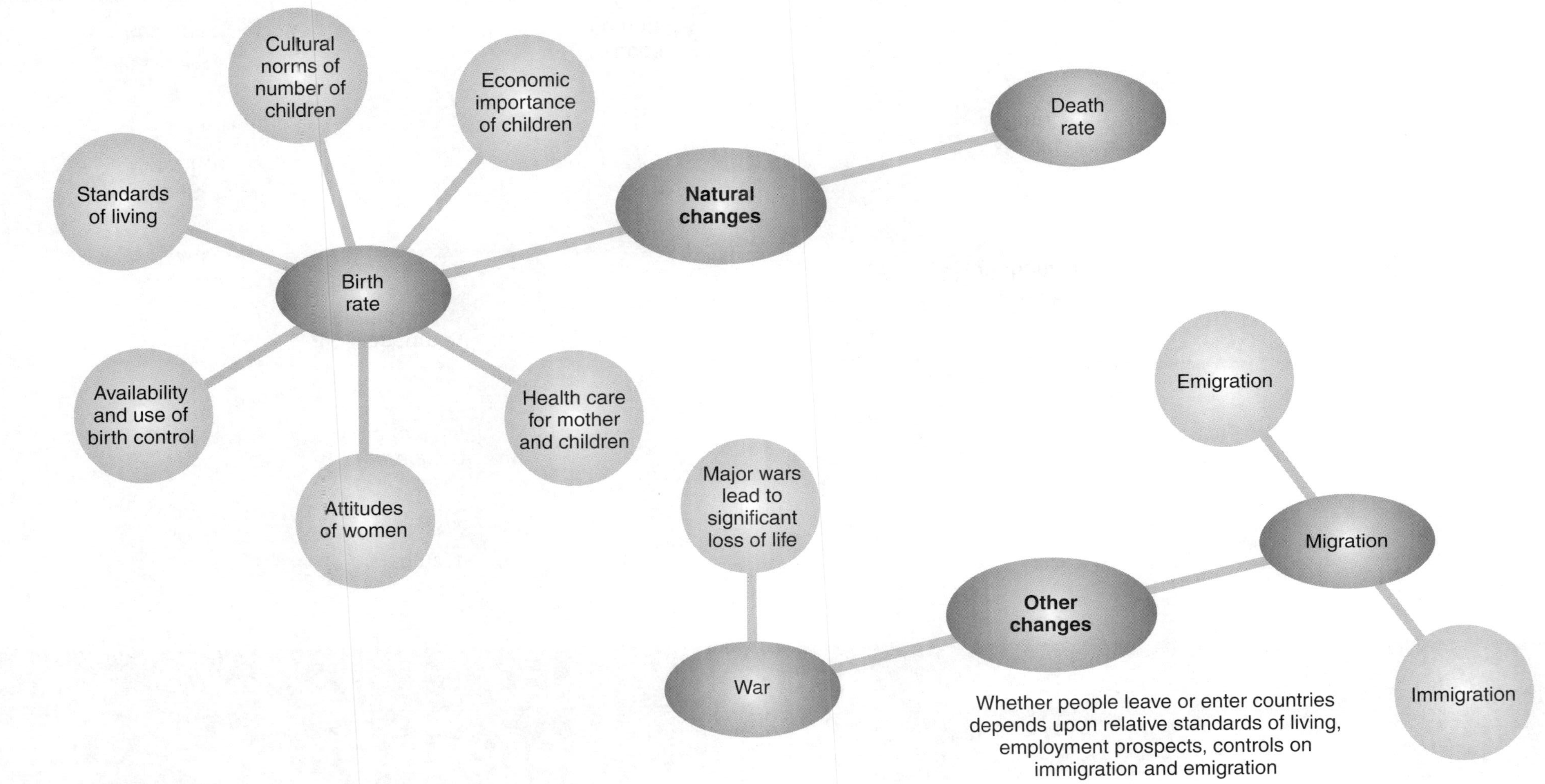
Cultural norms of number of children
Economic importance of children
Standards of living
Birth rate
Natural changes
Death rate
Availability and use of birth control
Attitudes of women
Health care for mother and children
Major wars lead to significant loss of life
War
Other changes
Migration
Emigration
Immigration
Whether people leave or enter countries depends upon relative standards of living, employment prospects, controls on immigration and emigration

OHT 5.2.1 THE STRUCTURE OF HEALTH AND SOCIAL CARE IN ENGLAND AND WALES

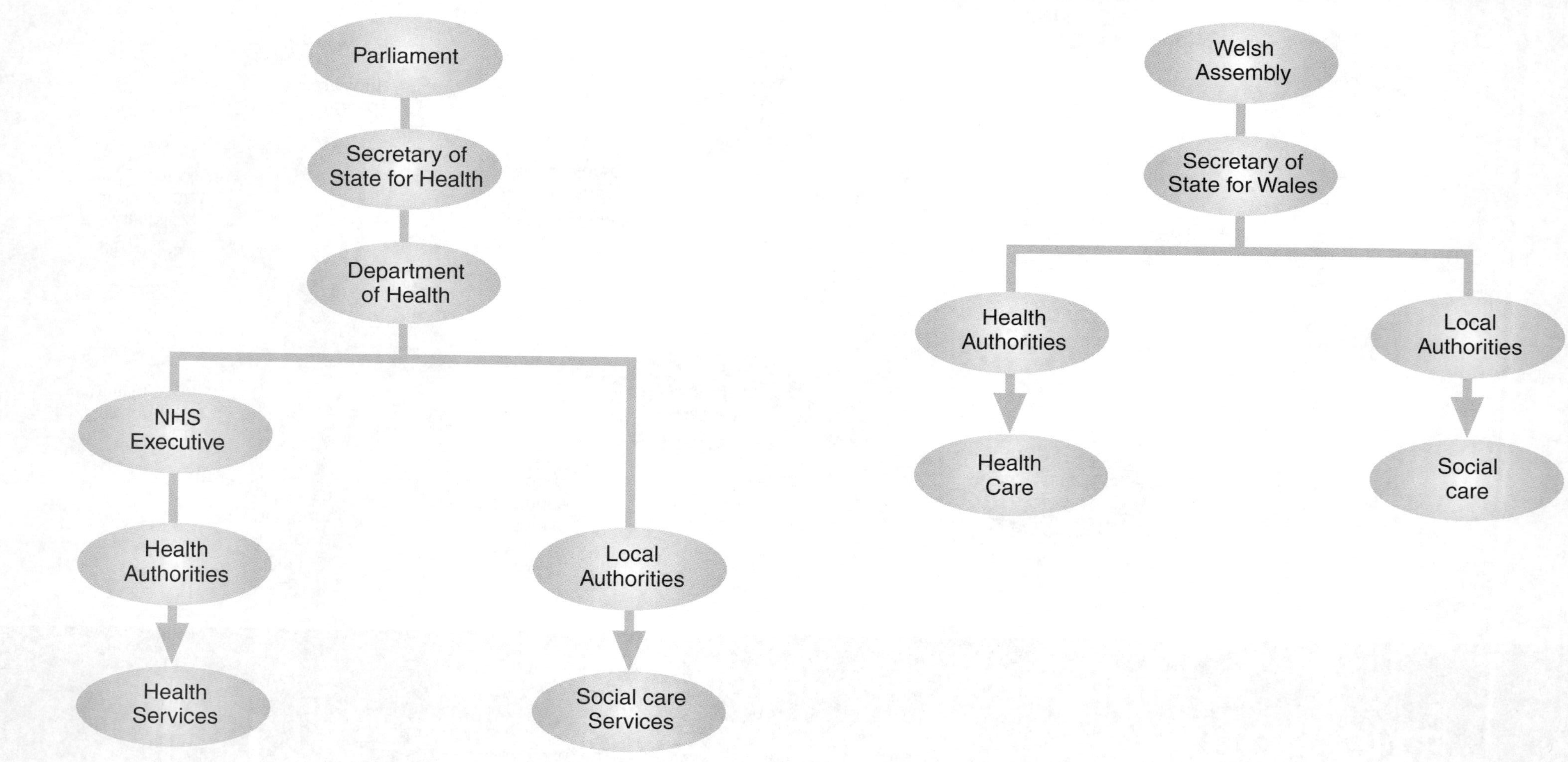
Parliament
Secretary of State for Health
Department of Health
NHS Executive
Health Authorities
Health Services
Local Authorities
Social care Services
Welsh Assembly
Secretary of State for Wales
Health Authorities
Health Care
Local Authorities
Social care

OHT 5.2.2 THE STRUCTURE OF HEALTH AND SOCIAL CARE IN SCOTLAND AND N. IRELAND

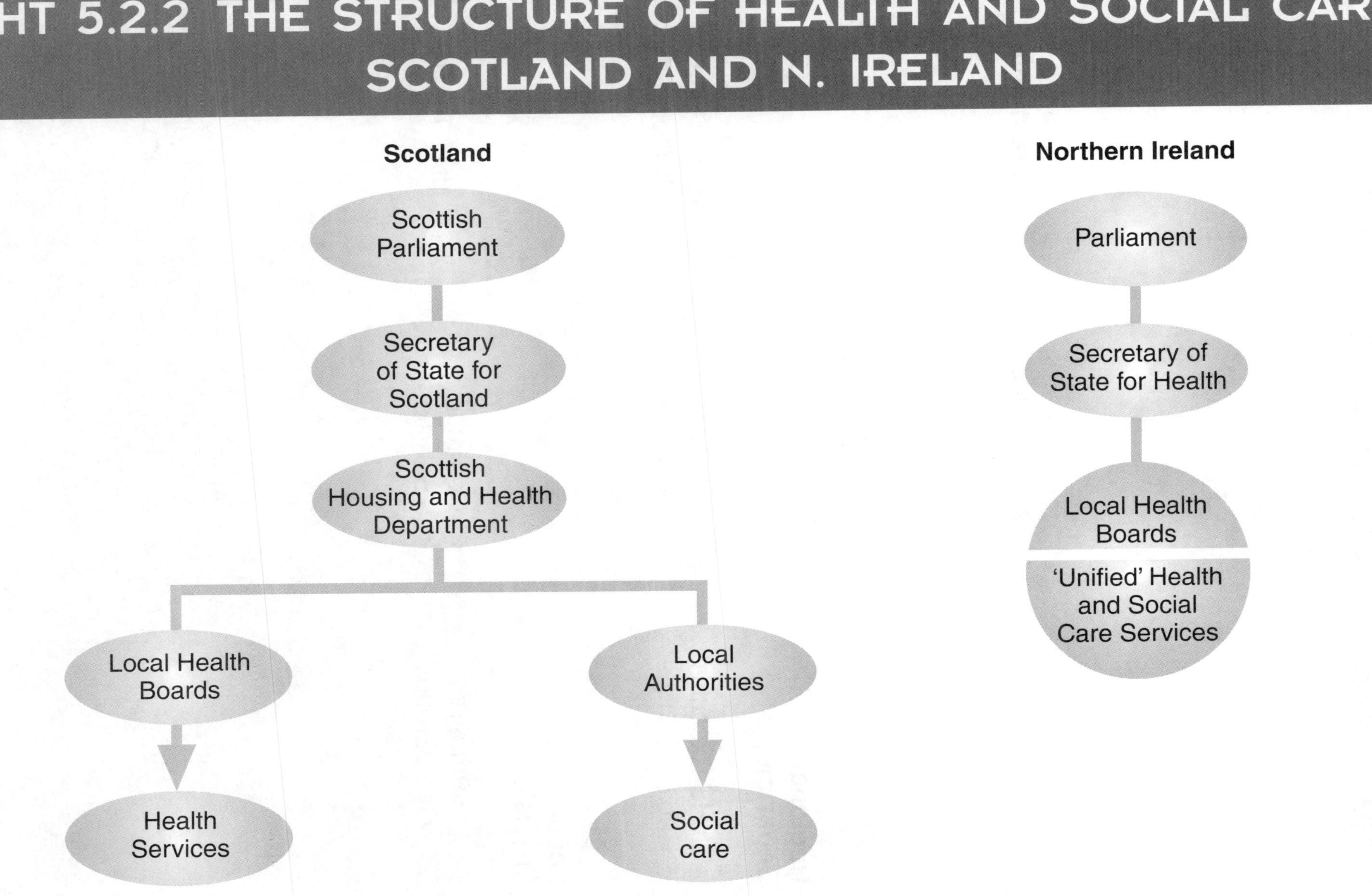

Scotland
Scottish Parliament
Secretary of State for Scotland
Scottish Housing and Health Department
Local Health Boards
Health Services
Local Authorities
Social care
Northern Ireland
Parliament
Secretary of State for Health
Local Health Boards
'Unified' Health and Social Care Services

OHT 5.2.3 STRUCTURE OF THE NHS (ENGLAND) LATE 1990s

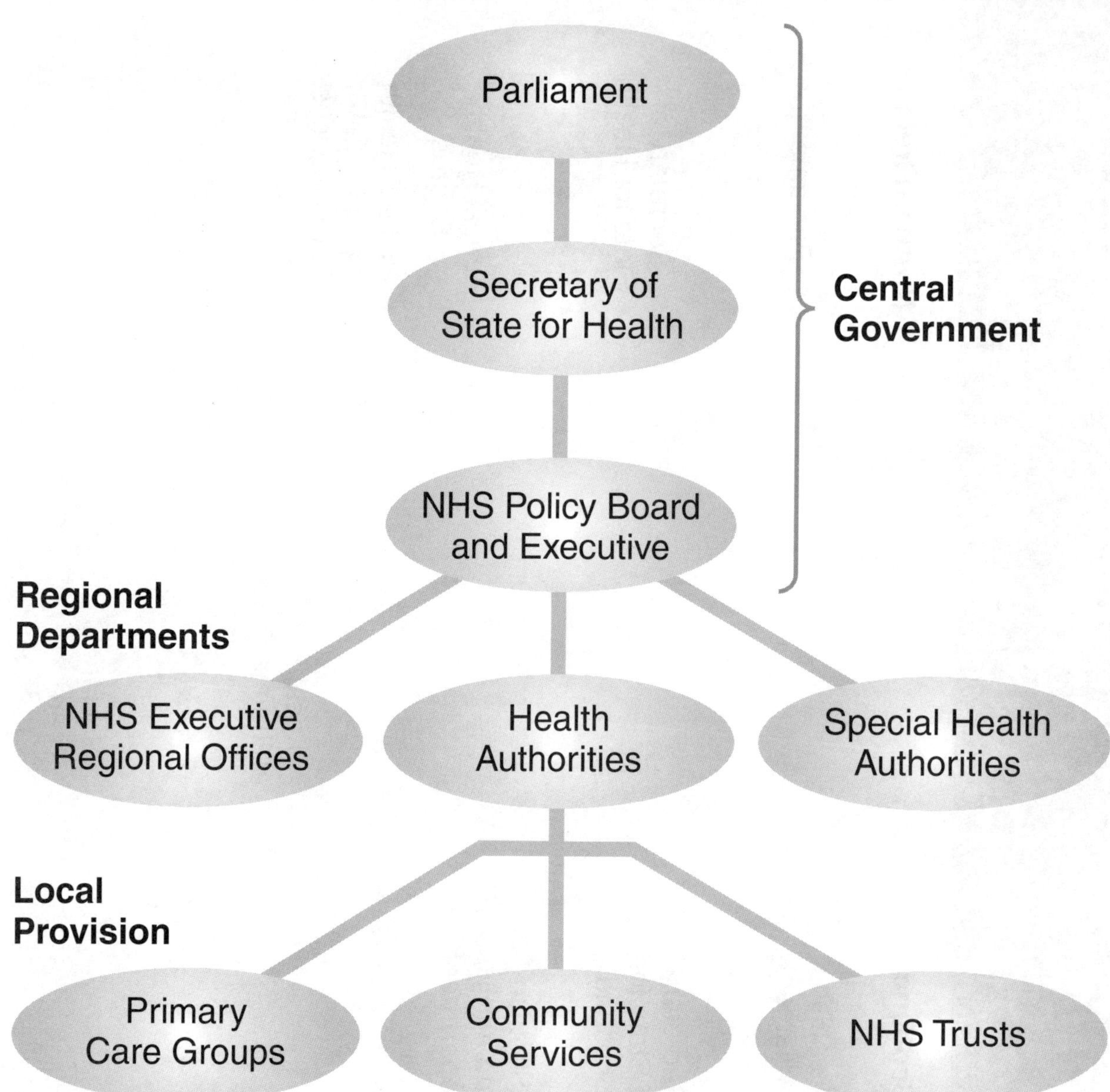
Parliament
Secretary of State for Health
NHS Policy Board and Executive
Central Government
Regional Departments
NHS Executive Regional Offices
Health Authorities
Special Health Authorities
Local Provision
Primary Care Groups
Community Services
NHS Trusts

OHT 5.2.4 STRUCTURE OF SOCIAL SERVICES

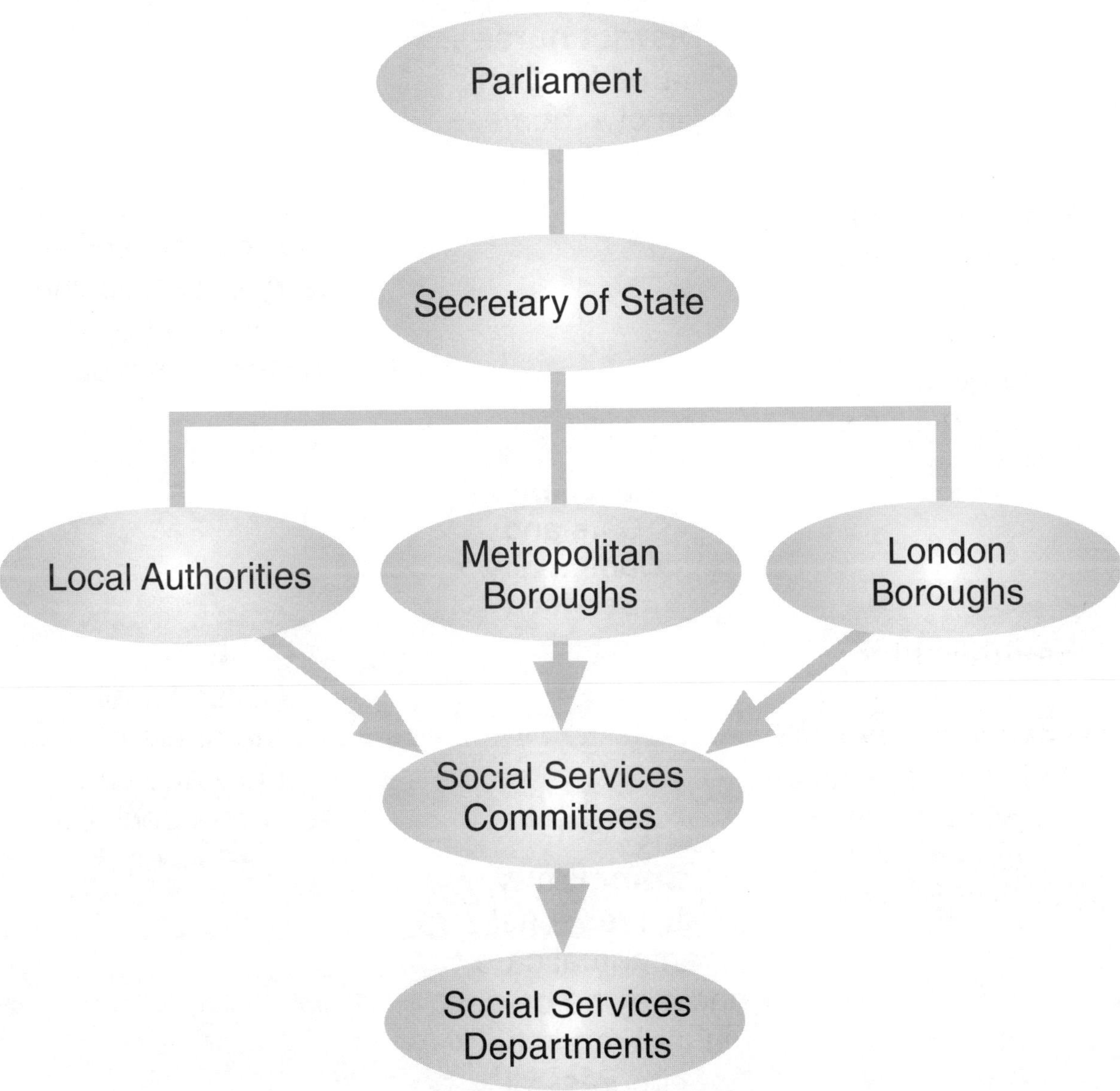
Parliament
Secretary of State
Local Authorities
Metropolitan Boroughs
London Boroughs
Social Services Committees
Social Services Departments

OHT 5.2.5 CHILD HEALTH CARE

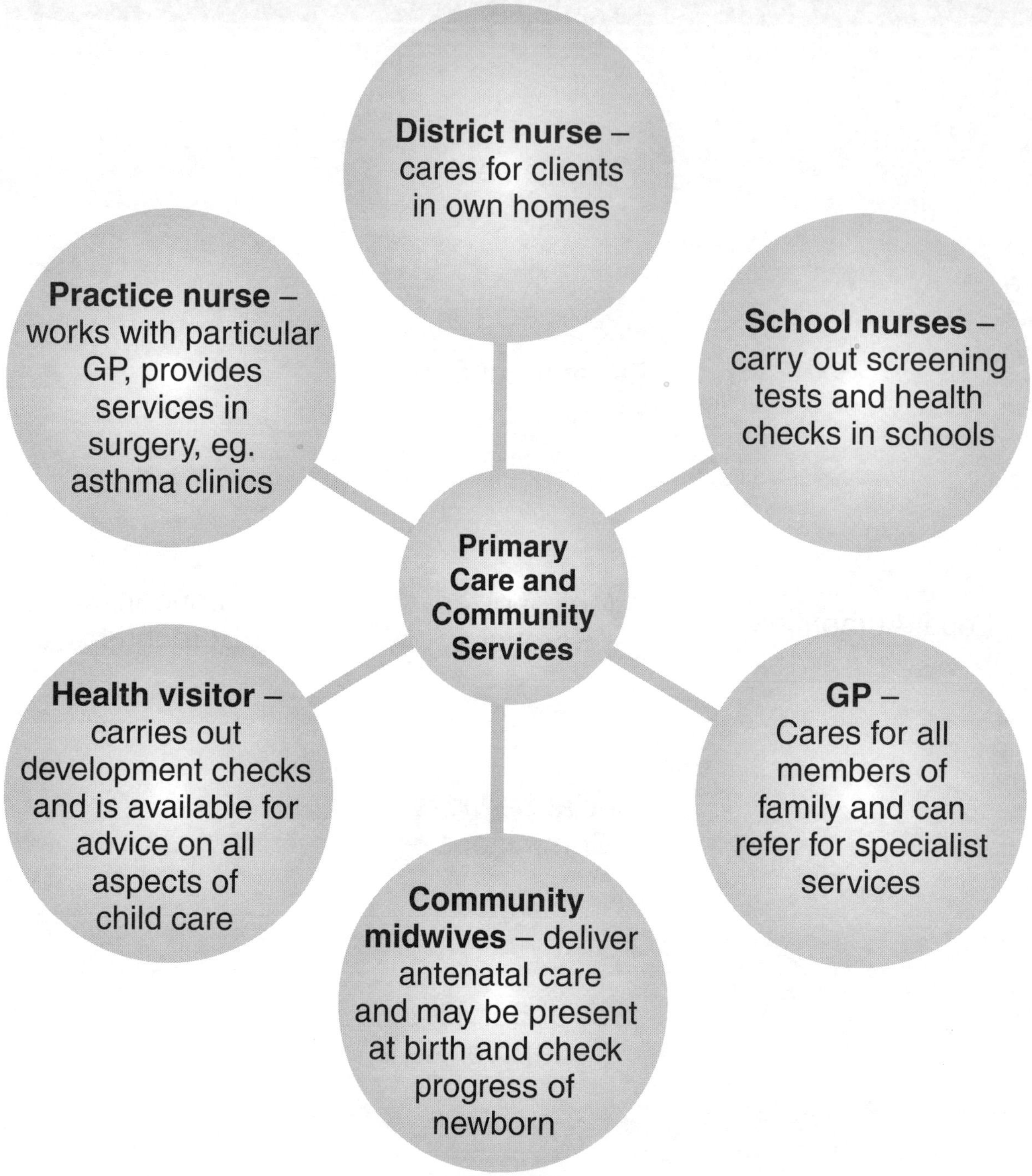

Primary Care and Community Services

District nurse – cares for clients in own homes

School nurses – carry out screening tests and health checks in schools

GP – Cares for all members of family and can refer for specialist services

Community midwives – deliver antenatal care and may be present at birth and check progress of newborn

Health visitor – carries out development checks and is available for advice on all aspects of child care

Practice nurse – works with particular GP, provides services in surgery, eg. asthma clinics

OHT 5.2.5 (continued)

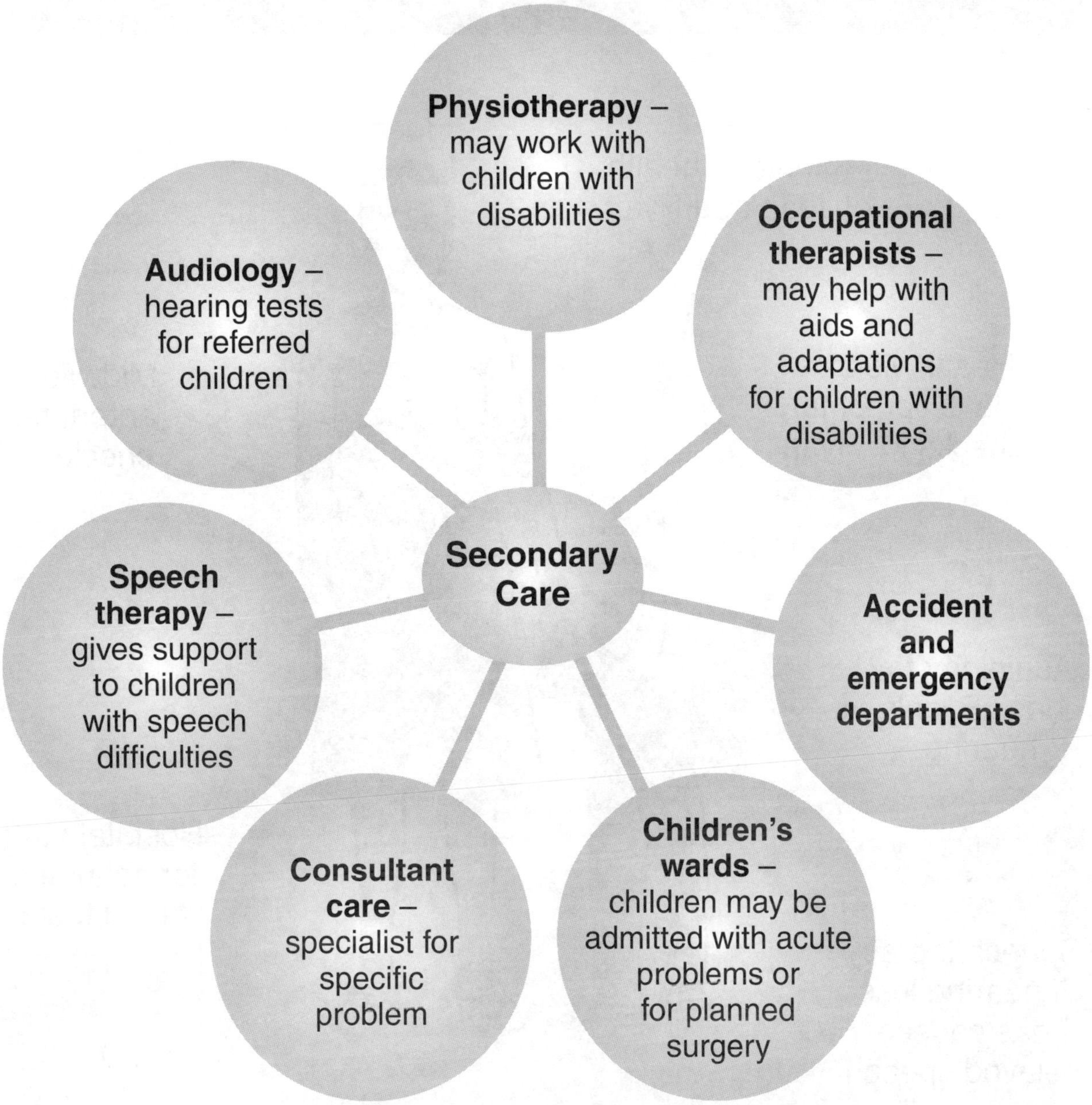

Secondary Care

Physiotherapy – may work with children with disabilities

Occupational therapists – may help with aids and adaptations for children with disabilities

Accident and emergency departments

Children's wards – children may be admitted with acute problems or for planned surgery

Consultant care – specialist for specific problem

Speech therapy – gives support to children with speech difficulties

Audiology – hearing tests for referred children

OHT 5.2.6 CHILD HEALTH CARE SERVICES

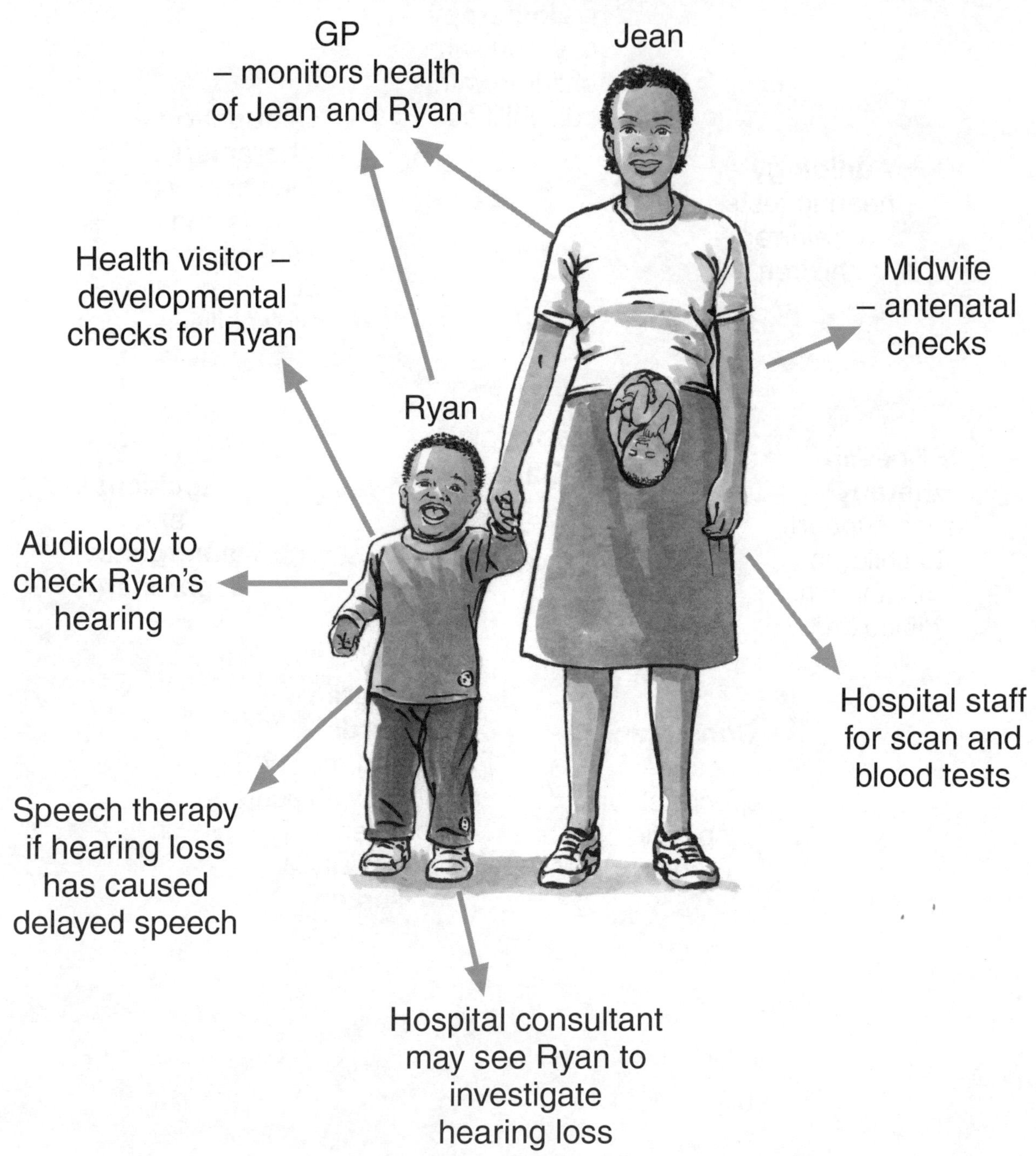
GP
– monitors health
of Jean and Ryan
Jean
Health visitor –
developmental
checks for Ryan
Midwife
– antenatal
checks
Ryan
Audiology to
check Ryan's
hearing
Hospital staff
for scan and
blood tests
Speech therapy
if hearing loss
has caused
delayed speech
Hospital consultant
may see Ryan to
investigate
hearing loss

OHT 5.2.7 THE FUTURE STRUCTURE OF HEALTH AND SOCIAL CARE

The government's new NHS Plan, published in 1999, proposes closer working relationships between the health and social care agencies. It is aimed at breaking down the barriers between health and social care.

Key points in the NHS Plan

- All social services to enter into a pooled budget arrangement with their local health authority.
- Where both agencies agree, new care trusts to be set up, bringing health and social services into one organisation.
- Where inspection indicates that agencies are not working effectively in partnerships, the government will require local health and social services to join together in a new care trust.

Services for older people

- By 2003/04 rapid response teams will be introduced to prevent unnecessary hospital admissions, and private nursing and residential homes will be used for rehabilitation to allow earlier discharge from hospital.
- Nursing care in residential and nursing homes to be funded by the NHS.
- In 2001 a new power will be introduced for government to give guidance on charges for home care services.

The Plan also aims to tackle health inequalities through the following

- Developing a set of national targets for reducing inequalities in health, including infant mortality rates.
- Developing new partnerships between health and local services to tackle the determinants of ill-health and inequality.
- By 2002 single integrated public health groups to be established across NHS regional offices and government offices for the regions.

OHT 5.2.8 UNDERSTANDING NEW TERMINOLOGY IN HEALTH AND SOCIAL CARE SERVICES

The NHS Plan could lead to major changes in the provision of health and social care, particularly for older people. Proposals have given rise to formalisation of many new ideas regarding services and this has resulted in lots of new terms being used. Here some of the main terms are explained:

Intermediate care

These are services which promote independence by:

- reducing avoidable admissions to acute beds
- facilitating timely discharge from acute beds
- promoting effective rehabilitation and minimising premature or avoidable dependence on long-term care in institutional settings

Some of the services include those listed below.

Community rehabilitation team

Specialist, multi-disciplinary teams that assess the needs of people at home, or who have just returned home from hospital, and organise packages of services to meet rehabilitation needs.

Rapid response team

These teams react to an event that could precipitate accident and emergency (A & E) attendance and aim to prevent acute hospital admission by providing assessment, diagnosis and immediate treatment in the patient's usual place of residence.

OHT 5.2.8 (continued)

Hospital-at-home

Provides active treatment by health care professionals at home for a condition that would otherwise require inpatient hospital admission.

Supported discharge

Medically stable patients able to finish recovering at home are discharged early with intensive support, such as continuing nursing care and therapy as well as personal care. Could be provided by a dedicated outreach team from a local rehabilitation unit.

Home-from-hospital scheme

Low-level, time-limited support for transition from hospital to home, designed to build patient and carer confidence. Current schemes are often provided by voluntary organisations and often don't include medical input.

Inpatient rehabilitation and recovery beds

Designed to help people who have been in acute care to make a rapid transition home.

Residential and day rehabilitation units

Intensive rehabilitation therapy for up to six weeks. Could take place in local authority or private residential homes or day centres.

OHT 5.2.9 PROVISION OF SOCIAL SERVICES FOR CHILDREN

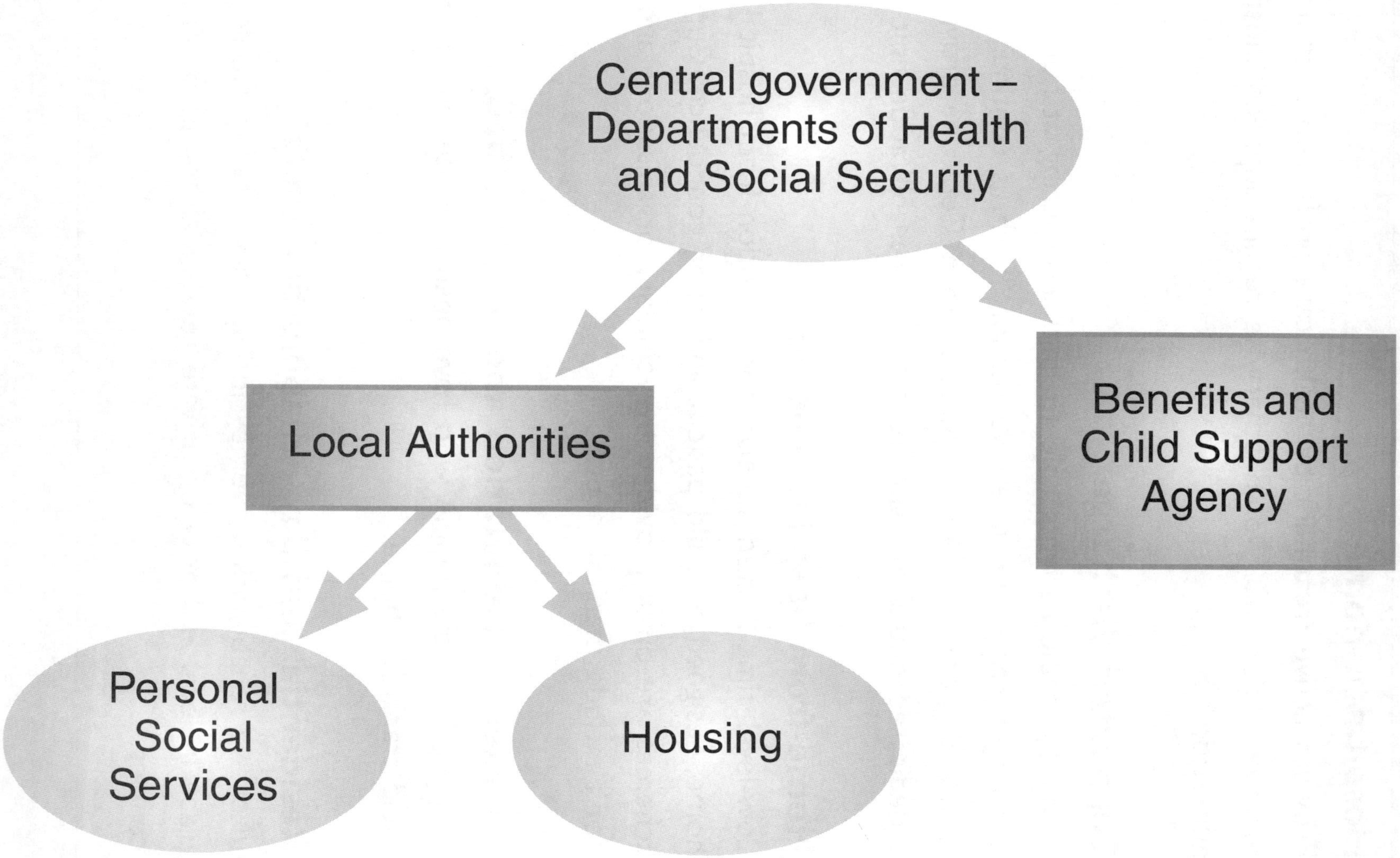

Central government – Departments of Health and Social Security

Local Authorities

Benefits and Child Support Agency

Personal Social Services

Housing

OHT 5.4.1 SERVICES FOR EARLY YEARS

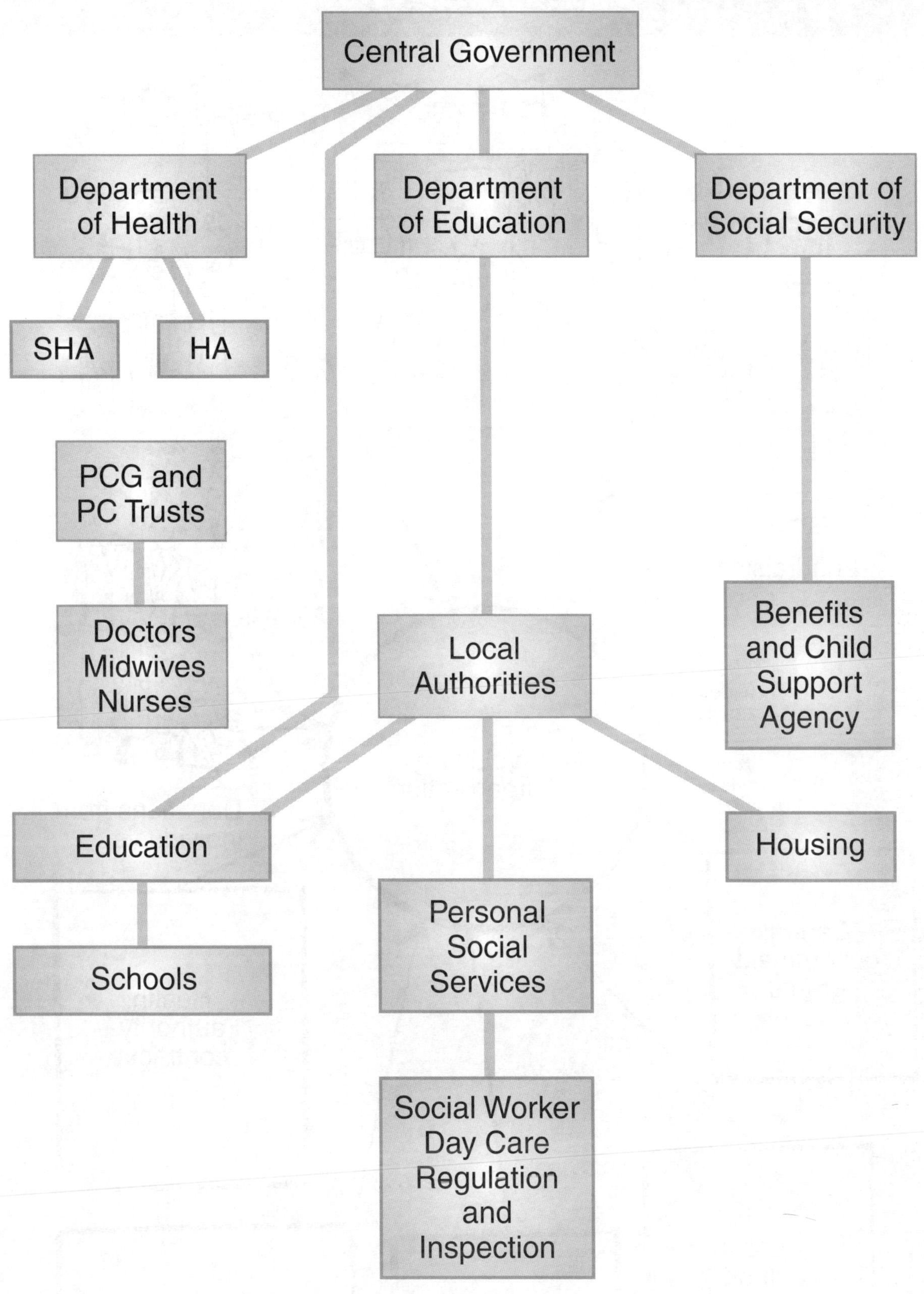
Central Government
Department of Health
Department of Education
Department of Social Security
SHA
HA
PCG and PC Trusts
Doctors Midwives Nurses
Local Authorities
Benefits and Child Support Agency
Education
Housing
Schools
Personal Social Services
Social Worker Day Care Regulation and Inspection

OHT 5.4.2 FINANCING VOLUNTARY ORGANISATIONS

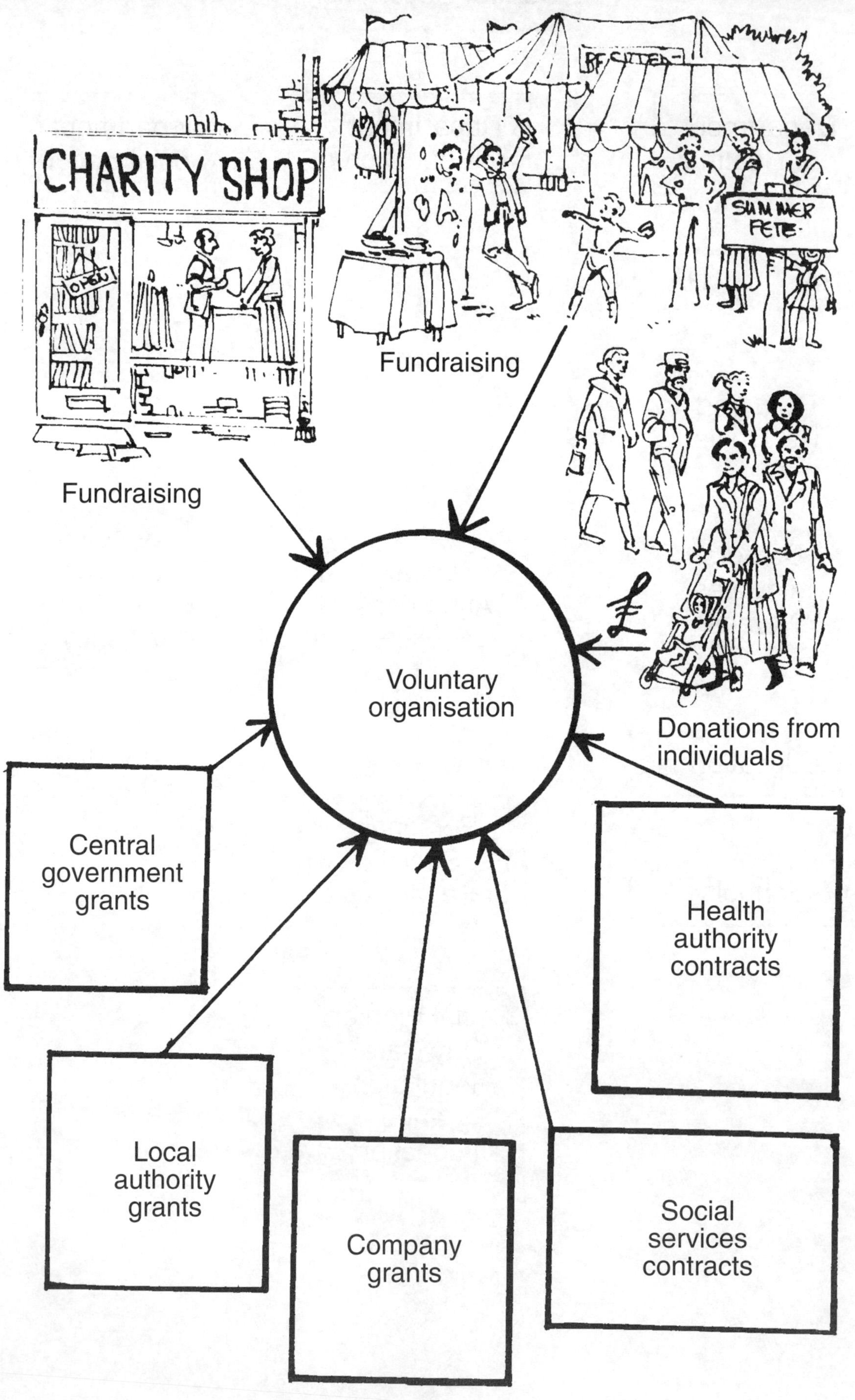
CHARITY SHOP
OPEN
SUMMER FETE
Fundraising
Fundraising
Voluntary organisation
Donations from individuals
Central government grants
Health authority contracts
Local authority grants
Company grants
Social services contracts

OHT 5.4.3 WELFARE BENEFITS

Here is more detailed information regarding some of the financial benefits that are available to people. This information can be used to do Activity 5.4.2.

Income Support

This is a 'safety-net' benefit for people who are exempt from work, or who are unable to sign on for work for health reasons, or are only able to work up to 16 hours a week. Individuals must have savings of no more than £8000. Premiums are added for families with children, pensioners, people with disabilities and carers.

Jobseekers Allowance

This is payable instead of Income Support for those people who are required to sign on for work. It is available as either contribution-based or income-based. Claimants must sign a jobseekers agreement specifying the conditions upon which they are available for work.

Incapacity Benefit

A short-term benefit payable at a lower rate for the first 28 weeks for people who are unable to work through sickness, but who are not entitled to Statutory Sick Pay. Long-term benefit is payable after one year of sickness. (Statutory Sick Pay is payable for up to 28 weeks and is paid by employers to people who are off work due to sickness.)

Disability Living Allowance

This benefit is paid to people under the age of 65 who need help with personal care because of illness or disability. There are two parts to this benefit – a care component for people who need supervision or attendance by another person – and a mobility component for people who need supervision when walking or who are unable, or virtually unable, to walk.

Attendance Allowance

This is payable to people aged over 65 who need regular assistance or supervision. A higher rate is payable for people who need attention or supervision 24 hours a day.

Invalid Care Allowance

This is payable to people between the age of 16 and 65 who care for someone who needs help and support for at least 35 hours a week. They must not be earning more than £50 per week after deduction of expenses or be in full-time education.

OHT 5.5.1 HEALTH IMPROVEMENT PROGRAMME TARGETS

HIP targets

These might include:

- the reduction of death rates by cancer in the under-65s
- the reduction of death rates from heart disease and strokes
- the improvement of the health, social functioning and quality of life for people with serious mental illness
- improving the life expectancy and quality of life for people with respiratory disease
- helping to reduce the accident rate
- the reduction of young people's misuse of drugs and alcohol
- reducing the rate of conceptions amongst the under-16s
- reducing the effects of diabetes
- helping to reduce the number of suicides.

OHT 5.5.2 HEALTHIER LIFESTYLES

New approaches in public health seek to improve health by preventing disease. One key element is to convince people to choose a healthier lifestyle and there are various health campaigns that promote this. A healthier lifestyle would include:

- exercise – preferably a minimum of 20 minutes vigorous exercise a week
- healthy diet – low in saturated fat, high in fibre, vegetables and fruit
- avoiding obesity
- moderate drinking of alcohol
- avoidance of smoking
- avoidance of drug misuse
- avoidance of stress.

OHT 5.5.3 CHILD POVERTY, PRESSURE GROUPS AND THE GOVERNMENT

In September 2000 leading children's charities called for a children's commissioner in each of the four UK countries and also called for a special cabinet ministry post to be set up to represent issues in respect of children.

Barnardo's, the Child Poverty Action Group and the NSPCC have developed a manifesto to help children escape from poverty. Fifty childrens' organisations have endorsed the manifesto. Child Poverty Action Group claimed that the number of children living in poverty increased by 1 million to 4.5 million in recent years. The NSPCC have called for the government's new children's unit to look at issues such as health, leisure, education, crime, child deaths and child killings.

These measure are being called for despite the government's recent report that:

- one million more people are in work than in 1997 – the lowest levels of unemployment for 20 years
- the number of children in workless households fell by more than 250,000 in the three years to spring 2000
- permanent school exclusions fell by 15% between 1997/8 and 1998/9.

The government has already added new indicators of child poverty, including one to monitor whether there is a reduction in the proportion of children registered on the child protection register. The aim is to reduce the proportion of children who are registered by 10 per cent by the year 2002.

The government has a target of eradicating child poverty within a generation. It is estimated that this could save the lives of about 1400 children under the age of 15 each year, according to a study for the Joseph Rowntree Foundation, published in September 2000.

Note: *Opportunity For All: One Year On* on www.dss.gov.uk

ACTIVITY 5.1.1 MIXED ECONOMY OF CARE

Read the case study below, then answer the questions that follow.

Mrs Williamson is a thirty-eight-year-old woman with three children aged three, nine and twelve. Her husband has a job with a computer company as a support worker. They live in a quiet residential area of Birmingham. Mr and Mrs Williamson's parents moved to England from Jamaica in the 1950s.

Eight months ago Mrs Williamson was diagnosed as having cancer of the breast. At the present time she is having a course of radiotherapy. This will be followed by a course of chemotherapy. She has to attend hospital once a week for six weeks. Following her treatment she often feels very sick and is unable to do anything for several days. As well as seeing a consultant at the hospital, she also sees her GP on a monthly basis, and the GP has arranged for a district nurse to visit her each week. A specialist nurse from the Macmillan Service, who has special knowledge of symptom and pain control in cancer care, also visits her from time to time, or when she is having particular problems.

To help the family the Social Services Department have arranged for Mrs Williamson's three-year-old daughter to attend day nursery. Mr Williamson takes her there each morning and has arranged for his mother to collect her in the afternoon and look after her until he gets home from work. Their nine-year-old son is taken to and from school by the mother of one of his friends. Their twelve-year-old daughter makes her own way to and from school, returning home to help her mother with getting the dinner ready for the rest of the family in the evening. She also helps her mother to get up and dressed in the mornings. The family have arranged for a private home help to do the housework once a week while Mrs Williamson is undergoing treatment.

QUESTIONS

1 Which of the following sorts of care do the Williamson family receive? Identify which services provide which type of care.

Services	Types of care
Statutory health care services	
Statutory social care services	
Voluntary health care services	
Voluntary social care services	
Private health care	
Private social care	
Informal carers	

ACTIVITY 5.1.1 (CONTINUED)

2 What other services might be of help to the family in the future, especially if Mrs Willamson needs to be hospitalised?

3 How might this additional support be provided? Could it be provided by statutory, voluntary or private organisations? What additional support might come from informal carers?

4 Could Mrs Williamson's older daughter be considered as being a 'young carer'?

5 Mrs Williamson and her family are receiving 'a mixed economy of care'. What is meant by this term? Give examples to show how this term relates to the Williamsons.

ACTIVITY 5.1.2 IMPROVING CHILD HEALTH CARE

Read the case study below and answer the following questions.

Katia is six years old and attends the local infant school. Her brother Benjamin is three and goes to the local nursery four mornings a week while his mother works part-time in the local newsagent shop. Benjamin has his breakfast and main meal of the day at the nursery. Katia and her mother do not have time for breakfast on the mornings that her mother works. Katia takes a packed lunch to school which usually includes a jam sandwich, a packet of crisps and a chocolate bar. Katia likes sweet things. After school she has a doughnut or some biscuits and then eats her main meal with her parents at about seven o'clock, after her brother has been put to bed. Katia is already overweight.

Katia sometimes has friends visit and they like playing various games, however she spends a lot of time watching the television and playing on the computer. At the weekends Katia's father takes her and her brother to the local playground, weather permitting.

Neither Katia nor her brother have been immunised. Katia catches cold quite easily and is allergic to a variety of food additives, animal fur and pollen. The family is on a very tight budget as neither of Katia's parents are very well paid. Her father works as a domestic in a general hospital. The only 'treat' Katia's parents have is a couple of packets of cigarettes a week.

QUESTIONS

1 How could Katia's diet be improved?

____

____

2 What other things could be done to improve Katia's weight problem?

____

____

3 What health problems might Katia encounter in the future as a result of her current lifestyle?

____

____

4 How might the family's circumstances be improved in order to improve Katia's health problems?

____

____

5 Put yourself in the position of adviser to Katia's family. You have been asked by them to provide them with a plan of action to improve Katia's health and weight. Using appropriate language, write out a health plan for Katia. You could do this exercise in pairs or groups.

ACTIVITY 5.3.1 THE NEEDS OF INFORMAL CARERS

Read the following case study, then answer the questions that follow.

Mrs Matthews has been looking after her 87-year-old father for the last ten years. Last year she felt that it was no longer possible for her father to continue to live alone and so he came to live with her and her husband. Her father, Mr Mazzibrada, has Parkinson's disease. This means that his walking is greatly reduced and he can only shuffle along. He is very slow in doing anything and needs a lot of encouragement and directions, even to get himself dressed. He seems to understand what is being said but does not respond either verbally or in any emotional way. Of late he has tended to wander off, both during the day and occasionally at night. His GP has been consulted and has prescribed medication, but whenever he asks Mrs Matthews if she is managing alright, she always says 'Yes'.

Mr and Mrs Matthews have not been able to go out together for many months. The only time that they have together is when one of their children come to 'grandad sit'. Mr Matthews stays with his father-in-law while his wife does the shopping and they share the household tasks between them. Their children are very worried about the situation, but both live more than fifty miles away, work full-time and have their own families to care for.

Mr and Mrs Matthews have often wondered if it would be possible to get any help, but are unsure of how to go about this. They have thought about buying in some private help, but all three of them only have their pensions, plus a small private pension that Mr Matthews receives from his previous employer. Fortunately they live in their own house, but still have two years before they pay off their mortgage.

QUESTIONS

1 Where might Mrs Matthews find out what sort of help is available? How would she go about accessing this?

___

___

2 What sort of help do you feel she and her father might need?

___

___

3 Who might provide this support – statutory, voluntary or private health or social care services?

___

___

4 Would Mrs Matthews, or her father, be entitled by law to any benefits to help pay for additional care?

___

___

5 What do carers need in order that they can continue to provide care?

___

___

ACTIVITY 5.3.2 THE NEEDS OF YOUNG CARERS

This is a role-play activity to help you understand the needs of young carers.

To help you think about the needs of young carers, work together in pairs using the role-play prompt cards on the following pages, with one person taking the role of the young carer and the other taking the role of the education welfare officer. The role of the education welfare officer is to find out what difficulties the young person is having and to discuss with them the kind of help that might be available to them and their family.

SCENARIO

Leon is 14 years old and has been missing from school at least one day a week for the past two terms. His mother was diagnosed as having breast cancer six months ago and has been having a course of chemotherapy. This was followed by a mastectomy operation two weeks ago which will be followed by a course of radiotherapy in a few weeks time. It is hoped that she will have recovered in about three to four months time. If the treatment is successful, then there is a very good chance that the cancer will not recur in the future. At the present time Leon's mother is unable to use her right arm and often feels too tired to get up in the mornings. The district nurse visits every other day, but apart from this the family has no help. Leon's father has to travel abroad a lot with his job, so Leon and his 12-year-old sister are having to do the housework, shopping, laundry and some of the cooking.

ACTIVITY 5.3.2 (CONTINUED) PROMPT CARDS

PROMPT CARD 1

Education Welfare Officer: Says that they are aware that Leon's mother has been unwell recently and asks him if he could tell them more about this.

PROMPT CARD 2

Leon: Leon explains about his mother's illness, including the operation, and that his mother will be having more treatment, which will mean that Leon is likely to need to continue helping in the home for the next three to four months.

PROMPT CARD 3

Education Welfare Officer : Asks Leon to describe a typical day and the things that he does during it.

PROMPT CARD 4

Leon: Described how he gets breakfast for the family; helps his mother to get washed and dressed (if she is feeling well enough to get up). He also has to make sure that his sister is ready for school and has all the right things. After school he sometimes has to do the shopping or fetch prescriptions for his mother. He usually prepares and cooks the evening meal although his sister helps with washing up. At the weekends he does the housework and the laundry and ironing.

PROMPT CARD 5

Education Welfare Officer: Asks what help he gets from other people and if there is anyone else who might help them.

PROMPT CARD 6

Leon: Explains that his father is away a lot of the time but does a lot of the housework and cooking when he is home. There are no other relatives living nearby except for a grandmother, but she is disabled. Leon's mother usually does the shopping for the grandmother and helps her with her housework. Leon and his sister are doing this at the moment. Leon does not know of anywhere else that he can get help.

ACTIVITY 5.3.2 (CONTINUED) PROMPT CARDS

PROMPT CARD 7

Education Welfare Officer: Tells Leon about the help that his grandmother could get from the local social services department and that his mother might also be able to get help especially with getting up and dressed, etc.

PROMPT CARD 8

Leon: Says he didn't know that his mother could get help, and in any case was afraid of contacting the social services department as he thought they would take his sister and himself into care.

PROMPT CARD 9

Education Welfare Officer: Explains that the social services department's aim would be to help the family cope in this difficult time. Then asks Leon what he finds most difficult at the moment.

PROMPT CARD 10

Leon: Talks about the practical problems of doing everything and then having to cope with school and homework. He talks about the emotional distress of having to help his mother with her personal care and his fear that the cancer will not be cured. He also talks about not having time to go out with his friends.

PROMPT CARD 11

Education Welfare Officer: Suggests that their first step might be to contact the social services' Young Carers' Officer who could talk with the family about the sort of help that is available and who would know how to get the help put in place.

ACTIVITY 5.4.1 SERVICES INVOLVED IN EARLY YEARS PROVISION

This activity gives you the opportunity to explore some of the services involved in early years provision and to write a report on one of them.

TASK 1

Below are a list of organisations that provide services for children and families. Find out, and write up, what they do.

- After Adoption,
  12–14 Chapel Street
  Manchester M3 7NN
  www.adoption@aol.com
- All Party Parliamentary Group for Children
  8 Wakely Street
  London SE1 2UF
  www.ncb.org.uk
- Children's Society
  The Edward Rudolf House
  Margery Street
  London WC1X 0JL
  www.the-childrens-society.org.uk
- Parents and Children Together (PACT)
  48 Bath Road
  Reading RG1 6PG
  www.pactcharity.co.uk
- Proadventure, 6 Bryntirion
  Llangollen
  Denbighshire
  NE Wales LL20 8LP
  www.proadventure.clara.net
- Ockendon International
  Constitution Hill
  Woking
  Surrey GU22 7UU
  Email:ov@ockendon.org.uk

TASK 2

Write a short report on one of these organisations. The headings that you might like to use may include:

- The year that they were started.
- How and why they were started.
- What they do.
- The geographical area that they cover.
- How they are staffed, e.g. paid staff and/or volunteers.
- How they are funded.

ACTIVITY 5.4.2 WELFARE BENEFITS

Read each of the following cases and answer the questions that follow each of them.

Read the information in OHT 5.4.3 to help you answer the questions below.

Aaron Glassman is a 67-year-old man. He has severe arthritis and now needs help each day to get up, washed and dressed. He also needs help getting back to bed each night, as well as with all household tasks.

- Is Aaron entitled to Attendance Allowance and if so, is he likely to get the higher or lower rate?

___

Thelma Glassman is Aaron's 44-year-old daughter. She works in a library each Saturday earning £60 a week. Each day she makes two 90p return bus journeys to help her father with his personal care. She spends about an hour with her father each morning and evening.

___

- Is Thelma entitled to Invalid Care Allowance? On what grounds?

___

Matthew Claydon is 22 years old and graduated from university about a year ago. He has been unable to find suitable employment so far. He is living at home and has no source of income.

___

- Is Matthew entitled to receive any benefits? Which?

___

___

Martina Southern is a single parent. She has three young children under the age of 10. She has no savings. Her eldest son has a severe disability and needs help with all his personal care on a regular basis throughout the day. He also needs help during the night to turn and to go to the toilet.

- Which of the benefits are Martina and her family likely to able to claim?

___

___

ACTIVITY 5.5.1 A HEALTHIER LIFESTYLE

Health improvement programmes (HIPs) are being developed by health and local authorities. In the past the government has developed special advertising campaigns in order to promote healthier lifestyles, for example the use of contraceptives for 'safe sex', in an attempt to raise awareness regarding the risk of AIDS.

Think about recent health promotion campaigns and then carry out the following tasks.

TASKS

1 Look for evidence of a current campaign. You may find this in a newspaper or magazine, on the television, in a cinema advertisement, on a poster in your GP's surgery, library or other public place.

2 Think about and make a list of some of the possible contributing causes of the following:

Problem	Contributing cause
Alcohol misuse	
Drug addiction	
Heart disease	
Lung cancer	
Road traffic accidents	
Suicide	

3 Choose one of the above problems and one of the contributing causes and design a poster aimed at warning teenagers about these dangers.

4 Where would you place the posters in order for them to be most effective?

5 What else could be done to promote your campaign?

6 How might campaigns aimed at teenagers differ from those aimed at elderly people?

ACTIVITY 5.6.1 ACCESSING SERVICES

TASKS

1 Collect some leaflets from your local health authority, social services department and voluntary and private organisations in your area and make up a **Resource File** of these. You may wish to work in small groups to do this.

Leaflets that you could collect might include information about:

- Local health clinics
- District nursing services
- Home care services
- Day care facilities for people with dementia
- Residential homes (either social services owned or private)
- Private nursing homes
- Private day nurseries
- Play groups

2 Select one of the leaflets that you collected. Choose one that you feel does not give very clear information and think of ways that it can be improved upon. Make a list of these improvements.

3 Re-design the leaflet.

4 Make a list of the places where the leaflet should be displayed in order for it to most effectively reach those people that it is aimed at.

ACTIVITY 5.6.2 CASE STUDY: ACCESSING SERVICES

Read the case study below then answer the following questions.

Mr Menzies is seventy years old. He lives in a privately rented cottage in a small village on the outskirts of Liverpool. Until recently he has been managing by himself with no help from health or social services. He has been in good health and rarely sees his GP. A few months ago he had a fall in the garden. Since then he has had a pain in his left hip and has had difficulty in getting about. He is now finding it difficult to do the household chores and has also noticed that he is becoming more and more forgetful and has to check over and over again to make sure he has done things, for example locking the doors at night or turning off the oven when he has cooked his meal. The cottage is in bad repair as the landlord will only do 'essential' repairs and Mr Menzies only has his state pension on which to live. Mr Menzies' only son and daughter-in-law live fifty miles away and can only visit at the weekend.

QUESTIONS

1 What are Mr Menzies' current health and social care needs?

___

___

2 What services does Mr Menzies need in order to meet those needs?

___

___

3 Where would Mr Menzies find information about those services?

___

___

4 Who would provide these services?

___

___

5 How would Mr Menzies access those services?

___

___

6 What barriers might there be for Mr Menzies in accessing these services?

___

___

UNIT 6 – RESEARCH PERSPECTIVES IN HEALTH AND SOCIAL CARE

OVERVIEW

This unit is about carrying out research, and both the unit content and the assessment requirements emphasise that research is an activity. Though students will need a theoretical understanding of research methods, and of other issues such as ethical considerations, this is in essence a practical unit.

The unit is divided into five sections:

6.1 Purpose of research in health and social care
6.2 Research methods
6.3 Planning research, methods of analysis and validation
6.4 Presenting research
6.5 Ethical issues

Aims and objectives

This unit covers:

- the purpose of research in health and social care
- research methods used in health and social care
- methods of analysis and validation
- presentation of results
- ethical issues during research.

Students should be able to:

- explain the different purposes of research carried out in health and social care
- investigate different methods of research which suit different purposes
- explain basic sampling techniques
- describe validity and reliability related to research projects
- record data accurately
- explain the problem and formulate a relevant hypothesis for research
- describe the purpose and relevance of the research
- identify variables that may impact on the research
- review the knowledge and publications applicable to the research
- explain and justify the chosen research methods
- describe different forms of sampling
- identify ways of checking research to comply with appropriate ethical standards
- recognise sources of bias and inaccuracy in collecting data
- explore and consider appropriate methods to analyse and present findings
- explain how conclusions are validated
- suggest recommendations for further development in the research study
- reference the research appropriately
- describe ethical issues that can arise during research and presentation of findings
- describe the management of the maintenance of clients' rights and confidentiality during research.

TEACHING NOTES

The order of the sections generally follows the order in which students are likely to deal with them. The exception is the consideration of ethical issues, which would be best introduced early in the course. Logically, students need to be aware of ethical considerations when they go about planning their own research, and ethical problems could be discussed as research methods are introduced.

One other issue is that the five sections are not equal divisions of the unit in terms of time and effort. Students will probably spend much more time on planning, carrying out, and presenting their research than they will on the other sections.

6.1 Purpose of research in health and social care

This section should serve as an introduction to research for students. The unit lists six purposes to which research can be put. These are examined in Section 6.1 of the textbook and are:

1 Plan service delivery by establishing the relevant demography.

2 Explore patterns of disease (epidemiology).

3 Obtain feedback on services for quality assurance.

4 Explore the use of hypothesis in social science.

5 Explore and improve individual and collective knowledge, understanding and practice.

6 Review and monitor changes in health and social care practice.

OHT 6.1.1 may be useful to have available for display whilst delivering this part of the course. It is likely that many students will begin the course with sketchy ideas about what research is, and how and why it is done. Their experience of research could be limited to articles published in newspapers and popular magazines. The **Try it out** exercise on page 424 of the textbook can help students understand the uses to which research can be put.

It may be a good idea to begin by exposing students to a variety of research reports and results. This will let them become familiar with how research reports are structured and how results are presented. Also it should form a good preparation for the process of secondary research. A collection of different materials can be chosen to provide examples of each of the categories of research mentioned above. *Social Trends* and the *Annual Abstract of Statistics* can provide examples of demographic data, and some epidemiological results. Similar publications should contain some examples of data giving feedback on services. Any recent example of social science research looking at social theory could be looked at, as can materials appearing in professional publications and focused on investigating changes in services and practices. Any locally based material, perhaps published by the local council or social services department, may be particularly useful as it could have increased relevance for students and so aid motivation.

Copies can be made of this collection of research materials so that each student can work from them, and useful activities based upon them can be devised. Students could be asked to identify examples of quantitative and qualitative data, and also identify the category from the list above that each piece of research most closely fits into. The activity could be extended by asking students to identify trends, peaks and other features from tables and charts amongst the provided data. This is a good introduction to the use of secondary sources and can clarify their ideas about quantitative and qualitative data.

The **Think it Over** activity on page 424 of the textbook also reinforces ideas about types of data. This could be extended using the research questions developed from the **Try it out** exercise on the same page.

This is also an opportunity to introduce the idea of reliability and validity. These terms are often misunderstood, and clarification may be more easily achieved with access to a varied range of types of research data. Students need to be aware that carefully collected quantitative data, such as official statistics, is generally reliable as it is scrupulously collected and presented. Qualitative data, obtained from in-depth interviews or open questions in surveys, is likely to display validity as people's authentic views and reasons for action emerge. The validity of official statistics is restricted since their function is to present a picture ready for interpretation, rather than demonstrate how that picture came about. The reliability of qualitative data is restricted since another sample could be chosen and present quite a different set of views and experiences.

Studies on divorce rates can provide a good example of the differences between reliability and validity, and of the way that complementary methods produce the best research. Official statistics on divorce are likely to be very reliable since they are compiled from a count of all divorces registered and no sampling is involved. But of themselves they tell nothing about why people get divorced, and do not give any clues as to why divorce rates have changed over time. Studies looking at these issues have generally carried out research on samples of divorced people and used questionnaire and/or interview methods to obtain data on individual experiences and feelings. They have tried to gain a valid picture of how divorces come about and tried to account for changes in patterns over time. Both these types of data are needed for a useful and complete impression of divorce trends to emerge.

One way to introduce the ideas of reliability and validity is to give an introductory explanation of the terms, and then ask students to work in small groups and attempt to rank the validity and reliability of the different examples of research you have provided for them. This could be done using a simple ten-point scale. More depth can be achieved if students are asked to provide an explanation of their decisions. Class discussion of these explanations during a feedback period could raise critical awareness of the issues they will face during their own secondary research.

To make this activity broader, and perhaps a bit more fun, a couple of examples of bad research could be included. These may be found in popular magazines and sometimes newspapers. Some pressure groups are also a useful source of poor research. Typical examples of bad research will make use of very small samples, case studies or anecdotal data, thus having low reliability, but make unrealistic claims for the broader applicability of the results. The validity of the research may be questionable where data has been carefully selected and presented so as to generate the result that is desired.

The section of the textbook on 'Sources of secondary data', starting on page 427, gives details of the strengths and weaknesses of different secondary data sources. This could equip students to carry out successfully the activities suggested above.

6.2 Research methods and 6.3 Planning research, methods of analysis and validation

These sections of the unit are probably the ones that demand most of the tutor. Students are faced with beginning to make decisions about the research question to pursue and the methods to use, whilst at the same time finding out about different methods of primary research and their suitability for different purposes. Students don't need in-depth knowledge of each method but they do need a basic understanding of them. For higher grades it is essential that the research report includes a consideration of the suitability of the methods chosen, better still a sound justification and explanation of other methods that could have been used. The delivery of a basic knowledge of each research method to all students will help with this.

Students will need a lot of support in making the right choices and thinking through the implications of the course of research that they choose to pursue. If unforeseen difficulties force students to abandon a research method that they have spent a lot of time developing it is likely to be extremely de-motivating for them. It is important that their research intentions will work. For these reasons it is worth spending time outlining different research methods.

Students might find it more interesting to learn about research methods in the context of practical projects, which they might undertake. Research methods might be introduced by discussing examples of projects that students could undertake. Methodologies such as questionnaires, interviewing and surveys could be introduced in the context of practical research projects. (See **Activity 6.3.1** and **OHT 6.3.1.**) It might therefore be appropriate to teach structured examples of research and planning research together.

Primary research methods

Students should have some knowledge of commonly used research methods including:

- Interviews: structured and in-depth.
- Self-completion questionnaires.
- Observation: direct and participant.
- Experiments.

For each method students will need to know:

- How it works, i.e. what the researcher actually does and how data is collected.
- The resources needed to carry it out.
- The type of data likely to be collected.
- The type of research question it is likely to be used for.

OHTs 6.2.1, 6.2.2 and **6.2.3** give basic comments about each research method in terms of the aspects listed above. Fuller details of the characteristics of different research methods are given in the textbook on pages 430–450.

Methods could be introduced by beginning with the students' own 'common knowledge' understanding of what they might entail. Lists made from their suggestions can stimulate discussion and lead into the OHTs. When delivering this section it is useful to show examples of published research that uses the research method under discussion. Examples could be drawn from the materials assembled for the activity in the previous section.

Differences between different methods should be related to the types of data that they are likely to collect and the types of research aims that they are associated with. This should again bring up differences between quantitative and qualitative data, and the relationship these have with the reliability and validity of results. It is worth looking at the reasons for the choices made by professional researchers and the relationship between the research methods used and the research constraints that they faced. Students need to make choices about which methods to use themselves. Their choice will be made in terms of the constraints imposed by:

- the research question and population of interest
- their own levels of skill and resources, including time available.

It may be reassuring for students to see how professionals have similar issues to consider when making their research decisions.

Students need to get some idea, at an early stage, of the type and amount of work they might be taking on when they choose a particular research method. Though research should begin with a research question rather than a choice of method, it is a good idea for students to begin to think through the amount and type of work they may be taking on. For instance, they should understand the high level of skill required for in-depth interviews and the possible problems with confidentiality that could arise with this method of research. Similarly, the difficulties of using participant observation in a student research project should be made clear.

A discussion of the characteristics of each research method should help reveal its strengths and its limitations. Ideas about the suitability of a method in different research situations should emerge. Again pages 430–450 of the textbook gives more detail. **OHTs 6.2.4, 6.2.5 and 6.2.6** show some of the 'pros and cons' of each research method. When using these OHTs it is worth stressing that the use of the term 'pros and cons' does not mean that one research method is better than another. They should be seen as pointers towards the type of research situation they are best fitted for.

Similarly, it is important for students to realise that quantitative research is not inherently better that qualitative research. If they have really understood the terms reliability and validity then this should be obvious to them. However, there is a general belief that useful and 'scientific' research should produce charts, graphs and numerical results. Above all, students need to realise that the quality of research is not measured by the quantity of graphical representations of results that are produced. The value of qualitative research data must be made clear to them, as must the dangers of trying to make research look scientific and accurate through the production of a large number of inappropriate charts.

Activity 6.2.1 is intended to give students some practice in assessing the usefulness of different research methods in a range of research situations. **OHT 6.2.7** consists of scenarios that need to be handed out to the students in order for them to do this activity and **OHT 6.2.8** is a table that students will also need for the activity.

This activity is intended to improve a student's understanding of different research methods and where they are most useful. It should give them practice in analysing the needs of a research question, and in deciding on an appropriate research method to address it. To access higher grades students need to consider how the use of alternative research methodologies could have affected the results of their research work. To support this the activity specifies that the reasons for rejecting or accepting each method should be given, along with any lingering reservations about the use of their preferred option.

6.4 Presenting Research

Once students have been introduced to the theory of research methods and how to plan research they should be advised of the issues involved in presenting research. One of the key things they will need to plan is the layout of a research report. **OHT 6.4.1** sets out the layout for a research report. Students should follow the main titles in bold and may also choose to include other titles depending on the nature of their project.

Referencing

Students should be advised to use a recommended referencing system. Many people choose the Harvard reference system as a basis for reporting references. A handout is supplied in this pack which students may find useful (see **OHT** 6.4.2).

Appropriate methods for presenting findings

Students must describe the use of appropriate methods to present their research findings. For a higher grade, accurate clear and coherent presentation methods must be used. Students' choice of presentational methods will naturally depend on their choice of project and research methodology. It will be important to introduce students to some of the options for presenting findings before they undertake their research. This pack lists some of the presentation methods relevant to quantitative data as handouts. (See **OHTs** 6.4.3–6.4.12.) There are also activities (**Activity** 6.4.1 and **Activity** 6.4.2) which might help students to understand some of the ways in which presentation can bias a report. At grade A, students should be able to justify their choice of presentational methods and explain some of the risks of bias that can arise when presenting data (Activity 6.4.1 and OHT 6.4.12).

Many students will find it difficult to write up a whole research project. It will be important to organise the students so that they write up their report in stages. It may be useful to set deadlines for the completion of the introduction and methodology, the completion of the results and the completion of the discussion and conclusions.

One possible way of assisting students to complete this work may be to organise small group peer assessment of one another's sections of work. Assuming that students in any given small group are working on different projects, and that they are used to working within supportive ground rules, students may gain a lot from learning to critique each other's research. It may be important to consider formative marking of draft sections of the research write up in order to guide student development in the development of this skill.

Diagrams can be used to make information obvious to anyone who looks at it. OHT 6.4.3, for example, provides a way of visually presenting the number of times that individuals contributed to a group discussion by being humorous. You can show how many times people asked questions, or gave long speeches, or any kind of behaviour that you can define, using this technique.

6.5 Ethical issues

Before students begin to plan any practical projects it will be vital to emphasise the importance of protecting other people's rights, obtaining other people's consent fairly and honestly and maintaining confidentiality. It will also be important to encourage students to develop an understanding of ways in which research and conclusions can be biased. Students will need to understand that biased and invalid research can cause harm to people. See **Activities** 6.5.1, 6.5.2 and 6.5.3, and **OHTs** 6.5.1 and 6.5.2.

Students should already have explored the care value base (OHT 1.3.1) and theories of ethical reasoning when they studied Unit 1. It will be important to remind students of the care value base and the need to promote other people's rights, including: physical and emotional safety, dignity and confidentiality. Unit 6 will also build on students' understanding of the ways in which culture, age, gender and ethnicity influence people's assumptions about what is right and what is real. If students are to achieve a C or an A grade they will need to be able to discuss ways in which bias can affect research outcomes. For example, questions can be biased because of assumptions, and research presentations can employ inappropriate methods that can lead to biased conclusions.

It may be appropriate to introduce the topic of ethical issues during the introduction to the research unit. The issue of bias and the importance of promoting client's rights might be integrated into the general teaching of research methods. Some specific teaching on ethical issues might be planned to follow the teaching on research methods and before students progress to complete their plans for the practical project.

Before students undertake any practical research it would be a good idea to ask them to produce a summary of what they intend to do. This summary should include examples of any questionnaires, interview schedules or other approaches they intend to take. Although the class teacher should take responsibility for checking students' plans, the students may be more likely to understand the importance of ethics if they are actively involved in checking their own and others' proposals.

One idea to promote the importance of ethical issues would be to ask students to 'peer assess' one another's proposals using a list of ethical criteria. A list of ethical criteria is published in this file as a handout (see **OHT 6.5.3**). Students might be asked to work in small groups (perhaps threes or fours) where each person presents an outline of their project and the other two or three students take turns in asking questions about ethical safeguards. Once the group is confident that all of their proposals are ethically sound the tutor might confirm the group's conclusion or offer further guidance.

ASSESSMENT SUMMARY

For this unit students need to design a research project, carry it out, and complete a research report. They can choose any research topic that is relevant to health, care or an early years setting. The assessment of the unit is based entirely on portfolio work, and this primarily consists of the student's research report.

The work that students do will involve:

- considering the purpose of research, and deriving a workable research question together with a rationale to support it
- carrying out secondary research
- looking at different research methods and choosing which to apply
- planning their primary research and designing suitable tools such as questionnaires or observation checklists
- collecting primary data
- collating and analysing of data collected
- drawing realistic conclusions that are related to the research question
- completing a research report which includes: details of the methodology used, findings and conclusions, appropriate data and statistics, relevant diagrams and charts, a bibliography, and an identification of ethical issues and how they were dealt with.

Grade E

To achieve a **grade E** you need to produce a report of a research project designed and carried out in a health, social care or early years setting which shows:

- An accurate description and application of an appropriate research methodology to a relevant issue in a health, social care or early years setting.
- A clear summary of a relevant literature search.
- An identification of relevant ethical issues.
- The uses of appropriate methods to present accurate clear findings, including appropriate data, statistics, diagrams, charts and bibliography.

Grade C

To achieve **grade C** the work must show the following:

- Students need to show independent selection and application of an appropriate research methodology, and clearly explain their decisions.
- They must assess the validity of the resources they use and show an understanding of the political and philosophical background of the authors.
- The effects of ethical considerations on the research project must be analysed.
- Possible sources of error must be identified and their effects evaluated.
- The research and findings are to be presented accurately, clearly and coherently.

Grade A

To achieve **grade A** the work must show the following:

- Students must show a comprehensive approach to the design of the research and to carrying out the methodology.
- Students must be able to draw and justify realistic conclusions, and make and justify recommendations for further research.
- They should justify their choice of research methodology and explain how their findings may have differed if other appropriate research methods had been used.

For the students this unit can be both eye-opening, and fun to carry out. The unit should give students skills and knowledge in research that they can apply to other areas of their studies. It can support research work carried out in other Advanced units. It can help students to understand where the knowledge and information they are finding out about in their studies comes from, and why it is believed to be correct. It could improve their understanding and use of secondary sources in their studies, and help them to approach information in a more critical and objective way.

OHTs

The OHTs to support reaching this unit are:

6.1.1 Purposes of research in health and social care
6.2.1 Research methods 1
6.2.2 Research methods 2
6.2.3 Research methods 3
6.2.4 Pros and cons of research methods 1
6.2.5 Pros and cons of research methods 2
6.2.6 Pros and cons of research methods 3
6.2.7 Handout – Scenarios for Activity 6.2.1
6.2.8 Handout – Table for Activity 6.2.1
6.3.1 Handout – Answers to Activity 6.3.1
6.4.1 Structure of a research report
6.4.2 Handout – How to use the Harvard reference system
6.4.3 Handout – Using diagrams to report observational data
6.4.4 Handout – Using tables to report observational data
6.4.5 Handout – Using tables to summarise rating scales
6.4.6 Handout – Summary sheets for questions
6.4.7 Handout – Using bar charts
6.4.8 Handout – Using pie charts
6.4.9 Handout – Using line graphs
6.4.10 Handout – Using scattergrams
6.4.11 Handout – Inventing diagrams to make your point
6.4.12 Handout – Answers to Activity 6.4.1
6.5.1 Handout to Activity 6.5.2
6.5.2 Handout to Activity 6.5.3
6.5.3 Handout – Ethical issues checklist

ACTIVITIES

The activities are designed to promote learning and understanding, provide consolidation and develop logical thinking and a national approach.

6.2.1 Choosing the best research method
6.3.1 What is wrong with this questionnaire?
6.4.1 Presentation of research
6.4.2 Choosing methods of presentation
6.5.1 Ethics and experimentation
6.5.2 Interviewing
6.5.3 Critiquing an interview

OHT 6.1.1 PURPOSES OF RESEARCH IN HEALTH AND SOCIAL CARE

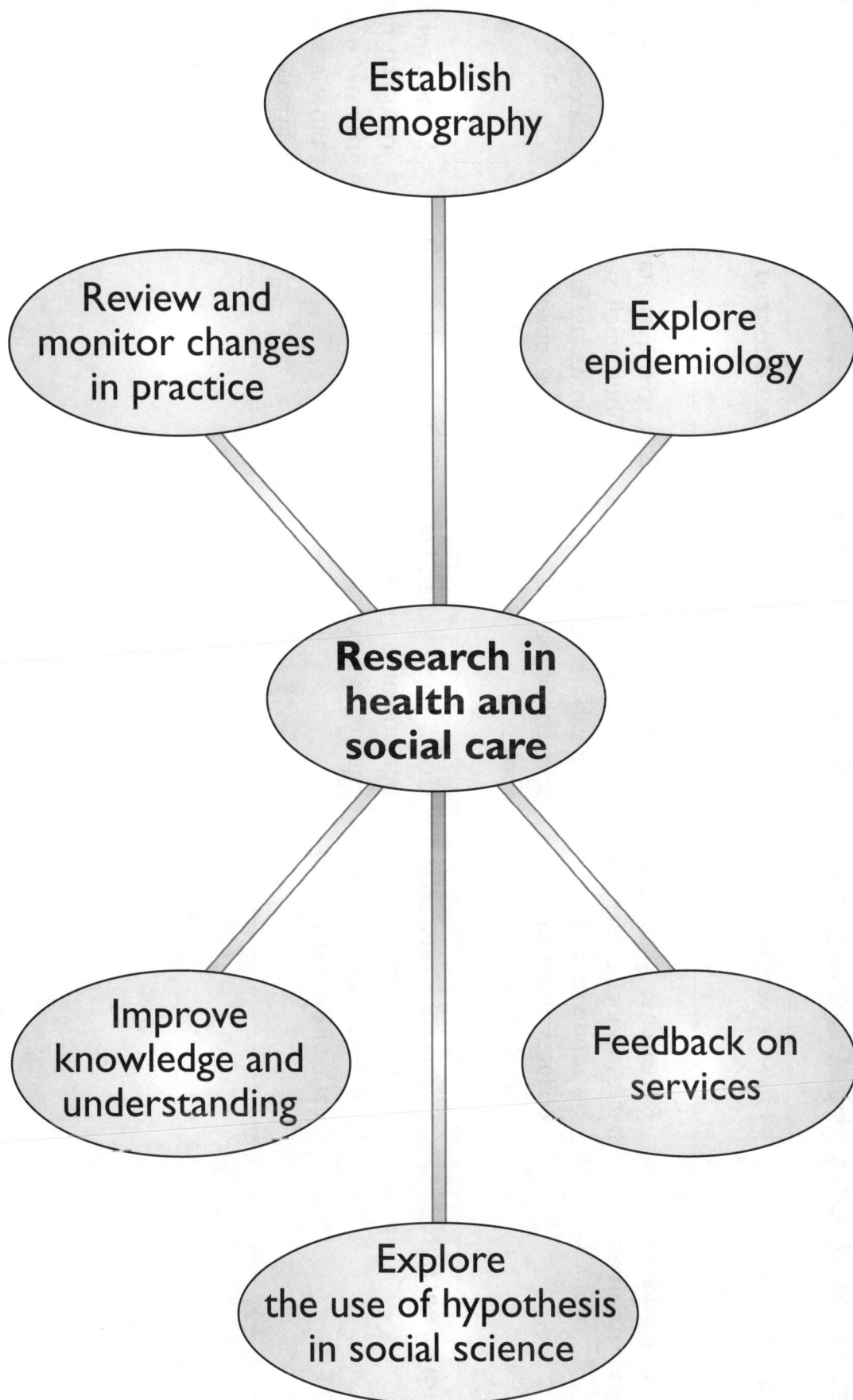
Establish demography
Review and monitor changes in practice
Explore epidemiology
Research in health and social care
Improve knowledge and understanding
Feedback on services
Explore the use of hypothesis in social science

OHT 6.2.1 RESEARCH METHODS 1

Method	How it works	Resources needed	Data collected	Likely to be used for:
Self-completion questionnaires	Researcher gives out questionnaire forms to respondents and collects them on completion.	Copies of a questionnaire form. A means of distributing and collecting the forms.	Can give quantitative data but small sample size limits usefulness. Can give quantitative and qualitative data.	Research needing data from a large or an inaccessible sample.
Experiments	Researcher sets up a controlled situation for subjects and records data of interest.	Could need expensive equipment or a few cheap resources	Only quantitative data is collected.	Studies where the research question is narrow enough to allow some control of variables.

OHT 6.2.2 RESEARCH METHODS 2

Method	How it works	Resources needed	Data collected	Likely to be used for:
Structured interviews	Researcher meets with respondents and asks a prepared list of questions.	Carefully prepared interview schedule. Somewhere to carry out a private interview. A carefully selected sample of respondents.	Particularly useful for quantitative data; can also give limited qualitative data.	Research needing quantifiable results, where results are analysed numerically and displayed graphically.
In-depth interviews	Researcher meets with respondents and stimulates them to comment freely on the issue of interest.	Privacy and time to carry out the interviews. Communication skills to enable a successful interview.	Most data likely to be qualitative.	Research aimed at getting people's true feelings and opinions. Studies where validity is important.

OHT 6.2.3 RESEARCH METHODS 3

Method	How it works	Resources needed	.Data collected	Likely to be used for:
Direct observation	Researcher watches subjects and records behaviour of interest.	Tick sheet or other data recording form.	Only quantitative data is collected.	Studies of group behaviour. Researching populations unable to be studied by other methods.
Participant observation	Researcher joins the group being studied and records data about them 'from the inside'.	Considerable time and commitment. Skills in remaining objective whilst being involved in a group. Depends on nature of planned experiment.	Mostly qualitative data is collected. Some quantitative data collected but small sample size limits comparability	Studies of groups inaccessible or hostile to outsiders. Situations where validity of data is important.

OHT 6.2.4 PROS AND CONS OF RESEARCH METHODS 1

Method	Pros	Cons
Experiments	The experimenter controls the experimental situation. Quantitative data collected can be analysed statistically. Other researchers can repeat the experiment to test the results.	Difficult for the experimenter to control all factors affecting the subjects. Experimental situation may distort subject's behaviour. 'Scientific' nature of experiments may lend false credibility to the work.
Self-completion questionnaires	Cheap and quick way to collect data. No problem with interviewer bias. Respondents can consider answers. Postal methods may be the only way to contact some respondents. May be more acceptable to some respondents than an interview.	Often suffer from a low response rate. No check on subject's understanding. No check on who completes the questionnaire. Can't observe respondents' reactions. Can't collect spontaneous answers. Answers limited to the options offered.

OHT 6.2.5 PROS AND CONS OF RESEARCH METHODS 2

Method	Pros	Cons
Structured interviews	Very good response rates possible. Interviewer can clarify questions and observe useful background data. Can induce spontaneous responses. You know who answers the questions. Probes allow extra lines of enquiry to be followed up.	Time-consuming, so only a small sample can be used. Interviewer/respondent bias can lead to distorted results. Respondents need to be easy to contact. Answers limited to the options offered.
In-depth interviews	Gets subjects' real opinions and feelings in their own terms. Respondents have time to 'open up' on sensitive issues. Interviewers are free to explore any interesting areas that arise.	Interviewer can affect answers given. Good communication skills needed. Privacy is needed for interviews. Time-consuming so small sample used, which limits broader applicability of the results.

OHT 6.2.6 PROS AND CONS OF RESEARCH METHODS 3

Method	Pros	Cons
Direct observation	Records what people actually do. Subjects in their natural environment. Can detect behaviour that subjects are unaware of. Can look at group behaviour. May be the only way with some subjects, e.g. small children.	Note-taking distracts the observer. Secretive observation leads to significant ethical problems. Lack of control over the sample. Gives no data on reasons for behaviour, and behaviour can be misinterpreted.
Participant observation	Can produce valid qualitative data. May be only method possible with closed or hostile groups. Little likelihood of serious misinterpretations of data.	Researcher needs time, commitment and high order social skills. Researchers influence on group behaviour almost inevitable. Secretive participant observation leads to serious ethical difficulties.

OHT 6.2.7 HANDOUT – SCENARIOS FOR ACTIVITY 6.2.1

Scenarios . . .

A

A local nursery caters for children up to 4 years old. A limited amount of money is available to update the play equipment. Staff want to make the best use of the money and choose items that the children will enjoy and use regularly.

The three full-time members of the nursery staff cannot agree on which types of play equipment the children prefer, so they decide to ask their part-time helper, Lucy, to look into it. Lucy is on an AVCE course in caring at the local college and helps at the nursery every Monday and Thursday. Mondays are the nursery's busiest day and all staff are kept very busy. Thursdays are much quieter.

Lucy is asked to find out what types of play equipment the children attending the nursery prefer, and report her findings to the staff team. She is expected to fit the work in with her normal duties. The staff do not need a full research report, but do want the result to be convincing and accurate so that money spent on new equipment is not wasted.

B

A GP's practice serves people living in a fairly well-off area of a small town. There are a larger than average number of older people living in the area, and the surgery sees many regular patients. The practice manager is concerned that the current system used for making appointments and managing waiting times is not working well enough. Her main aim is to maximise patient satisfaction and she has received complaints from patients about the system now in use.

She is considering adopting the system used by a practice in a neighbouring area. Their patients tend to be less well-off, and they have many young families on their books. Their practice manager receives few complaints about appointments.

Both practice managers are keen to improve their services and they want to work together to achieve this. They decide to carry out research themselves to find out more about patient satisfaction. They want to find out the views of a wide range of patients at both surgeries and get an accurate picture of patient satisfaction levels. Both are very busy people. They intend to try to fit the work into their normal duties, but are aware that this will severely limit the time that they can give to the research.

C

A number of homeless people live in a large town and a voluntary organisation intends to set up a drop-in centre to help them. The organisation wants to offer facilities and support that the homeless really need. Also they want to be sure that the homeless are not put off from attending the centre due to the way it is organised or the systems that are set up to run it.

It is decided that research into the needs and the attitudes of local homeless people is required. A worker employed by the voluntary organisation in a nearby town has had experience of carrying out social research and has worked with homeless people in the past. He is given four weeks to do the research and report back to the team that is planning the centre. The team do not need detailed statistics. They do need the views and feelings of the homeless people about their own needs, so that the centre that is set up will be well attended and genuinely helpful.

OHT 6.2.7 HANDOUT (CONTINUED)

D

Staff at a residential home have complained to the management that recent increases in the number of residents has made it difficult for them to complete all the tasks required of them. They are particularly concerned that the time taken to clean residents' rooms is causing problems, and that extra staff hours are needed to deal with this.

The management is sympathetic, but it is unsure how many staff hours are needed to deal with the extra rooms now being cleaned. It decides to do research into the problem so that it can accurately assess how many staff hours are now needed.

E

A 'meals on wheels' service delivers meals to a large number of clients. The service covers a wide area and serves clients in many different neighbourhoods. The service organisers are reviewing the menus and the type of food provided. They want to make the food appealing to as many of their clients as possible. Also they want to assess the need for alternative diets, such as vegetarian food and cuisine suitable for members of different cultures in the community.

They need information from as wide a range of their clients as possible, but staff time to carry out the research is limited. As well as finding out about the dietary preferences of their clients, the service organisers would also like to know how clients feel about the way the service operates, and how well it meets their needs.

F

A health promotion exhibition focusing on the dangers of cigarette smoking has been set up in a busy shopping centre. The exhibition is attracting a lot of visitors with many different types of people attending. The organisers are particularly interested in the impact of the exhibition on teenage girls, as there are concerns about increases in the level of smoking amongst this group. There are a number of teenage girls amongst the visitors to the exhibition.

It is decided to do research to find out how well the exhibition is working to deter teenage girls from smoking. There are three staff based at the exhibition, and they can make time between them to allow one person to carry out the research during periods when the exhibition is open. The staff will have time to deal with the data they collect when the three-week run of the exhibition is over.

OHT 6.2.8 HANDOUT – TABLE FOR ACTIVITY 6.2.1

Scenario:		
Method	**Advantages**	**Disadvantages**
Experiment		
Questionnaires		
Structured interviews		
In-depth interviews		
Direct observation		
Participant observation		
Chosen method(s)		
Resources needed		

OHT 6.3.1 HANDOUT – ANSWERS TO ACTIVITY 6.3.1

The points below correspond to the sections in the questionnaire.

1 The questionnaire does not:
- explain the purpose of the research
- make a polite request to fill in the questionnaire
- explain how the information will be used.

2
- There is no guarantee of confidentiality, so the questionnaire fails to meet a requirement of the care value base.
- Because of this fewer people are likely to fill it in.

3
- The question is framed so that the respondents have only one choice, when in fact they could find the job both interesting and tiring, for example.
- There is no 'Don't know' option.

4
- This is a closed question to which respondents have to answer Yes or No.
- The respondents should be given the choice of agreeing or not agreeing, as in 'Would you agree, or would you not agree'.

5
- This is also a closed question.
- It asks the respondent to quantify something, which many would not be able to do.
- Also many respondents may not be clear as to what consitutes an employee: whether it is someone who works full-time, part-time, or voluntarily, for example.

6
- This is also a closed question.
- The question is too personal and confidential and may cause offence and not be answered.

7
- This creates an ethical problem in that it is open to labelling or stereotyping vulnerable clients, and may offend respondents.
- It is too difficult to answer. Many respondents will not know the basis on which to classify people in this way, and may fall into giving a stereotyped answer, making the result biased and meaningless.

8 • The rating scale limits responses to True or False, when actually many respondents don't know or have mixed views.
- As a result the data may be biased.

(a) It is impossible to rate this, as it poses a double question that requires a limited response. It doesn't allow for the work to be easy and interesting or boring and hard, for example.

(b) This is likely to produce a biased response, as most people will tend to answer it positively, even if it isn't true.

(c) • This is not an appropriate research situation for such accusations to be made.
- The issue is too complex to be answered through such a questionnaire.
- There is a danger of violating the rights of clients and staff.

(d) The question forces a biased response, as people will almost always say that they are not paid enough and will invariably say they enjoy working with people, particularly in care work.

General points

- The questionnaire doesn't have a strategy.
- It isn't clear what is being researched or how information could be analysed to produce results.
- Questions are biased, unclear and could be offensive.
- It illustrates the need to spend time in careful planning of a questionnaire.

OHT 6.4.1 THE STRUCTURE OF A RESEARCH REPORT

1 Title	
2 Contents	Most published works have a contents page.
3 Summary	Sometimes called an Abstract.
4 Introduction	This may include a literature review. The introduction must also explain why the project was worth doing and may state objectives for the project.
5 Method	The research methods that were used.
6 Results	The research findings – data.
7 Discussion	Discussion of the research findings.
8 Conclusions and recommendations	These are sometimes included in the discussion section but there must be conclusions at the end of the project.
9 Bibliography and/or references	The bibliography is a list of written works that you have found useful, references are works that you have actually quoted in the project.
10 Appendices	You may have details of practical work that you wish to include but which do not form part of the report.

OHT 6.4.2 HANDOUT – HOW TO USE THE HARVARD REFERENCE SYSTEM

Throughout your studies you will be doing written work to show that you have a good grasp of the knowledge for your course. This is a great opportunity for you to 'show what you know'. You can do this in your written work by quoting small amounts of text that you have read. This is called referencing.

So how do you do referencing? Here is a step-by-step guide.

Harvard referencing

Most courses ask students to reference using the Harvard System. It is used when you provide a **full book reference list** at the end of your piece of work, and you make references to specific pages from those books in your text. There are 2 parts to this system.

Part 1. You write your quote out, and in brackets put the author name, date and page.
Part 2. Then you provide a list of books you have referenced from at the end of your written work.

Here is an example.
You have read about Piaget's cognitive development theory in *Child Care and Education* by Penny Tassoni. It is on pages 136 to 138.

This is what you put in your written work:

'Michael seems to be using his experiences to help him in his work. This links to Piaget's theory that "children develop logic based on their experiences and try to draw conclusions from these experiences".'

Tassoni, (1998) P.136

Author name — *Year of publication* — *page number*

This is what you put at the end of your written work:
References
Tassoni, P. (1998) Child Care and Education. Heinemann

Author's surname and initials — *Date of publication* — *Full title of the book* — *Name of the publisher*

You will find the year of publication and the name of the publisher in the front of the book.

OHT 6.4.3 HANDOUT – USING DIAGRAMS TO REPORT OBSERVATIONAL DATA

Key:
A to F = Each of 6 people
Numbers in brackets = the number of times each person contributed to a 20-minute group discussion.

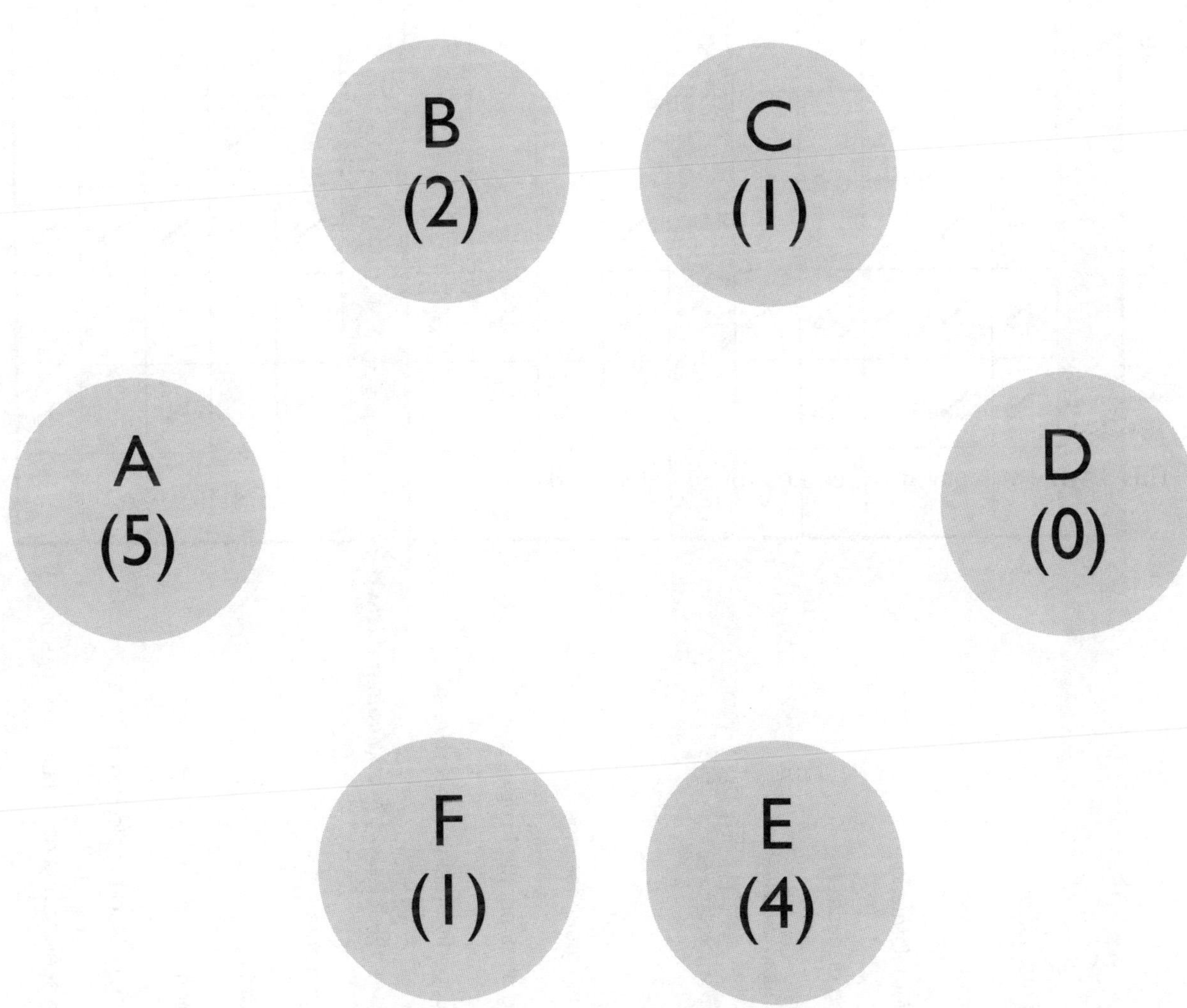

B
(2)
C
(1)
A
(5)
D
(0)
F
(1)
E
(4)

OHT 6.4.4 HANDOUT – USING TABLES TO REPORT OBSERVATIONAL DATA

Tables and grids can be used to report observational data. This table is adapted from OHT 2.3.1 and shows how summary data can be presented.

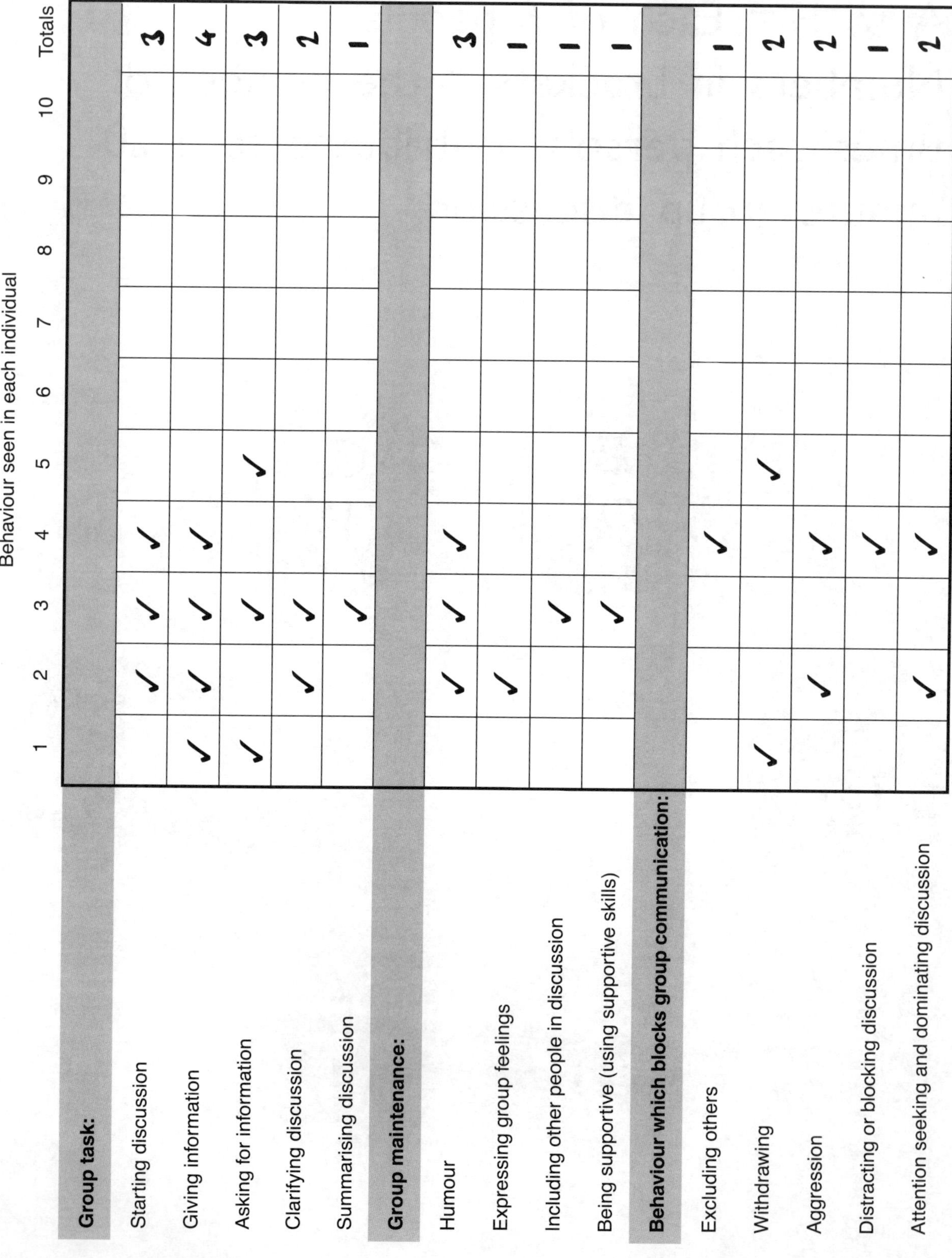

	Behaviour seen in each individual: 1	2	3	4	5	6	7	8	9	10	Totals
Group task:											
Starting discussion		✓	✓	✓							3
Giving information	✓	✓	✓	✓							4
Asking for information	✓		✓		✓						3
Clarifying discussion		✓	✓								2
Summarising discussion			✓								1
Group maintenance:											
Humour		✓	✓	✓							3
Expressing group feelings		✓									1
Including other people in discussion			✓								1
Being supportive (using supportive skills)			✓								1
Behaviour which blocks group communication:											
Excluding others				✓							1
Withdrawing	✓				✓						2
Aggression		✓		✓							2
Distracting or blocking discussion				✓							1
Attention seeking and dominating discussion		✓		✓							2

OHT 6.4.5 HANDOUT – USING TABLES TO SUMMARISE RATING SCALES

Barriers in the environment	**Rating scale**				
Lighting	1	2	3	4	5
Results on lighting (from a sample of 10 people)	4 40%	1 10%	1 10%	2 20%	2 20%
Noise levels	1	2	3	4	5
Results on noise levels	2 20%	1 10%	3 30%	4 40%	0 0%
Opportunity to communicate	1	2	3	4	5
Results on opportunity to communicate	1 10%	2 20%	3 30%	0 0%	4 40%
You can adapt any rating scale you use to record the results. Part of Activity 2.4.1 is shown above with totals from observational research added in.					

OHT 6.4.6 HANDOUT – SUMMARY SHEETS FOR QUESTIONS

The table shows how structured questions might be reported using percentages of respondents who agreed to create a summary sheet.

Attitudes towards grandparenting[1], 1998 (Great Britain)

Attitudes	Percentages			
	Respondent			
	Grand-parent	Grand-child	Linking parent	All[2]
With so many working mothers, families need grandparents to help more and more	79	72	74	74
People today don't place enough value on the part grandparents play in family life	50	50	51	51
Many parents today do not appreciate the help that grandparents give	40	31	41	41
In most families, grandparents should be closely involved in deciding how their grandchildren are brought up	24	19	16	20
Grandparents tend to interfere too much with the way their grandchildren are brought up	9	10	8	11
Grandparents have little to teach the grandchildren of today	13	8	6	9

[1]Percentage aged 18 and over who agreed with each statement.
[2]Includes respondents who do not fall into the first three categories.

Source: British Social Attitudes Survey, National Centre for Social Research, *Social Trends 2001*

OHT 6.4.7 HANDOUT – USING BAR CHARTS

Bar charts (also known as histograms) are a popular way of displaying information.

Pupils achieving five or more GCSE grades A* to C or equivalent[1]: by parents' socio-economic group, 1989 and 2000, England and Wales

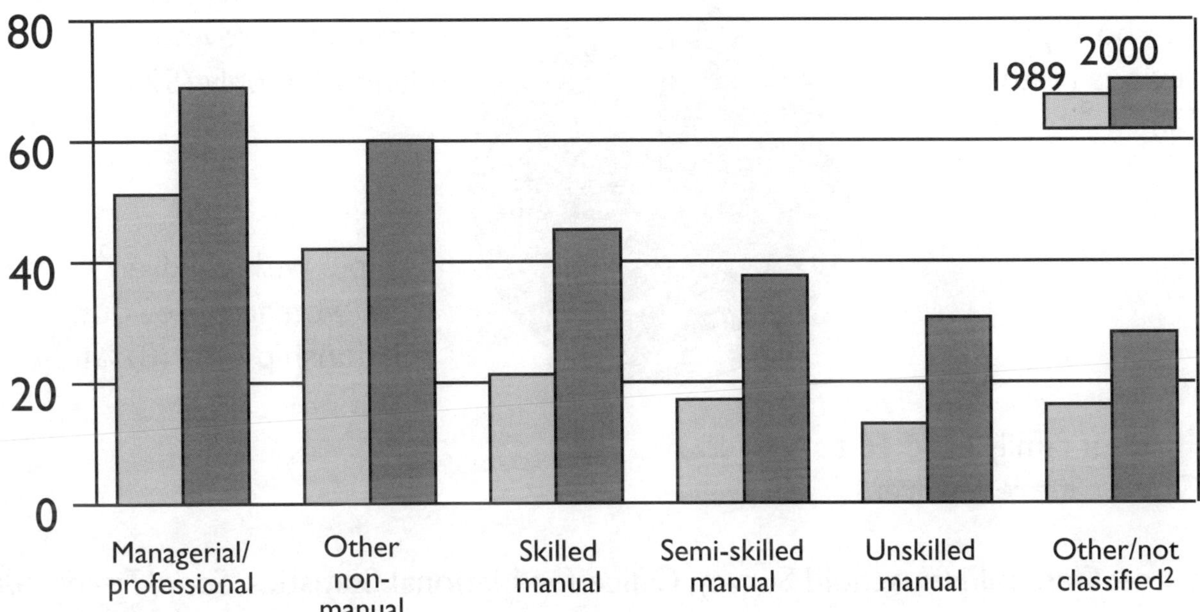
Percentages
80
60
40
20
0
1989
2000
Managerial/ professional
Other non-manual
Skilled manual
Semi-skilled manual
Unskilled manual
Other/not classified2

[1] Includes equivalent GNVQ qualifications achieved in Year 11.
[2] Includes a high percentage of respondents who had neither parent in a full-time job.

Source: Youth Cohort Study, Department for Education and Employment, *Social Trends 2001*

OHT 6.4.8 HANDOUT – USING PIE CHARTS

The pie chart illustrated below is another popular way of showing proportions that exist within a data set

Stepfamilies[1] with dependent children[2]: by family type, 1998–99, Great Britain

Percentages

Couple with children[2] from both partners' previous relationship (7%)

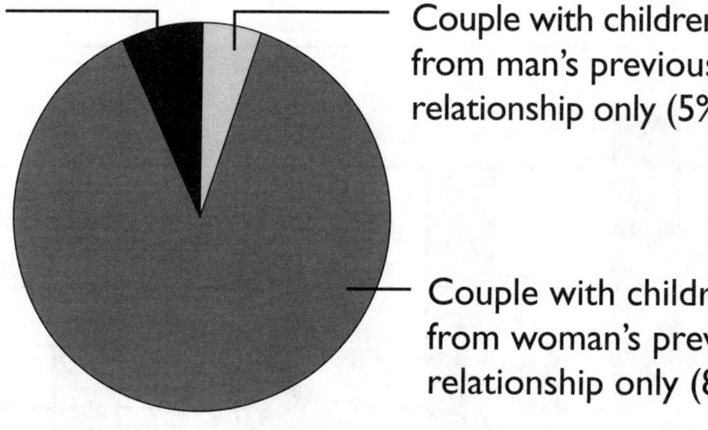

Couple with children[2] from man's previous relationship only (5%)

Couple with children[2] from woman's previous relationship only (87%)

[1] Head of family aged 16 to 59.
[2] One or more children.

Source: General Household Survey, Office for National Statistics, *Social Trends 2001*

OHT 6.4.9 HANDOUT – USING LINE GRAPHS

Line graphs are often used to show relationships over time between variables.

Achievement at GCSE A level or equivalent[1]: by gender, United Kingdom

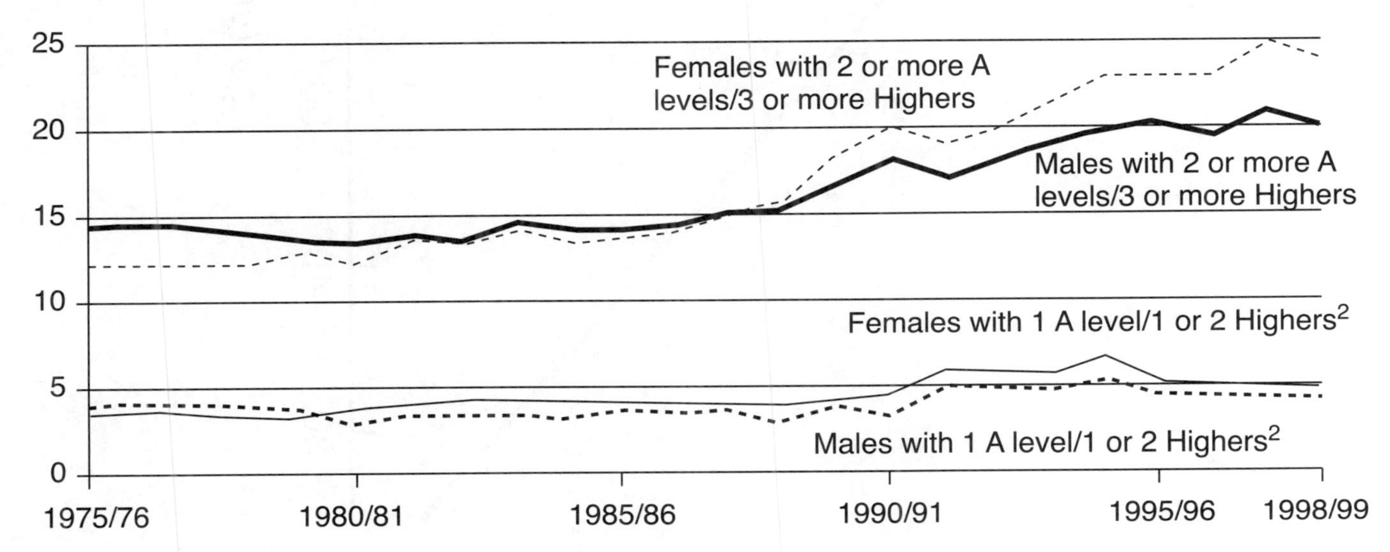

Percentages
25
20
15
10
5
0
Females with 2 or more A levels/3 or more Highers
Males with 2 or more A levels/3 or more Highers
Females with 1 A level/1 or 2 Highers²
Males with 1 A level/1 or 2 Highers²
1975/76
1980/81
1985/86
1990/91
1995/96
1998/99

[1]Based on population aged 17 at the start of the academic year. Data to 1990/91 (1991/92 in Northern Ireland) relate to school leavers. From 1991/92 data relate to any age for Great Britain while school performance data are used in Northern Ireland from 1992/93. Figures exclude sixth form colleges in England and Wales which were reclassified as FE colleges from 1 April 1993. Excludes GNVQ Advanced qualifications throughout.

[2]From 1996/97, figures only include two SCE Highers.

Source: Department for Education and Employment; National Assembly for Wales; Scottish Executive; Northern Ireland Department of Education, *Social Trends 2001*

OHT 6.4.10 HANDOUT – USING SCATTERGRAMS

Scattergrams give a visual impression of relationships within data by showing patterns that emerge when data points are plotted.

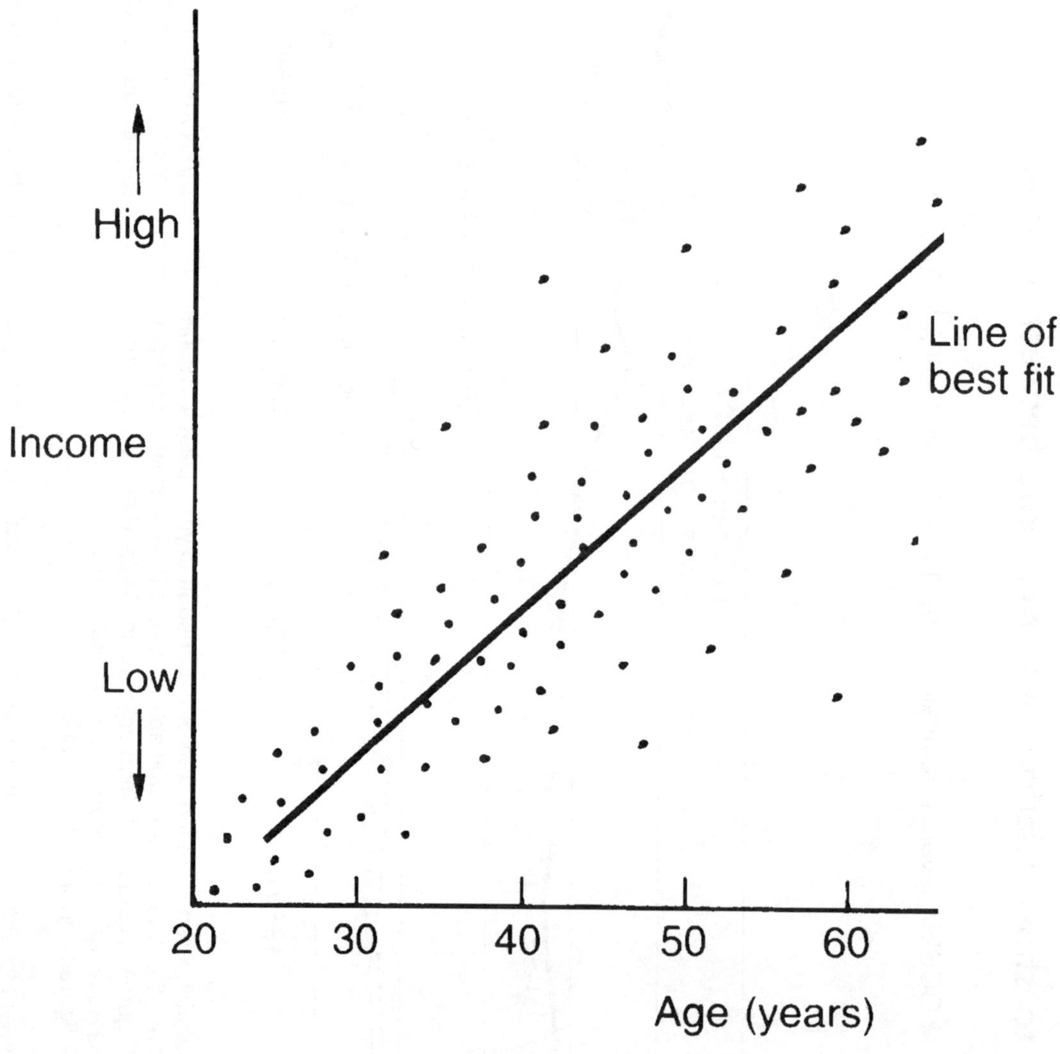

High
Income
Low
Line of best fit
20
30
40
50
60
Age (years)

OHT 6.4.11 HANDOUT – INVENTING DIAGRAMS TO MAKE YOUR POINT

It can be worth being creative and trying to display processes or procedures that you have become aware of. The diagram below is a flow diagram which shows causes and the influences on the outcome of a group.

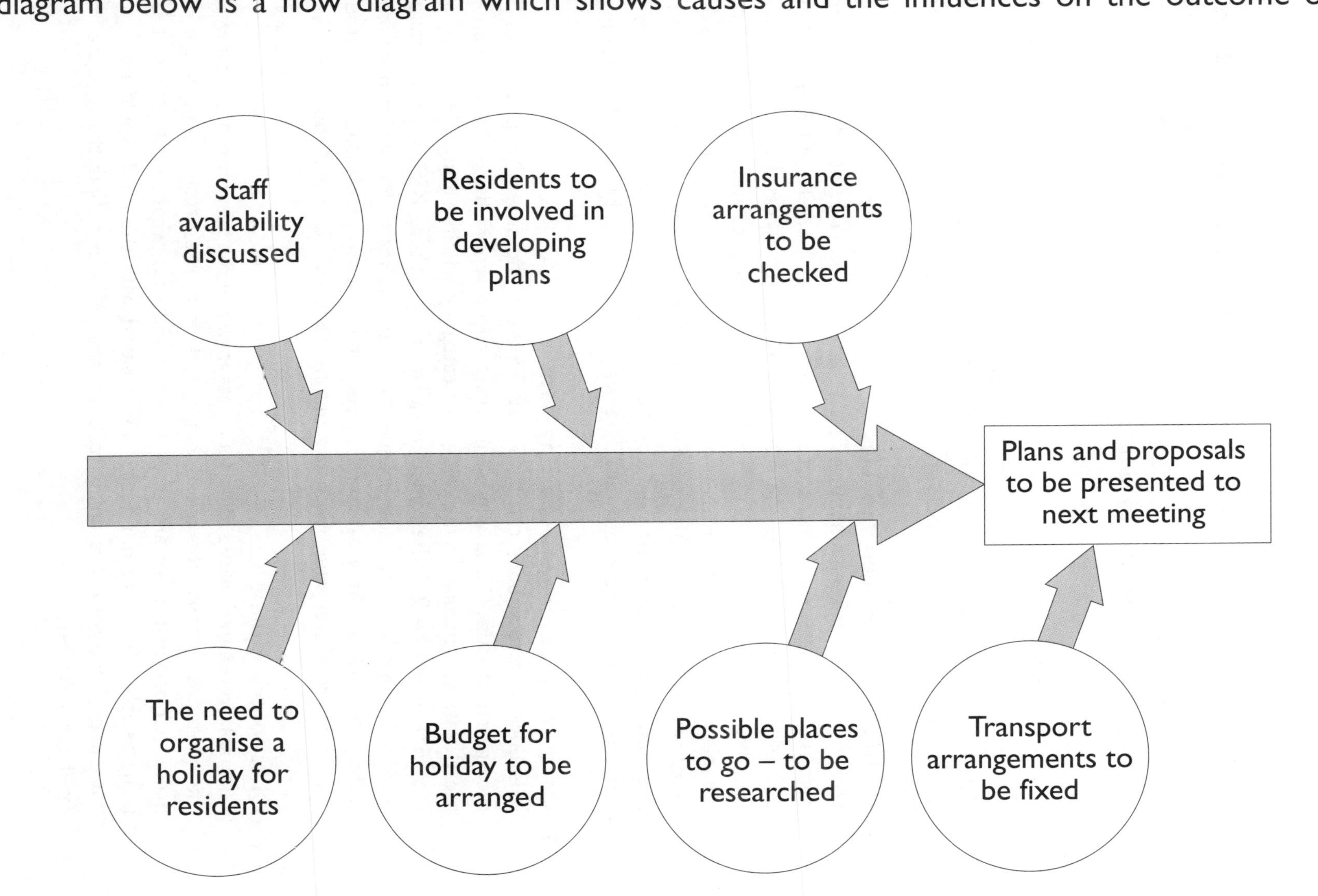

Staff availability discussed
Residents to be involved in developing plans
Insurance arrangements to be checked
The need to organise a holiday for residents
Budget for holiday to be arranged
Possible places to go – to be researched
Transport arrangements to be fixed
Plans and proposals to be presented to next meeting

OHT 6.4.12 HANDOUT – ANSWERS TO ACTIVITY 6.4.1

1 **Bar graphs**
The scale has being cut off on this graph to give the impression of large differences when in fact the differences are quite small. This is a biased way of presenting information to make it look more significant than it really is.

2 **Line graphs**
There is no data which suggests that it is reasonable to extend a trend from only two points. The trend displayed is called an extrapolation. In this situation it is unreasonable to extrapolate from the data provided in the graph. Trends should only be projected when there is a large amount of information to suggest that a trend is reasonable.

3 **Pie charts**
When there are only a few people it is unreasonable to present this information as percentages in a pie chart. The conclusion is completely unreasonable; a sample of just three people will be too small to enable generalisable conclusions to be made. It is inappropriate to use pie charts for such a small sample.

4 **Relationships between variables**
Looking at how different measures relate to each other is called correlation. Just because two measures relate to each other (or are 'correlated') does not mean that one of the variables causes the other. The rule is that 'correlation never proves causality'. The conclusions about cold weather leading to the death of older people are completely unjustified. There is probably a common factor that is associated with the weather and with the death rate. For example, there may be more flu and respiratory infections about during the cold weather. Flu and respiratory infections may be the cause of the increased death rate. The weather may not be directly responsible.

5 **Using the mean when reporting data**
It is obvious that nobody can have 1.66 brothers and sisters! It is inappropriate to average some data. This is why some researchers report using the **median** rather than the **mean**. The median is the mid-point category within a range. Here the median category would be 2 – the midpoint of the range. There is also a term called the **mode**. The mode is the most frequently occurring term in a series of numbers. In the series it would not be very useful to report that two people had no brothers and sisters whereas everyone else had a number between one and four.

6 **Questionnaire data**
The table presented allows only four categories, three of which are positive. By asking the questions this way the questionnaire is biased. The presentation of the questions makes it clear that there are three positive and one negative categories. It is likely that many people who were not really very pleased with the food would have opted for the 'satisfactory' category. It is unfair to claim that 90% of people thought that the food was satisfactory or better.

OHT 6.5.1 HANDOUT – ANSWERS TO ACTIVITY 6.5.2

INTERVIEW 1

The first interview represents a series of closed questions. It is never appropriate to ask a series of closed questions in a research interview. The focus of the interview is not particularly clear. The informant has given very little information and the interview has a jerky and unpleasant feel to it. When preparing to interview it is a good idea to follow the guideline that 'every closed question should start as an open one!' This interview should have used a range of open questions. These questions might lead in to a specific closed question.

INTERVIEW 2

This second interview is an example of a biased interview. The way the interviewer asks questions leads the informant to agree with their line of thinking. There are many leading questions.

IMPROVING A BIASED INTERVIEW

Questions should be asked in an unbiased way. The outline below provides an example of a balanced interview.

Balanced interview

Interviewer: So how did you feel when you were made redundant?

Informant: Well, I was shocked at first. It was unexpected, but then I thought, well, when one door shuts, another one opens.

Interviewer: Could you explain about the doors – I didn't really understand.

Informant: Yes, I was upset, but then I thought well, I've just got to find another job – there must be something.

Interviewer: So what did you do then?

Informant: Well, I went to the job centre and all that, but then a friend said that there was this job going at the home where she worked and she wondered whether I could do that kind of job.

Interviewer: So how do you feel now?

Informant: Oh well, now I've found this work I'm really happy. I look back on the redundancy and I think – best thing that ever happened to me.

OHT 6.5.2 HANDOUT – ANSWERS TO ACTIVITY 6.5.3

If this had been a formal structured interview it would have been important to organise the questions more carefully. Questions might have been structured so that open questions funnelled into specific or closed questions that needed clear answers. The questions are not sufficiently clearly organised in order to collect useful data across a sample of interviewees. In this situation the informant had some problems working out what to say.

In a formal structured interview the researcher should have prepared fixed probes and prompts that might be used to follow up their questions. The student has invented their own supplementary questions in order to keep the interview going. If this happens during structured interview research different informants will give quite different responses to the structured interview – because of the different questions.

The transcripts contain no evidence of a warm up or conclusion to the interview. It would be good practice to introduce the purpose of the interview and guarantee anonymity and confidentiality before the interview begins. It would also be good practice to thank the informant for their time at the end of the interview.

OHT 6.5.3 HANDOUT – AN ETHICAL ISSUES CHECKLIST

Questions to help check the ethical nature of research proposals
• What is the stated purpose of the research – are there any biased assumptions in this purpose?
• What sampling methods have been chosen and what assumptions are involved in the choice of sampling and methods? How will conclusions be restricted by the choice of sampling methods?
• Have questions that will be asked been checked for cultural assumptions which may bias people's responses?
• Have questions that will be asked been checked for technical problems which may bias people's responses?
• Will every person who may be involved in the research be given a clear and honest explanation of what the research is about?
• Will every person who may be involved in the research be given a real choice as to whether to participate in the research or not? How will consent be obtained?
• Is the project free of any form of deception?
• How will people's rights to confidentiality be protected? Is there a statement about confidentiality that is given or read out to participants?
• Is there anything about the research project which might threaten the physical or emotional safety of participants?
• Is there any possibility that any participant might be disadvantaged because they take part in the research?
• How will the project safeguard clients' rights as set out in the care value base?
• Will methods chosen to present the project provide a clear and accurate account of findings; will presentation methods be free of bias?

ACTIVITY 6.2.1 CHOOSING THE BEST RESEARCH METHOD

This activity is about choosing research methods in different research situations. It involves thinking about the strengths and weaknesses of each main research method if it were to be applied in a range of different research situations. Remember that the reasons for *not* using a particular method are just as important here as the reasons for choosing another. Thinking about how research may have been affected by the use of different research methods is one of the criteria for higher grades in this unit.

TASK 1

In the scenarios you will be given (OHT 6.2.7) are brief descriptions of different research situations. Each situation has a different research population and different aims for the research. Your task is to decide which research method, or combination of methods, the researchers should use.

The research methods that could be used are:

- Experiment
- Questionnaires
- Structured interviews
- In-depth interviews
- Direct observation
- Participant observation

1 Read carefully through each research situation and think about the problems and opportunities it presents to researchers. Also, think about the researchers themselves and the resources they have available to them.

2 Next think about how each of the research methods listed above could be applied to the research situations. What are the advantages and disadvantages of using each method in the research situations? While doing this think about:

   - The type of data the researchers intend to collect.
   - The characteristics of the research population.
   - The resources that the researchers have available to them.

3 Make a record of your thinking, showing the advantages and disadvantages of each method. A table, such as the one provided (OHT 6.2.8), can be used for this. Complete a table for each of the research situations. Your tables should contain comments on the advantages and disadvantages of each of the research methods. Even if it seems obvious that a particular method will not work, or that one method stands out as the best one to use, make sure that you note down why this is the case.

4 Decide which research method seems to be the most appropriate, taking into account all the pros and cons you have identified. Note your result on the form, and write a short explanation of your final decision. You may well decide that a combination of methods would get the best results. This is often how researchers work. If so, explain how the methods would work together to produce the results you are looking for.

5 Write down the resources that your chosen method will require. These could include things like questionnaire forms, structured interview schedules, or observation checklists.

ACTIVITY 6.2.1 (CONTINUED)

TASK 2

Each of the research projects described in the scenarios could make use of secondary data. Look again at each scenario and answer the following questions.

1 What type of secondary data is needed, or would be helpful, taking into account the aims of the research and the population it is concerned with?

2 Where could the researchers obtain the secondary data you have suggested?

3 How would the secondary data you have suggested support and complement the primary research work?

ACTIVITY 6.3.1 WHAT IS WRONG WITH THIS QUESTIONNAIRE?

Badly designed questionnaires will fail to gain any worthwhile information and may also fail to be ethical.

Almost everything is wrong with the questionnaire set out below. A questionnaire like this would fail to collect useful information, it is biased and it might even offend some respondents. A questionnaire like this should never be used in practice. Can you detect what is wrong with this questionnaire and explain what the problems are with the way questions are worded and laid out?

Questionnaire on working in Health and Social Care

1 Please answer the following questions – your answers will be discussed with other people to help understand attitudes about working in care.

2 Please state your Name ....

Please state your Job Title..

Please give the name and address of the organisation you work for ....

....

3 What is it like to work in your job? Would you say it was (a) very interesting, (b) interesting, (c) tiring or (d) very tiring?

4 Would you agree that your work is enjoyable?

5 How many other people are employed by your organisation?

6 How much money do you get each week?

7 What would you say is the average social class of the clients that you work with?

8 Please rate how true or false the following statements are of the organisation that you work in. Please use the scale below:

True

Mainly true

Mainly false

False

(a) The work is very hard, but it is very interesting to do.

(b) I get on well with other staff members.

(c) Clients are sometimes abused by staff in my setting.

(d) I enjoy working with people but we are never paid enough.

ACTIVITY 6.4.1 PRESENTATION OF RESEARCH

What is wrong with the methods of presentation and the assumptions made in the diagrams below?

1 **Using bar graphs to show differences between variables**

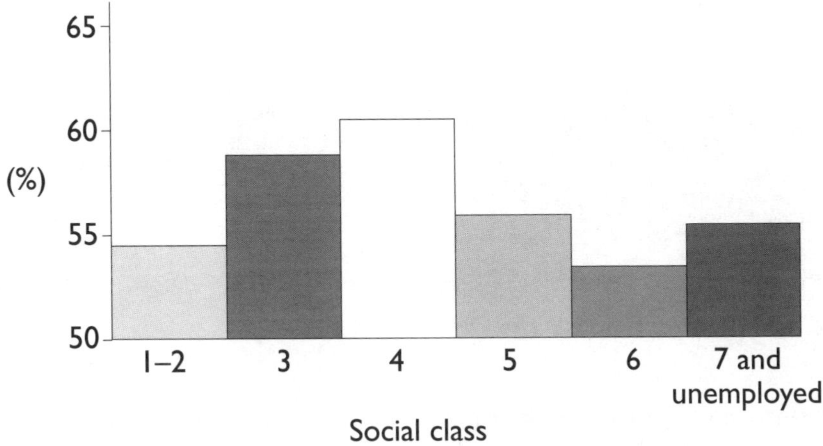
65
60
(%)
55
50
1–2
3
4
5
6
7 and unemployed
Social class

The graph above shows the dramatic differences that research found between the percentage of people in different social class groups who were willing to pay extra income tax in order to improve schools and hospitals.

2 **Using line graphs to display a trend**

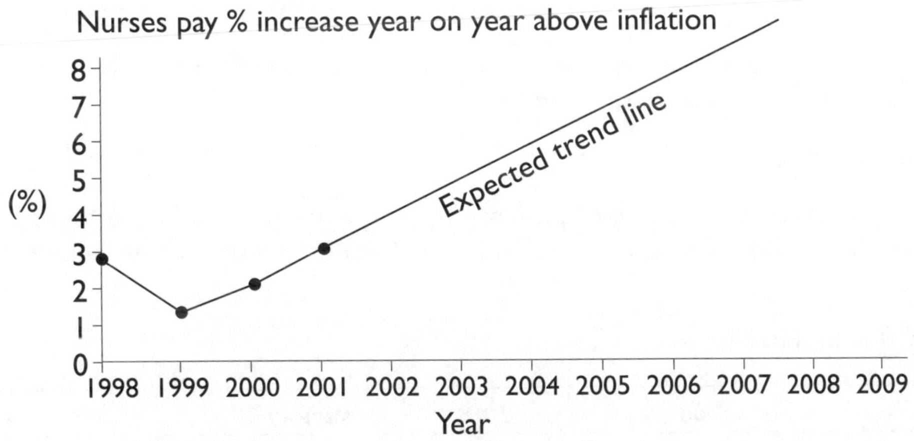
Nurses pay % increase year on year above inflation
8
7
6
5
(%)
4
3
2
1
0
Expected trend line
1998 1999 2000 2001 2002 2003 2004 2005 2006 2007 2008 2009
Year

The graph above shows how nurses' pay will increase in the next eight years

3 **Using pie charts to display information**

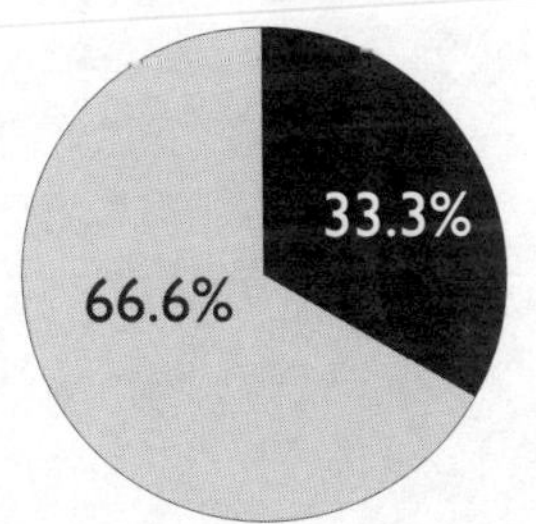
33.3%
66.6%

Our research interviewed three people about smoking. 66.6% of people interviewed said that they enjoyed smoking, this suggests that most people enjoy smoking.

ACTIVITY 6.4.1 PRESENTATION OF RESEARCH (CONTINUED)

4 **Displaying relationships between variables**

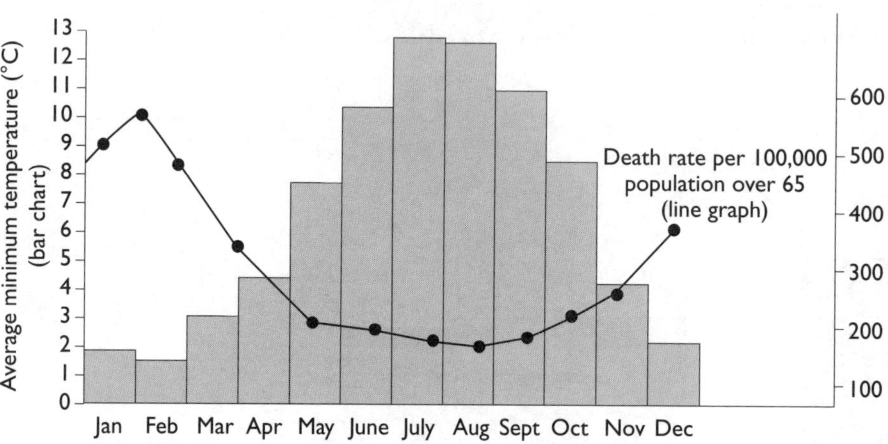
Average minimum temperature (°C) (bar chart)
13
12
11
10
9
8
7
6
5
4
3
2
1
0
Jan Feb Mar Apr May June July Aug Sept Oct Nov Dec
Death rate per 100,000 population over 65 (line graph)
600
500
400
300
200
100

As can be seen from the graphs, more 'older people' died when the weather was cold. Cold weather is clearly responsible for the deaths of many older people. Perhaps the government should do more to protect people from the cold.

5 **Using the mean when reporting data**

Person number	1	2	3	4	5	6
Number of brothers or sisters each person has	1	3	2	0	4	0

The table above shows that the average number of brothers and sisters in this group is 1.66. Each person has a mean number of 1.66 brothers and sisters.

6 **Interpreting questionnaire data**

A sample of 20 people were asked to give their opinions on the quality of food in the hospital. They were asked to rate the quality of food on a scale of four. Detailed results are set out in the table below.

The quality of food in this hospital is:

Statement	Very good	Good	Satisfactory	Bad
Number of responses	1	2	15	2

As can be seen, 90% of people thought that the food was satisfactory or better within the hospital.

ACTIVITY 6.4.2 CHOOSING METHODS OF PRESENTATION

Working in groups of two or three, study the table below. Using the handouts, OHTs 6.4.2–6.4.12, on presentational methods, decide on an alternative way of displaying the data in this table.

Percentage of dependent children[1] living in different family types (Great Britain)

Family types	Percentages			
	1972	1981	1991–92	2000[2]
Couple families				
1 child	16	18	17	17
2 children	35	41	37	38
3 or more children	41	29	28	26
Lone mother families				
1 child	2	3	5	6
2 children	2	4	7	7
3 or more children	2	3	6	6
Lone father families				
1 child	–	1	–	1
2 or more children	1	1	1	1
All dependent children[3]	100	100	100	100

[1]See Appendix, Part 2: Families.

[2]At Spring 2000.

[3]In Spring 2000, includes cases where the dependent child is a family unit, for example a foster child.

Source: General Household Survey and Labour Force Survey, Office for National Statistics, *Social Trends 2001*.

ACTIVITY 6.5.1 ETHICS AND EXPERIMENTATION

The importance of ethics in research might be highlighted with reference to real research. The summary below provides a brief outline of some famous research first published in 1963. It is very unlikely that this kind of research would be permitted today.

Obedience to Authority – Stanley Milgram's famous research

Stanley Milgram, a Professor in the USA, wanted to understand how far people were willing to obey authority figures. He set up an experiment which offered to pay volunteers for an hour of their time to help research memory and learning. When the volunteers arrived they met with an experimenter and with a second person who was introduced as another volunteer. The second person took the role of an actor – in fact really they were not a volunteer but pretending to be one, due to the need to deceive the real volunteer.

The real volunteer and the actor drew cards from a hat in order to decide which of them would be the teacher and which the learner in the experiment that they were to perform. The system was fixed so that the real volunteer always became the teacher.

The experiment involved electric shock apparatus. The actor was wired up to an electric shock generator and the real volunteer was asked to operate equipment which would deliver electric shocks to the actor. The real volunteer was given a small electric shock to convince them that the situation was real.

In reality the actor never received electric shocks – but the volunteer was led to believe that he or she were delivering ever increasing electric shocks to the other person. The real volunteer had to deliver a shock every time the actor made a mistake. These electric shocks increased by 15 volts each time. The experiment was designed so that the actor made lots of mistakes. In one experiment the actor banged on the wall at 300 volts and then after a shock of 315 volts everything went quiet – as if the person had become unconscious or died.

Milgram discovered that 65% of the volunteers were prepared to keep giving shocks up to 415 volts (a point where the other person might have died if the experiment had been real). In one of Milgram's experiments the actor was asked to cry out at 120 volts and refuse to continue at 150 volts, however the actor remained wired to the apparatus and volunteers were told to continue the experiment. Volunteers were told statements such as 'The experiment requires you to continue' or 'You have no other choice you must go on'. Under these conditions 62.5% of the volunteers gave shocks up to 450 volts.

While the volunteers were pressured to continue to give electric shocks many of them showed signs of nervousness, sweating, trembling, biting their lips, and so on. One real volunteer suffered a convulsive fit during the experiment.

All the volunteers were debriefed after the experiment and discovered that they hadn't really harmed anyone. The volunteers were sent questionnaires a year later to try and check that they had not suffered long-term emotional harm.

QUESTIONS

If this kind of experiment were to be done nowadays, it would raise serious ethical problems.

In groups of two or three, work out exactly what the ethical issues might be, by discussing questions such as these:

1 Do you believe that peoples' rights would be infringed in any way? If so what rights may be infringed?

2 Do you believe that there could be any risk of harm to the volunteers' self-esteem or emotional well-being?

3 Does the deception involved in this kind of experiment breach ethical principles or could it be acceptable?

4 Can you explain why it is important to check even simple interviews and questionnaires for ethical issues before using them with other people.

ACTIVITY 6.5.2 INTERVIEWING

Explain what is wrong in the following two interviews.

INTERVIEW 1

Interviewer: How long have you worked here?

Informant: 12 years.

Interviewer: Do you like it here?

Informant: Yes.

Interviewer: If you had the chance would you like to work with children?

Informant: Yes.

Interviewer: Do you get paid well?

Informant: No.

Interviewer: Do you think it's a good job?

Informant: Not really.

Interviewer: Anything else you would like to say?

Informant: No!

INTERVIEW 2

Interviewer: So was it terrible when you were made redundant?

Informant: Well, in a way I suppose it was.

Interviewer: What was the worst thing about it?

Informant: Well, it was the shock – one minute everything was going OK and the next minute – I'd lost my job.

Interviewer: Did you feel sad and angry about that?

Informant: Yes, I suppose I did at the time.

Interviewer So were you treated unfairly?

Informant: Yes, that's right, I did feel it was unfair.

How should the questions have been asked in the second interview?

ACTIVITY 6.5.3 CRITIQUING AN INTERVIEW

A student prepared the following questions to ask a care worker on placement. A transcript of the interview that followed from these questions is provided below. If the student had been trying to design a structured interview what changes would be necessary to the planning and practice of this interview?

PLANNED QUESTIONS

Career routes

- Could you tell me how long you have worked as a senior care worker?
- What work did you do before this?
- Why did you decide to work in social care in the first place?
- Would you like promotion? What other jobs could you go on to?

Day-to-day work

- What hours do you normally have to work?
- What does your work with clients involve?
- Please could you describe how you work with other staff, for example do you work as a team, with people of the same or other disciplines?

Stereotypes of role

- Do you think there is a stereotype of people who work with older people? If there is, could you tell me about it?

THE INTERVIEW

Interviewer: Could you tell me what hours you have to work?

Carer: Yes, a 39-hour week.

Interviewer: Oh, I see – but what about shifts?

Carer: Oh, you want to know about times of the day. Well, they change from week to week. I do early mornings through to 2 pm some weeks and then afternoons and later on other weeks. Shall I show you the rota?

Interviewer: Oh, that's OK, I really just wanted to learn about the kind of work that you do – what does your work with clients involve?

Carer: Well, physical care, emotional care, everything really.

Interviewer: Could you tell me about a typical day at work?

Carer: Yes – take yesterday… [*The senior carer gives a full description of yesterday's work events.*]

Interviewer: Thanks, that was really helpful. I can understand what the job involves now. Could you tell me about working with other staff?

Carer: Yes – do you mean how do I get on with them?

Interviewer: Well, what work do you have to do?

ACTIVITY 6.5.3 CRITIQUING AN INTERVIEW (CONTINUED)

Carer: Ah well, I'll show you my job description. I'll get you a copy of it. Basically, I do everything. I have to hold the home when the manager and assistant manager aren't here. I have to know all the residents and I'm responsible for the care-plan records.

Interviewer: What does 'hold the home' mean?

Carer: That I'm in charge. I have to take over and make decisions until the manager returns.

Interviewer: That sounds like a lot of work.

Carer: It is! I feel exhausted at the end of the day. I really wonder if it's all worth it sometimes.

[*The Interviewer hasn't looked at his notes and can't remember what to ask next so he quickly thinks of something.*]

Interviewer: Why did you come into care work, I mean, why did you choose it in the first place?

Carer: Now that's a difficult one! Let's see, well, I suppose I'd always enjoyed looking after people. I used to look after my gran you know, and when a job as a care assistant came up I went for it.

Interviewer: So you worked as a care assistant first?

Carer: Yes, for eight years, then I did an in-service course at college one day a week. After that I became a senior care worker. I've worked for four years as a senior care worker.

Interviewer: What's an in-service course?

Carer: Oh, it's a certificate for a one-year part-time course. It's not run any longer. We did three assignments and a couple of residential courses in a hotel. You have to achieve an 80 per cent attendance rate. It was great fun, I enjoyed it.

[*The Interviewer forgets what he was going to ask and can't check with his notes in time; but he keeps the conversation going.*]

Interviewer: Umm, do you think there are stereotypes of people who work with older people?

Carer: Well, I expect so, what do you really want to know?

Interviewer: Well, I just thought that the work you do might not be how relatives and the public imagine it.

Carer: Right, that's absolutely right. A lot of people imagine it's all serving tea to nice old ladies and sitting around having chats. Well, you've seen what it's like – you never sit down, or if you do you can't stand up again; and that's just the easy bit. All the paperwork, the phone calls, it never used to be so bad.

Interviewer: Why has it become more difficult?

Carer: Well, more regulations, more work – like care plans – but fewer staff to do the work and the clients are much more demanding. When I started, only six or seven residents had dementia, now most of them do.

Interviewer: I guess I'm running out of time, but could I just ask about career routes? Would you like promotion? What jobs could you go on to?

Carer: Oh, I don't think I'd want to be a manager – no, life's hard enough, but some people go on to management. It helps if you can get the right qualifications – there are Diplomas in Management Studies, HNCs, a City and Guilds Management qualification.

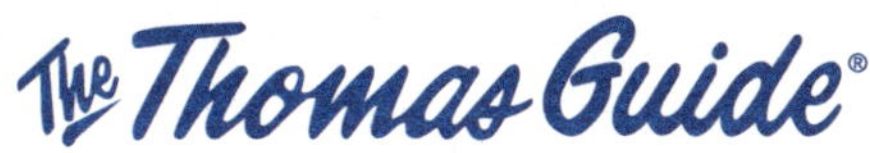
The Thomas Guide®

Y0-DOI-493

Easy-to-Read Santa Barbara & San Luis Obispo Counties street guide

TELL US WHAT YOU THINK

comment card on last page

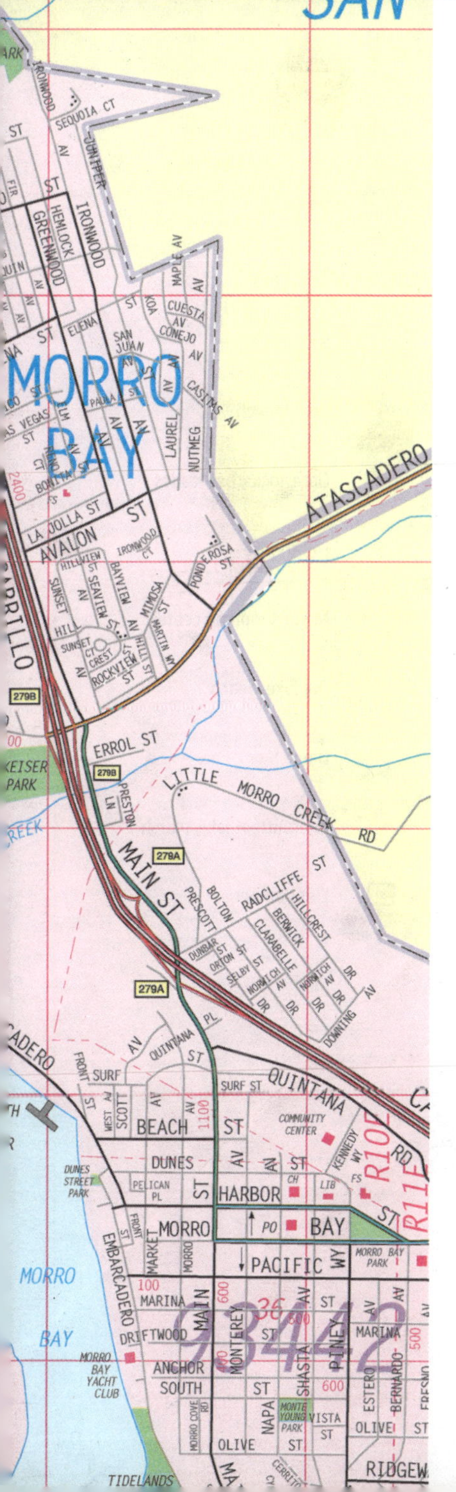
MORRO BAY
ATASCADERO
MAIN ST
LITTLE MORRO CREEK RD
ERROL ST
QUINTANA
BEACH
HARBOR
MORRO
PACIFIC
MARINA
DRIFTWOOD
ANCHOR
SOUTH
OLIVE
EMBARCADERO
MORRO BAY YACHT CLUB
MORRO BAY PARK
MONTE YOUNG PARK
COMMUNITY CENTER
DUNES STREET PARK
KEISER PARK
93442

Contents

Introduction

Using Your Street Guide	A
PageFinder™ Map	B
Legend	D
We've Got You Covered	E

Maps

Downtown Map	F
Street Guide Detail Maps	453-1018
Vicinity Map	Inside back cover

Lists and Indexes

Cities & Communities Index	1019
List of Abbreviations	1020
Street Index and Points of Interest Index	1021
Comment Card	Last page

PageFinder™ Map U.S. Patent No. 5,419,586
Canadian Patent No. 2,116,425
Patente Mexicana No. 188186

Published in U.S.A. Printed in U.S.A.

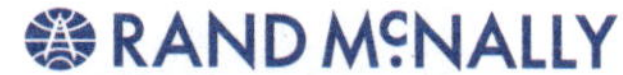
RAND McNALLY

Rand McNally Consumer Affairs
P.O. Box 7600
Chicago, IL 60680-9915
randmcnally.com
For comments or suggestions, please call (800) 777-MAPS (-6277)
or email us at:
consumeraffairs@randmcnally.com

Legend

Freeway
Interchange/ramp
Highway
Primary road
Secondary road
Minor road
Restricted road
Alley
Unpaved road
Tunnel
Toll road
High occupancy vehicle lane
Stacked multiple roadways
Proposed road
Proposed freeway
Freeway under construction
One-way road
Two-way road
Trail, walkway
Stairs
Railroad
Rapid transit
Rapid transit, underground

Ferry
City boundary
County boundary
State boundary
International boundary
Military base, Indian reservation
Township, range, rancho
River, creek, shoreline
98607 ZIP code boundary, ZIP code
5 Interstate
5 Interstate (Business)
3 U.S. highway
1 4 8 9 State highways
Carpool lane
A Street list marker
Street name continuation
Street name change
Station (train, bus)
Building (see List of Abbreviations page)
Building footprint
Public elementary school
Public high school

Private elementary school
Private high school
Fire station
Library
Mission
Winery
Campground
H Hospital
Mountain
Section corner
Boat launch
Gate, locks, barricades
Lighthouse
Major shopping center
Dry lake, beach
Dam
Intermittent lake, marsh
29 Exit number

we've got you COVERED

Rand McNally's broad selection of products is perfect for your every need. Whether you're looking for the convenience of write-on wipe-off laminated maps, extra maps for every car, or a Road Atlas to plan your next vacation or to use as a reference, Rand McNally has you covered.

Street Guides

- Los Angeles & Orange Counties
- Los Angeles & Orange Counties - Pro Series Laminated Edition
- Los Angeles & San Bernardino Counties
- Los Angeles & Ventura Counties
- Los Angeles County
- Los Angeles County - Easy to Read
- Orange County
- Orange County - Easy to Read
- Riverside & Orange Counties
- Riverside & San Diego Counties
- Riverside County
- Riverside County - Easy to Read
- San Bernardino & Riverside Counties
- San Bernardino & Riverside Counties - Pro Series Laminated Edition
- San Bernardino County
- San Bernardino County - Easy to Read
- San Diego & Orange Counties
- San Diego County
- Santa Barbara & San Luis Obispo Counties - Easy to Read
- Santa Barbara, San Luis Obispo & Ventura Counties - Easy to Read
- Ventura County - Easy to Read

Folded Maps

EasyFinder Laminated Maps:

- Los Angeles & Vicinity
- Los Angeles to San Diego Regional
- Los Angeles/ Hollywood
- Palm Springs
- Pomona/Ontario
- Riverside
- San Diego
- San Diego & Vicinity
- Southern California
- West LA/ Santa Monica

Paper Maps:

- Anaheim/ Fullerton
- Hemet/ Perris
- Lancaster/ Palmdale
- Long Beach/ Carson/ Torrance
- Los Angeles
- Los Angeles & Vicinity
- Moreno Valley/ Banning
- North San Diego/ Encinitas
- Oceanside/ Escondido
- Ontario/ Pomona
- Orange County, Central
- Orange County, Northern
- Orange County, Southern
- Palm Springs/ Desert Cities
- River Cities
- Riverside
- San Bernardino/ Fontana
- San Diego
- San Fernando Valley
- San Gabriel Valley/ Pasadena
- Santa Clarita Valley
- Southern California Freeways
- Temecula/ Murrieta
- Thousand Oaks/ Simi Valley
- Ventura/ Oxnard
- Victorville/ Barstow

Wall Maps

- California State
- Southern California Arterial

Road Atlases

- California Road Atlas
- Road Atlas
- Road Atlas & Travel Guide
- Large Scale Road Atlas
- Midsize Road Atlas
- Deluxe Midsize Road Atlas
- Pocket Road Atlas

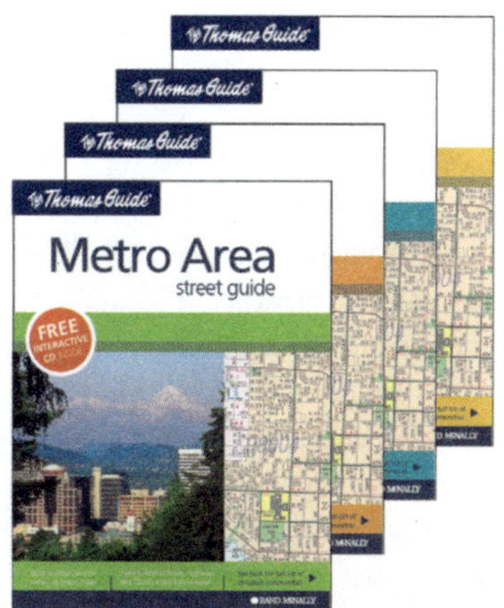
Thomas Guide
Metro Area
street guide
FREE

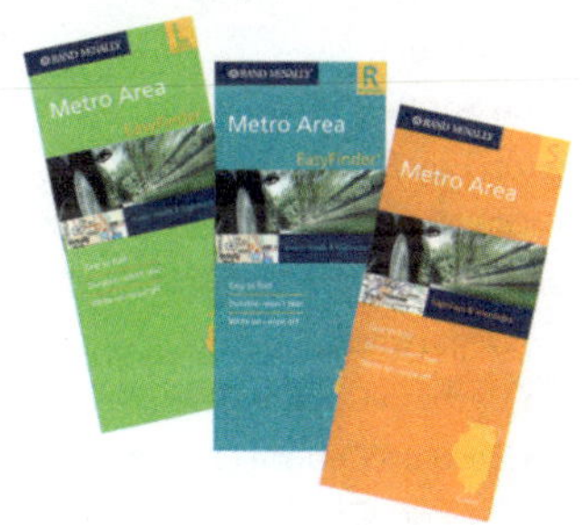
Metro Area
Metro Area
Metro Area

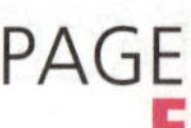
PAGE
F

Downtown Santa Barbara

Points of Interest

1	Amtrak Santa Barbara Station	D5
2	Arlington Theatre	B3
3	Bus Station	B4
4	Casa De Covarrubias & Lugo Adobe	C4
5	Casa De La Guerra	C4
6	City Public Works	D4
7	County Welfare Department	C4
8	De La Guerra Plaza	C4
9	El Presidio De Santa Barbara State Historic Park	C4
10	Fernald Mansion & Trussell-Winchester Adobe	C6
11	Granada Theater	B4
12	Guardhouse & Miranda Adobe	C4
13	Hastings Adobe	C6
14	Historical Society Museum	C4
15	Lobero Theater	C4
16	Mission Santa Barbara	A1
17	Moreton Bay Fig Tree	C5
18	Museum of Art	B4
19	Museum of Natural History	A1
20	Police Department	C3
21	Santa Barbara County Bowl	C2
22	Santa Barbara Central Library	B4
23	Santa Barbara City Hall	C4
24	Santa Barbara Co Adminstration & Board of Supervisors	B3
25	Santa Barbara County Courthouse	B3
26	Santa Barbara Harbor	D7
27	Santa Barbara News - Press	C4
28	Stearns Wharf	E6
29	Upham Hotel	A4
30	Victoria Court	B4
31	Visitors & Convention Bureau	C4
32	Visitors Center	D5
33	Waterfront Department	D7

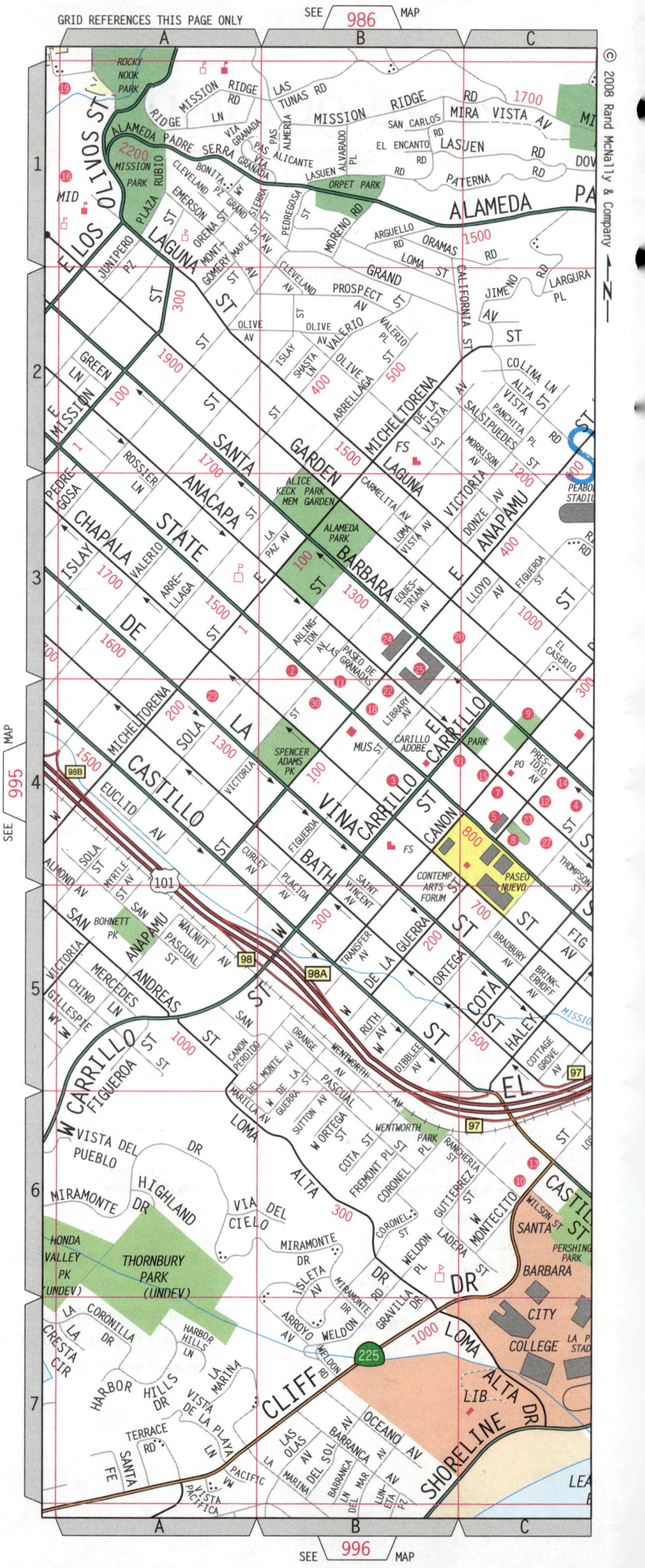

Map Scale

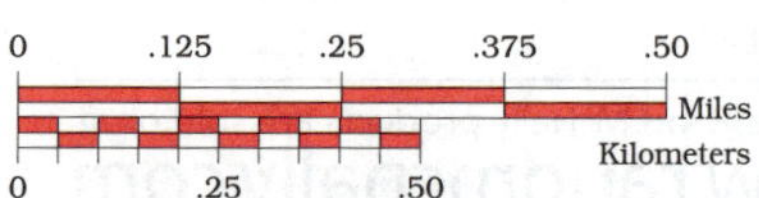
0
.125
.25
.375
.50
Miles
Kilometers
0
.25
.50

GRID REFERENCES THIS PAGE ONLY

SEE 986 MAP

SEE 995 MAP

SEE 996 MAP

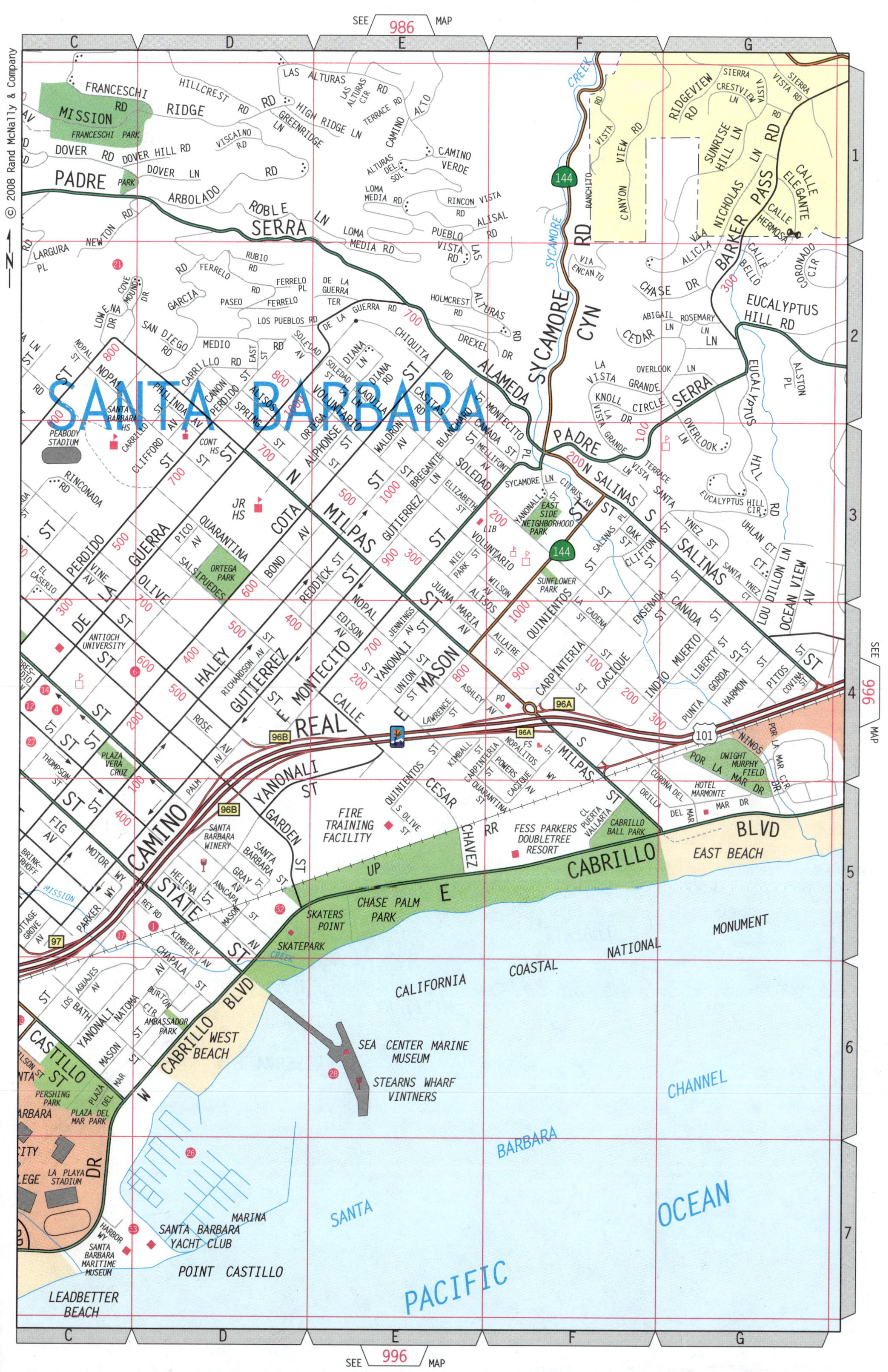

SEE 986 MAP
SEE 996 MAP
© 2008 Rand McNally & Company
SANTA BARBARA
MISSION
FRANCESCHI PARK
FRANCESCHI RD
HILLCREST RD
RIDGE RD
LAS ALTURAS RD
HIGH RIDGE LN
GREENRIDGE LN
DOVER RD
DOVER HILL RD
DOVER LN
PADRE
ARBOLADO RD
ROBLE LN
SERRA
LOMA MEDIA RD
PUEBLO VISTA RD
ALISAL RD
RINCON VISTA RD
CAMINO VERDE
SYCAMORE CYN RD
SYCAMORE CREEK
RIDGEVIEW RD
SUNRISE HILL LN
NICHOLAS LN
BARKER PASS RD
CALLE ELEGANTE
EUCALYPTUS HILL RD
CHASE DR
ALAMEDA PADRE SERRA
SANTA BARBARA HS
PEABODY STADIUM
JR HS
ORTEGA PARK
EAST SIDE NEIGHBORHOOD PARK
SUNFLOWER PARK
DE LA GUERRA
GUERRA ST
COTA ST
MILPAS ST
SALINAS ST
VOLUNTARIO ST
QUINIENTOS ST
CARPINTERIA ST
MASON ST
HALEY ST
GUTIERREZ ST
MONTECITO ST
ANTIOCH UNIVERSITY
PLAZA VERA CRUZ
CAMINO REAL
YANONALI ST
CESAR CHAVEZ
FIRE TRAINING FACILITY
FESS PARKERS DOUBLETREE RESORT
CABRILLO BALL PARK
DWIGHT MURPHY FIELD
HOTEL MARMONTE
CABRILLO BLVD
EAST BEACH
CHASE PALM PARK
SKATERS POINT
SKATEPARK
STATE ST
SANTA BARBARA WINERY
CALIFORNIA COASTAL NATIONAL MONUMENT
WEST BEACH
SEA CENTER MARINE MUSEUM
STEARNS WHARF VINTNERS
AMBASSADOR PARK
PERSHING PARK
PLAZA DEL MAR PARK
CASTILLO ST
LA PLAYA STADIUM
CITY COLLEGE
MARINA
SANTA BARBARA YACHT CLUB
SANTA BARBARA MARITIME MUSEUM
POINT CASTILLO
LEADBETTER BEACH
SANTA BARBARA CHANNEL
PACIFIC OCEAN
101
144
96A
96B
97

SEE B MAP

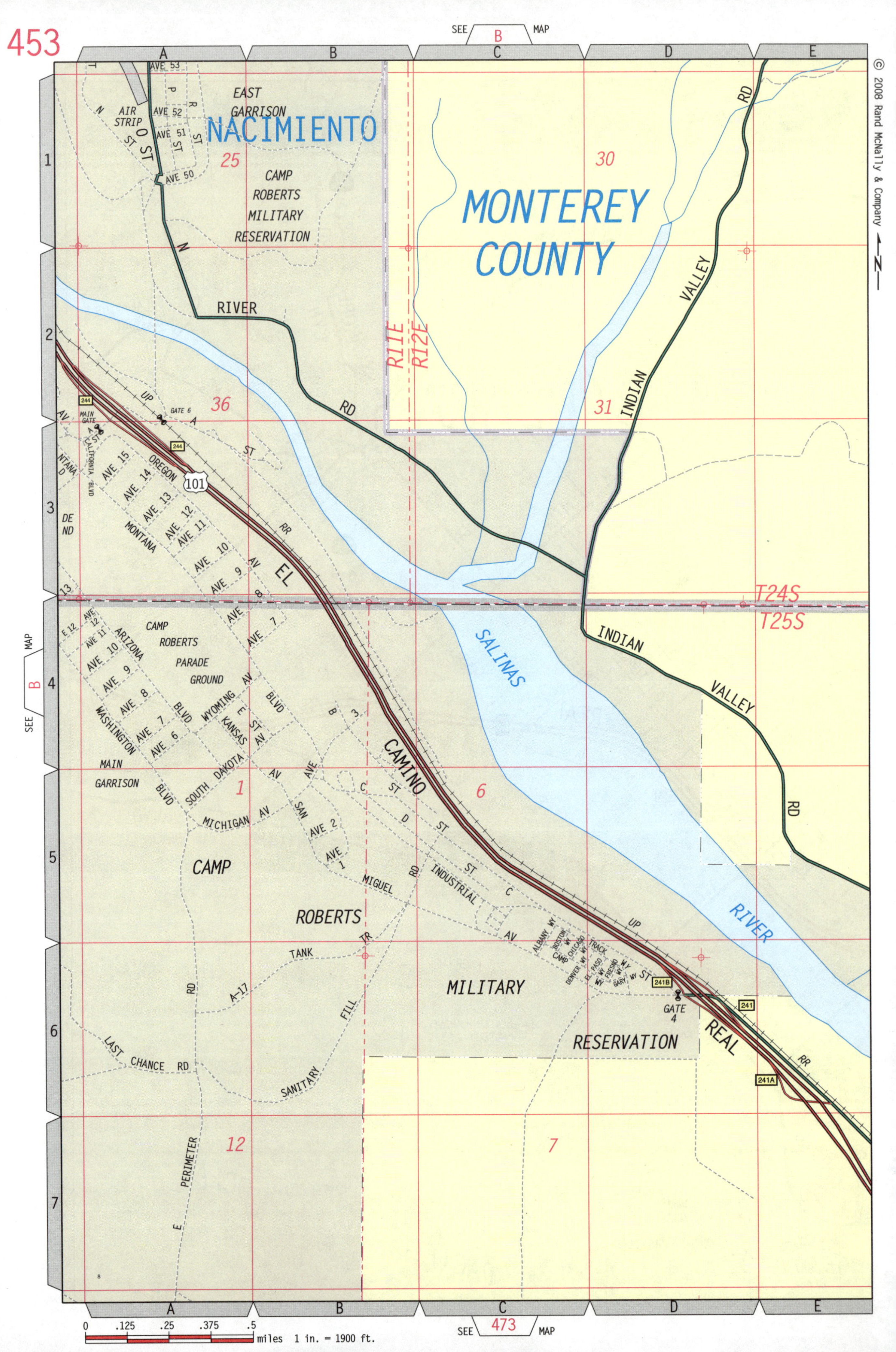

NACIMIENTO
EAST GARRISON
CAMP ROBERTS MILITARY RESERVATION
MONTEREY COUNTY
AIR STRIP
AVE 53
AVE 52
AVE 51
AVE 50
N ST
O ST
P ST
R ST
RIVER RD
R11E
R12E
INDIAN VALLEY RD
T24S
T25S
SALINAS RIVER
EL CAMINO REAL
101
244
241
241A
241B
GATE 6
MAIN GATE
GATE 4
UP RR
CALIFORNIA BLVD
OREGON
MONTANA
AVE 15
AVE 14
AVE 13
AVE 12
AVE 11
AVE 10
AVE 9
AVE 8
AVE 7
CAMP ROBERTS PARADE GROUND
ARIZONA
WASHINGTON
WYOMING BLVD
KANSAS AV
SOUTH DAKOTA AV
MAIN GARRISON BLVD
MICHIGAN AV
SAN MIGUEL RD
INDUSTRIAL AV
TANK TR
A-17
LAST CHANCE RD
SANITARY FILL
PERIMETER RD
ALBANY WY
BOSTON WY
CHICAGO WY
DENVER WY
EL PASO WY
FRESNO WY
GARY WY
CAMP TRACK ST
25
30
36
31
1
6
12
7

0 .125 .25 .375 .5 miles 1 in. = 1900 ft.

SEE 473 MAP

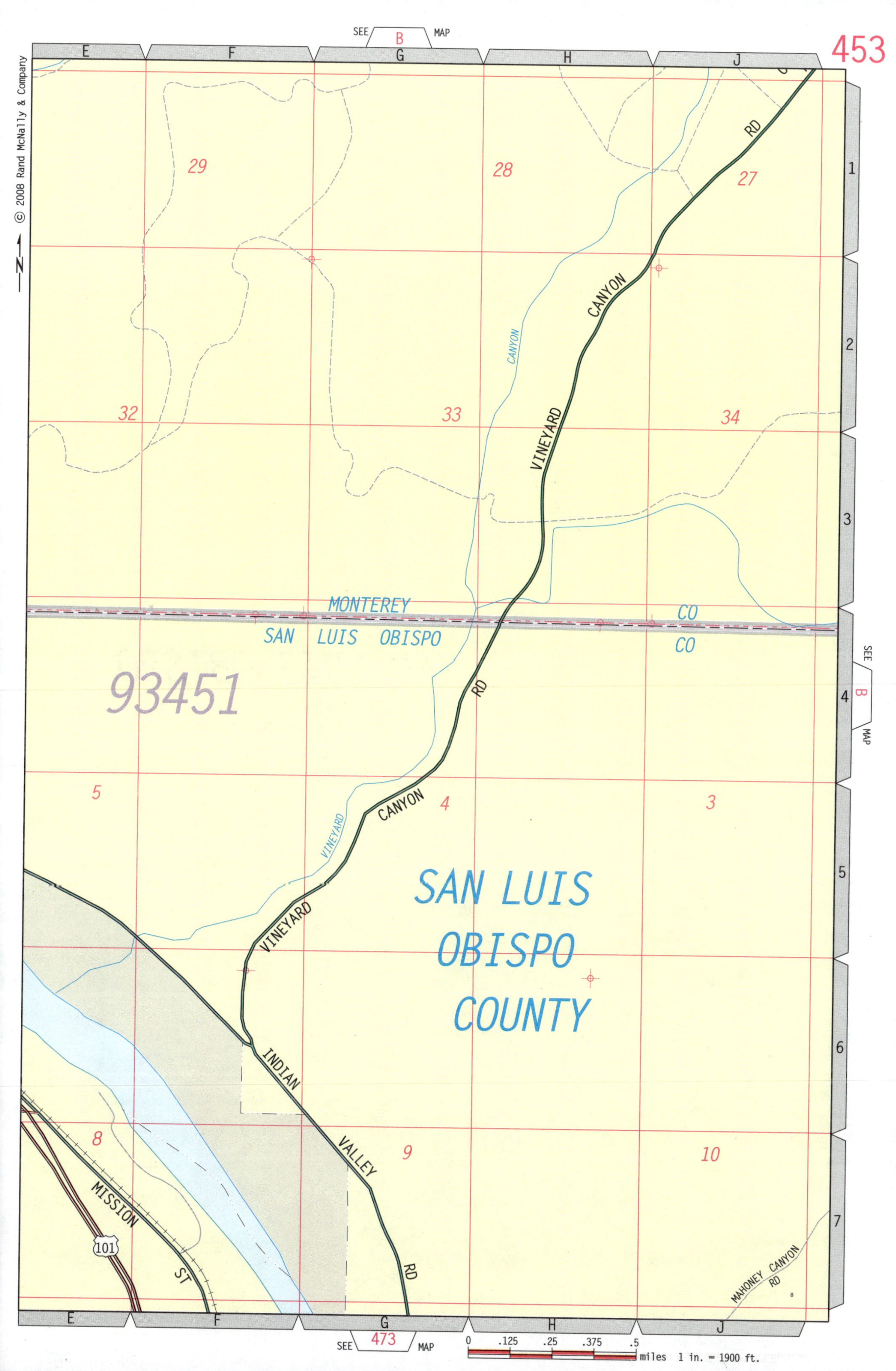
SEE B MAP
E
F
G
H
J
1
2
3
4
5
6
7
29
28
27
32
33
34
5
4
3
8
9
10
VINEYARD CANYON RD
CANYON
MONTEREY CO
SAN LUIS OBISPO CO
93451
VINEYARD
SAN LUIS OBISPO COUNTY
INDIAN VALLEY RD
MISSION ST
101
MAHONEY CANYON RD
SEE B MAP
SEE 473 MAP
0 .125 .25 .375 .5 miles 1 in. = 1900 ft.

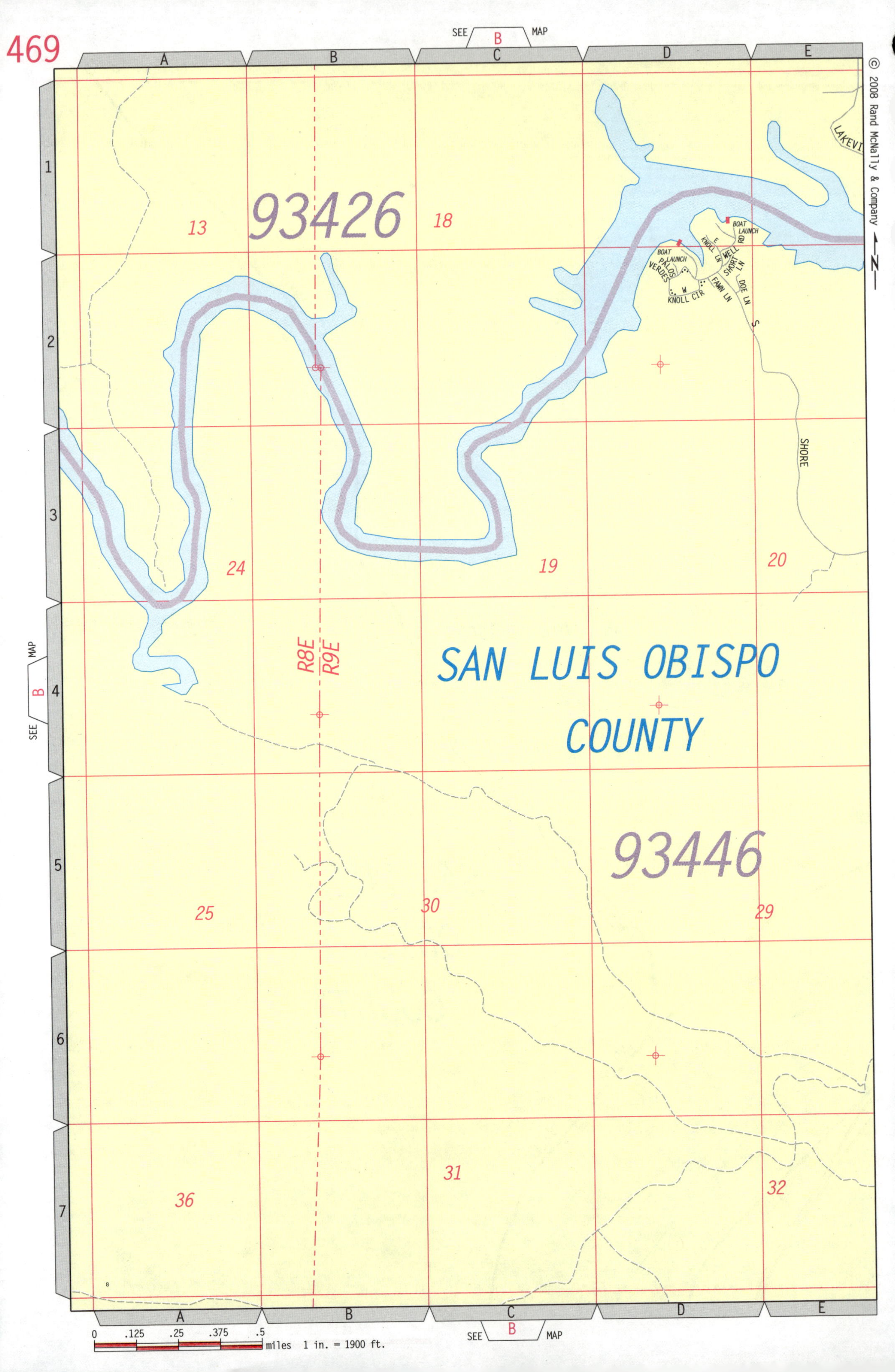

SEE B MAP
A
B
C
D
E
1
2
3
4
5
6
7
93426
13
18
24
19
20
BOAT LAUNCH
BOAT LAUNCH
PALOS VERDES
W KNOLL CIR
E KNOLL LN
WELL RD
SHORT LN
FAWN LN
DOE LN
S SHORE
LAKEVI
R8E
R9E
SAN LUIS OBISPO COUNTY
93446
25
30
29
36
31
32
SEE B MAP
SEE B MAP
0 .125 .25 .375 .5 miles 1 in. = 1900 ft.

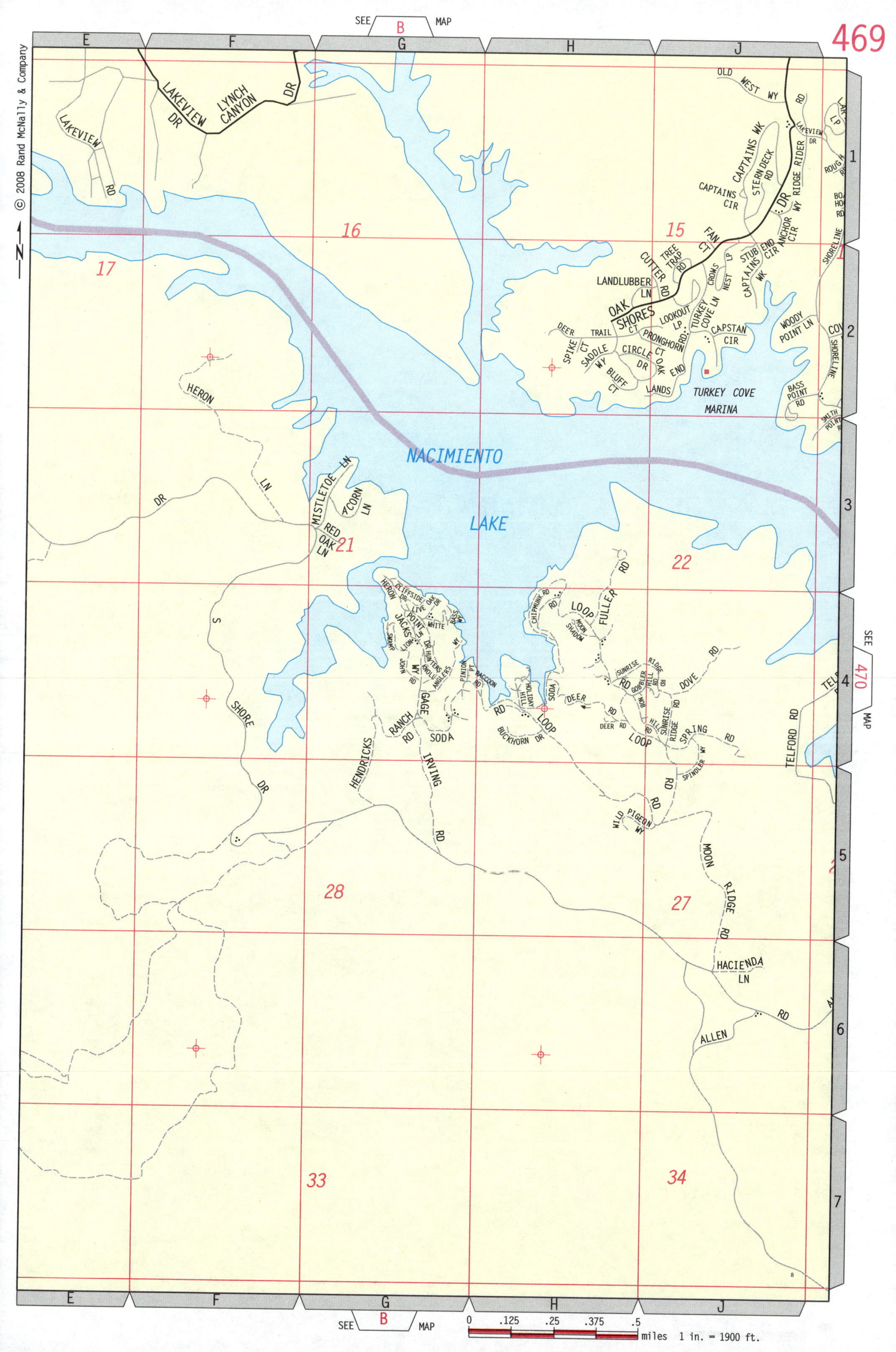

SEE B MAP
E
F
G
H
J
1
2
3
4
5
6
7
NACIMIENTO
LAKE
LAKEVIEW DR
LYNCH CANYON DR
LAKEVIEW RD
OLD WEST WY
CAPTAINS WK
STERN DECK RD
CAPTAINS CIR
RIDGE RIDER WY
DR
ANCHOR CIR
END CIR
STUB
CAPTAINS WK
FAN CT
TREE TRAP RD
CUTTER RD
LANDLUBBER LN
OAK SHORES
CROWS NEST LP
TURKEY COVE LN
LOOKOUT LP
DEER TRAIL CT
SPIKE CT
SADDLE WY
PRONGHORN RD
CIRCLE DR
OAK END
BLUFF CT
LANDS
CAPSTAN CIR
TURKEY COVE MARINA
WOODY POINT LN
BASS POINT RD
SMITH POINT
SHORELINE
HERON LN
DR
MISTLETOE LN
ACORN LN
RED OAK LN
CLIFFSIDE DR
HERON DR
LIVE OAK DR
POINT
WHITE
BASS WY
JACKS
HUNTERS DR
KNOLL
ANGLERS
WY
JOHN RD
GAGE
RANCH RD
SODA
IRVING RD
HENDRICKS
PINION PT
RACCOON RD
HOLIDAY HILL
SODA
LOOP
BUCKHORN DR
RD
CHIPMUNK RD
LOOP
MOON SHADOW
FULLER RD
SUNRISE RIDGE RD
GOBBLER HILL RD
DEER RD
DEER RD
SUNRISE RIDGE RD
SPRING RD
SPINDLER WY
DOVE RD
LOOP
RD
WILD PIGEON WY
S SHORE DR
MOON RIDGE RD
HACIENDA LN
ALLEN RD
TELFORD RD
16
15
17
21
22
28
27
33
34
SEE 470 MAP
SEE B MAP
0 .125 .25 .375 .5 miles 1 in. = 1900 ft.

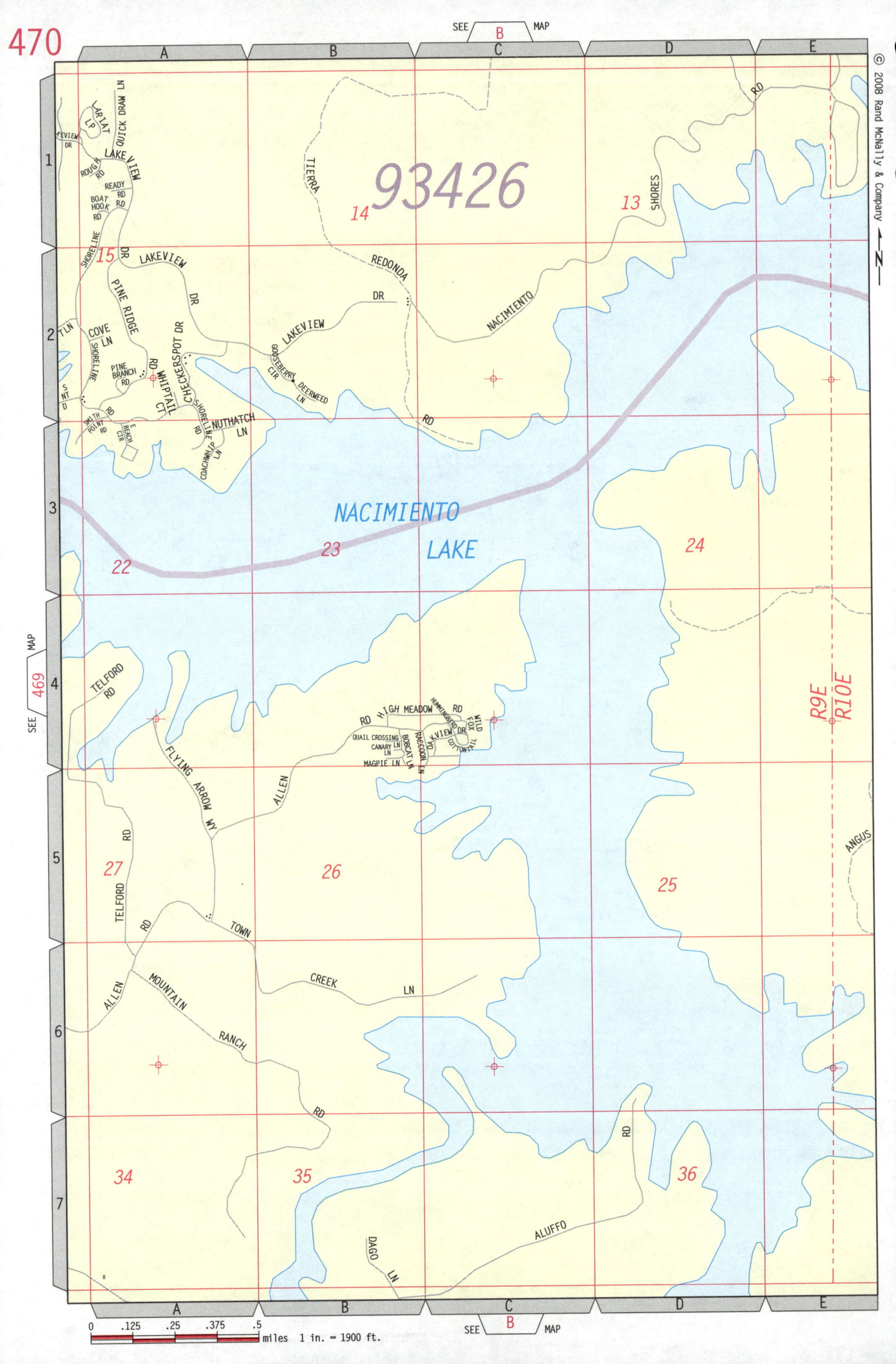

SEE B MAP
93426
NACIMIENTO LAKE
LARIAT LP
QUICK DRAW LN
LAKEVIEW
ROUGH RD
READY RD
BOAT HOOK RD
SHORELINE DR
LAKEVIEW DR
PINE RIDGE RD
COVE LN
SHORELINE
PINE BRANCH RD
WHIPTAIL CT
CHECKERSPOT DR
SMITH POINT RD
E BEACH CIR
SHORELINE
NUTHATCH LN
COACHWHIP LN
GOOSEBERRY CIR
DEERWEED LN
LAKEVIEW
TIERRA REDONDA DR
RD
NACIMIENTO
SHORES RD
TELFORD RD
FLYING ARROW WY
ALLEN
HIGH MEADOW RD
HUMMINGBIRD RD
WILD FOX
OAKVIEW DR
COTTONTAIL
QUAIL CROSSING
CANARY LN
BOBCAT LN
RACCOON LN
MAGPIE LN
TELFORD RD
TOWN CREEK LN
ALLEN
MOUNTAIN RANCH RD
ANGUS
ALUFFO RD
DAGO LN
R9E
R10E
SEE 469 MAP
13
14
15
22
23
24
25
26
27
34
35
36

0 .125 .25 .375 .5 miles 1 in. = 1900 ft.

SEE B MAP

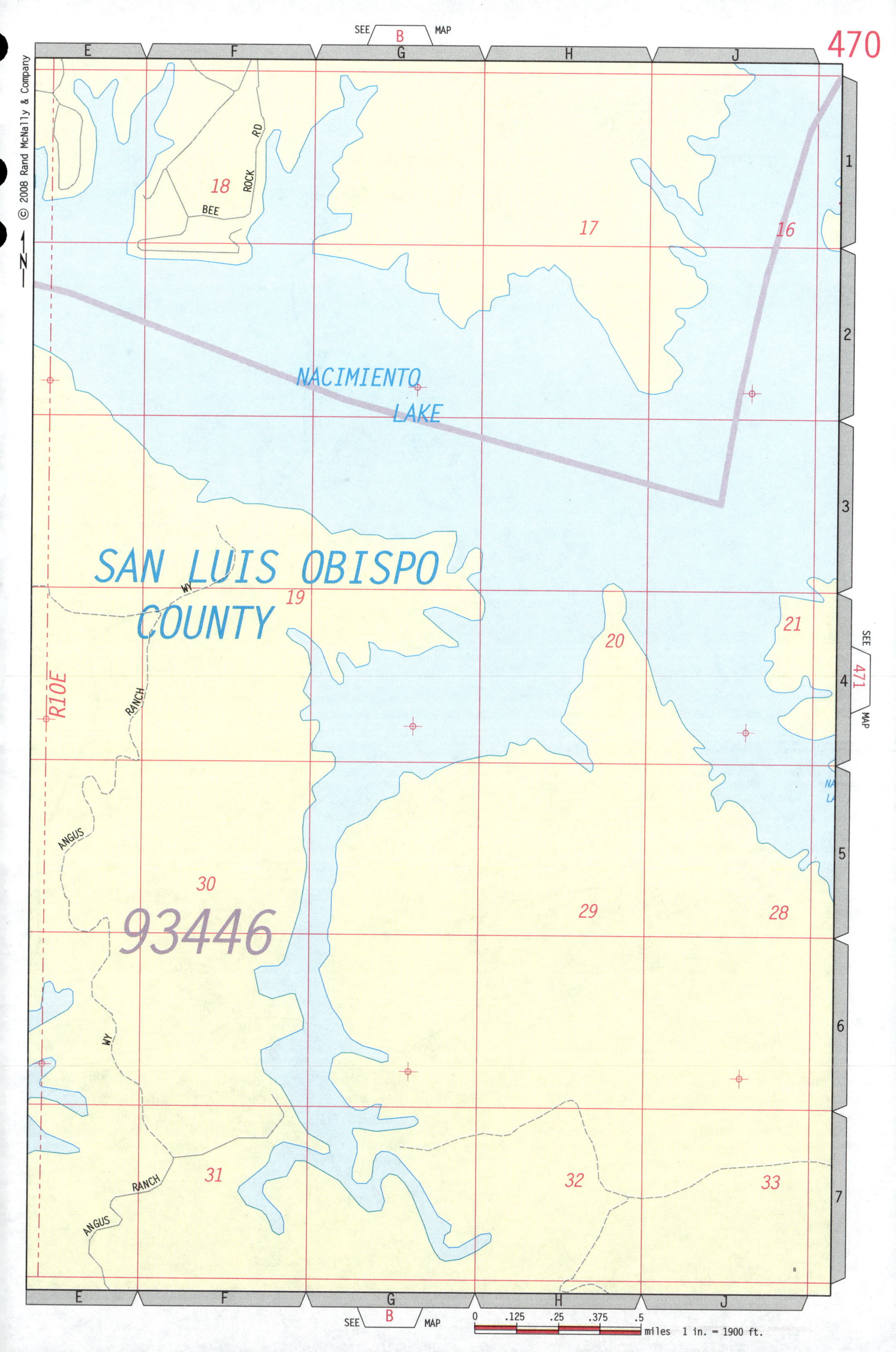
SEE B MAP
E
F
G
H
J
1
2
3
4
5
6
7
18
17
16
19
20
21
30
29
28
31
32
33
ROCK RD
BEE
NACIMIENTO LAKE
SAN LUIS OBISPO COUNTY
93446
WY
RANCH
ANGUS
WY
RANCH
ANGUS
R10E
SEE 471 MAP
0 .125 .25 .375 .5 miles 1 in. = 1900 ft.

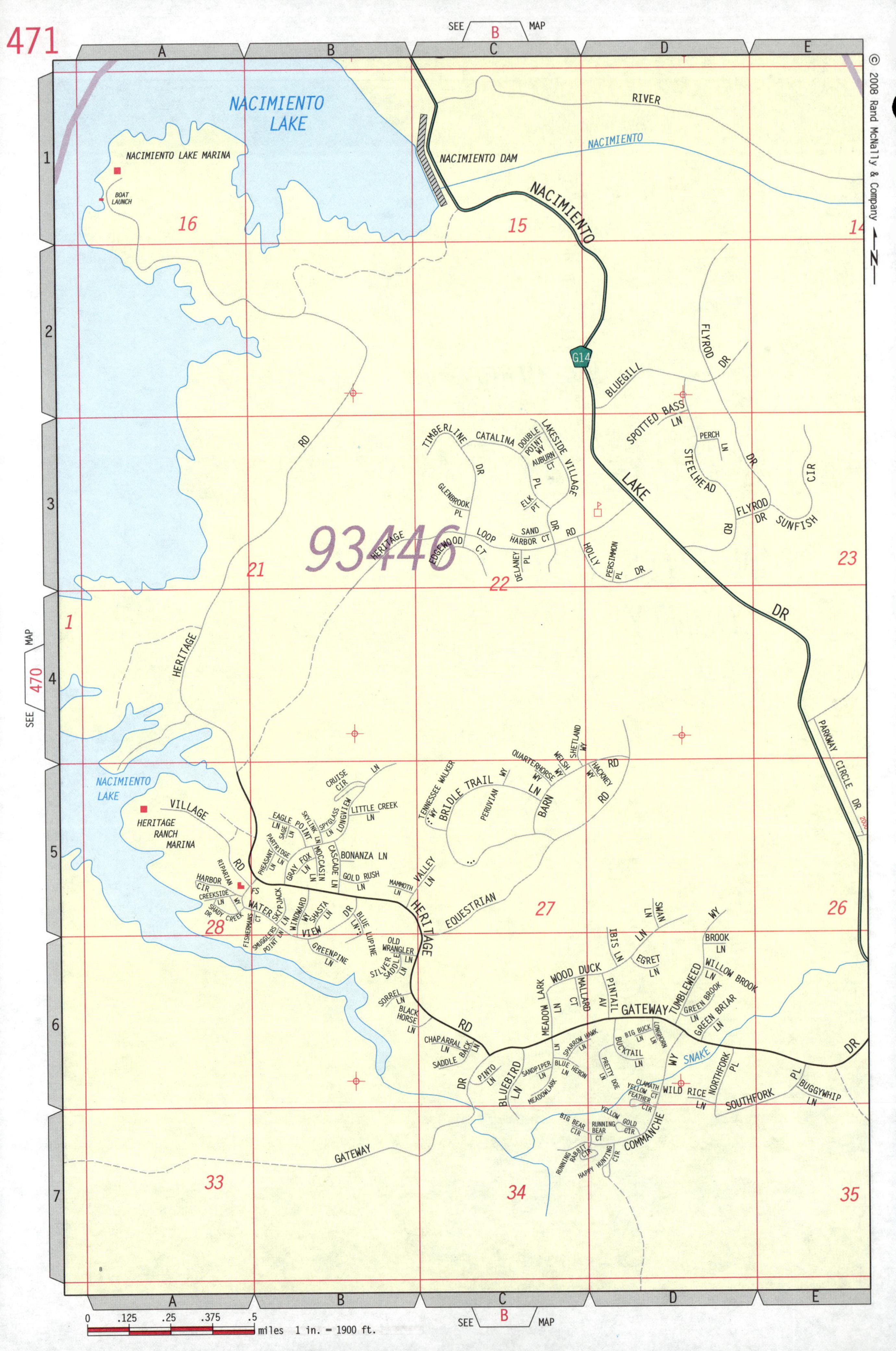
SEE B MAP
NACIMIENTO LAKE
NACIMIENTO LAKE MARINA
BOAT LAUNCH
NACIMIENTO DAM
RIVER
NACIMIENTO
NACIMIENTO
LAKE
DR
G14
93446
BLUEGILL
FLYROD DR
SPOTTED BASS LN
PERCH LN
STEELHEAD
FLYROD DR
SUNFISH CIR
TIMBERLINE DR
CATALINA
DOUBLE POINT WY
AUBURN CT
LAKESIDE VILLAGE
ELK PT
GLENBROOK PL
LOOP
SAND HARBOR CT
EDGEWOOD CT
DELANEY PL
HOLLY
PERSIMMON PL
DR
RD
HERITAGE
RD
HERITAGE
NACIMIENTO LAKE
VILLAGE
HERITAGE RANCH MARINA
RD
RIPARIAN
HARBOR CIR
CREEKSIDE LN
SHADY CREEK DR
WATER
FISHERMANS CT
SMUGGLERS POINT LN
SKYPJACK
WINDWARD
VIEW
SHASTA
GREENPINE LN
PHEASANT LN
PARTRIDGE
EAGLE POINT LN
SAGE LN
GRAY FOX LN
SKYLINK LN
SPYGLASS LN
MOCCASIN LN
CASCADE LN
LONGVIEW
CRUISE CIR
LITTLE CREEK LN
BONANZA LN
GOLD RUSH LN
MAMMOTH LN
VALLEY LN
BLUE LUPINE LN
DR
OLD WRANGLER LN
SILVER SADDLE LN
SORREL LN
BLACK HORSE LN
CHAPARRAL LN
SADDLE BACK LN
RD
HERITAGE
EQUESTRIAN
TENNESSEE WALKER WY
BRIDLE TRAIL
PERUVIAN
QUARTERHORSE WY
LN
BARN
WELSH WY
SHETLAND WY
HACKNEY WY
RD
RD
PARKWAY CIRCLE DR
SWAN LN
IBIS LN
EGRET LN
BROOK LN
WILLOW BROOK LN
WY
WOOD DUCK
MEADOW LARK LN
MALLARD CT
PINTAIL AV
GATEWAY
TUMBLEWEED
GREEN BROOK LN
GREEN BRIAR LN
BIG BUCK LN
LONGHORN LN
SPARROW HAWK LN
BUCKTAIL LN
WY
SNAKE
DR
BLUE HERON LN
SANDPIPER LN
MEADOWLARK
PRETTY DOE LN
PINTO LN
BLUEBIRD LN
DR
CLAMATH CT
YELLOW FEATHER CIR
WILD RICE LN
NORTHFORK PL
SOUTHFORK
PL
BUGGYWHIP LN
BIG BEAR CIR
RUNNING BEAR CT
YELLOW GOLD CIR
COMMANCHE
RUNNING RABBIT CIR
HAPPY HUNTING CIR
GATEWAY
SEE 470 MAP
A B C D E
1 2 3 4 5 6 7
16 15 14 21 22 23 1 28 27 26 33 34 35
0 .125 .25 .375 .5 miles 1 in. = 1900 ft.
SEE B MAP

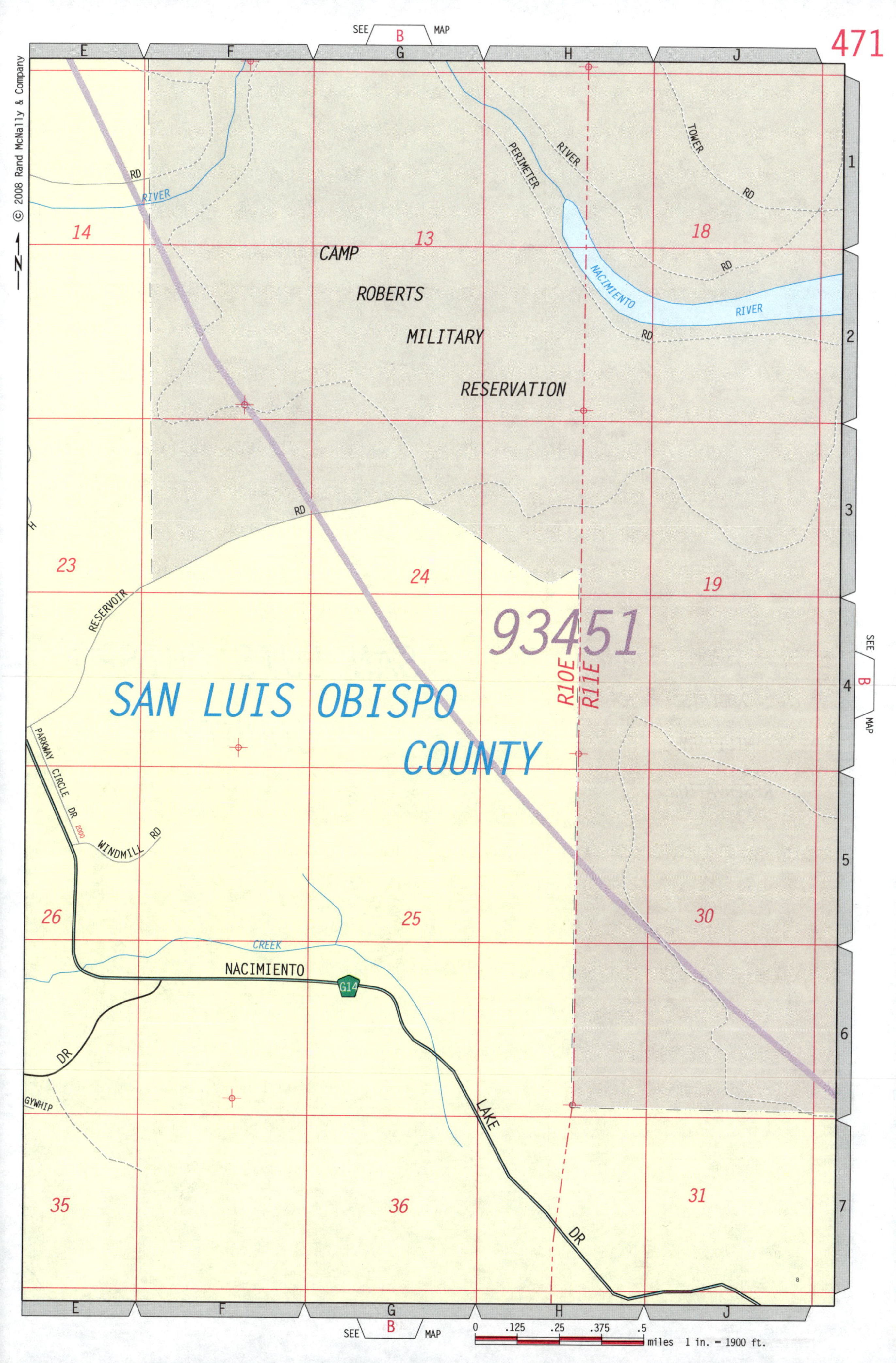

SEE B MAP
E
F
G
H
J
1
2
3
4
5
6
7
© 2008 Rand McNally & Company
RD
RIVER
14
13
18
CAMP
ROBERTS
MILITARY
RESERVATION
PERIMETER
RIVER
TOWER
RD
RD
NACIMIENTO
RIVER
RD
RD
23
24
19
RESERVOIR
93451
R10E
R11E
SAN LUIS OBISPO
COUNTY
SEE B MAP
PARKWAY
CIRCLE
DR
2000
WINDMILL RD
26
25
30
CREEK
NACIMIENTO
G14
DR
LAKE
GYWHIP
35
36
31
DR
SEE B MAP
0 .125 .25 .375 .5 miles 1 in. = 1900 ft.

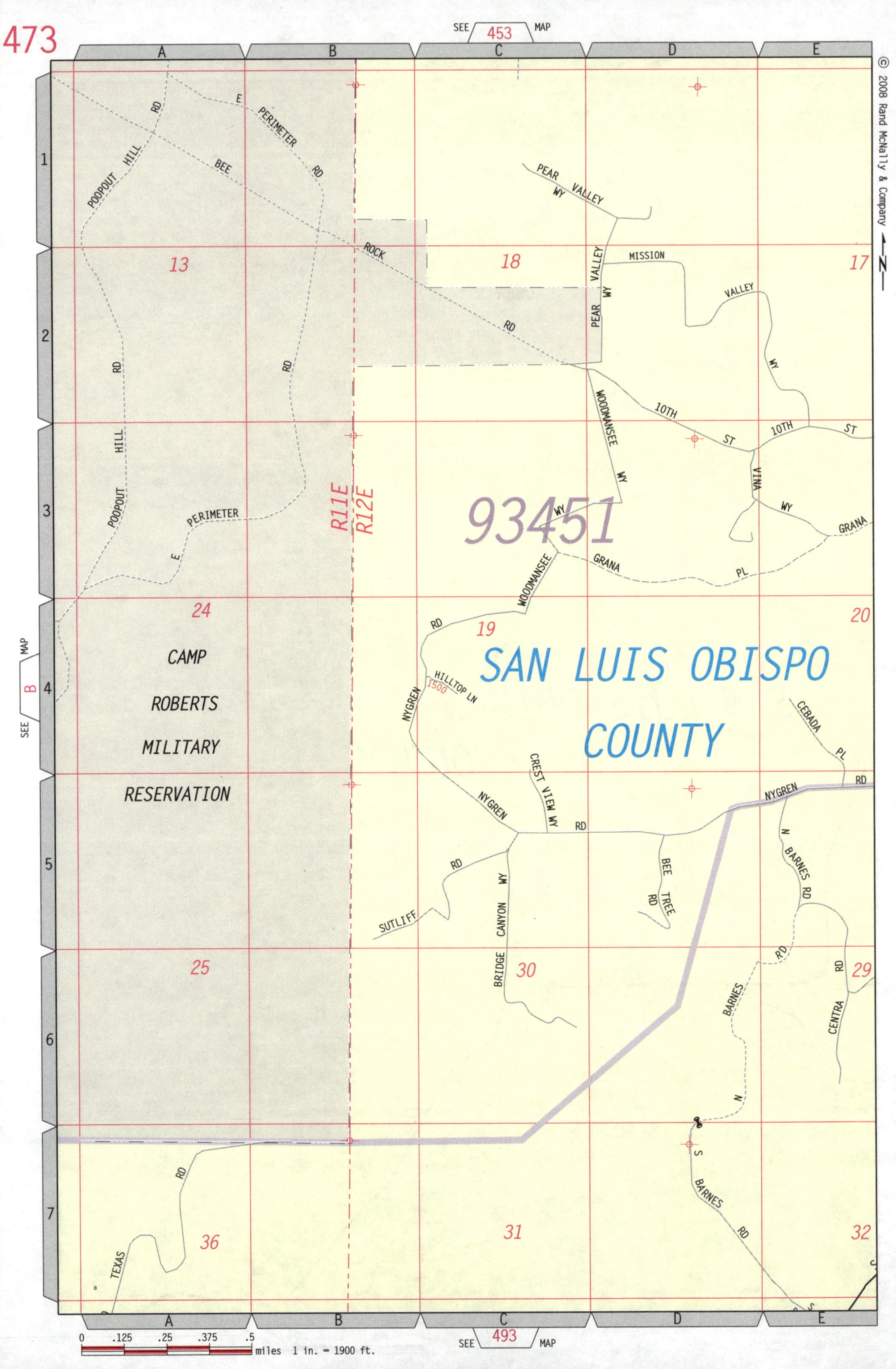

SEE 453 MAP
A
B
C
D
E
1
2
3
4
5
6
7
E PERIMETER RD
POOPOUT HILL RD
BEE ROCK RD
PEAR VALLEY WY
MISSION
VALLEY WY
10TH ST
VINA WY
GRANA PL
WOODMANSEE WY
WOODMANSEE RD
R11E
R12E
93451
13
18
17
24
19
20
25
30
29
36
31
32
CAMP ROBERTS MILITARY RESERVATION
SAN LUIS OBISPO COUNTY
HILLTOP LN
1500
NYGREN RD
CEBADA PL
CREST VIEW WY
BEE TREE RD
N BARNES RD
SUTLIFF RD
BRIDGE CANYON WY
CENTRA RD
S BARNES RD
TEXAS RD
SEE B MAP
SEE 493 MAP
0 .125 .25 .375 .5
miles 1 in. = 1900 ft.

SEE 453 MAP

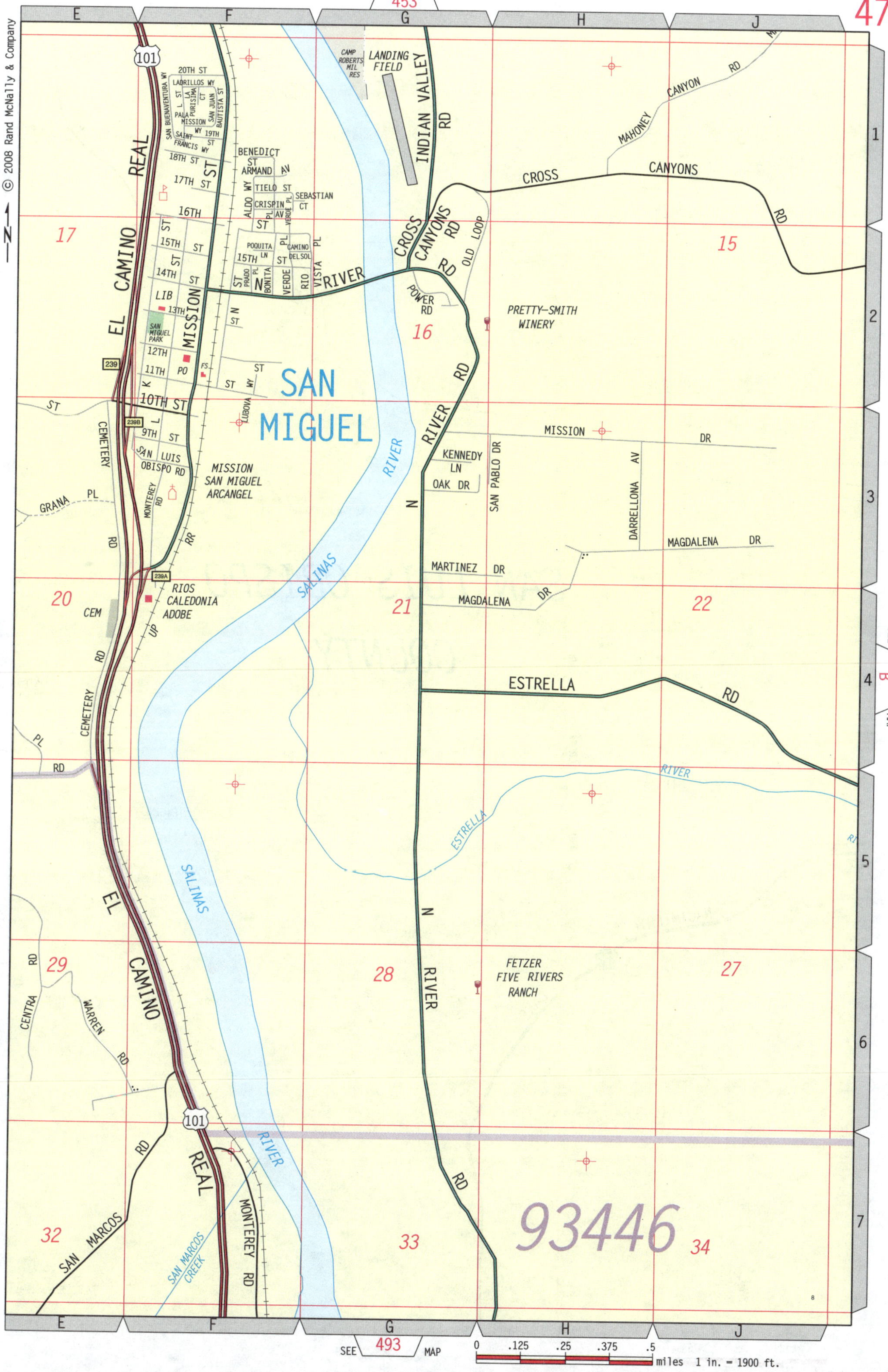

E F G H J

1 2 3 4 5 6 7

SAN MIGUEL

EL CAMINO REAL
101
20TH ST
LADRILLOS WY
SAN BUENAVENTURA WY
L ST
LA PURISIMA CT
PALA
MISSION WY
SAN JUAN BAUTISTA ST
19TH ST
SAINT FRANCIS WY
18TH ST
17TH ST
16TH
15TH ST
14TH ST
LIB
13TH
SAN MIGUEL PARK
12TH
11TH
PO
FS
10TH ST
9TH ST
SAN LUIS OBISPO RD
MISSION ST
BENEDICT ST
ARMAND AV
ALDO WY
TIELO ST
SEBASTIAN CT
CRISPIN PL
AV
VERDE PL
ST
POQUITA PL
CAMINO DEL SOL
15TH LN
ST
PRADO PL
BONITA
VERDE
RIO
VISTA PL
N RIVER RD
N ST
ST
LUBOVA WY
ST
239
239B
239A
ST
CEMETERY RD
GRANA PL
MONTEREY RD
MISSION SAN MIGUEL ARCANGEL
UP RR
RIOS CALEDONIA ADOBE
CEM
CEMETERY RD
PL
RD
CAMP ROBERTS MIL RES
LANDING FIELD
INDIAN VALLEY RD
CROSS CANYONS RD
OLD LOOP
POWER RD
MAHONEY CANYON RD
CROSS CANYONS RD
PRETTY-SMITH WINERY
MISSION DR
KENNEDY LN
OAK DR
SAN PABLO DR
DARRELLONA AV
MAGDALENA DR
MARTINEZ DR
MAGDALENA DR
SALINAS RIVER
ESTRELLA RD
ESTRELLA RIVER
FETZER FIVE RIVERS RANCH
CENTRA RD
WARREN RD
SAN MARCOS RD
SAN MARCOS CREEK
MONTEREY RD
93446

17 15 16 20 21 22 29 28 27 32 33 34

SEE B MAP

SEE 493 MAP

0 .125 .25 .375 .5 miles 1 in. = 1900 ft.

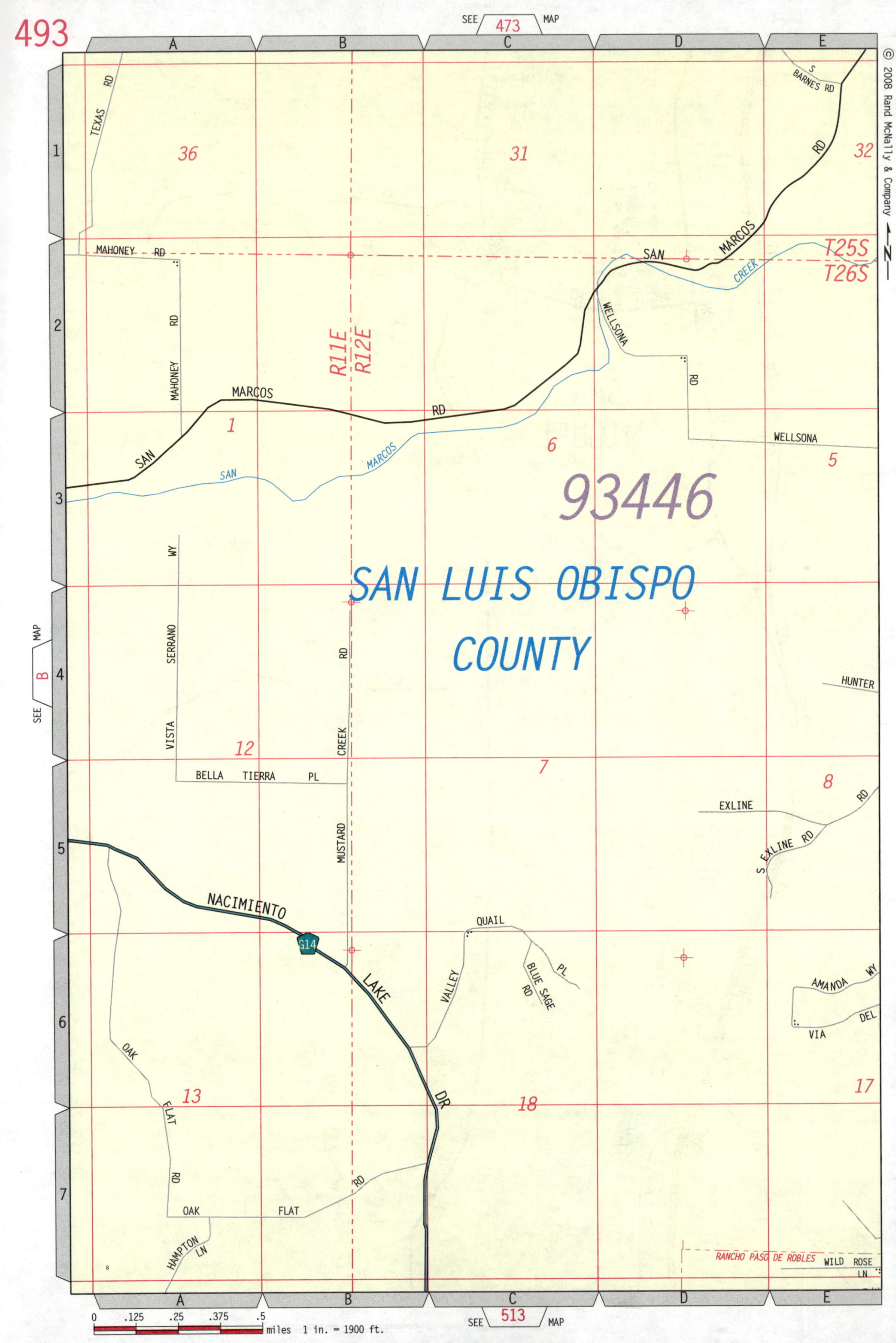

SEE 473 MAP
SAN LUIS OBISPO COUNTY
93446
TEXAS RD
MAHONEY RD
SAN MARCOS RD
SAN MARCOS CREEK
WELLSONA RD
WELLSONA
S BARNES RD
T25S
T26S
R11E
R12E
VISTA SERRANO WY
MUSTARD CREEK RD
BELLA TIERRA PL
HUNTER
EXLINE RD
S EXLINE RD
NACIMIENTO LAKE DR
G14
QUAIL VALLEY
BLUE SAGE RD
PL
AMANDA WY
VIA DEL
OAK FLAT RD
HAMPTON LN
RANCHO PASO DE ROBLES
WILD ROSE LN
36
31
32
1
6
5
12
7
8
13
18
17
SEE B MAP
SEE 513 MAP
0 .125 .25 .375 .5 miles 1 in. = 1900 ft.

SEE 473 MAP

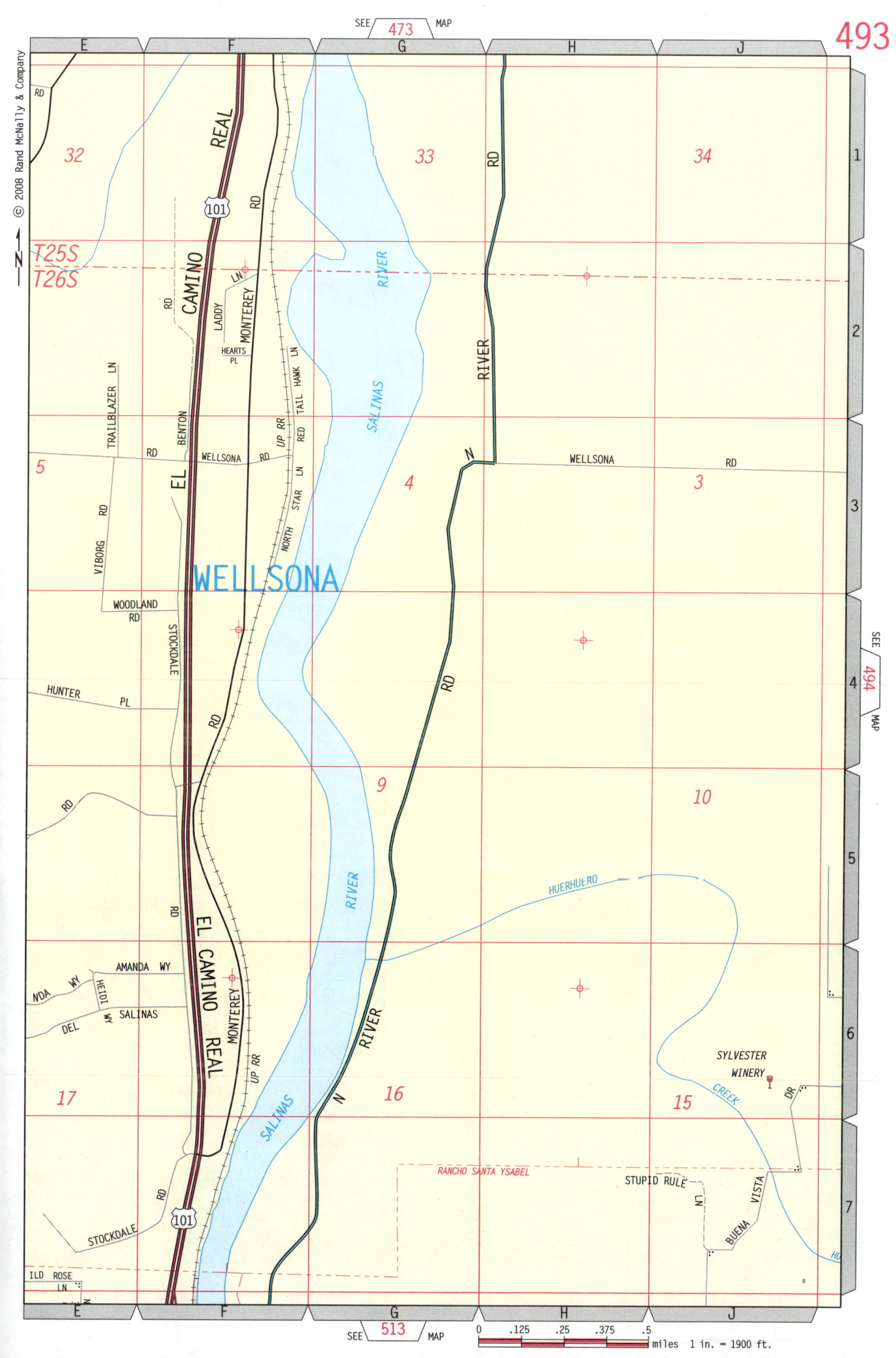
E
F
G
H
J
1
2
3
4
5
6
7
32
33
34
5
4
3
9
10
17
16
15
T25S
T26S
EL CAMINO REAL
101
MONTEREY RD
LADDY LN
HEARTS PL
TAIL HAWK LN
RED STAR LN
NORTH
UP RR
TRAILBLAZER LN
BENTON RD
WELLSONA RD
VIBORG RD
WELLSONA
WOODLAND RD
STOCKDALE RD
HUNTER PL
SALINAS RIVER
N RIVER RD
HUERHUERO CREEK
AMANDA WY
HEIDI WY
DEL SALINAS
SYLVESTER WINERY
DR
RANCHO SANTA YSABEL
STUPID RULE LN
BUENA VISTA
ROSE LN
SEE 494 MAP
© 2008 Rand McNally & Company
0 .125 .25 .375 .5 miles 1 in. = 1900 ft.

SEE 513 MAP

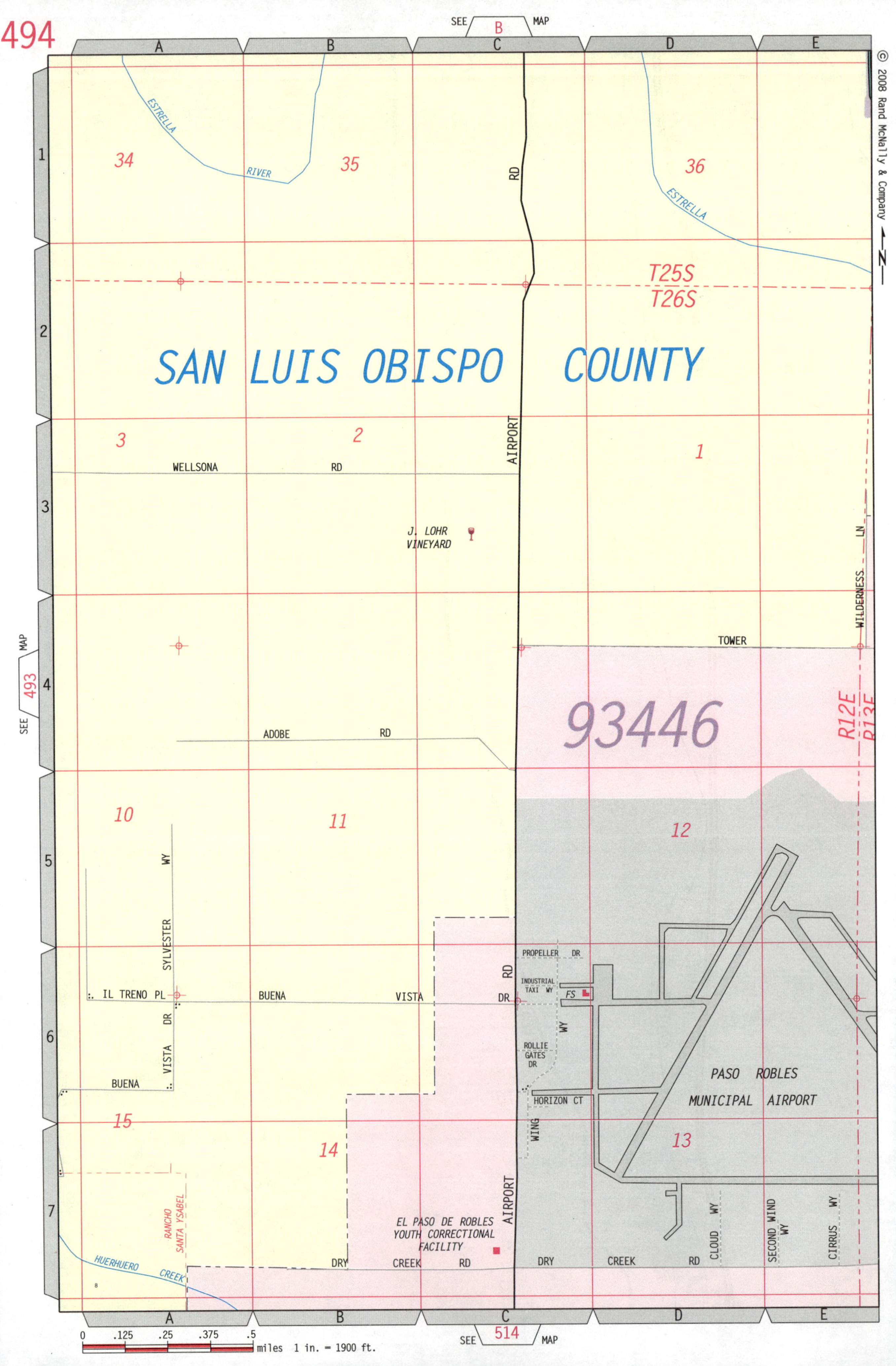
SEE B MAP
A
B
C
D
E
1
2
3
4
5
6
7
© 2008 Rand McNally & Company
34
35
36
ESTRELLA
RIVER
ESTRELLA
RD
T25S
T26S
SAN LUIS OBISPO COUNTY
3
2
1
AIRPORT
WELLSONA RD
J. LOHR VINEYARD
WILDERNESS LN
TOWER
SEE 493 MAP
93446
R12E
R13E
ADOBE RD
10
11
12
SYLVESTER WY
PROPELLER DR
INDUSTRIAL TAXI WY
FS
IL TRENO PL
BUENA VISTA DR
RD
VISTA DR
WY
ROLLIE GATES DR
BUENA
HORIZON CT
PASO ROBLES MUNICIPAL AIRPORT
15
14
13
WING
RANCHO SANTA YSABEL
AIRPORT
EL PASO DE ROBLES YOUTH CORRECTIONAL FACILITY
CLOUD WY
SECOND WIND WY
CIRRUS WY
HUERHUERO CREEK
DRY CREEK RD
DRY CREEK RD
0 .125 .25 .375 .5
miles 1 in. = 1900 ft.
SEE 514 MAP

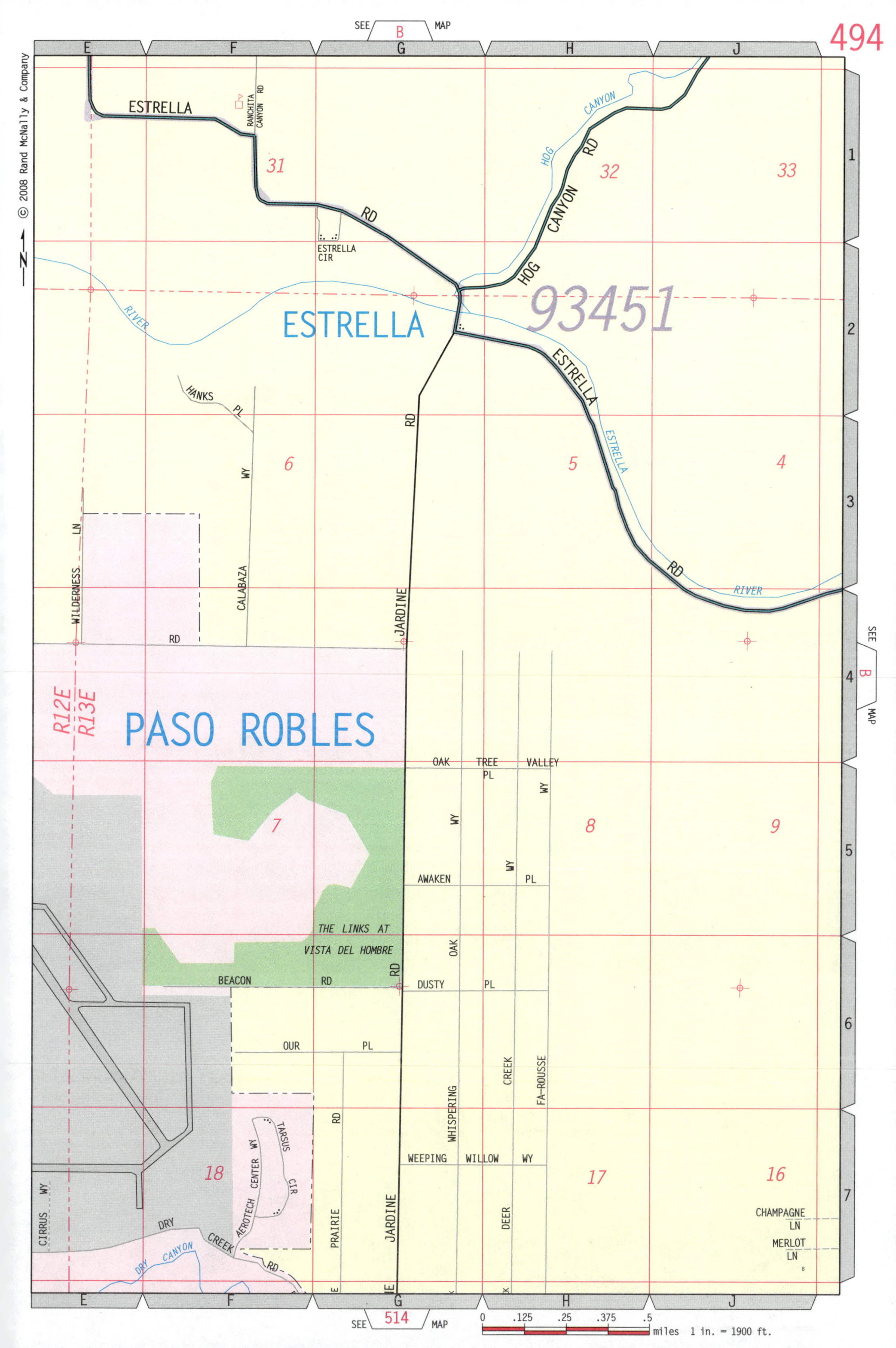
SEE B MAP
E
F
G
H
J
ESTRELLA
RANCHITA CANYON RD
31
32
33
RD
HOG CANYON
HOG CANYON RD
ESTRELLA CIR
RIVER
ESTRELLA
93451
ESTRELLA
RD
HANKS PL
6
5
4
WY
CALABAZA
WILDERNESS LN
JARDINE RD
RIVER
RD
SEE B MAP
R12E
R13E
PASO ROBLES
OAK TREE VALLEY
PL
WY
WY
7
8
9
AWAKEN
WY
PL
THE LINKS AT
VISTA DEL HOMBRE
BEACON RD
RD
DUSTY PL
OAK
OUR PL
CREEK
FA-ROUSSE
WHISPERING
TARSUS CIR
WY
AEROTECH CENTER
RD
WEEPING WILLOW WY
18
17
16
CIRRUS WY
DRY CREEK RD
DRY CANYON
PRAIRIE
JARDINE
DEER
CHAMPAGNE LN
MERLOT LN
1
2
3
4
5
6
7
© 2008 Rand McNally & Company
SEE 514 MAP
0 .125 .25 .375 .5
miles 1 in. = 1900 ft.

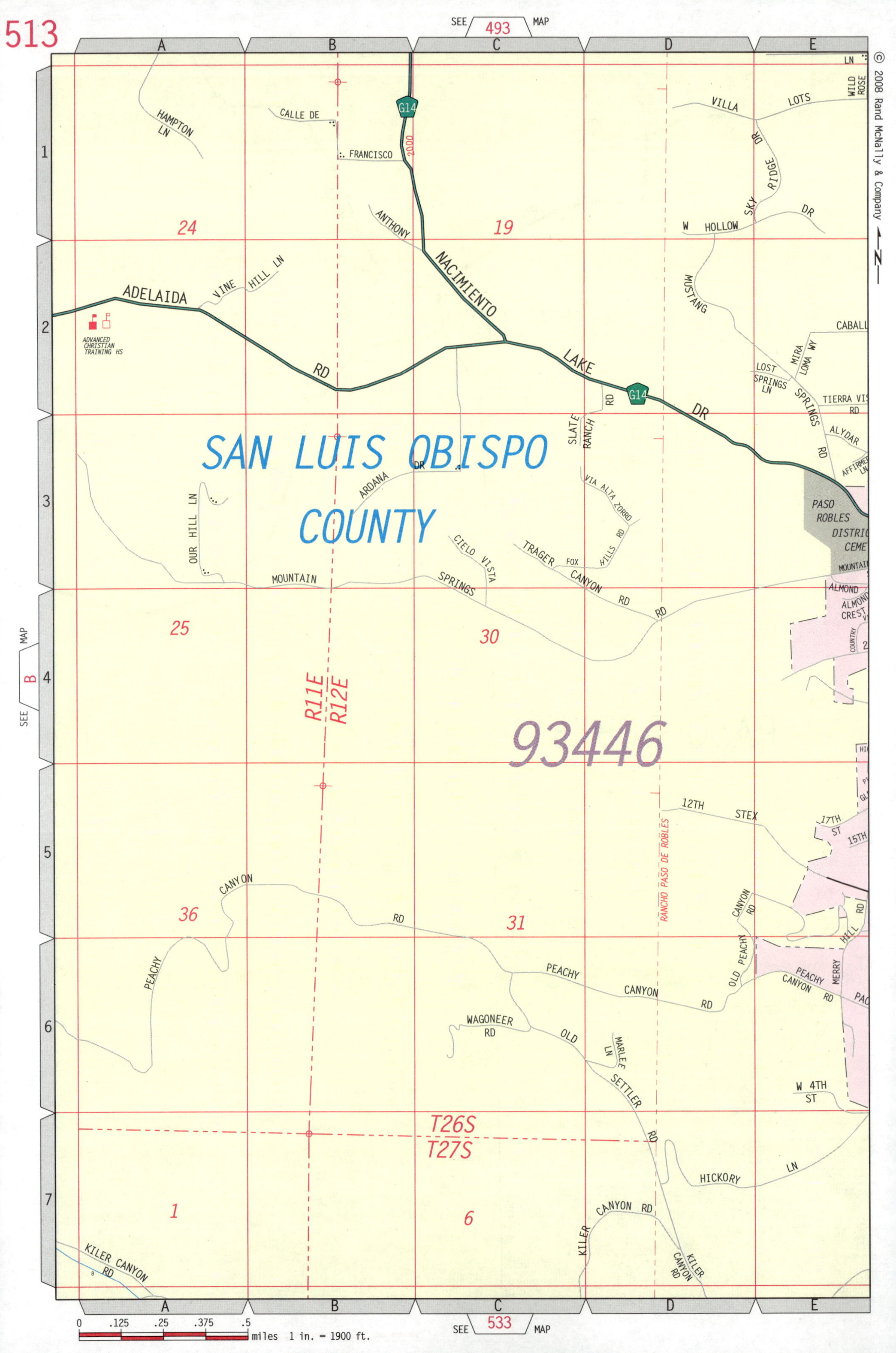
SEE 493 MAP
SAN LUIS OBISPO
COUNTY
93446
ADELAIDA RD
NACIMIENTO LAKE DR
G14
HAMPTON LN
CALLE DE FRANCISCO
ANTHONY
VINE HILL LN
ADVANCED CHRISTIAN TRAINING HS
VILLA LOTS DR
SKY RIDGE DR
W HOLLOW
MUSTANG
LOST SPRINGS LN
MIRA LOMA WY
SPRINGS RD
TIERRA VIS RD
ALYDAR
SLATE RANCH RD
ARDANA DR
OUR HILL LN
VIA ALTA ZORRO
HILLS RD
CIELO VISTA
TRAGER FOX CANYON RD
MOUNTAIN SPRINGS RD
PASO ROBLES DISTRIC CEME
ALMOND
ALMOND CREST
R11E
R12E
12TH STEX
17TH ST
15TH
RANCHO PASO DE ROBLES
CANYON RD
PEACHY CANYON RD
OLD PEACHY CANYON RD
HILL RD
PEACHY CANYON RD
MERRY
WAGONEER RD
OLD SETTLER RD
MARLEE LN
W 4TH ST
T26S
T27S
HICKORY LN
KILER CANYON RD
24
19
25
30
36
31
1
6
2000
SEE B MAP
0 .125 .25 .375 .5 miles 1 in. = 1900 ft.
SEE 533 MAP

SEE 493 MAP

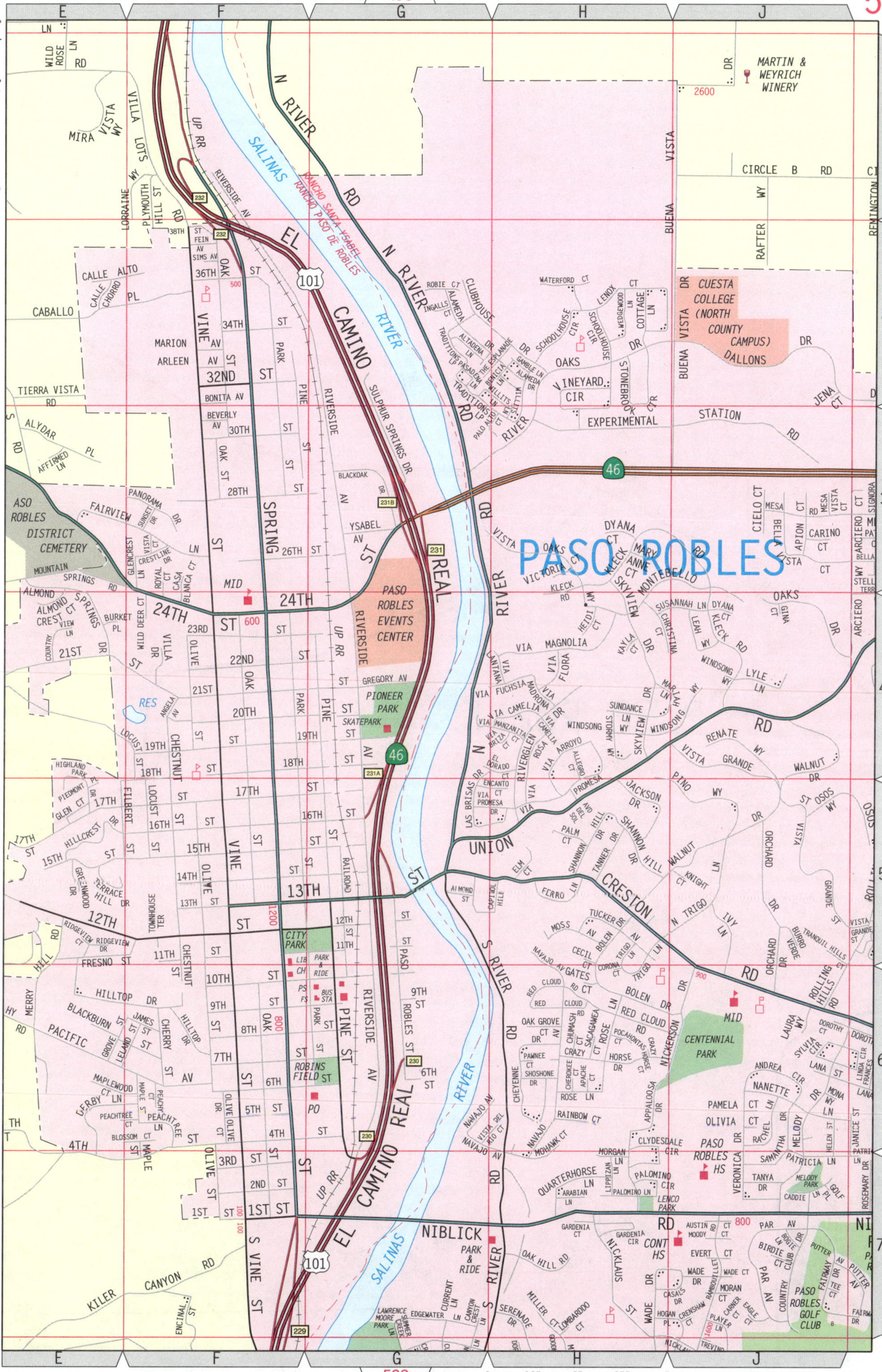

E F G H J

PASO ROBLES

SALINAS RIVER
RANCHO SANTA YSABEL
RANCHO PASO DE ROBLES
N RIVER RD
EL CAMINO REAL
101
46
SPRING ST
VINE ST
PINE ST
PARK ST
OAK ST
RIVERSIDE AV
UP RR
24TH ST
13TH ST
UNION RD
CRESTON RD
NIBLICK RD
S RIVER RD
EXPERIMENTAL STATION RD
BUENA VISTA DR
CIRCLE B RD
MARTIN & WEYRICH WINERY
CUESTA COLLEGE (NORTH COUNTY CAMPUS)
PASO ROBLES EVENTS CENTER
PIONEER PARK
SKATEPARK
CITY PARK
ROBINS FIELD
PASO ROBLES DISTRICT CEMETERY
CENTENNIAL PARK
PASO ROBLES HS
CONT HS
PASO ROBLES GOLF CLUB
PARK & RIDE
KILER CANYON RD
S VINE ST
PO

SEE 514 MAP

1 2 3 4 5 6 7

SEE 533 MAP

0 .125 .25 .375 .5 miles 1 in. = 1900 ft.

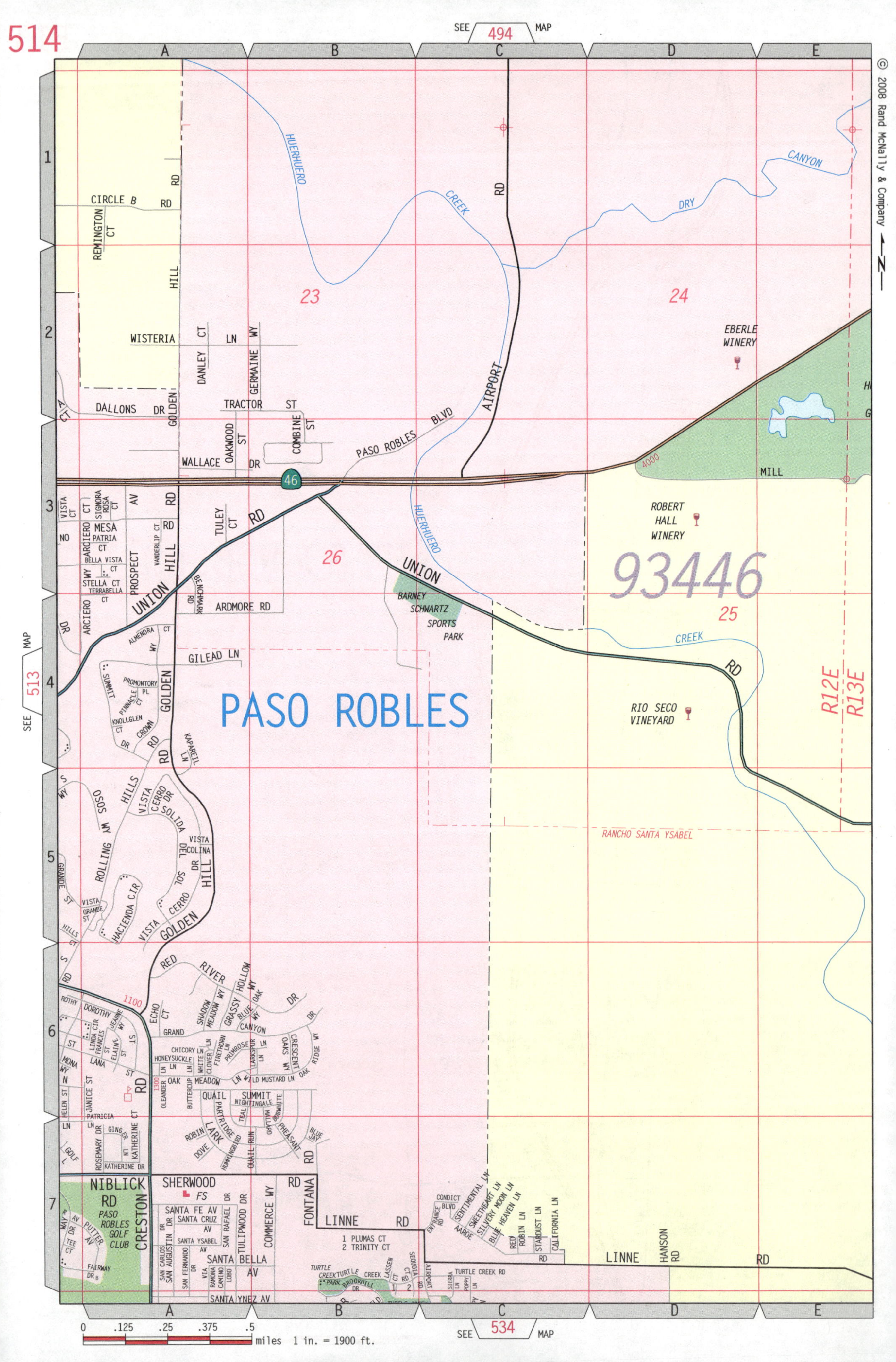
SEE 494 MAP
SEE 513 MAP
SEE 534 MAP
© 2008 Rand McNally & Company
PASO ROBLES
93446
HUERHUERO CREEK
DRY CANYON CREEK
AIRPORT RD
PASO ROBLES BLVD
UNION RD
GOLDEN HILL RD
MILL
LINNE RD
CRESTON RD
NIBLICK RD
EBERLE WINERY
ROBERT HALL WINERY
RIO SECO VINEYARD
BARNEY SCHWARTZ SPORTS PARK
PASO ROBLES GOLF CLUB
RANCHO SANTA YSABEL
R12E
R13E
23
24
25
26
46
WISTERIA LN
DANLEY CT
GERMAINE WY
TRACTOR ST
COMBINE ST
OAKWOOD ST
WALLACE DR
DALLONS DR
CIRCLE B RD
REMINGTON CT
TULEY CT
BENCHMARK RD
ARDMORE RD
GILEAD LN
PROSPECT AV
FONTANA RD
HANSON RD
SHERWOOD
TULIPWOOD DR
COMMERCE WY
SANTA BELLA AV
SANTA YNEZ AV
1 PLUMAS CT
2 TRINITY CT
TURTLE CREEK RD
0 .125 .25 .375 .5 miles 1 in. = 1900 ft.

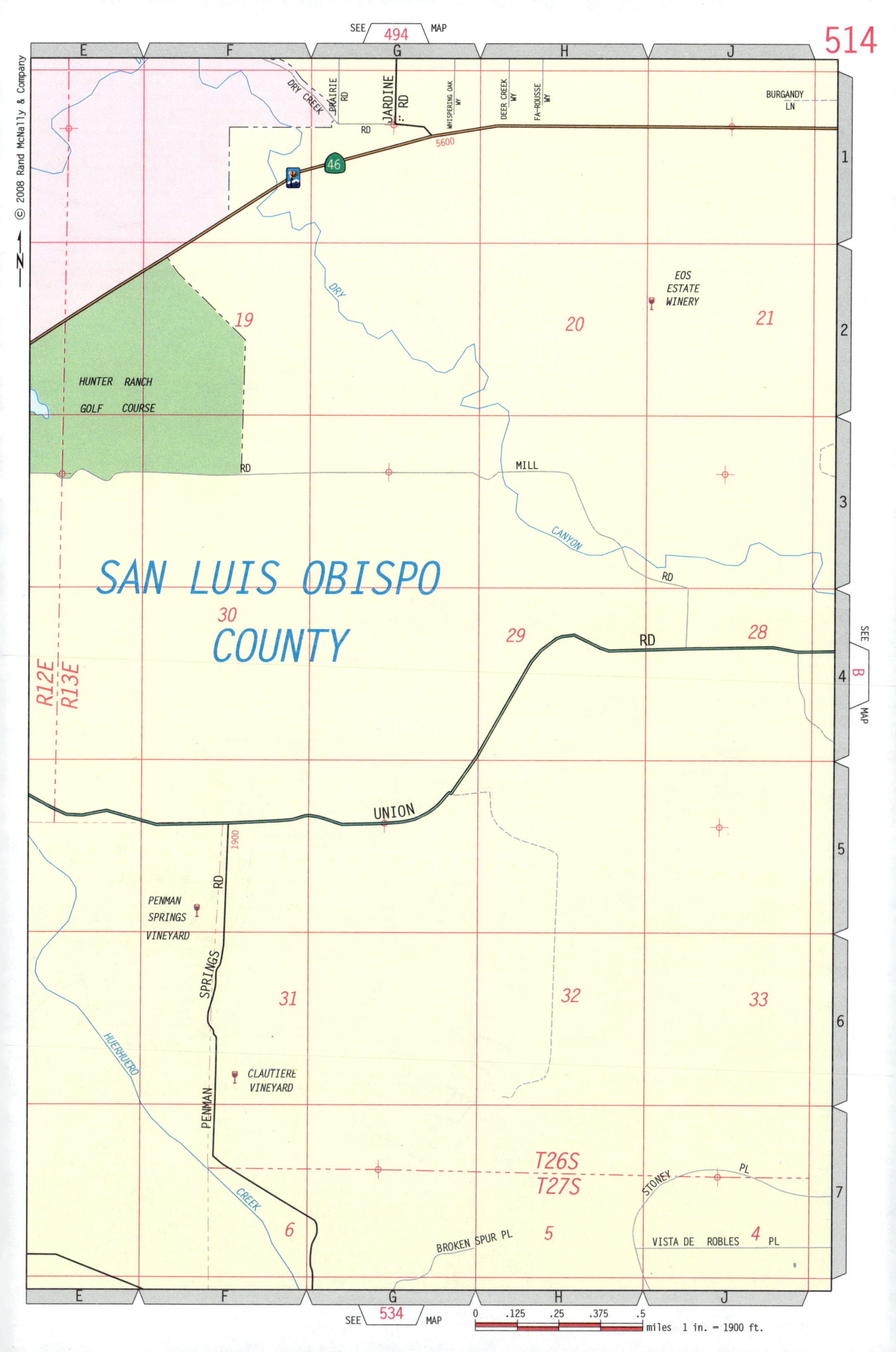
SEE 494 MAP
E
F
G
H
J
DRY CREEK
PRAIRIE RD
JARDINE RD
RD
WHISPERING OAK WY
DEER CREEK WY
FA-ROUSSE WY
BURGANDY LN
5600
46
1
DRY
19
20
21
EOS ESTATE WINERY
2
HUNTER RANCH GOLF COURSE
RD
MILL
3
CANYON
RD
SAN LUIS OBISPO COUNTY
30
29
RD
28
R12E
R13E
4
SEE B MAP
UNION
1900
RD
5
PENMAN SPRINGS VINEYARD
SPRINGS
31
32
33
6
HUERHUERO
CLAUTIERE VINEYARD
PENMAN
T26S
T27S
STONEY
PL
7
CREEK
6
BROKEN SPUR PL
5
VISTA DE ROBLES
4
PL
SEE 534 MAP
0 .125 .25 .375 .5
miles 1 in. = 1900 ft.

SEE B MAP

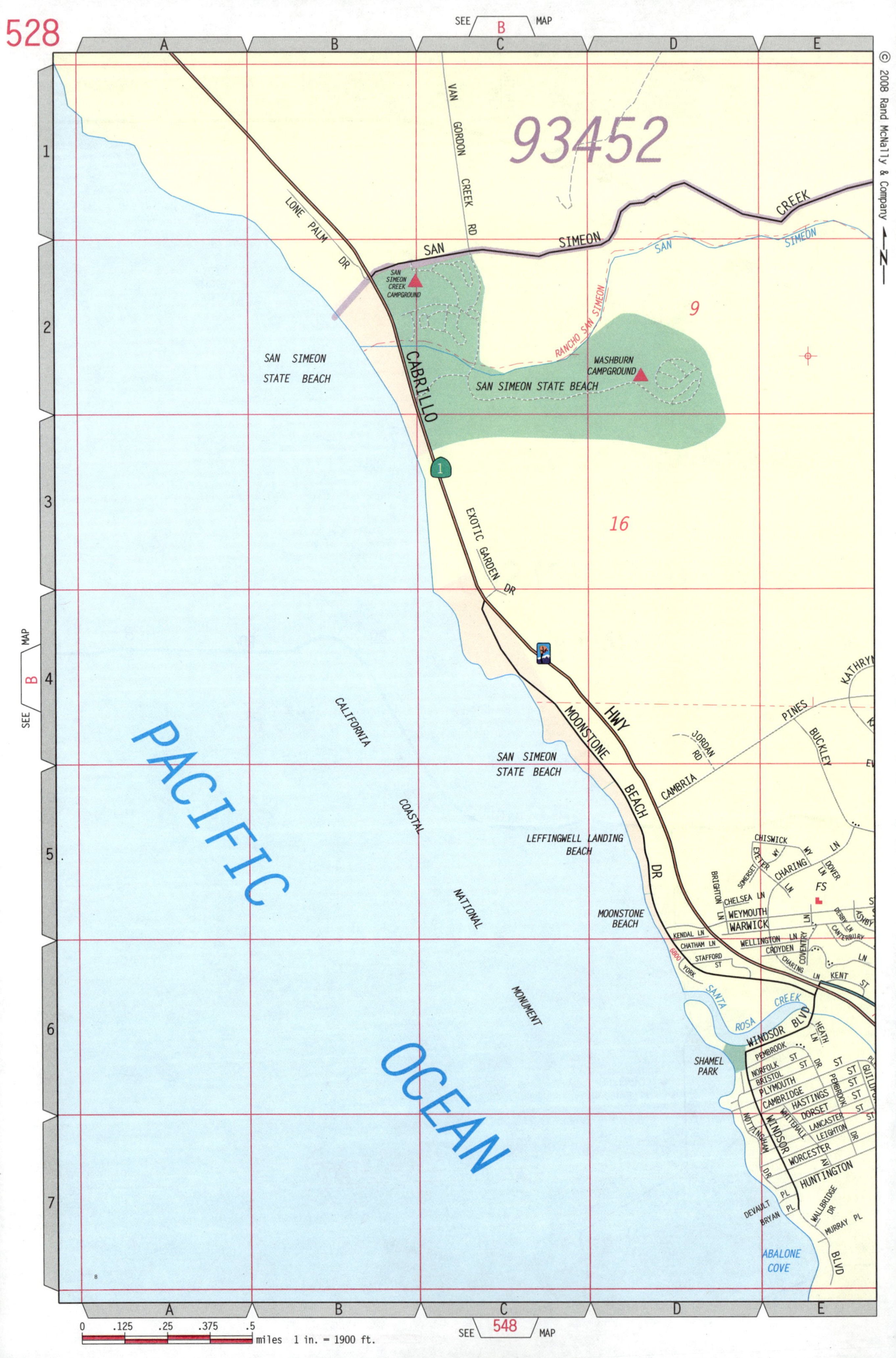
93452
SAN SIMEON CREEK
VAN GORDON CREEK RD
LONE PALM DR
SAN SIMEON CREEK CAMPGROUND
RANCHO SAN SIMEON
WASHBURN CAMPGROUND
SAN SIMEON STATE BEACH
CABRILLO
9
16
EXOTIC GARDEN DR
MOONSTONE BEACH DR
HWY
JORDAN RD
CAMBRIA
PINES
BUCKLEY
KATHRYN
PACIFIC OCEAN
CALIFORNIA COASTAL NATIONAL MONUMENT
LEFFINGWELL LANDING BEACH
MOONSTONE BEACH
CHISWICK
EXETER
SOMERSET
CHARING LN
DOVER LN
BRIGHTON LN
CHELSEA LN
WEYMOUTH
WARWICK
FS
KENDAL LN
CHATHAM LN
STAFFORD ST
YORK
WELLINGTON LN
CROYDEN
COVENTRY
CANTERBURY
KENT ST
SANTA ROSA CREEK
WINDSOR BLVD
HEATH LN
SHAMEL PARK
PEMBROOK
NORFOLK ST
BRISTOL ST
PLYMOUTH
CAMBRIDGE
HASTINGS
DORSET
LANCASTER
LEIGHTON
WORCESTER
HUNTINGTON
NOTTINGHAM DR
WHITEHALL
DEVAULT PL
BRYAN PL
WALLBRIDGE DR
MURRAY PL
ABALONE COVE
A B C D E
1 2 3 4 5 6 7

SEE B MAP

0 .125 .25 .375 .5 miles 1 in. = 1900 ft.

SEE 548 MAP

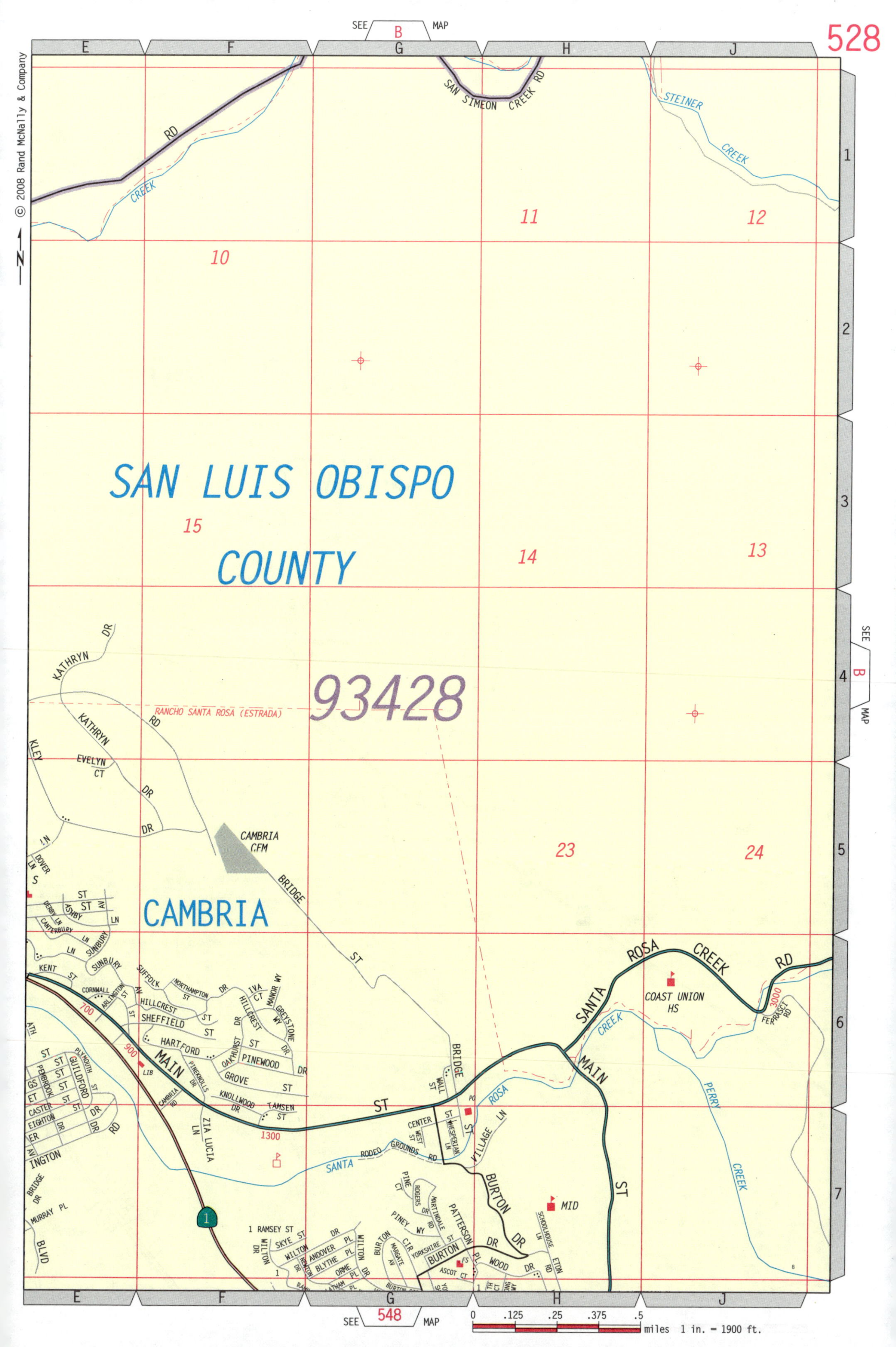
SEE B MAP
SEE B MAP
SEE 548 MAP
SAN LUIS OBISPO COUNTY
93428
CAMBRIA
SAN SIMEON CREEK RD
STEINER CREEK
CREEK
RD
RANCHO SANTA ROSA (ESTRADA)
KATHRYN DR
EVELYN CT
CAMBRIA CEM
BRIDGE ST
SANTA ROSA CREEK RD
COAST UNION HS
FERRASCI RD
PERRY CREEK
MAIN ST
SANTA ROSA
RODEO GROUNDS RD
BURTON DR
PATTERSON PL
VILLAGE LN
MID
SCHOOLHOUSE LN
EATON RD
WOOD DR
SANTA ROSA CREEK
KENT ST
SUNBURY
SUFFOLK ST
NORTHAMPTON DR
HILLCREST
SHEFFIELD ST
HARTFORD
OAKHURST DR
PINEWOOD DR
GROVE ST
KNOLLWOOD DR
TAMSEN ST
GREYSTONE
MANOR WY
IVA CT
ZIA LUCIA LN
GUILDFORD DR
PLYMOUTH ST
PEMBROOK
CASTER
BRIDGE DR
MURRAY PL
BLVD
RAMSEY ST
SKYE ST
WILTON DR
ANDOVER PL
BLYTHE PL
ORME
MARGATE AV
YORKSHIRE
BURTON
ASCOT CT
PINE CT
ROGERS DR
MARTINDALE RD
PINEY WY
CENTER ST
WEST ST
HESPERIAN LN
WALL ST
LIB
PO
FS
700
900
1300
3000
10 11 12 14 13 15 23 24
0 .125 .25 .375 .5 miles 1 in. = 1900 ft.

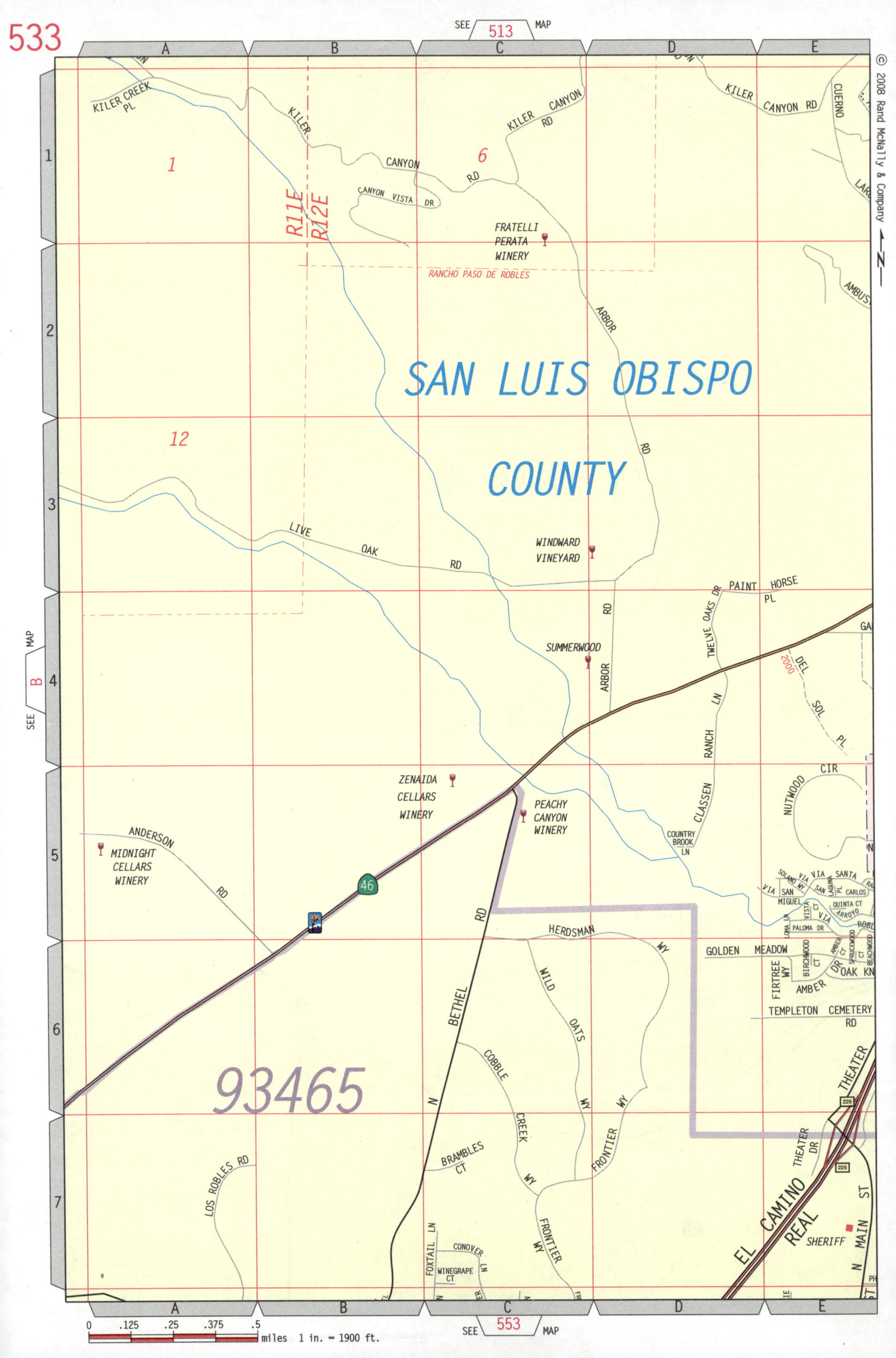
SEE 513 MAP
SAN LUIS OBISPO COUNTY
KILER CREEK PL
KILER CANYON RD
CANYON VISTA DR
FRATELLI PERATA WINERY
RANCHO PASO DE ROBLES
R11E
R12E
ARBOR RD
LIVE OAK RD
WINDWARD VINEYARD
SUMMERWOOD
TWELVE OAKS DR
PAINT HORSE PL
DEL SOL PL
RANCH LN
CLASSEN
COUNTRY BROOK LN
NUTWOOD CIR
ZENAIDA CELLARS WINERY
PEACHY CANYON WINERY
ANDERSON RD
MIDNIGHT CELLARS WINERY
46
N BETHEL RD
HERDSMAN WY
WILD OATS WY
GOLDEN MEADOW
FIRTREE WY
BIRCHWOOD CT
AMBER DR
OAK KN
TEMPLETON CEMETERY RD
PALOMA DR
VIA SAN MIGUEL
SANTA
QUINTA CT
COBBLE CREEK WY
FRONTIER WY
BRAMBLES CT
LOS ROBLES RD
FOXTAIL LN
CONOVER LN
WINEGRAPE CT
THEATER DR
EL CAMINO REAL
N MAIN ST
SHERIFF
226
93465
SEE B MAP
SEE 553 MAP
miles 1 in. = 1900 ft.

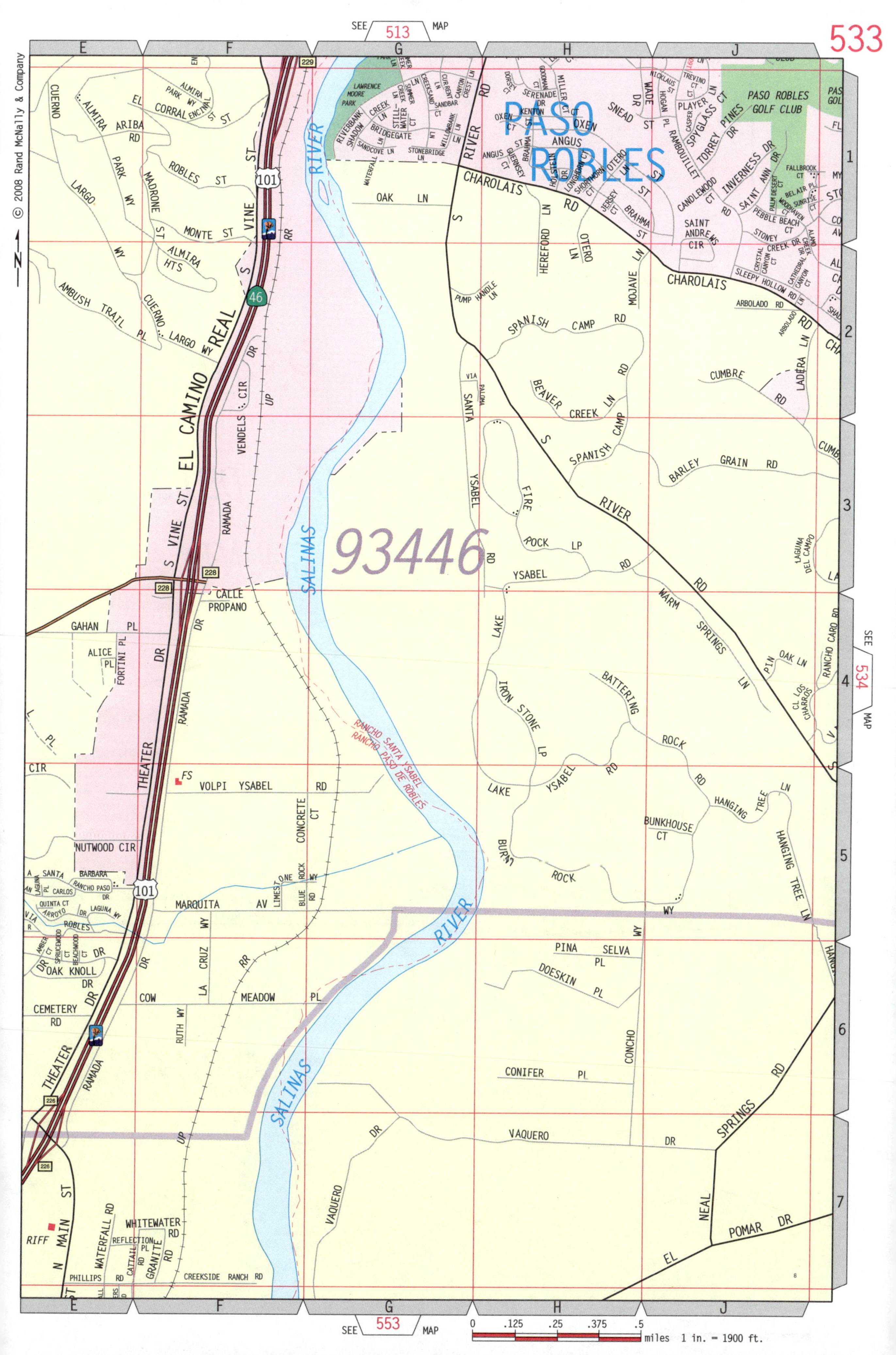
SEE 513 MAP
PASO ROBLES
PASO ROBLES GOLF CLUB

CUERNO
ALMIRA
ARIBA RD
EL CORRAL ENCINAL ST
ALMIRA ST
PARK WY
ENCINAL ST
ROBLES ST
MADRONE ST
MONTE ST
VINE ST
ALMIRA HTS
AMBUSH TRAIL PL
CUERNO LARGO WY
LARGO
PARK WY

S VINE ST
VENDELS CIR
RAMADA
UP
DR

RIVER
SALINAS

CHAROLAIS
CHAROLAIS RD
OAK LN
PUMP HANDLE LN
HEREFORD LN
OTERO LN
MOJAVE LN

SPANISH CAMP RD
BEAVER CREEK LN
VIA PALOMA
VIA SANTA YSABEL
SPANISH CAMP RD
BARLEY GRAIN RD
CUMBRE RD
LADERA LN
ARBOLADO RD

FIRE ROCK LP
YSABEL
RIVER
WARM SPRINGS LN
PIN OAK LN
LAGUNA DEL CAMPO
RANCHO CARO RD

LAKE YSABEL RD
IRON STONE LP
BATTERING ROCK RD
HANGING TREE LN
BUNKHOUSE CT
CL LOS CHARROS

LAKE YSABEL
BURN ROCK
HANGING TREE LN

GAHAN PL
ALICE PL
FORTINI PL
CALLE PROPANO
THEATER DR
RAMADA DR

FS
VOLPI YSABEL RD
CONCRETE CT
LIMESTONE WY
BLUE ROCK RD

CIR
NUTWOOD CIR
SANTA
LAGUNA
BARBARA
RANCHO PASO DR
QUINTA CT
MARQUITA AV
ROBLES DR
OAK KNOLL DR
SPRUCEWOOD
BEACHWOOD
LA CRUZ WY
RR
MEADOW PL
COW DR
RUTH WY

PINA SELVA PL
DOESKIN PL
CONCHO
CONIFER PL
VAQUERO DR

CEMETERY RD
THEATER DR
RAMADA
UP
NEAL
POMAR DR
EL SPRINGS RD

RIFF
N MAIN ST
WATERFALL RD
WHITEWATER RD
REFLECTION
CATTAIL
GRANITE
CREEKSIDE RANCH RD
PHILLIPS RD
VAQUERO

RANCHO SANTA YSABEL
RANCHO PASO DE ROBLES

0 .125 .25 .375 .5
93446
SALINAS RIVER
EL CAMINO REAL
SEE 534 MAP
SEE 553 MAP
miles 1 in. = 1900 ft.

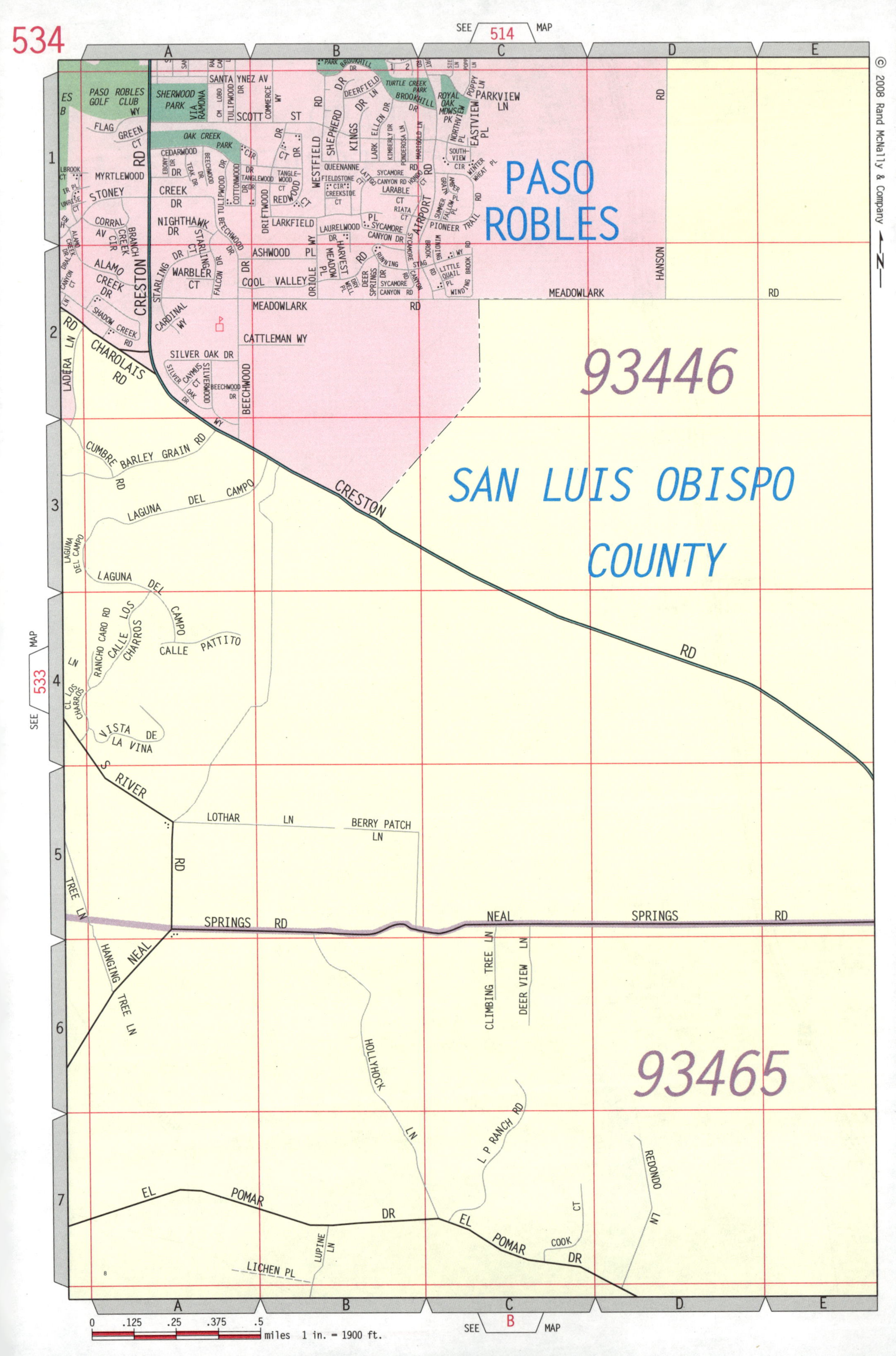
SEE 514 MAP
PASO ROBLES
SAN LUIS OBISPO COUNTY
93446
93465
CRESTON RD
MEADOWLARK RD
NEAL SPRINGS RD
EL POMAR DR
S RIVER RD
LAGUNA DEL CAMPO
LOTHAR LN
BERRY PATCH LN
HOLLYHOCK LN
L P RANCH RD
REDONDO LN
CLIMBING TREE LN
DEER VIEW LN
HANGING TREE LN
LUPINE LN
LICHEN PL
COOK CT
CHAROLAIS RD
BARLEY GRAIN RD
PASO ROBLES GOLF CLUB
SHERWOOD PARK
OAK CREEK PARK
AIRPORT RD
SEE 533 MAP
SEE B MAP
0 .125 .25 .375 .5 miles 1 in. = 1900 ft.

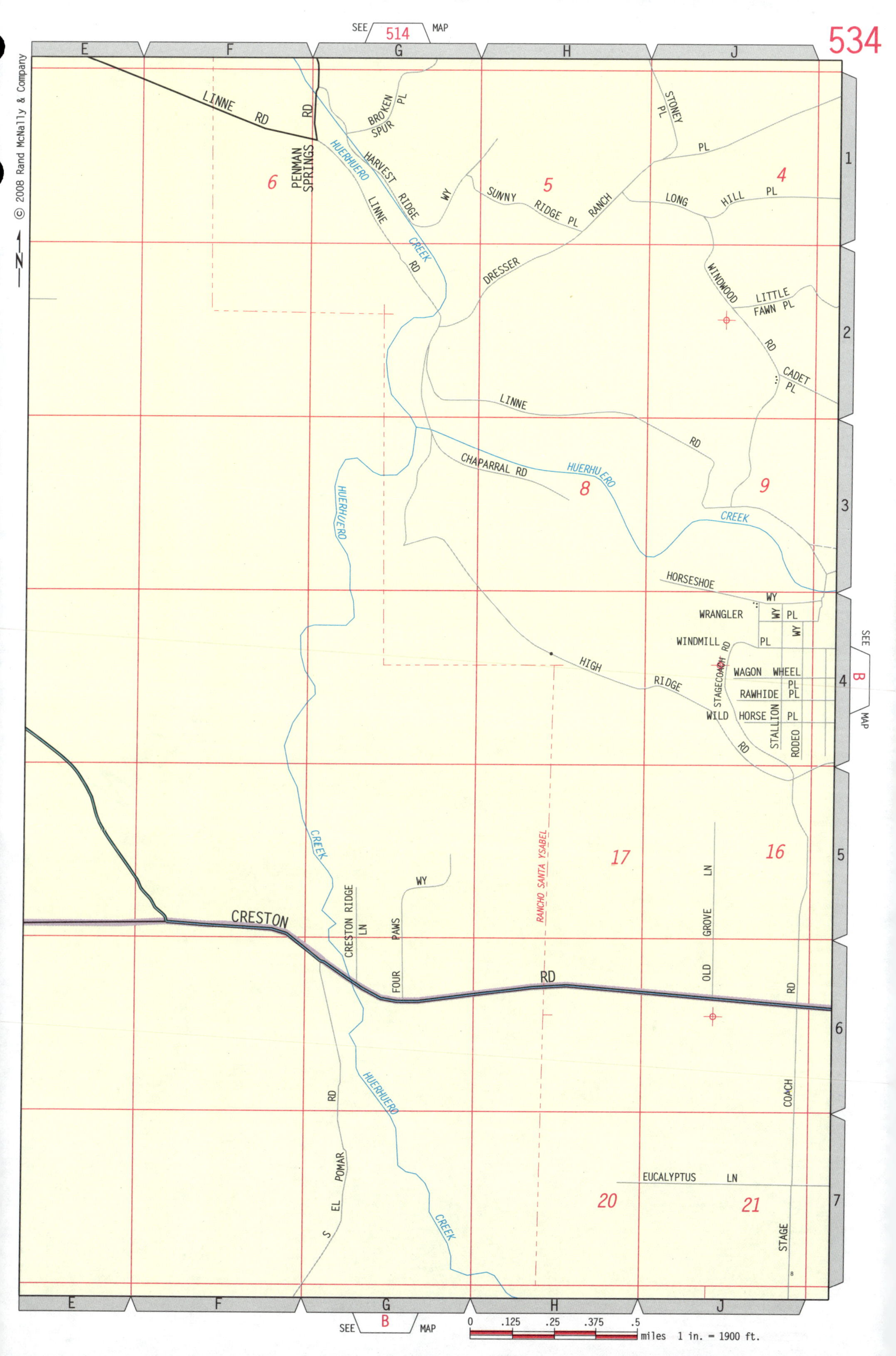

SEE 514 MAP
E
F
G
H
J
LINNE RD
RD
PENMAN SPRINGS
BROKEN SPUR PL
HUERHUERO CREEK
HARVEST RIDGE WY
LINNE RD
STONEY PL
PL
SUNNY RIDGE PL
RANCH
LONG HILL PL
DRESSER
WINDWOOD RD
LITTLE FAWN PL
CADET PL
LINNE RD
CHAPARRAL RD
HUERHUERO CREEK
HUERHUERO
HORSESHOE WY
WRANGLER WY PL
WINDMILL PL WY
WAGON WHEEL PL
RAWHIDE PL
HORSE PL
STAGECOACH RD
WILD
STALLION
RODEO
HIGH RIDGE RD
RANCHO SANTA YSABEL
CREEK
CRESTON RD
CRESTON RIDGE LN
FOUR PAWS WY
OLD GROVE LN
RD
COACH
STAGE
S EL POMAR RD
HUERHUERO CREEK
EUCALYPTUS LN
1
2
3
4
5
6
7
4
5
6
8
9
16
17
20
21
SEE B MAP
0 .125 .25 .375 .5
miles 1 in. = 1900 ft.

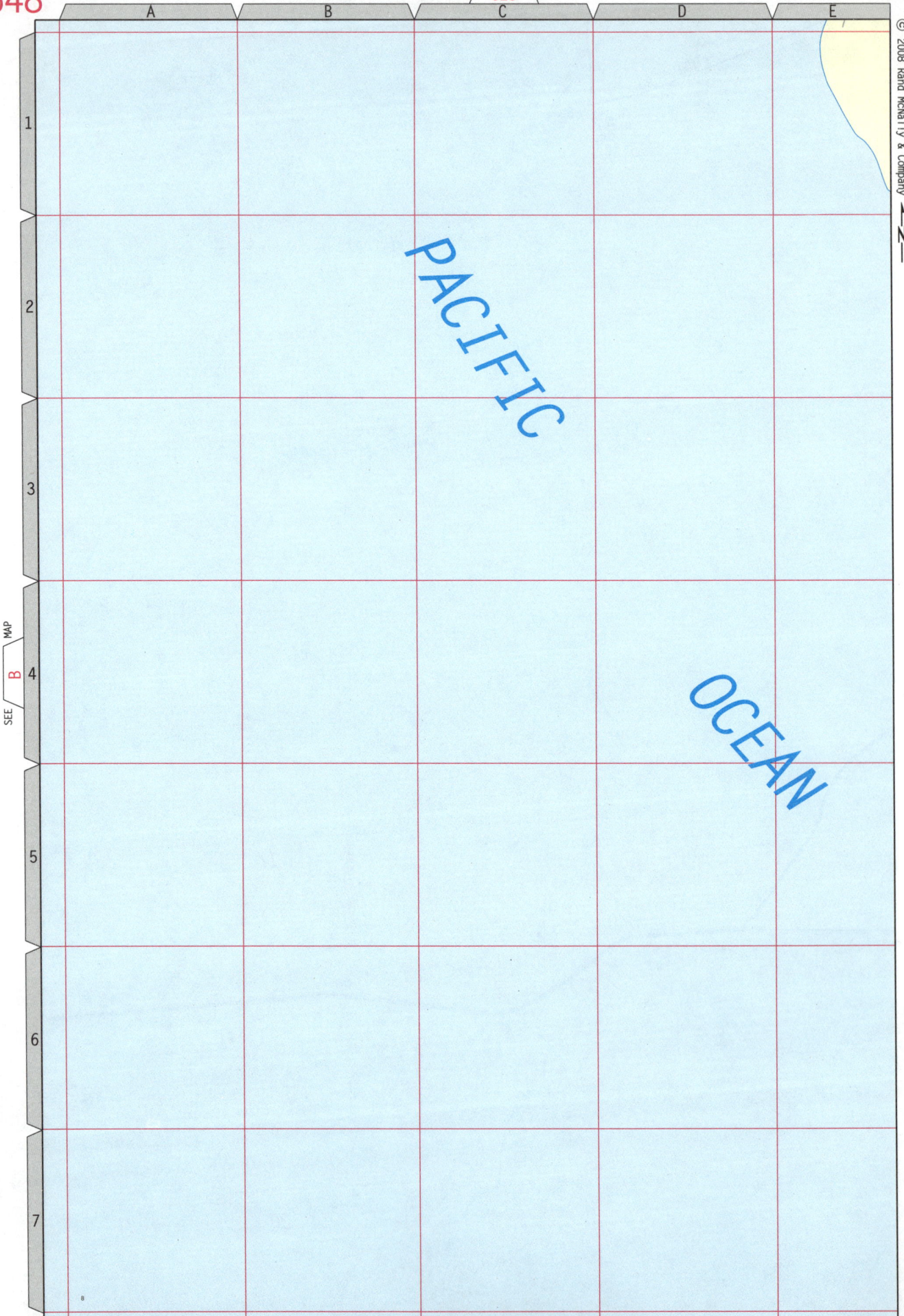

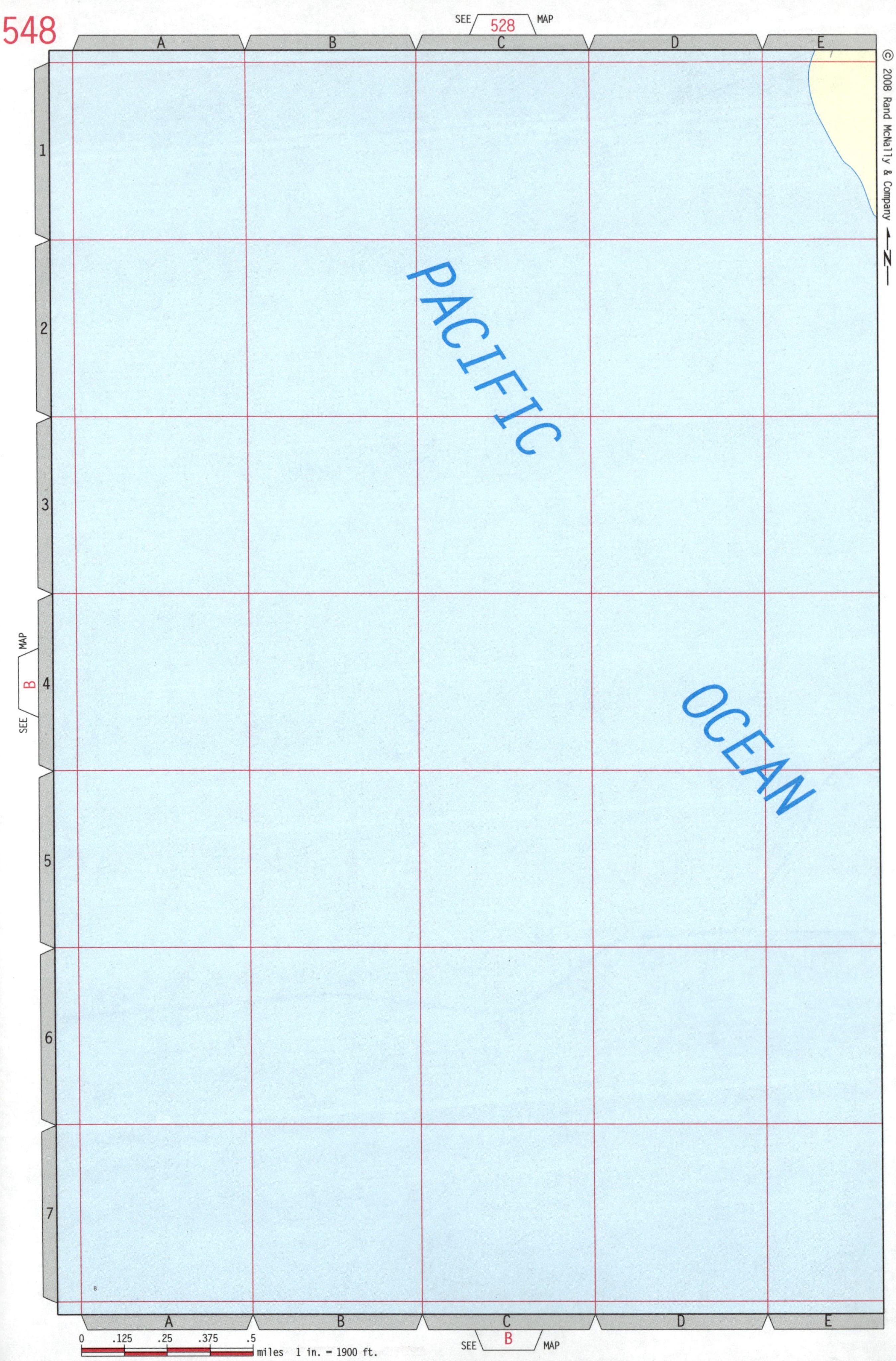

SEE 528 MAP
A
B
C
D
E
1
2
3
4
5
6
7
SEE B MAP
PACIFIC
OCEAN
0
.125
.25
.375
.5
miles 1 in. = 1900 ft.

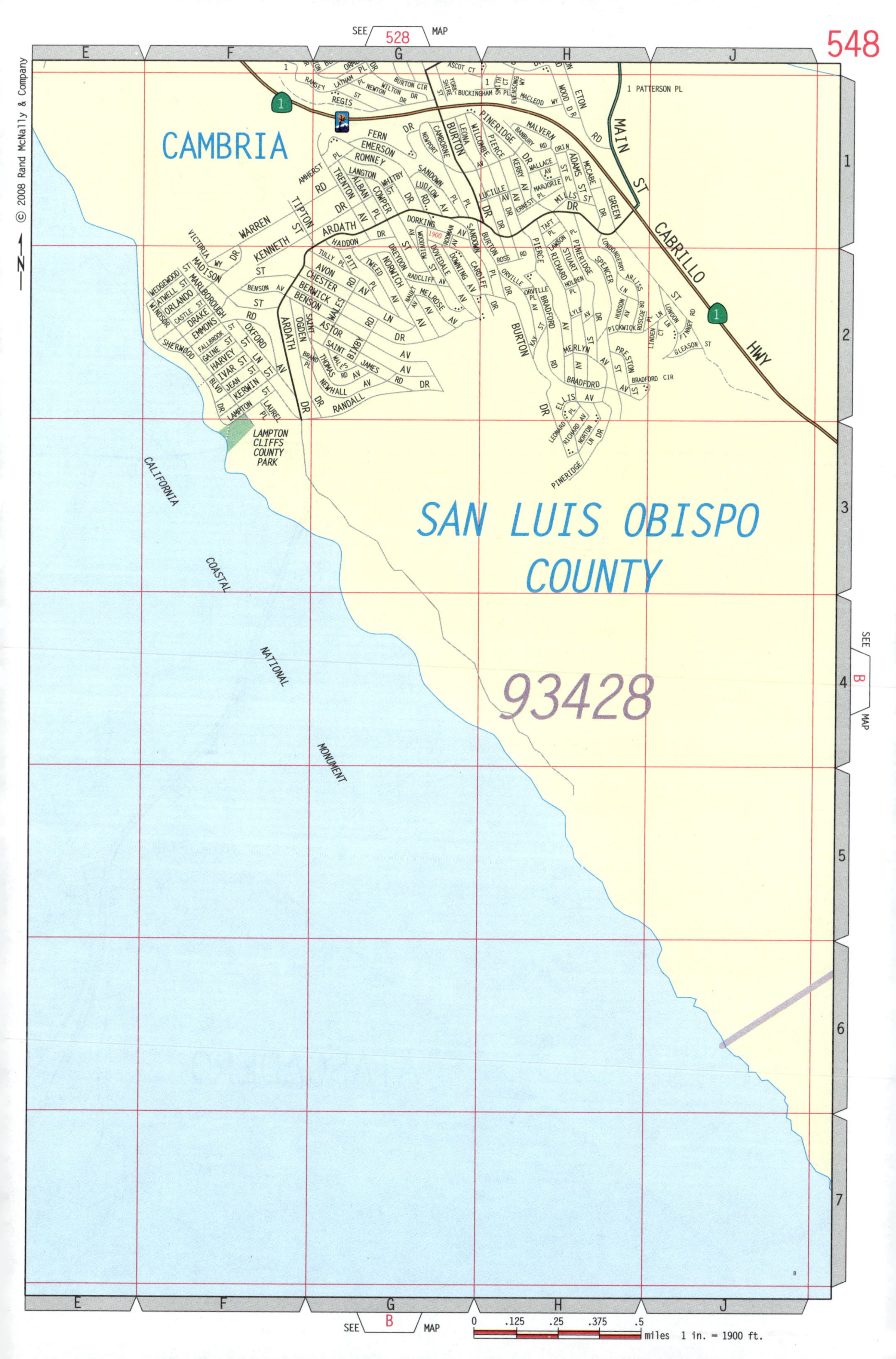
SEE 528 MAP
E
F
G
H
J
1
2
3
4
5
6
7
© 2008 Rand McNally & Company
CAMBRIA
SAN LUIS OBISPO
COUNTY
93428
CALIFORNIA
COASTAL
NATIONAL
MONUMENT
LAMPTON
CLIFFS
COUNTY
PARK
1 PATTERSON PL
MAIN ST
CABRILLO HWY
1
BURTON DR
PINERIDGE DR
ARDATH DR
WARREN
TIPTON ST
KENNETH ST
MADISON ST
MARLBOROUGH
WINDSOR BLVD
SHERWOOD
OXFORD AV
EMERSON
ROMNEY
FERN DR
TRENTON
ALBAN
COWPER
WHITBY
SANDOWN
LUDLOW RD
CAMBORNE
LEONA
WILLCOMBE
PIERCE
KERRY AV
LUCILLE AV
MALVERN
ADAMS ST
MCCABE
GREEN DR
MILLS ST
CARDIFF PL
DOWNING AV
DOVEDALE
NORWICH AV
DREYDON
TWEED
PITT
AVON
CHESTER
BERWICK
BENSON
WALES
ASTOR
BIXBY
JAMES AV
NEWHALL AV
RANDALL DR
RICHARD AV
STUART
SPENCER
BRADFORD RD
MERLYN
PRESTON ST
BRADFORD CIR
ELLIS AV
NORTON LN
GLEASON ST
FINNEY RD
LONDON CT
HUDSON AV
ROSCOE DR
LONDONDERRY LN
ETON RD
WOOD DR
REGIS
RAMSEY
LATHAM PL
NEWTON DR
WILTON
BURTON CIR
BUCKINGHAM PL
ASCOT CT
MACLEOD WY
EVENSONG WY
SEE B MAP
0 .125 .25 .375 .5
miles 1 in. = 1900 ft.

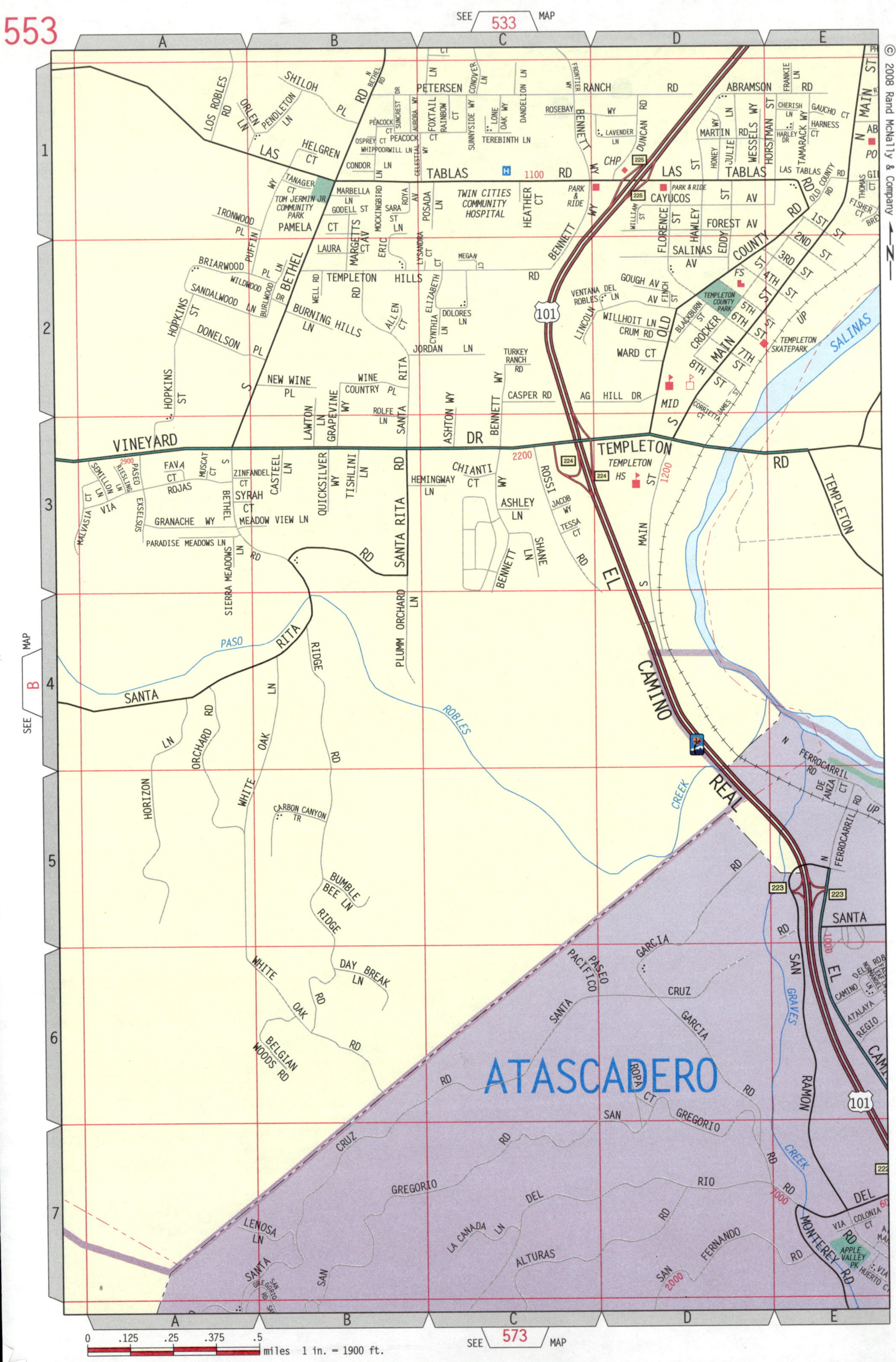
SEE 533 MAP
SEE B MAP
SEE 573 MAP
A
B
C
D
E
1
2
3
4
5
6
7
ATASCADERO
TWIN CITIES COMMUNITY HOSPITAL
TOM JERMIN JR COMMUNITY PARK
TEMPLETON COUNTY PARK
TEMPLETON SKATEPARK
TEMPLETON HS
APPLE VALLEY PK
SALINAS
PASO ROBLES CREEK
GRAVES CREEK
VINEYARD DR
TEMPLETON RD
LAS TABLAS RD
EL CAMINO REAL
S BETHEL RD
SANTA RITA RD
PETERSEN RANCH RD
S MAIN ST
OLD COUNTY RD
TEMPLETON HILLS RD
BURNING HILLS LN
NEW WINE PL
WINE COUNTRY PL
HOPKINS ST
DONELSON PL
SHILOH PL
HELGREN CT
PAMELA CT
JORDAN LN
AG HILL DR
CASPER RD
CHIANTI CT
ASHLEY LN
ROSSI RD
WHITE OAK LN
WHITE OAK RD
HORIZON LN
ORCHARD RD
PLUMM ORCHARD LN
RIDGE RD
BUMBLE BEE LN
DAY BREAK LN
BELGIAN WOODS RD
CARBON CANYON TR
SAN RAMON RD
N FERROCARRIL RD
SANTA CRUZ RD
SAN GREGORIO RD
DEL RIO RD
SAN FERNANDO RD
MONTEREY RD
LENOSA LN
ALTURAS RD
LA CANADA LN
PASEO PACIFICO
GARCIA RD
101
223
224
225
1100
1200
2200
2900
1000
2000
0 .125 .25 .375 .5 miles 1 in. = 1900 ft.

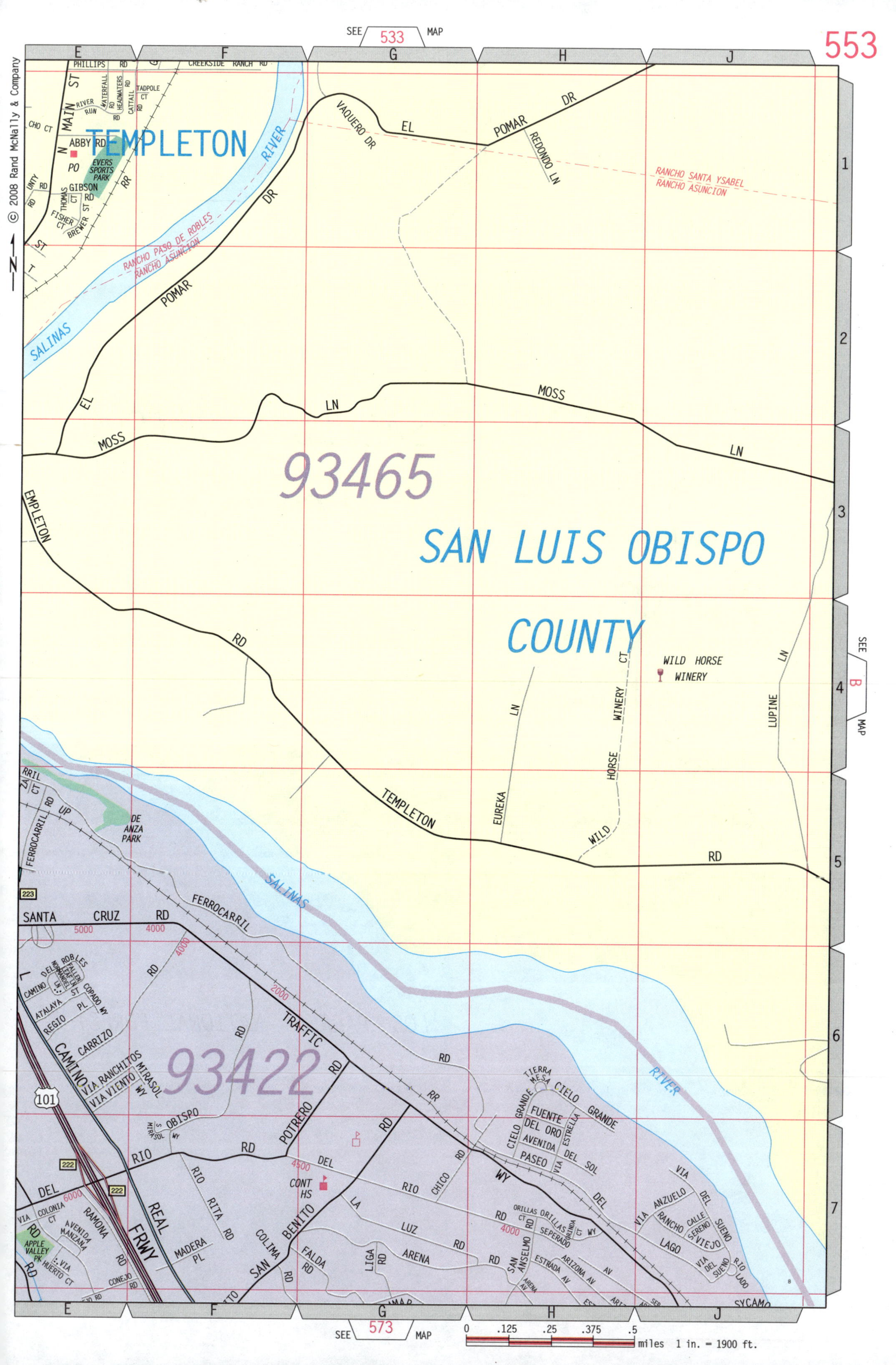
SEE 533 MAP
E
F
G
H
J
1
2
3
4
5
6
7
TEMPLETON
PHILLIPS RD
CREEKSIDE RANCH RD
N MAIN ST
WATERFALL RD
HEADWATERS RD
CATTAIL RD
TADPOLE CT
RIVER RUN RD
CHO CT
ABBY RD
PO
EVERS SPORTS PARK
UNTY RD
GIBSON RD
THOMAS CT
FISHER CT
BREWER ST
RR
SALINAS RIVER
RANCHO PASO DE ROBLES
RANCHO ASUNCION
RANCHO SANTA YSABEL
RANCHO ASUNCION
VAQUERO DR
EL POMAR DR
REDONDO LN
MOSS LN
93465
SAN LUIS OBISPO COUNTY
TEMPLETON RD
WILD HORSE WINERY
WILD HORSE WINERY CT
EUREKA LN
LUPINE LN
SEE B MAP
FERROCARRIL RD
DE ANZA PARK
223
SANTA CRUZ RD
5000
4000
TRAFFIC WY
93422
CAMINO REAL
101
RIO RD
POTRERO RD
CONT HS
DEL RIO RD
CHICO RD
LA LUZ RD
ARENA RD
SAN BENITO RD
COLIMA RD
FALDA RD
LIGA RD
SAN ANSELMO
ESTRADA AV
ARIZONA AV
MADERA PL
RITA RD
RAMONA RD
AVENIDA MANZANA
APPLE VALLEY PK
VIA HUERTO CT
CONEJO RD
FRWY
222
CARRIZO
REGIO PL
ATALAYA ST
COPADO WY
VIA RANCHITOS
VIA VIENTO
MIRASOL WY
OBISPO
CIELO GRANDE
TIERRA MESA
FUENTE DEL ORO
AVENIDA ESTRELLA
PASEO DEL SOL
VIA DEL SOL
ORILLAS CT
ORILLAS WY
SEPERADO CT
VIA ANZUELO
RANCHO LAGO
CALLE SERENO
VIA DEL SUENO
VIA VIEJO
RIO LADO
SYCAMO
SEE 573 MAP
0 .125 .25 .375 .5 miles 1 in. = 1900 ft.

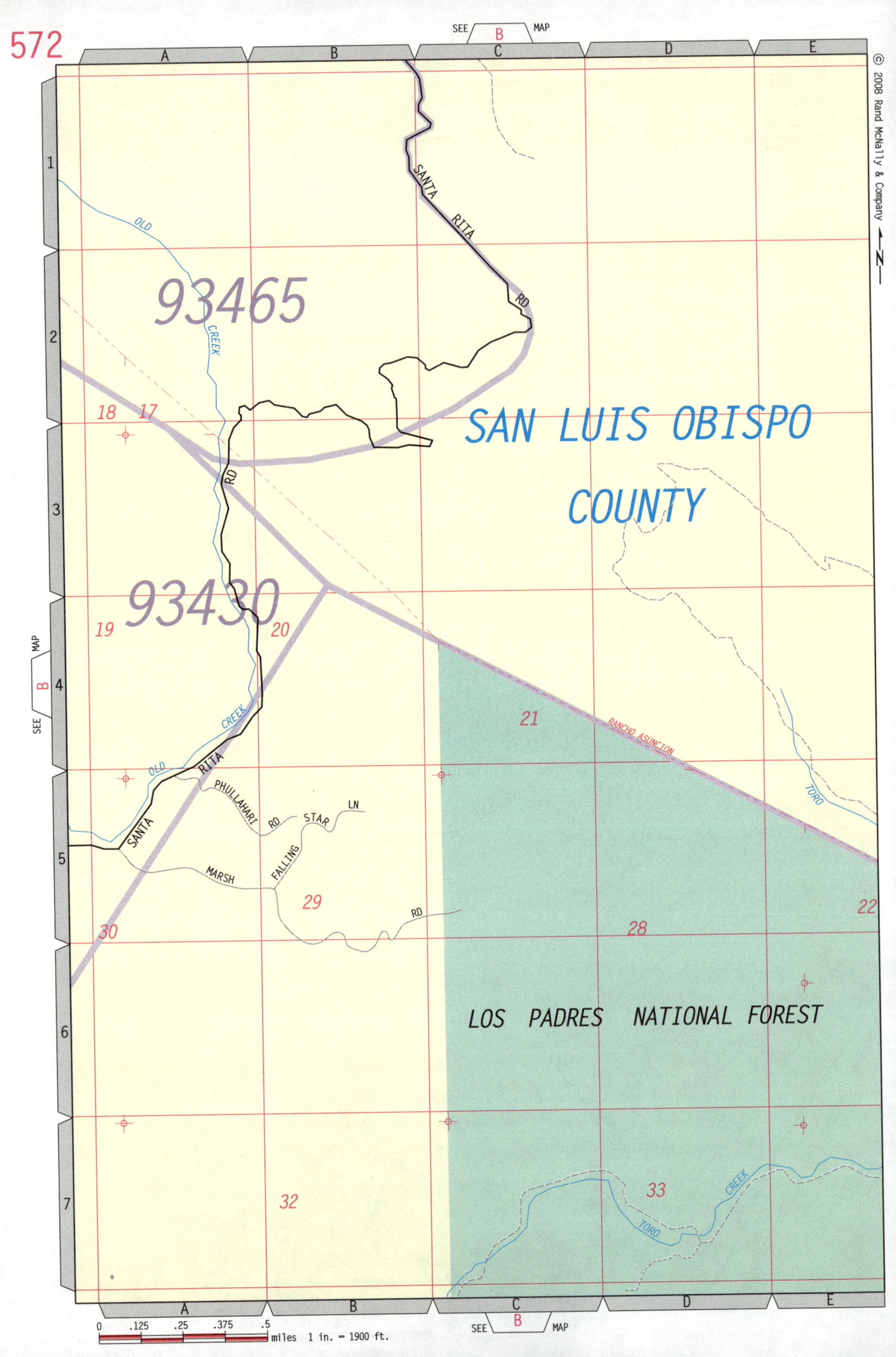
SEE B MAP
A
B
C
D
E
1
2
3
4
5
6
7
SANTA RITA RD
OLD CREEK
93465
93430
18
17
19
20
21
22
28
29
30
32
33
SAN LUIS OBISPO
COUNTY
RANCHO ASUNCION
TORO
PHULLAHARI RD
STAR LN
FALLING
MARSH
RD
LOS PADRES NATIONAL FOREST
TORO CREEK
0 .125 .25 .375 .5
miles 1 in. = 1900 ft.

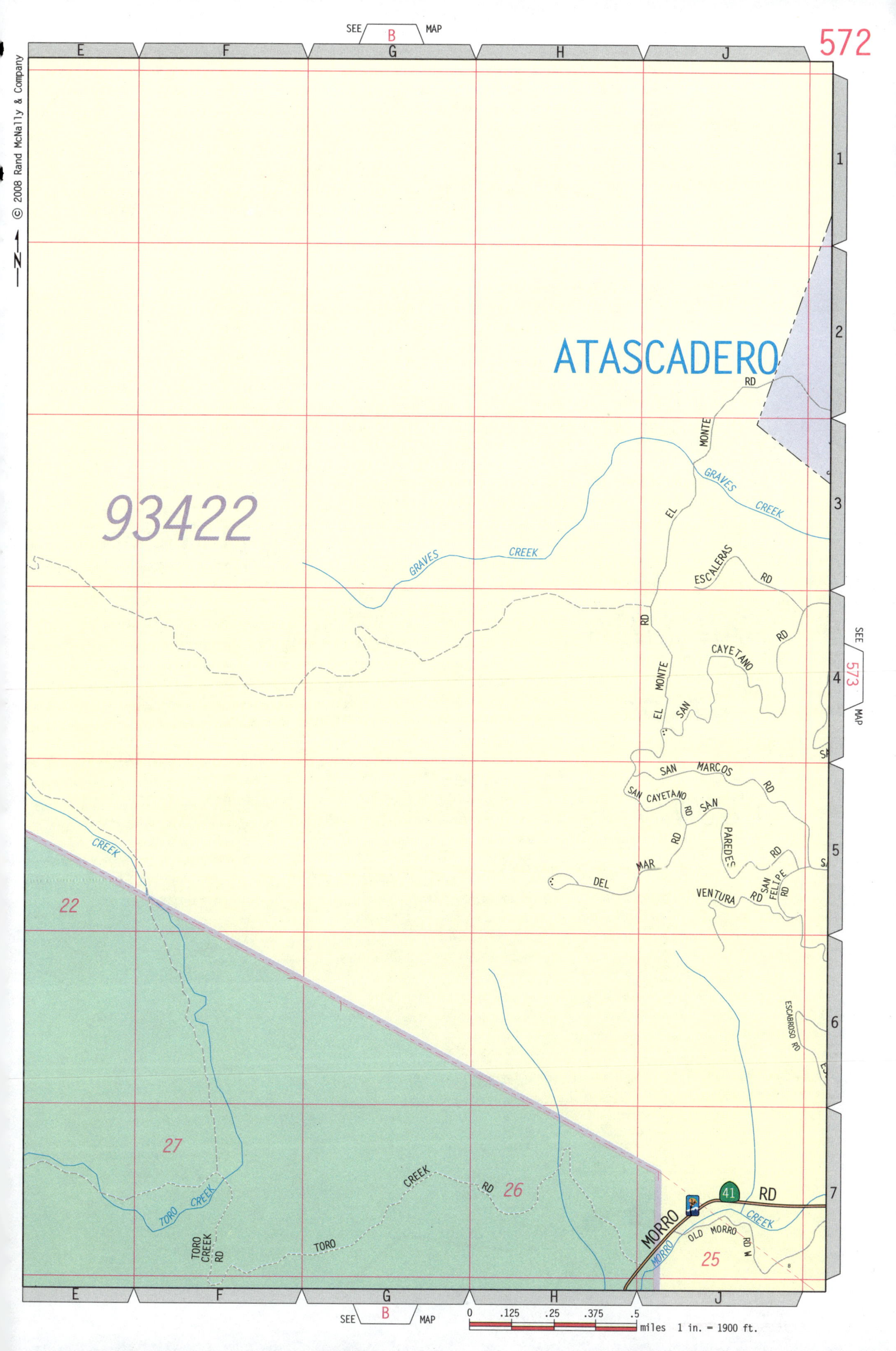
SEE B MAP
E
F
G
H
J
1
2
3
4
5
6
7
ATASCADERO
93422
GRAVES CREEK
MONTE
EL
RD
ESCALERAS
CAYETANO
EL MONTE
SAN
SEE 573 MAP
SAN MARCOS RD
SAN CAYETANO RD
SAN PAREDES RD
DEL MAR RD
VENTURA RD
SAN FELIPE RD
ESCABROSO RD
CREEK
22
27
26
25
TORO CREEK
TORO CREEK RD
CREEK RD
TORO
41
MORRO RD
MORRO CREEK
OLD MORRO RD W
0 .125 .25 .375 .5 miles 1 in. = 1900 ft.

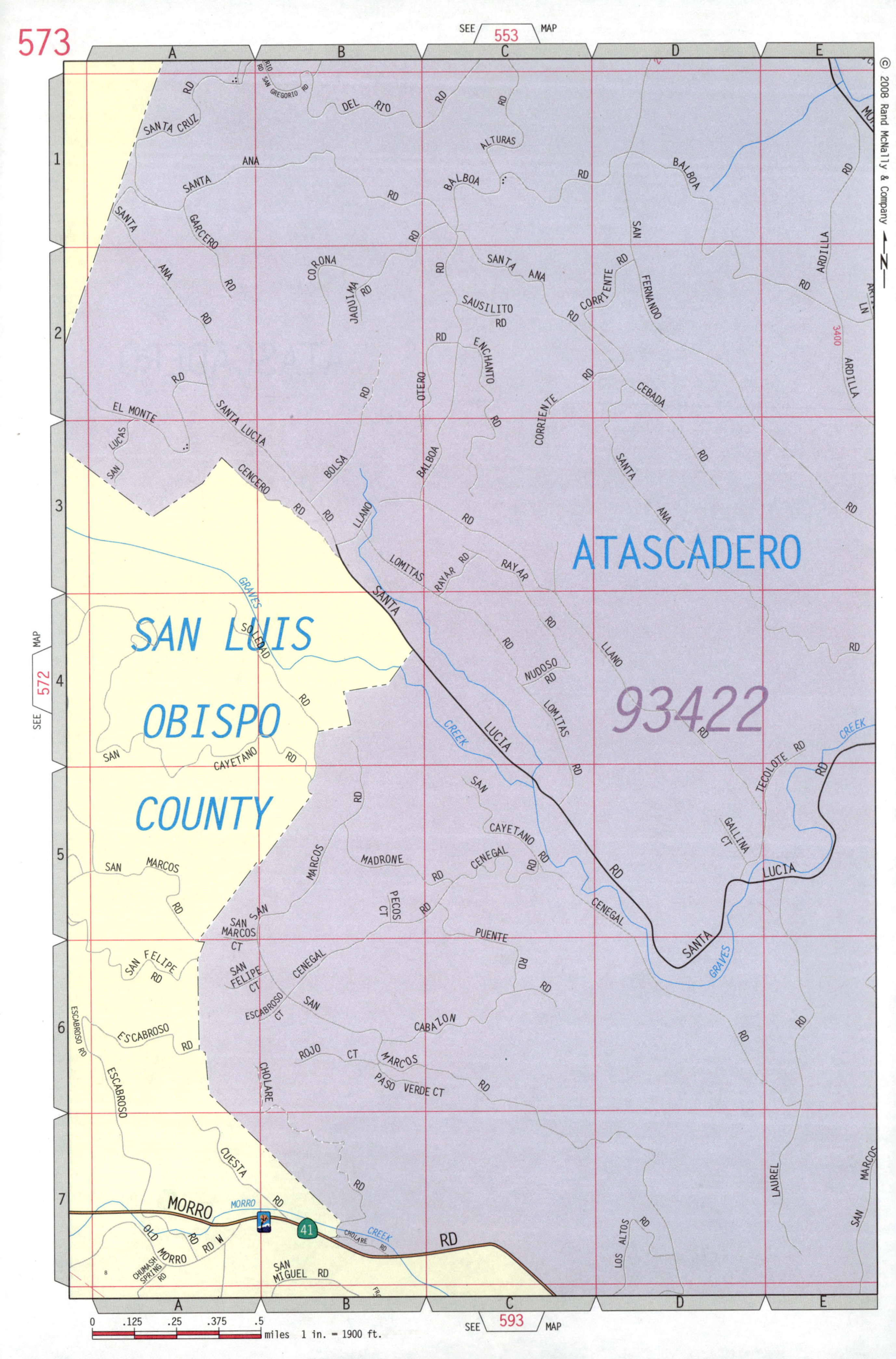
SEE 553 MAP
SEE 572 MAP
SEE 593 MAP
A
B
C
D
E
1
2
3
4
5
6
7
ATASCADERO
93422
SAN LUIS OBISPO COUNTY
SANTA CRUZ RD
DEL RIO RD
SAN GREGORIO RD
RIO RD
SANTA ANA RD
ALTURAS RD
BALBOA RD
GARCERO RD
CORONA RD
JAQUIMA RD
SAUSILITO RD
CORRIENTE RD
SAN FERNANDO RD
ARDILLA RD
ENCHANTO RD
OTERO RD
CEBADA RD
EL MONTE RD
LUCAS
SANTA LUCIA RD
CENCERO RD
BOLSA RD
LLANO RD
LOMITAS RD
RAYAR RD
NUDOSO RD
SOLEDAD RD
GRAVES CREEK
SAN CAYETANO RD
TECOLOTE RD
GALLINA CT
MADRONE RD
CENEGAL RD
PECOS CT
PUENTE RD
SAN MARCOS RD
SAN MARCOS CT
SAN FELIPE RD
SAN FELIPE CT
ESCABROSO RD
ESCABROSO CT
CABAZON RD
ROJO CT
PASO VERDE CT
CHOLARE RD
CUESTA RD
MORRO RD
MORRO CREEK
OLD MORRO RD W
CHUMASH SPRING RD
SAN MIGUEL RD
LOS ALTOS RD
LAUREL RD
41
3400
0 .125 .25 .375 .5 miles 1 in. = 1900 ft.

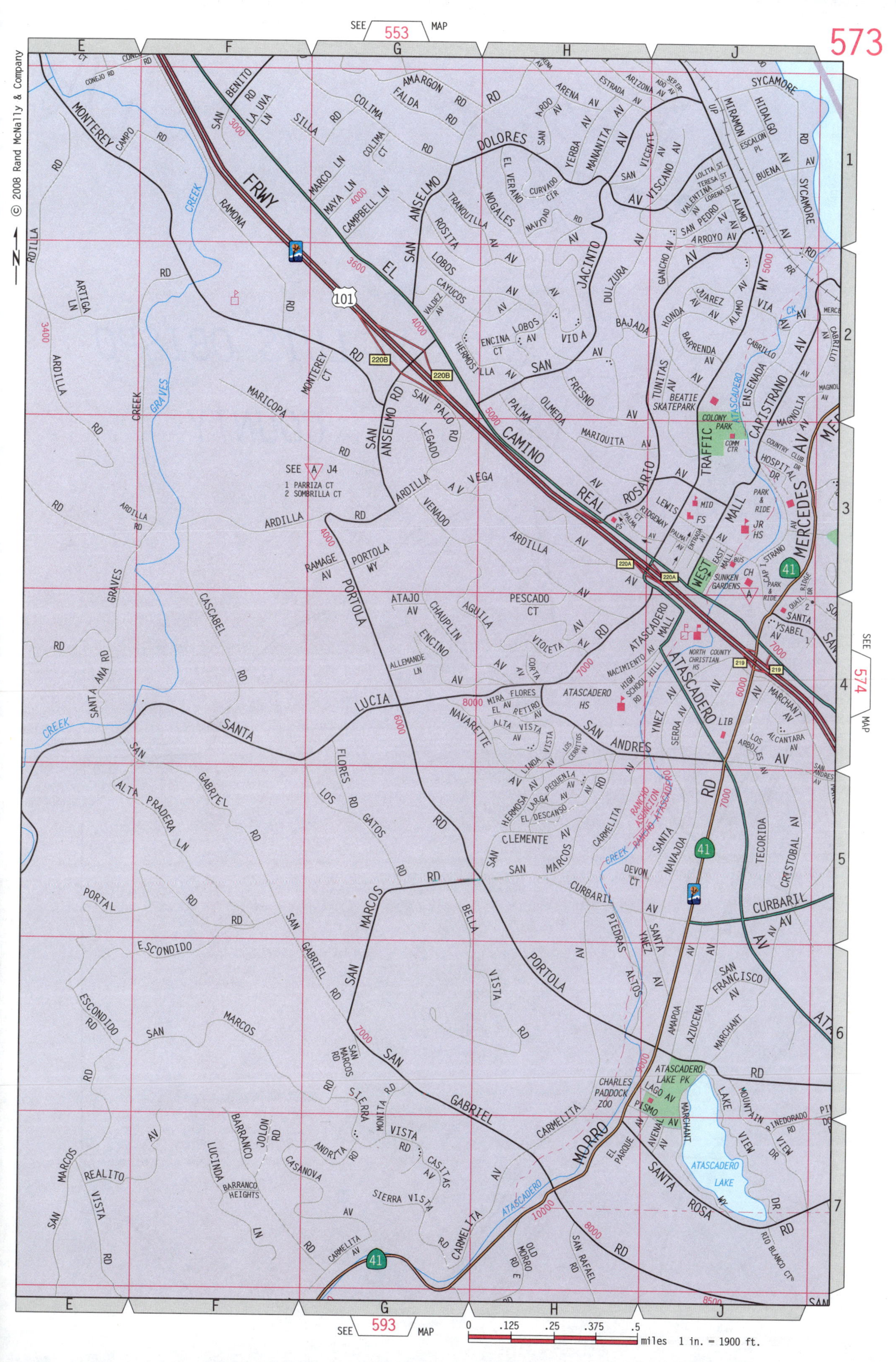
573
© 2008 Rand McNally & Company
SEE 553 MAP
SEE 574 MAP
SEE 593 MAP
E
F
G
H
J
1
2
3
4
5
6
7
MONTEREY RD
CONEJO RD
CAMPO RD
ARTIGA LN
ARDILLA
GRAVES CREEK
MARICOPA RD
MONTEREY CT
RAMONA
FRWY
101
220B
220A
219
41
EL CAMINO REAL
SAN BENITO RD
LA UVA LN
SILLA RD
COLIMA CT
AMARGON RD
FALDA RD
MARCO LN
MAYA LN
CAMPBELL LN
SAN ANSELMO RD
DOLORES RD
EL VERANO
NOGALES AV
TRANQUILLA AV
ROSITA AV
LOBOS AV
CAYUCOS AV
VALDEZ AV
HERMOSILLA AV
ENCINA CT
VIDA AV
SAN JACINTO AV
ARENA AV
ARDO AV
YERBA AV
MANANITA AV
ESTRADA AV
ARIZONA AV
SAN VICENTE AV
VISCANO AV
DULZURA AV
BAJADA AV
SYCAMORE RD
HIDALGO AV
MIRAMON
ESCALON PL
BUENA AV
LOLITA ST
TERESA ST
VALENTINA AV
LORENA ST
ALAMO AV
SAN PEDRO AV
ARROYO AV
GANCHO AV
JUAREZ AV
HONDA AV
BARRENDA AV
TUNITAS AV
BEATIE SKATEPARK
COLONY PARK
COMM CTR
TRAFFIC WY
CAPISTRANO AV
ENSENADA AV
CABRILLO
MAGNOLIA AV
COUNTRY CLUB DR
HOSPITAL DR
MERCEDES AV
ATASCADERO
SAN PALO RD
LEGADO
VEGA AV
VENADO
ARDILLA AV
PALMA AV
OLMEDA AV
FRESNO AV
MARIQUITA AV
ROSARIO AV
LEWIS AV
MALL
PARK & RIDE
JR HS
FS
WEST MALL
EAST MALL
SUNKEN GARDENS
CH
STRANO
QUAIL RIDGE DR
SANTA YSABEL AV
SEE A J4
1 PARRIZA CT
2 SOMBRILLA CT
RAMAGE AV
PORTOLA WY
PORTOLA RD
ATAJO AV
CHAUPLIN
AGUILA
PESCADO CT
ENCINO
ALLEMANDE LN
VIOLETA AV
ATASCADERO MALL
NACIMIENTO AV
HIGH SCHOOL HILL RD
NORTH COUNTY CHRISTIAN HS
ATASCADERO HS
ATASCADERO RD
LIB
MARCHANT AV
ALCANTARA AV
LOS ARBOLES AV
CASCABEL RD
SANTA ANA RD
SANTA LUCIA RD
FLORES
MIRA
EL RETIRO AV
ALTA VISTA AV
NAVARETTE
SAN ANDRES AV
YNEZ AV
SERRA AV
CREEK
SAN GABRIEL RD
ALTA PRADERA LN
FLORES RD
LOS GATOS RD
HERMOSA
LARGA
PEQUENIA
EL DESCANSO
CLEMENTE AV
SAN MARCOS RD
CARMELITA
RANCHO ASUNCION
RANCHO ATASCADERO
SANTA NAVAJOA
DEVON CT
TECORIDA
CRISTOBAL AV
CURBARIL AV
PORTAL
ESCONDIDO RD
BELLA VISTA RD
PIEDRAS ALTOS
SANTA YNEZ AV
AMAPOA
AZUCENA
SAN FRANCISCO AV
MARCHANT
ATASCADERO LAKE PK
CHARLES PADDOCK ZOO
LAGO AV
PISMO AV
AVENAL AV
ATASCADERO LAKE
LAKE VIEW DR
MOUNTAIN VIEW DR
PINEDORADO RD
SIERRA VISTA RD
MONITA RD
CASITAS AV
ANDRITA RD
CASANOVA
BARRANCO RD
JOLON RD
LUCINDA LN
BARRANCO HEIGHTS
REALITO
SAN MARCOS
VISTA RD
CARMELITA AV
MORRO RD
EL PARQUE
SANTA ROSA RD
OLD MORRO RD E
SAN RAFAEL RD
RIO BLANCO CT
0 .125 .25 .375 .5 miles 1 in. = 1900 ft.

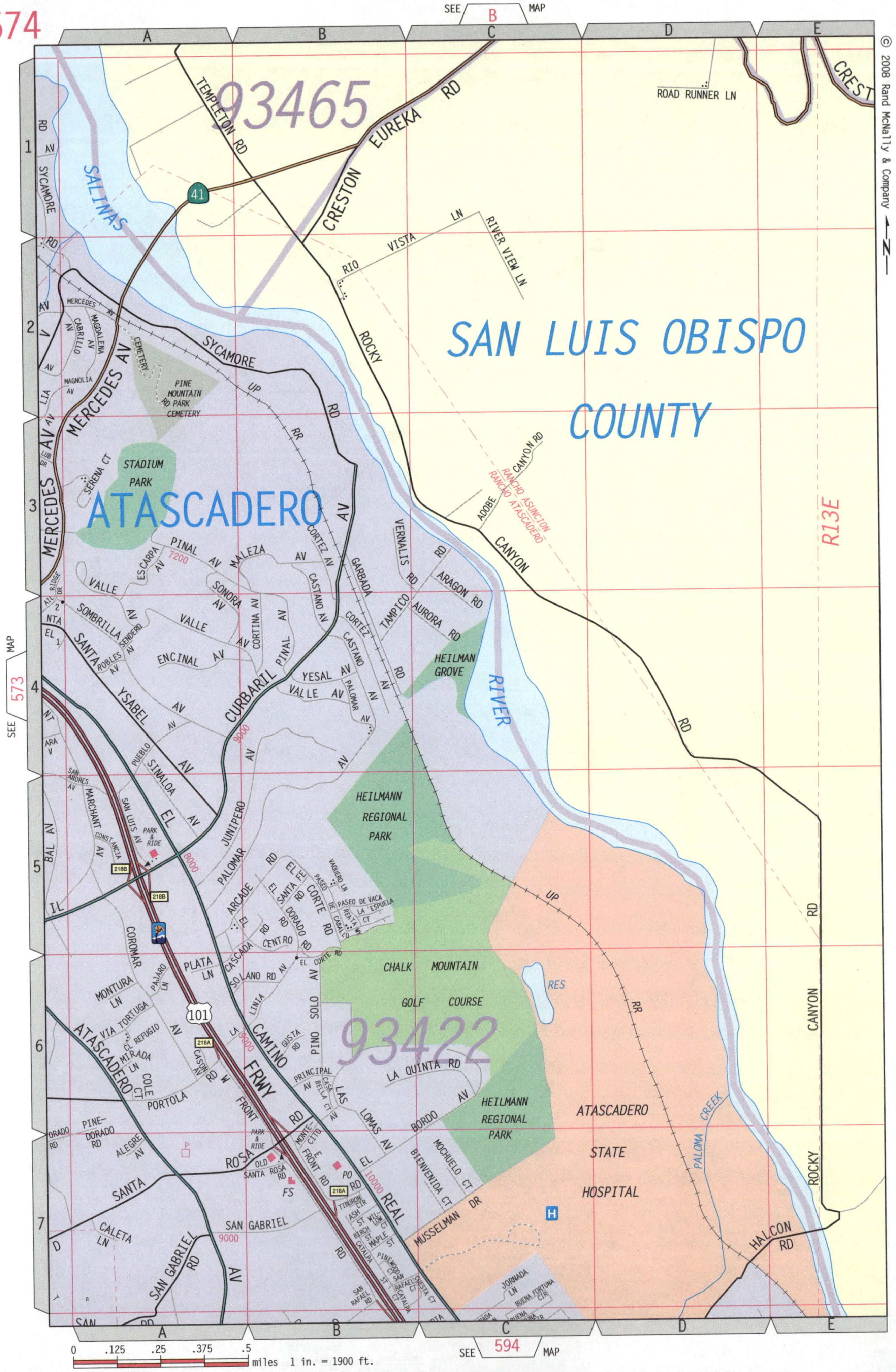

SEE B MAP

SEE 573 MAP

SEE 594 MAP

A B C D E
1 2 3 4 5 6 7

SAN LUIS OBISPO COUNTY

ATASCADERO

93465

93422

R13E

SALINAS RIVER

TEMPLETON RD
CRESTON EUREKA RD
CRESTON RD
41
ROAD RUNNER LN
CREST
RIO VISTA LN
RIVER VIEW LN
ROCKY CANYON RD
SYCAMORE RD
MERCEDES AV
MAGDALENA AV
CABRILLO AV
MAGNOLIA AV
CEMETERY RD
PINE MOUNTAIN PARK CEMETERY
STADIUM PARK
SERENA CT
LUB DR
UP RR
ADOBE CANYON RD
RANCHO ASUNCION
RANCHO ATASCADERO
CANYON RD
PINAL AV
ESCARPA AV
MALEZA AV
VALLE AV
SONORA AV
CORTEZ AV
CASTANO AV
GARBADA RD
VERNALIS RD
ARAGON RD
TAMPICO
AURORA RD
HEILMAN GROVE
RIDGE DR
SOMBRILLA AV
SENDERO
ROBLES AV
ENCINAL AV
CORTINA AV
PINAL AV
CURBARIL AV
YESAL AV
VALLE AV
PALOMAR AV
SANTA YSABEL AV
PUEBLO
SINALOA AV
7200
9000
8000
SAN ANDRES AV
MARCHANT AV
SAN LUIS AV
CONSTANCIA AV
PARK & RIDE
218B
JUNIPERO AV
PALOMAR AV
HEILMANN REGIONAL PARK
EL CAMINO REAL
ARCADE RD
EL SANTA FE RD
CORTE RD
VAQUERO LN
PASEO DE CABALLO
PASEO DE VACA
LA ESPUELA CT
RENATA
EL DORADO RD
CENTRO RD
CASCADA RD
EL CORTE RD
PLATA LN
SOLANO RD
COROMAR AV
MONTURA LN
PAJARO LN
VIA TORTUGA
CL REFUGIO
MIRADA LN
COLE CT
ATASCADERO AV
LINIA
PINO SOLO AV
CHALK MOUNTAIN GOLF COURSE
RES
101
218A
LA 9600
CASON RD
GUSTA RD
FRWY
PRINCIPAL AV
CASA BELLA CT
LAS LOMAS AV
LA QUINTA RD
BORDO AV
HEILMANN REGIONAL PARK
ATASCADERO STATE HOSPITAL
PALOMA CREEK
PORTOLA
W FRONT RD
PINE-DORADO RD
ORADO RD
ALEGRE AV
SANTA ROSA RD
OLD SANTA ROSA RD
MONTE CITO
E FRONT RD
PO
FS
10000
BIENVENIDA CT
MOCHUELO CT
MUSSELMAN DR
H
TIBURON CIR
ASH ST
WILLOW LN
BIRCH ST
MAPLE ST
CATALPA ST
PINEWOOD CT
SAN RAFAEL CT
SAN RAFAEL RD
CUESTA CT
CATALPA CT
JORNADA LN
BUENA FORTUNA CIR
SAN GABRIEL RD
9000
CALETA LN
HALCON RD

0 .125 .25 .375 .5 miles 1 in. = 1900 ft.

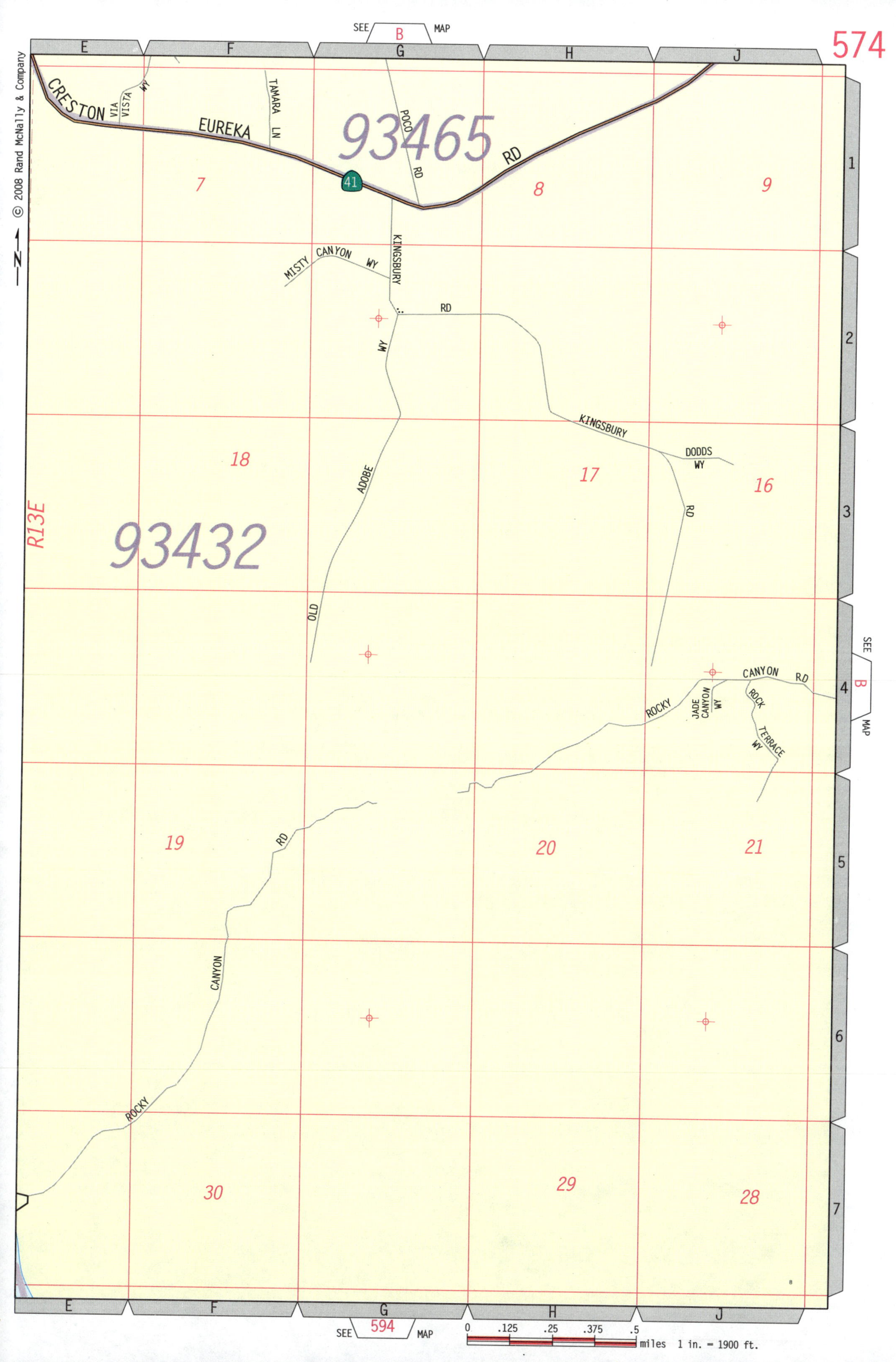
SEE B MAP
E
F
G
H
J
1
2
3
4
5
6
7
© 2008 Rand McNally & Company
CRESTON
EUREKA
RD
VIA VISTA WY
TAMARA LN
POCO RD
41
93465
93432
R13E
7
8
9
KINGSBURY
MISTY CANYON WY
RD
WY
KINGSBURY
DODDS WY
RD
18
17
16
ADOBE
OLD
SEE B MAP
CANYON RD
ROCKY
JADE CANYON WY
ROCK TERRACE WY
19
20
21
RD
CANYON
ROCKY
30
29
28
SEE 594 MAP
0 .125 .25 .375 .5 miles 1 in. = 1900 ft.

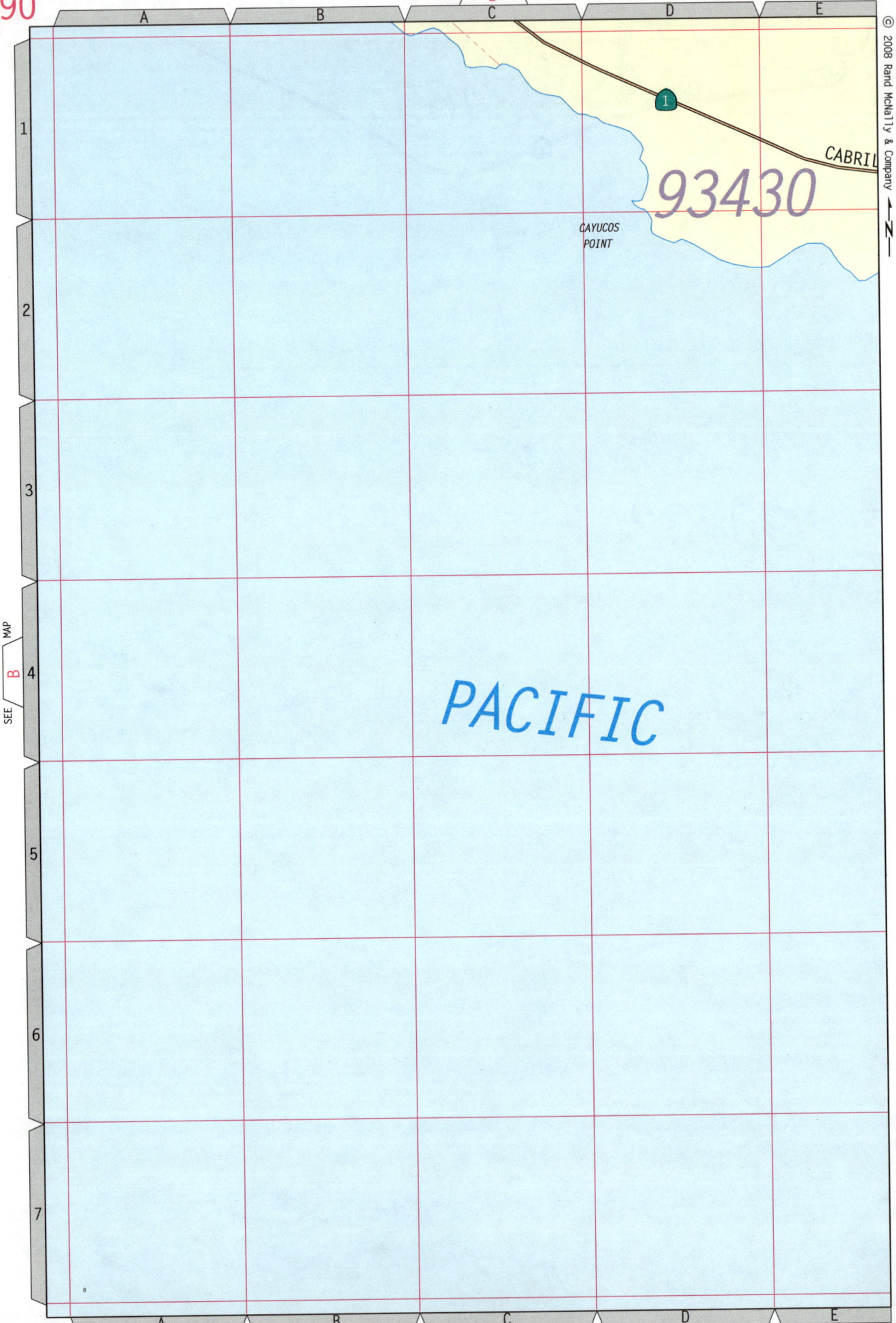

SEE B MAP
A
B
C
D
E
1
2
3
4
5
6
7
SEE B MAP
1
CABRIL
93430
CAYUCOS POINT
PACIFIC
0 .125 .25 .375 .5 miles 1 in. = 1900 ft.
SEE B MAP
© 2008 Rand McNally & Company
N

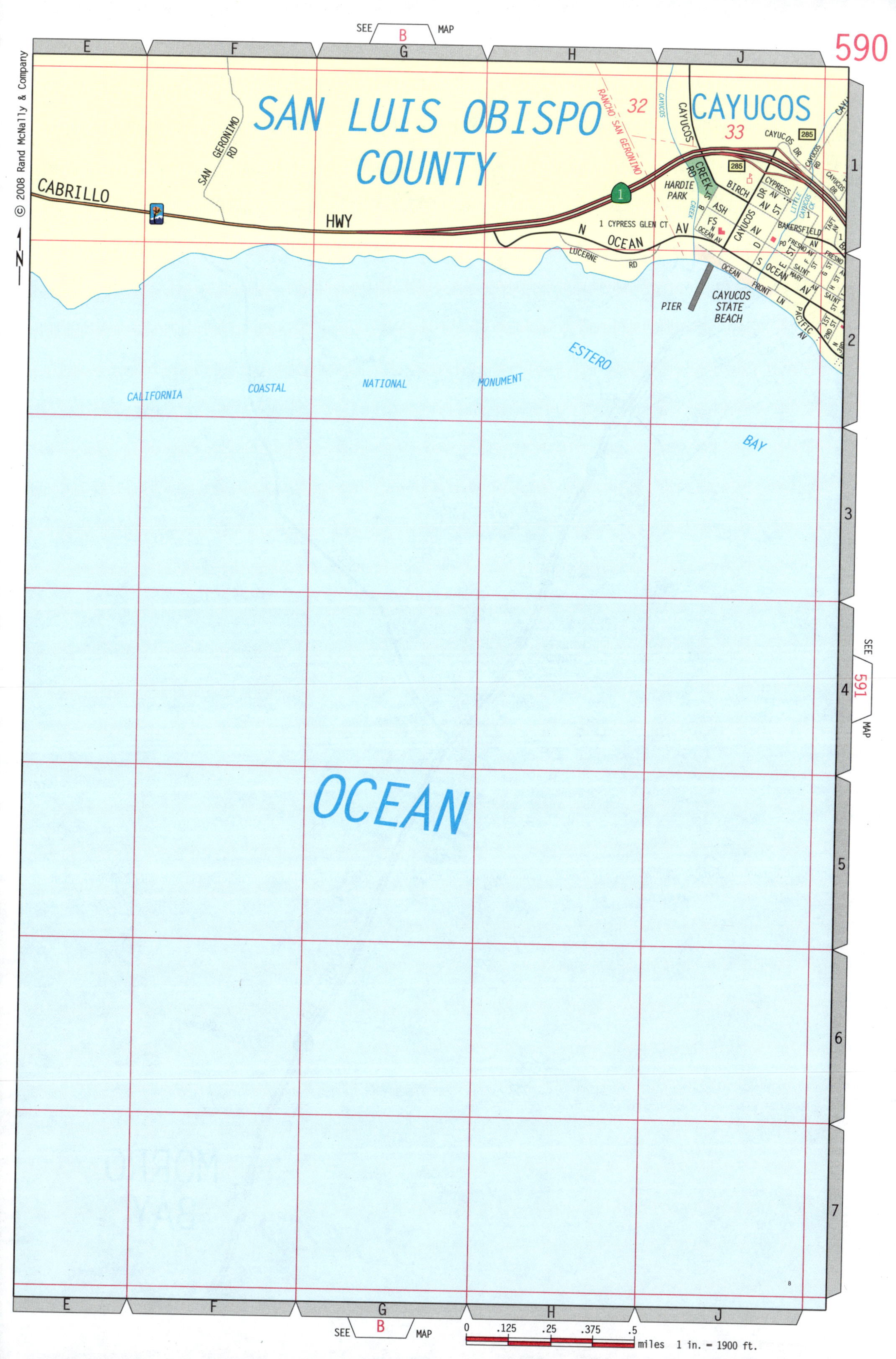
SEE B MAP
E
F
G
H
J
SAN LUIS OBISPO
COUNTY
CAYUCOS
32
33
CABRILLO
HWY
SAN GERONIMO RD
RANCHO SAN GERONIMO
CAYUCOS
CAYUCOS DR
285
1
HARDIE PARK
CREEK RD
BIRCH
ASH
CYPRESS
1 CYPRESS GLEN CT
N OCEAN AV
LUCERNE RD
BAKERSFIELD
PIER
CAYUCOS STATE BEACH
OCEAN FRONT LN
PACIFIC AV
ESTERO
CALIFORNIA
COASTAL
NATIONAL
MONUMENT
BAY
OCEAN
SEE 591 MAP
1
2
3
4
5
6
7
0
.125
.25
.375
.5
miles 1 in. = 1900 ft.

SEE B MAP

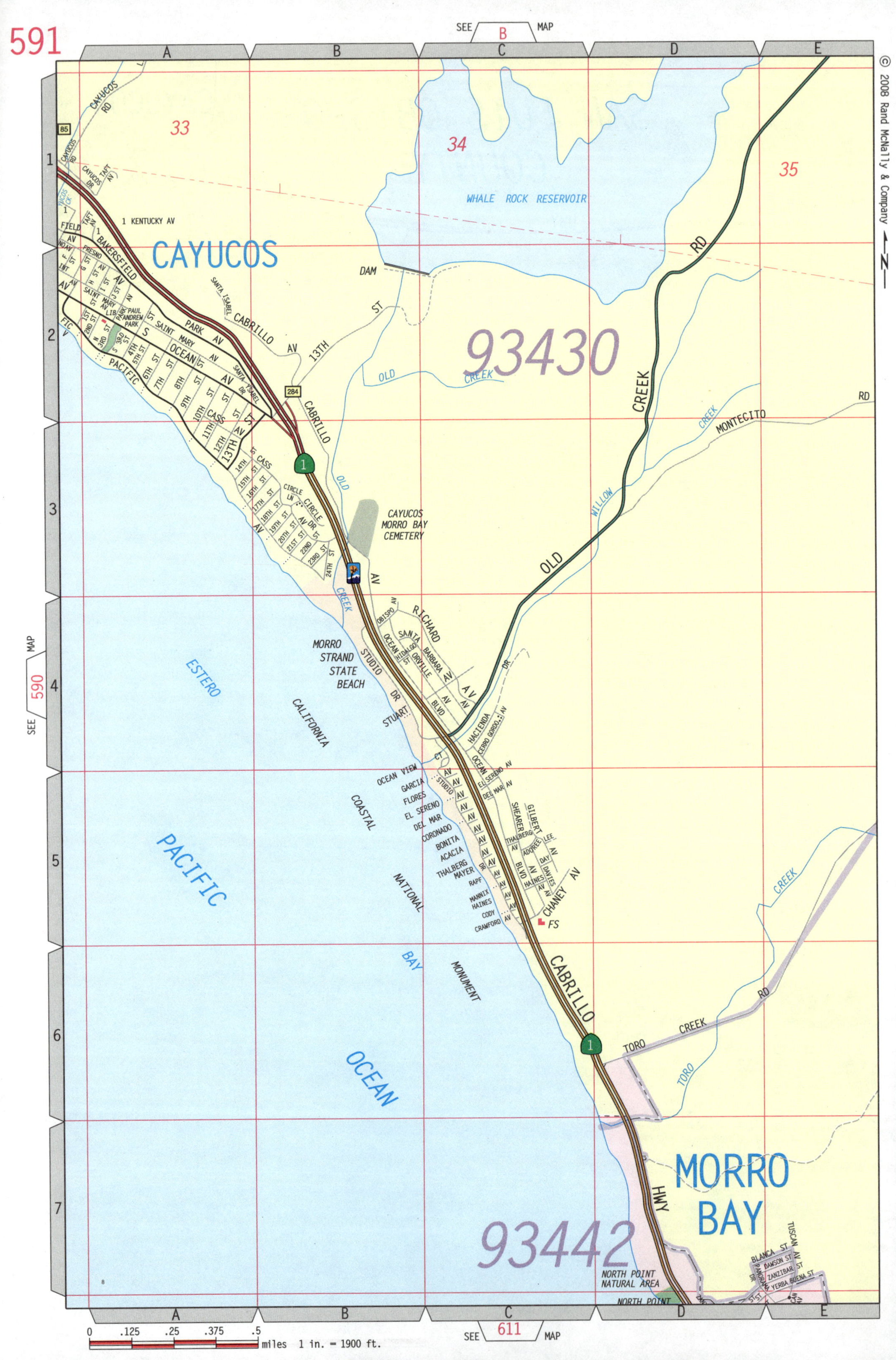

CAYUCOS
WHALE ROCK RESERVOIR
93430
93442
MORRO BAY
PACIFIC OCEAN
ESTERO
CALIFORNIA COASTAL NATIONAL MONUMENT
MORRO STRAND STATE BEACH
CAYUCOS MORRO BAY CEMETERY
NORTH POINT NATURAL AREA
OLD CREEK RD
TORO CREEK RD
MONTECITO RD
CABRILLO HWY
DAM
SEE B MAP
SEE 590 MAP
SEE 611 MAP
0 .125 .25 .375 .5 miles 1 in. = 1900 ft.

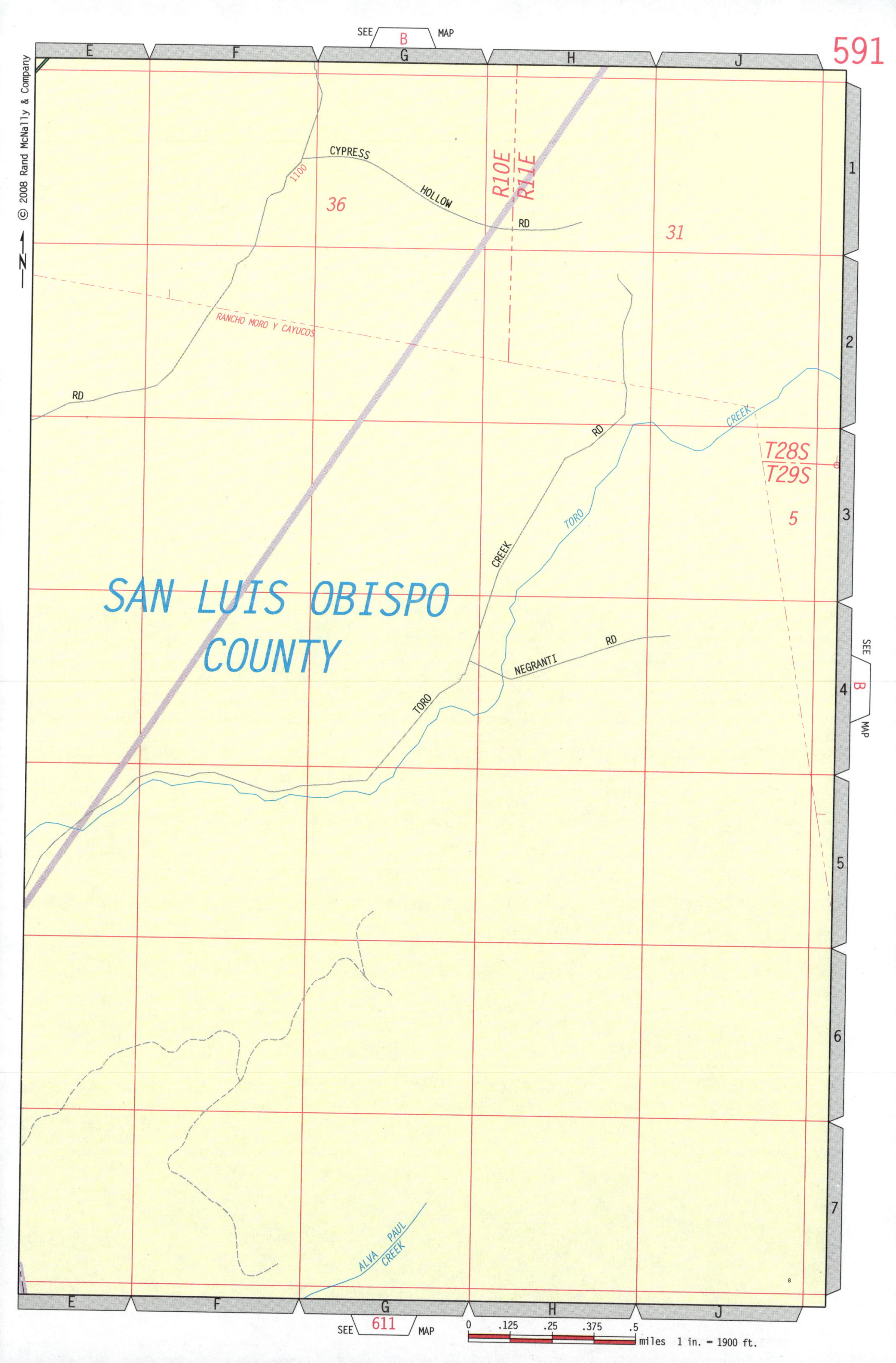
SEE B MAP
E
F
G
H
J
1
2
3
4
5
6
7
CYPRESS
HOLLOW
RD
1100
36
R10E
R11E
31
RANCHO MORO Y CAYUCOS
RD
RD
CREEK
T28S
T29S
5
TORO
CREEK
SAN LUIS OBISPO
COUNTY
NEGRANTI
RD
TORO
SEE B MAP
ALVA PAUL CREEK
SEE 611 MAP
0 .125 .25 .375 .5
miles 1 in. = 1900 ft.

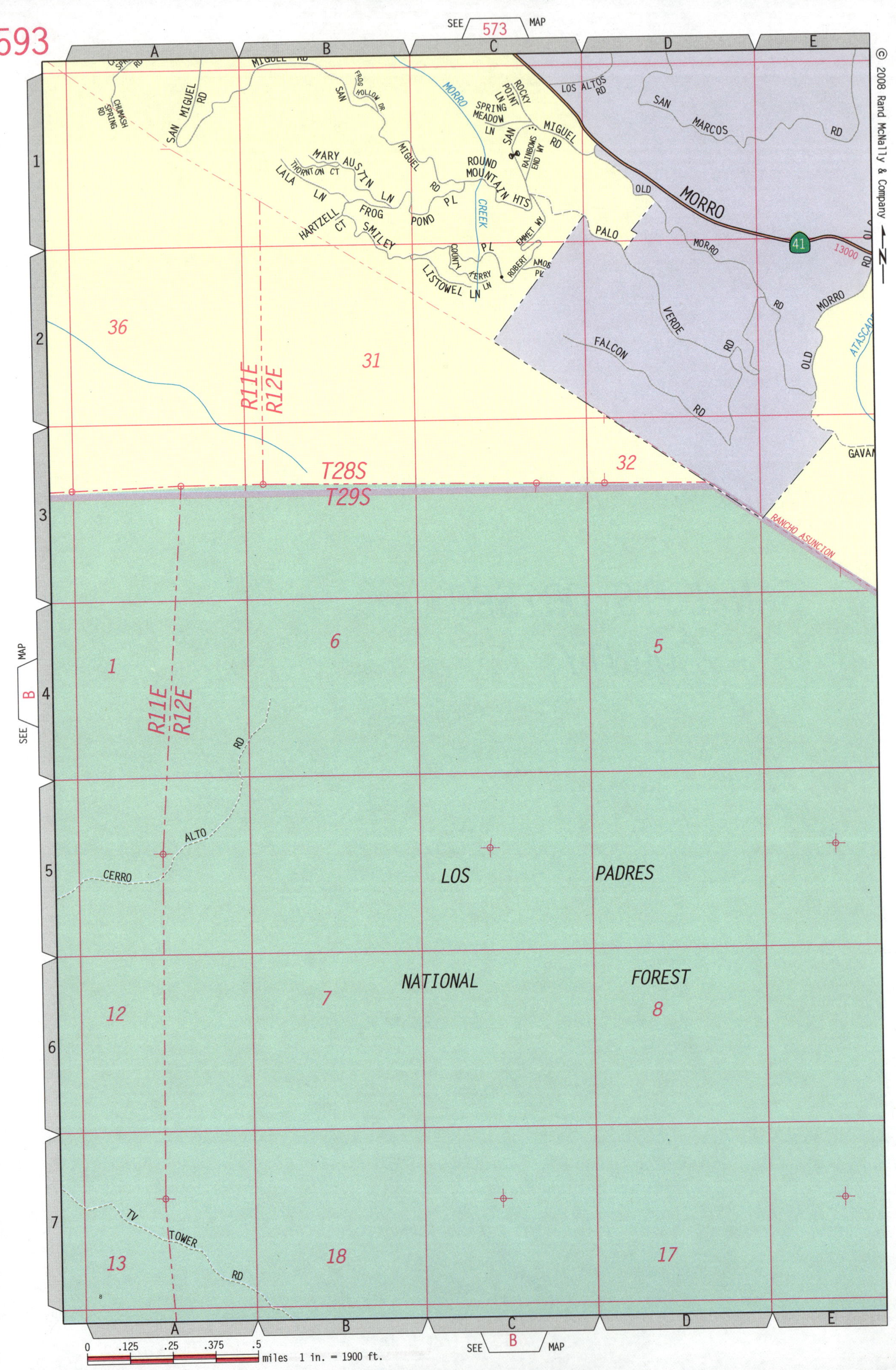
SEE 573 MAP
SAN MIGUEL RD
CHUMASH SPRING RD
FROG HOLLOW DR
MORRO CREEK
ROCKY POINT LN
SPRING MEADOW LN
SAN MIGUEL RD
LOS ALTOS RD
SAN MARCOS RD
MARY AUSTIN LN
THORNTON CT
LALA LN
HARTZELL CT
FROG POND PL
SMILEY
ROUND MOUNTAIN HTS
RAINBOWS END WY
EMMET WY
COUNTY
KERRY LN
LISTOWEL LN
ROBERT
AMOS PL
PALO
OLD MORRO
MORRO
41
13000
VERDE RD
FALCON RD
OLD MORRO RD
ATASCADERO
GAVAN
36
31
32
R11E
R12E
T28S
T29S
RANCHO ASUNCION
1
6
5
CERRO ALTO RD
LOS PADRES NATIONAL FOREST
12
7
8
13
18
17
TV TOWER RD
SEE B MAP
0 .125 .25 .375 .5 miles 1 in. = 1900 ft.

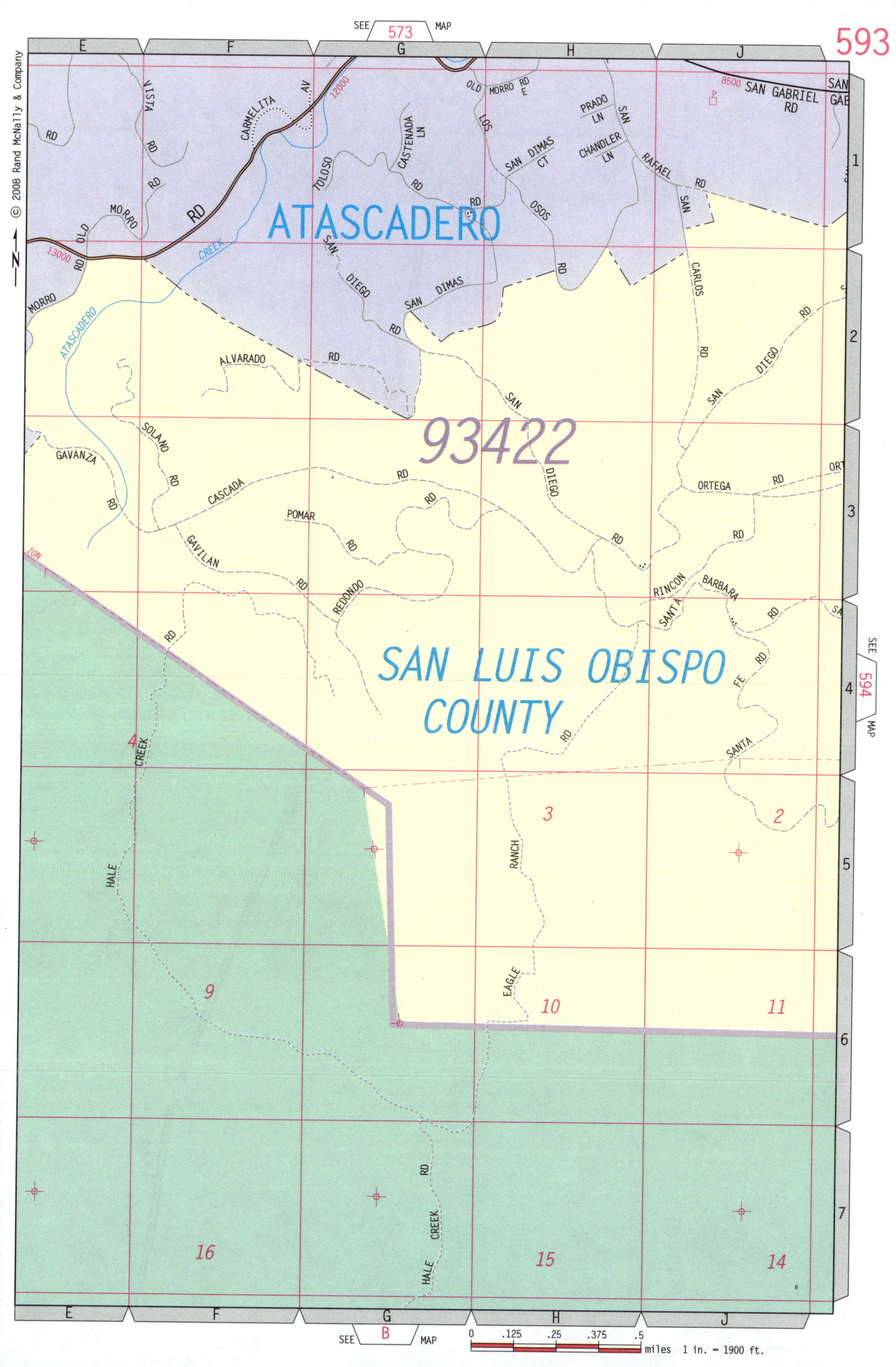

SEE 573 MAP
E
F
G
H
J
ATASCADERO
93422
SAN LUIS OBISPO COUNTY
SAN GABRIEL RD
8500
CARMELITA AV
12000
13000
OLD MORRO RD
OLD MORRO RD E
VISTA RD
TOLOSO RD
CASTENADA LN
LOS OSOS RD
SAN DIMAS CT
PRADO LN
CHANDLER LN
SAN RAFAEL RD
SAN CARLOS RD
SAN DIEGO RD
SAN DIMAS RD
ATASCADERO CREEK
ALVARADO RD
SOLANO RD
GAVANZA RD
CASCADA RD
POMAR RD
GAVILAN RD
REDONDO RD
ORTEGA RD
RINCON RD
SANTA BARBARA RD
SANTA FE RD
RANCH
EAGLE
HALE CREEK RD
1
2
3
4
5
6
7
2
3
4
9
10
11
14
15
16
SEE 594 MAP
SEE B MAP
0 .125 .25 .375 .5 miles 1 in. = 1900 ft.

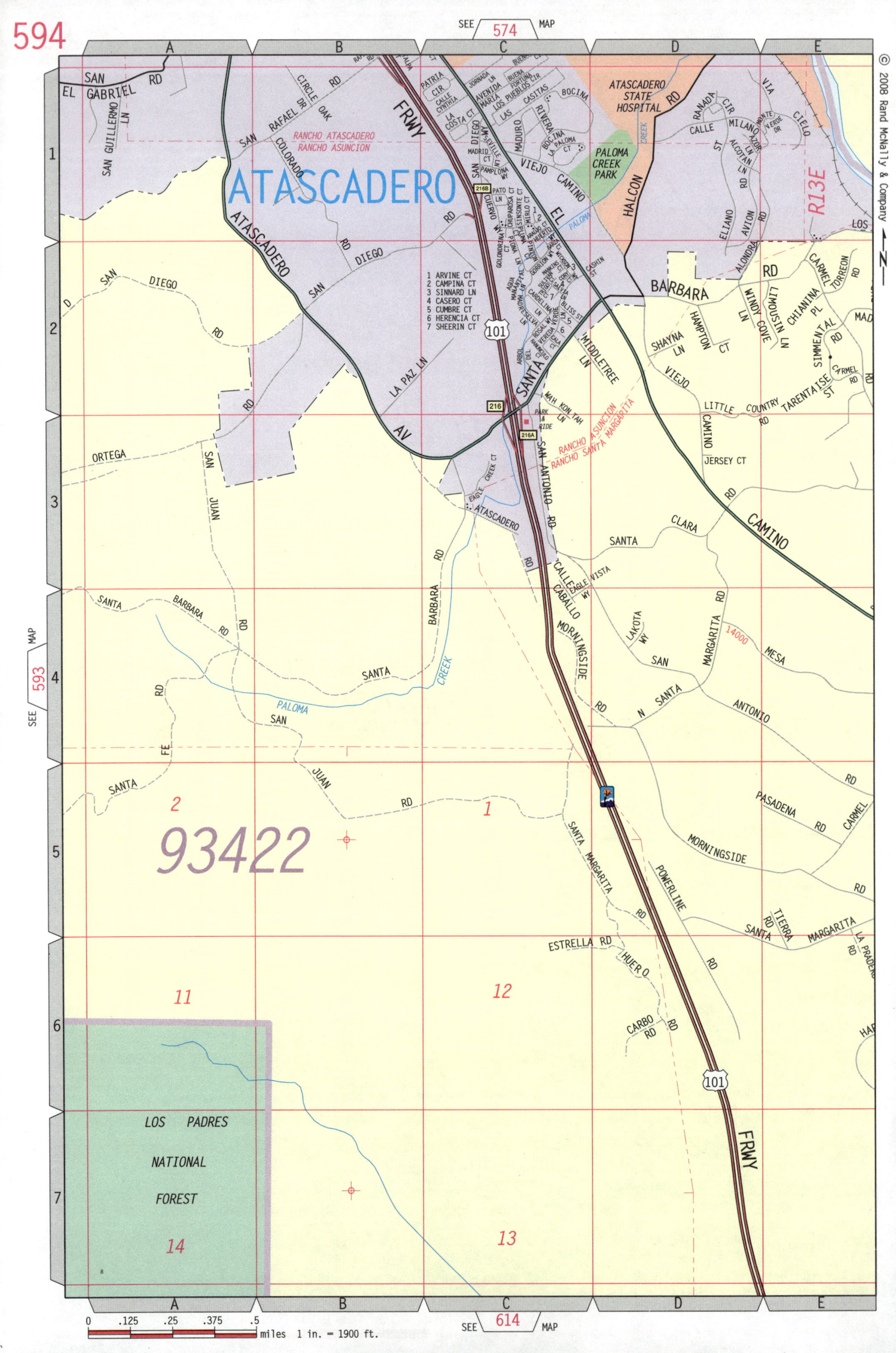
594
SEE 574 MAP
SEE 593 MAP
SEE 614 MAP
A
B
C
D
E
1
2
3
4
5
6
7
© 2008 Rand McNally & Company
ATASCADERO
93422
ATASCADERO STATE HOSPITAL
PALOMA CREEK PARK
RANCHO ATASCADERO
RANCHO ASUNCION
RANCHO SANTA MARGARITA
LOS PADRES NATIONAL FOREST
R13E
FRWY
101
216
216A
216B
14000
PARK & RIDE
SAN GABRIEL RD
EL GABRIEL
SAN GUILLERMO LN
SAN RAFAEL DR
CIRCLE OAK RD
COLORADO
ATASCADERO AV
SAN DIEGO RD
LA PAZ LN
ORTEGA
SAN JUAN RD
SANTA BARBARA RD
SANTA FE RD
PALOMA CREEK
SANTA ROSA
EL CAMINO REAL
VIEJO CAMINO
HALCON RD
BARBARA RD
SAN ANTONIO RD
SANTA CLARA RD
SANTA MARGARITA RD
MORNINGSIDE RD
POWERLINE RD
ESTRELLA RD
HUERO
CARBO RD
PASADENA RD
CARMEL RD
MESA
N SANTA
LAKOTA WY
EAGLE VISTA WY
CALLE CABALLO
MIDDLETREE LN
WAH KON TAH LN
SHAYNA LN
HAMPTON CT
WINDY COVE LN
LIMOUSIN LN
CHIANINA PL
SIMMENTAL RD
TARENTAISE ST
LITTLE COUNTRY RD
CAMINO
JERSEY CT
TORREON
ELIANO
AVION
ALONDRA
ALCOTAN LN
MILANO
RANADA CIR
CALLE
VIA CIELO
LOS
BOCINA
LA PALOMA CT
RIVERA
CASITAS
LOS PUEBLOS CIR
MADURO
LAS
LA COSTA CT
CALLE CYNTHIA
PATRIA CIR
JORNADA
AVENIDA MARIA
SAN DIEGO
PAMPLONA WY
MADRID CT
PATO LN
CUERVO
EAGLE CREEK CT
1 ARVINE CT
2 CAMPINA CT
3 SINNARD LN
4 CASERO CT
5 CUMBRE CT
6 HERENCIA CT
7 SHEERIN CT
LA PRADERA
2
1
11
12
13
14
0 .125 .25 .375 .5 miles 1 in. = 1900 ft.

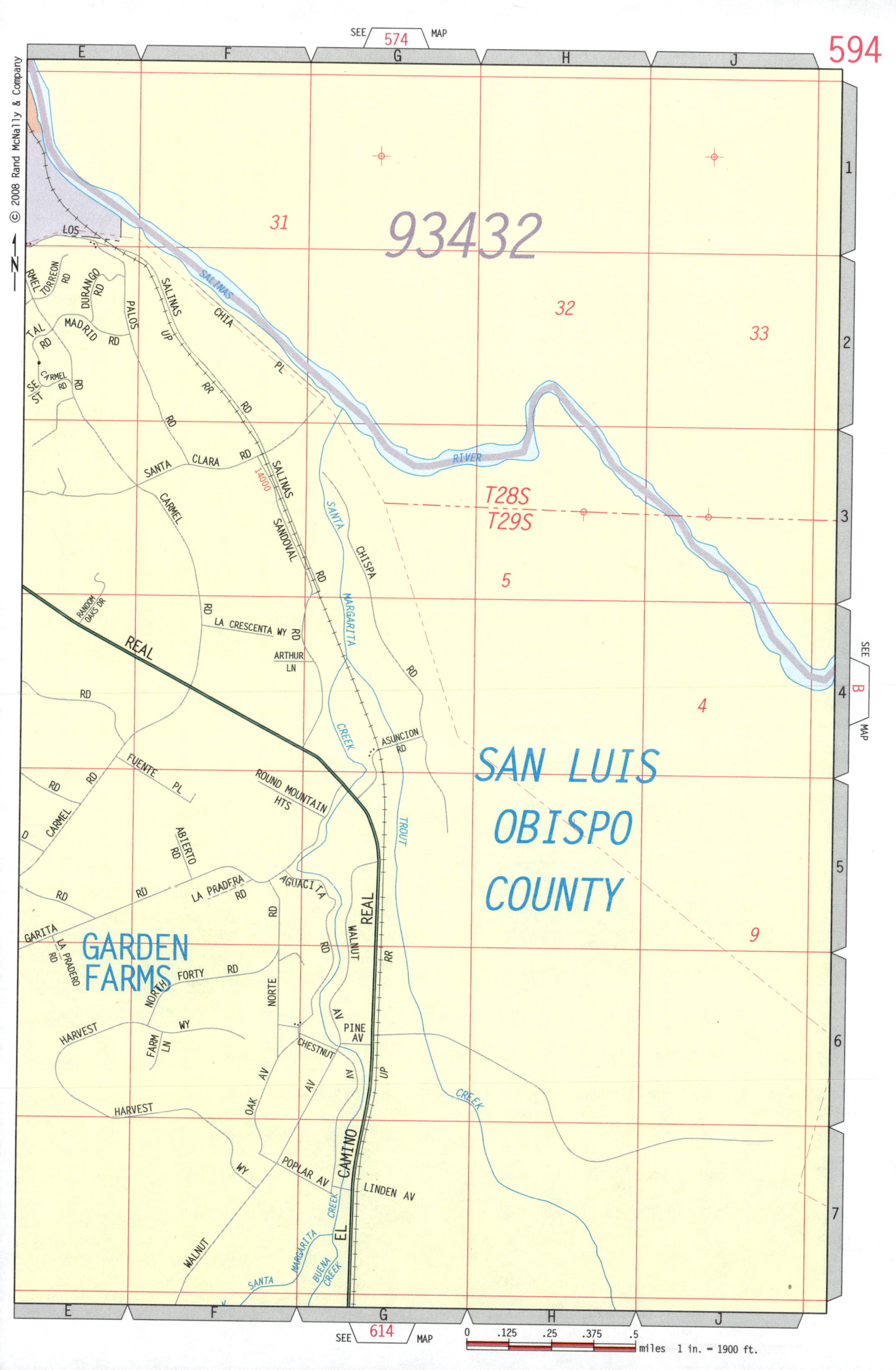
SEE 574 MAP
E
F
G
H
J
1
2
3
4
5
6
7
93432
31
32
33
T28S
T29S
5
4
9
SALINAS RIVER
SAN LUIS OBISPO COUNTY
GARDEN FARMS
LOS
TORREON RD
DURANGO RD
MADRID RD
PALOS
SALINAS UP RR
CHIA PL
RD
SANTA CLARA RD
14000
SALINAS
SANDOVAL RD
CARMEL
SANTA MARGARITA CREEK
CHISPA RD
RANDOM OAKS DR
REAL
LA CRESCENTA WY
RD
ARTHUR LN
ASUNCION RD
FUENTE PL
ROUND MOUNTAIN HTS
TROUT CREEK
ABIERTO RD
LA PRADERA RD
AGUACITA RD
GARITA
LA PRADERO RD
NORTH FORTY RD
NORTE
WALNUT
REAL
UP RR
HARVEST WY
FARM LN
PINE AV
CHESTNUT AV
OAK AV
POPLAR AV
LINDEN AV
EL CAMINO
SANTA MARGARITA
BUENA CREEK
CREEK
SEE B MAP
SEE 614 MAP
0 .125 .25 .375 .5
miles 1 in. = 1900 ft.

SEE 591 MAP

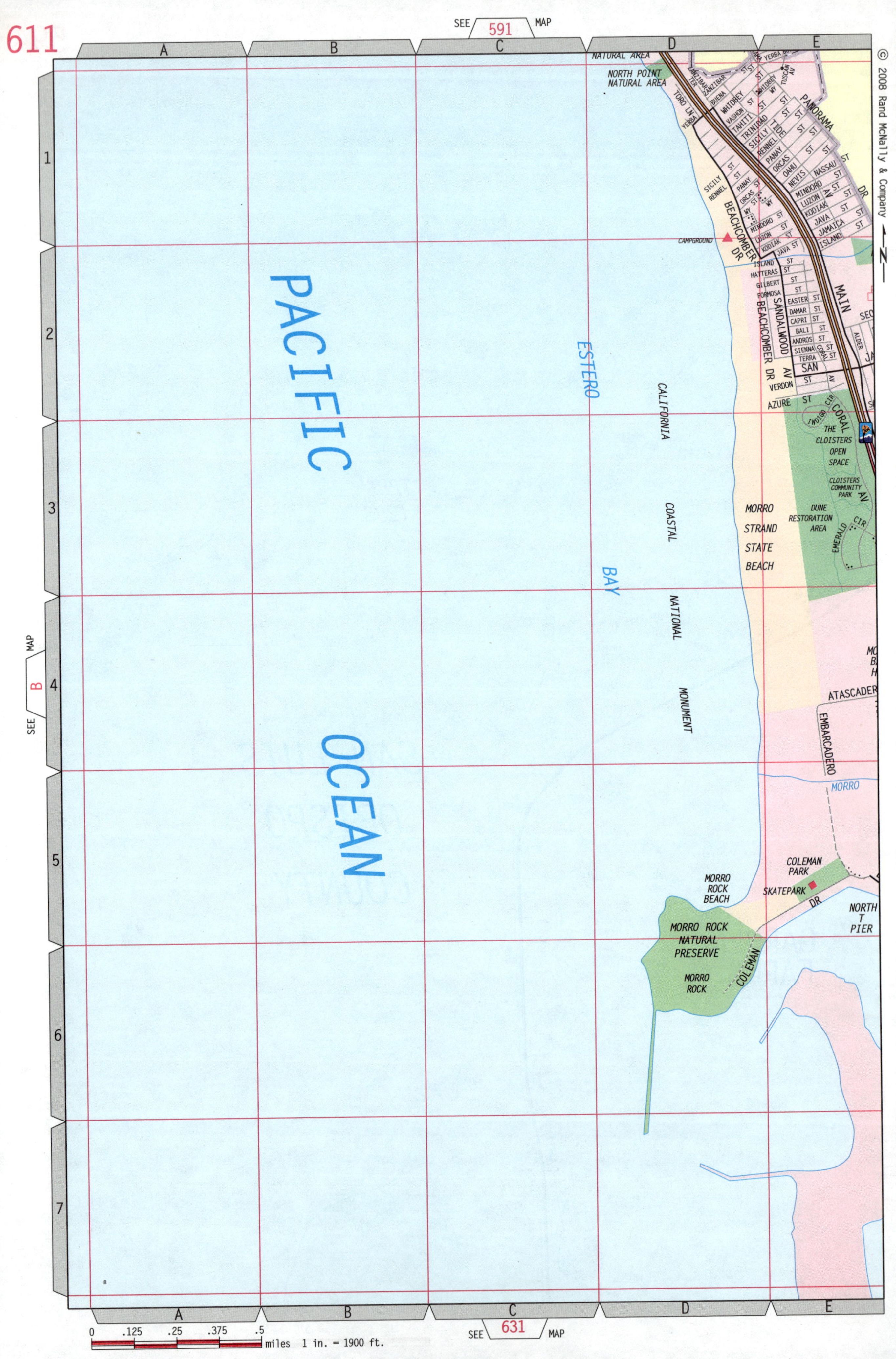
PACIFIC
OCEAN
ESTERO
BAY
CALIFORNIA
COASTAL
NATIONAL
MONUMENT
NORTH POINT
NATURAL AREA
CAMPGROUND
MORRO
STRAND
STATE
BEACH
THE
CLOISTERS
OPEN
SPACE
CLOISTERS
COMMUNITY
PARK
DUNE
RESTORATION
AREA
MORRO
ROCK
BEACH
MORRO ROCK
NATURAL
PRESERVE
MORRO
ROCK
COLEMAN
PARK
SKATEPARK
NORTH
T
PIER
BEACHCOMBER DR
SANDALWOOD
MAIN
PANORAMA DR
ATASCADERO
EMBARCADERO
COLEMAN
DR
AZURE ST
VERDON
SAN
INDIGO CIR
CORAL AV
EMERALD CIR
SICILY
RENNEL
ISLAND
HATTERAS
GILBERT
FORMOSA
EASTER
DAMAR
CAPRI
BALI
ANDROS
SIENNA
TERRA
MINDORO
LUZON
KODIAK
JAVA
JAMAICA
NASSAU
NEVIS
OAHU
PANAY
ORCAS
TRINIDAD
TAHITI
VASHON
WHIDBEY
BUENA
ZANZIBAR
TORO LN
YERBA
TUSCAN AV
© 2008 Rand McNally & Company
A
B
C
D
E
1
2
3
4
5
6
7
0
.125
.25
.375
.5
miles 1 in. = 1900 ft.

SEE B MAP

SEE 631 MAP

SEE 591 MAP

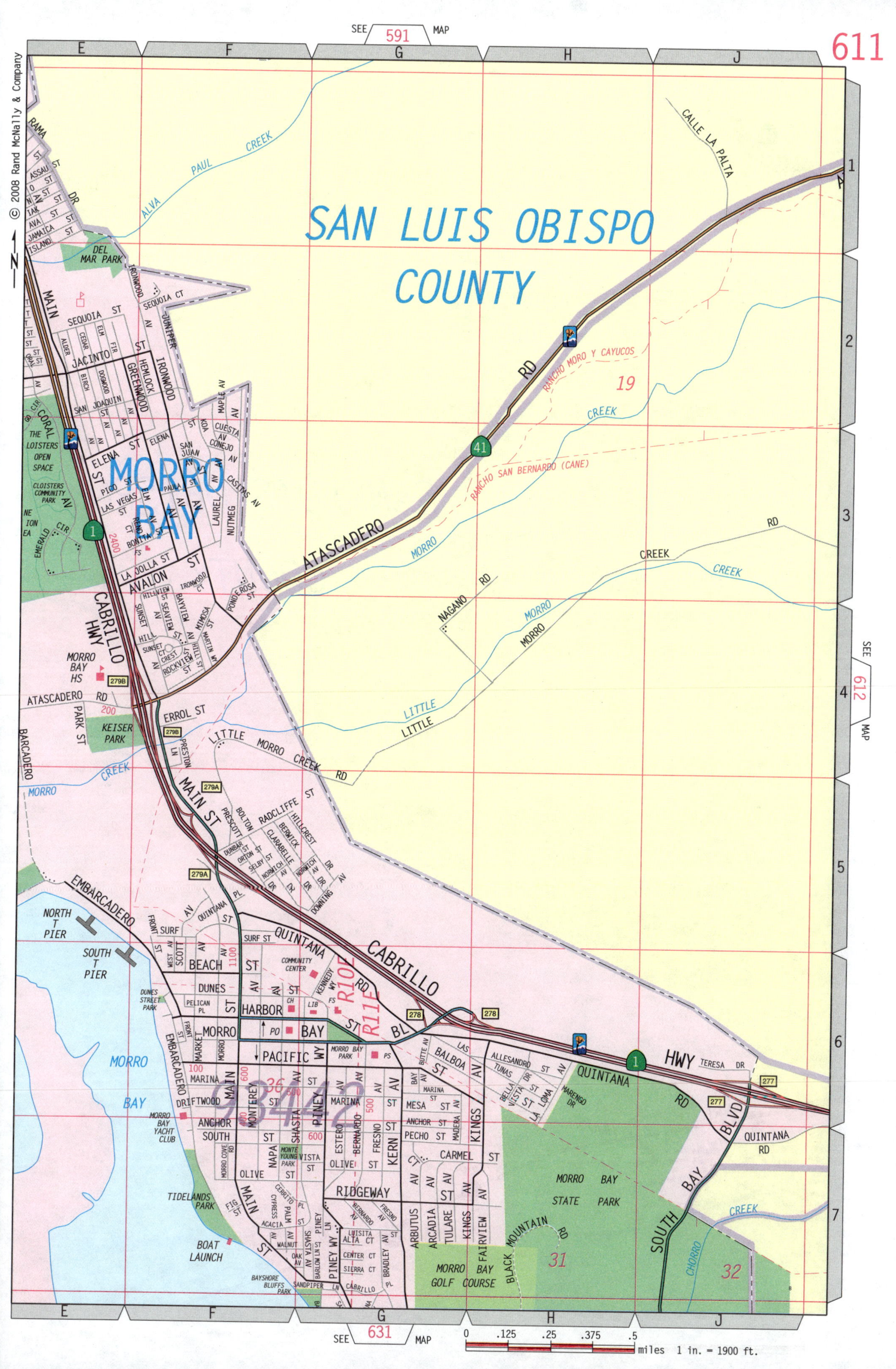

SAN LUIS OBISPO COUNTY
MORRO BAY
93442
E
F
G
H
J
1
2
3
4
5
6
7
ALVA PAUL CREEK
CALLE LA PALTA
DEL MAR PARK
MAIN
RAMA
SEQUOIA ST
SEQUOIA CT
JACINTO ST
SAN JOAQUIN ST
HEMLOCK
GREENWOOD
IRONWOOD
JUNIPER
ALDER
CEDAR
ELM
FIR
BIRCH
DOGWOOD
CORAL AV
THE LOISTERS OPEN SPACE
CLOISTERS COMMUNITY PARK
EMERALD CIR
ELENA ST
PICO ST
LAS VEGAS ST
BONITA ST
LA JOLLA ST
AVALON ST
SAN JUAN ST
PAULA
CUESTA AV
CONEJO AV
KOA AV
MAPLE AV
CASITAS AV
LAUREL AV
NUTMEG
PONDEROSA ST
HILLVIEW
SUNSET AV
SEAVIEW AV
BAYVIEW
MIMOSA ST
MARTIN WY
ROCKVIEW ST
HILL ST
CABRILLO HWY
1
41
ATASCADERO RD
RANCHO MORO Y CAYUCOS
19
RANCHO SAN BERNARDO (CANE)
MORRO CREEK
NAGANO RD
MORRO CREEK RD
LITTLE MORRO CREEK RD
MORRO BAY HS
279B
ATASCADERO RD
200
PARK ST
KEISER PARK
ERROL ST
PRESTON LN
BARCADERO
MORRO CREEK
279A
MAIN ST
BOLTON
PRESCOTT
RADCLIFFE ST
HILLCREST
BERWICK
CLARABELLE
DUNBAR ST
ORTON ST
SELBY ST
NORWICH AV
DOWNING AV
EMBARCADERO
NORTH T PIER
SOUTH T PIER
QUINTANA PL
SURF ST
FRONT ST
WEST AV
SCOTT AV
BEACH ST
1100
DUNES ST
DUNES STREET PARK
PELICAN PL
HARBOR ST
MORRO ST
PACIFIC ST
BAY ST
MORRO BAY PARK
QUINTANA RD
COMMUNITY CENTER
KENNEDY WY
LIB
FS
PO
PS
R10E
R11E
CABRILLO ST
278
BALBOA ST
LAS TUNAS
ALLESANDRO ST
BELLA VISTA DR
LA LOMA AV
MARENGO DR
TERESA DR
277
QUINTANA RD
SOUTH BAY BLVD
MORRO BAY
MORRO BAY YACHT CLUB
MARINA ST
DRIFTWOOD ST
ANCHOR ST
SOUTH ST
MONTEREY AV
SHASTA AV
PINEY WY
ESTERO
BERNARDO
FRESNO
KERN AV
BUTTE AV
MESA ST
PECHO ST
MADERA AV
KINGS AV
CARMEL ST
OLIVE ST
NAPA
MONTE YOUNG VISTA PARK
RIDGEWAY
MORRO COVE RD
TIDELANDS PARK
FIG ST
CERRITO PL
CYPRESS
ACACIA AV
PALM AV
WALNUT
OAK AV
BARLOW LN
LUISITA CT
ALTA CT
CENTER CT
SIERRA CT
BRADLEY AV
ARBUTUS AV
ARCADIA AV
TULARE AV
FAIRVIEW AV
BLACK MOUNTAIN RD
MORRO BAY STATE PARK
MORRO BAY GOLF COURSE
BOAT LAUNCH
BAYSHORE BLUFFS PARK
SANDPIPER LN
CABRILLO PL
CHORRO CREEK
31
32

SEE 612 MAP

SEE 631 MAP

0 .125 .25 .375 .5 miles 1 in. = 1900 ft.

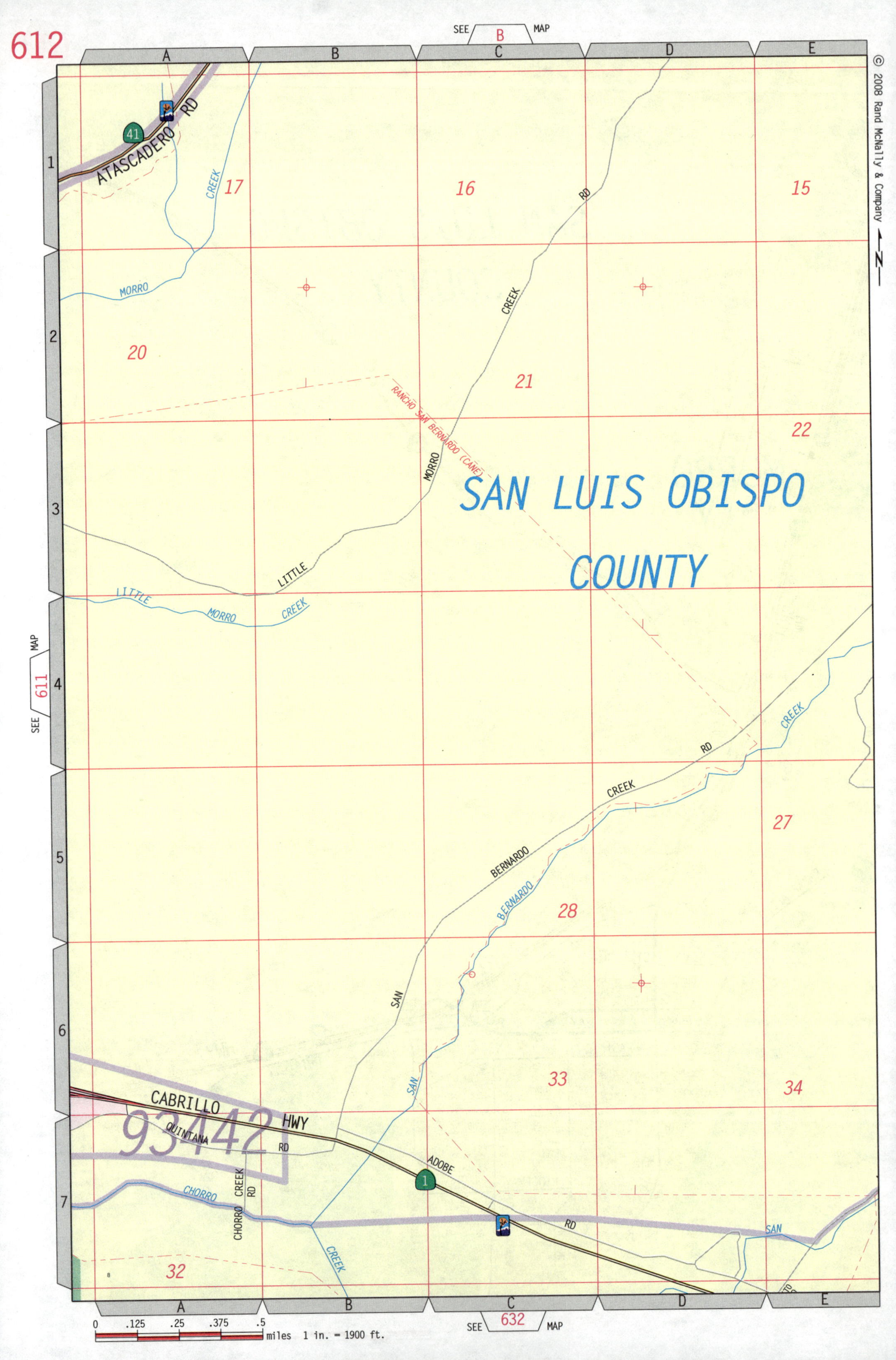
SEE B MAP
A
B
C
D
E
1
2
3
4
5
6
7
ATASCADERO RD
41
CREEK
17
16
15
RD
MORRO
20
CREEK
21
RANCHO SAN BERNARDO (CANE)
22
MORRO
SAN LUIS OBISPO
COUNTY
LITTLE
LITTLE
MORRO
CREEK
SEE 611 MAP
CREEK
RD
CREEK
27
BERNARDO
BERNARDO
28
SAN
SAN
33
34
CABRILLO
HWY
93442
QUINTANA
RD
ADOBE
1
CHORRO
CREEK
RD
CHORRO
RD
SAN
CREEK
CHORRO
32
0
.125
.25
.375
.5
miles 1 in. = 1900 ft.
SEE 632 MAP

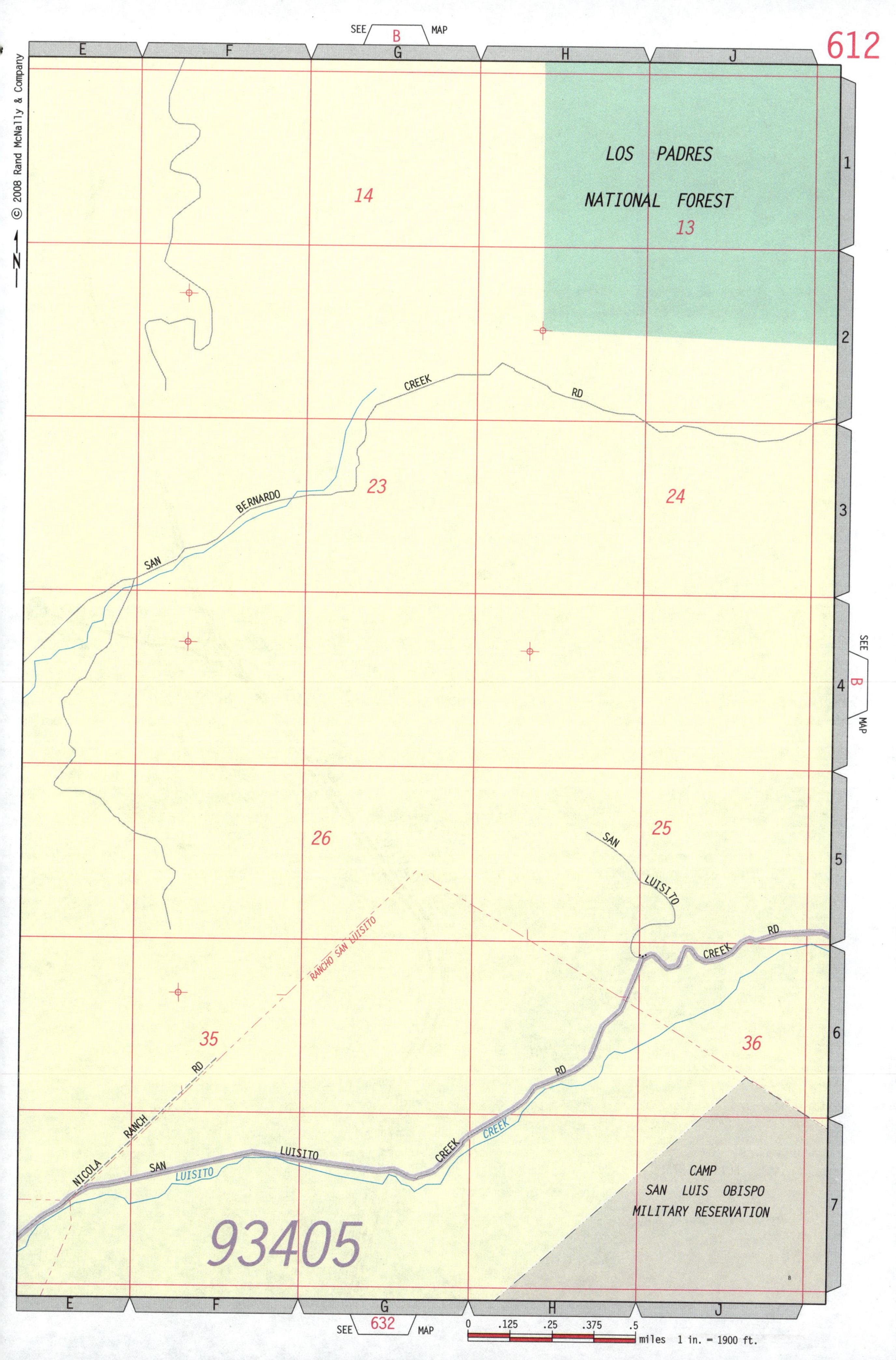
SEE B MAP
E
F
G
H
J
LOS PADRES
NATIONAL FOREST
14
13
1
2
CREEK
RD
23
24
BERNARDO
SAN
3
SEE B MAP
4
26
25
SAN
LUISITO
5
RANCHO SAN LUISITO
CREEK
RD
35
36
RD
6
RD
RANCH
NICOLA
SAN
LUISITO
LUISITO
CREEK
CREEK
CAMP
SAN LUIS OBISPO
MILITARY RESERVATION
7
93405
SEE 632 MAP
0
.125
.25
.375
.5
miles 1 in. = 1900 ft.
N

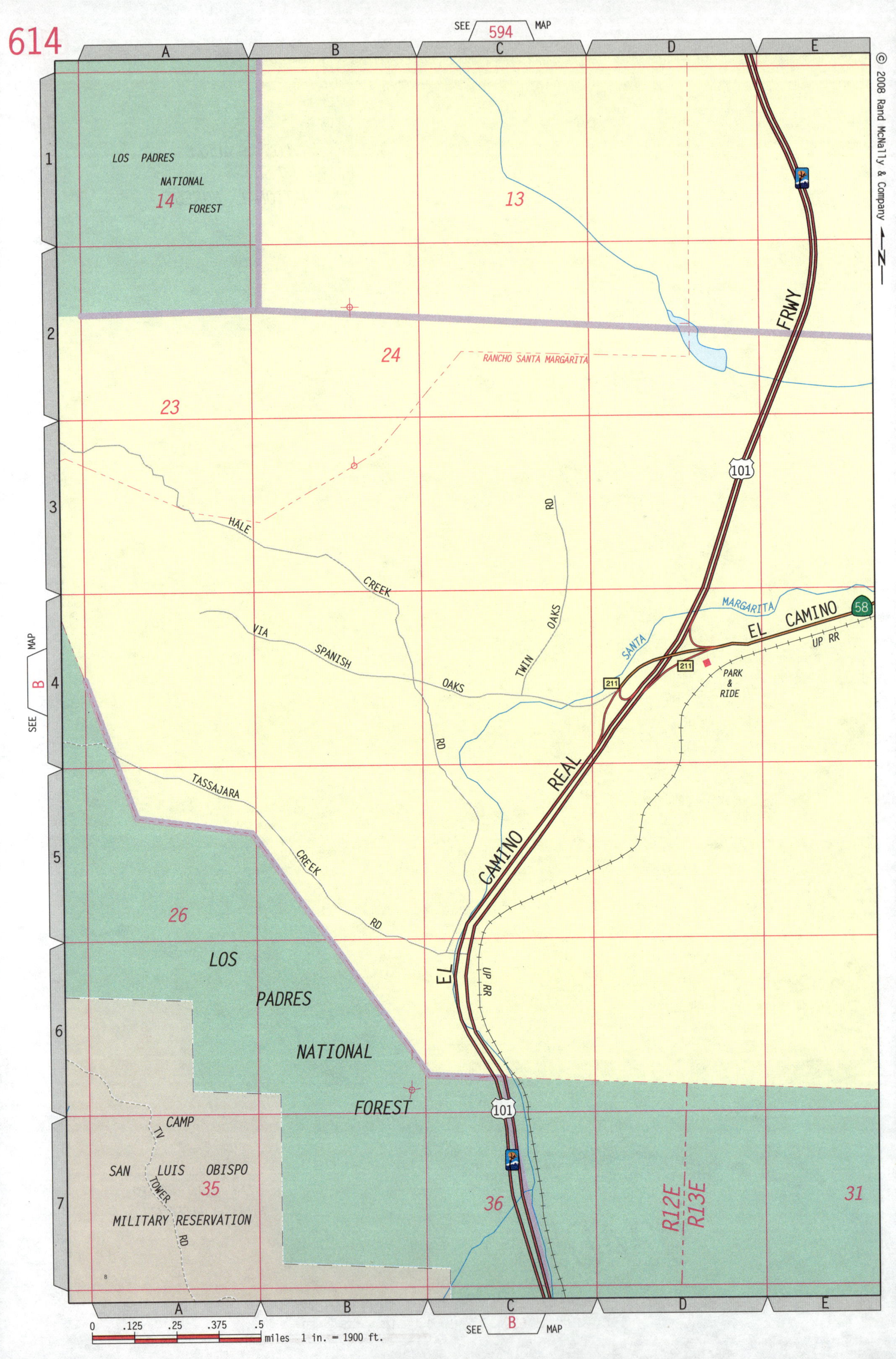
SEE 594 MAP
A
B
C
D
E
1
2
3
4
5
6
7
LOS PADRES NATIONAL FOREST
14
13
24
23
RANCHO SANTA MARGARITA
FRWY
101
HALE CREEK
RD
TWIN OAKS
VIA SPANISH OAKS RD
SANTA MARGARITA
EL CAMINO
58
UP RR
211
PARK & RIDE
EL CAMINO REAL
TASSAJARA CREEK RD
26
LOS PADRES NATIONAL FOREST
EL CAMINO REAL
UP RR
CAMP SAN LUIS OBISPO MILITARY RESERVATION
TV TOWER RD
35
36
R12E
R13E
31
SEE B MAP
0 .125 .25 .375 .5 miles 1 in. = 1900 ft.

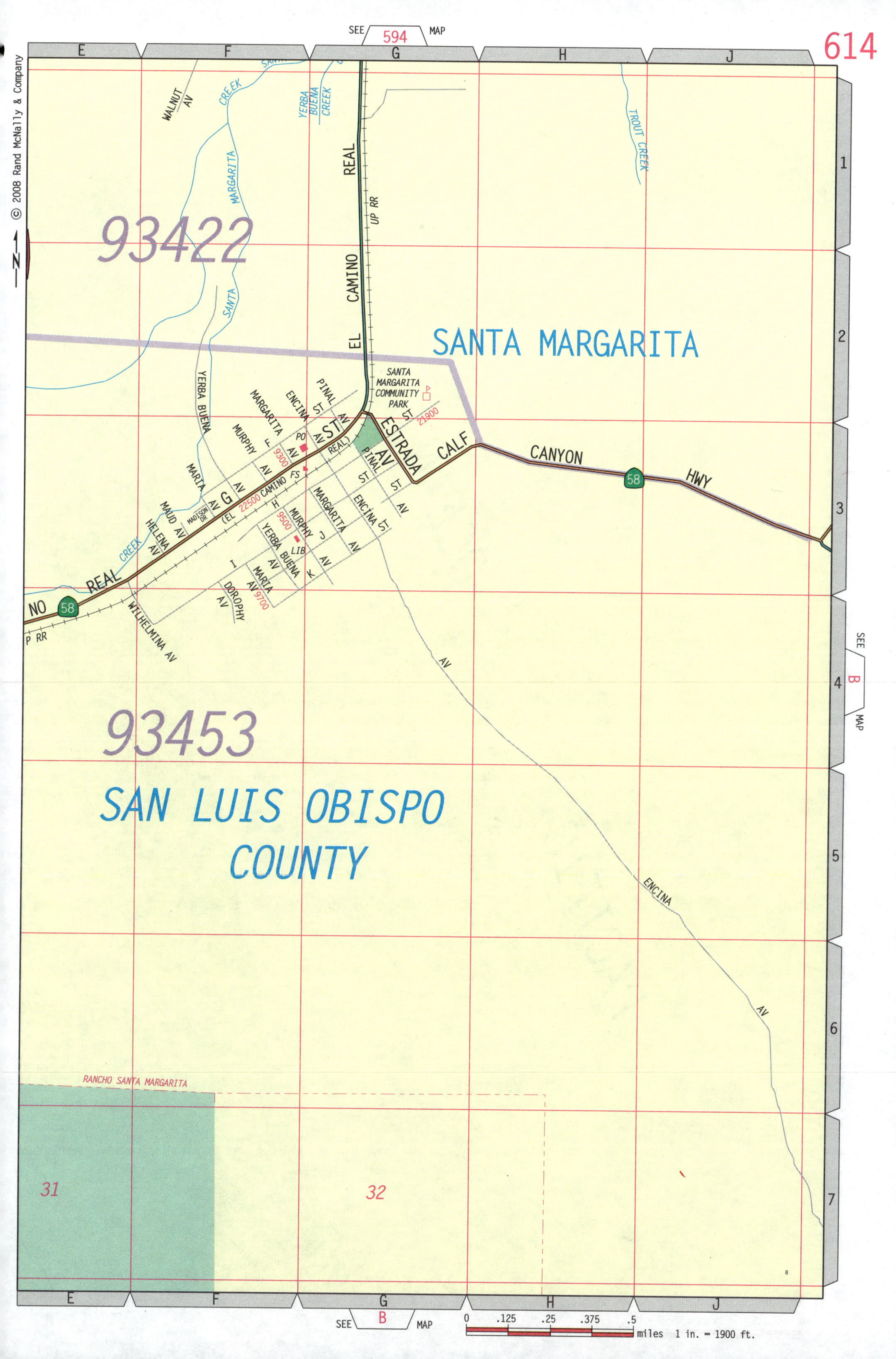
SEE 594 MAP
E
F
G
H
J
1
2
3
4
5
6
7
WALNUT AV
SANTA MARGARITA CREEK
YERBA BUENA CREEK
TROUT CREEK
EL CAMINO REAL
UP RR
93422
SANTA MARGARITA
SANTA MARGARITA COMMUNITY PARK
YERBA BUENA
MARGARITA
ENCINA
PINAL
ST
AV
ESTRADA AV
ST
21900
CALF CANYON HWY
58
MURPHY
MARIA
MAUD AV
HELENA AV
MADISON DR
G
(EL CAMINO REAL)
22500
9300
9500
9700
PO
FS
LIB
H
I
J
K
F
DOROPHY AV
REAL
NO
P RR
WILHELMINA AV
SEE B MAP
93453
SAN LUIS OBISPO COUNTY
ENCINA AV
RANCHO SANTA MARGARITA
31
32
0
.125
.25
.375
.5
miles 1 in. = 1900 ft.

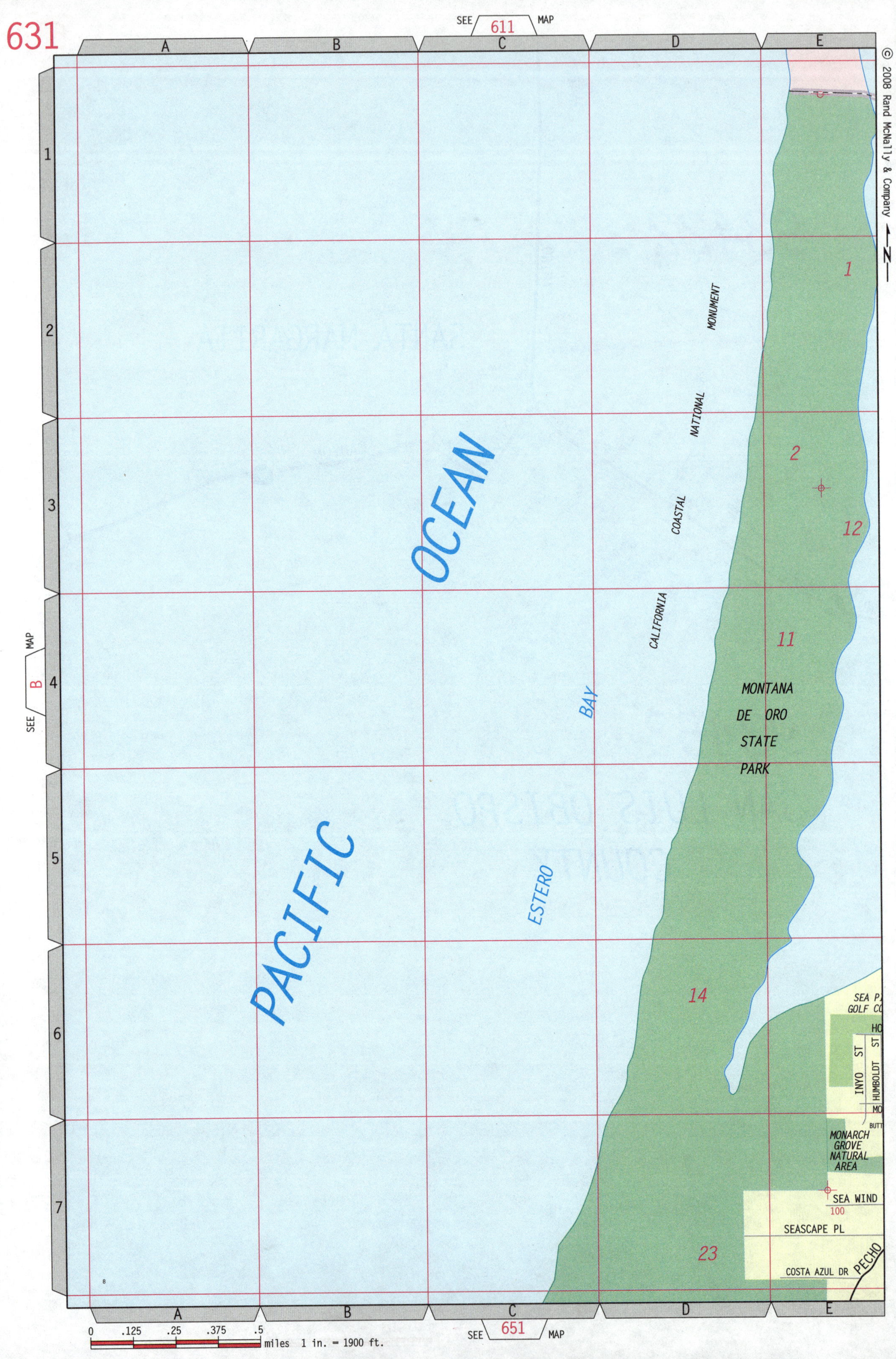

SEE 611 MAP
SEE B MAP
SEE 651 MAP
PACIFIC
OCEAN
ESTERO
BAY
CALIFORNIA
COASTAL
NATIONAL
MONUMENT
MONTANA
DE ORO
STATE
PARK
MONARCH
GROVE
NATURAL
AREA
INYO ST
HUMBOLDT ST
SEA WIND
SEASCAPE PL
COSTA AZUL DR
PECHO
0 .125 .25 .375 .5 miles 1 in. = 1900 ft.

SEE 611 MAP

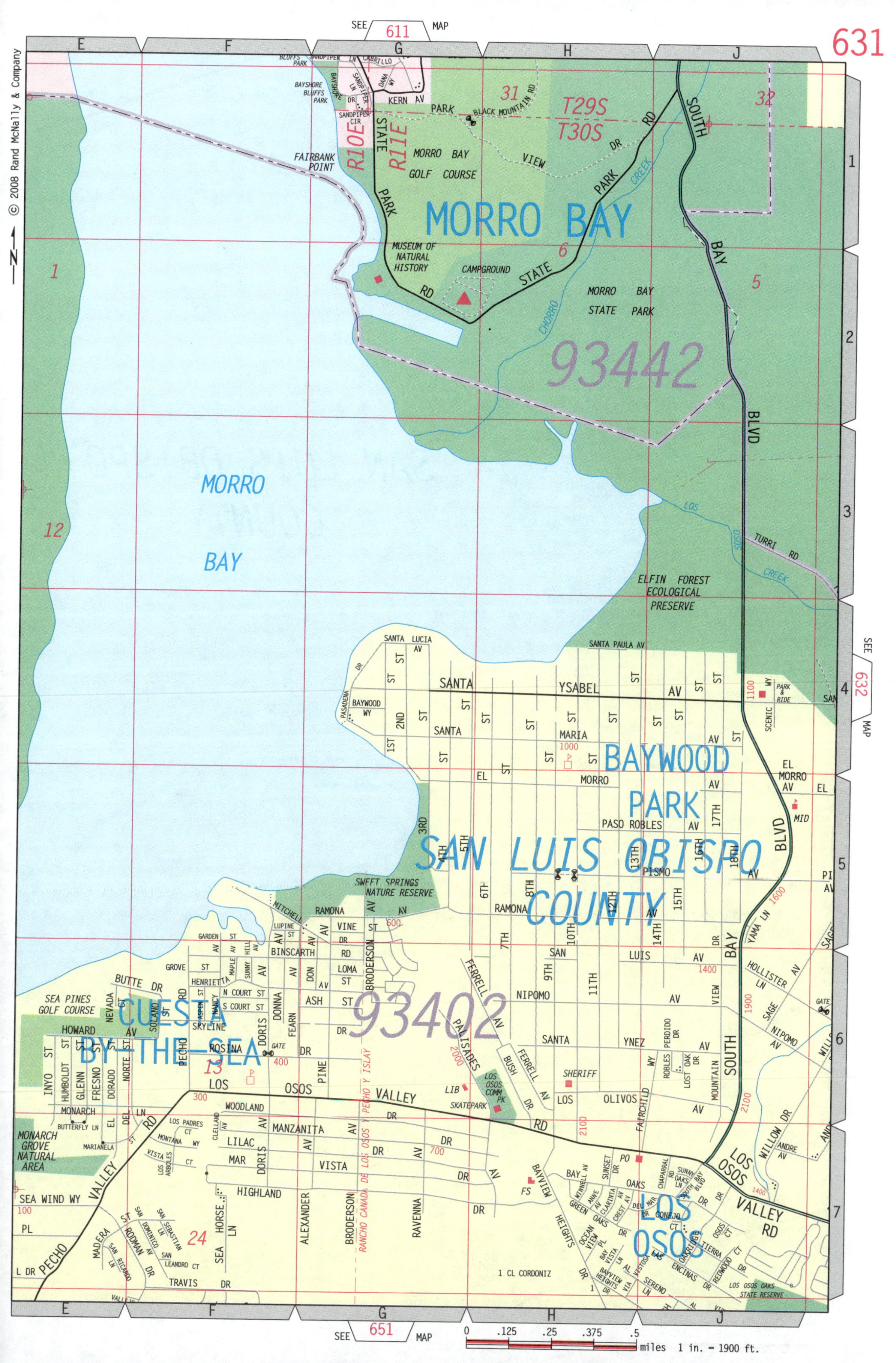
MORRO BAY
MORRO BAY STATE PARK
MORRO BAY GOLF COURSE
MUSEUM OF NATURAL HISTORY
CAMPGROUND
STATE PARK RD
BLACK MOUNTAIN RD
PARK VIEW DR
SOUTH BAY BLVD
FAIRBANK POINT
BAYSHORE BLUFFS PARK
KERN AV
T29S
T30S
R10E
R11E
CHORRO CREEK
93442
MORRO
BAY
LOS OSOS CREEK
TURRI RD
ELFIN FOREST ECOLOGICAL PRESERVE
SANTA LUCIA AV
SANTA PAULA AV
SANTA YSABEL AV
SANTA MARIA AV
BAYWOOD PARK
SAN LUIS OBISPO COUNTY
EL MORRO AV
PASO ROBLES AV
PISMO AV
RAMONA AV
SWEET SPRINGS NATURE RESERVE
SAN LUIS AV
NIPOMO AV
SANTA YNEZ AV
HOLLISTER LN
YAMA LN
SAGE AV
WILLOW DR
CUESTA BY-THE-SEA
SEA PINES GOLF COURSE
BUTTE DR
HOWARD AV
ROSINA DR
93402
LOS OSOS VALLEY RD
LOS OSOS COMM PK
SKATEPARK
LIB
SHERIFF
FS
PO
LOS OSOS
MONARCH GROVE NATURAL AREA
SEA WIND WY
PECHO VALLEY RD
RANCHO CANADA DE LOS OSOS Y PECHO Y ISLAY
HIGHLAND DR
TRAVIS DR
BAYVIEW HEIGHTS DR
LOS OSOS OAKS STATE RESERVE
1 CL CORDONIZ
PARK & RIDE
SEE 632 MAP
© 2008 Rand McNally & Company
0 .125 .25 .375 .5 miles 1 in. = 1900 ft.

SEE 651 MAP

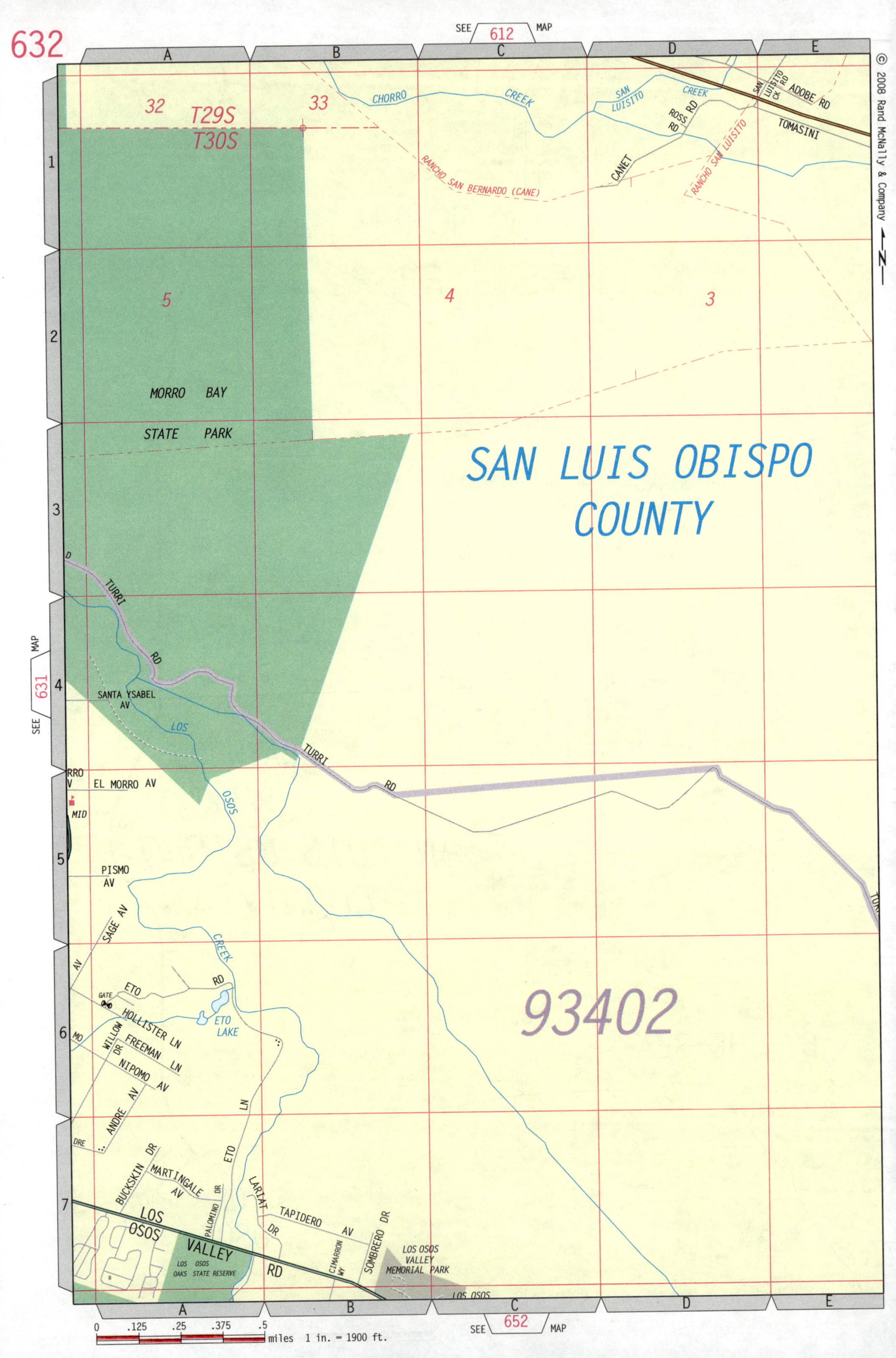
SEE 612 MAP
A
B
C
D
E
1
2
3
4
5
6
7
32
33
T29S
T30S
CHORRO CREEK
SAN LUISITO CREEK
ROSS RD
SAN LUISITO CK RD
ADOBE RD
TOMASINI
CANET
RANCHO SAN BERNARDO (CANE)
RANCHO SAN LUISITO
5
4
3
MORRO BAY STATE PARK
SAN LUIS OBISPO COUNTY
TURRI RD
SANTA YSABEL AV
LOS OSOS CREEK
EL MORRO AV
MID
PISMO AV
SAGE AV
ETO RD
GATE
HOLLISTER LN
ETO LAKE
WILLOW DR
FREEMAN LN
NIPOMO AV
ANDRE AV
ETO LN
93402
BUCKSKIN DR
MARTINGALE AV
PALOMINO DR
LARIAT DR
TAPIDERO AV
SOMBRERO DR
CIMARRON WY
LOS OSOS VALLEY RD
LOS OSOS OAKS STATE RESERVE
LOS OSOS VALLEY MEMORIAL PARK
SEE 631 MAP
SEE 652 MAP
0 .125 .25 .375 .5 miles 1 in. = 1900 ft.

SEE 612 MAP

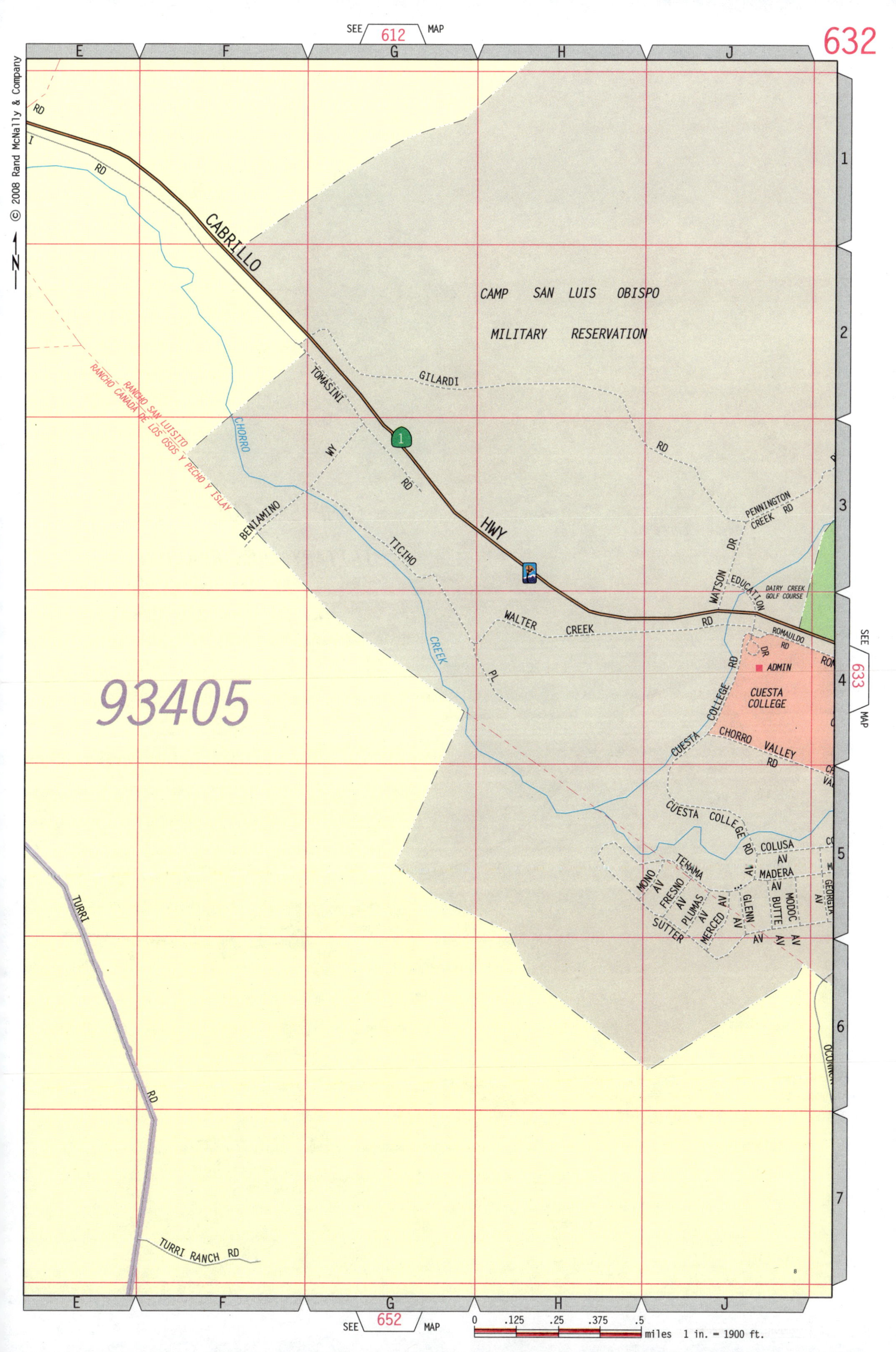

E
F
G
H
J
1
2
3
4
5
6
7
CAMP SAN LUIS OBISPO
MILITARY RESERVATION
CABRILLO
HWY
GILARDI
RD
TOMASINI
RD
WY
BENIAMINO
TICIHO
PL
WALTER CREEK RD
CHORRO
CREEK
RANCHO SAN LUISITO
RANCHO CANADA DE LOS OSOS Y PECHO Y ISLAY
PENNINGTON CREEK RD
WATSON DR
EDUCATION DR
DAIRY CREEK GOLF COURSE
ROMAULDO RD
ADMIN
CUESTA COLLEGE
CUESTA COLLEGE RD
CHORRO VALLEY RD
COLUSA AV
MADERA AV
TEHAMA
MONO AV
FRESNO AV
PLUMAS AV
MERCED AV
GLENN AV
BUTTE AV
MODOC AV
GEORGIA AV
SUTTER AV
93405
TURRI RD
TURRI RANCH RD
OCONNOR

SEE 633 MAP

SEE 652 MAP

0 .125 .25 .375 .5 miles 1 in. = 1900 ft.

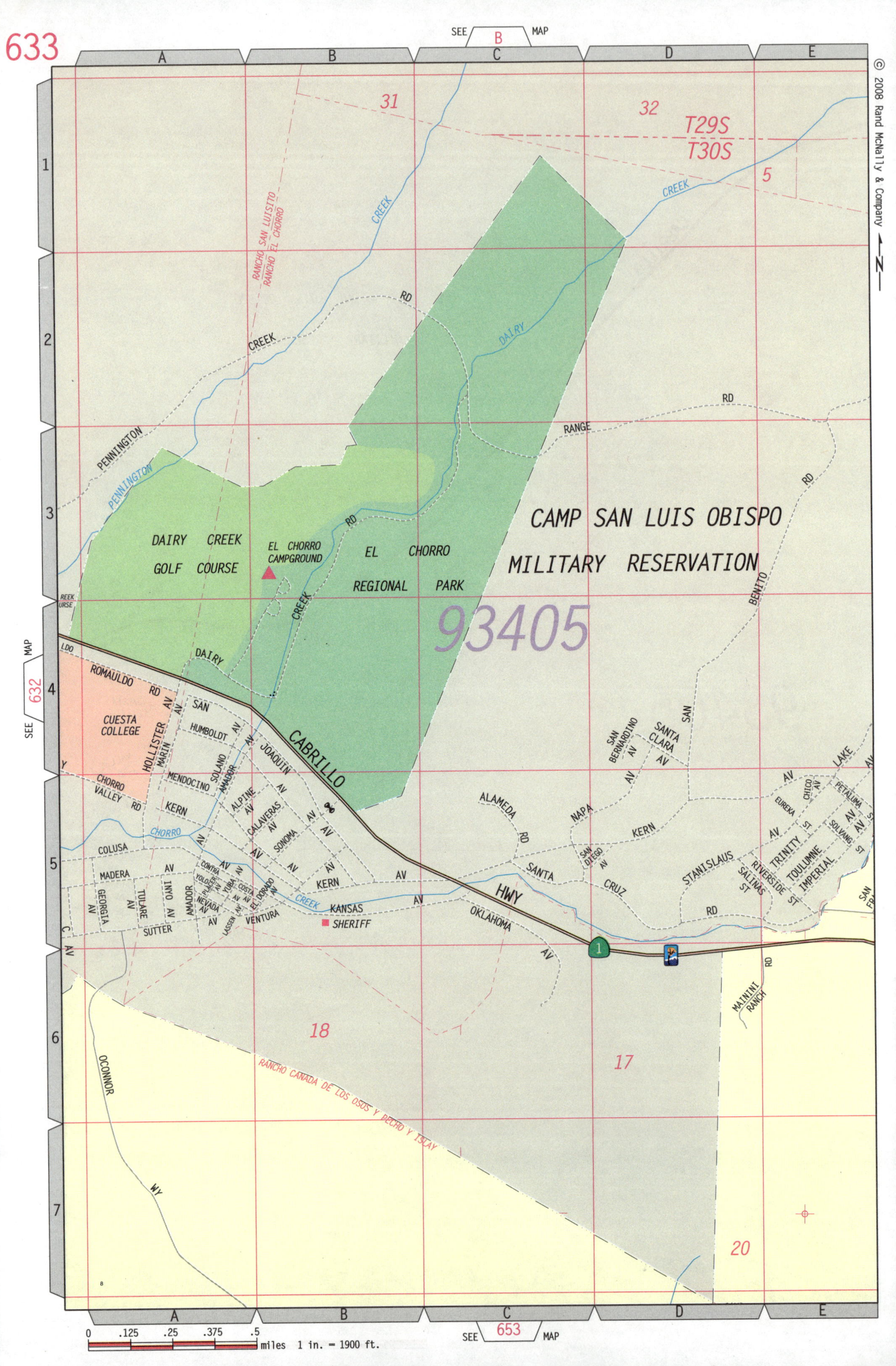
SEE B MAP
SEE 632 MAP
SEE 653 MAP
CAMP SAN LUIS OBISPO
MILITARY RESERVATION
DAIRY CREEK
GOLF COURSE
EL CHORRO
CAMPGROUND
EL CHORRO
REGIONAL PARK
CUESTA
COLLEGE
93405
T29S
T30S
RANCHO SAN LUISITO
RANCHO EL CHORRO
RANCHO CANADA DE LOS OSOS Y PECHO Y ISLAY
CABRILLO HWY
SHERIFF
PENNINGTON CREEK
DAIRY CREEK
CHORRO CREEK
RANGE RD
BENITO RD
OCONNOR WY
MAININI RANCH RD
0 .125 .25 .375 .5 miles 1 in. = 1900 ft.

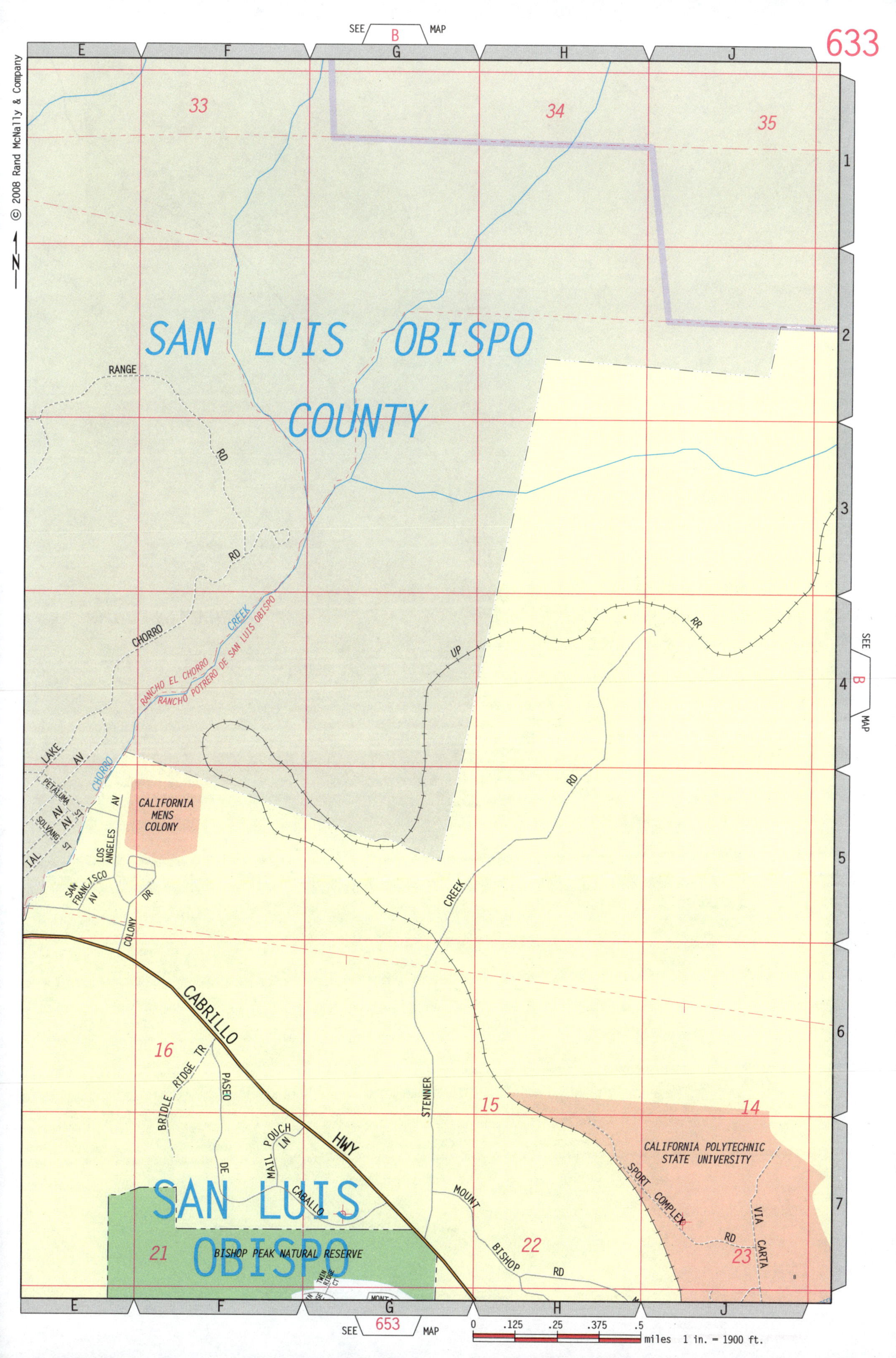

SEE B MAP
E
F
G
H
J
1
2
3
4
5
6
7
33
34
35
SAN LUIS OBISPO
COUNTY
RANGE
RD
RD
CHORRO
CREEK
RANCHO EL CHORRO
RANCHO POTRERO DE SAN LUIS OBISPO
CHORRO
LAKE
AV
PETALUMA
AV
AV
SOLVANG
ST
ST
AV
LOS ANGELES
CALIFORNIA MENS COLONY
SAN FRANCISCO
AV
DR
COLONY
UP
RR
RD
CREEK
SEE B MAP
CABRILLO
HWY
16
BRIDLE RIDGE TR
PASEO
DE
MAIL POUCH LN
CABALLO
STENNER
15
14
CALIFORNIA POLYTECHNIC STATE UNIVERSITY
SPORT COMPLEX
RD
VIA CARTA
23
MOUNT
BISHOP
RD
22
SAN LUIS OBISPO
21
BISHOP PEAK NATURAL RESERVE
TWIN RIDGE CT

SEE 653 MAP

0 .125 .25 .375 .5 miles 1 in. = 1900 ft.

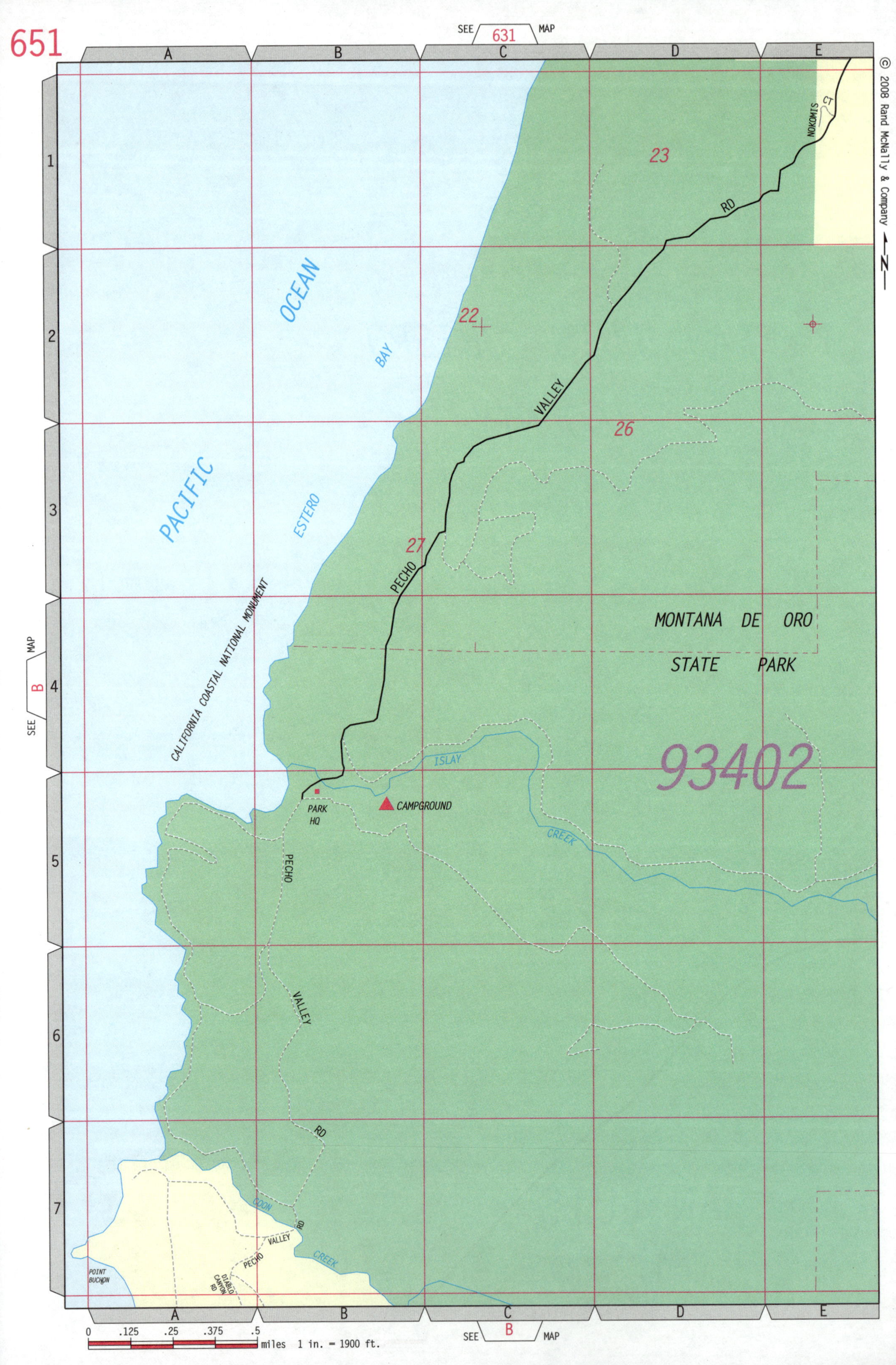
SEE 631 MAP
A
B
C
D
E
1
2
3
4
5
6
7
PACIFIC
OCEAN
ESTERO
BAY
CALIFORNIA COASTAL NATIONAL MONUMENT
NOKOMIS CT
23
22
26
27
PECHO
VALLEY
RD
MONTANA DE ORO
STATE PARK
93402
ISLAY
CREEK
PARK HQ
CAMPGROUND
PECHO
VALLEY
RD
COON
CREEK
PECHO VALLEY RD
DIABLO CANYON RD
POINT BUCHON
SEE B MAP
0 .125 .25 .375 .5 miles 1 in. = 1900 ft.

SEE 631 MAP

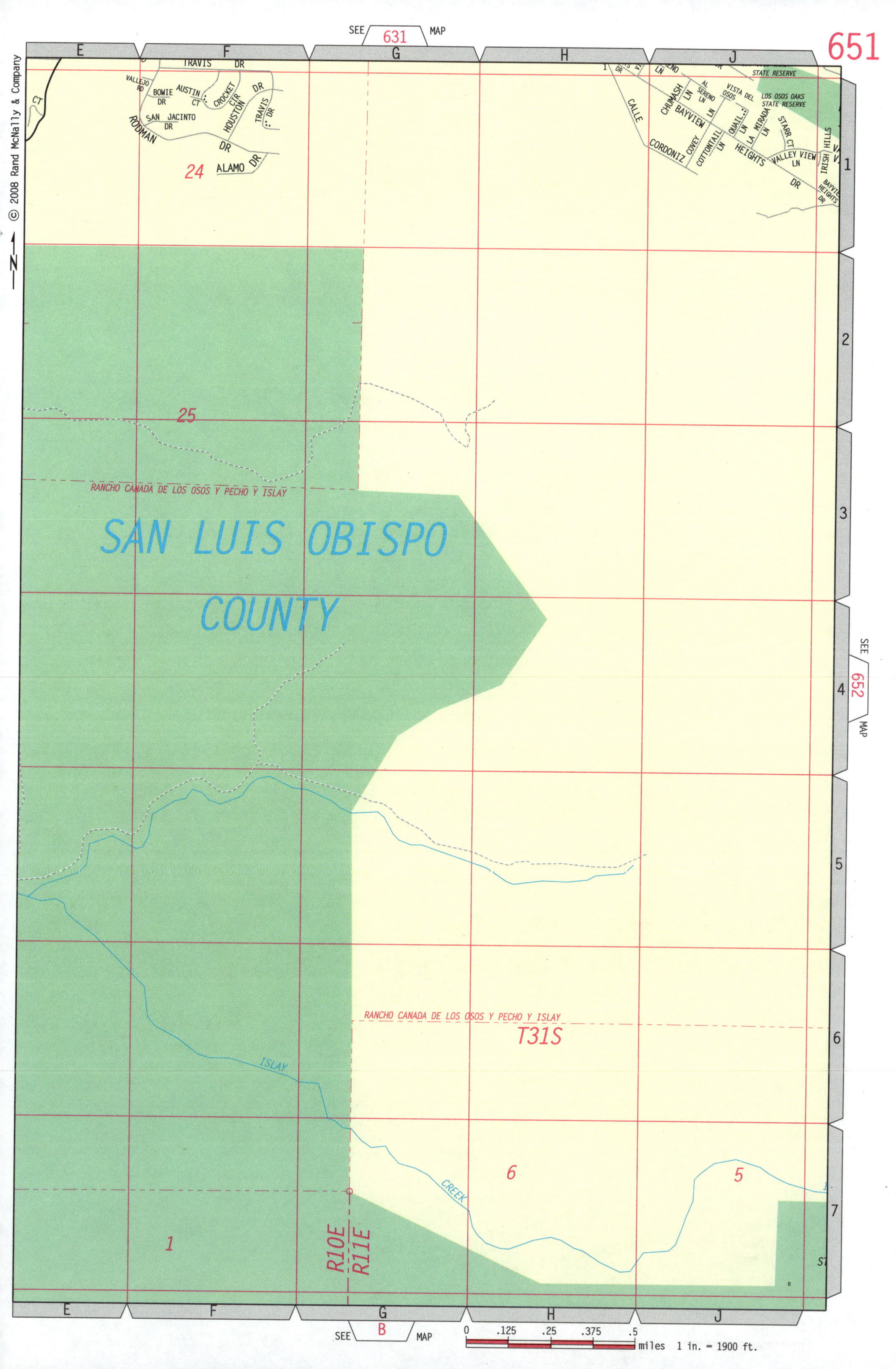
E
F
G
H
J
TRAVIS DR
VALLEJO RD
BOWIE DR
AUSTIN CT
CROCKET CIR
DR
TRAVIS DR
SAN JACINTO DR
RODMAN DR
HOUSTON
ALAMO DR
24
CALLE
CHUMASH LN
AL SERENO LN
VISTA DEL OSOS
BAYVIEW LN
LOS OSOS OAKS STATE RESERVE
STATE RESERVE
QUAIL LN
LA MIRADA LN
STARR CT
CORDONIZ
COVEY LN
COTTONTAIL LN
HEIGHTS
VALLEY VIEW LN
DR
IRISH HILLS
BAYVIEW HEIGHTS DR
1
2
3
4
5
6
7
25
RANCHO CANADA DE LOS OSOS Y PECHO Y ISLAY
SAN LUIS OBISPO
COUNTY
SEE 652 MAP
RANCHO CANADA DE LOS OSOS Y PECHO Y ISLAY
T31S
ISLAY
CREEK
6
5
1
R10E
R11E
0
.125
.25
.375
.5
miles 1 in. = 1900 ft.

SEE B MAP

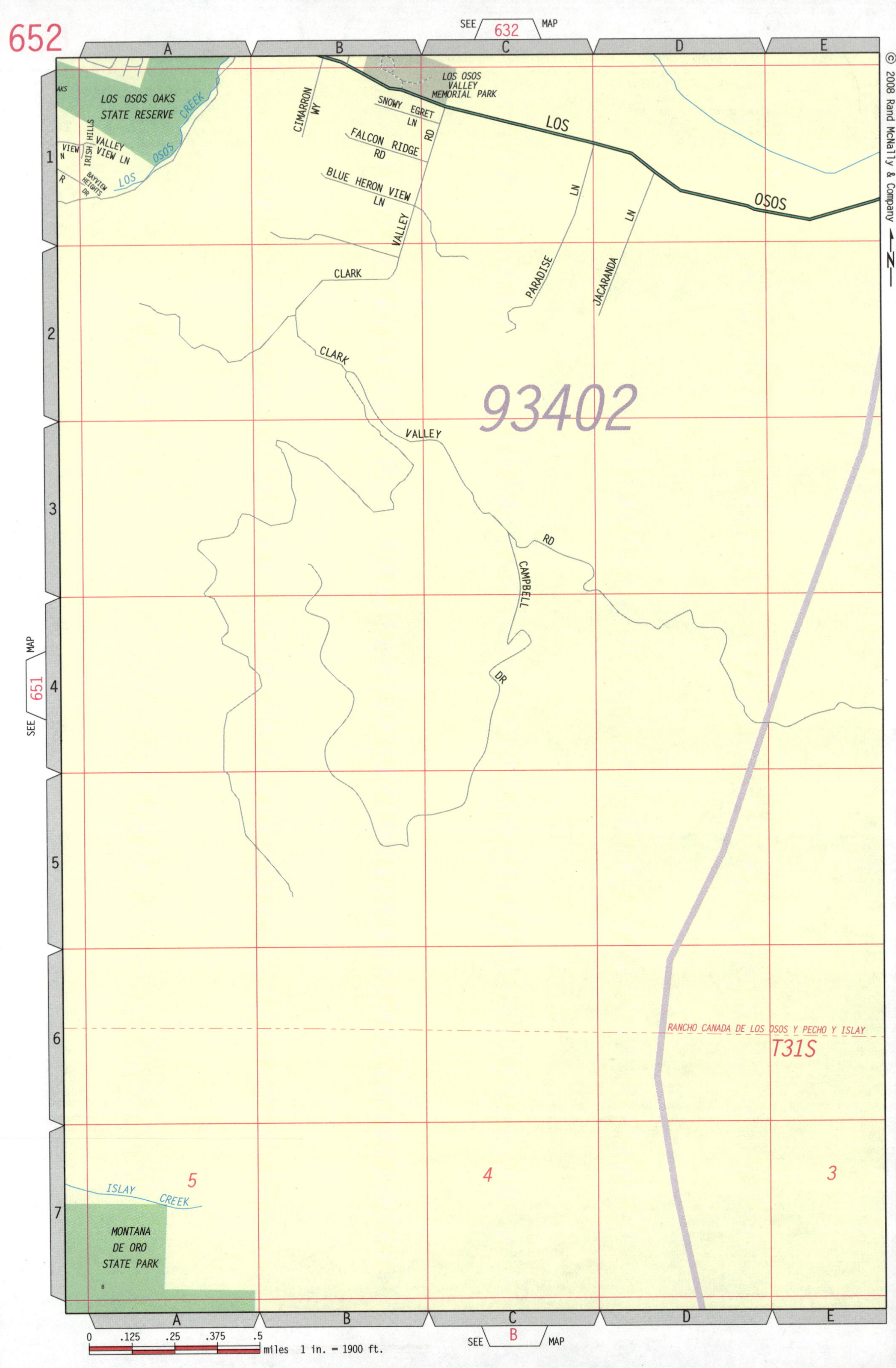
SEE 632 MAP
LOS OSOS OAKS STATE RESERVE
LOS OSOS CREEK
LOS OSOS VALLEY MEMORIAL PARK
CIMARRON WY
SNOWY EGRET LN
FALCON RIDGE RD
BLUE HERON VIEW LN
VALLEY VIEW LN
IRISH HILLS
BAYVIEW HEIGHTS DR
LOS OSOS
VALLEY RD
CLARK
CLARK
VALLEY
RD
PARADISE LN
JACARANDA LN
93402
CAMPBELL DR
SEE 651 MAP
RANCHO CANADA DE LOS OSOS Y PECHO Y ISLAY
T31S
ISLAY CREEK
MONTANA DE ORO STATE PARK
5
4
3
SEE B MAP
0 .125 .25 .375 .5 miles 1 in. = 1900 ft.

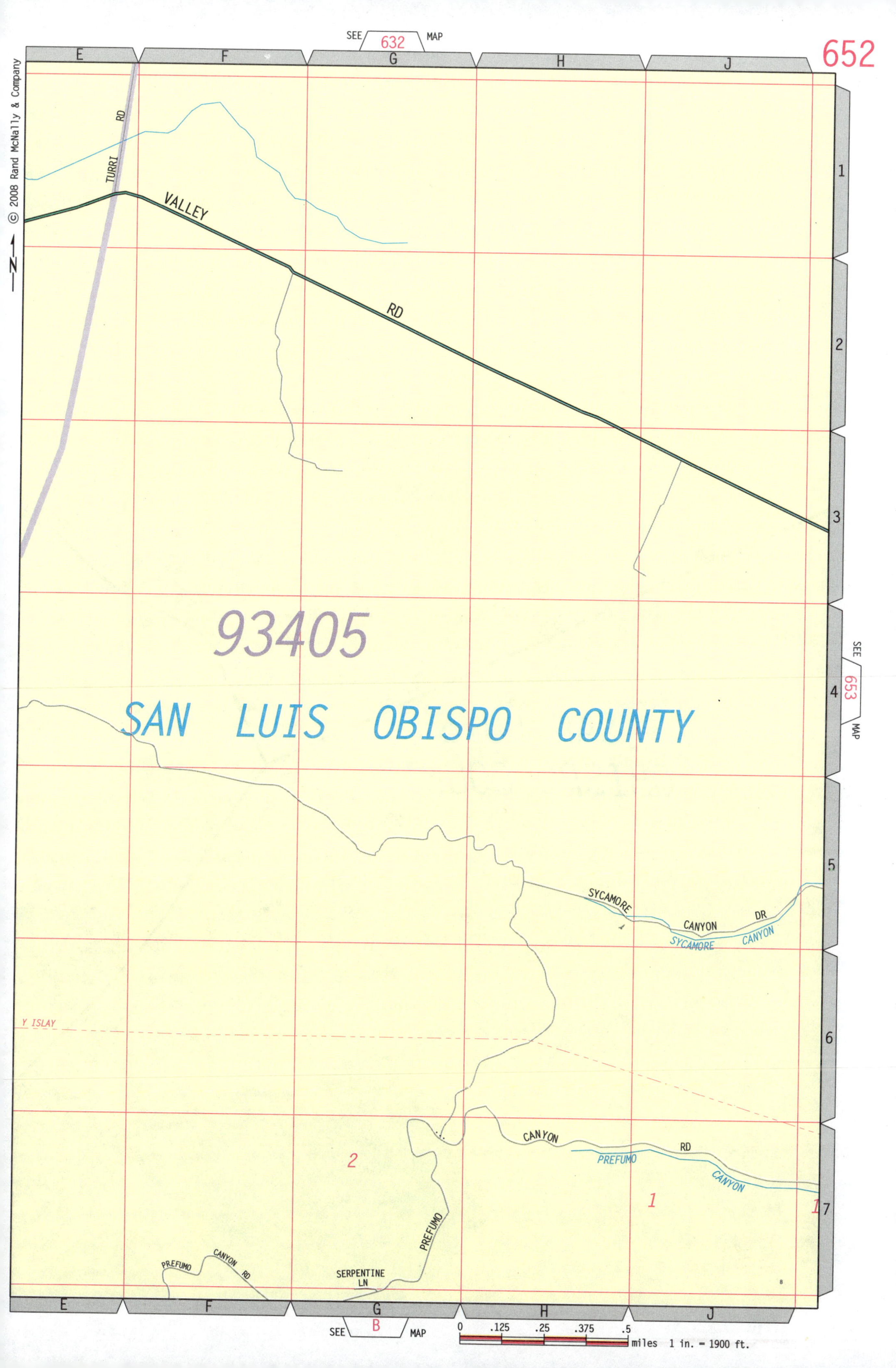

SEE 632 MAP
E
F
G
H
J
1
2
3
4
5
6
7
SEE 653 MAP
TURRI RD
VALLEY RD
93405
SAN LUIS OBISPO COUNTY
SYCAMORE CANYON DR
SYCAMORE CANYON
Y ISLAY
CANYON RD
PREFUMO CANYON
PREFUMO
PREFUMO CANYON RD
SERPENTINE LN
2
1
SEE B MAP
0 .125 .25 .375 .5
miles 1 in. = 1900 ft.
© 2008 Rand McNally & Company

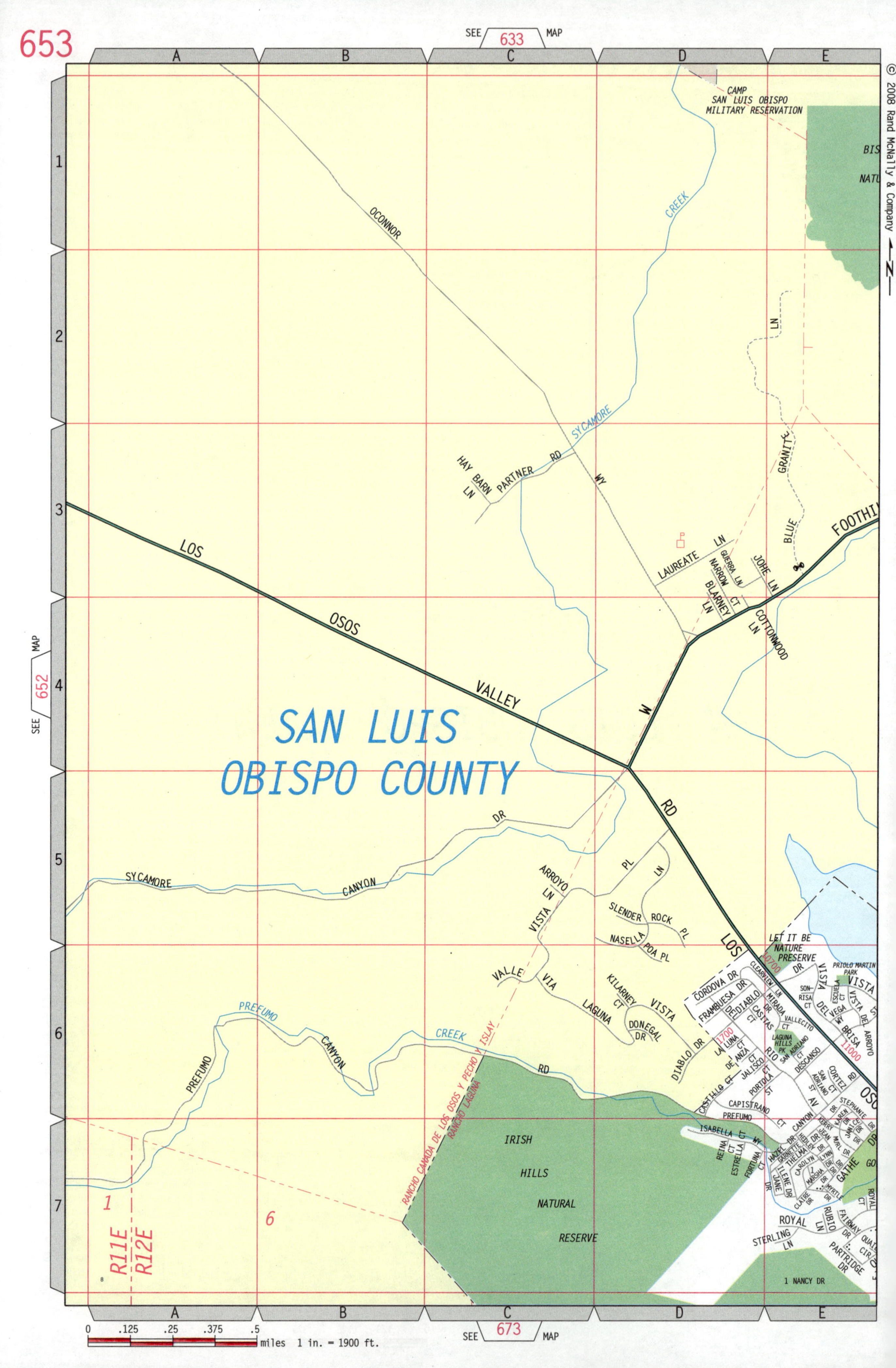
SEE 633 MAP
SEE 673 MAP
SEE 652 MAP
A
B
C
D
E
1
2
3
4
5
6
7
CAMP SAN LUIS OBISPO MILITARY RESERVATION
SAN LUIS OBISPO COUNTY
LOS OSOS VALLEY RD
OCONNOR WY
SYCAMORE CREEK
HAY BARN LN
PARTNER RD
LAUREATE LN
GUERBA LN
MARROW CT
BLARNEY LN
JOHE LN
COTTONWOOD LN
BLUE GRANITE LN
FOOTHILL
SYCAMORE CANYON DR
ARROYO LN
VISTA PL
SLENDER ROCK PL
NASELLA
POA PL
VALLE VIA
KILARNEY CT
VISTA LAGUNA
DONEGAL DR
DIABLO DR
PREFUMO CREEK
PREFUMO CANYON RD
RANCHO CANADA DE LOS OSOS Y PECHO Y ISLAY
RANCHO LAGUNA
IRISH HILLS NATURAL RESERVE
LET IT BE NATURE PRESERVE
PRIOLO MARTIN PARK
CORDOVA DR
FRAMBUESA DR
CLEARVIEW LN
MIRADA DR
CASITAS CT
VISTA DEL VEGA
VISTA DEL ARROYO
BRISA
LAGUNA HILLS PK
VALLECITO CT
SAN ADRIANO CT
DESCANSO
CORTEZ
CAPISTRANO
PREFUMO
ISABELLA WY
REINA CT
ESTRELLA CT
FORTUNA CT
HAZEL DR
JANE
ILENE DR
CAROLYN
MARSHA
MYRTLE
GATHE DR
ROYAL
STERLING LN
RUBIO LN
FAIRWAY DR
PARTRIDGE DR
1 NANCY DR
10700
1700
11000
R11E
R12E
1
6
0 .125 .25 .375 .5 miles 1 in. = 1900 ft.

SEE 633 MAP

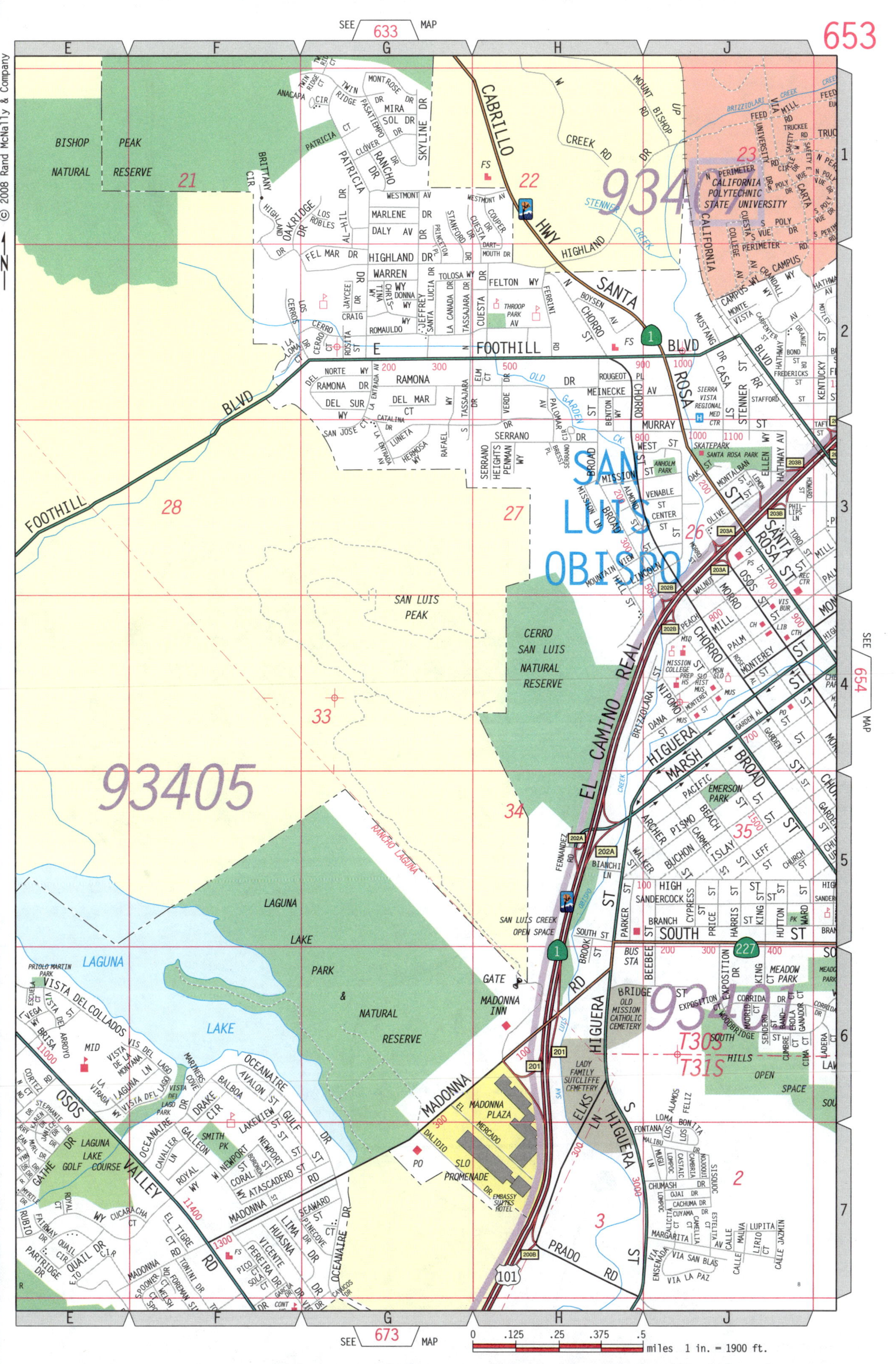
E
F
G
H
J
1
2
3
4
5
6
7
BISHOP PEAK NATURAL RESERVE
21
22
23
CABRILLO HWY
CREEK RD
MOUNT BISHOP RD
93407
CALIFORNIA POLYTECHNIC STATE UNIVERSITY
HIGHLAND DR
FOOTHILL BLVD
SANTA ROSA
28
27
26
SAN LUIS OBISPO
SAN LUIS PEAK
CERRO SAN LUIS NATURAL RESERVE
33
34
35
93405
EL CAMINO REAL
HIGUERA ST
MARSH ST
BROAD ST
MONTEREY ST
EMERSON PARK
LAGUNA LAKE PARK & NATURAL RESERVE
LAGUNA LAKE
LAGUNA LAKE GOLF COURSE
MADONNA INN
MADONNA PLAZA
SLO PROMENADE
EMBASSY SUITES HOTEL
SAN LUIS CREEK OPEN SPACE
OLD MISSION CATHOLIC CEMETERY
LADY FAMILY SUTCLIFFE CEMETERY
93401
T30S
T31S
SOUTH HILLS OPEN SPACE
LOS OSOS VALLEY RD
MADONNA RD
PRADO RD
SOUTH ST
2
3
101
1
227
0
.125
.25
.375
.5
miles 1 in. = 1900 ft.

SEE 654 MAP

SEE 673 MAP

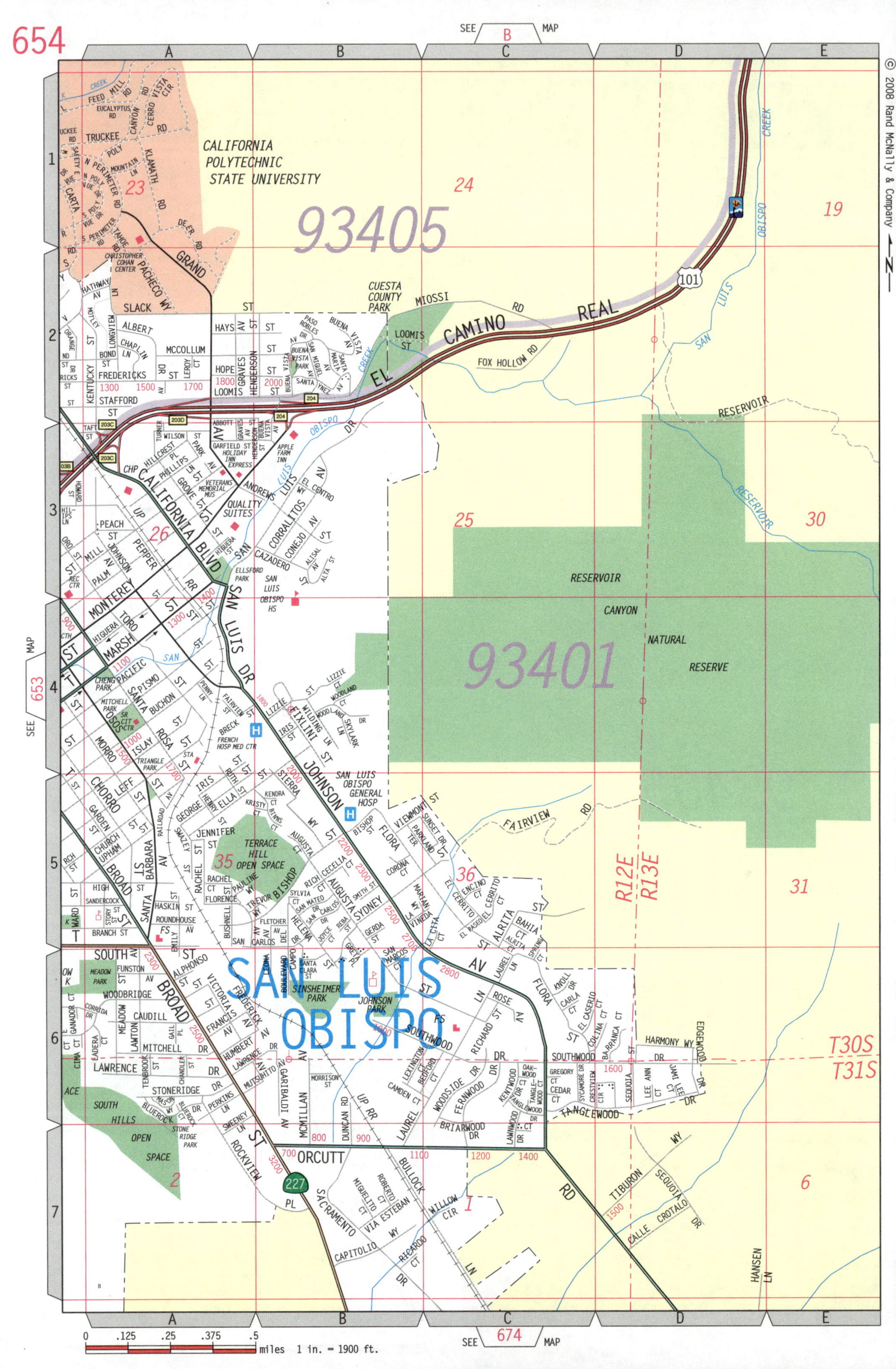

SEE B MAP
A
B
C
D
E
1
2
3
4
5
6
7
CALIFORNIA POLYTECHNIC STATE UNIVERSITY
93405
93401
24
23
19
25
26
30
35
36
31
1
2
6
CHRISTOPHER COHAN CENTER
GRAND
SLACK
PACHECO WY
CUESTA COUNTY PARK
MIOSSI
EL CAMINO REAL
101
FOX HOLLOW RD
LOOMIS ST
RESERVOIR
SAN LUIS CREEK
OBISPO CREEK
RESERVOIR CANYON NATURAL RESERVE
CALIFORNIA BLVD
SAN LUIS DR
JOHNSON AV
MONTEREY
MARSH
HIGUERA
SAN LUIS OBISPO HS
FRENCH HOSP MED CTR
SAN LUIS OBISPO GENERAL HOSP
TERRACE HILL OPEN SPACE
FAIRVIEW RD
R12E
R13E
T30S
T31S
SAN LUIS OBISPO
SINSHEIMER PARK
JOHNSON PARK
MEADOW PARK
SOUTH HILLS OPEN SPACE
STONERIDGE PARK
BROAD ST
ORCUTT RD
227
TANGLEWOOD
TIBURON WY
SEQUOIA
CALLE CROTALO DR
HANSEN LN
SEE 653 MAP
SEE 674 MAP
0 .125 .25 .375 .5 miles 1 in. = 1900 ft.

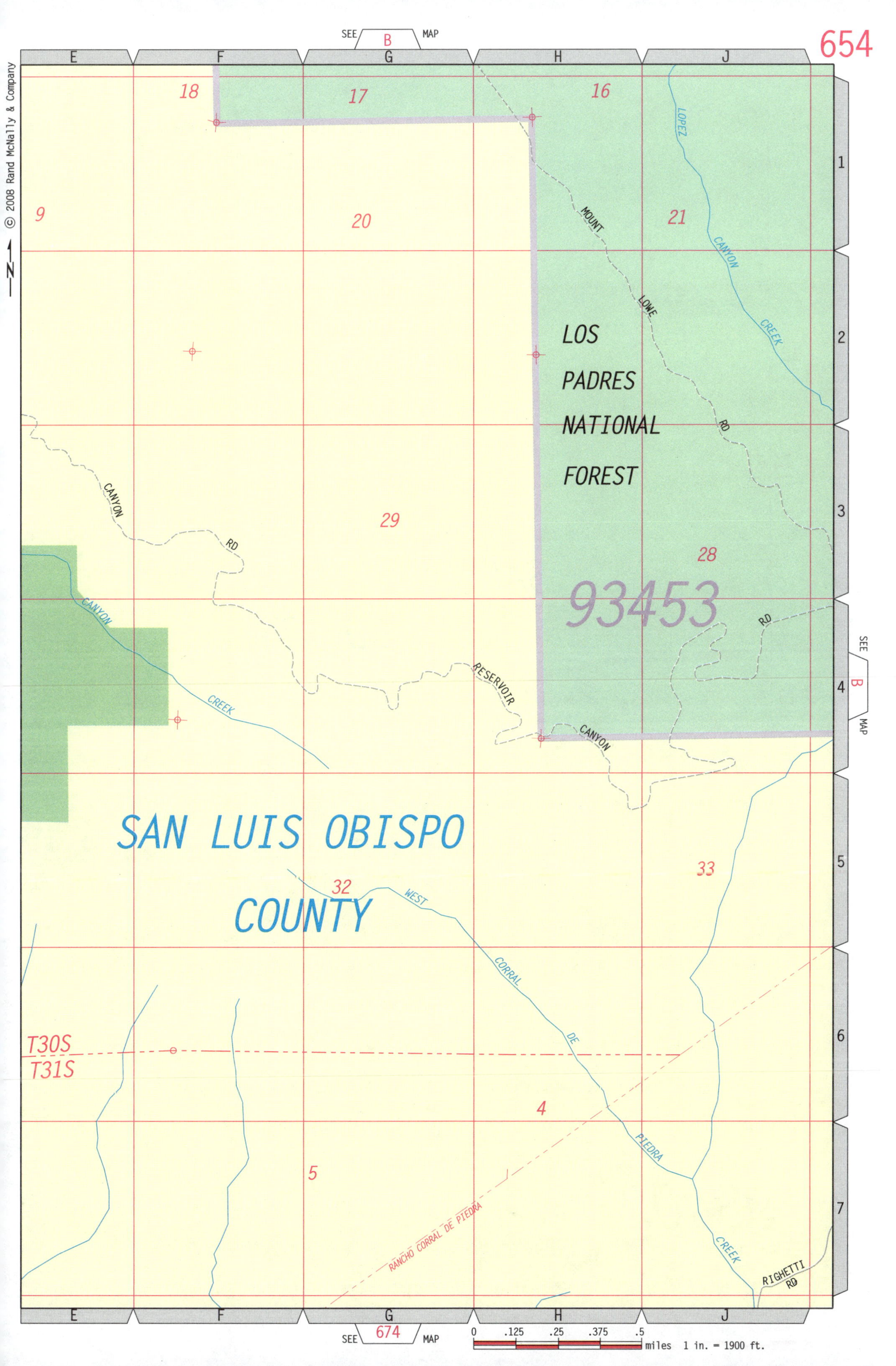
SEE B MAP
E
F
G
H
J
18
17
16
9
20
21
LOPEZ
CANYON
CREEK
MOUNT
LOWE
RD
LOS
PADRES
NATIONAL
FOREST
CANYON
RD
29
28
93453
RD
CANYON
CREEK
RESERVOIR
CANYON
SEE B MAP
SAN LUIS OBISPO
COUNTY
32
33
WEST
CORRAL
DE
PIEDRA
CREEK
T30S
T31S
4
5
RANCHO CORRAL DE PIEDRA
RIGHETTI
RD
1
2
3
4
5
6
7
SEE 674 MAP
0 .125 .25 .375 .5
miles 1 in. = 1900 ft.

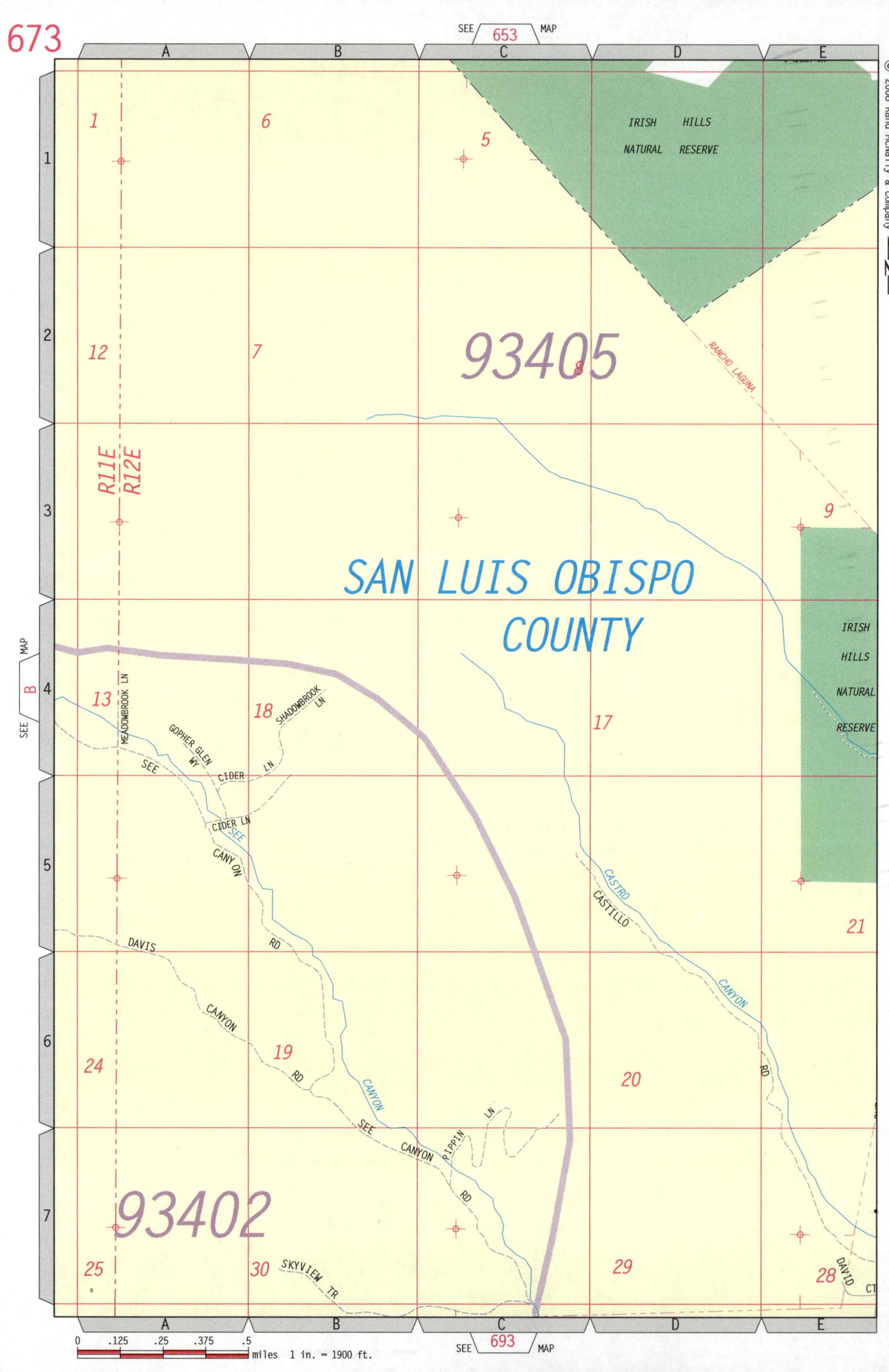
SEE 653 MAP
IRISH HILLS
NATURAL RESERVE
93405
RANCHO LAGUNA
R11E
R12E
SAN LUIS OBISPO
COUNTY
IRISH
HILLS
NATURAL
RESERVE
SEE B MAP
MEADOWBROOK LN
SHADOWBROOK LN
GOPHER GLEN WY
CIDER LN
SEE
CIDER LN
SEE
CANYON
RD
CASTRO
CASTILLO
CANYON
RD
DAVIS
CANYON
RD
CANYON
SEE
CANYON
PIPPIN
LN
RD
93402
SKYVIEW TR
DAVID
CT
1
6
5
12
7
8
9
13
18
17
21
24
19
20
25
30
29
28
0 .125 .25 .375 .5
miles 1 in. = 1900 ft.
SEE 693 MAP

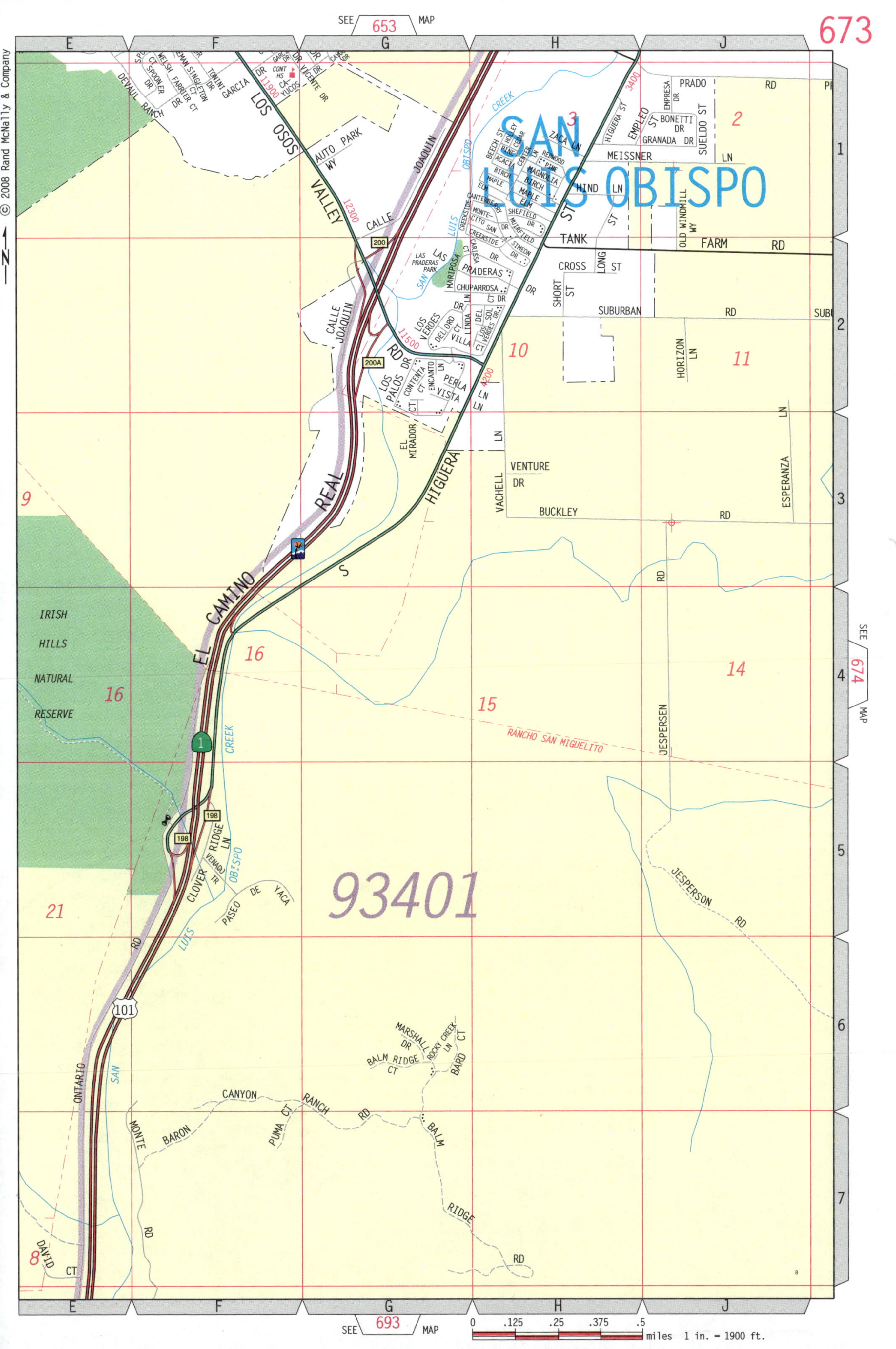
SEE 653 MAP
SAN LUIS OBISPO
93401
LOS OSOS VALLEY RD
EL CAMINO REAL
JOAQUIN
HIGUERA ST
S HIGUERA
AUTO PARK WY
CALLE JOAQUIN
TANK FARM RD
MEISSNER LN
HIND LN
PRADO RD
SUBURBAN RD
CROSS ST
LONG ST
SHORT ST
HORIZON LN
VENTURE DR
VACHELL LN
BUCKLEY RD
ESPERANZA LN
JESPERSEN RD
JESPERSON RD
RANCHO SAN MIGUELITO
IRISH HILLS NATURAL RESERVE
SAN LUIS OBISPO CREEK
CLOVER RIDGE LN
VENADO TR
PASEO DE YACA
ONTARIO RD
MONTE RD
BARON CANYON RANCH RD
PUMA CT
BALM RIDGE CT
BALM RIDGE RD
MARSHALL DR
ROCKY CREEK LN
BARD CT
DAVID CT
EL MIRADOR
LAS PRADERAS PARK
LAS PRADERAS DR
CHUPARROSA
MARIPOSA
LOS VERDES DR
LOS PALOS DR
PERLA VISTA LN
DEVAUL RANCH DR
SEE 674 MAP
SEE 693 MAP
0 .125 .25 .375 .5 miles 1 in. = 1900 ft.

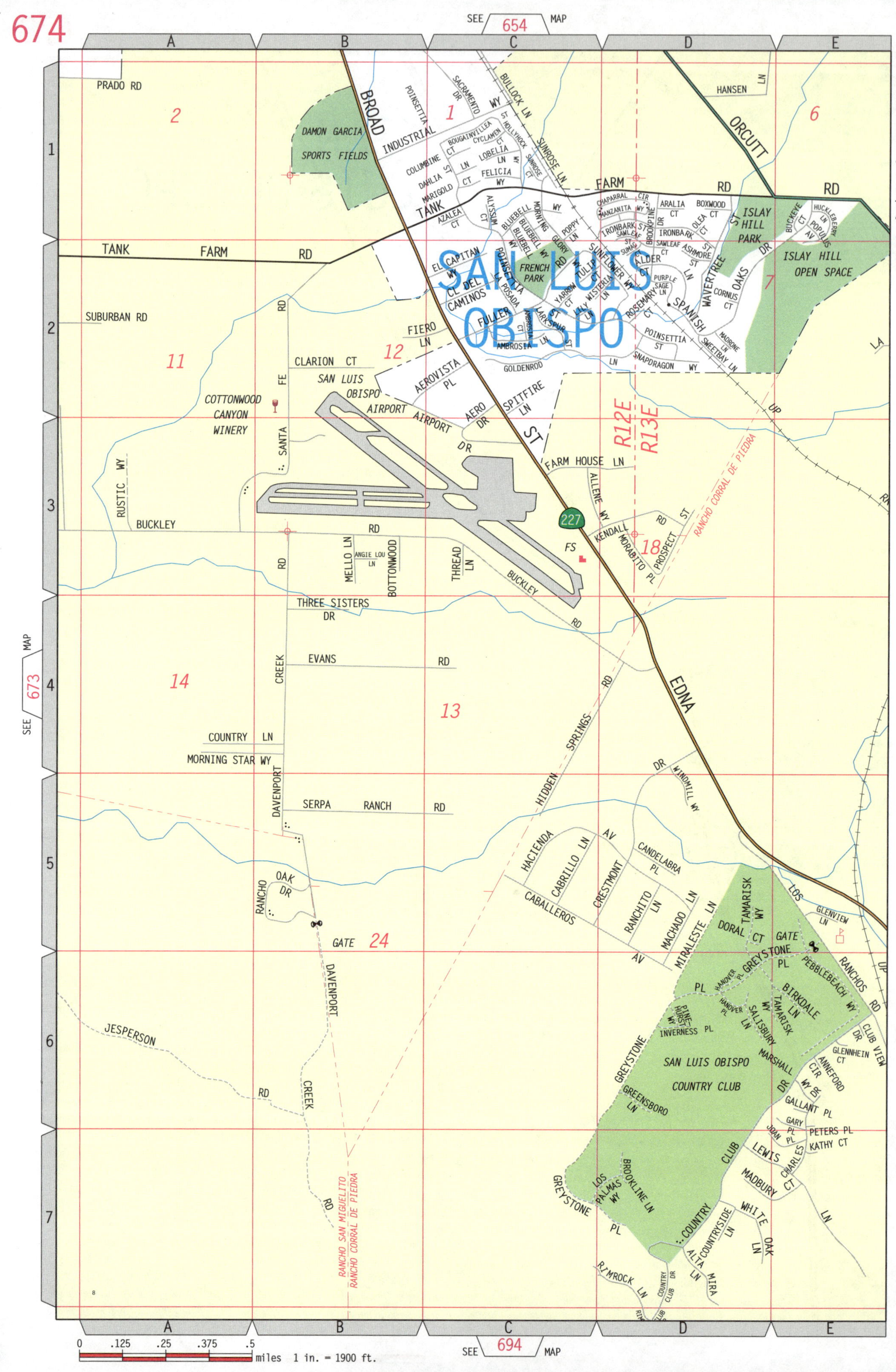
SEE 654 MAP
SEE 673 MAP
SEE 694 MAP
SAN LUIS OBISPO
DAMON GARCIA SPORTS FIELDS
FRENCH PARK
ISLAY HILL PARK
ISLAY HILL OPEN SPACE
SAN LUIS OBISPO AIRPORT
COTTONWOOD CANYON WINERY
SAN LUIS OBISPO COUNTRY CLUB
TANK FARM RD
BROAD ST
EDNA
ORCUTT RD
BUCKLEY RD
SANTA FE RD
CREEK RD
DAVENPORT CREEK RD
HIDDEN SPRINGS RD
THREE SISTERS DR
EVANS RD
SERPA RANCH RD
COUNTRY LN
MORNING STAR WY
PRADO RD
SUBURBAN RD
RUSTIC WY
JESPERSON RD
GREYSTONE PL
RANCHOS RD
R12E
R13E
RANCHO CORRAL DE PIEDRA
RANCHO SAN MIGUELITO
GATE
227
FS
miles 1 in. = 1900 ft.

SEE 654 MAP

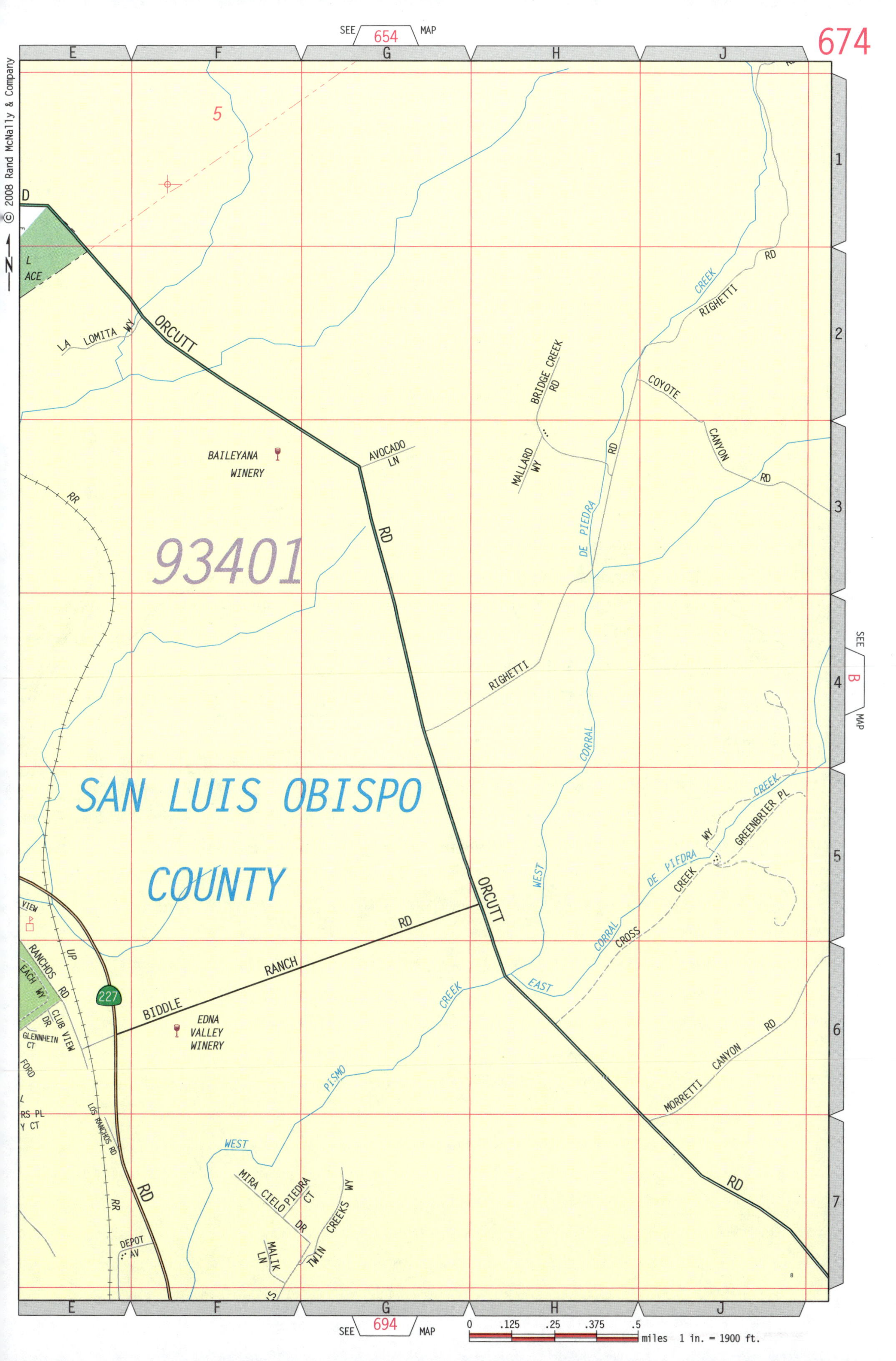

E
F
G
H
J
1
2
3
4
5
6
7
ORCUTT
RD
LA LOMITA WY
AVOCADO LN
BAILEYANA WINERY
93401
RR
BRIDGE CREEK RD
MALLARD WY
RIGHETTI RD
COYOTE CANYON RD
CREEK
DE PIEDRA
CORRAL
WEST
SAN LUIS OBISPO
COUNTY
BIDDLE RANCH RD
EDNA VALLEY WINERY
227
LOS RANCHOS RD
CLUB VIEW DR
GLENNHEIN CT
PISMO
CREEK
EAST
CROSS CREEK
GREENBRIER PL
WY
MORRETTI CANYON RD
MIRA CIELO
PIEDRA CT
DR
TWIN CREEKS WY
MALIK LN
DEPOT AV
UP
SEE B MAP

SEE 694 MAP

0 .125 .25 .375 .5 miles 1 in. = 1900 ft.

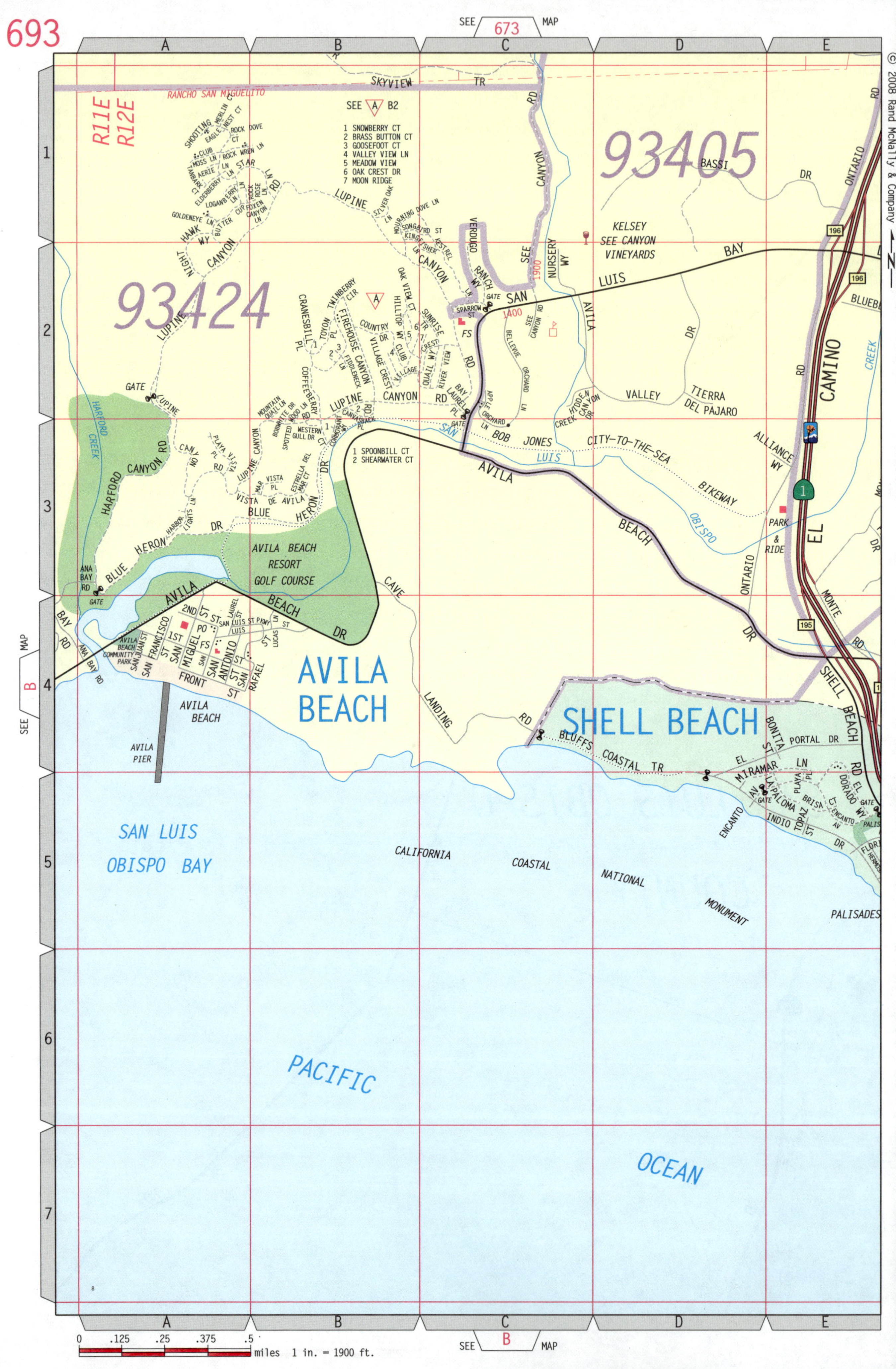
SEE 673 MAP
A
B
C
D
E
1
2
3
4
5
6
7
SKYVIEW TR
RANCHO SAN MIGUELITO
R11E
R12E
SEE A B2
1 SNOWBERRY CT
2 BRASS BUTTON CT
3 GOOSEFOOT CT
4 VALLEY VIEW LN
5 MEADOW VIEW
6 OAK CREST DR
7 MOON RIDGE
93405
93424
BASSI DR
ONTARIO RD
SEE CANYON RD
KELSEY SEE CANYON VINEYARDS
SAN LUIS BAY DR
NURSERY WY
VERDUGO RANCH WY
LUPINE CANYON RD
HARFORD CANYON RD
HARFORD CREEK
GATE
1900
1400
SPARROW ST
FS
AVILA VALLEY DR
TIERRA DEL PAJARO
HIDDEN CANYON DR
CREEK
BOB JONES CITY-TO-THE-SEA BIKEWAY
ALLIANCE WY
SAN LUIS OBISPO CREEK
EL CAMINO RD
PARK & RIDE
1 SPOONBILL CT
2 SHEARWATER CT
AVILA BEACH DR
BLUE HERON DR
AVILA BEACH RESORT GOLF COURSE
CAVE LANDING RD
ANA BAY RD
AVILA BEACH
AVILA BEACH COMMUNITY PARK
FRONT ST
AVILA PIER
SHELL BEACH
SHELL BEACH RD
BLUFFS COASTAL TR
EL MIRAMAR
PORTAL DR
BONITA ST
SAN LUIS OBISPO BAY
CALIFORNIA COASTAL NATIONAL MONUMENT
PALISADES
PACIFIC OCEAN
MONTE RD
196
195
1
© 2008 Rand McNally & Company
0 .125 .25 .375 .5 miles 1 in. = 1900 ft.
SEE B MAP

SEE 673 MAP

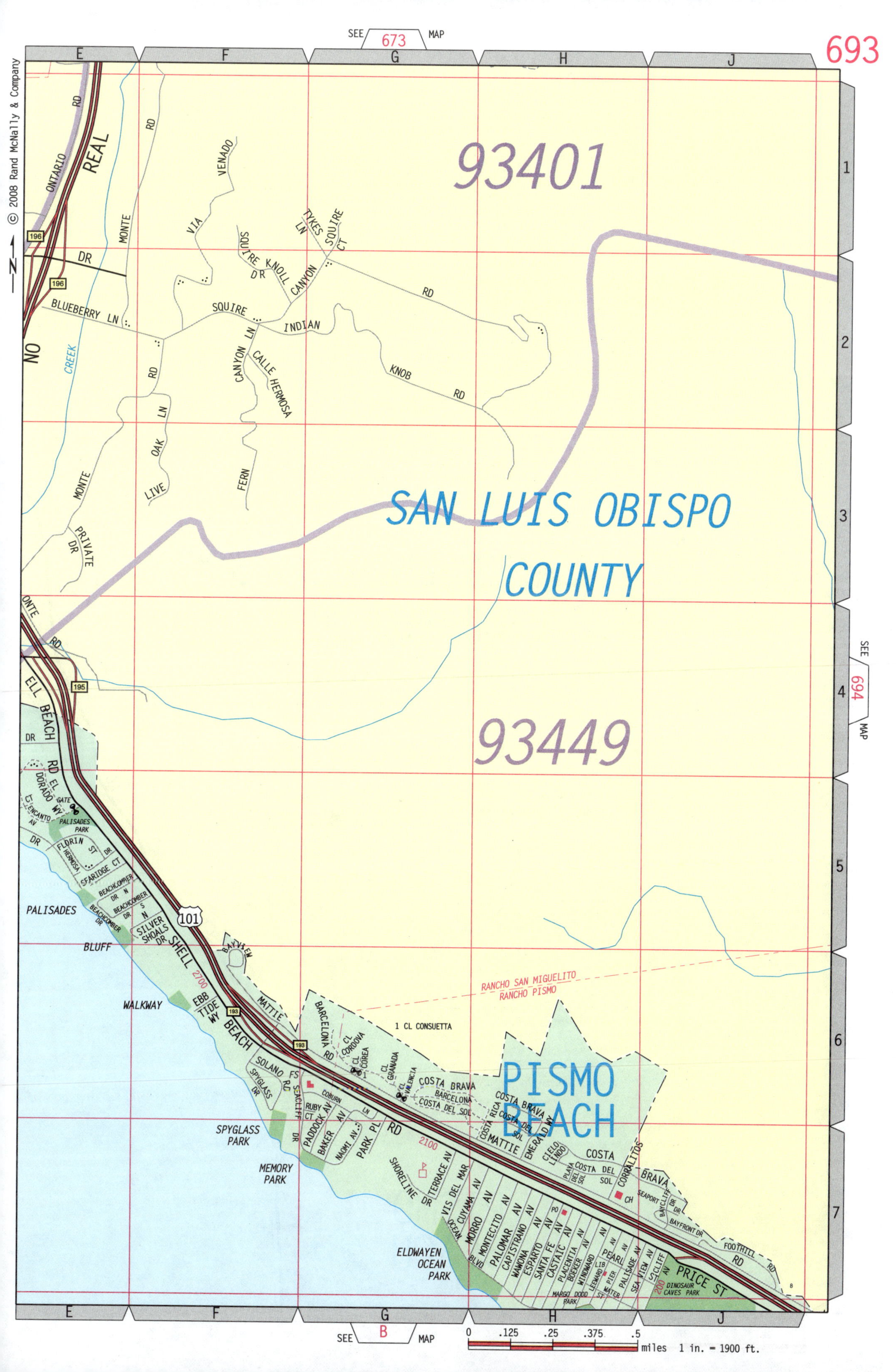
93401
SAN LUIS OBISPO COUNTY
93449
PISMO BEACH
ONTARIO RD
NO REAL
MONTE RD
VIA VENADO
TYKES LN
SQUIRE CT
SQUIRE KNOLL DR
CANYON
RD
BLUEBERRY LN
SQUIRE
INDIAN
CANYON LN
CALLE HERMOSA
KNOB RD
RD
LIVE OAK LN
FERN
MONTE
PRIVATE DR
CREEK
DR
ONTE RD
SHELL BEACH RD
EL DORADO WY
GATE
ENCANTO AV
CT
PALISADES PARK
FLORIN ST
HERMOSA DR
SEAFARIDGE CT
BEACHCOMBER DR N
BEACHCOMBER DR S
BEACHCOMBER DR
N SILVER SHOALS DR
PALISADES
BLUFF
WALKWAY
BAYVIEW
2700
EBB TIDE WY
MATTIE
BARCELONA RD
CL CORDOVA
CL COREA
CL GRANADA
CL VALENCIA
1 CL CONSUETTA
RANCHO SAN MIGUELITO
RANCHO PISMO
SOLANO RD
FS
SPYGLASS DR
SEACLIFF DR
COBURN LN
RUBY CT
PADDOCK AV
BAKER AV
NAOMI AV
PARK PL
RD
2100
COSTA BRAVA
BARCELONA
COSTA DEL SOL
COSTA RICA
COSTA BRAVA
COSTA DEL SOL
MATTIE
EMERALD WY
CIELO LINDO
PLAYA DEL SOL
COSTA DEL SOL
COSTA BRAVA
CORRALITOS
CH
SEAPORT DR
BAYCLIFF DR
BAYFRONT DR
FOOTHILL RD
SPYGLASS PARK
MEMORY PARK
SHORELINE DR
TERRACE AV
VIS DEL MAR
CUYAMA AV
OCEAN BLVD
MORRO AV
MONTECITO AV
PALOMAR AV
CAPISTRANO AV
WAWONA AV
ESPARTO AV
SANTA FE AV
PO
CASTAIC AV
PLACENTIA AV
BOEKER AV
WINDWARD AV
LEONARD AV
LIB
PIER AV
PEARL AV
PALISADE AV
SEA VIEW AV
SEACLIFF AV
200
PRICE ST
DINOSAUR CAVES PARK
MARGO DODD PARK
ELDWAYEN OCEAN PARK
101
193
195
196
E F G H J
1 2 3 4 5 6 7
0 .125 .25 .375 .5 miles 1 in. = 1900 ft.

SEE 694 MAP

SEE B MAP

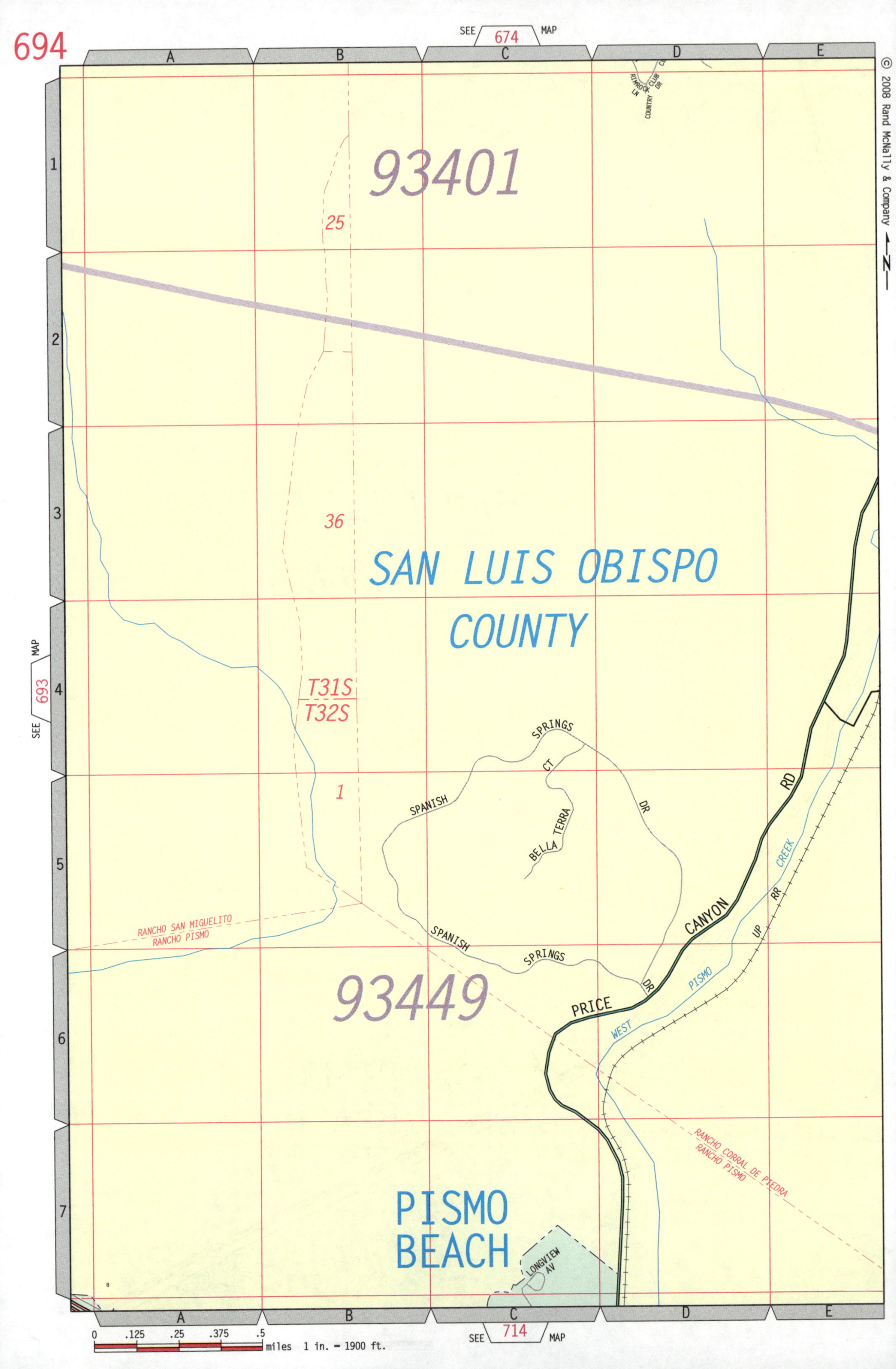

SEE 674 MAP
A
B
C
D
E
1
2
3
4
5
6
7
RIMROCK LN
COUNTRY CLUB DR
93401
25
36
SAN LUIS OBISPO
COUNTY
T31S
T32S
SEE 693 MAP
SPANISH
SPRINGS
CT
DR
BELLA TERRA
1
RANCHO SAN MIGUELITO
RANCHO PISMO
SPANISH
SPRINGS
DR
CANYON
RD
PRICE
CREEK
PISMO
West
UP
RR
93449
RANCHO CORRAL DE PIEDRA
RANCHO PISMO
PISMO
BEACH
LONGVIEW AV
SEE 714 MAP
0 .125 .25 .375 .5
miles 1 in. = 1900 ft.

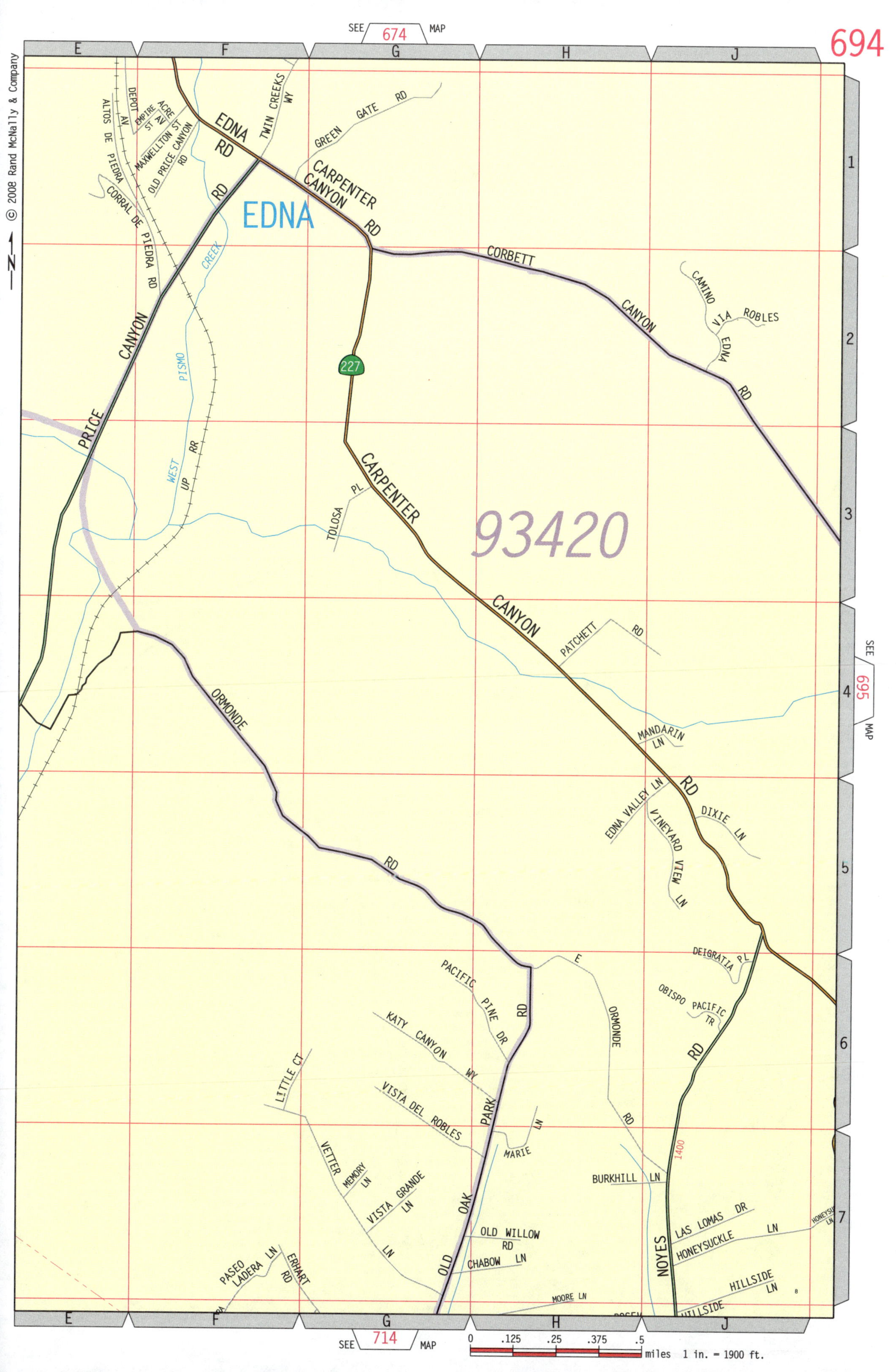

SEE 674 MAP
E
F
G
H
J
1
2
3
4
5
6
7
SEE 695 MAP
SEE 714 MAP
EDNA
93420
EDNA RD
CARPENTER CANYON RD
CORBETT CANYON RD
PRICE CANYON RD
ORMONDE RD
TWIN CREEKS WY
GREEN GATE RD
ALTOS DE PIEDRA AV
DEPOT ST
EMPIRE AV
ACRE AV
MAXWELLTON ST
OLD PRICE CANYON RD
CORRAL DE PIEDRA RD
PISMO CREEK
WEST
UP RR
227
TOLOSA PL
CAMINO VIA ROBLES
EDNA RD
PATCHETT RD
MANDARIN LN
EDNA VALLEY LN
VINEYARD VIEW LN
DIXIE LN
DEIGRATIA PL
OBISPO PACIFIC TR
E ORMONDE RD
NOYES RD
1400
PACIFIC PINE DR
KATY CANYON WY
OLD OAK PARK RD
LITTLE CT
VISTA DEL ROBLES
MARIE LN
VETTER LN
MEMORY LN
VISTA GRANDE LN
BURKHILL LN
LAS LOMAS DR
HONEYSUCKLE LN
OLD WILLOW RD
CHABOW LN
PASEO LADERA LN
ERHART RD
MOORE LN
HILLSIDE LN
0 .125 .25 .375 .5 miles 1 in. = 1900 ft.

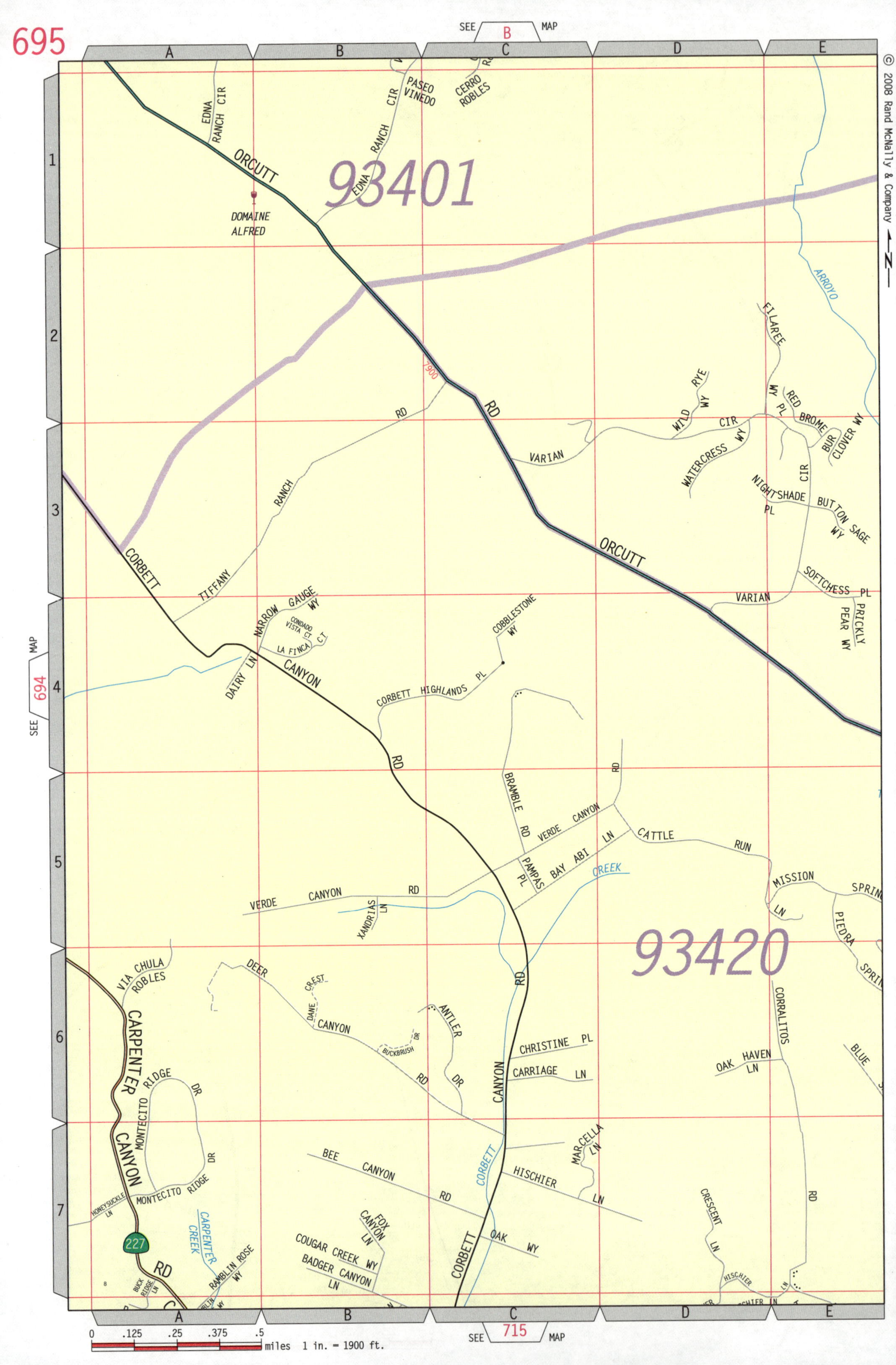

SEE B MAP
SEE 694 MAP
SEE 715 MAP
93401
93420
ORCUTT RD
EDNA RANCH CIR
PASEO VINEDO
CERRO ROBLES
DOMAINE ALFRED
ARROYO
FILAREE WY
RYE WY
WILD CIR
RED PL
BROME
BUR
CLOVER WY
WATERCRESS WY
CIR
NIGHTSHADE PL
BUTTON SAGE WY
VARIAN
SOFTCHESS PL
PRICKLY PEAR WY
1900
RANCH RD
TIFFANY
CORBETT CANYON RD
NARROW GAUGE WY
CONDADO VISTA CT
LA FINCA CT
DAIRY LN
COBBLESTONE WY
CORBETT HIGHLANDS PL
BRAMBLE RD
VERDE CANYON RD
CATTLE RUN
BAY ABI LN
PAMPAS PL
CREEK
MISSION LN
SPRING
PIEDRA
XANDRIAS LN
VIA CHULA ROBLES
DEER CANYON RD
CREST
DANE
BUCKBRUSH DR
ANTLER DR
CORRALITOS RD
CARPENTER CANYON RD
MONTECITO RIDGE DR
CHRISTINE PL
CARRIAGE LN
OAK HAVEN LN
BLUE
MARCELLA LN
HISCHIER LN
CORBETT
BEE CANYON RD
CRESCENT LN
HONEYSUCKLE LN
227
CARPENTER CREEK
FOX CANYON LN
COUGAR CREEK WY
BADGER CANYON LN
OAK WY
RAMBLIN ROSE WY
BUCK RIDGE LN
HISCHIER
0 .125 .25 .375 .5 miles 1 in. = 1900 ft.

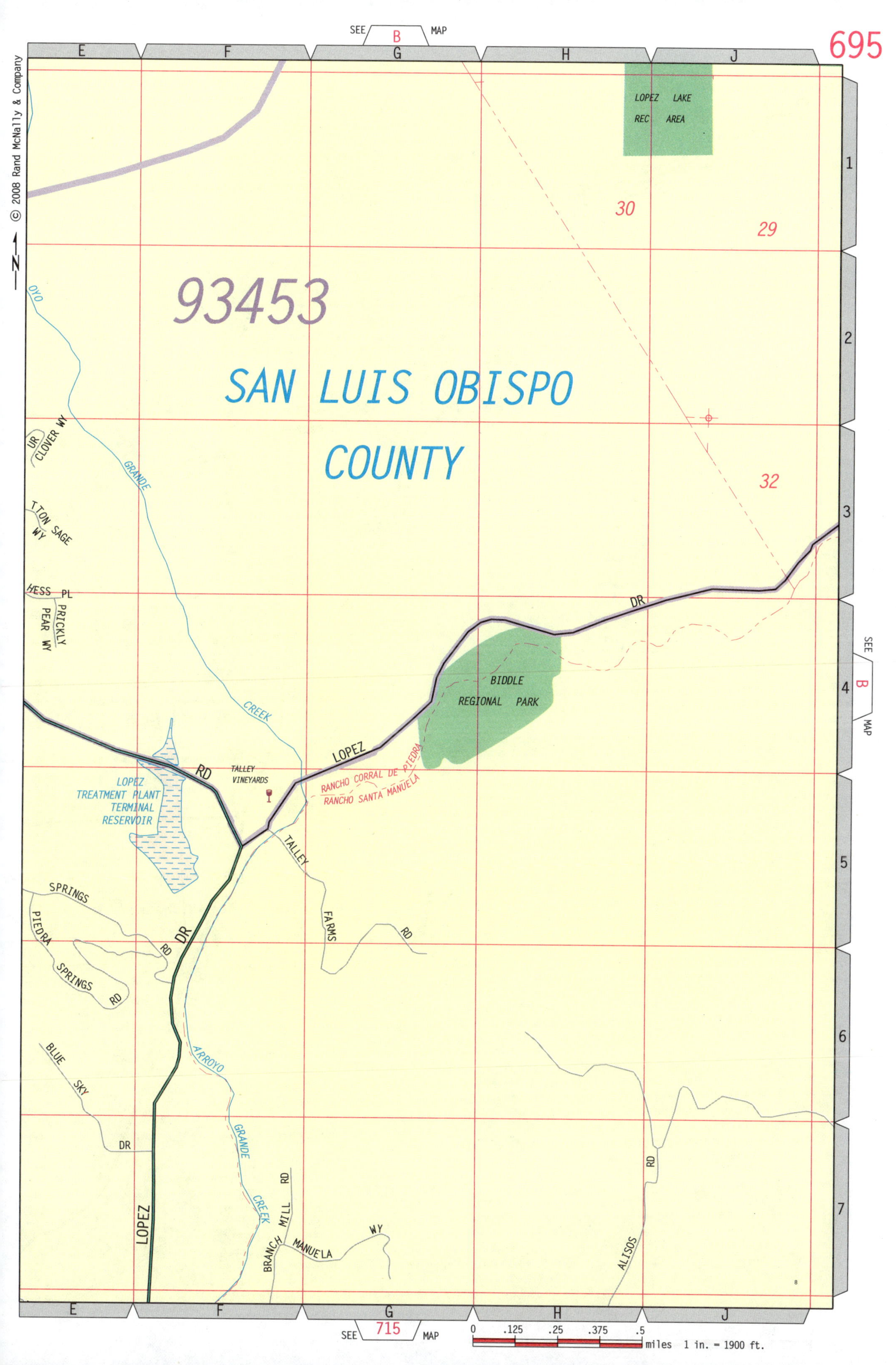
SEE B MAP
E
F
G
H
J
1
2
3
4
5
6
7
LOPEZ LAKE REC AREA
30
29
32
93453
SAN LUIS OBISPO
COUNTY
CLOVER WY
GRANDE
SAGE
WY
HESS PL
PRICKLY PEAR WY
DR
BIDDLE REGIONAL PARK
CREEK
LOPEZ
RD
TALLEY VINEYARDS
LOPEZ TREATMENT PLANT TERMINAL RESERVOIR
RANCHO CORRAL DE PIEDRA
RANCHO SANTA MANUELA
TALLEY
FARMS
RD
SPRINGS
PIEDRA
SPRINGS
RD
DR
ARROYO
BLUE
SKY
DR
GRANDE
CREEK
LOPEZ
BRANCH MILL RD
MANUELA
WY
RD
ALISOS
SEE B MAP
SEE 715 MAP
0 .125 .25 .375 .5 miles 1 in. = 1900 ft.

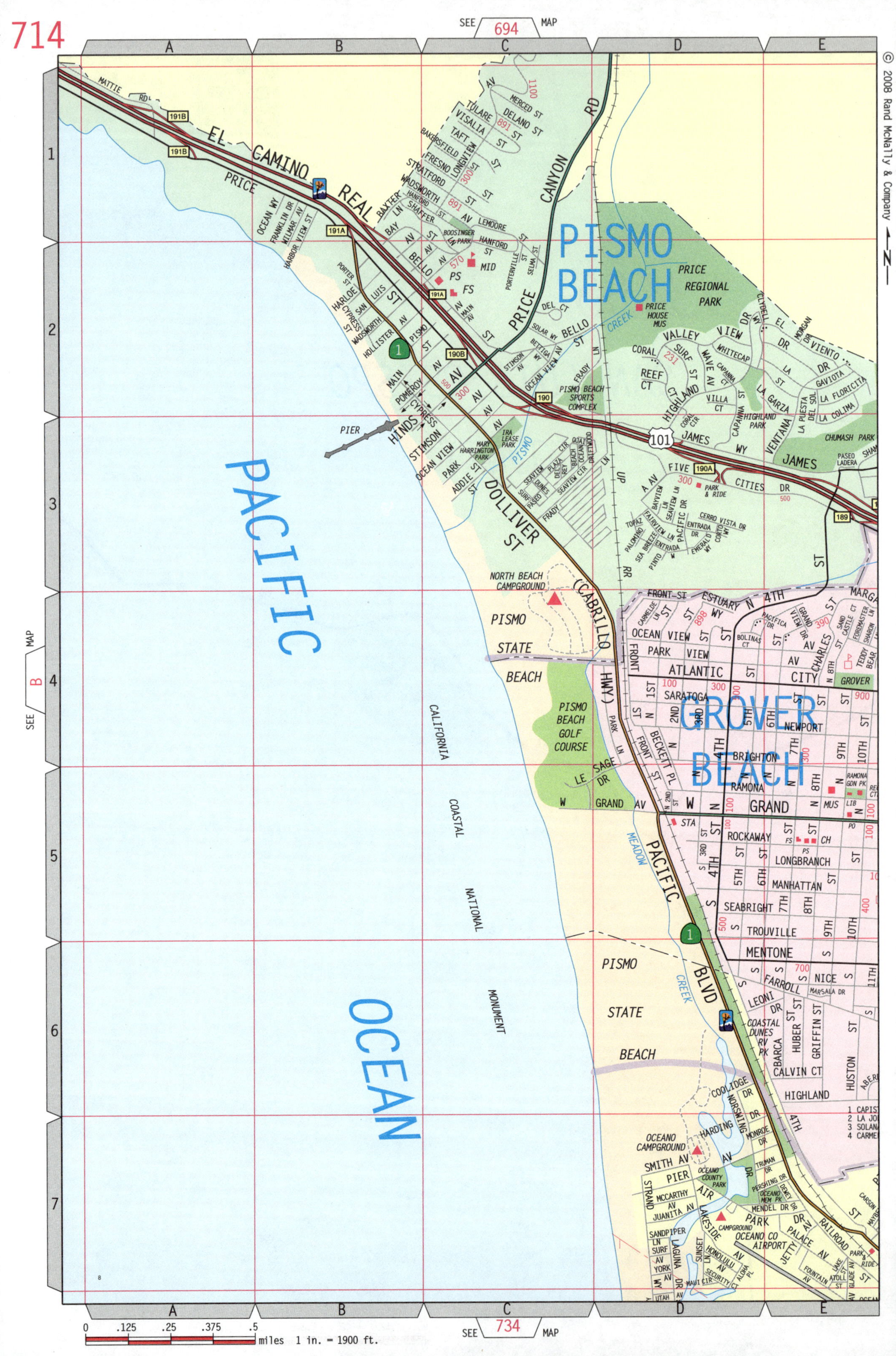

SEE 694 MAP
SEE 734 MAP
SEE B MAP
A
B
C
D
E
1
2
3
4
5
6
7
PACIFIC
OCEAN
PISMO BEACH
GROVER BEACH
PRICE REGIONAL PARK
PRICE HOUSE MUS
PISMO BEACH SPORTS COMPLEX
IRA LEASE PARK
MARY HARRINGTON PARK
CHUMASH PARK
PASEO LADERA
HIGHLAND PARK
PIER
NORTH BEACH CAMPGROUND
PISMO STATE BEACH
PISMO BEACH GOLF COURSE
CALIFORNIA COASTAL NATIONAL MONUMENT
OCEANO CAMPGROUND
OCEANO COUNTY PARK
OCEANO CO AIRPORT
OCEANO MEM PK
COASTAL DUNES RV PK
RAMONA GDN PK
EL CAMINO REAL
PRICE CANYON RD
PRICE ST
DOLLIVER ST
(CABRILLO HWY)
PACIFIC BLVD
JAMES WY
FIVE CITIES DR
VALLEY VIEW DR
ATLANTIC CITY AV
GRAND AV
W GRAND AV
PISMO CREEK
MEADOW CREEK
UP RR
MATTIE RD
101
1
191A
191B
190A
190B
190
189
PS
FS
MID
MUS
LIB
PO
STA
CH
PARK & RIDE
1 CAPIST
2 LA JO
3 SOLANA
4 CARME
0 .125 .25 .375 .5 miles 1 in. = 1900 ft.

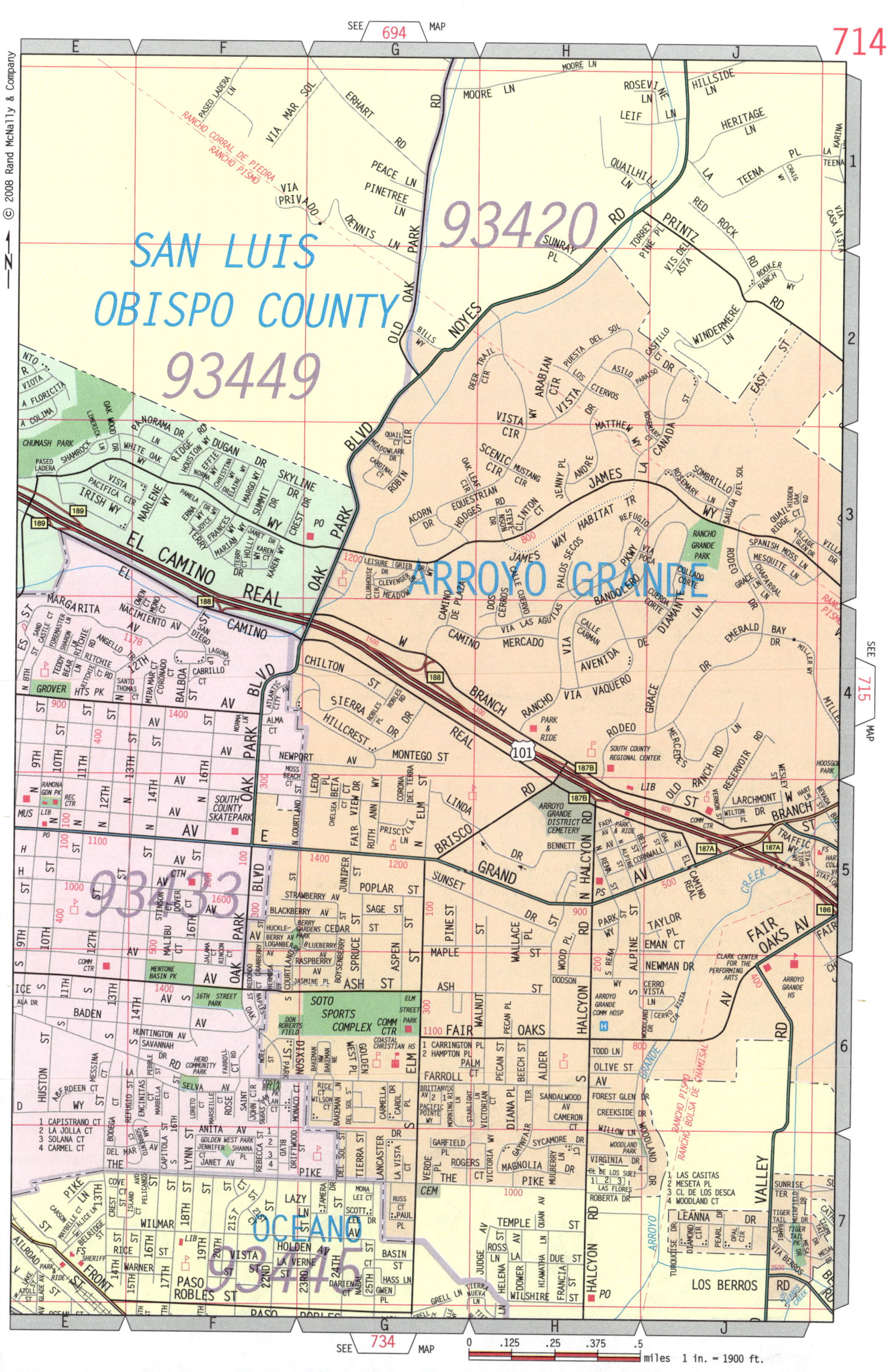

SEE 694 MAP
SEE 715 MAP
SEE 734 MAP
SAN LUIS OBISPO COUNTY
93449
93420
ARROYO GRANDE
93433
OCEANO
93445
RANCHO CORRAL DE PIEDRA
RANCHO PISMO
RANCHO BOLSA DE CHAMISAL
CHUMASH PARK
GROVER HTS PK
SOUTH COUNTY SKATEPARK
SOTO SPORTS COMPLEX
ARROYO GRANDE DISTRICT CEMETERY
RANCHO GRANDE PARK
SOUTH COUNTY REGIONAL CENTER
CLARK CENTER FOR THE PERFORMING ARTS
ARROYO GRANDE HS
ARROYO GRANDE COMM HOSP
HOOSGOW PARK
MENTONE BASIN PK
16TH STREET PARK
HERO COMMUNITY PARK
ELM STREET PARK
LOS BERROS
EL CAMINO REAL
OAK PARK BLVD
OLD OAK PARK RD
NOYES RD
JAMES WY
GRAND AV
FAIR OAKS AV
HALCYON RD
PRINTZ RD
BRANCH ST
VALLEY RD
THE PIKE
ARROYO GRANDE CREEK
LOS BERROS CREEK
101
miles 1 in. = 1900 ft.
0 .125 .25 .375 .5

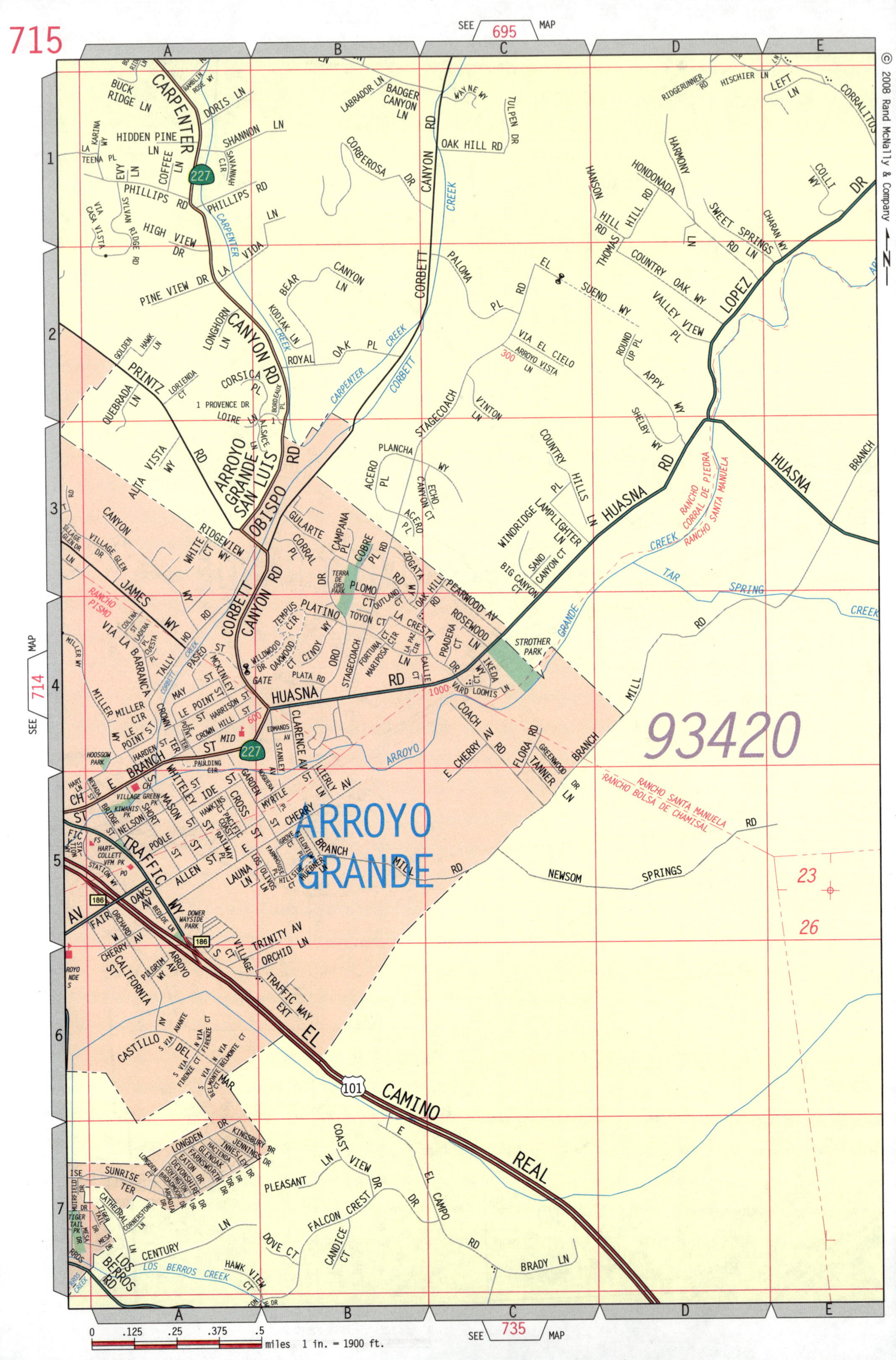

SEE 695 MAP
A
B
C
D
E
1
2
3
4
5
6
7
© 2008 Rand McNally & Company
CARPENTER
CANYON RD
BUCK RIDGE LN
DORIS LN
SHANNON LN
HIDDEN PINE LN
COFFEE LN
SAVANNAH CIR
227
PHILLIPS RD
HIGH VIEW DR
LA VIDA LN
PINE VIEW DR
LABRADOR LN
BADGER CANYON LN
WAYNE WY
TULPEN DR
OAK HILL RD
CORBEROSA DR
CANYON RD
CORBETT
CREEK
BEAR CANYON LN
KODIAK LN
ROYAL OAK PL
PALOMA PL
EL SUENO WY
VIA EL CIELO
ARROYO VISTA LN
300
RIDGERUNNER RD
HISCHIER LN
LEFT LN
CORRALITOS
HARMONY
HANSON HILL RD
HONDONADA
THOMAS HILL RD
SWEET SPRINGS RD LN
CHARAN WY
COLLI WY
COUNTRY OAK WY
VALLEY VIEW PL
LOPEZ DR
ROUND UP PL
APPY WY
SHELBY WY
GOLDEN HAWK LN
LONGHORN LN
PRINTZ RD
LORIENDA CT
QUEBRADA LN
CORSICA PL
1 PROVENCE DR
LOIRE LN
ALSACE LN
ARROYO GRANDE SAN LUIS OBISPO RD
ALTA VISTA WY
STAGECOACH
VINTON LN
PLANCHA WY
ACERO PL
ECHO CANYON CT
COUNTRY HILLS LN
LAMPLIGHTER LN
WINDRIDGE PL
HUASNA RD
HUASNA
BRANCH
RANCHO CORRAL DE PIEDRA
RANCHO SANTA MANUELA
CANYON
VILLAGE GLEN DR
JAMES WY
RIDGEVIEW WY
WHITE CT
GULARTE
CORRAL PL
CAMPANA PL
COBRE PL
TERRA DE ORO PARK
PLOMO CT
ZOGATA WY
OAK HILL RD
PEARWOOD AV
ROSEWOOD LN
PRADERA CT
BIG CANYON CT
SAND CANYON CT
TAR SPRING CREEK
GRANDE
STROTHER PARK
RANCHO PISMO
VIA LA BARRANCA
TALLY HO RD
PLATINO
TEMPUS CIR
CINDY WY
TOYON CT
LA CRESTA
OUTLAND CT
ORO
STAGECOACH RD
FORTUNA
MARIPOSA CIR
LA PAZ CIR
CALLIE CT
IKEDA
VARD LOOMIS LN
WILDWOOD DR
OAKWOOD CT
GATE
PLATA RD
PASEO ST
MCKINLEY ST
MAY ST
LE POINT ST
HARRISON ST
CROWN HILL ST
CROWN TER
MILLER WY
MILLER CIR
LE POINT ST
HUASNA RD
1000
600
MID ST
EDMANDS
STANLEY AV
CLARENCE AV
COACH AV
E CHERRY AV
FLORA RD
GREENWOOD
TANNER LN
BRANCH DR
MILL RD
93420
HOOSGOW PARK
HARDEN ST
E BRANCH ST
PAULDING CIR
WHITELEY ST
MASON ST
IDE ST
HAWKINS
CROSS ST
GARDEN ST
MYRTLE
LIERLY AV
ARROYO
RANCHO SANTA MANUELA
RANCHO BOLSA DE CHAMISAL
NELSON ST
SHORT ST
POOLE ST
KIWANIS PK
VILLAGE GREEN PK
TRAFFIC WY
HART-COLLETT VFM PK
ALLEN ST
RAILWAY PL
PACIFIC COAST
LAUNA LN
LOS OLIVOS LN
CHERRY
BRANCH MILL RD
ARROYO GRANDE
NEWSOM SPRINGS RD
23
26
186
FAIR OAKS AV
ORCHARD
BEDLOE LN
DOWER WAYSIDE PARK
TRINITY AV
ORCHID LN
W CHERRY AV
CALIFORNIA ST
PILGRIM AV
ARROYO
S VILLAGE CT
TRAFFIC WAY EXT
EL CAMINO REAL
101
CASTILLO DEL MAR
VIA AVANTE
VIA FIRENZE CT
BELMONTE CT
LONGDEN DR
KINGSBURY DR
JENNINGS DR
INNESLEY DR
HACIENDA
GLENOAK
EATON DR
FARNSWORTH DR
DEVONSHIRE DR
SUNRISE TER
CATHEDRAL
CORNERSTONE LN
TIGER TAIL PK
MUIRFIELD DR
MESA DR
COAST VIEW DR
PLEASANT LN
E EL CAMPO RD
FALCON CREST DR
CANDICE CT
DOVE CT
CENTURY LN
LOS BERROS RD
LOS BERROS CREEK
HAWK VIEW CT
BRADY LN
SEE 714 MAP
SEE 735 MAP
0 .125 .25 .375 .5 miles 1 in. = 1900 ft.

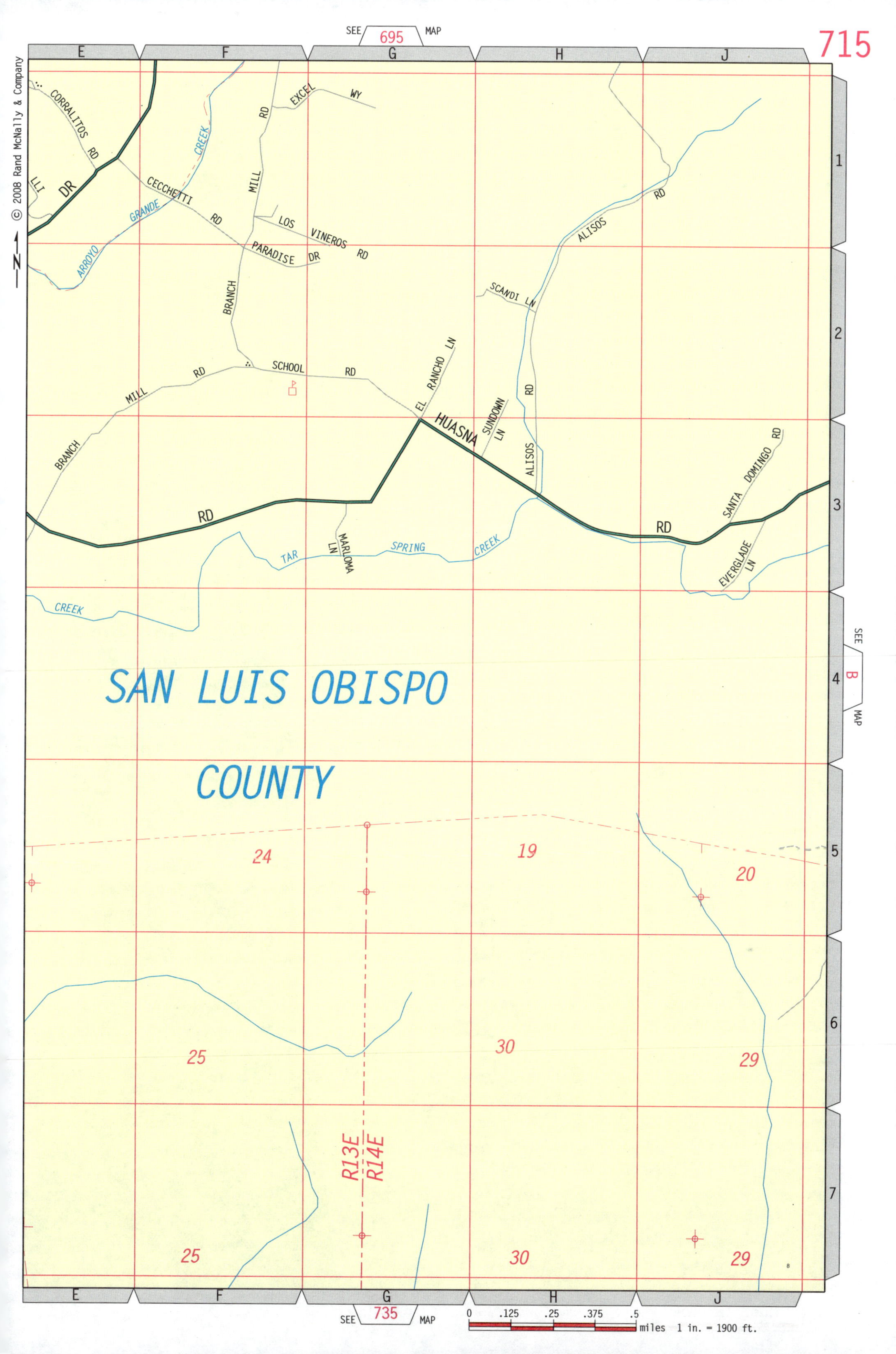
SEE 695 MAP
E
F
G
H
J
1
2
3
4
5
6
7
CORRALITOS RD
DR
CECCHETTI RD
ARROYO GRANDE CREEK
MILL RD
EXCEL WY
LOS VINEROS RD
PARADISE DR
BRANCH
ALISOS RD
SCANDI LN
SCHOOL RD
BRANCH MILL RD
EL RANCHO LN
HUASNA RD
SUNDOWN LN
ALISOS RD
SANTA DOMINGO RD
TAR SPRING CREEK
MARLOMA LN
EVERGLADE LN
CREEK
SEE B MAP
SAN LUIS OBISPO COUNTY
24
19
20
25
30
29
R13E
R14E
25
30
29
SEE 735 MAP
0 .125 .25 .375 .5 miles 1 in. = 1900 ft.

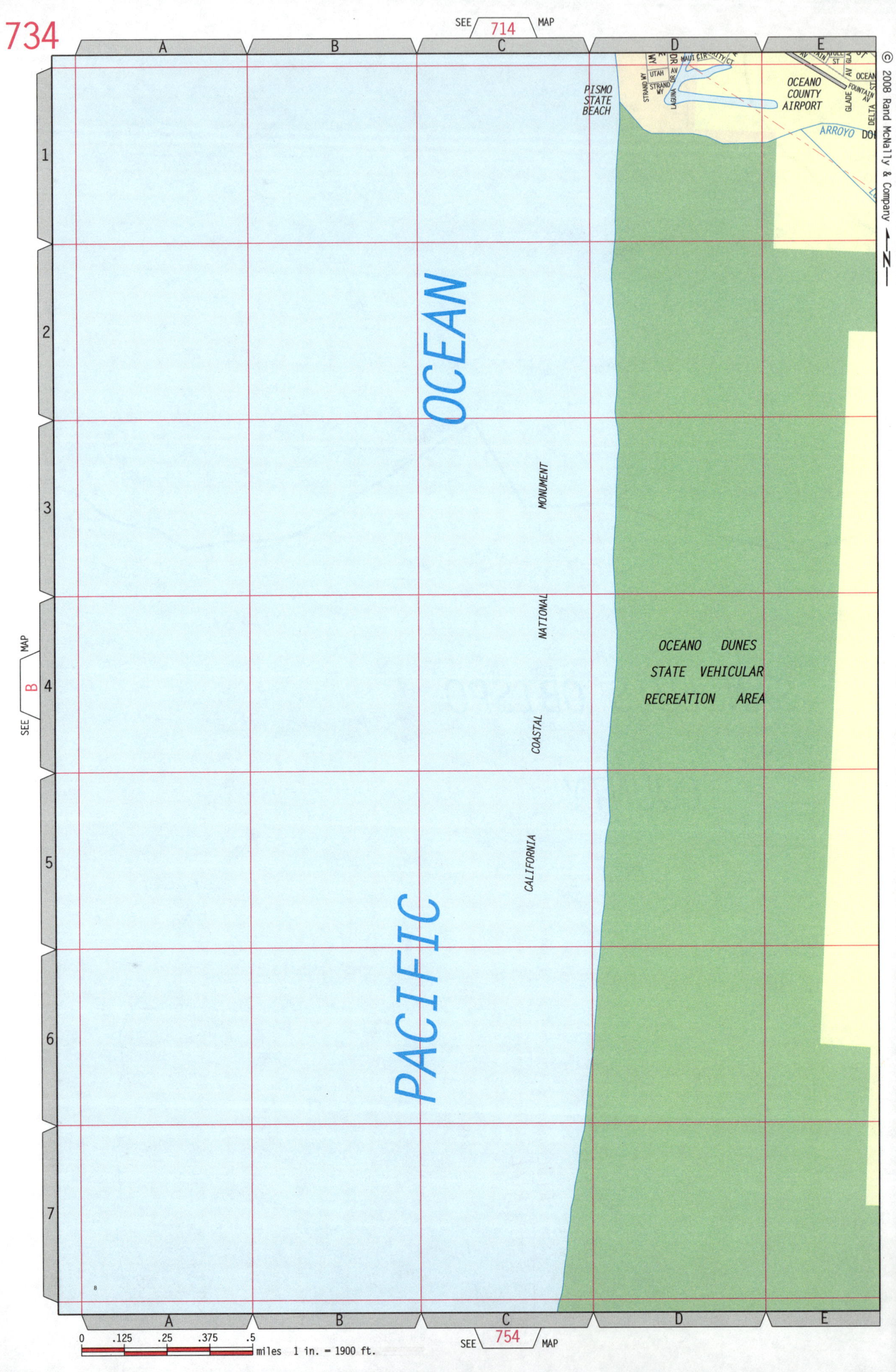

SEE 714 MAP
A
B
C
D
E
1
2
3
4
5
6
7
PISMO
STATE
BEACH
OCEANO
COUNTY
AIRPORT
ARROYO
STRAND WY
UTAH
STRAND WY
LAGUNA DR
MAUI CIR
GLADE AV
FOUNTAIN AV
DELTA
OCEAN
PACIFIC
OCEAN
CALIFORNIA
COASTAL
NATIONAL
MONUMENT
OCEANO DUNES
STATE VEHICULAR
RECREATION AREA
SEE B MAP
SEE 754 MAP
0 .125 .25 .375 .5
miles 1 in. = 1900 ft.

SEE 714 MAP

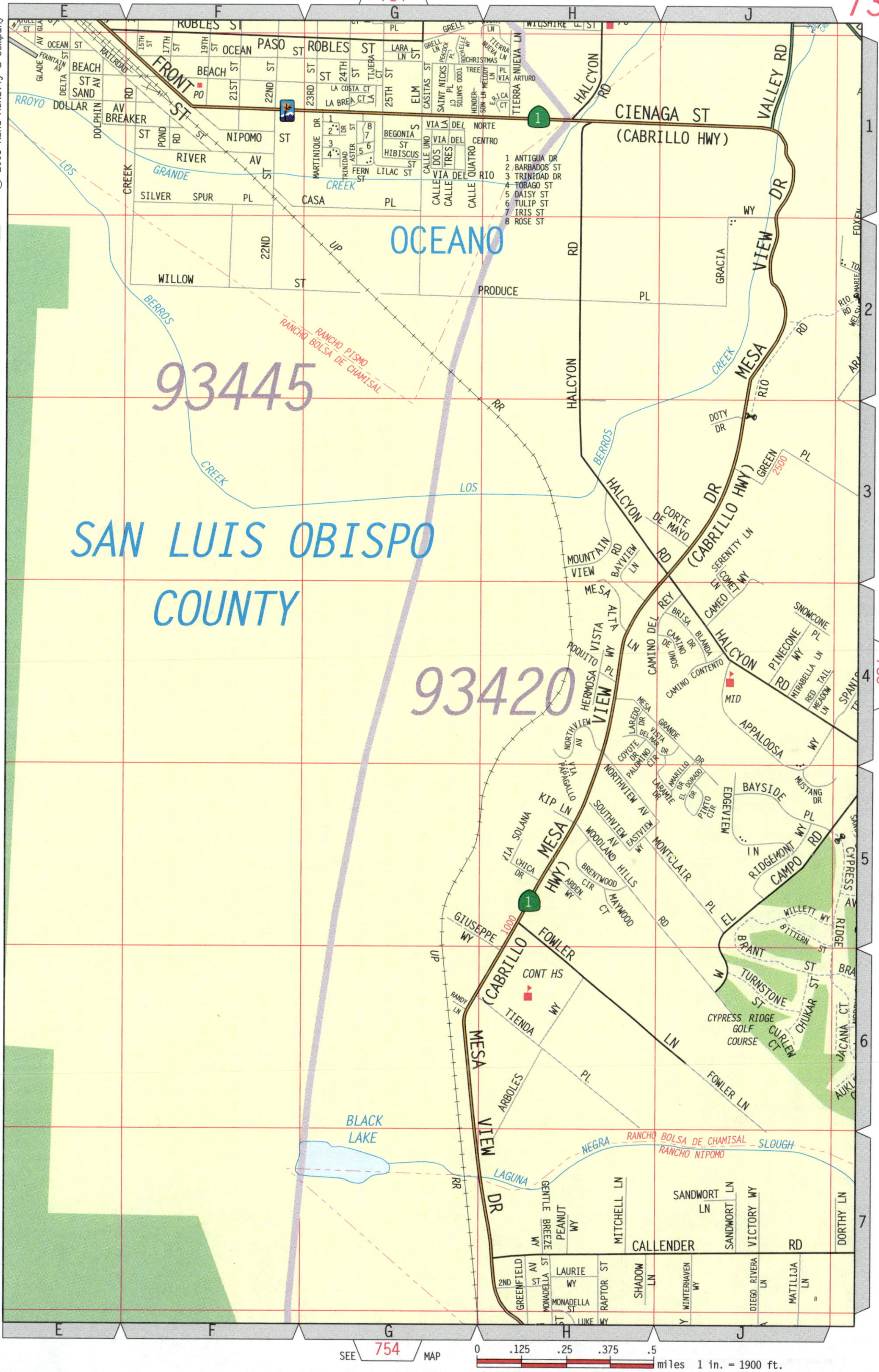

OCEANO

SAN LUIS OBISPO COUNTY

93445

93420

CIENAGA ST (CABRILLO HWY)

MESA VIEW DR (CABRILLO HWY)

HALCYON RD

VALLEY RD

FRONT ST

ROBLES ST

OCEAN ST

PASO ROBLES ST

BEACH ST

DOLLAR AV

BREAKER

NIPOMO ST

RIVER AV

SILVER SPUR PL

CASA PL

WILLOW ST

PRODUCE PL

LOS BERROS CREEK

ARROYO GRANDE CREEK

RANCHO PISMO

RANCHO BOLSA DE CHAMISAL

1 ANTIGUA DR
2 BARBADOS ST
3 TRINIDAD DR
4 TOBAGO ST
5 DAISY ST
6 TULIP ST
7 IRIS ST
8 ROSE ST

MID

CONT HS

FOWLER LN

TIENDA WY

ARBOLES PL

BLACK LAKE

LAGUNA NEGRA

RANCHO BOLSA DE CHAMISAL

RANCHO NIPOMO

SLOUGH

CALLENDER RD

CYPRESS RIDGE GOLF COURSE

SEE 735 MAP

SEE 754 MAP

0 .125 .25 .375 .5 miles 1 in. = 1900 ft.

SEE 715 MAP

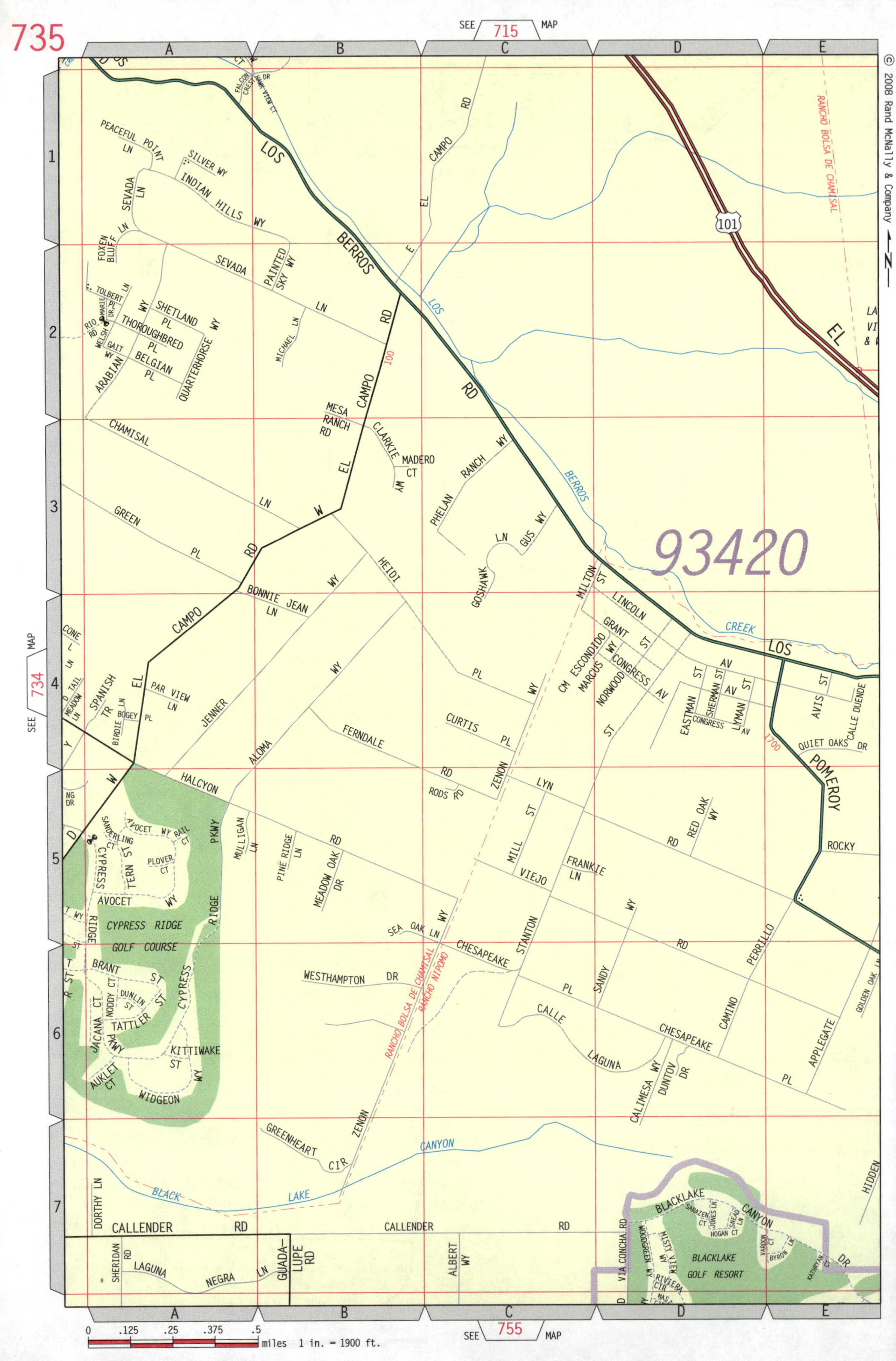

LOS BERROS RD
EL CAMPO RD
W EL CAMPO RD
93420
PEACEFUL POINT LN
SILVER WY
INDIAN HILLS WY
SEVADA LN
FOXEN BLUFF LN
PAINTED SKY WY
SHETLAND PL
THOROUGHBRED PL
BELGIAN PL
QUARTERHORSE WY
ARABIAN WY
TOLBERT LN
MICHAEL LN
CHAMISAL LN
GREEN PL
MESA RANCH RD
CLARKIE WY
MADERO CT
PHELAN RANCH WY
GOSHAWK LN
GUS WY
HEIDI PL
BONNIE JEAN LN
JENNER WY
ALOMA WY
SPANISH TR
PAR VIEW LN
BOGEY PL
BIRDIE LN
FERNDALE RD
CURTIS PL
ZENON WY
RODS RD
HALCYON PKWY
MILTON ST
LINCOLN ST
GRANT ST
CM ESCONDIDO
MARCUS WY
CONGRESS AV
NORWOOD ST
EASTMAN AV
SHERMAN ST
LYMAN AV
AVIS ST
CALLE DUENDE
QUIET OAKS DR
POMEROY
ROCKY
LYN RD
RED OAK WY
MILL ST
VIEJO RD
FRANKIE LN
SANDY WY
PERRILLO
STANTON
CHESAPEAKE PL
CALLE LAGUNA
CAMINO
APPLEGATE
GOLDEN OAK LN
CALIMESA WY
DUNTOV DR
MULLIGAN LN
PINE RIDGE LN
MEADOW OAK DR
SEA OAK LN
WESTHAMPTON DR
CYPRESS RIDGE GOLF COURSE
CYPRESS RIDGE PKWY
AVOCET WY
SANDERLING CT
RAIL CT
TERN ST
PLOVER CT
BRANT ST
DUNLIN ST
NODDY CT
JACANA CT
TATTLER
KITTIWAKE ST
AUKLET CT
WIDGEON WY
RANCHO BOLSA DE CHAMISAL
RANCHO NIPOMO
GREENHEART CIR
BLACK LAKE CANYON
DORTHY LN
CALLENDER RD
SHERIDAN RD
LAGUNA NEGRA LN
GUADALUPE RD
ALBERT WY
VIA CONCHA RD
BLACKLAKE CANYON DR
BLACKLAKE GOLF RESORT
SARAZEN CT
JONES LN
HOGAN CT
SNEAD LN
VARDON CT
BYRON LN
KATHRYN CT
WOODGREEN WY
MISTY VIEW WY
RIVIERA CIR
HIDDEN
CREEK
101
100
1700
SEE 734 MAP
© 2008 Rand McNally & Company

0 .125 .25 .375 .5 miles 1 in. = 1900 ft.

SEE 755 MAP

SEE 715 MAP

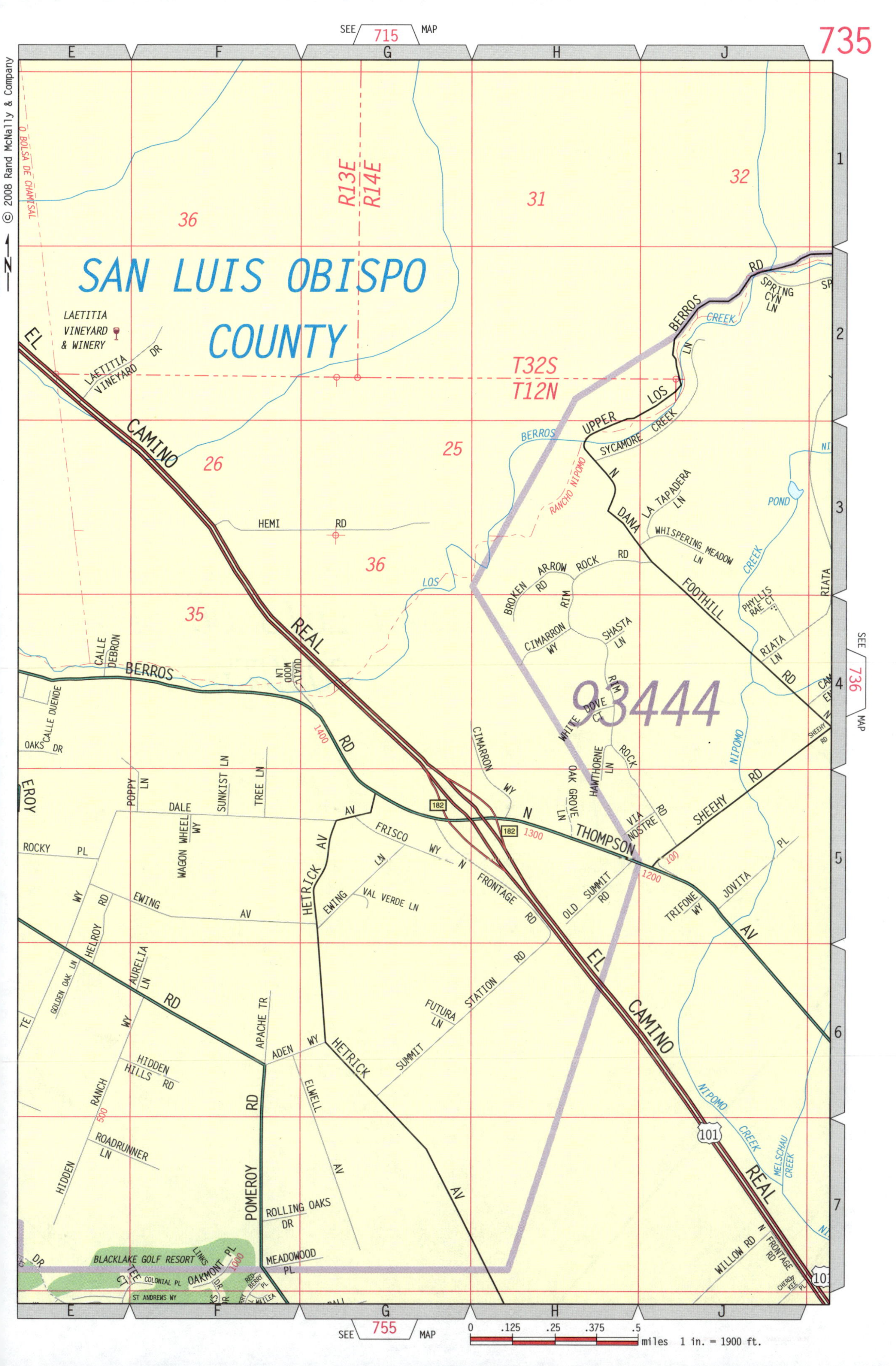
SAN LUIS OBISPO
COUNTY
LAETITIA
VINEYARD
& WINERY
LAETITIA VINEYARD DR
EL CAMINO REAL
HEMI RD
BERROS RD
UPPER LOS BERROS RD
SYCAMORE CREEK
N DANA FOOTHILL
LA TAPADERA LN
WHISPERING MEADOW LN
BROKEN ARROW RD
ROCK RD
RIM ROCK RD
CIMARRON WY
SHASTA LN
WHITE DOVE CT
HAWTHORNE LN
OAK GROVE LN
VIA NOSTRE RD
N THOMPSON AV
SHEEHY RD
TRIFONE WY
JOVITA PL
PHYLLIS RAE CT
RIATA LN
POND
NIPOMO CREEK
MELSCHAU CREEK
93444
CALLE DEBRON
CALLE DUENDE
OAKS DR
QUAIL WOOD LN
POPPY LN
SUNKIST LN
TREE LN
DALE AV
WAGON WHEEL WY
ROCKY PL
EWING AV
HETRICK AV
FRISCO WY
N FRONTAGE RD
VAL VERDE LN
OLD SUMMIT RD
HELROY RD
GOLDEN OAK LN
AURELIA LN
RANCH WY
HIDDEN HILLS RD
ROADRUNNER LN
HIDDEN
APACHE TR
ADEN WY
ELMWELL AV
FUTURA LN
SUMMIT STATION RD
POMEROY RD
ROLLING OAKS DR
MEADOWOOD PL
BLACKLAKE GOLF RESORT
LINKS
OAKMONT PL
COLONIAL PL
ST ANDREWS WY
WILLOW RD
N FRONTAGE RD
CHEROKEE PL
RANCHO NIPOMO
R13E
R14E
T32S
T12N
O BOLSA DE CHAMISAL
182
101
36
31
32
26
25
35
1400
1300
1200
100
500
1000

SEE 736 MAP

SEE 755 MAP

0 .125 .25 .375 .5 miles 1 in. = 1900 ft.

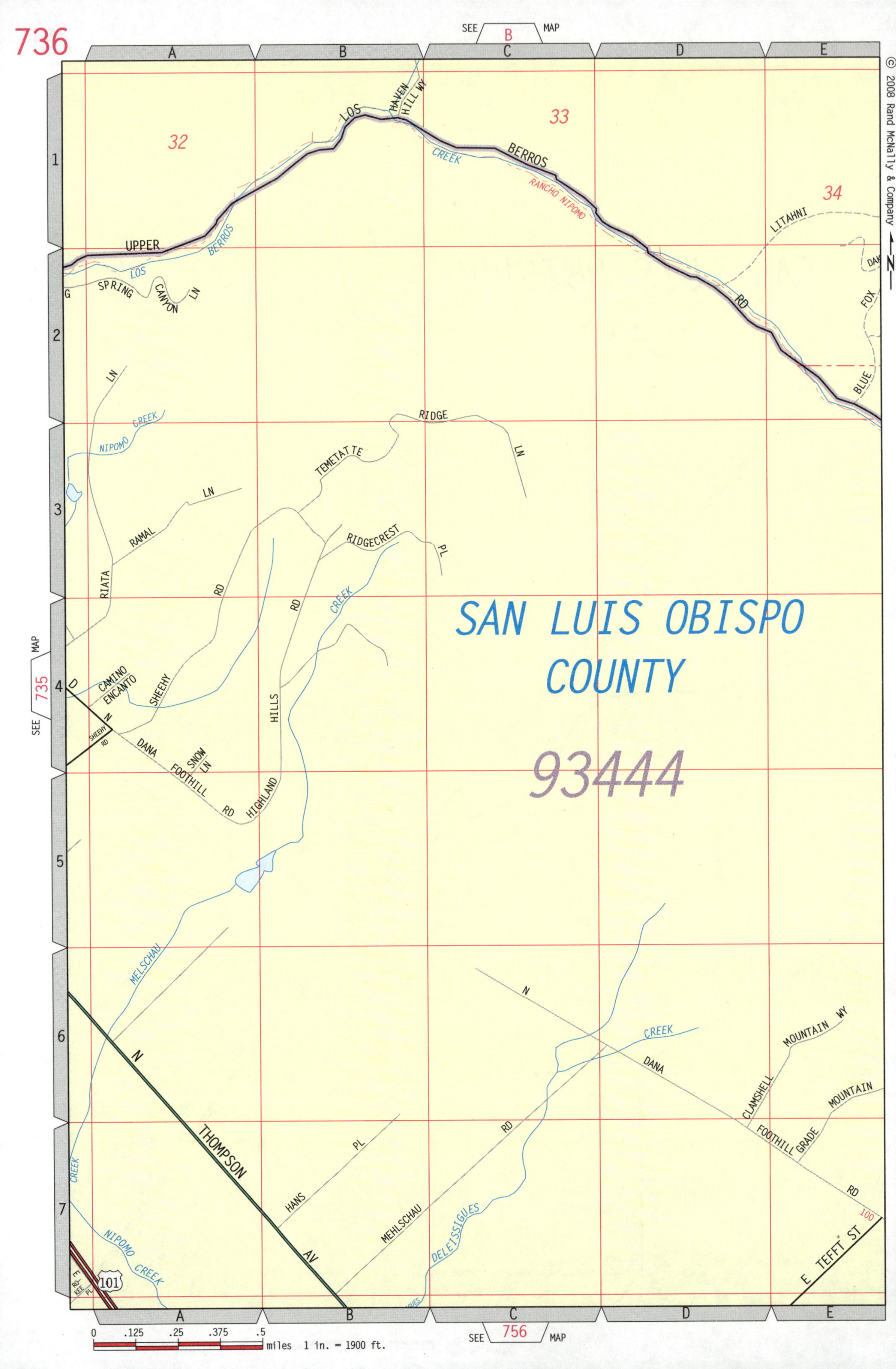
SEE B MAP
SEE 735 MAP
SEE 756 MAP
32
33
34
UPPER LOS BERROS RD
LOS BERROS CREEK
RANCHO NIPOMO
HAVEN
HILL WY
LITAHNI
FOX
BLUE
SPRING CANYON LN
NIPOMO CREEK
RIDGE
TEMETATE
LN
RAMAL LN
RIATA LN
RIDGECREST PL
RD
RD
CREEK
CAMINO ENCANTO
SHEEHY
SHEEHY RD
DANA FOOTHILL RD
SNOW LN
HILLS
HIGHLAND
SAN LUIS OBISPO COUNTY
93444
MELSCHAU
N THOMPSON AV
HANS PL
MEHLSCHAU RD
DELEISSIGUES
CREEK
N DANA FOOTHILL RD
CLAMSHELL
MOUNTAIN WY
GRADE
MOUNTAIN
E TEFFT ST
100
NIPOMO CREEK
101
miles 1 in. = 1900 ft.

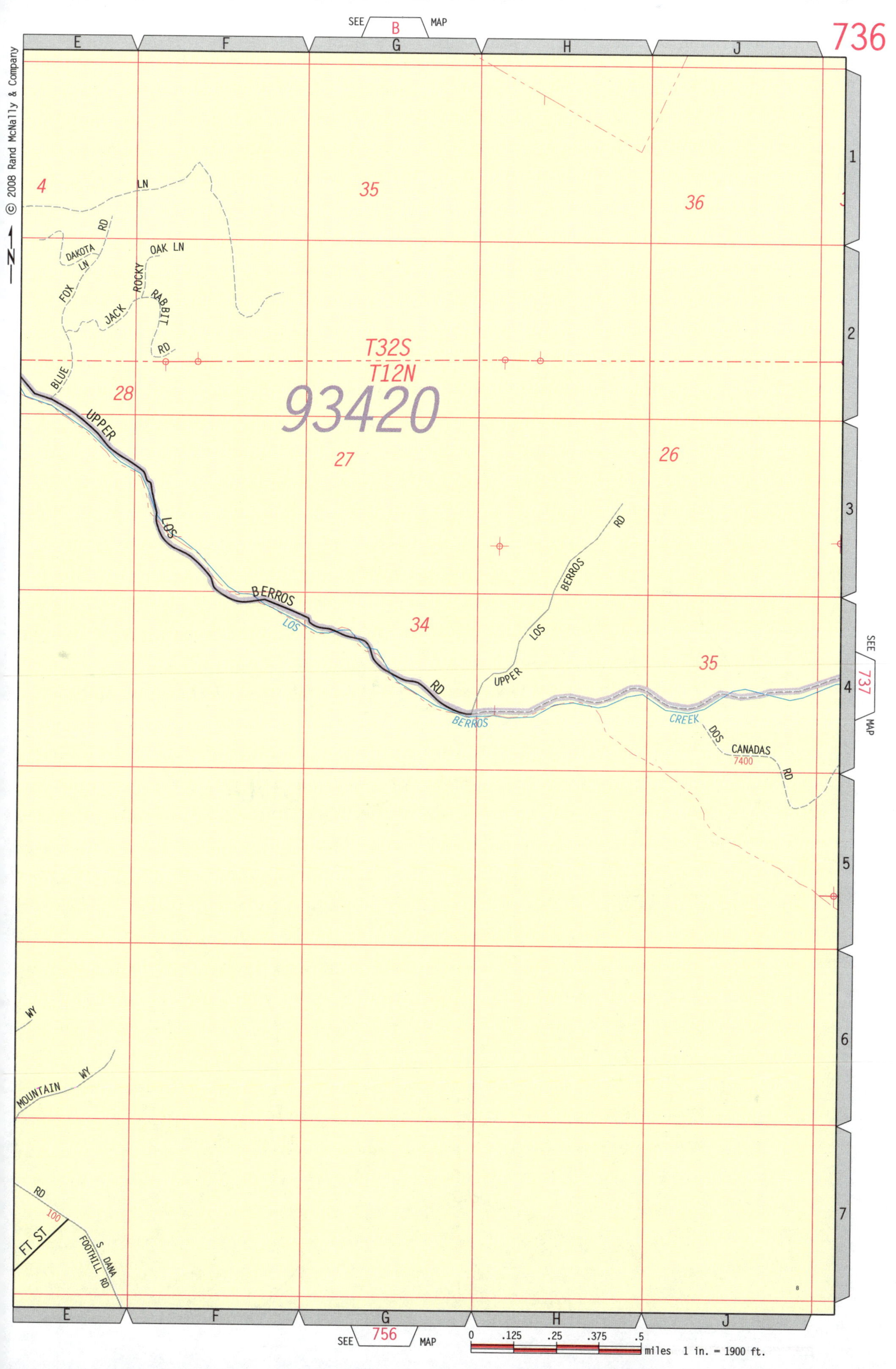

SEE B MAP
E
F
G
H
J
1
2
3
4
5
6
7
4
35
36
LN
DAKOTA
LN
RD
FOX
OAK LN
ROCKY
RABBIT
JACK
RD
BLUE
T32S
T12N
28
93420
UPPER
27
26
LOS
BERROS
LOS
34
RD
BERROS
LOS
UPPER
RD
35
SEE 737 MAP
BERROS
CREEK
DOS
CANADAS
7400
RD
WY
MOUNTAIN
WY
RD
100
FT ST
S DANA
FOOTHILL RD
SEE 756 MAP
0
.125
.25
.375
.5
miles 1 in. = 1900 ft.

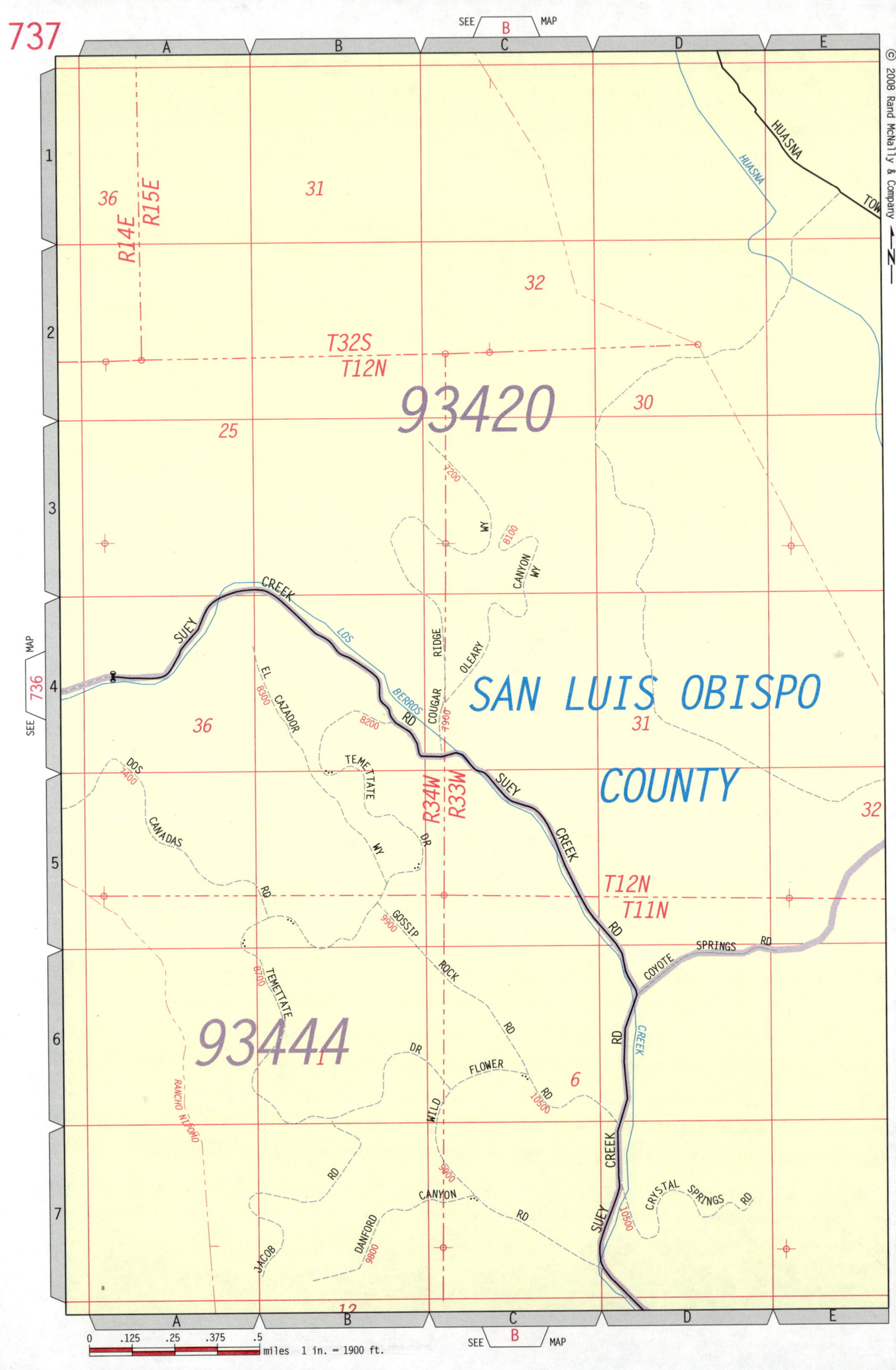
SEE B MAP
A
B
C
D
E
1
2
3
4
5
6
7
SEE 736 MAP
93420
93444
SAN LUIS OBISPO
COUNTY
SUEY CREEK RD
LOS BERROS
COYOTE SPRINGS RD
HUASNA
HUASNA
TOW
EL CAZADOR
TEMETTATE DR
TEMETTATE WY
COUGAR RIDGE
OLEARY
CANYON WY
DOS CANADAS RD
GOSSIP ROCK RD
WILD FLOWER RD
DANFORD CANYON RD
JACOB RD
CRYSTAL SPRINGS RD
CREEK
RANCHO NIPOMO
R14E
R15E
R34W
R33W
T32S
T12N
T12N
T11N
36
31
32
25
30
36
31
32
1
6
12
0
.125
.25
.375
.5
miles 1 in. = 1900 ft.

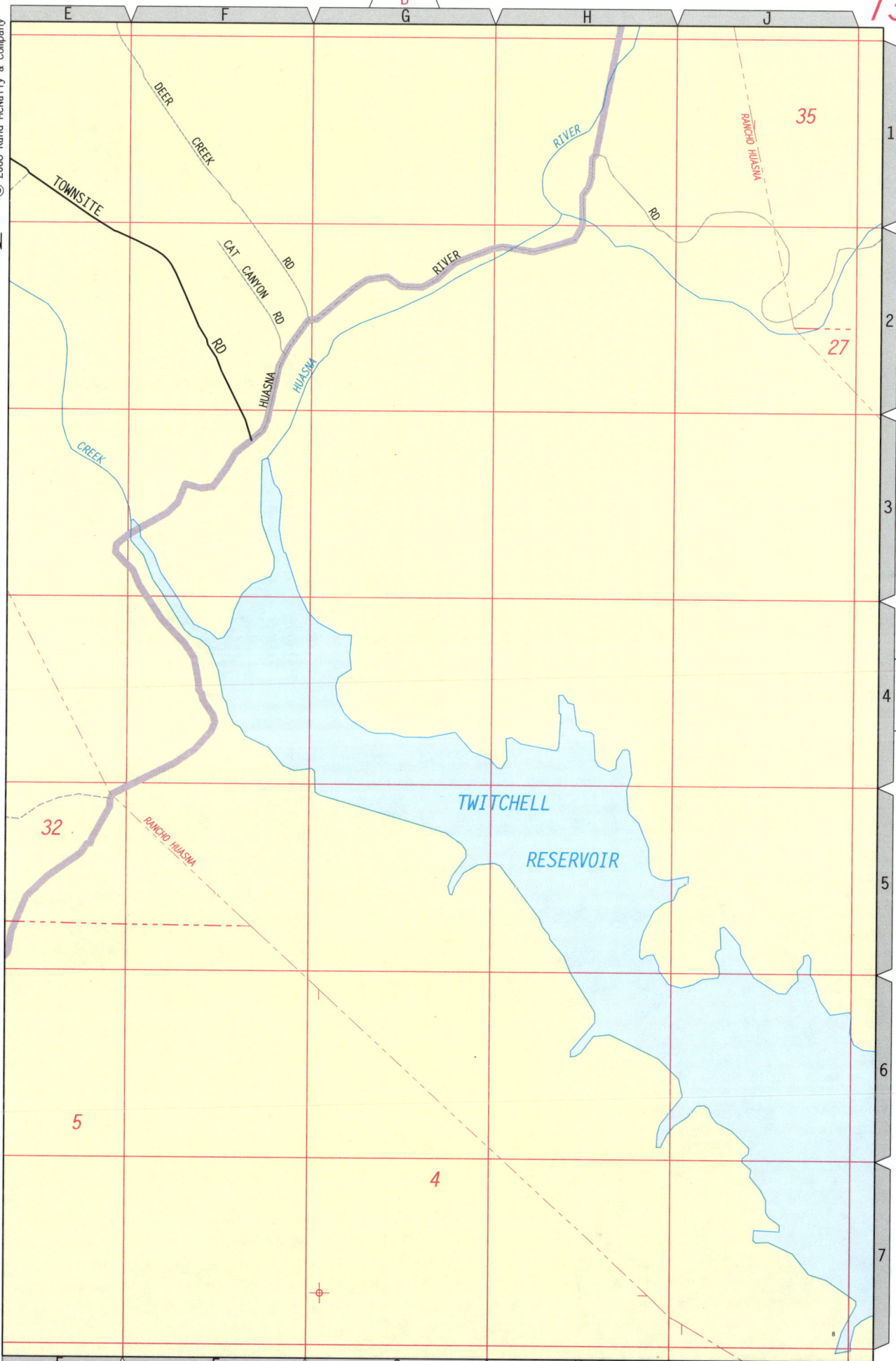

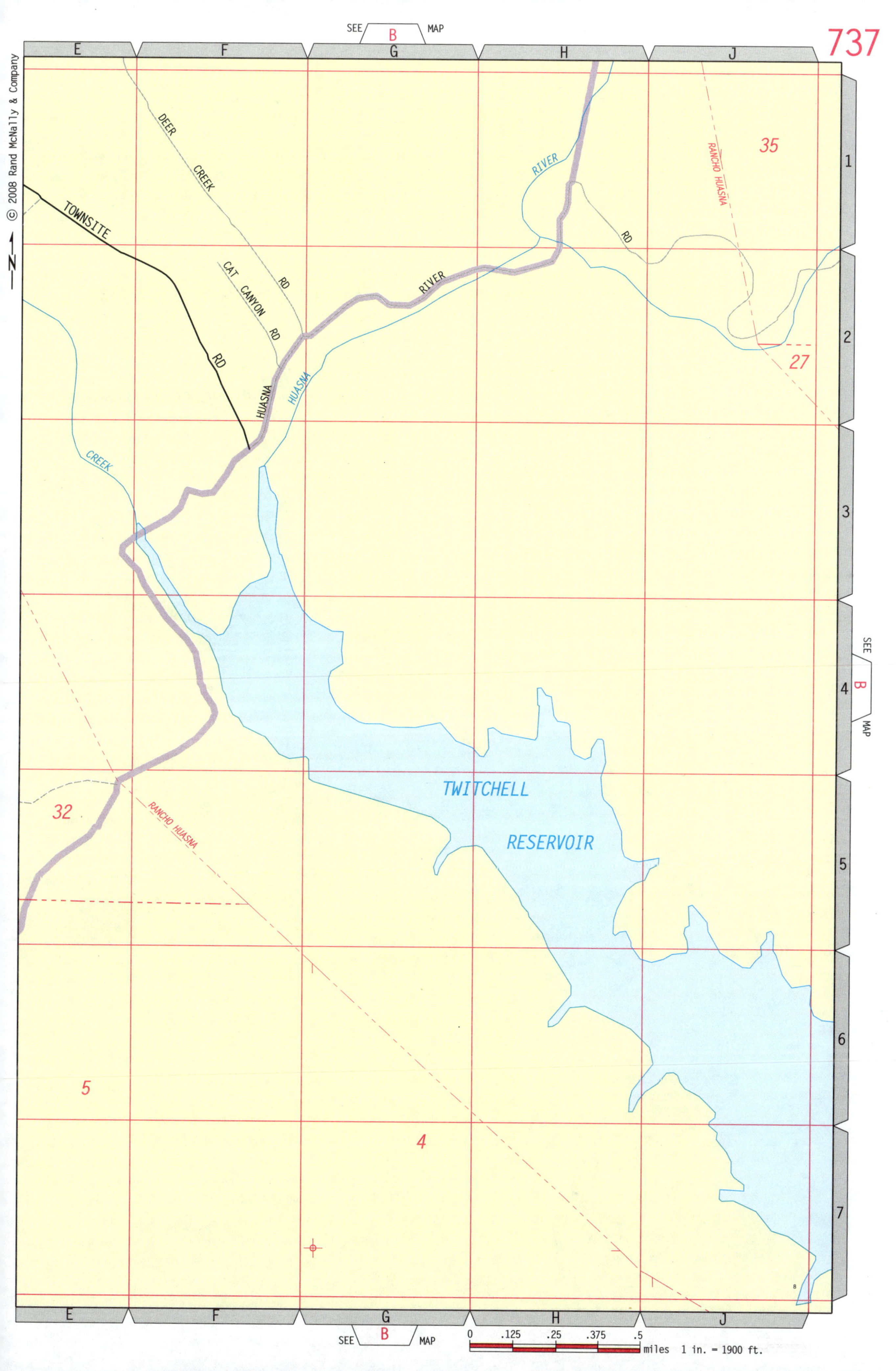
SEE B MAP
E
F
G
H
J
1
2
3
4
5
6
7
SEE B MAP
© 2008 Rand McNally & Company
N
DEER CREEK RD
TOWNSITE RD
CAT CANYON RD
HUASNA RIVER
HUASNA CREEK
RIVER
RD
RANCHO HUASNA
35
27
32
5
4
TWITCHELL RESERVOIR
0 .125 .25 .375 .5
miles 1 in. = 1900 ft.

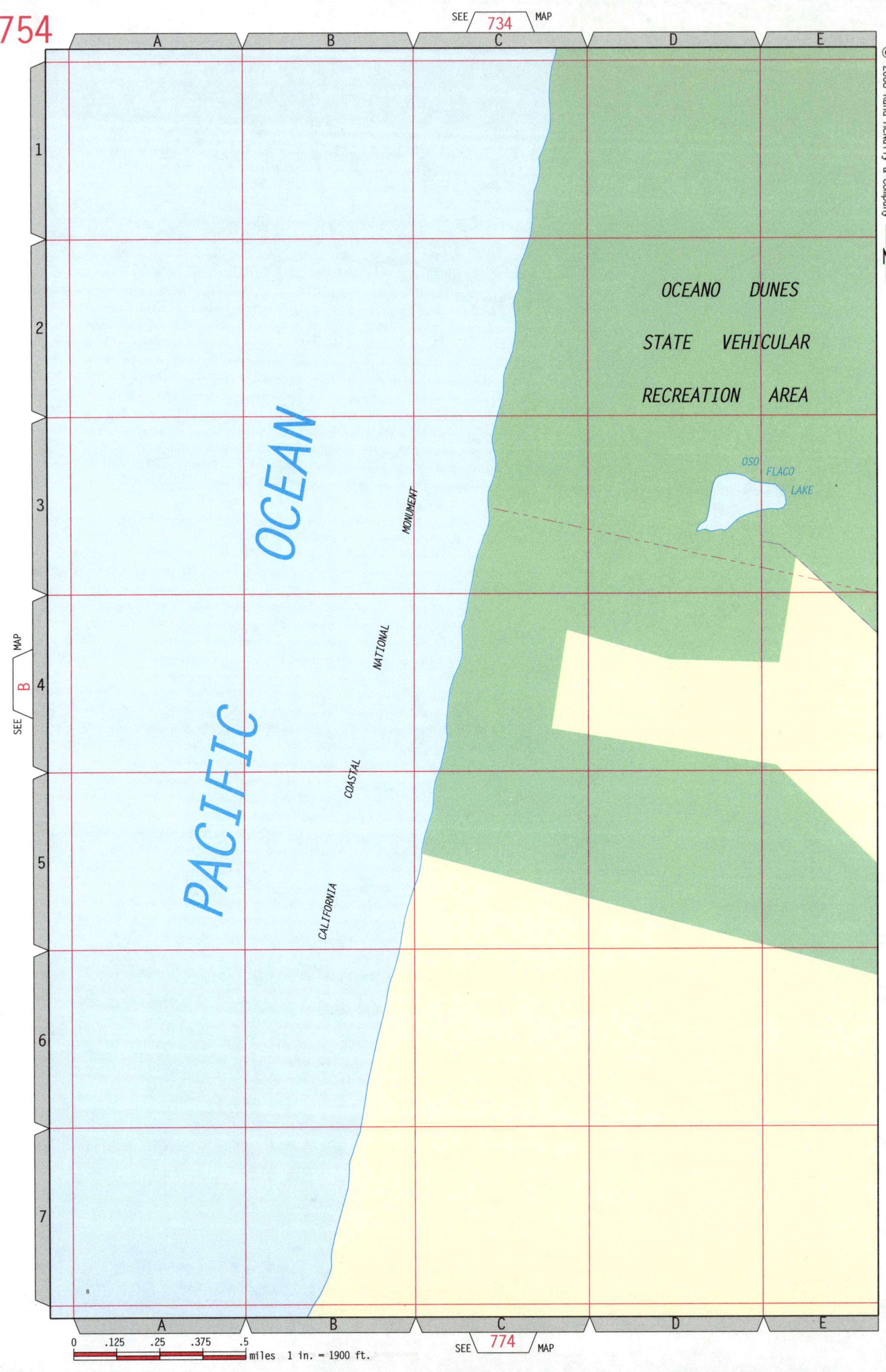
SEE 734 MAP
A
B
C
D
E
1
2
3
4
5
6
7
SEE B MAP
PACIFIC OCEAN
CALIFORNIA COASTAL NATIONAL MONUMENT
OCEANO DUNES STATE VEHICULAR RECREATION AREA
OSO FLACO LAKE
SEE 774 MAP
0 .125 .25 .375 .5
miles 1 in. = 1900 ft.

SEE 734 MAP

E F G H J

3RD ST
CABRILLO HWY
MONADELLA ST
LUKE WY
MONADELLA ST
RAPTOR ST
AUTUMN PL
WINTERHAVEN WY
2400 600
JAMESON CT
DIEGO RIVERA LN
MATILIJA LN
600
IDYLLWILD PL
700 2300 700
WY
WILLOW RD
(CABRILLO HWY)
1
2300 2200
FS
GARRETT LN
RALCOA
CALLE BENDITA
RANCHO NIPOMO
RANCHO BOLSA DE CHAMISAL
ALLEY OOP WY
OOP CT
GASOLINE ALLEY PL

93420

UP RR

RANCHO BOLSA DE CHAMISAL
RANCHO GUADALUPE

OSO FLACO LAKE RD

93445

SAN LUIS OBISPO COUNTY

1 2 3 4 5 6 7

SEE 755 MAP

SEE 774 MAP

0 .125 .25 .375 .5 miles 1 in. = 1900 ft.

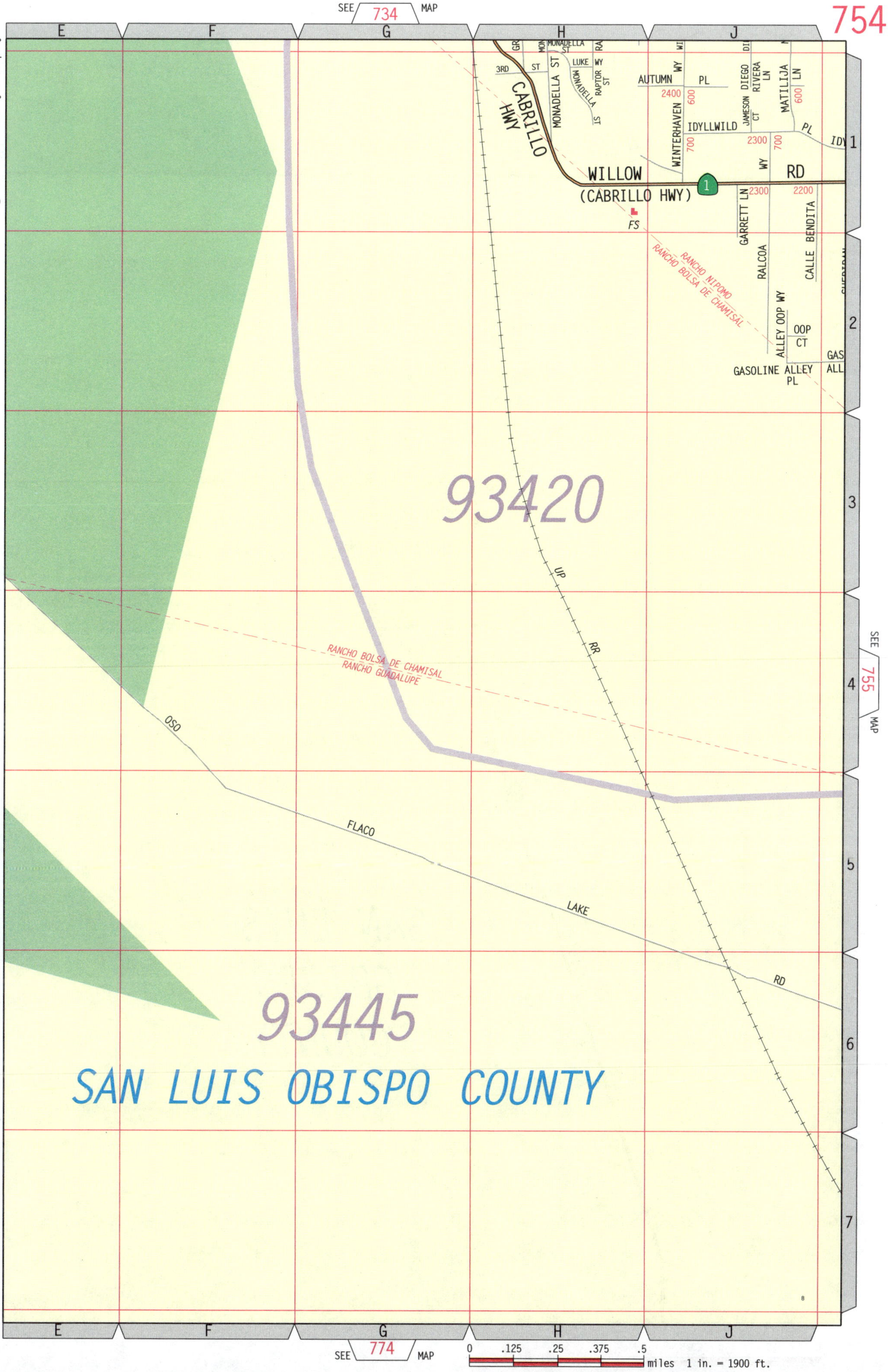

SEE 735 MAP

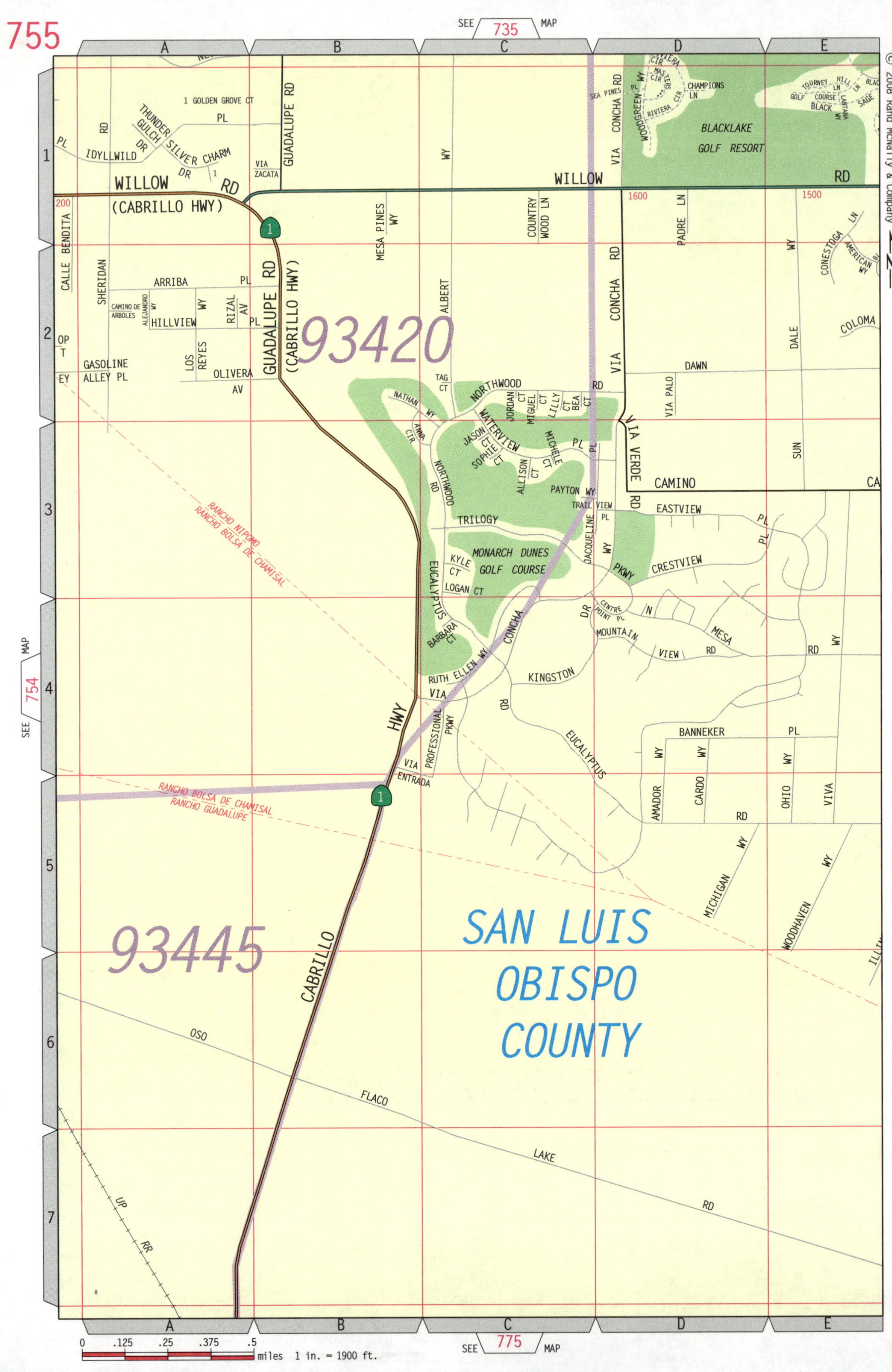

93420
93445
SAN LUIS OBISPO COUNTY
BLACKLAKE GOLF RESORT
MONARCH DUNES GOLF COURSE
WILLOW RD
(CABRILLO HWY)
GUADALUPE RD
VIA CONCHA RD
CABRILLO HWY
OSO FLACO LAKE RD
UP RR
RANCHO NIPOMO
RANCHO BOLSA DE CHAMISAL
RANCHO GUADALUPE
THUNDER GULCH DR
SILVER CHARM DR
IDYLLWILD
1 GOLDEN GROVE CT
VIA ZACATA
CALLE BENDITA
SHERIDAN
ARRIBA PL
CAMINO DE ARBOLES
ALEJANDRO WY
HILLVIEW WY
RIZAL AV
LOS REYES
OLIVERA AV
GASOLINE ALLEY PL
MESA PINES WY
COUNTRY WOOD LN
ALBERT
TAG CT
NORTHWOOD RD
NATHAN WY
ANNA CIR
JORDAN CT
MIGUEL CT
LILLY CT
BEA CT
JASON CT
SOPHIE CT
WATERVIEW PL
MICHELE CT
ALLISON CT
PAYTON WY
TRAIL VIEW PL
TRILOGY
KYLE CT
LOGAN CT
EUCALYPTUS RD
BARBARA CT
RUTH ELLEN WY
JACQUELINE WY
CONCHA
VIA VERDE RD
CAMINO
EASTVIEW PL
CRESTVIEW PKWY
CENTRE POINT PL
MOUNTAIN VIEW RD
MESA RD
KINGSTON
PROFESSIONAL PKWY
VIA ENTRADA
BANNEKER PL
AMADOR WY
CARDO WY
OHIO WY
VIVA
MICHIGAN WY
WOODHAVEN WY
PADRE LN
VIA PALO
DAWN
DALE
SUN
COLOMA
CONESTOGA LN
AMERICAN WY
SEA PINES
WOODGREEN WY
MASTERS CIR
RIVIERA CIR
CHAMPIONS LN
TOURNEY HILL LN
GOLF COURSE LN
BLACK SAGE
LANTANA WY
1600
1500
200

SEE 754 MAP

0 .125 .25 .375 .5 miles 1 in. = 1900 ft.

SEE 775 MAP

SEE 735 MAP

E F G H J
1 2 3 4 5 6 7
GOLF BALL RD
HETRICK AV
WILLOW RD
CHEROKEE PL
FEIJOA PL
WILLOW RD
AUGUSTA
LINKS DR
ST ANDREWS WY
SUNDAY
REDBERRY PL
REDBERRY
SHELTER RIDGE
MISTY GLEN PL
MIDDLE RIDGE PL
SOUTHRIDGE LN
BLACKLAKE CIR
SAGE
BARBERRY WY
POMEROY RD
LIVE OAK RIDGE RD
VIA SECO
VILLA NONA
BLACK OAK LN
CALLE TIO
AMBER WY
RIDGE RD
GLENHAVEN PL
TEN OAKS WY
CALIMEX PL
HETRICK AV
JENNIE LN
HANA LN
SAN YSIDRO LN
POMEROY RD
STOGA LN
BLACKLAKE CANYON DR
AMERICAN WY
BLACK LAKE CIR
OLD RANCH LN
COLOMA LN
BLACKLAKE CANYON DR
WESTWIND WY
WHISPER LN
CALLE FRESA
CABALLO
PEGGY LEE CT
HUNTER RIDGE LN
TALL TREE DR
WAYPOINT DR
PATTY KAY CT
BLUE GUM LN
WHIMBREL CT
CASCADA LN
SILVER DOLLAR LN
RED GUM LN
SWEET GUM LN
CALIMEX PL
CALLE DE TOPO
MILES OAK LN
OAKS LN
QUAIL CT
SANDRA CT
KARL CT
CAMINO
SANDY OAKS LN
SANDYDALE DR
CORY WY
INGA RD
CABALLO
1 HIBISCUS CT
2 ALYSSUM CIR
NIPOMO COMMUNITY PARK
SUMMER LN
PATRICIO LN
CHEYENNE CT
MANDI CT
CEDAR GREEN CT
EVERGREEN WY
GEORGE WY
OLYMPIC
LA SERENATA WY
CAMINO CODORNIZ
CAMINO ROBLE
SWEET DONNA PL
EASY LN
CHARRO WY
N TEJAS PL
AMIGO PL
N TEJAS WY
CALLE FRESA
N MESA RD
ESTATE WY
KIWI LN
N MESA RD
SERENA
MIMOSA CT
LA ST
LANTANA
VERBENA
ZINNIA CT
AZALEA CT
93444
VIVA WY
EUCALYPTUS RD
OSAGE ST
VIA VICENTE WY
VIA MAXWELL
EUCALYPTUS RD
VIA PROMESA
SUNRIDGE LN
ROSE DR
LA CAMARILLA PL
CAMINO MARIPOSA
PARK
VILLA
ILLINOIS WY
INDIANA WY
SCENIC VIEW WY
DOOLITTLE WY
MESA
PAJARO LN
MESA VERDE LN
TEFFT
CALICO CT
QUINTA DR
PALOMA ST
N LAS FLORES DR
LA SERENA
ALTA
PABLO ORO
CASA DEL REAL PL
LA LN
VIA CALLE CIELO
VIA MIRA VALLE
CAMINO
CALLE DEL SOL
LA CUMBRE
TRES CASA LN
EL CERRITO DR
LA MIRADA DR
S LAS FLORES DR
LA LOMA DR
LA JOYA DR
COUNTRY
RIVERSIDE RD
RANCHO NIPOMO
RANCHO GUADALUPE
DIVISION ST
BONITA SCHOOL RD
1100 900 700 500 800 300 1400 1300 1500

SEE 756 MAP

SEE 775 MAP

0 .125 .25 .375 .5 miles 1 in. = 1900 ft.

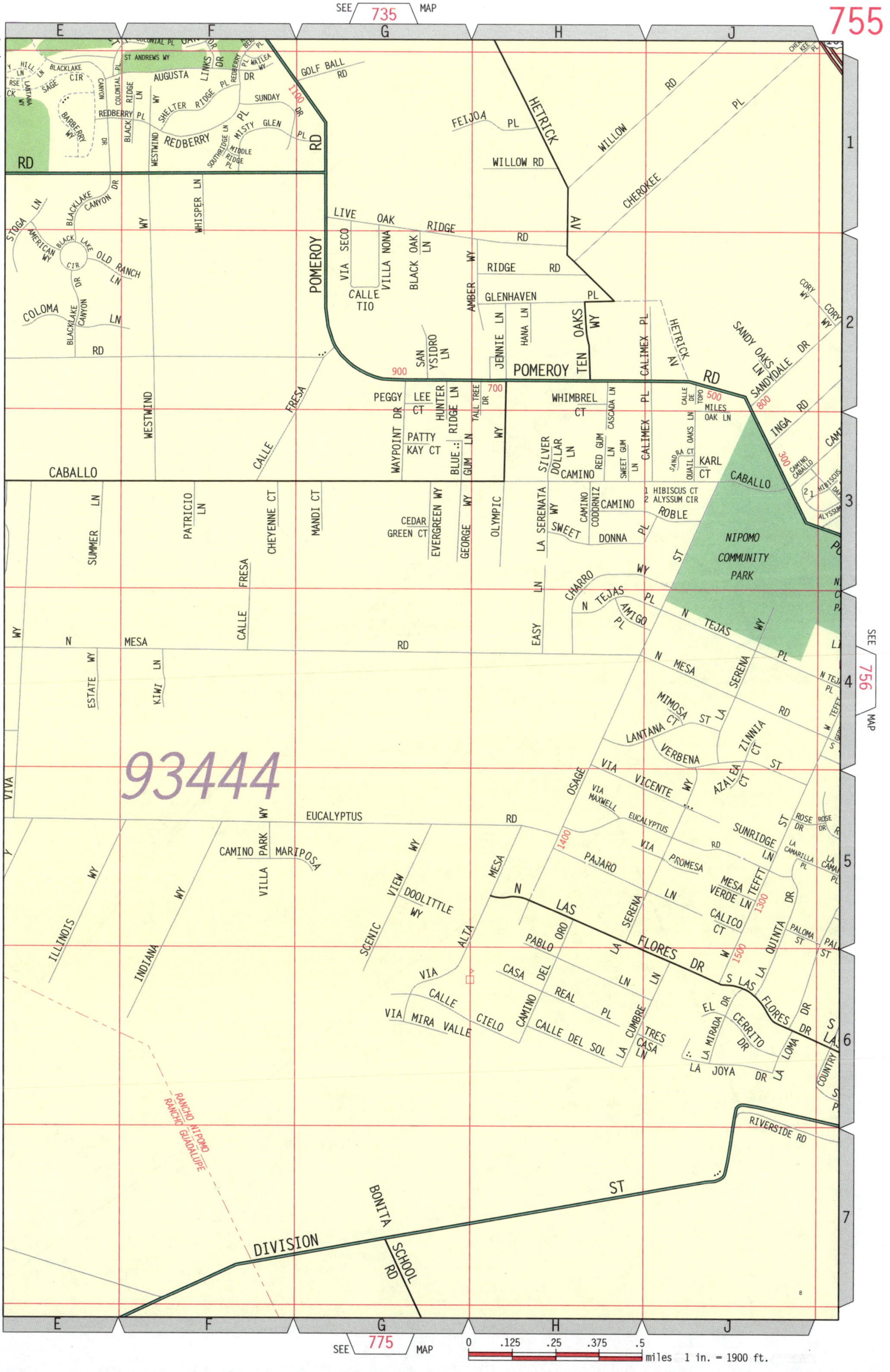

SEE 736 MAP

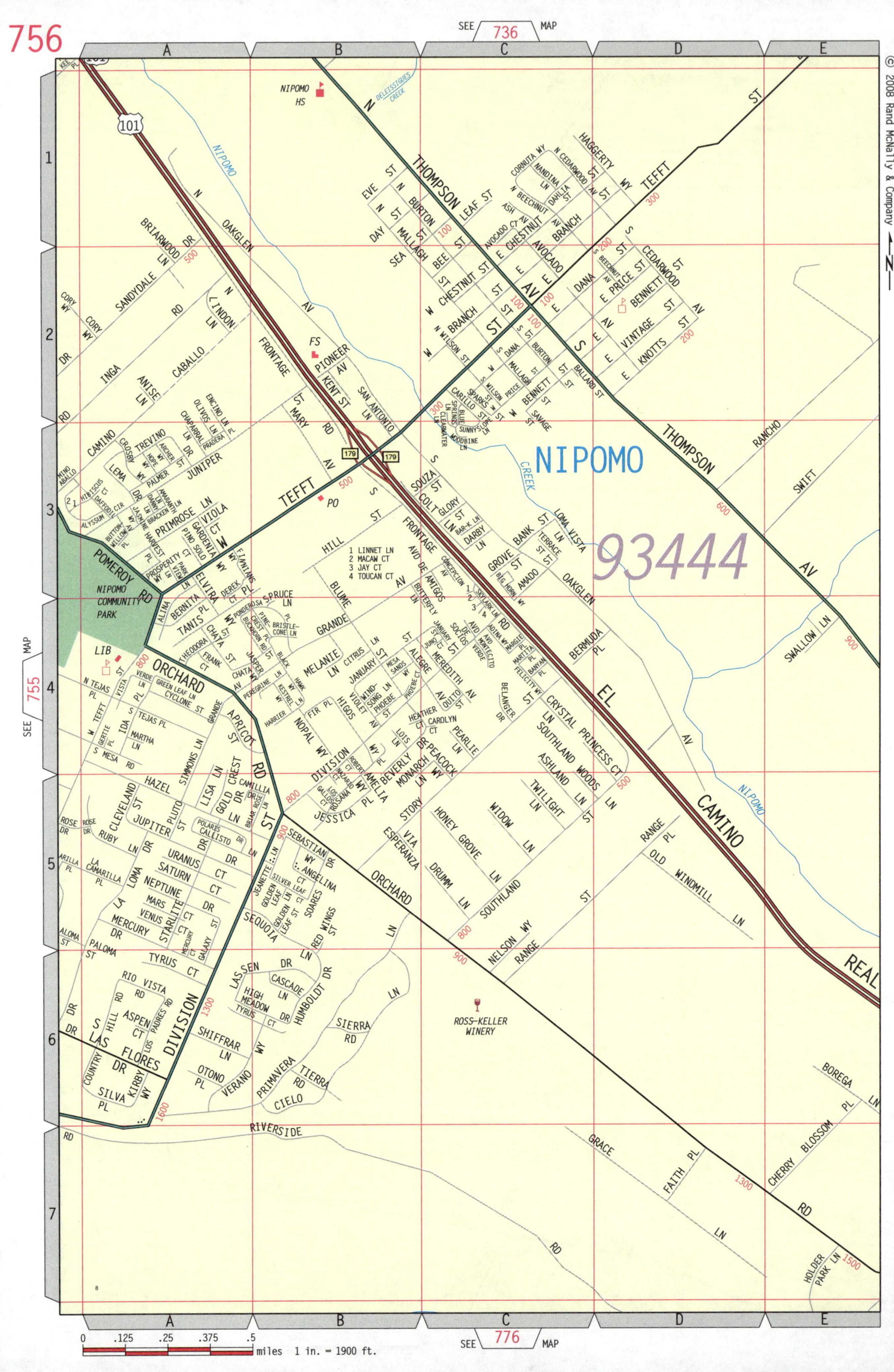
NIPOMO
93444
NIPOMO HS
NIPOMO COMMUNITY PARK
ROSS-KELLER WINERY
THOMPSON AV
EL CAMINO REAL
TEFFT ST
ORCHARD RD
DIVISION ST
FRONTAGE RD
OAKGLEN AV
RIVERSIDE RD
NIPOMO CREEK
DELEISSIGUES CREEK
1 LINNET LN
2 MACAW CT
3 JAY CT
4 TOUCAN CT
0 .125 .25 .375 .5 miles 1 in. = 1900 ft.

SEE 755 MAP

SEE 776 MAP

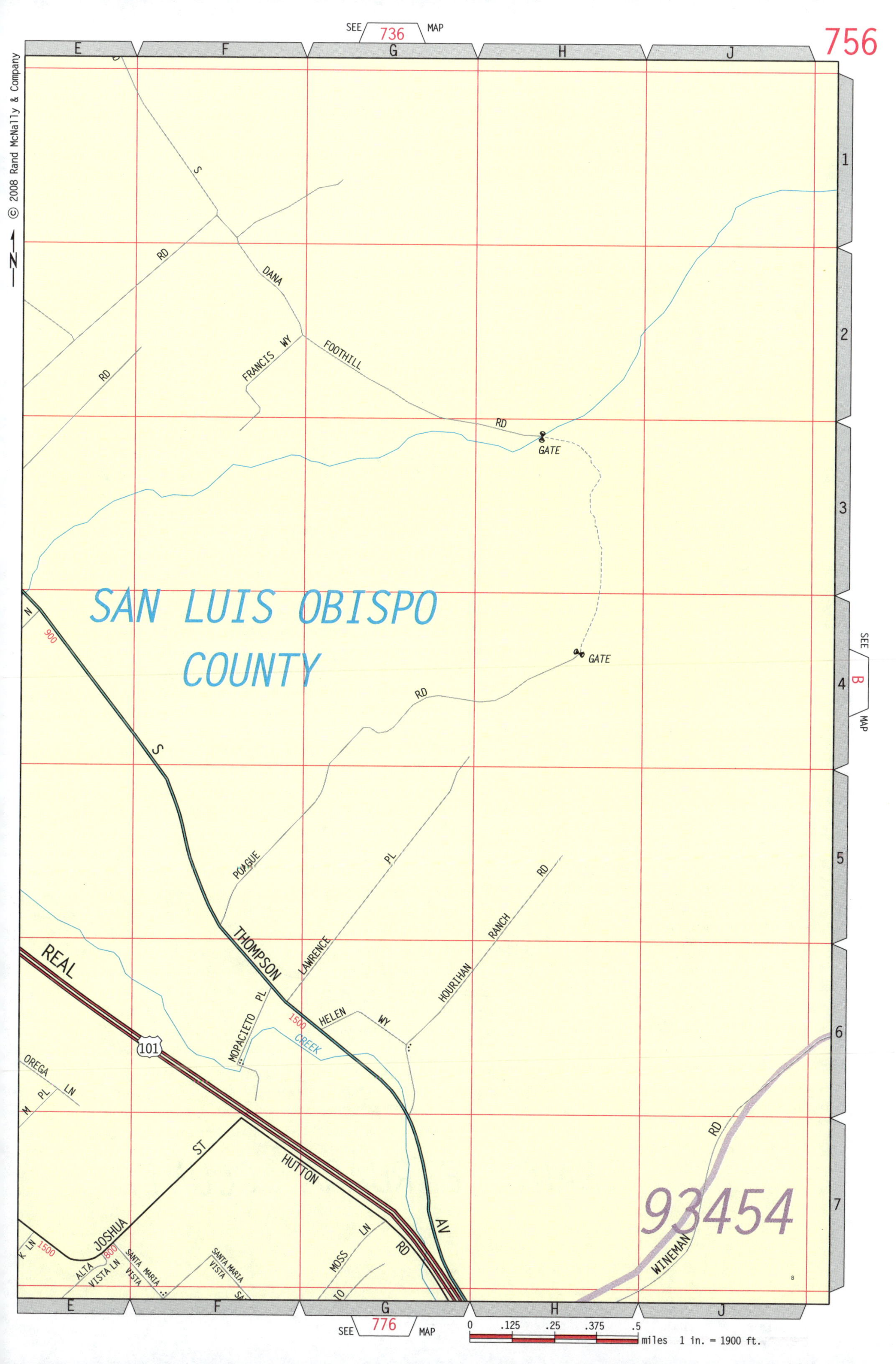
SEE 736 MAP
E
F
G
H
J
1
2
3
4
5
6
7
SEE B MAP
SAN LUIS OBISPO
COUNTY
S
RD
DANA
FRANCIS WY
FOOTHILL
RD
RD
GATE
GATE
RD
N
900
S
POLGUE
PL
LAWRENCE
RD
RANCH
HOURIHAN
THOMPSON
REAL
101
MOPACIETO
PL
1500
HELEN
WY
CREEK
OREGA
PL
LN
M
ST
HUTTON
JOSHUA
K LN
1500
800
ALTA
VISTA LN
SANTA MARIA
VISTA
SANTA MARIA
VISTA
MOSS
LN
RD
TO
AV
RD
WINEMAN
93454
SEE 776 MAP
0
.125
.25
.375
.5
miles 1 in. = 1900 ft.

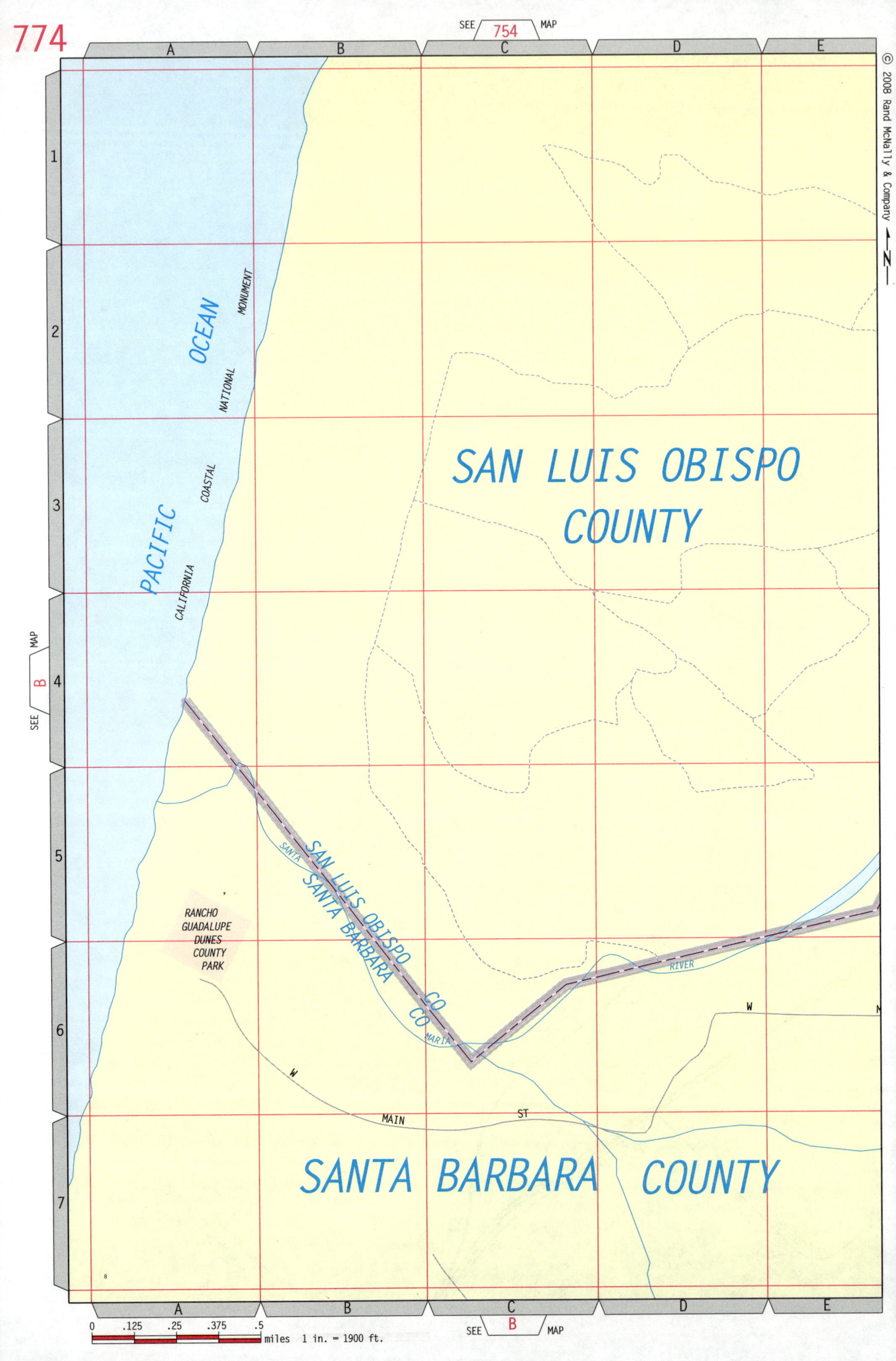
SEE 754 MAP
A
B
C
D
E
1
2
3
4
5
6
7
SEE B MAP
PACIFIC
OCEAN
CALIFORNIA
COASTAL
NATIONAL
MONUMENT
SAN LUIS OBISPO
COUNTY
SAN LUIS OBISPO CO
SANTA BARBARA CO
SANTA
MARIA
RIVER
RANCHO
GUADALUPE
DUNES
COUNTY
PARK
W
MAIN
ST
SANTA BARBARA COUNTY
0
.125
.25
.375
.5
miles 1 in. = 1900 ft.

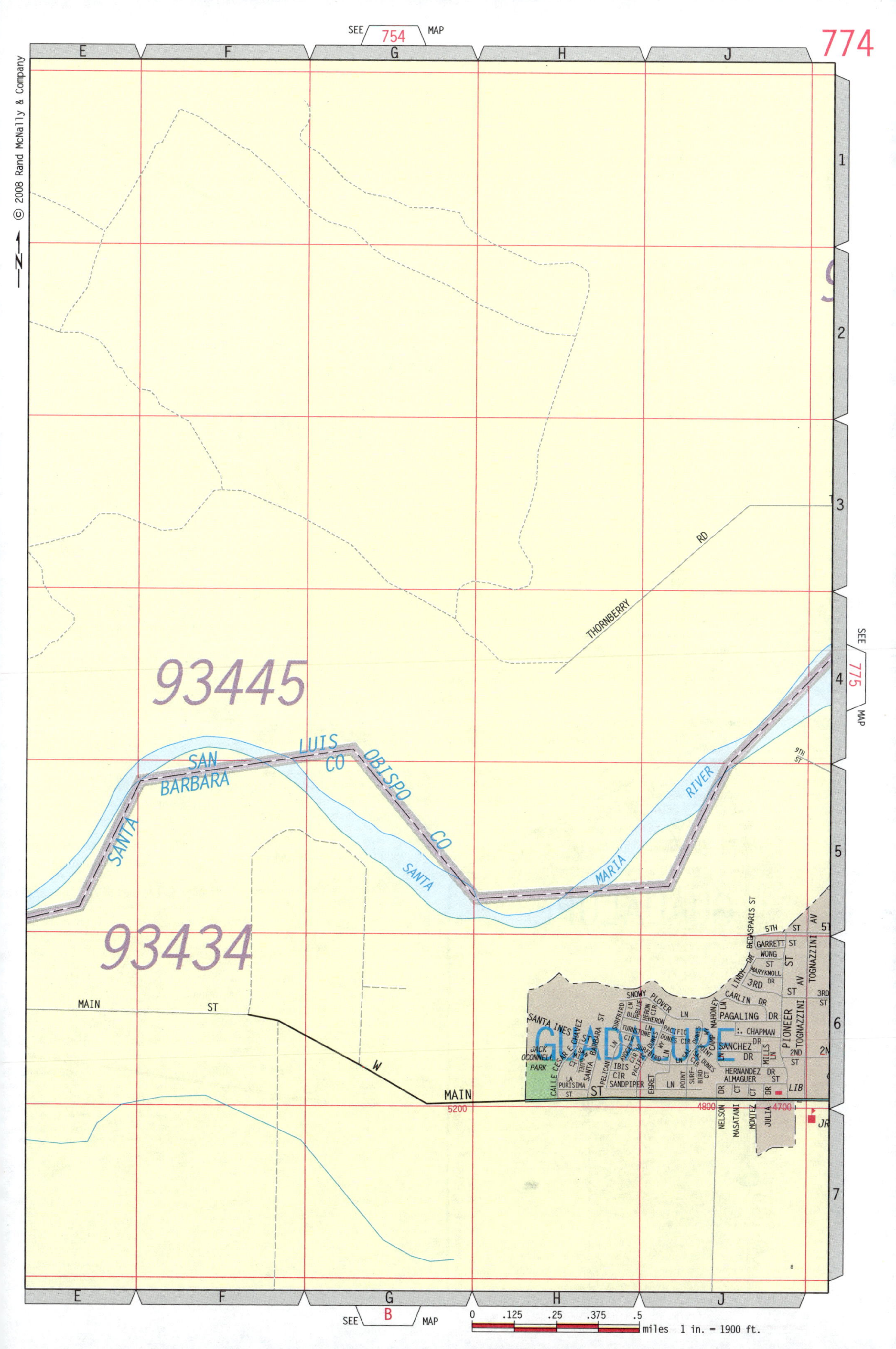

SEE 754 MAP
E
F
G
H
J
1
2
3
4
5
6
7
THORNBERRY RD
SEE 775 MAP
93445
93434
SAN LUIS OBISPO CO
SANTA BARBARA CO
SANTA MARIA RIVER
MAIN ST
W MAIN
5200
4800
4700
GUADALUPE
JACK OCONNELL PARK
SANTA INES ST
CALLE CESAR E CHAVEZ
SANTA BARBARA ST
LA PURISIMA ST
SNOWY PLOVER LN
PELICAN
IBIS CIR
SANDPIPER
EGRET
TURNSTONE
PACIFIC DUNES CIR
SURFBIRD
MAHONEY
PAGALING DR
CHAPMAN
SANCHEZ DR
HERNANDEZ DR
ALMAGUER ST
PIONEER
TOGNAZZINI AV
MILLS LN
CARLIN DR
3RD DR
LINDY DR
GARRETT ST
WONG ST
MARYKNOLL DR
5TH ST
OBEGASPARIS ST
NELSON DR
MASATANI CT
MONTEZ CT
JULIA DR
LIB
9TH ST
2ND ST
3RD ST
SEE B MAP
0 .125 .25 .375 .5
miles 1 in. = 1900 ft.

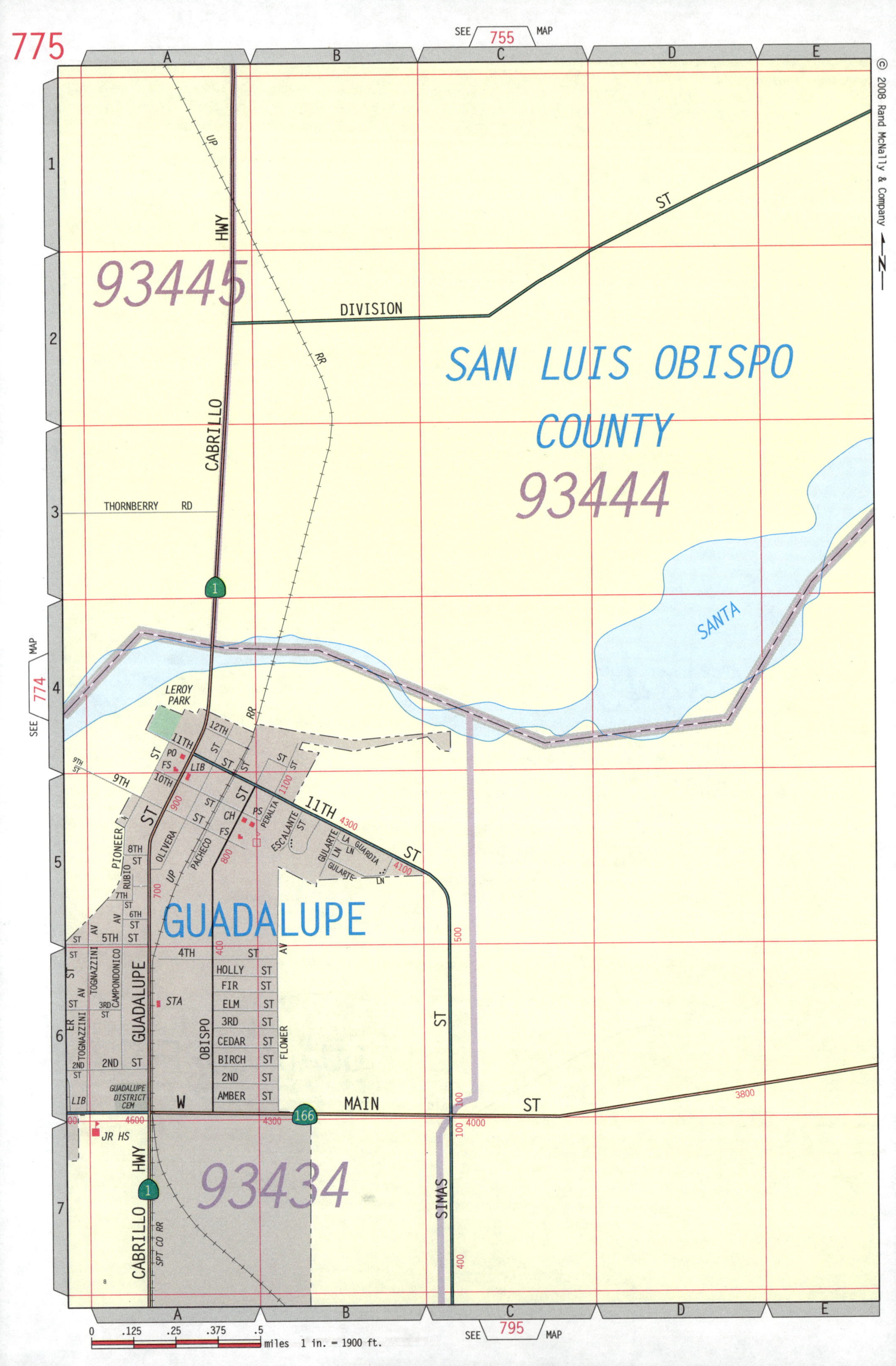

SEE 755 MAP
SAN LUIS OBISPO COUNTY
93444
93445
93434
GUADALUPE
CABRILLO HWY
DIVISION
ST
THORNBERRY RD
SANTA
LEROY PARK
11TH ST
MAIN ST
W
SIMAS ST
OBISPO ST
GUADALUPE ST
FLOWER AV
HOLLY ST
FIR ST
ELM ST
3RD ST
CEDAR ST
BIRCH ST
2ND ST
AMBER ST
4TH ST
5TH ST
6TH ST
7TH
8TH ST
9TH
10TH
12TH ST
PIONEER
OLIVERA
PACHECO
PERALTA
ESCALANTE ST
GULARTE LN
LA GUARDIA LN
TOGNAZZINI AV
CAMPONDONICO
RUBIO
JR HS
GUADALUPE DISTRICT CEM
LIB
STA
SPT CO RR
UP RR
SEE 774 MAP
SEE 795 MAP
miles 1 in. = 1900 ft.

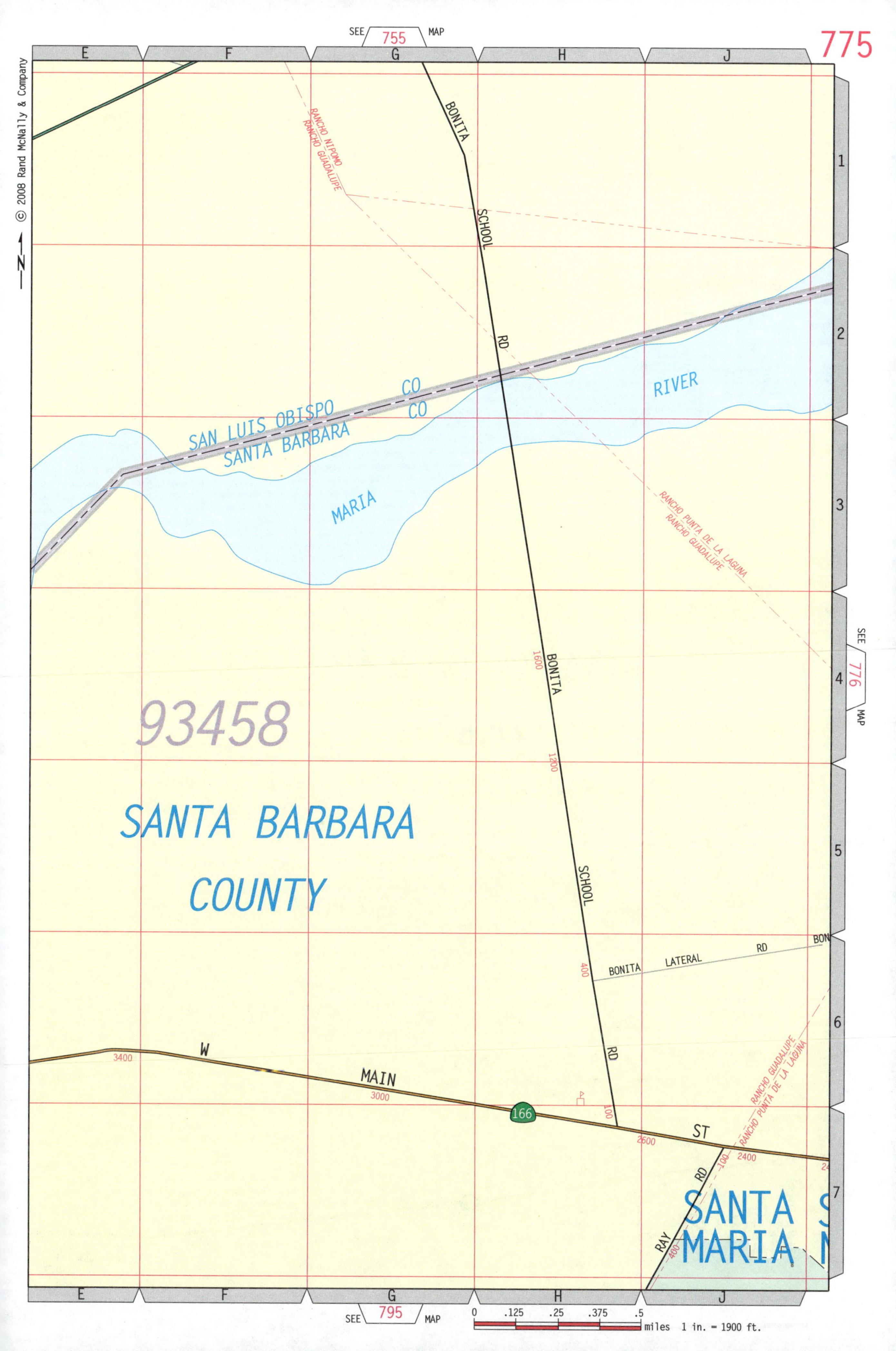
SEE 755 MAP
E
F
G
H
J
BONITA
RANCHO NIPOMO
RANCHO GUADALUPE
SCHOOL
RD
SAN LUIS OBISPO
SANTA BARBARA
CO
CO
RIVER
MARIA
RANCHO PUNTA DE LA LAGUNA
RANCHO GUADALUPE
1600
BONITA
93458
1200
SANTA BARBARA
COUNTY
SCHOOL
BONITA
LATERAL
RD
400
RD
W
MAIN
3400
3000
166
100
2600
ST
2400
RANCHO GUADALUPE
RANCHO PUNTA DE LA LAGUNA
RD
RAY
400
SANTA
MARIA
1
2
3
4
5
6
7
SEE 776 MAP
SEE 795 MAP
0 .125 .25 .375 .5
miles 1 in. = 1900 ft.

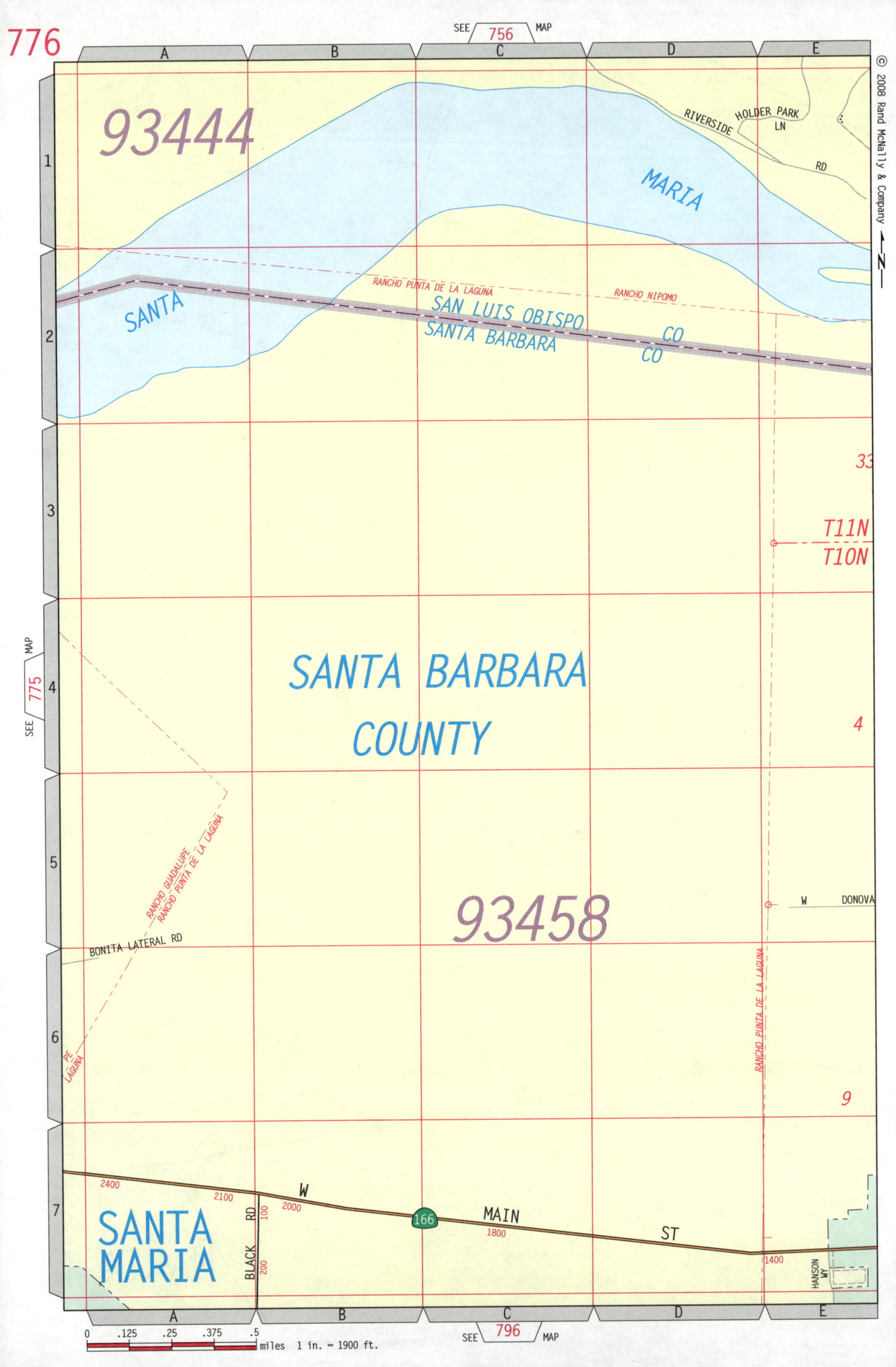

SEE 756 MAP
A
B
C
D
E
1
2
3
4
5
6
7
93444
RIVERSIDE
HOLDER PARK
LN
RD
MARIA
SANTA
RANCHO PUNTA DE LA LAGUNA
RANCHO NIPOMO
SAN LUIS OBISPO
SANTA BARBARA
CO
CO
33
T11N
T10N
SEE 775 MAP
SANTA BARBARA
COUNTY
4
RANCHO GUADALUPE
RANCHO PUNTA DE LA LAGUNA
W
DONOVA
93458
BONITA LATERAL RD
PE
LAGUNA
RANCHO PUNTA DE LA LAGUNA
9
2400
2100
W
2000
166
MAIN
1800
ST
1400
BLACK
RD
100
200
SANTA
MARIA
HANSON
WY
0
.125
.25
.375
.5
miles 1 in. = 1900 ft.
SEE 796 MAP

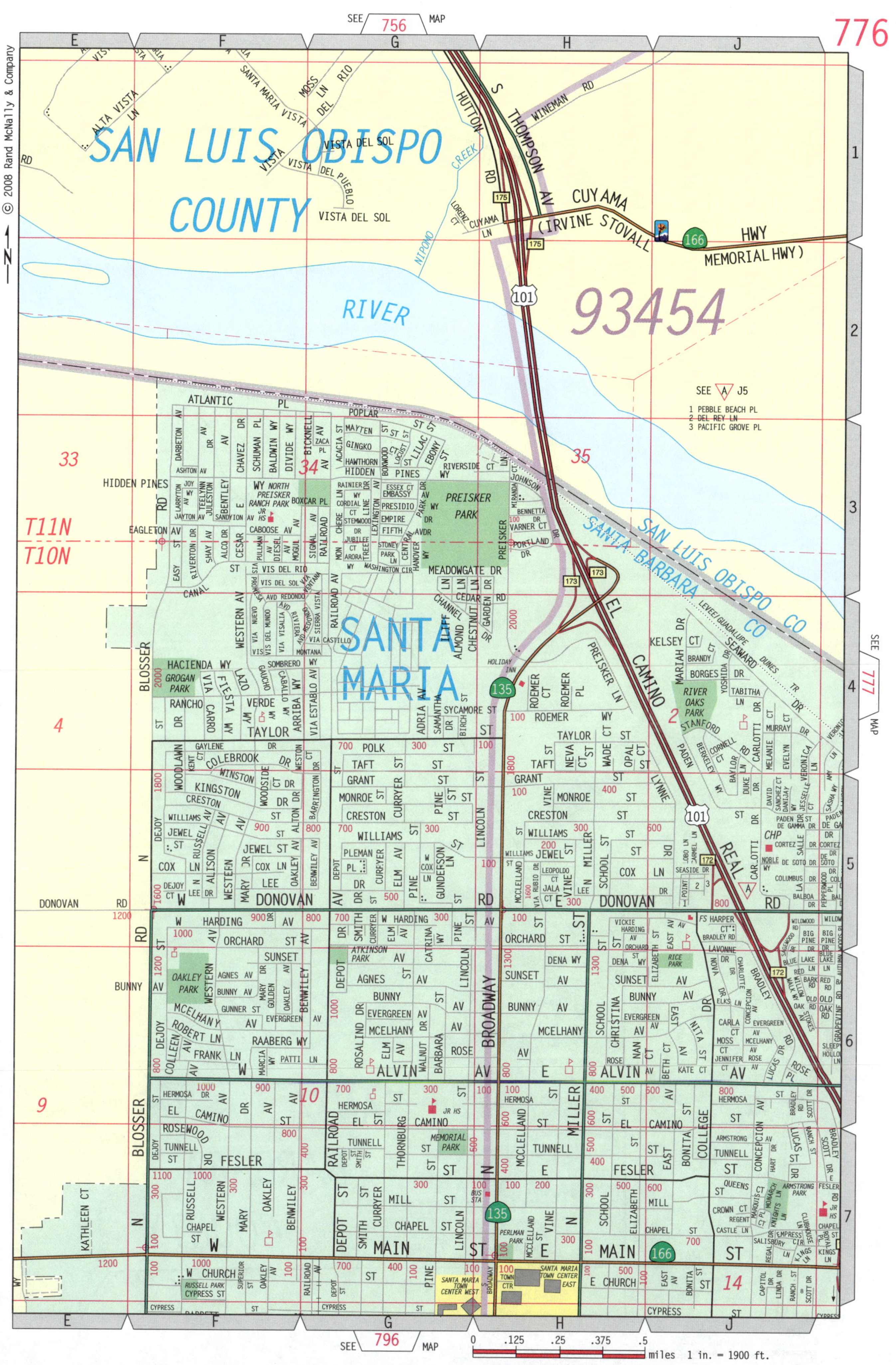
SEE 756 MAP
SAN LUIS OBISPO
COUNTY
RIVER
93454
SANTA
MARIA
SANTA BARBARA CO
SAN LUIS OBISPO CO
CUYAMA (IRVINE STOVALL HWY MEMORIAL HWY)
S THOMPSON AV
HUTTON RD
WINEMAN RD
NIPOMO CREEK
VISTA DEL SOL
ALTA VISTA LN
SANTA MARIA VISTA
MOSS LN
DEL RIO
PREISKER PARK
GROGAN PARK
OAKLEY PARK
ATKINSON PARK
MEMORIAL PARK
RIVER OAKS PARK
RICE PARK
ARMSTRONG PARK
PERLMAN PARK
RUSSELL PARK
NORTH PREISKER RANCH PARK
SANTA MARIA TOWN CENTER WEST
SANTA MARIA TOWN CENTER EAST
HOLIDAY INN
SEE A J5
1 PEBBLE BEACH PL
2 DEL REY LN
3 PACIFIC GROVE PL
T11N
T10N
33
34
35
4
2
9
10
14
BROADWAY
EL CAMINO REAL
BLOSSER RD
DONOVAN RD
MAIN ST
ATLANTIC PL
TAYLOR ST
POLK ST
ALVIN AV
FESLER ST
CHURCH ST
CYPRESS ST
MILLER ST
SEE 777 MAP
SEE 796 MAP
0 .125 .25 .375 .5
miles 1 in. = 1900 ft.

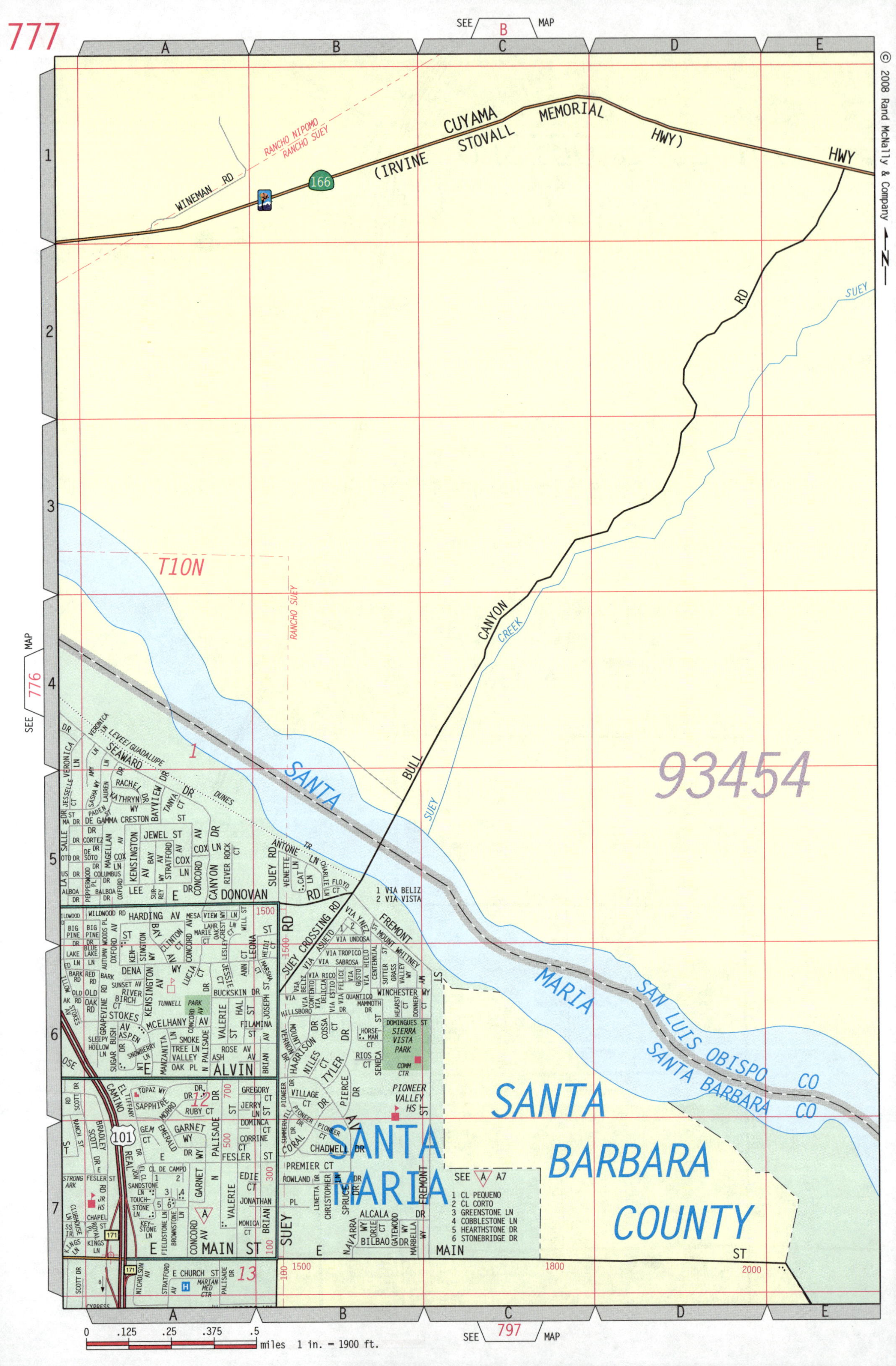
SEE B MAP
SEE 776 MAP
SEE 797 MAP
CUYAMA MEMORIAL HWY
(IRVINE STOVALL HWY)
166
WINEMAN RD
RANCHO NIPOMO
RANCHO SUEY
BULL CANYON RD
SUEY CREEK
T10N
RANCHO SUEY
SANTA MARIA
93454
SAN LUIS OBISPO CO
SANTA BARBARA CO
SANTA BARBARA COUNTY
SANTA MARIA
SUEY RD
SUEY CROSSING RD
E DONOVAN RD
ALVIN AV
E MAIN ST
FREMONT ST
HARDING AV
CONCORD AV
PALISADE ST
SIERRA VISTA PARK
PIONEER VALLEY HS
E CHURCH ST
MARIAN MED CTR
101
171
SEE A7
1 CL PEQUENO
2 CL CORTO
3 GREENSTONE LN
4 COBBLESTONE LN
5 HEARTHSTONE DR
6 STONEBRIDGE DR
1 VIA BELIZ
2 VIA VISTA
1500
1800
2000
0 .125 .25 .375 .5 miles 1 in. = 1900 ft.

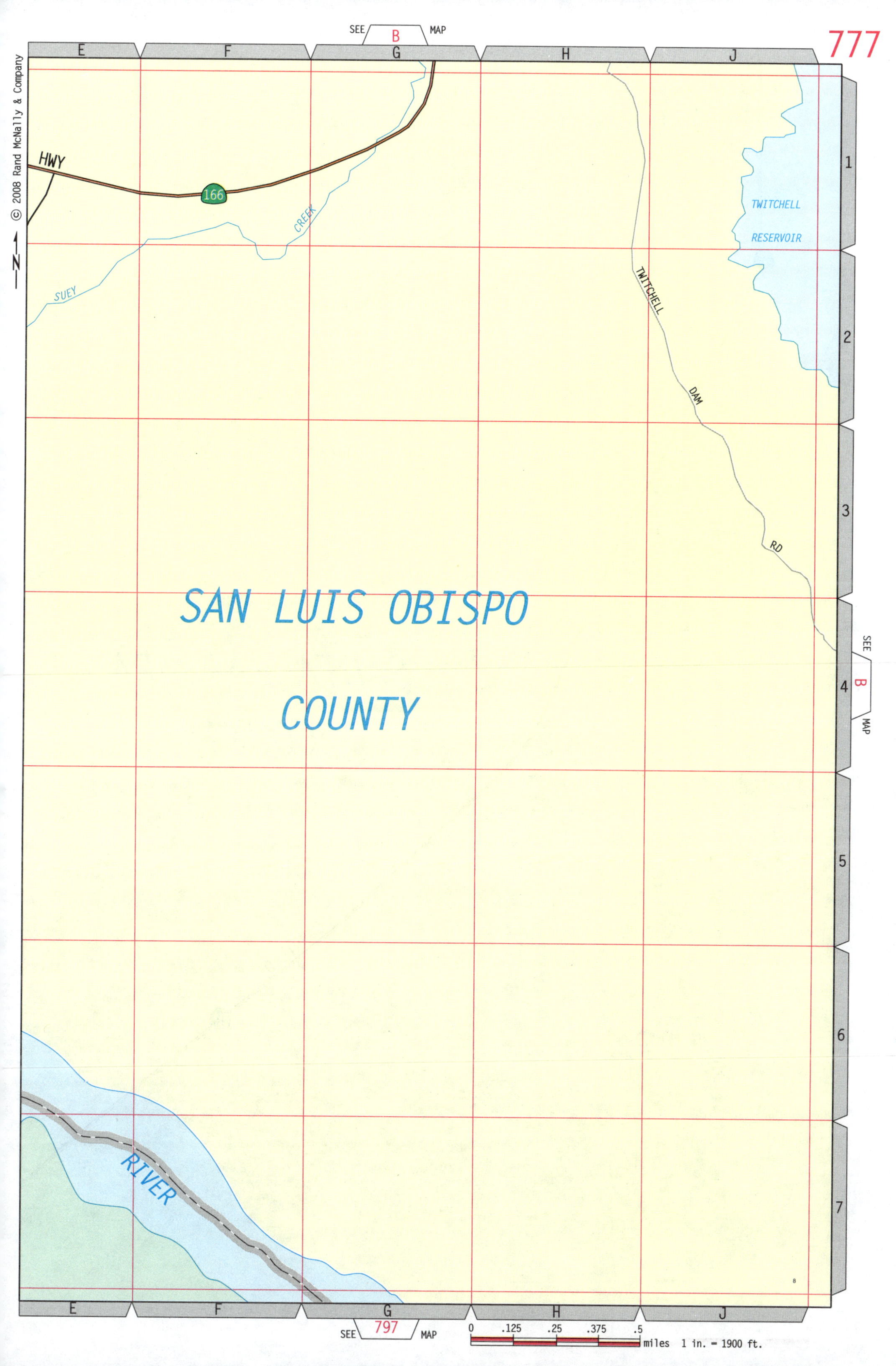

SEE B MAP
E
F
G
H
J
HWY
166
CREEK
SUEY
TWITCHELL RESERVOIR
TWITCHELL
DAM
RD
SAN LUIS OBISPO
COUNTY
RIVER
1
2
3
4
5
6
7
SEE B MAP
SEE 797 MAP
0
.125
.25
.375
.5
miles 1 in. = 1900 ft.

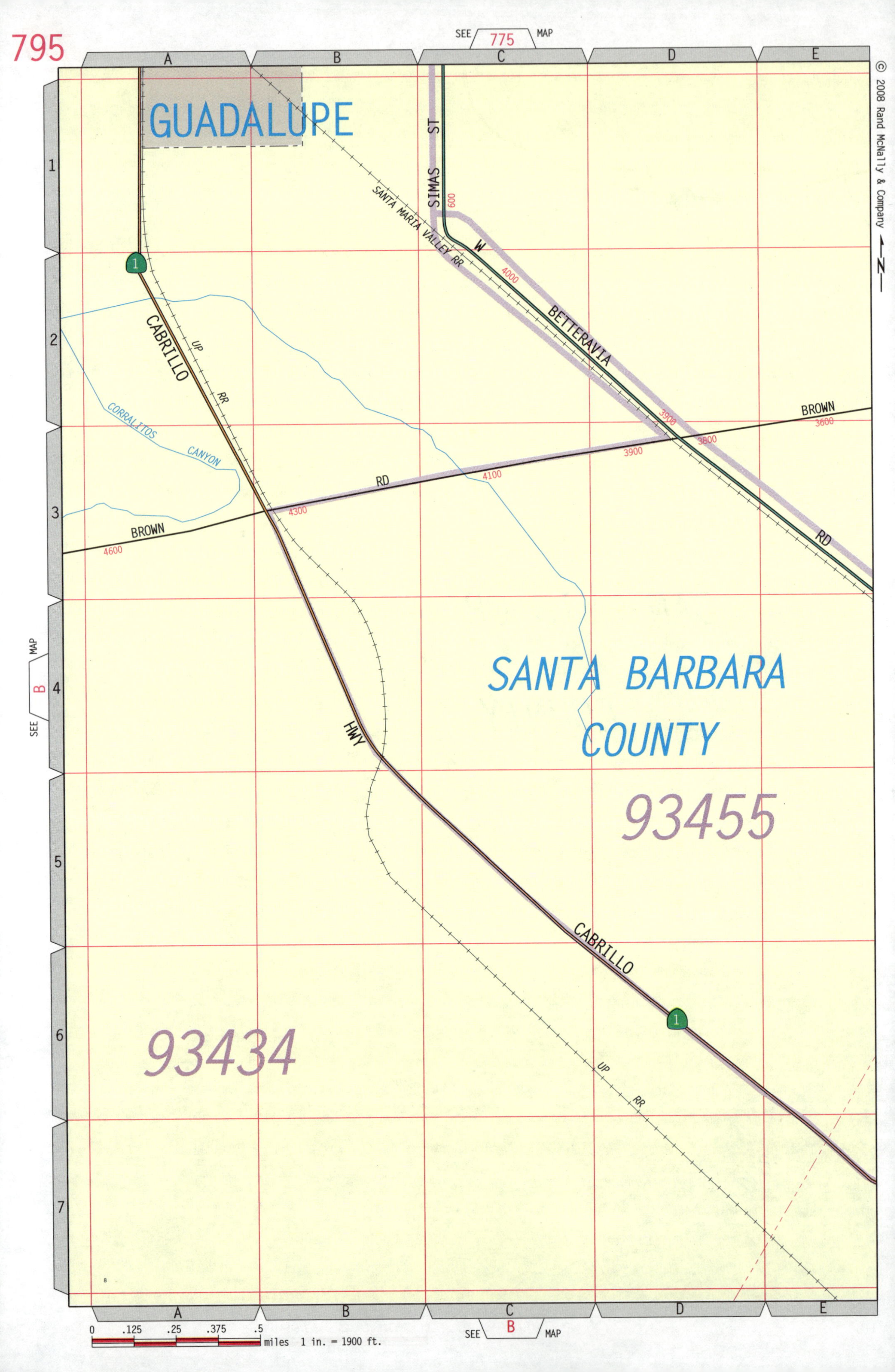
SEE 775 MAP
A
B
C
D
E
1
2
3
4
5
6
7
GUADALUPE
SIMAS ST
600
SANTA MARIA VALLEY RR
W
4000
BETTERAVIA
RD
3900
3800
BROWN
3600
CABRILLO
UP
RR
CORRALITOS
CANYON
RD
4100
3900
4300
BROWN
4600
SEE B MAP
SANTA BARBARA
COUNTY
HWY
93455
CABRILLO
93434
UP
RR
SEE B MAP
0 .125 .25 .375 .5
miles 1 in. = 1900 ft.

SEE 775 MAP

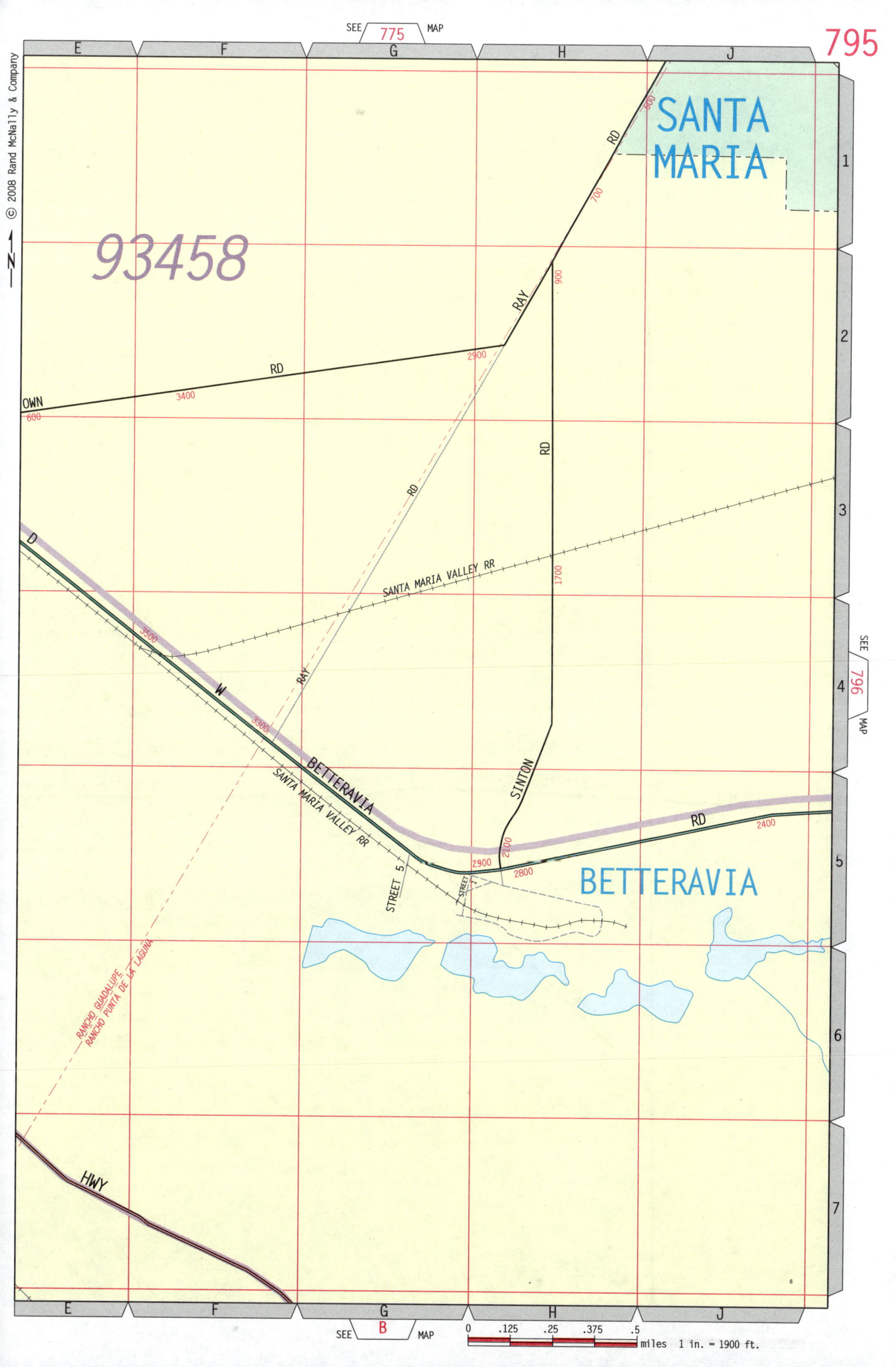
SANTA
MARIA
93458
RAY
RD
OWN
RD
SINTON
RD
SANTA MARIA VALLEY RR
W
BETTERAVIA
RD
SANTA MARIA VALLEY RR
STREET 5
STREET 1
BETTERAVIA
RANCHO GUADALUPE
RANCHO PUNTA DE LA LAGUNA
HWY
E
F
G
H
J
1
2
3
4
5
6
7
0
.125
.25
.375
.5
miles 1 in. = 1900 ft.

SEE 796 MAP
SEE B MAP

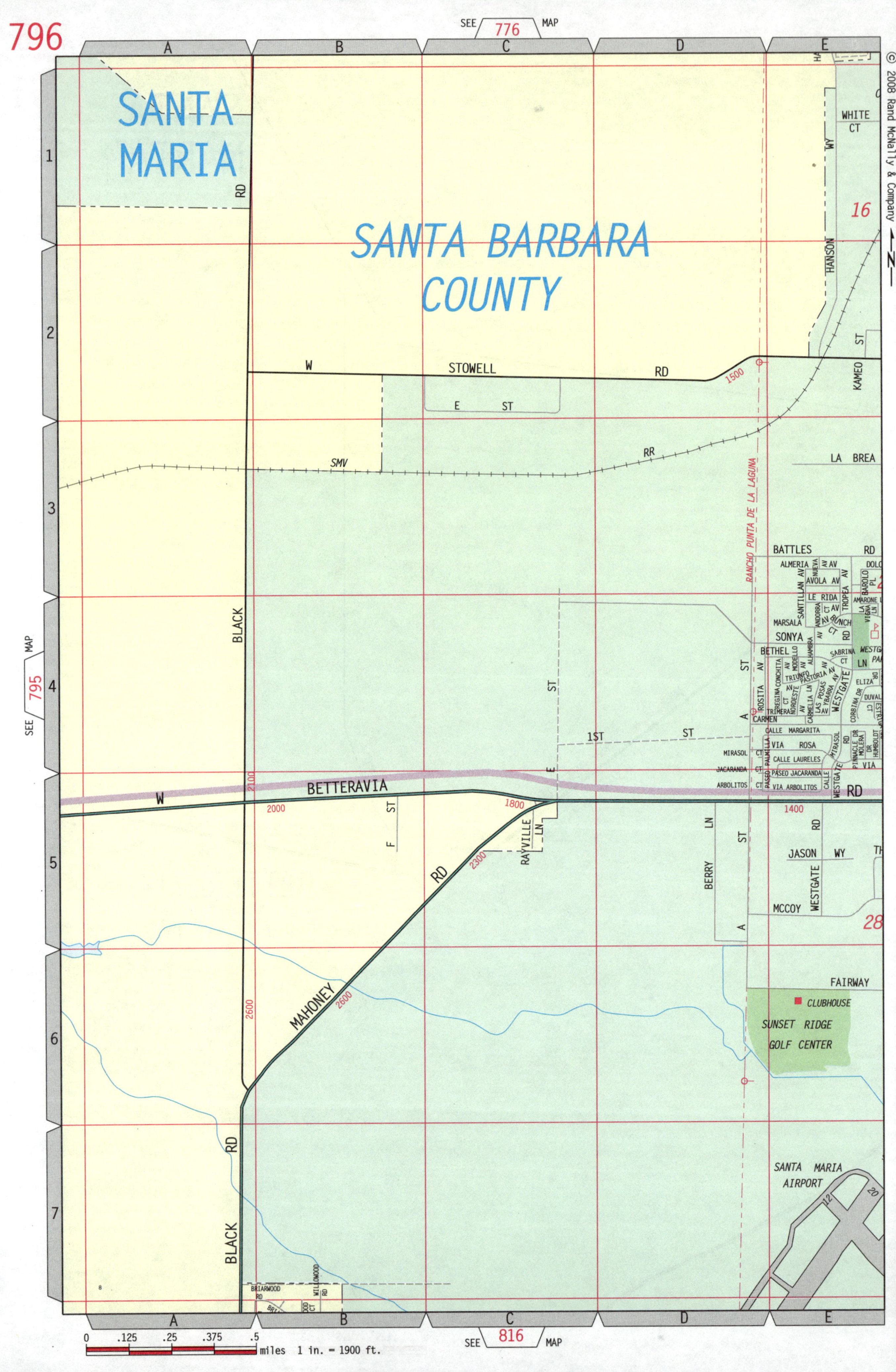
SEE 776 MAP
SANTA MARIA
SANTA BARBARA COUNTY
W STOWELL RD
E ST
SMV RR
LA BREA
KAMEO ST
HANSON WY
WHITE CT
16
RANCHO PUNTA DE LA LAGUNA
BATTLES RD
BLACK RD
W BETTERAVIA RD
E ST
1ST ST
A ST
F ST
RAYVILLE LN
MAHONEY RD
BERRY LN
JASON WY
WESTGATE RD
MCCOY
28
FAIRWAY
CLUBHOUSE
SUNSET RIDGE GOLF CENTER
SANTA MARIA AIRPORT
BRIARWOOD RD
WILLOWOOD RD
SEE 795 MAP
SEE 816 MAP
0 .125 .25 .375 .5 miles 1 in. = 1900 ft.

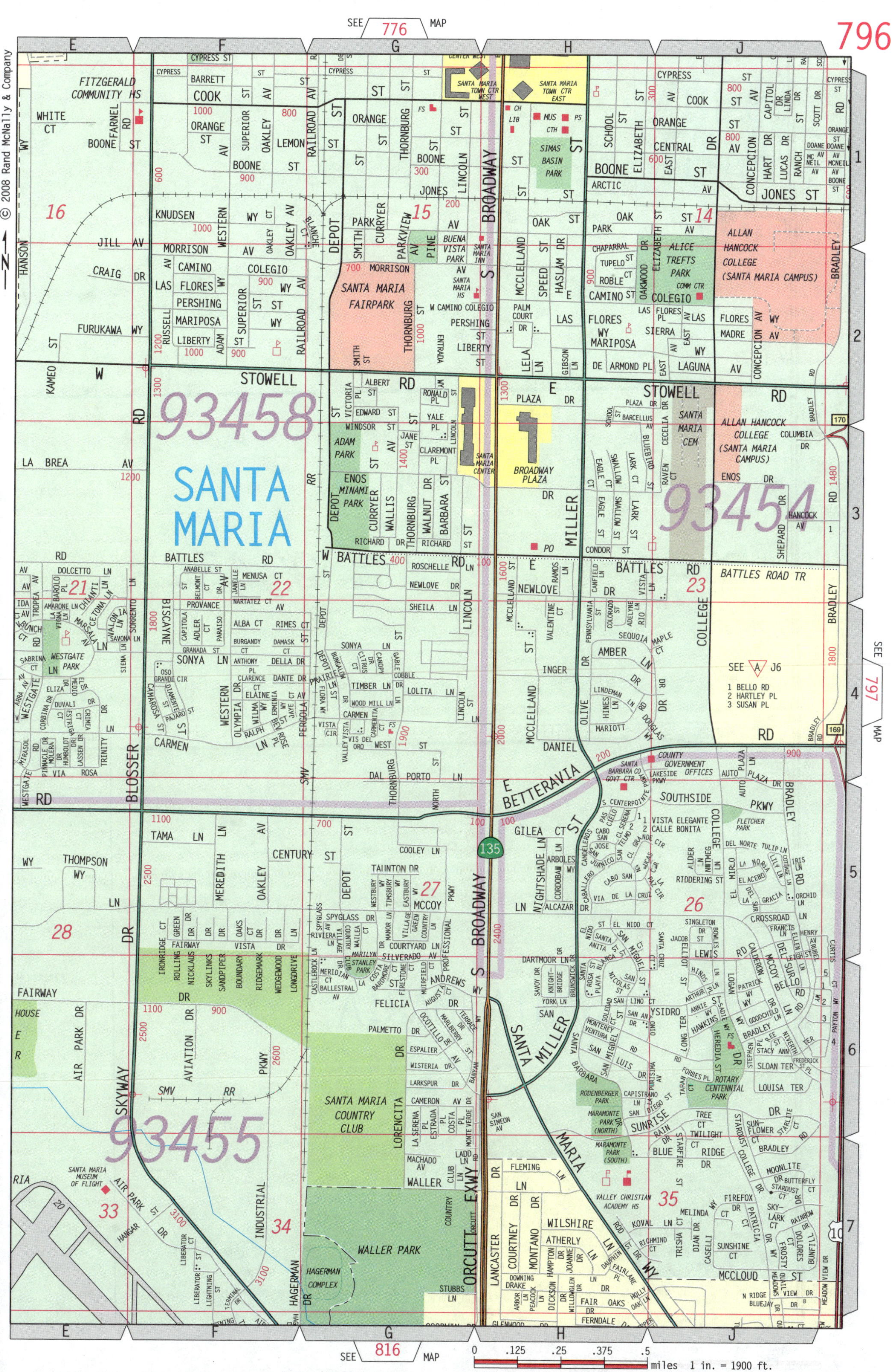
SEE 776 MAP
SANTA MARIA
93458
93454
93455
FITZGERALD COMMUNITY HS
ALLAN HANCOCK COLLEGE (SANTA MARIA CAMPUS)
SANTA MARIA FAIRPARK
ALICE TREFTS PARK
SIMAS BASIN PARK
SANTA MARIA TOWN CTR WEST
SANTA MARIA TOWN CTR EAST
SANTA MARIA CEM
BROADWAY PLAZA
ADAM PARK
ENOS MINAMI PARK
WESTGATE PARK
BATTLES ROAD TR
SEE 797 MAP
SANTA MARIA COUNTRY CLUB
WALLER PARK
HAGERMAN COMPLEX
SANTA MARIA MUSEUM OF FLIGHT
VALLEY CHRISTIAN ACADEMY HS
CENTENNIAL PARK
RODENBERGER PARK
COUNTY GOVERNMENT OFFICES
SANTA BARBARA CO GOVT CTR
BROADWAY
STOWELL RD
BATTLES RD
BETTERAVIA
SKYWAY
BLOSSER
SEE 816 MAP
miles 1 in. = 1900 ft.

SEE 777 MAP

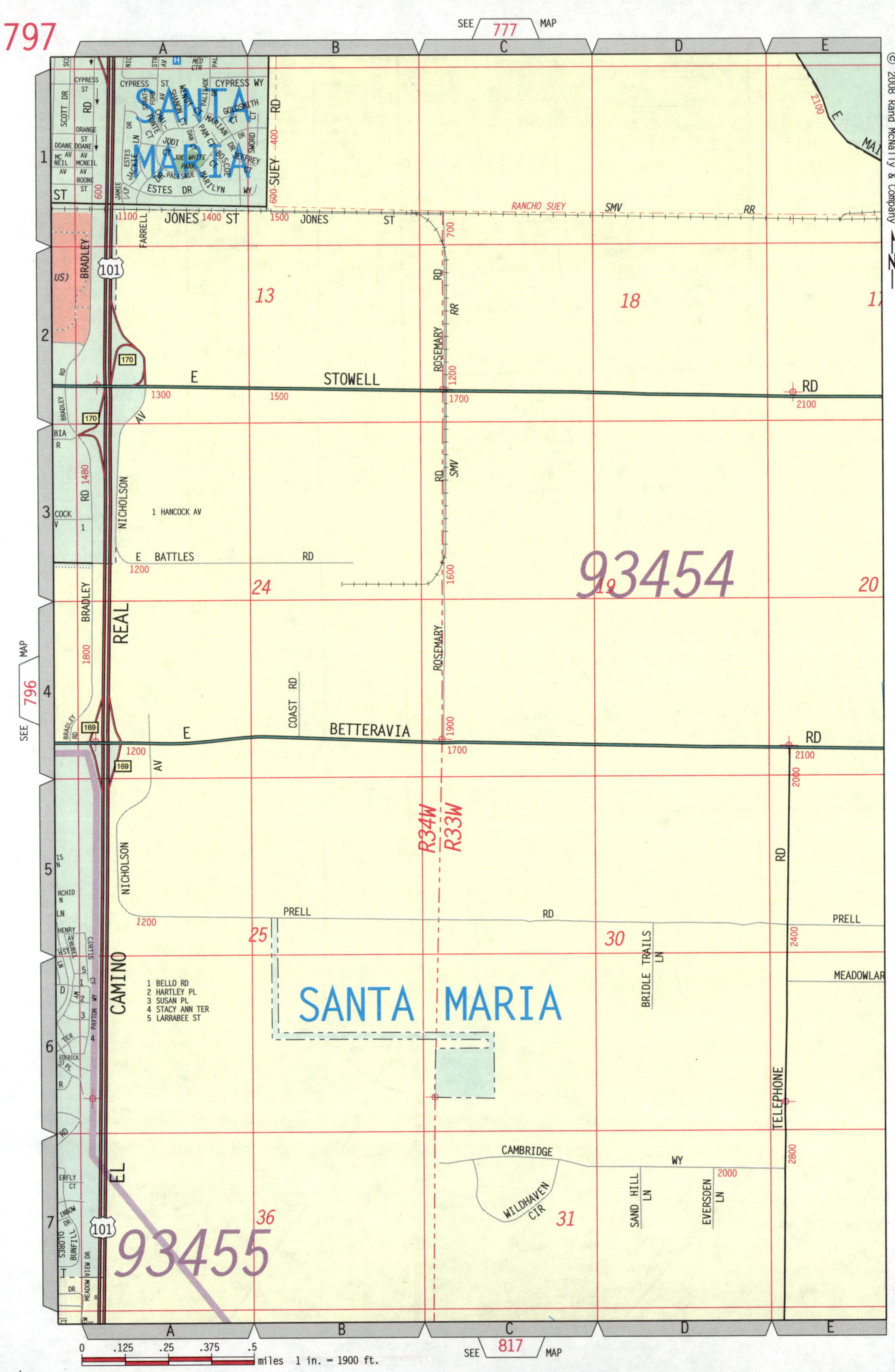
SANTA MARIA
CYPRESS ST
CYPRESS WY
JONES ST
SUEY RD
RANCHO SUEY SMV RR
E STOWELL RD
ROSEMARY RD
NICHOLSON AV
E BATTLES RD
1 HANCOCK AV
EL CAMINO REAL
BRADLEY RD
E BETTERAVIA RD
COAST RD
PRELL RD
BRIDLE TRAILS LN
TELEPHONE RD
MEADOWLAR
1 BELLO RD
2 HARTLEY PL
3 SUSAN PL
4 STACY ANN TER
5 LARRABEE ST
CAMBRIDGE WY
WILDHAVEN CIR
SAND HILL LN
EVERSDEN LN
R34W
R33W
93454
93455
13
18
24
19
20
25
30
36
31
© 2008 Rand McNally & Company

SEE 796 MAP

SEE 817 MAP

0 .125 .25 .375 .5 miles 1 in. = 1900 ft.

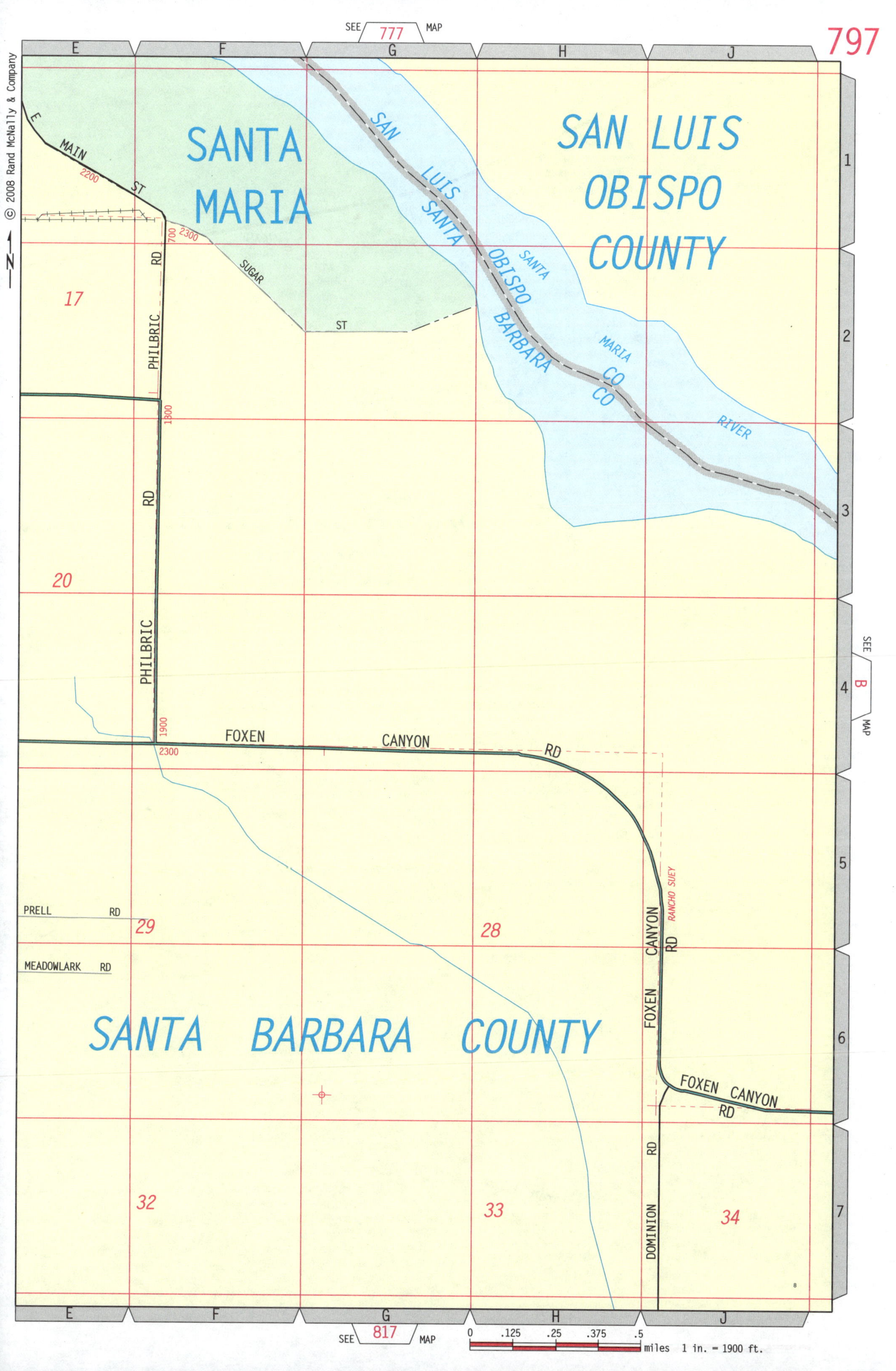
SEE 777 MAP
E
F
G
H
J
1
2
3
4
5
6
7
SANTA MARIA
SAN LUIS OBISPO COUNTY
SAN LUIS OBISPO CO
SANTA BARBARA CO
SANTA MARIA RIVER
E MAIN ST
2200
2300
700
SUGAR ST
PHILBRIC RD
1300
1900
17
20
FOXEN CANYON RD
2300
RANCHO SUEY
FOXEN CANYON RD
PRELL RD
MEADOWLARK RD
29
28
SANTA BARBARA COUNTY
DOMINION RD
32
33
34
SEE B MAP
SEE 817 MAP
0 .125 .25 .375 .5 miles 1 in. = 1900 ft.

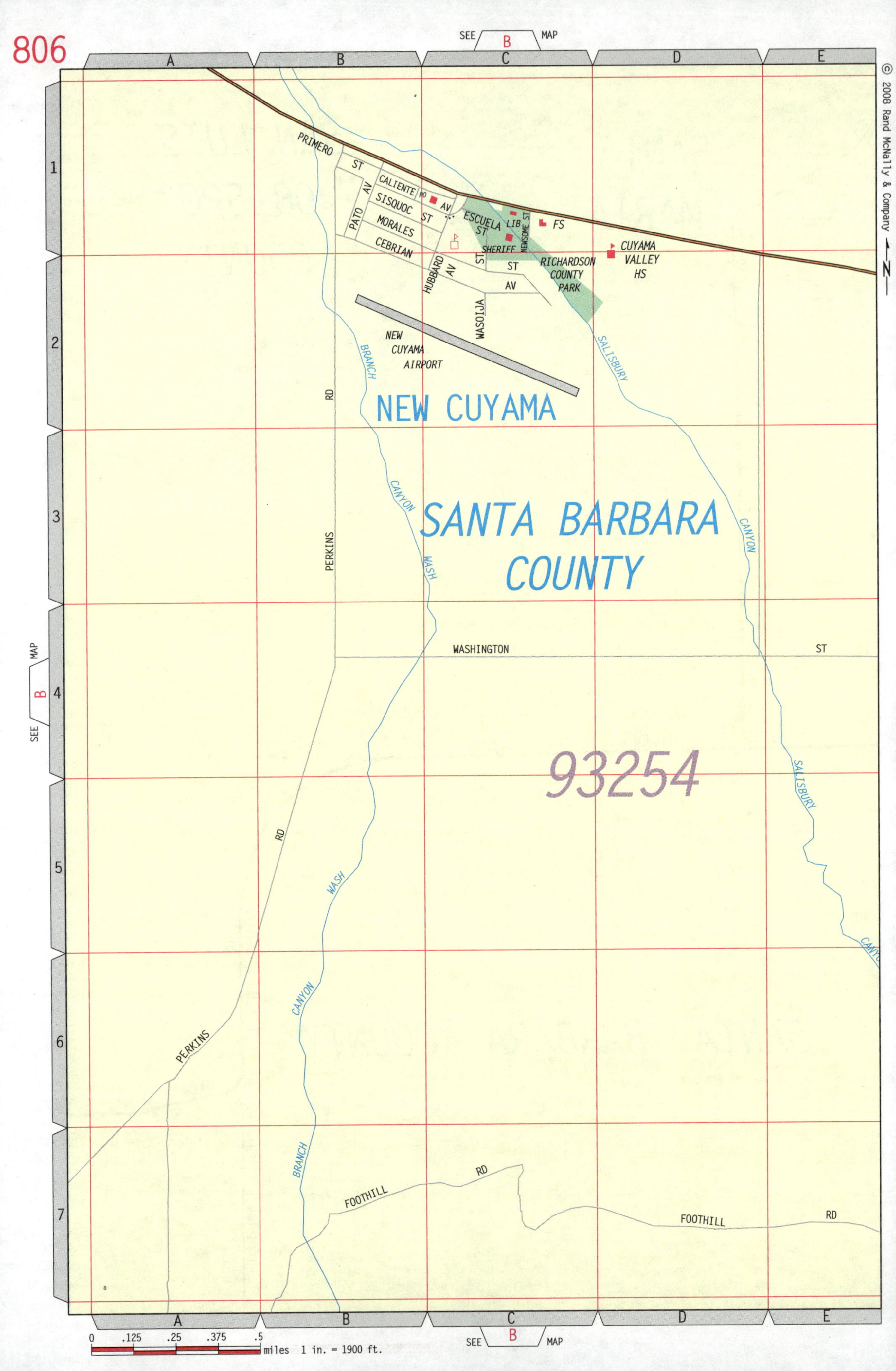

SEE B MAP
A
B
C
D
E
1
2
3
4
5
6
7
PRIMERO
ST
CALIENTE
PO
AV
SISQUOC
ST
PATO
AV
MORALES
CEBRIAN
ESCUELA
ST
LIB
NEWSOME ST
FS
SHERIFF
CUYAMA
VALLEY
HS
RICHARDSON
COUNTY
PARK
HUBBARD
AV
ST
ST
AV
WASOIJA
NEW
CUYAMA
AIRPORT
BRANCH
SALISBURY
RD
NEW CUYAMA
CANYON
SANTA BARBARA
COUNTY
CANYON
PERKINS
WASH
WASHINGTON
ST
93254
SALISBURY
RD
WASH
CANYON
CANYON
PERKINS
BRANCH
RD
FOOTHILL
FOOTHILL
RD
0
.125
.25
.375
.5
miles 1 in. = 1900 ft.

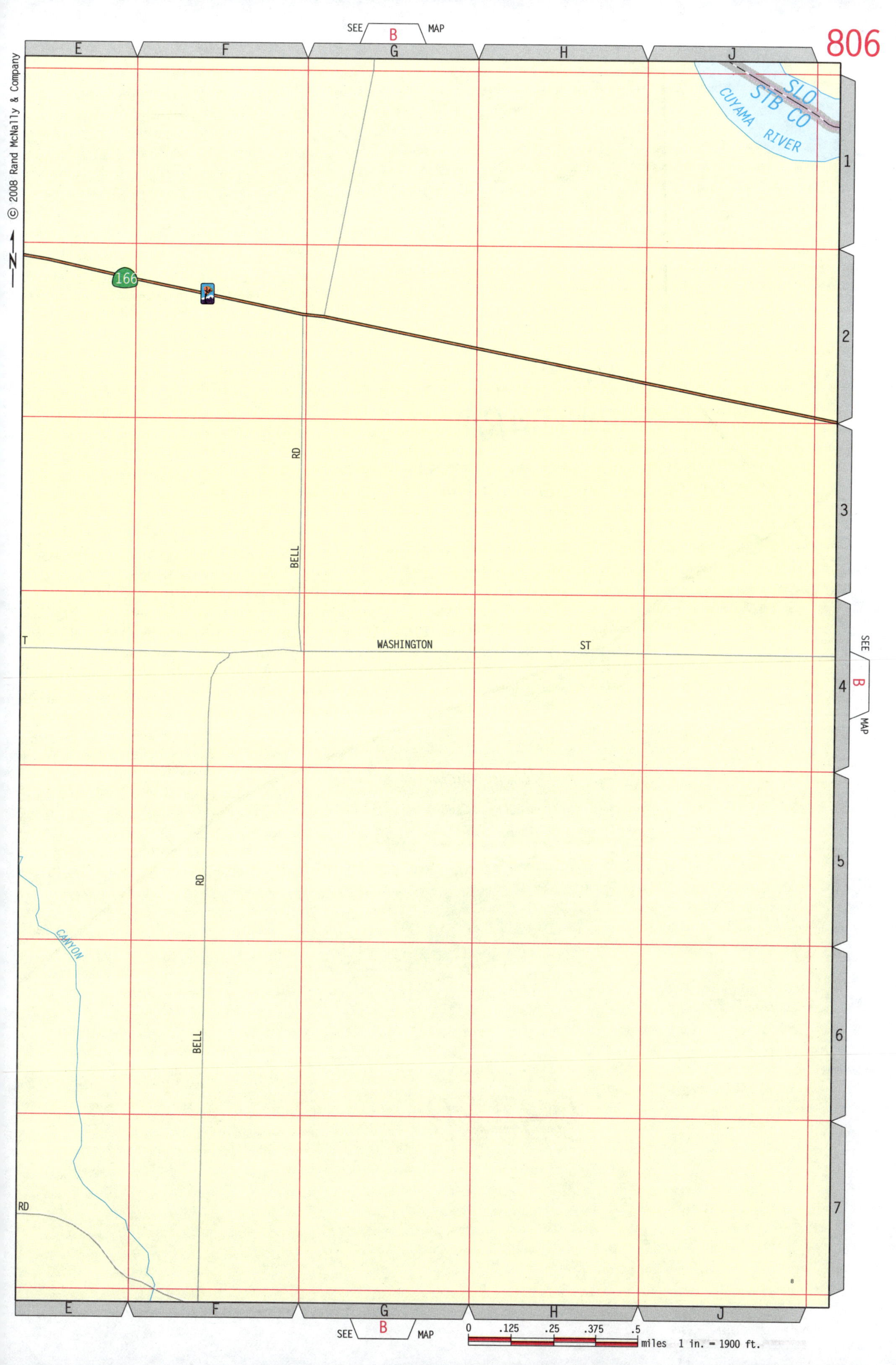
SEE B MAP
E
F
G
H
J
SLO
STB CO
CUYAMA RIVER
1
2
3
4
5
6
7
166
BELL RD
WASHINGTON ST
T
SEE B MAP
CANYON
RD
BELL RD
E
F
G
H
J
SEE B MAP
0 .125 .25 .375 .5
miles 1 in. = 1900 ft.

SEE 796 MAP

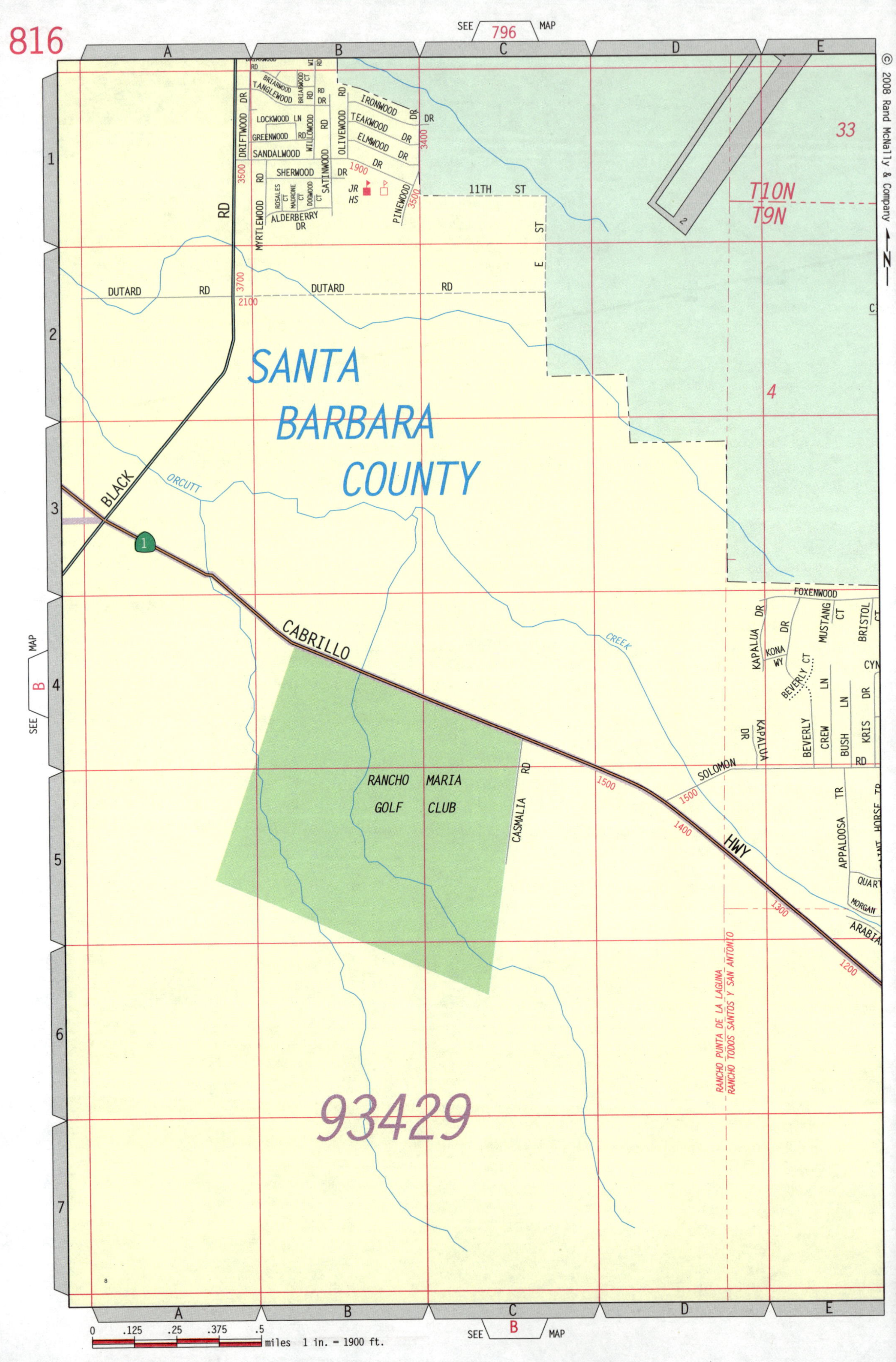
SANTA
BARBARA
COUNTY
93429
RANCHO MARIA
GOLF CLUB
CABRILLO HWY
BLACK RD
DUTARD RD
ORCUTT CREEK
11TH ST
E ST
CASMALIA RD
SOLOMON RD
FOXENWOOD
KAPALUA DR
KONA WY
BEVERLY CT
BEVERLY LN
CREW LN
BUSH LN
KRIS DR
MUSTANG CT
BRISTOL
APPALOOSA TR
MORGAN
ARABIAN
DRIFTWOOD DR
MYRTLEWOOD RD
IRONWOOD DR
TEAKWOOD DR
ELMWOOD DR
OLIVEWOOD DR
PINEWOOD
SATINWOOD
SHERWOOD DR
SANDALWOOD
GREENWOOD
LOCKWOOD LN
TANGLEWOOD
BRIARWOOD
ALDERBERRY DR
ROSALES CT
MADRONE CT
DOGWOOD CT
JR HS
T10N
T9N
33
4
RANCHO PUNTA DE LA LAGUNA
RANCHO TODOS SANTOS Y SAN ANTONIO
0 .125 .25 .375 .5 miles 1 in. = 1900 ft.

SEE B MAP

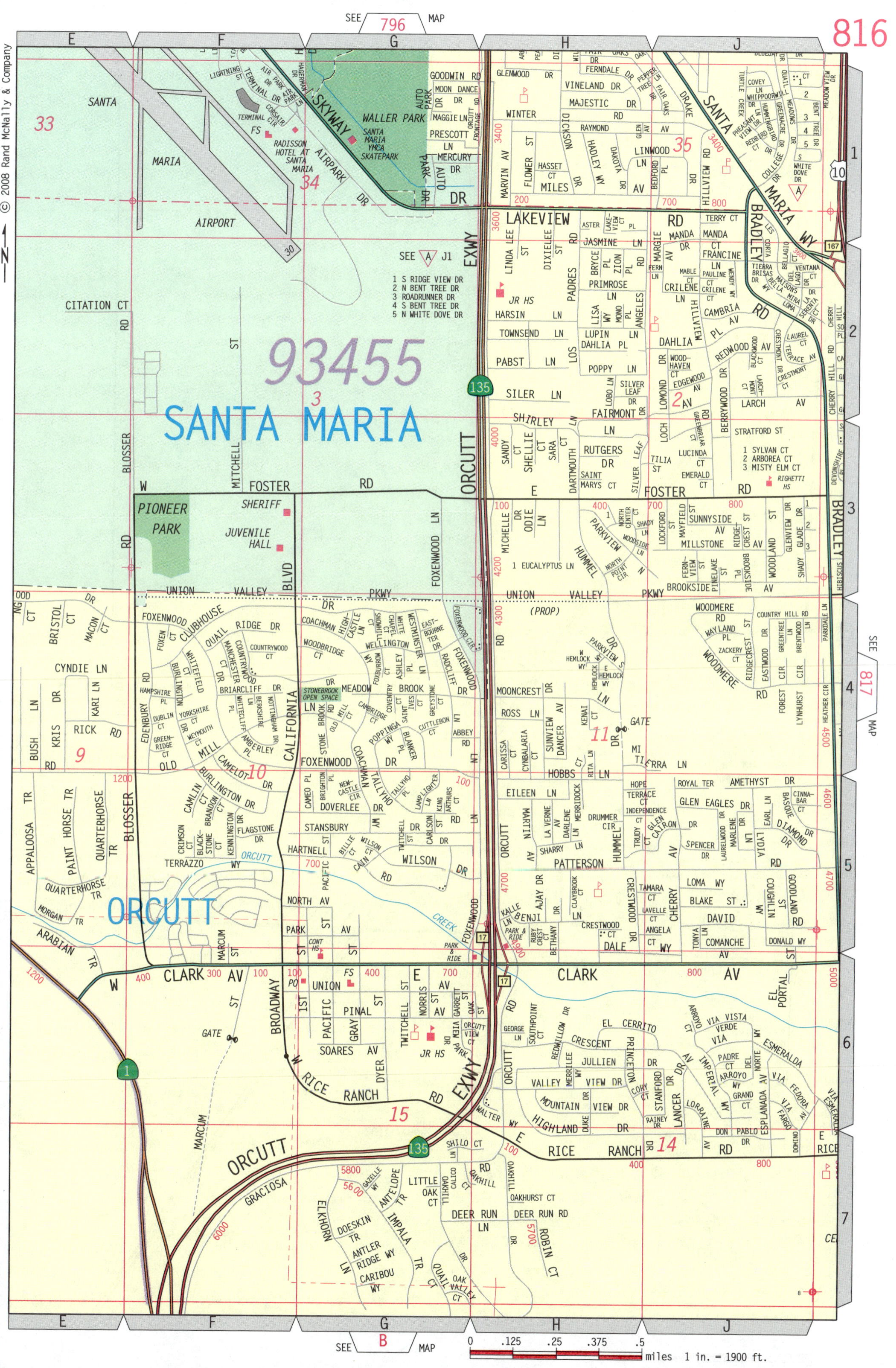
SEE 796 MAP
SANTA MARIA
93455
SANTA MARIA
ORCUTT
SANTA MARIA AIRPORT
WALLER PARK
SANTA MARIA YMCA SKATEPARK
RADISSON HOTEL AT SANTA MARIA
PIONEER PARK
SHERIFF
JUVENILE HALL
STONEBROOK OPEN SPACE
JR HS
RIGHETTI HS
CONT HS
SKYWAY
AIRPARK DR
LAKEVIEW RD
FOSTER RD
UNION VALLEY PKWY
CLARK AV
RICE RANCH RD
ORCUTT EXWY
BLOSSER RD
CALIFORNIA BLVD
BROADWAY
BRADLEY RD
SANTA MARIA WY
FOXENWOOD LN
ORCUTT CREEK
GRACIOSA
135
1
SEE A J1
1 S RIDGE VIEW DR
2 N BENT TREE DR
3 ROADRUNNER DR
4 S BENT TREE DR
5 N WHITE DOVE DR
1 SYLVAN CT
2 ARBOREA CT
3 MISTY ELM CT
SEE 817 MAP
SEE B MAP
0 .125 .25 .375 .5 miles 1 in. = 1900 ft.

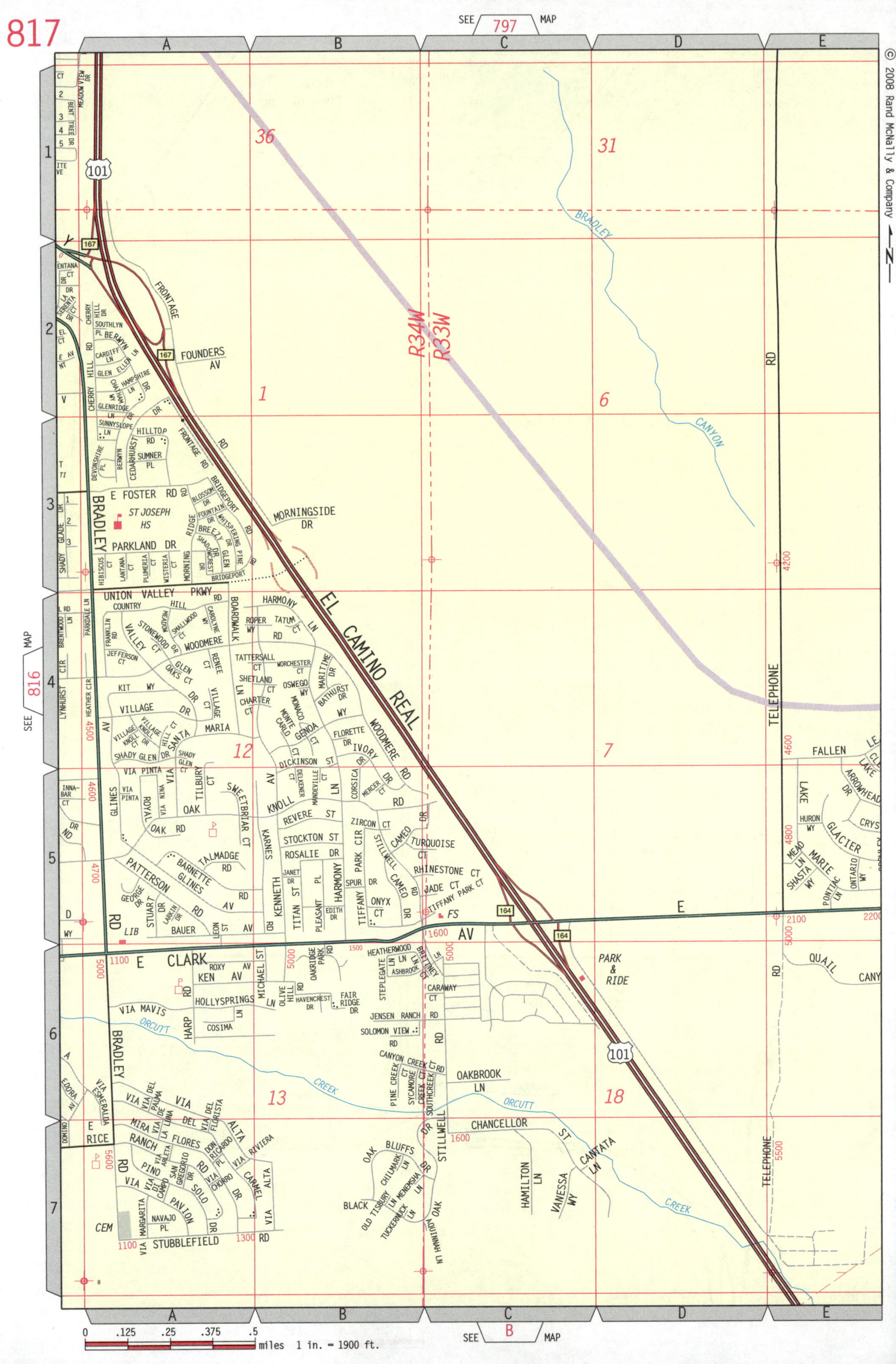
SEE 797 MAP
SEE 816 MAP
SEE B MAP
EL CAMINO REAL
TELEPHONE RD
BRADLEY RD
E CLARK AV
UNION VALLEY PKWY
E FOSTER RD
STILLWELL RD
ORCUTT CREEK
BRADLEY CANYON
ST JOSEPH HS
PARK & RIDE
CEM
LIB
FS
R34W
R33W
STUBBLEFIELD RD
CHANCELLOR ST
OAKBROOK LN
FOUNDERS AV
MORNINGSIDE DR
0 .125 .25 .375 .5 miles 1 in. = 1900 ft.

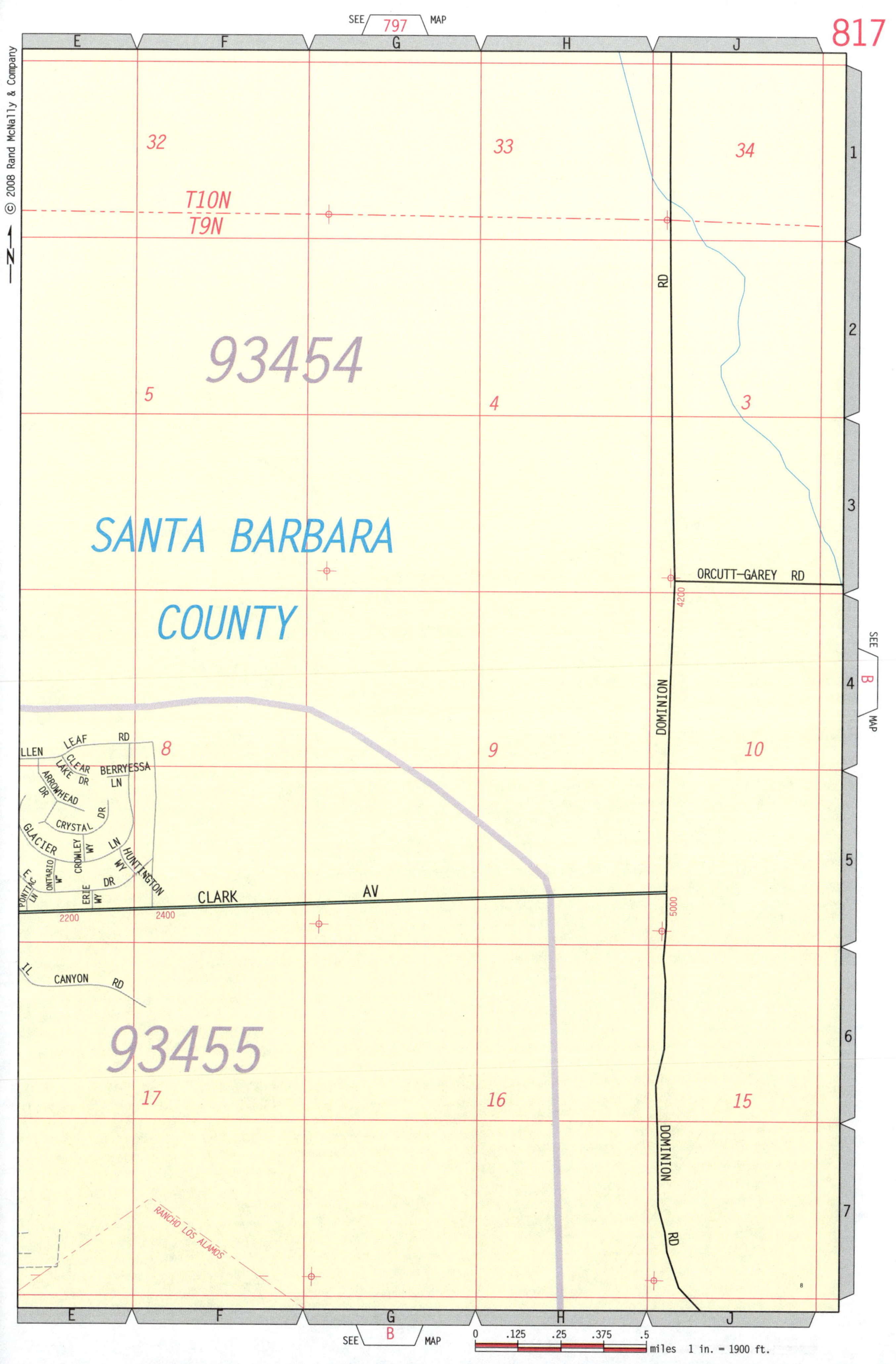
SEE 797 MAP
E
F
G
H
J
1
2
3
4
5
6
7
32
33
34
T10N
T9N
RD
93454
5
4
3
SANTA BARBARA
COUNTY
ORCUTT-GAREY RD
4200
SEE B MAP
DOMINION
LEAF RD
LLEN
CLEAR LAKE DR
BERRYESSA LN
ARROWHEAD DR
CRYSTAL DR
GLACIER
CROWLEY WY
LN
HUNTINGTON
WY
ONTARIO WY
PONTIAC LN
ERIE WY
DR
8
9
10
CLARK AV
2200
2400
5000
CANYON RD
93455
17
16
15
DOMINION RD
RANCHO LOS ALAMOS
SEE B MAP
0 .125 .25 .375 .5 miles 1 in. = 1900 ft.

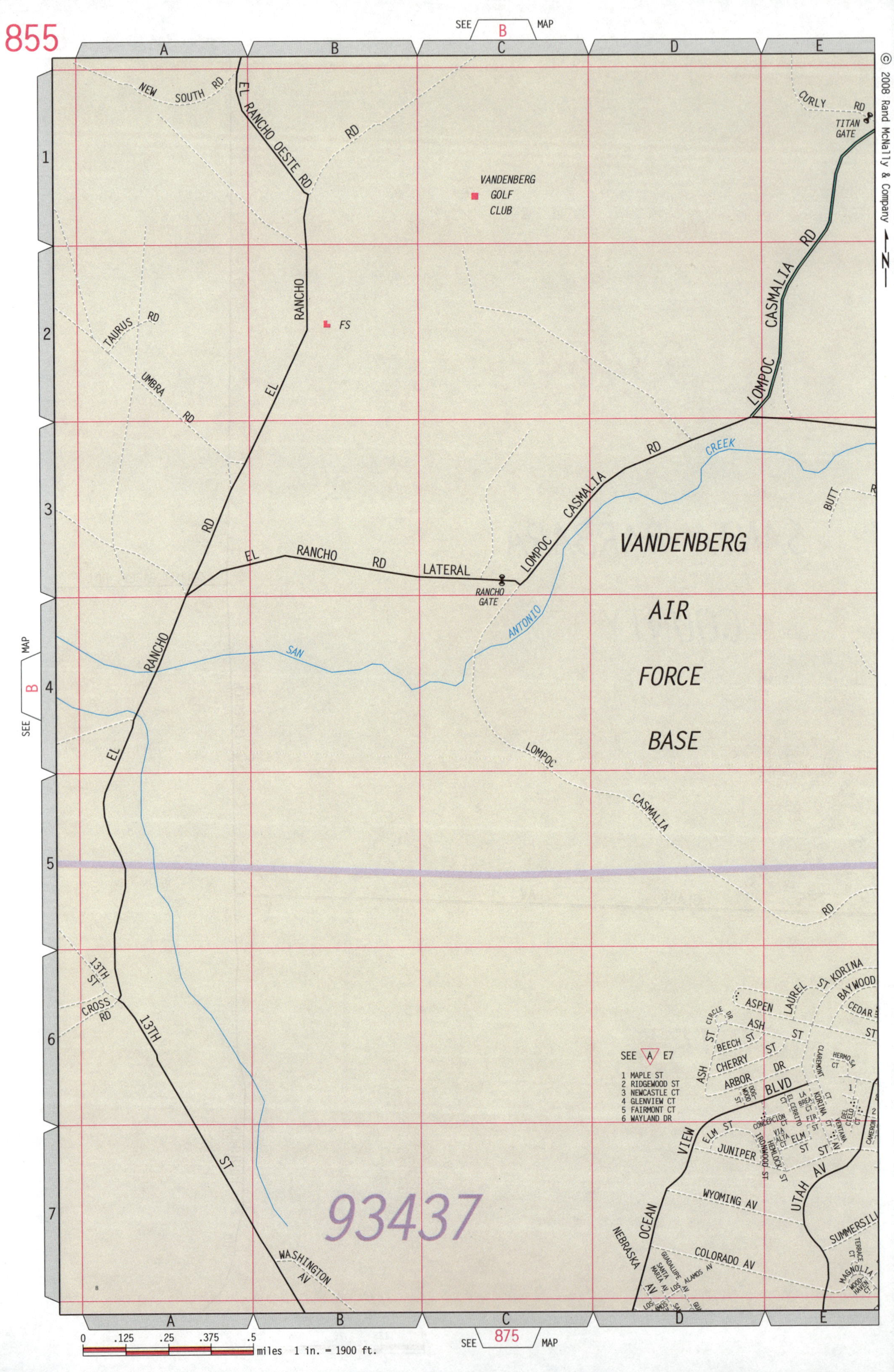

SEE B MAP
A
B
C
D
E
1
2
3
4
5
6
7
NEW SOUTH RD
EL RANCHO OESTE RD
RD
VANDENBERG GOLF CLUB
CURLY RD
TITAN GATE
LOMPOC CASMALIA RD
TAURUS RD
EL RANCHO RD
FS
UMBRA RD
CREEK
BUTT
EL RANCHO RD LATERAL
RANCHO GATE
VANDENBERG AIR FORCE BASE
SAN ANTONIO
SEE B MAP
EL RANCHO
LOMPOC CASMALIA RD
13TH ST
CROSS RD
13TH ST
ASPEN
LAUREL ST
KORINA
BAYWOOD
CEDAR
CIRCLE DR
ASH ST
BEECH ST
CHERRY ST
ARBOR DR
CLAREMONT
HERMOSA CT
BLVD
SEE A E7
1 MAPLE ST
2 RIDGEWOOD ST
3 NEWCASTLE CT
4 GLENVIEW CT
5 FAIRMONT CT
6 WAYLAND DR
ELM ST
JUNIPER
IRONWOOD ST
HEMLOCK ST
ELM ST
UTAH AV
VIEW
WYOMING AV
OCEAN
NEBRASKA AV
COLORADO AV
SUMMERSILL
MAGNOLIA
93437
WASHINGTON AV
SEE 875 MAP
0 .125 .25 .375 .5 miles 1 in. = 1900 ft.

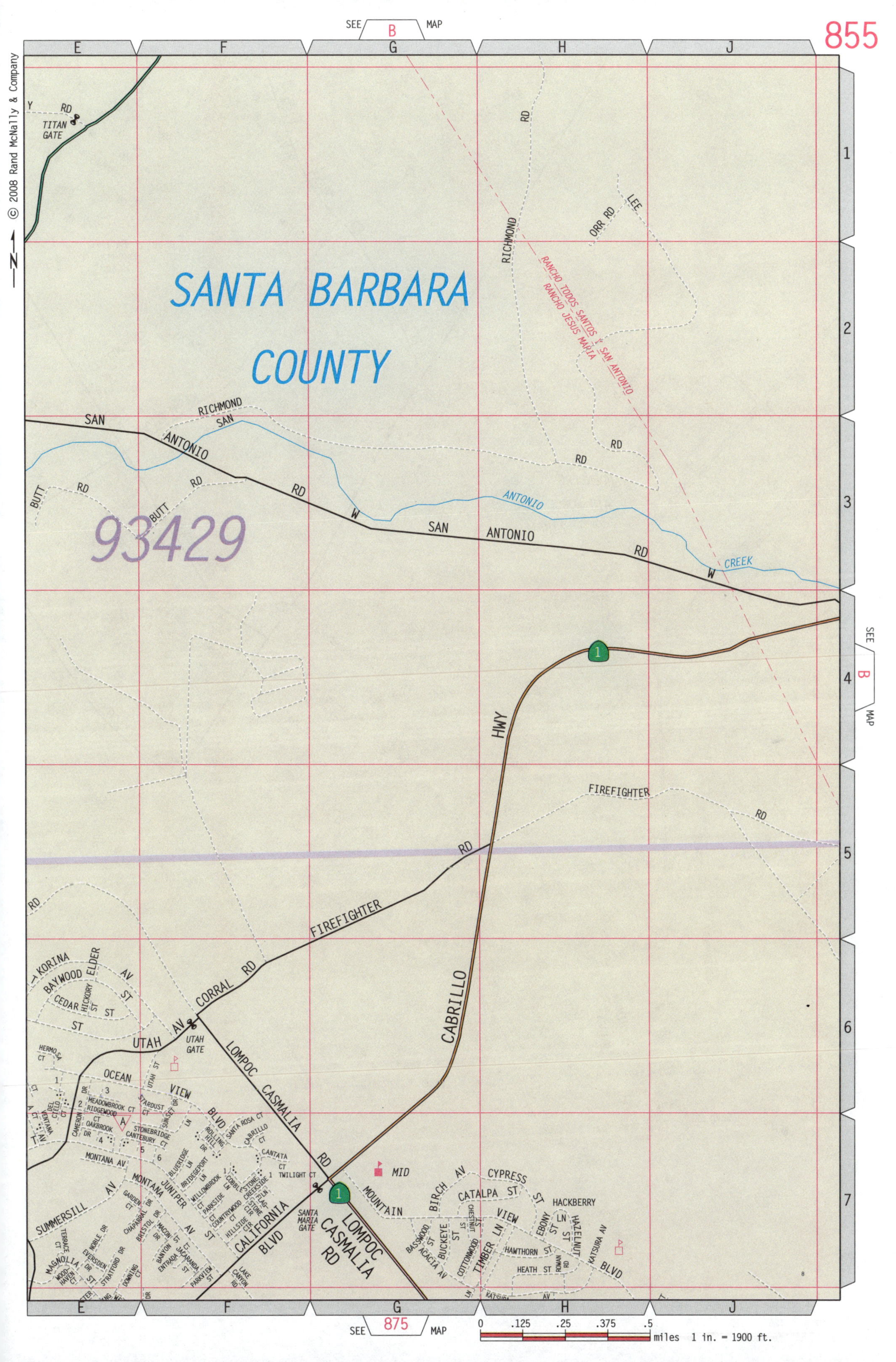

855
© 2008 Rand McNally & Company
SEE B MAP
SEE 875 MAP
SANTA BARBARA COUNTY
93429
TITAN GATE
RICHMOND RD
ORR RD
LEE
RANCHO TODOS SANTOS Y SAN ANTONIO
RANCHO JESUS MARIA
SAN ANTONIO RD
W SAN ANTONIO RD
SAN ANTONIO CREEK
BUTT RD
CABRILLO HWY
FIREFIGHTER RD
CORRAL RD
UTAH AV
UTAH GATE
LOMPOC CASMALIA RD
OCEAN VIEW BLVD
CALIFORNIA BLVD
SANTA MARIA GATE
MOUNTAIN VIEW BLVD
CYPRESS ST
CATALPA ST
HACKBERRY
BIRCH AV
MID
SUMMERSILL AV
MONTANA AV
KORINA
BAYWOOD
ELDER AV
CEDAR ST
HICKORY ST
HAWTHORN ST
HEATH ST
TIMBER LN
KATSURA AV
miles 1 in. = 1900 ft.

SEE 855 MAP

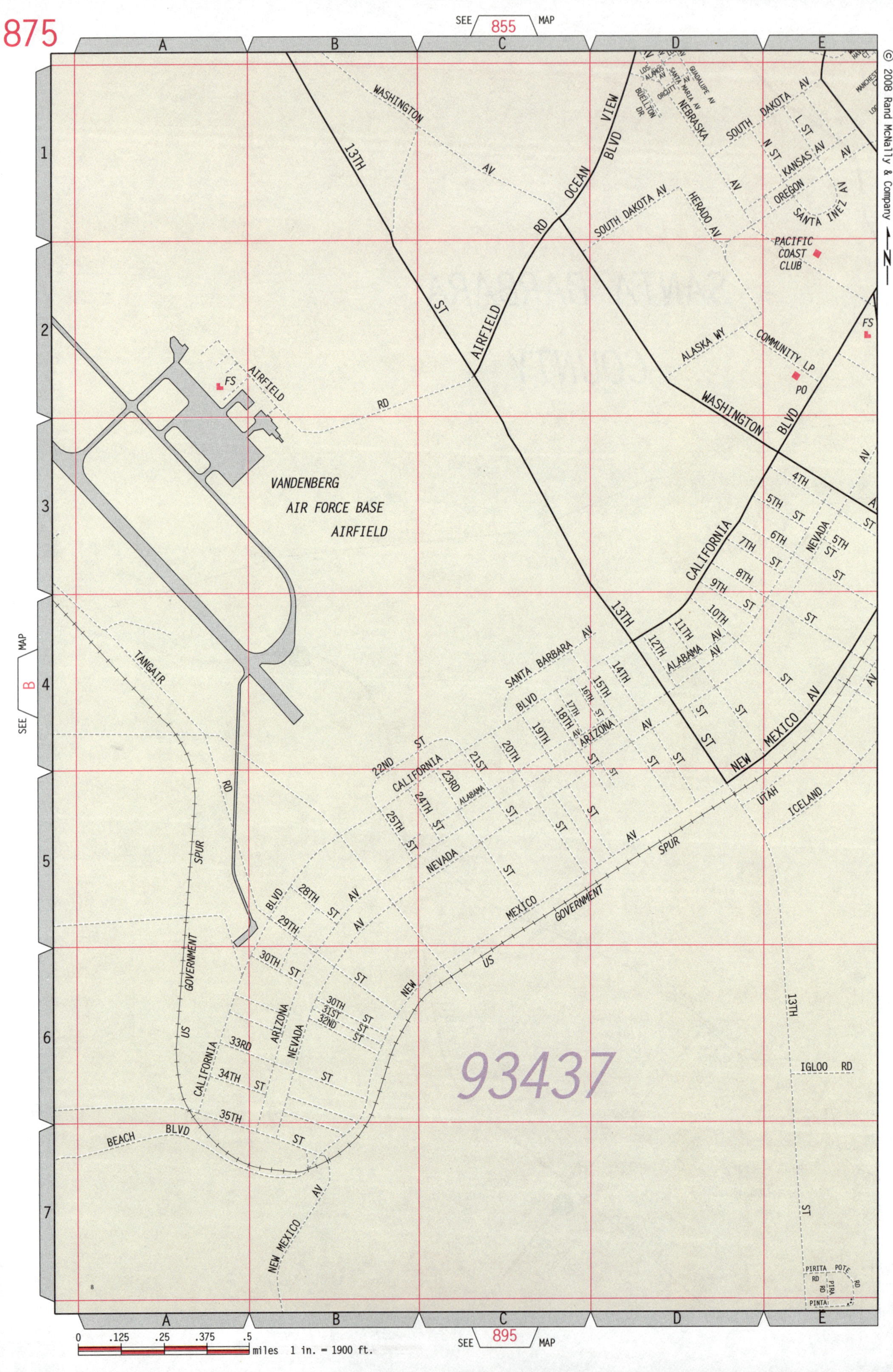
VANDENBERG
AIR FORCE BASE
AIRFIELD
93437
PACIFIC COAST CLUB
FS
PO
WASHINGTON AV
13TH ST
OCEAN VIEW BLVD
AIRFIELD RD
SOUTH DAKOTA AV
HERADO AV
NEBRASKA AV
KANSAS AV
OREGON AV
SANTA INEZ AV
ALASKA WY
COMMUNITY LP
WASHINGTON BLVD
CALIFORNIA BLVD
NEVADA AV
ALABAMA AV
ARIZONA AV
NEW MEXICO AV
SANTA BARBARA AV
UTAH
ICELAND
US GOVERNMENT SPUR
TANGAIR RD
BEACH BLVD
IGLOO RD
PIRITA RD
POTE RD
PINTA
© 2008 Rand McNally & Company

SEE B MAP

0 .125 .25 .375 .5 miles 1 in. = 1900 ft.

SEE 895 MAP

SEE 855 MAP

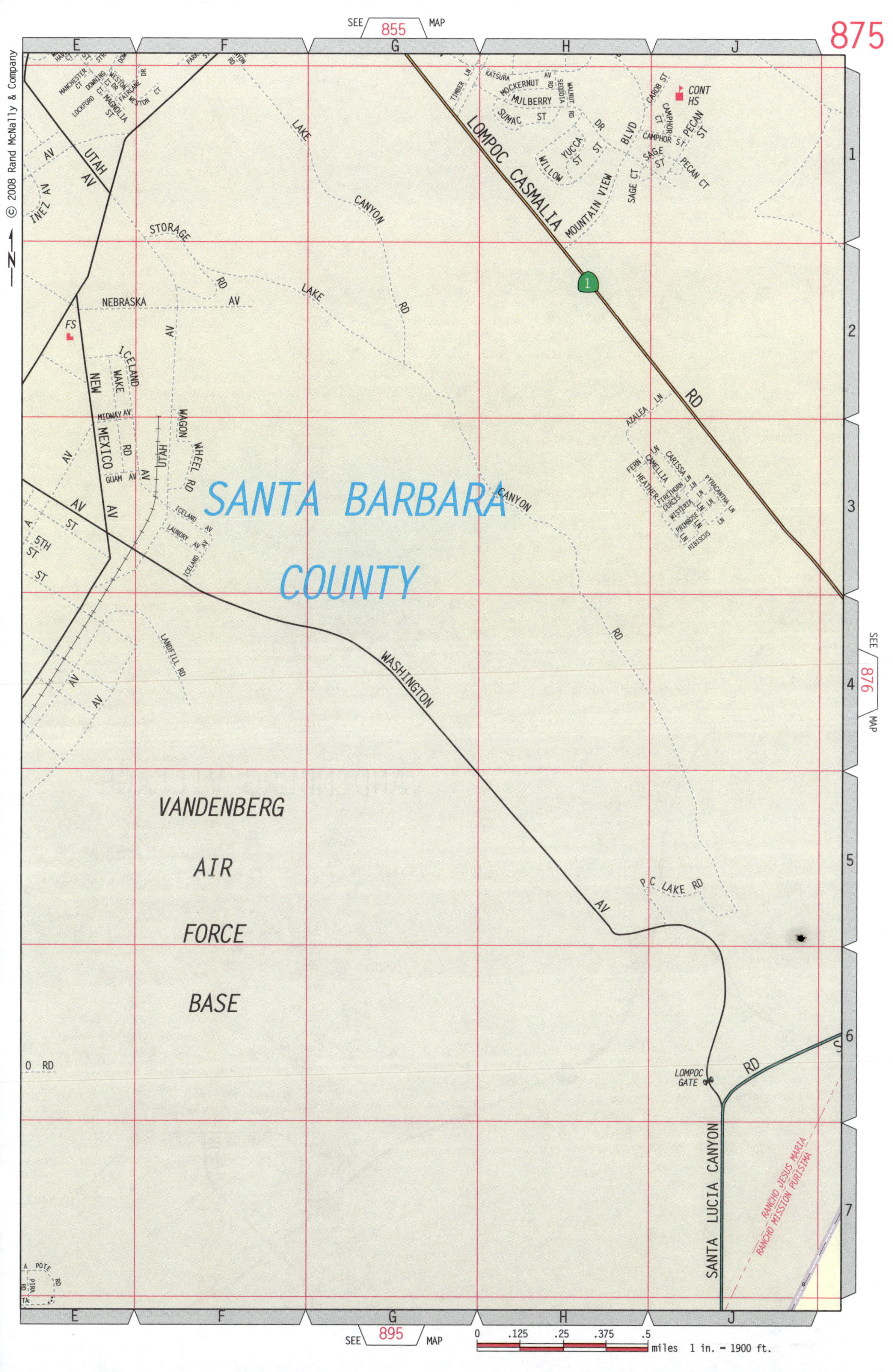
SANTA BARBARA
COUNTY
VANDENBERG
AIR
FORCE
BASE
LOMPOC CASMALIA RD
WASHINGTON AV
SANTA LUCIA CANYON RD
LOMPOC GATE
CONT HS
FS
STORAGE RD
NEBRASKA AV
LAKE CANYON RD
MOUNTAIN VIEW BLVD
P C LAKE RD
LANDFILL RD
WAGON WHEEL RD
NEW MEXICO AV
UTAH AV
ICELAND AV
LAUNDRY AV
RANCHO JESUS MARIA
RANCHO MISSION PURISIMA
miles 1 in. = 1900 ft.

SEE 876 MAP

SEE 895 MAP

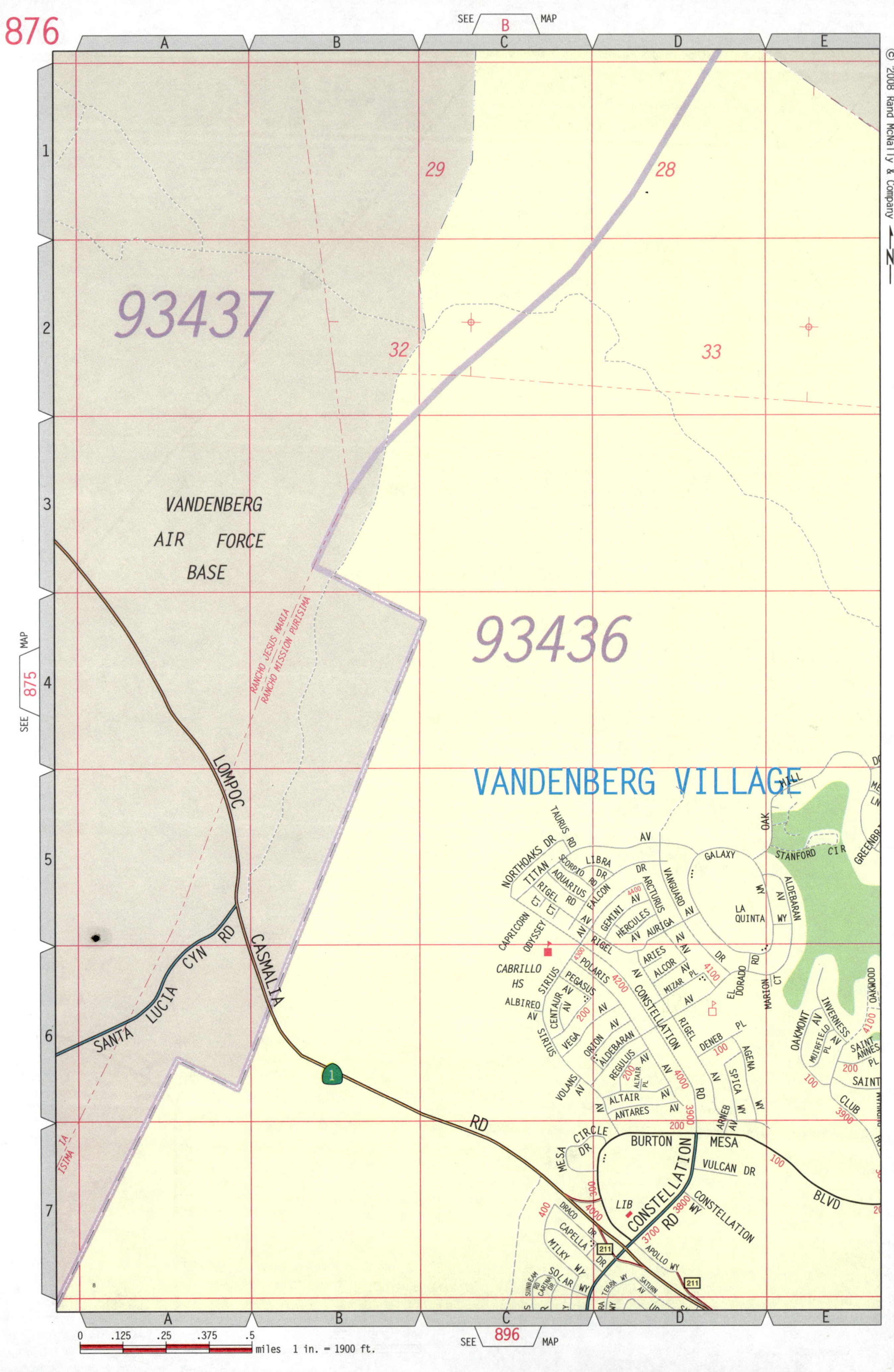
SEE B MAP
A
B
C
D
E
1
2
3
4
5
6
7
29
28
32
33
93437
93436
VANDENBERG
AIR FORCE
BASE
RANCHO JESUS MARIA
RANCHO MISSION PURISIMA
SEE 875 MAP
LOMPOC
CASMALIA
RD
SANTA LUCIA CYN RD
1
VANDENBERG VILLAGE
CABRILLO
HS
LIB
BURTON MESA BLVD
CONSTELLATION RD
CONSTELLATION WY
VULCAN DR
MESA CIRCLE DR
APOLLO WY
211
LA QUINTA WY
STANFORD CIR
OAK HILL
GALAXY
VANGUARD AV
TAURUS RD
NORTHOAKS DR
TITAN
SCORPIO RD
LIBRA DR
AQUARIUS RD
FALCON AV
ARCTURUS DR
GEMINI AV
HERCULES AV
AURIGA AV
RIGEL CT
RIGEL AV
RIGEL RD
CAPRICORN CT
ODYSSEY
POLARIS AV
ARIES AV
ALCOR AV
MIZAR PL
EL DORADO DR
MARION CT
ALDEBARAN AV
ALDEBARAN
SIRIUS AV
PEGASUS
CENTAUR AV
ALBIREO AV
VEGA AV
ORION AV
REGULUS AV
ALTAIR PL
ALTAIR AV
ANTARES AV
VOLANS AV
DENEB PL
DENEB AV
AGENA
SPICA WY
ARNEB AV
DRACO DR
CAPELLA DR
MILKY WY
SOLAR WY
SUNBEAM RD
CARINA DR
TERRA WY
SATURN AV
OAKMONT AV
INVERNESS
MUIRFIELD PL
SAINT ANNES PL
SAINT
CLUB
OAKWOOD
GREENBRIAR
4400
4300
4200
4100
4000
3900
3800
3700
400
300
200
100
3900
0 .125 .25 .375 .5 miles 1 in. = 1900 ft.
SEE 896 MAP

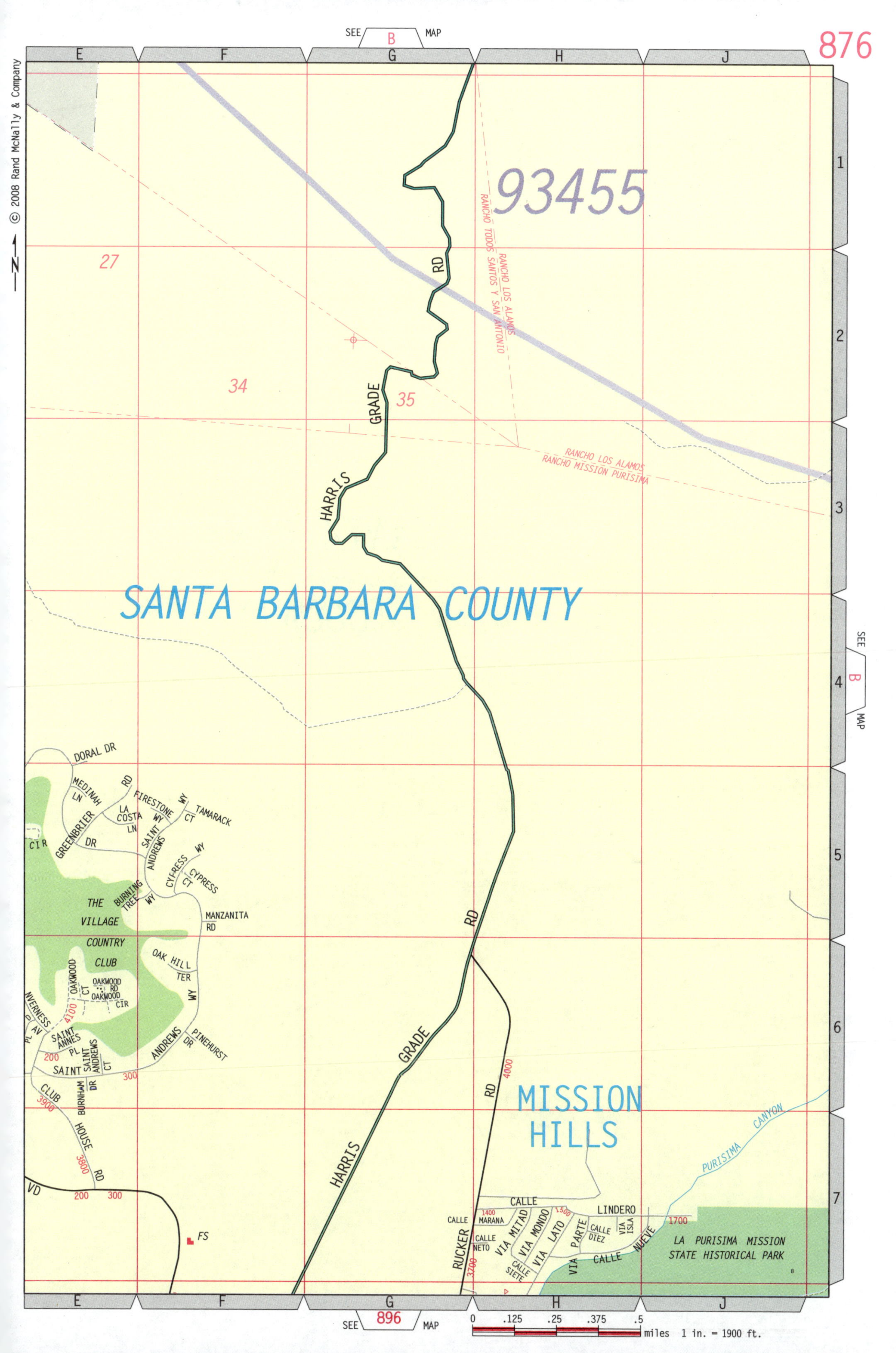

SEE B MAP
E
F
G
H
J
93455
RANCHO TODOS SANTOS Y SAN ANTONIO
RANCHO LOS ALAMOS
27
34
35
HARRIS GRADE RD
RANCHO LOS ALAMOS
RANCHO MISSION PURISIMA
SANTA BARBARA COUNTY
DORAL DR
MEDINAH LN
GREENBRIER DR
FIRESTONE RD
LA COSTA LN
WY
TAMARACK CT
SAINT ANDREWS WY
CIR
CYPRESS WY
CYPRESS CT
BURNING TREE WY
THE VILLAGE COUNTRY CLUB
MANZANITA RD
OAK HILL TER
OAKWOOD CT
OAKWOOD RD
OAKWOOD CIR
INVERNESS PL
AV
4100
SAINT ANNES PL
SAINT ANDREWS CT
SAINT ANDREWS WY
PINEHURST DR
200
300
BURNHAM DR
CLUB HOUSE RD
3900
3800
VD
FS
RUCKER RD
4000
3700
MISSION HILLS
CALLE LINDERO
CALLE MARANA
1400
1500
VIA MITAD
VIA MONDO
VIA LATO
VIA PARTE
CALLE DIEZ
VIA ISLA
CALLE NETO
CALLE SIETE
CALLE NUEVE
1700
PURISIMA CANYON
LA PURISIMA MISSION STATE HISTORICAL PARK
1
2
3
4
5
6
7
SEE B MAP
SEE 896 MAP
0 .125 .25 .375 .5 miles 1 in. = 1900 ft.

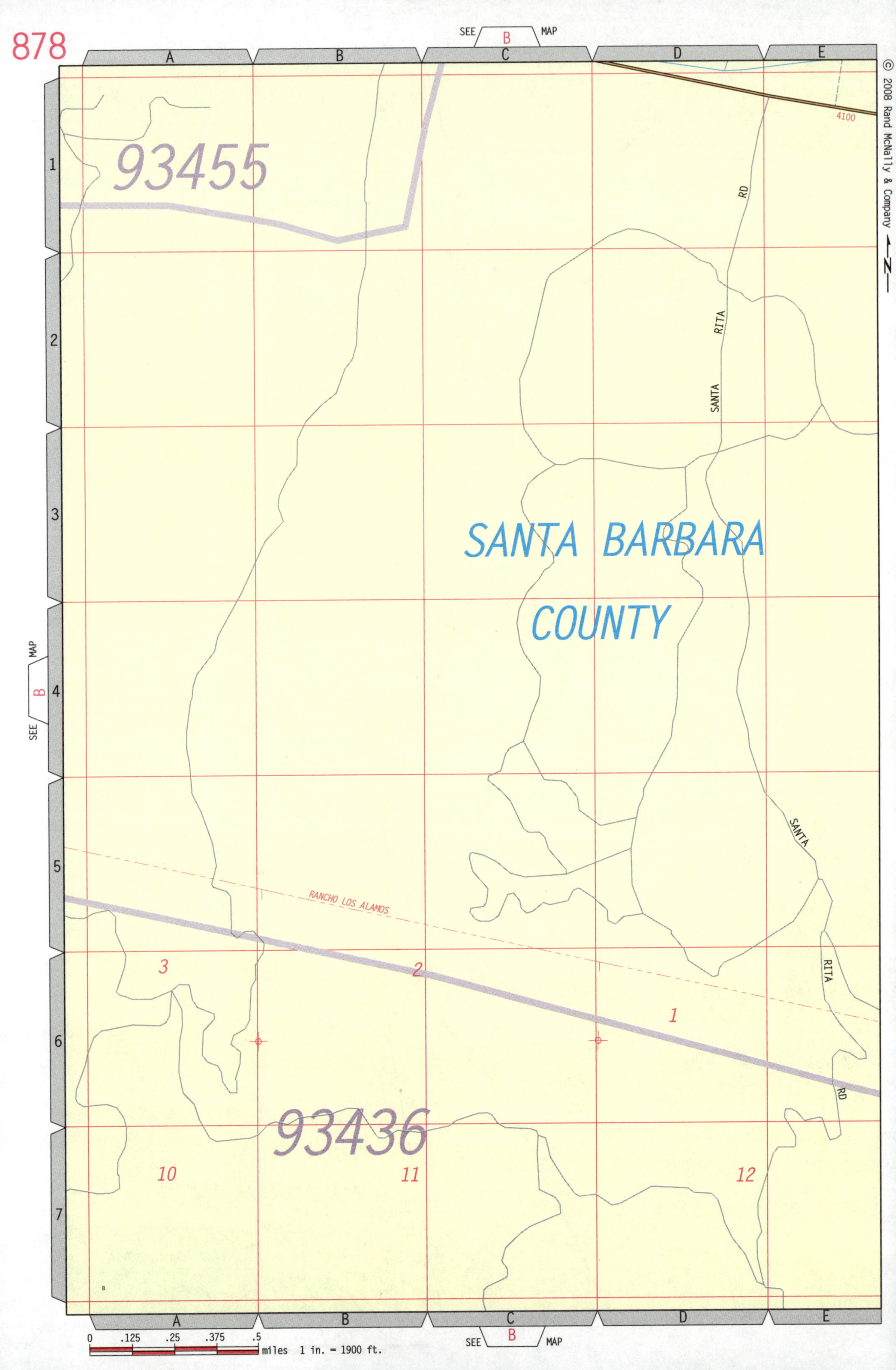
SEE B MAP
A
B
C
D
E
1
2
3
4
5
6
7
93455
4100
RD
RITA
SANTA
SANTA BARBARA
COUNTY
SEE B MAP
RANCHO LOS ALAMOS
SANTA
RITA
RD
3
2
1
93436
10
11
12
0 .125 .25 .375 .5
miles 1 in. = 1900 ft.
SEE B MAP

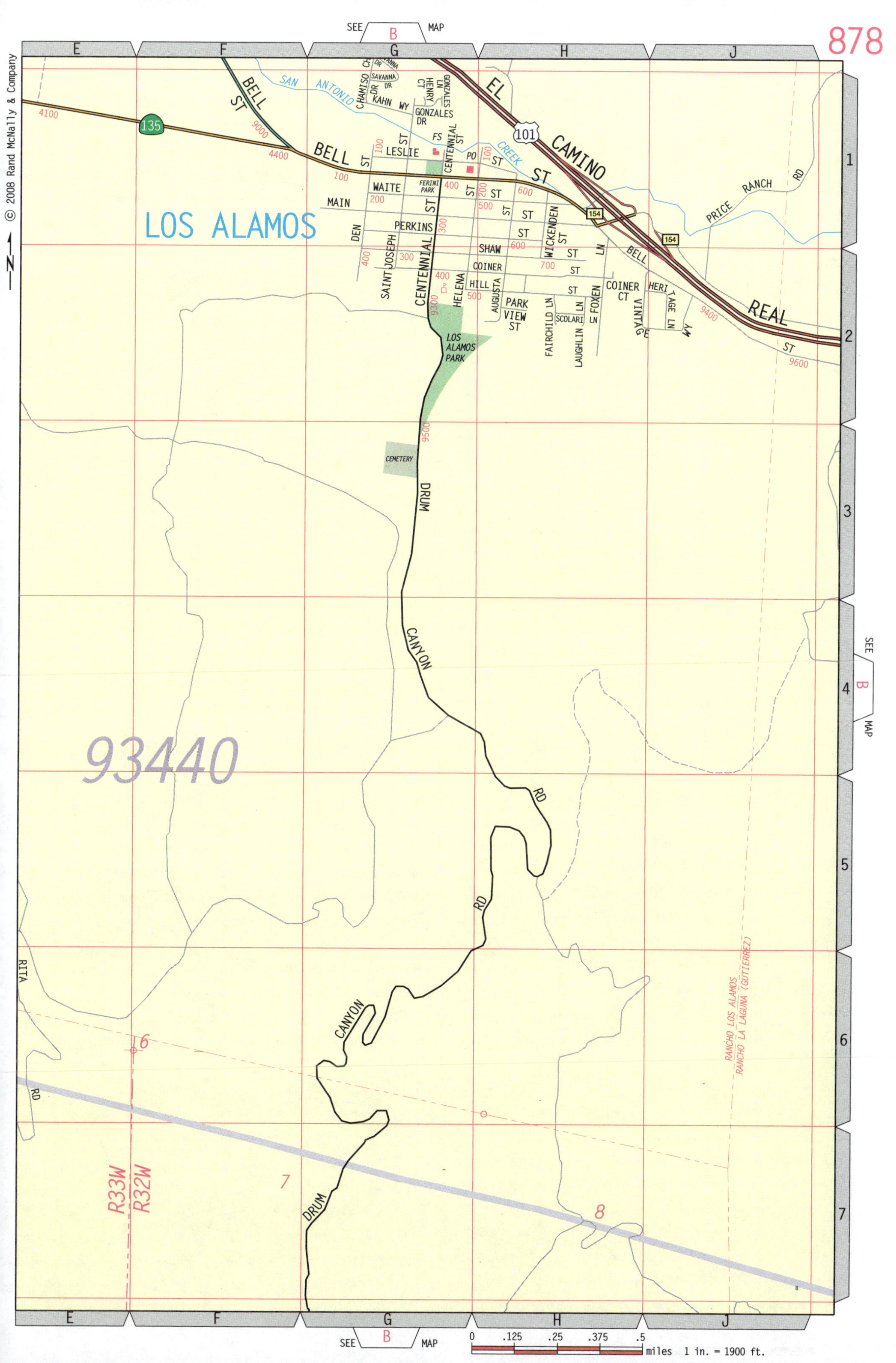
SEE B MAP
LOS ALAMOS
93440
BELL ST
SAN ANTONIO CREEK
EL CAMINO REAL
101
135
154
BELL ST
LESLIE
WAITE
MAIN
PERKINS
SHAW
COINER
HILL
PARK VIEW ST
CENTENNIAL ST
SAINT JOSEPH
HELENA
AUGUSTA
WICKENDEN ST
FAIRCHILD LN
SCOLARI
LAUGHLIN LN
FOXEN LN
COINER CT
HERITAGE LN
VINTAGE WY
GONZALES DR
KAHN WY
CHAMISO CT
SAVANNA DR
HENRY CT
GONZALES LN
FERINI PARK
FS
PO
PRICE RANCH RD
LOS ALAMOS PARK
CEMETERY
DRUM CANYON RD
RITA RD
RANCHO LOS ALAMOS
RANCHO LA LAGUNA (GUTIERREZ)
R33W
R32W
6
7
8
SEE B MAP
0 .125 .25 .375 .5 miles 1 in. = 1900 ft.

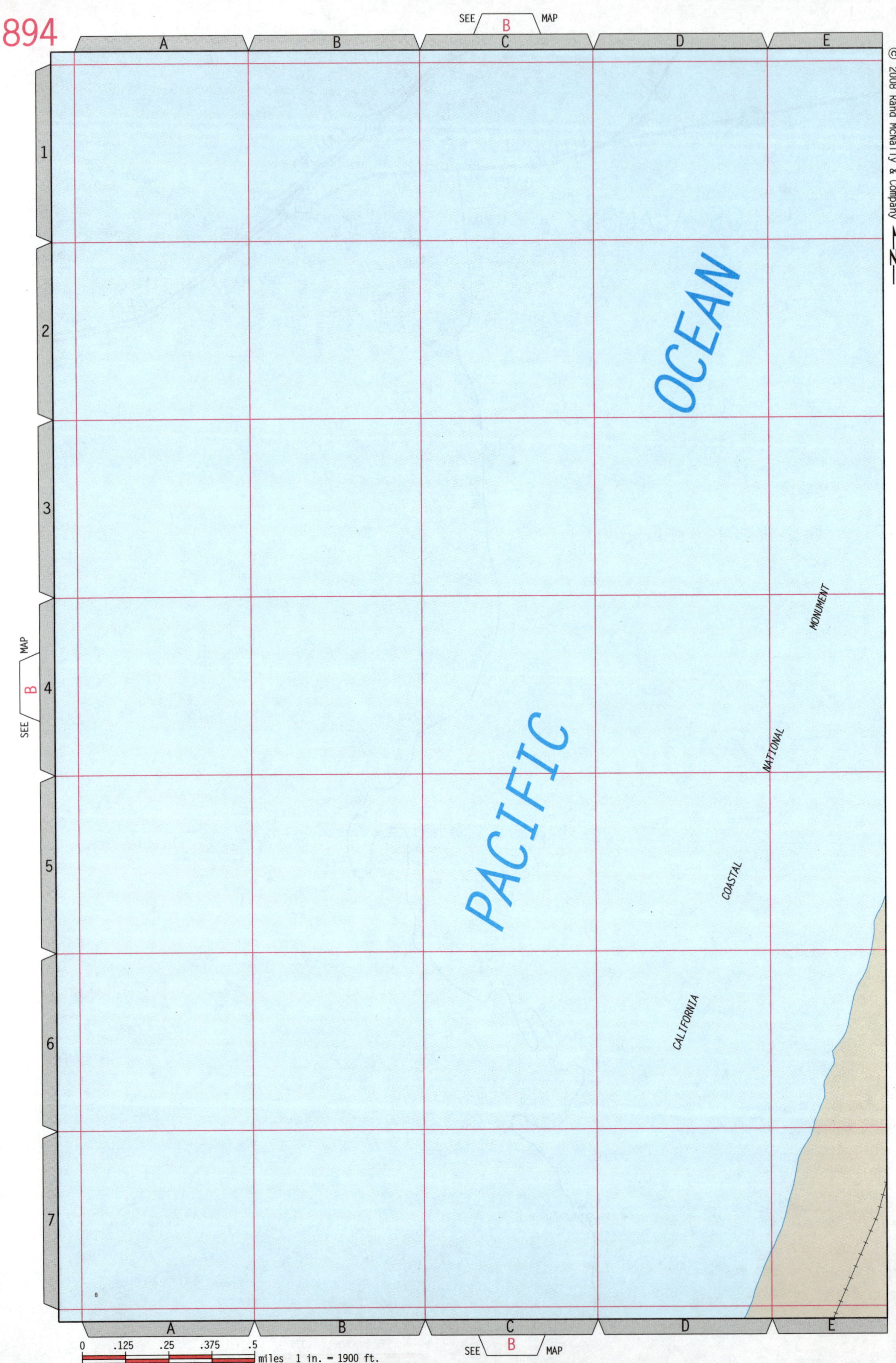

SEE B MAP
A
B
C
D
E
1
2
3
4
5
6
7
SEE B MAP
PACIFIC
OCEAN
CALIFORNIA
COASTAL
NATIONAL
MONUMENT
0
.125
.25
.375
.5
miles 1 in. = 1900 ft.

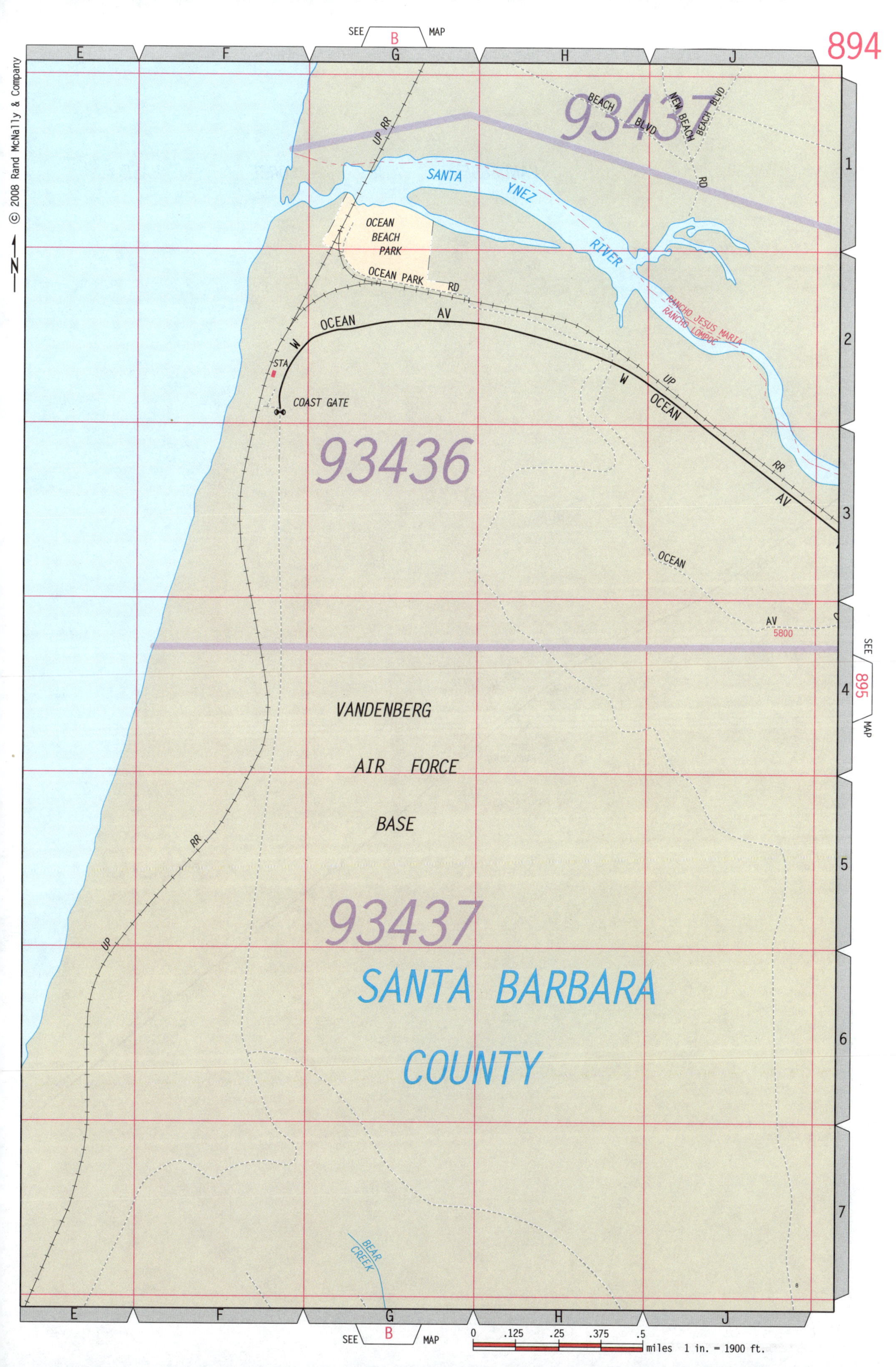
SEE B MAP
E
F
G
H
J
1
2
3
4
5
6
7
93437
BEACH BLVD
NEW BEACH
BEACH BLVD
RD
UP RR
SANTA YNEZ RIVER
OCEAN BEACH PARK
OCEAN PARK RD
RANCHO JESUS MARIA
RANCHO LOMPOC
OCEAN AV
W
STA
COAST GATE
W OCEAN
UP RR
AV
93436
OCEAN
AV
5800
SEE 895 MAP
VANDENBERG
AIR FORCE
BASE
RR
UP
93437
SANTA BARBARA
COUNTY
BEAR CREEK
0 .125 .25 .375 .5
miles 1 in. = 1900 ft.

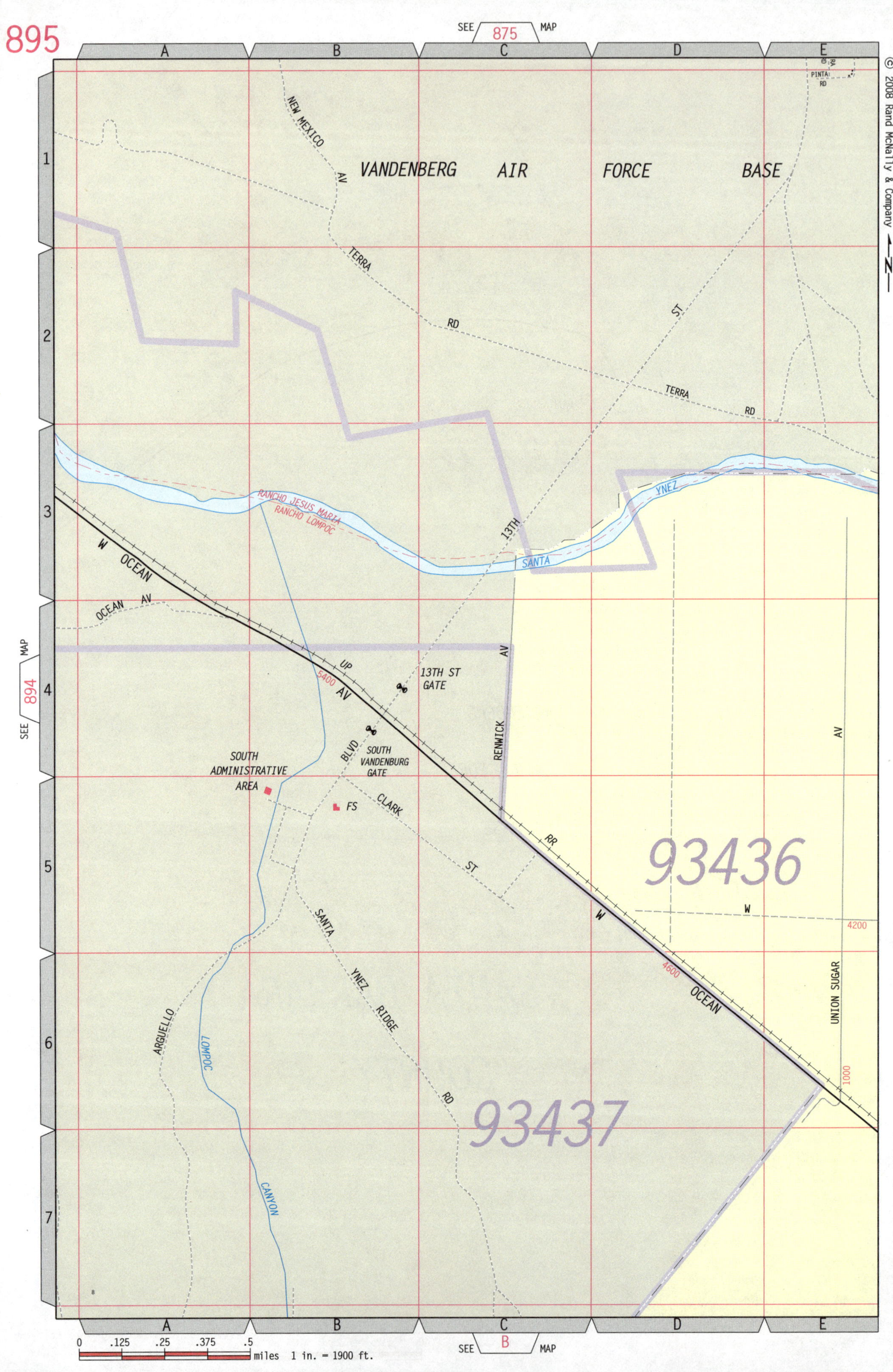

SEE 875 MAP
VANDENBERG AIR FORCE BASE
NEW MEXICO AV
TERRA RD
TERRA RD
ST
13TH
RANCHO JESUS MARIA
RANCHO LOMPOC
SANTA YNEZ
W OCEAN AV
OCEAN AV
UP
5400
13TH ST GATE
SOUTH VANDENBURG GATE
BLVD
SOUTH ADMINISTRATIVE AREA
FS
CLARK ST
RENWICK AV
RR
W OCEAN
4600
4200
93436
W
AV
UNION SUGAR
1000
SANTA YNEZ RIDGE RD
ARGUELLO
LOMPOC CANYON
93437
PINTA RD
SEE 894 MAP
SEE B MAP
0 .125 .25 .375 .5 miles 1 in. = 1900 ft.

SEE 875 MAP

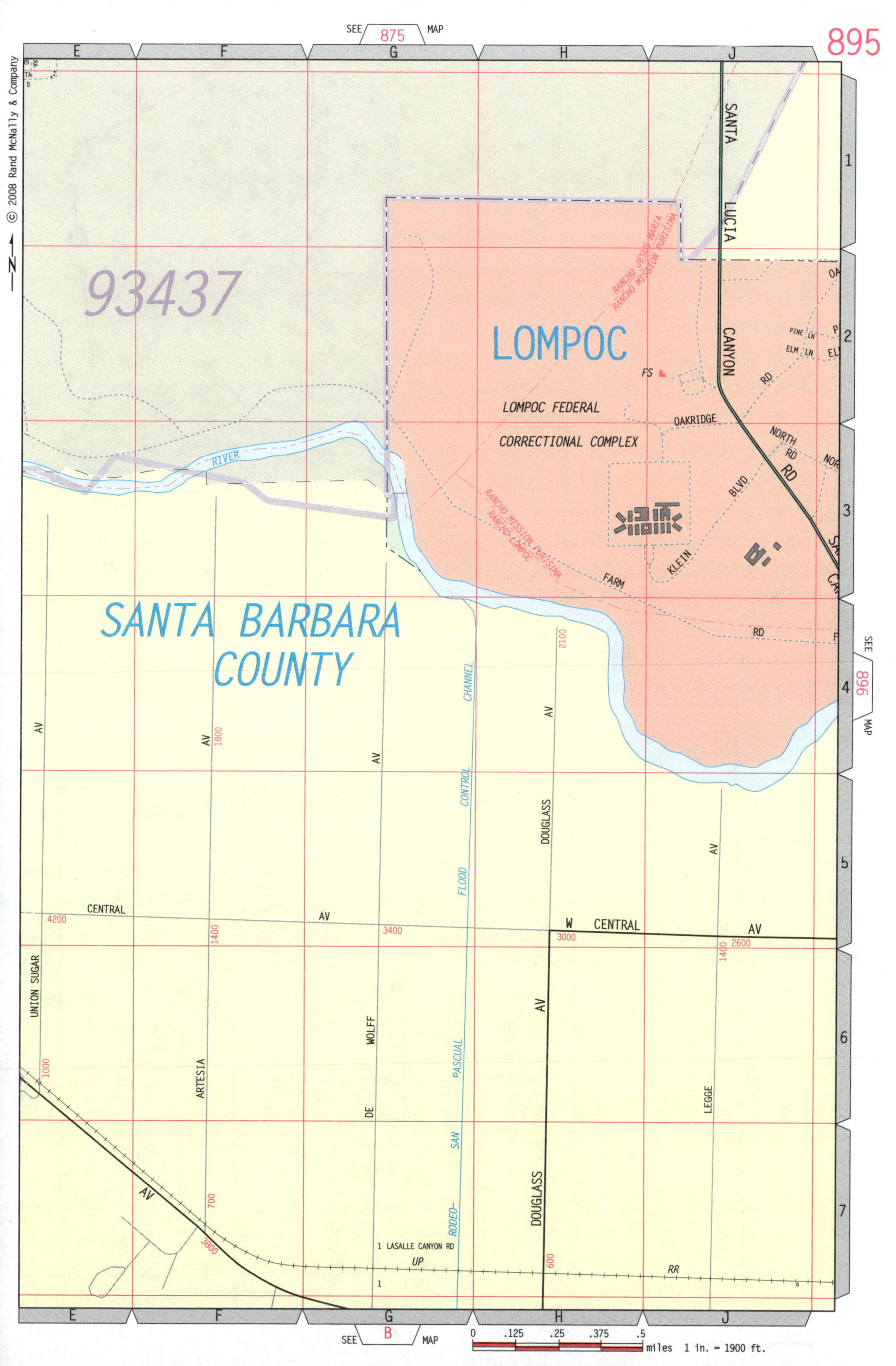
93437
LOMPOC
LOMPOC FEDERAL
CORRECTIONAL COMPLEX
SANTA BARBARA
COUNTY
SANTA
LUCIA
CANYON
RD
OAKRIDGE
NORTH
RD
KLEIN
BLVD
FARM
RD
FS
PINE LN
ELM LN
RANCHO JESUS MARIA
RANCHO MISSION PURISIMA
RANCHO LOMPOC
RIVER
CENTRAL
AV
W CENTRAL AV
UNION SUGAR AV
ARTESIA AV
DE WOLFF AV
DOUGLASS AV
LEGGE AV
SAN PASCUAL FLOOD CONTROL CHANNEL
RODEO-SAN
1 LASALLE CANYON RD
UP RR
4200
3400
3000
2600
2100
1800
1400
1000
700
3800
600

SEE 896 MAP
SEE B MAP
0 .125 .25 .375 .5 miles 1 in. = 1900 ft.

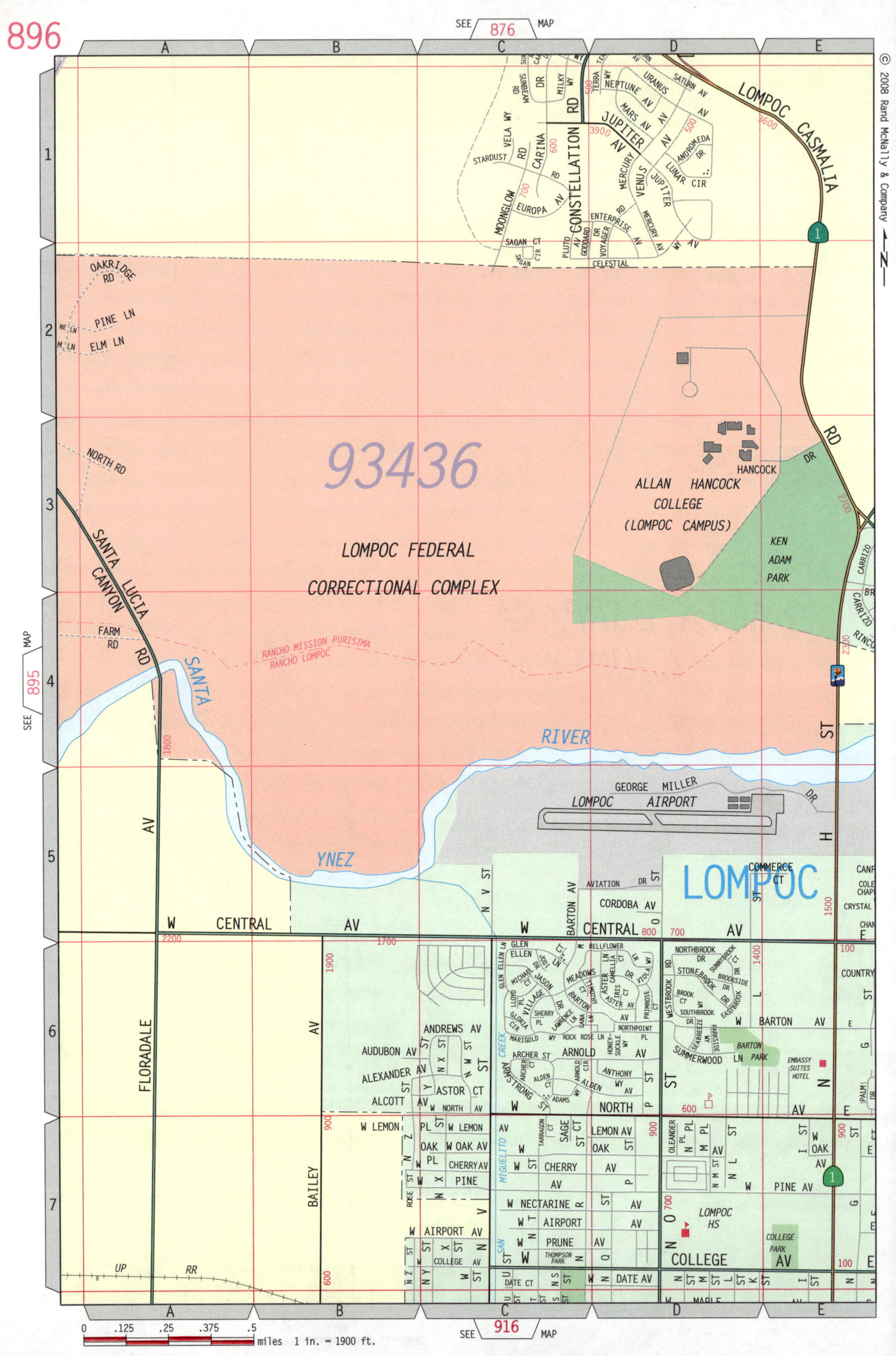
SEE 876 MAP
SEE 895 MAP
SEE 916 MAP
93436
LOMPOC FEDERAL
CORRECTIONAL COMPLEX
ALLAN HANCOCK
COLLEGE
(LOMPOC CAMPUS)
KEN
ADAM
PARK
LOMPOC CASMALIA RD
SANTA LUCIA CANYON RD
SANTA YNEZ RIVER
RANCHO MISSION PURISIMA
RANCHO LOMPOC
GEORGE MILLER DR
LOMPOC AIRPORT
LOMPOC
W CENTRAL AV
FLORADALE AV
BAILEY AV
CONSTELLATION RD
JUPITER AV
OAKRIDGE RD
PINE LN
ELM LN
NORTH RD
FARM RD
LOMPOC HS
BARTON PARK
EMBASSY SUITES HOTEL
UP RR
COLLEGE AV
0 .125 .25 .375 .5 miles 1 in. = 1900 ft.

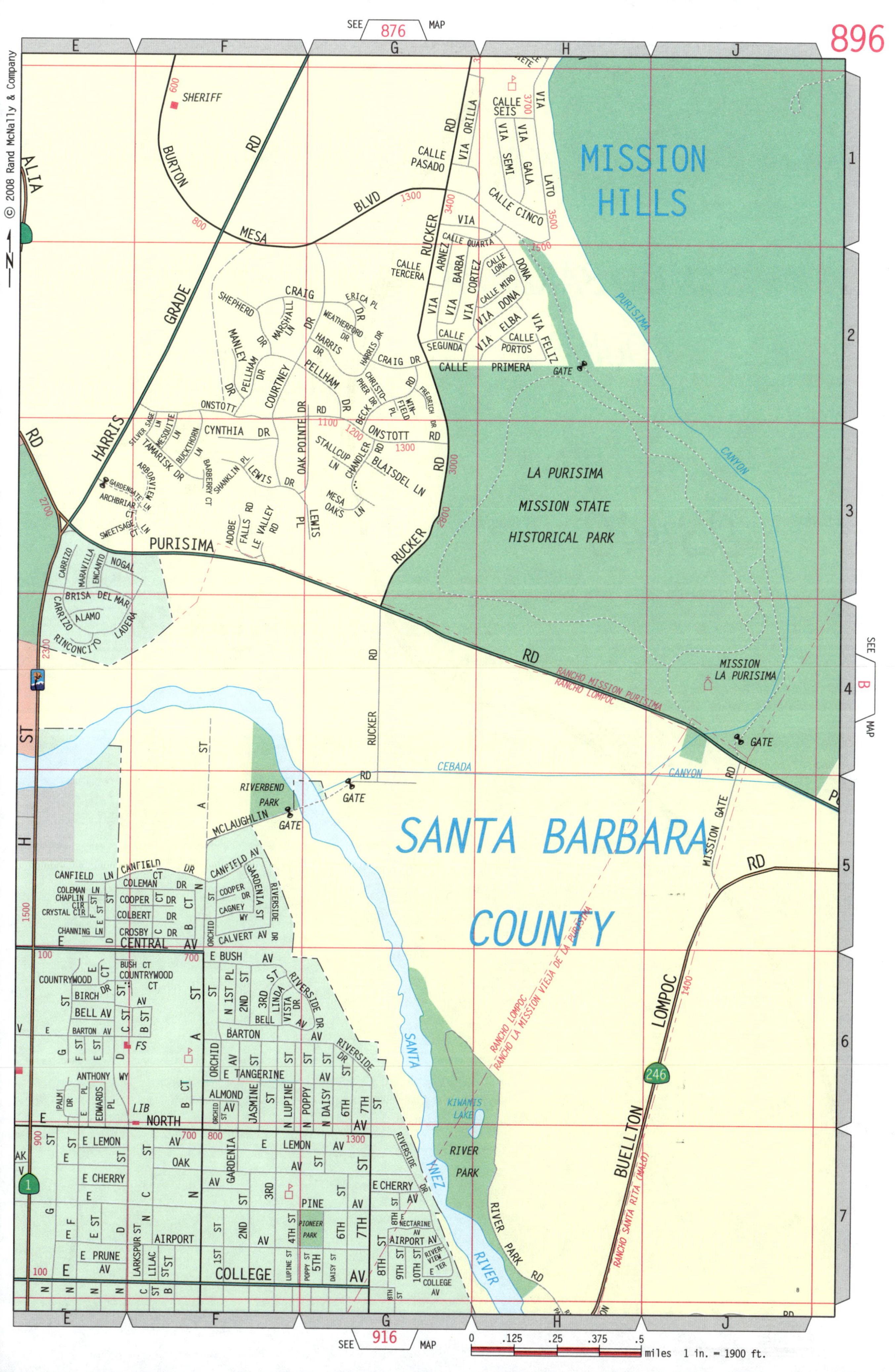

MISSION HILLS
LA PURISIMA MISSION STATE HISTORICAL PARK
SANTA BARBARA COUNTY
MISSION LA PURISIMA
RIVERBEND PARK
RIVER PARK
KIWANIS LAKE
PIONEER PARK
SHERIFF
BURTON MESA BLVD
HARRIS GRADE RD
RUCKER RD
PURISIMA RD
ONSTOTT RD
CRAIG DR
CYNTHIA DR
OAK POINTE DR
CENTRAL AV
NORTH AV
COLLEGE AV
MCLAUGHLIN
CEBADA CANYON RD
MISSION GATE RD
BUELLTON LOMPOC RD
RIVERSIDE DR
RIVER PARK RD
SANTA YNEZ RIVER
PURISIMA CANYON
RANCHO MISSION PURISIMA
RANCHO LOMPOC
RANCHO LA MISSION VIEJA DE LA PURISIMA
RANCHO SANTA RITA (MALO)
GATE

SEE 876 MAP
SEE B MAP
SEE 916 MAP

0 .125 .25 .375 .5 miles 1 in. = 1900 ft.

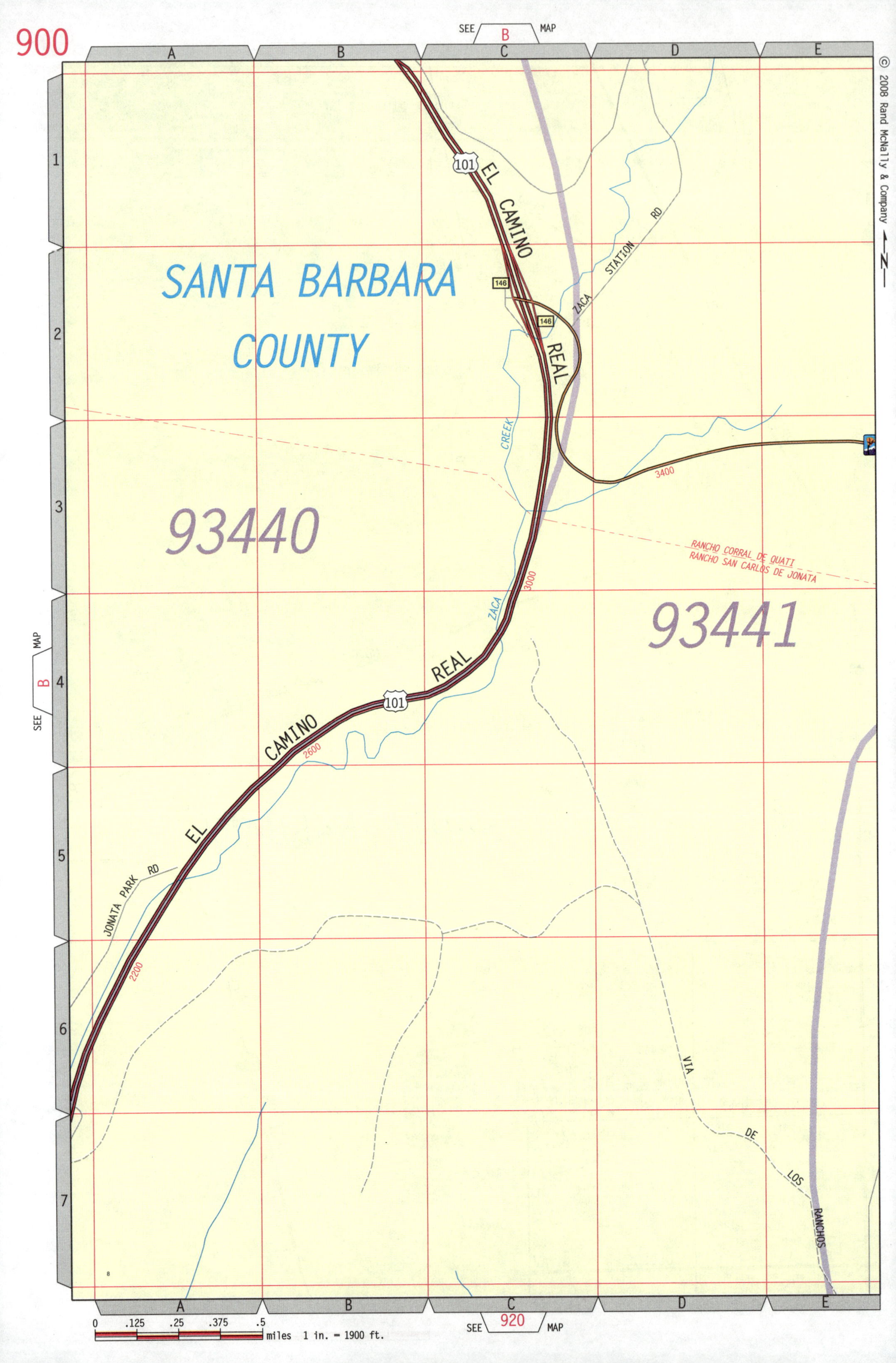
SEE B MAP
A
B
C
D
E
1
2
3
4
5
6
7
SANTA BARBARA
COUNTY
93440
93441
101
EL CAMINO REAL
146
ZACA STATION RD
ZACA CREEK
3400
3000
2600
2200
RANCHO CORRAL DE QUATI
RANCHO SAN CARLOS DE JONATA
JONATA PARK RD
VIA DE LOS RANCHOS
SEE B MAP
SEE 920 MAP
0 .125 .25 .375 .5
miles 1 in. = 1900 ft.

SEE B MAP 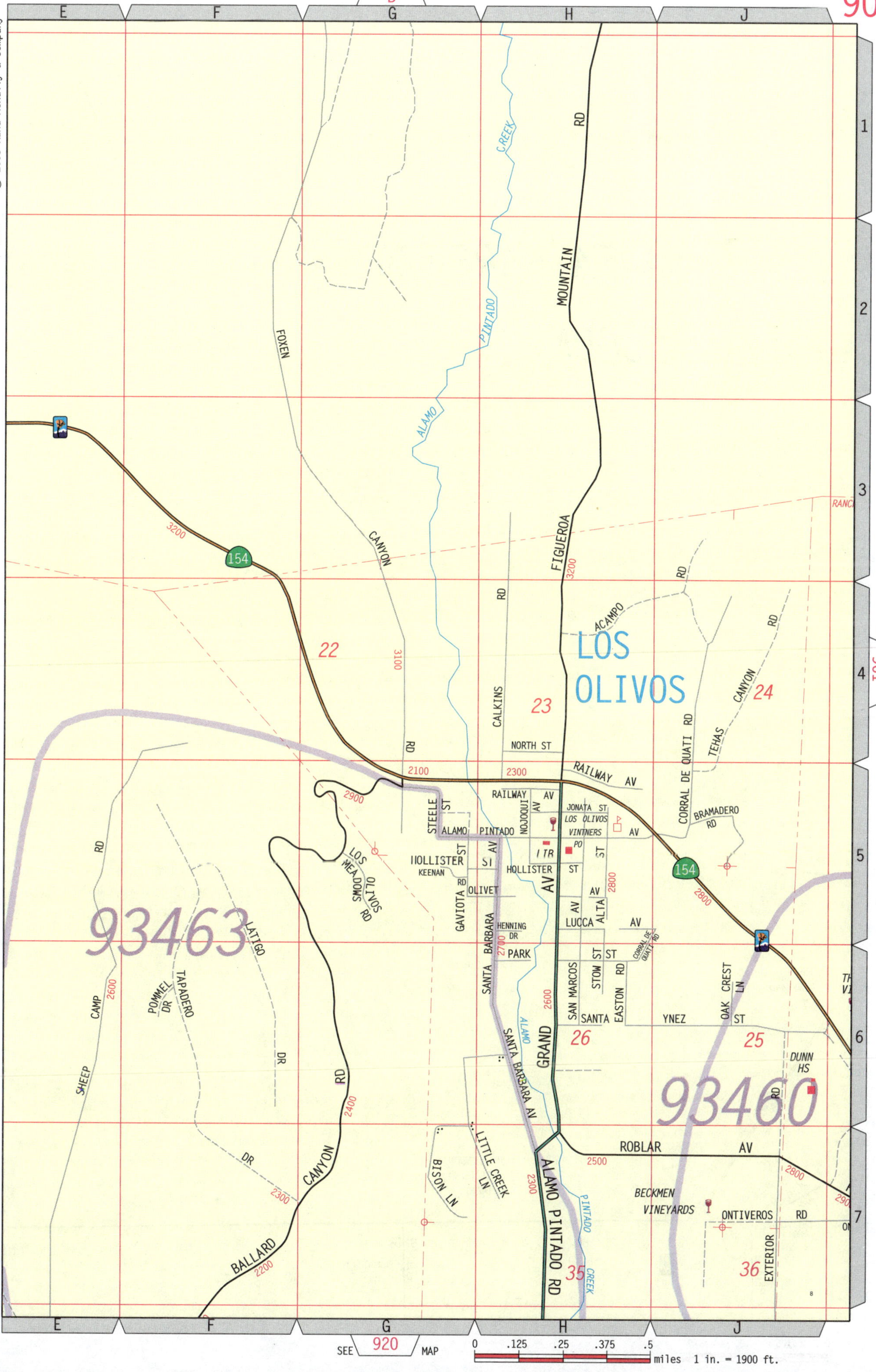
SEE 901 MAP
SEE 920 MAP
E F G H J
1 2 3 4 5 6 7
LOS OLIVOS
93463
93460
154
FOXEN CANYON RD
FIGUEROA MOUNTAIN RD
ALAMO PINTADO CREEK
CALKINS RD
ACAMPO RD
CORRAL DE QUATI RD
TEHAS CANYON RD
NORTH ST
RAILWAY AV
BRAMADERO RD
STEELE ST
ALAMO PINTADO AV
NOJOQUI AV
JONATA ST
LOS OLIVOS
VINTNERS AV
HOLLISTER ST
KEENAN RD
GAVIOTA ST
OLIVET
LOS OLIVOS MEADOWS RD
HENNING DR
SANTA BARBARA AV
PARK
GRAND AV
ALTA ST
LUCCA AV
STOW ST
SAN MARCOS
EASTON RD
SANTA YNEZ ST
OAK CREST LN
DUNN HS
ROBLAR AV
LITTLE CREEK LN
BISON LN
ALAMO PINTADO RD
BECKMEN VINEYARDS
ONTIVEROS RD
EXTERIOR RD
LATIGO DR
POMMEL DR
TAPADERO DR
SHEEP CAMP RD
BALLARD CANYON RD
PO
TR
22 23 24 25 26 35 36
3200 3100 2100 2300 2900 2800 2700 2600 2500 2400 2300 2200
0 .125 .25 .375 .5 miles 1 in. = 1900 ft.

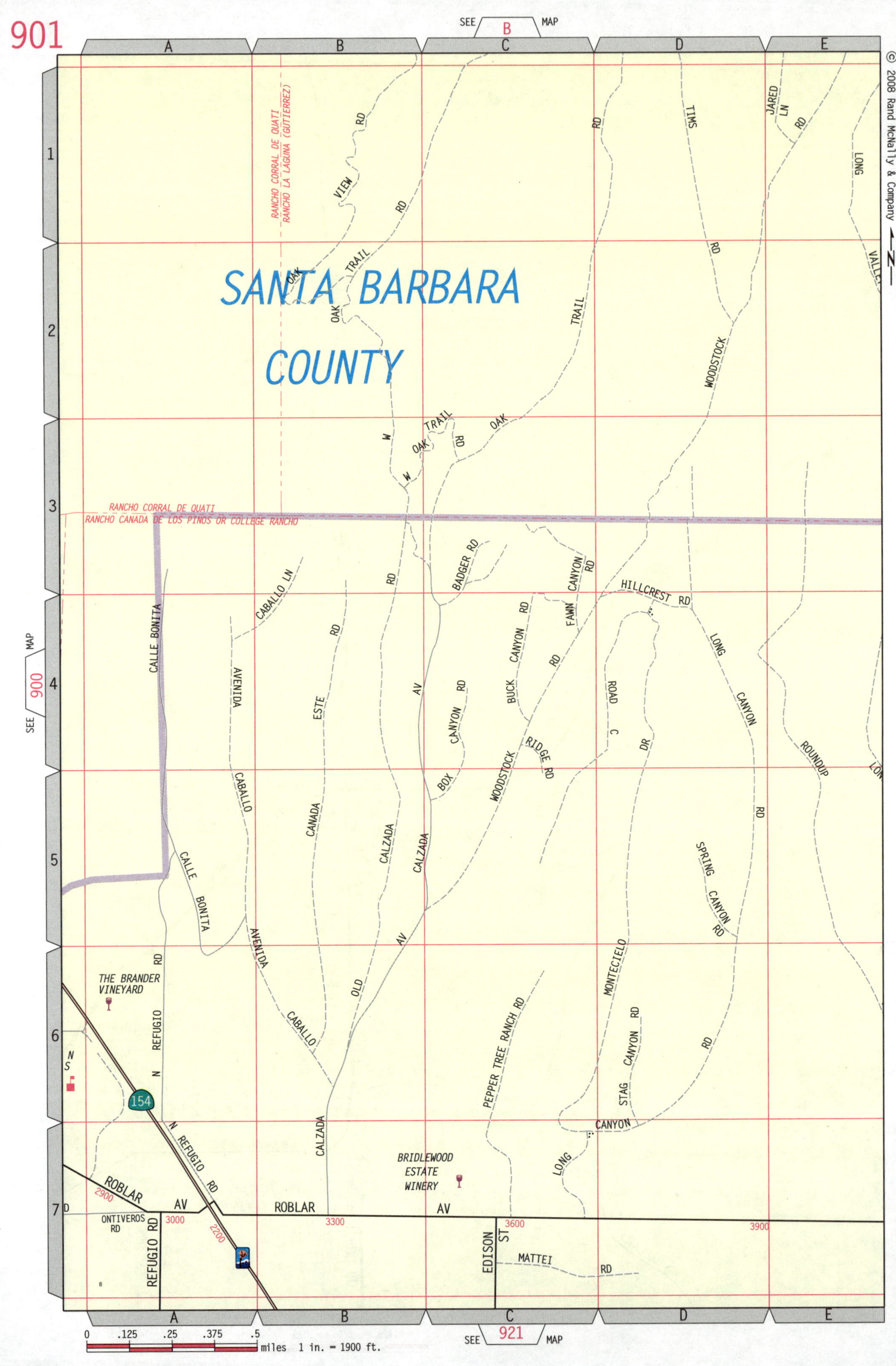
SANTA BARBARA
COUNTY
RANCHO CORRAL DE QUATI
RANCHO LA LAGUNA (GUTIERREZ)
RANCHO CORRAL DE QUATI
RANCHO CANADA DE LOS PINOS OR COLLEGE RANCHO
VIEW RD
TRAIL RD
OAK TRAIL
OAK
W OAK TRAIL RD
W OAK
TRAIL RD
TIMS RD
JARED LN
RD
LONG VALLEY
WOODSTOCK RD
BADGER RD
CABALLO LN
FAWN CANYON RD
HILLCREST RD
CALLE BONITA
AVENIDA CABALLO
ESTE RD
CANADA
CALZADA AV
BUCK CANYON RD
BOX CANYON RD
RIDGE RD
WOODSTOCK
ROAD C DR
LONG CANYON RD
ROUNDUP
SPRING CANYON RD
CALZADA AV
OLD
THE BRANDER VINEYARD
N REFUGIO RD
154
N REFUGIO RD
CALZADA
PEPPER TREE RANCH RD
MONTECIELO RD
STAG CANYON RD
CANYON
LONG
BRIDLEWOOD ESTATE WINERY
ROBLAR AV
2900
ONTIVEROS RD
REFUGIO RD
3000
2200
3300
3600
3900
EDISON ST
MATTEI RD
N S
0 .125 .25 .375 .5 miles 1 in. = 1900 ft.

SEE B MAP
SEE 900 MAP
SEE 921 MAP

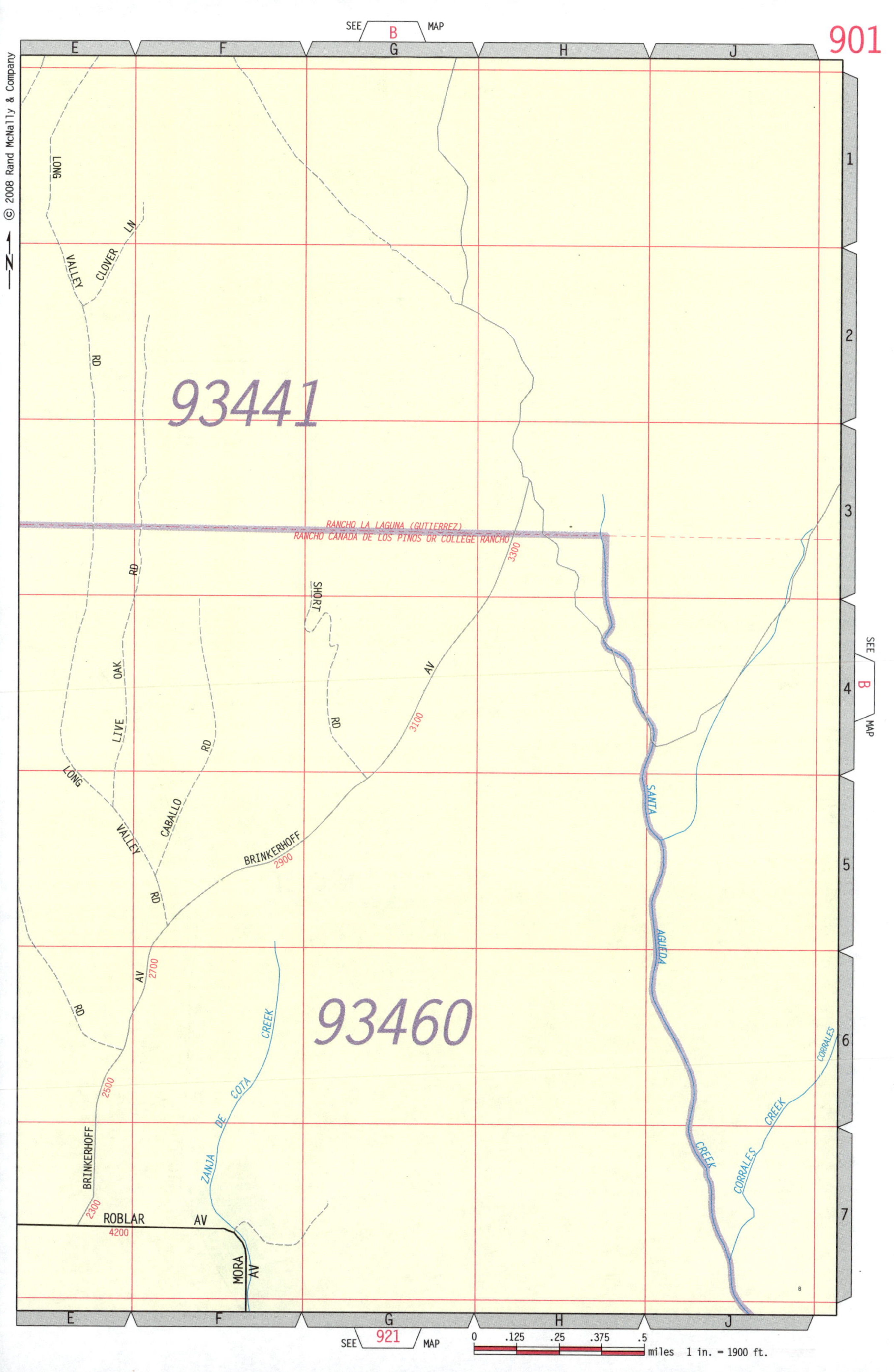

SEE B MAP
E
F
G
H
J
1
2
3
4
5
6
7
© 2008 Rand McNally & Company
LONG
VALLEY
CLOVER
LN
RD
93441
RANCHO LA LAGUNA (GUTIERREZ)
RANCHO CANADA DE LOS PINOS OR COLLEGE RANCHO
3300
RD
SHORT
RD
LIVE
OAK
AV
3100
RD
CABALLO
LONG
VALLEY
RD
BRINKERHOFF
2900
SANTA
AGUEDA
CREEK
AV
2700
RD
93460
CREEK
COTA
DE
ZANJA
2500
BRINKERHOFF
2300
ROBLAR
AV
4200
MORA
AV
CORRALES
CREEK
CORRALES
SEE B MAP
SEE 921 MAP
0
.125
.25
.375
.5
miles 1 in. = 1900 ft.

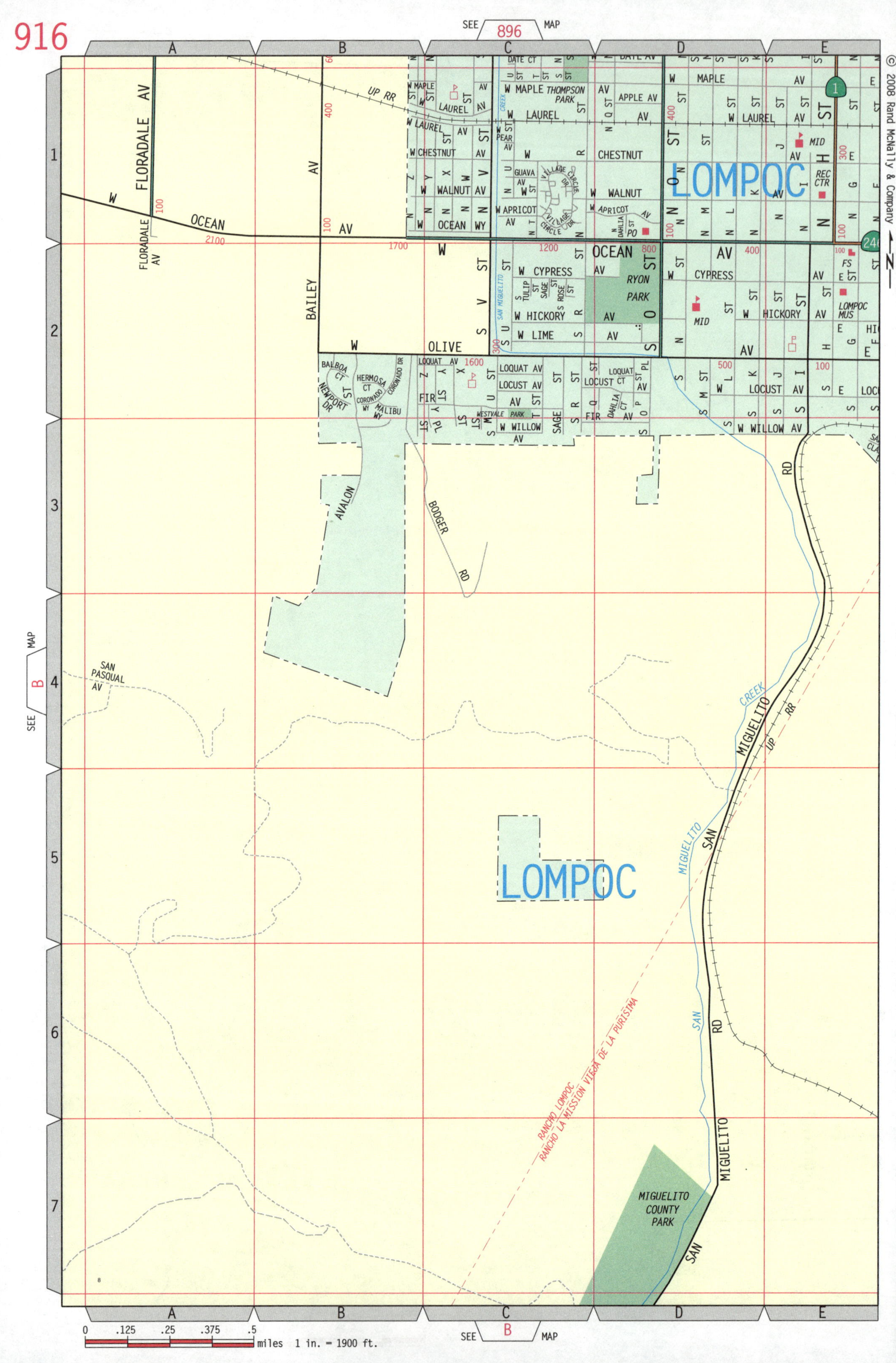

SEE 896 MAP
SEE B MAP
LOMPOC
LOMPOC
FLORADALE AV
W OCEAN AV
BAILEY AV
W OLIVE
UP RR
RYON PARK
THOMPSON PARK
WESTVALE PARK
MIGUELITO COUNTY PARK
SAN MIGUELITO RD
SAN MIGUELITO CREEK
AVALON
BODGER RD
SAN PASQUAL AV
RANCHO LOMPOC
RANCHO LA MISSION VIEJA DE LA PURISIMA
LOMPOC MUS
REC CTR

0 .125 .25 .375 .5 miles 1 in. = 1900 ft.

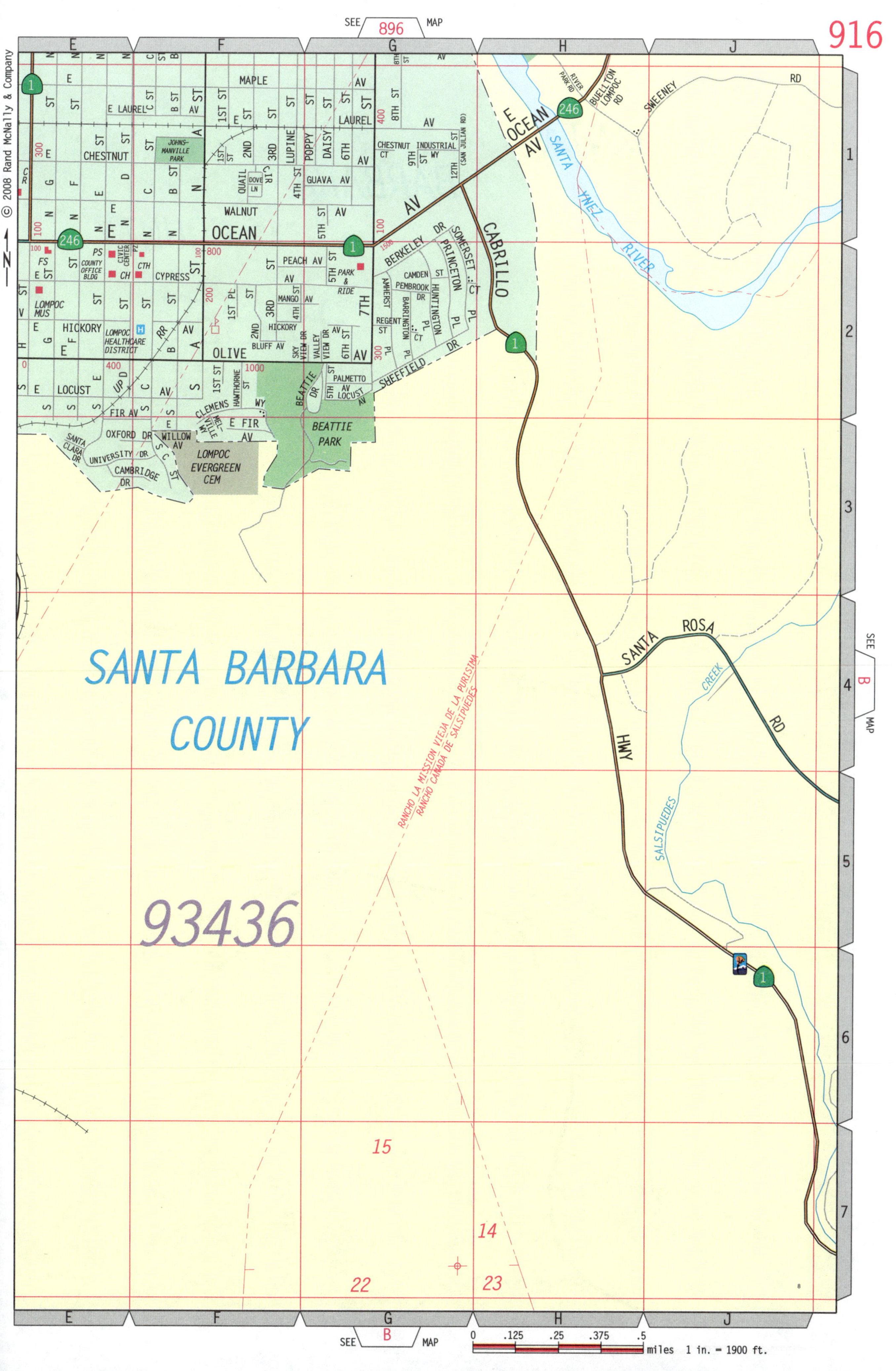
SEE 896 MAP
SEE B MAP
SANTA BARBARA
COUNTY
93436
OCEAN AV
E OCEAN AV
CABRILLO HWY
SANTA ROSA RD
SANTA YNEZ RIVER
SALSIPUEDES CREEK
BUELLTON LOMPOC RD
RIVER PARK RD
SWEENEY RD
RANCHO LA MISION VIEJA DE LA PURISIMA
RANCHO CANADA DE SALSIPUEDES
JOHNS-MANVILLE PARK
BEATTIE PARK
LOMPOC EVERGREEN CEM
LOMPOC HEALTHCARE DISTRICT
LOMPOC MUS
COUNTY OFFICE BLDG
CIVIC CENTER
PARK & RIDE
MAPLE
CHESTNUT
WALNUT
CYPRESS
HICKORY
OLIVE
LOCUST
FIR AV
LAUREL
GUAVA AV
PEACH AV
MANGO AV
PALMETTO
SHEFFIELD DR
BERKELEY DR
PRINCETON
SOMERSET
CAMDEN
PEMBROOK DR
HUNTINGTON PL
BARRINGTON PL
AMHERST
REGENT ST
INDUSTRIAL WY
12TH ST (SAN JULIAN RD)
OXFORD DR
UNIVERSITY DR
CAMBRIDGE DR
SANTA CLARA DR
WILLOW AV
CLEMENS WY
HAWTHORNE ST
BLUFF AV
SKY VIEW DR
VALLEY VIEW DR
15
14
22
23
0 .125 .25 .375 .5 miles 1 in. = 1900 ft.

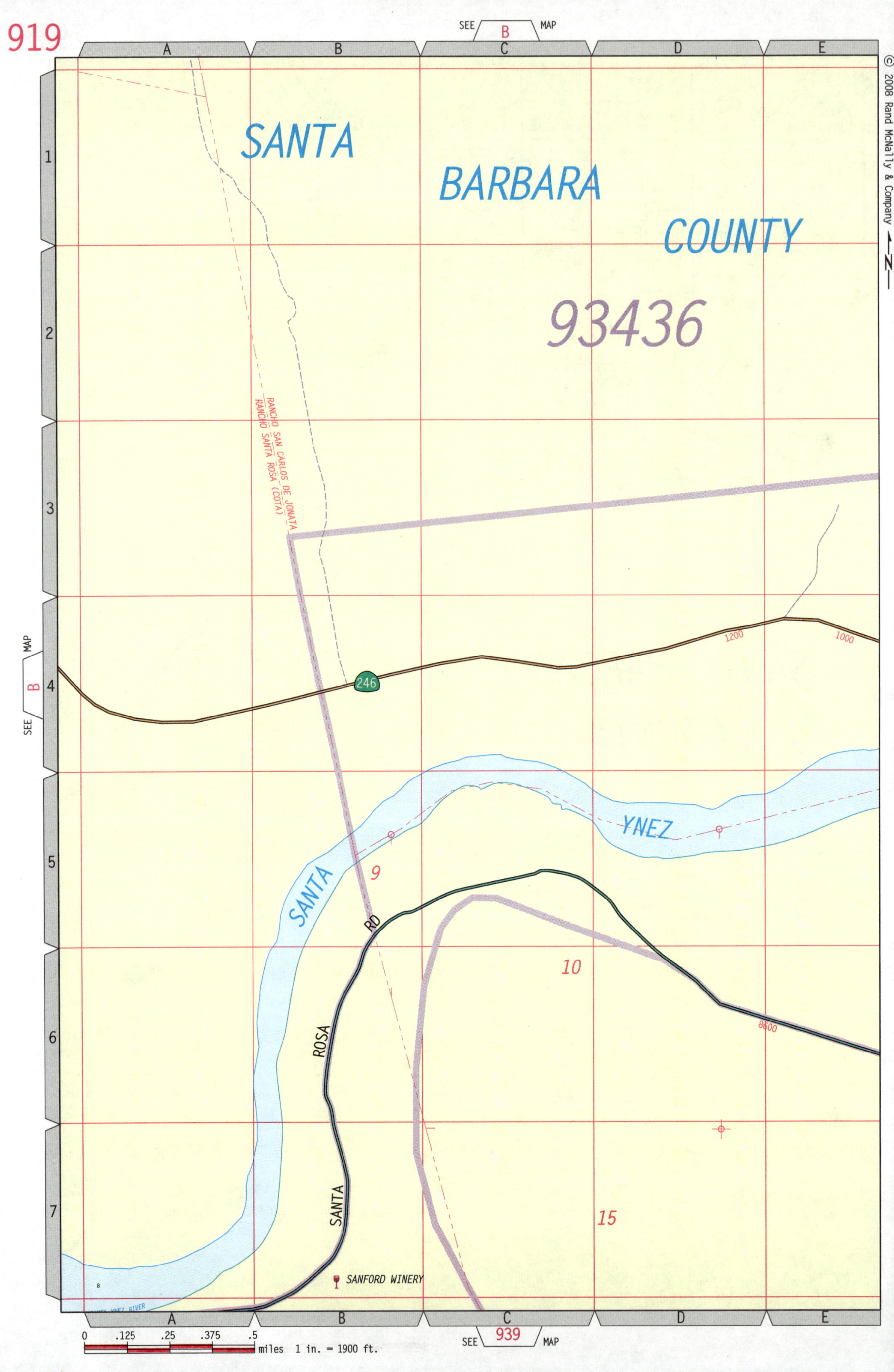

SEE B MAP
A
B
C
D
E
1
2
3
4
5
6
7
SEE B MAP
SANTA
BARBARA
COUNTY
93436
RANCHO SAN CARLOS DE JONATA
RANCHO SANTA ROSA (COTA)
246
1200
1000
SANTA
YNEZ
9
10
15
RD
ROSA
SANTA
8600
SANFORD WINERY
0
.125
.25
.375
.5
miles 1 in. = 1900 ft.
SEE 939 MAP

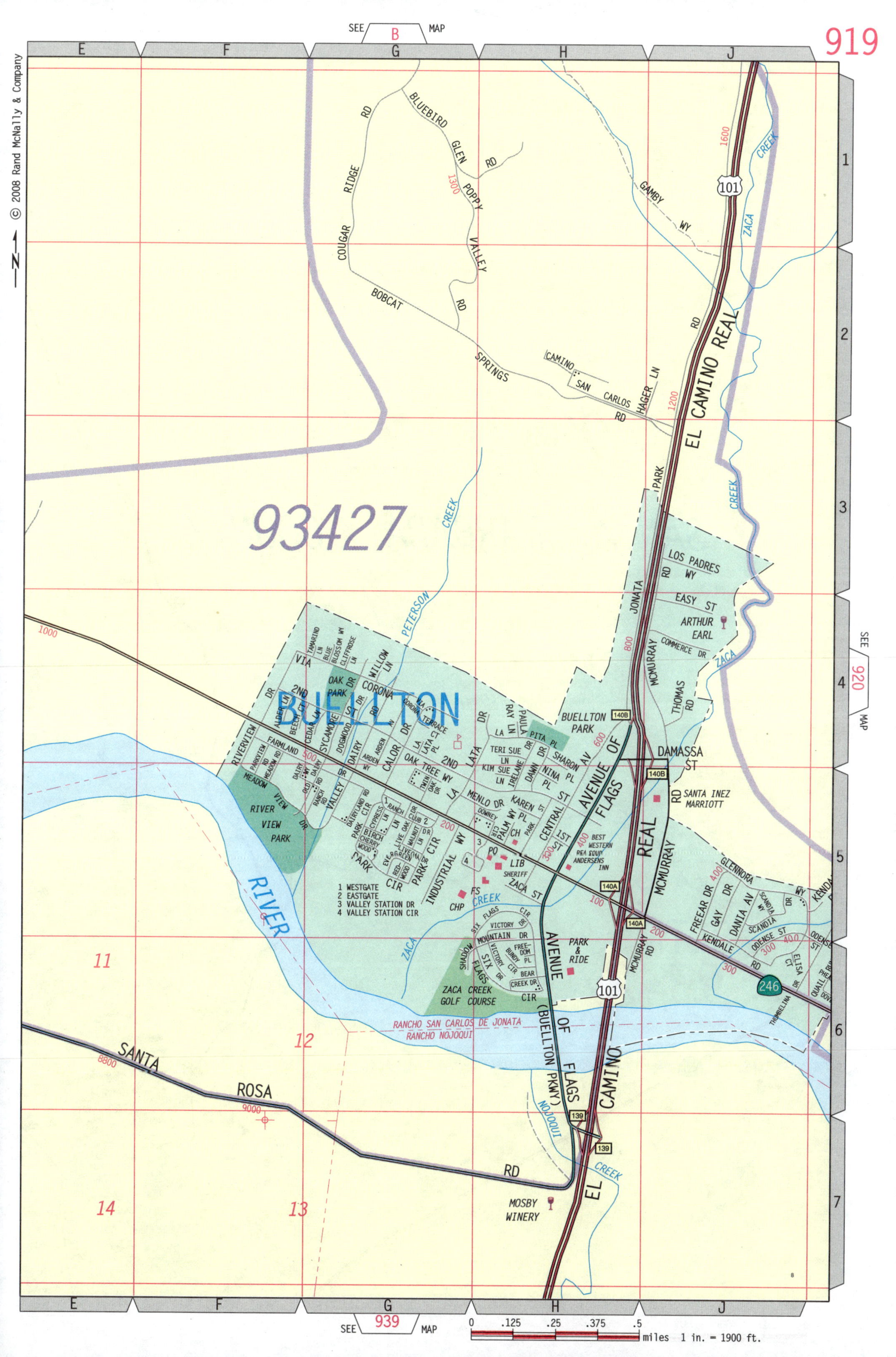
SEE B MAP
E
F
G
H
J
© 2008 Rand McNally & Company
N
1
2
3
4
5
6
7
SEE 920 MAP
BLUEBIRD
GLEN
RD
RIDGE
RD
COUGAR
POPPY
VALLEY
RD
1300
BOBCAT
SPRINGS
CAMINO
SAN
CARLOS
RD
HAGER LN
1200
1600
GAMBY
WY
101
ZACA
CREEK
RD
EL CAMINO REAL
PARK
93427
PETERSON
CREEK
LOS PADRES
RD
WY
EASY ST
ARTHUR
EARL
COMMERCE DR
JONATA
800
MCMURRAY
THOMAS
RD
ZACA
1000
BUELLTON
VIA
TAMARIND LN
BLUE BLOSSOM WY
CLIFFROSE LN
WILLOW LN
OAK PARK
CORONA
2ND
DR
ALDER LN
BEECH CT
CEDAR LN
SYCAMORE
DOGWOOD
ST
RD
DR
TERRACE
RAY LN
PAULA
PITA PL
BUELLTON PARK
140B
600
RIVERVIEW
FARMLAND
PARKVIEW
RD
MEADOW RD
500
DAIRY
ARDEN
CALOR
DR
LA LATA CT
PL
2ND
LA LATA
TERI SUE
LN
KIM SUE
LN
IRELAND
DAWN
DR
NINA PL
SHARON
PL
AV
AVENUE OF FLAGS
DAMASSA ST
140B
SANTA INEZ MARRIOTT
RD
OAK TREE WY
TWIN OAK DR
MEADOW
VIEW
DR
RIVER
VIEW
PARK
VALLEY
RANCH
RD
DAIRYLAND RD
PARK CIR
CYPRESS
BIRCH
CHERRY WOOD
RANCH
CLUB
LIVE OAK LN
WALNUT LN
EVERGREEN
PARK CIR
PARK CIR
200
LA
MENLO DR
DOWNEY
KAREN PL
ST
CENTRAL
1ST
400
300
BEST WESTERN PEA SOUP ANDERSENS INN
REAL
MCMURRAY
GLENNORA
400
WY
KENDALL
INDUSTRIAL WY
PALM WY
CH
PO
LIB
SHERIFF
ZACA ST
140A
100
140A
FREEAR DR
GAY DR
DANIA AV
SCANDIA WY
DR
SCANDIA
ODENSE ST
400
300
KENDALE
RD
ELISA CT
QUAIL
1 WESTGATE
2 EASTGATE
3 VALLEY STATION DR
4 VALLEY STATION CIR
FS
CHP
CREEK
SIX FLAGS CIR
VICTORY DR
MOUNTAIN DR
FREEDOM PL
SHADOW
VICTORY CIR
BUNDY
SIX FLAGS DR
BEAR CREEK DR
CIR
ZACA CREEK GOLF COURSE
AVENUE
PARK & RIDE
MCMURRAY RD
200
300
246
THUMBELINA
RIVER
ZACA
11
12
RANCHO SAN CARLOS DE JONATA
RANCHO NOJOQUI
SANTA
ROSA
8800
9000
RD
OF
(BUELLTON PKWY)
FLAGS
CAMINO
EL
139
139
NOJOQUI
CREEK
MOSBY WINERY
14
13
SEE 939 MAP
0 .125 .25 .375 .5
miles 1 in. = 1900 ft.

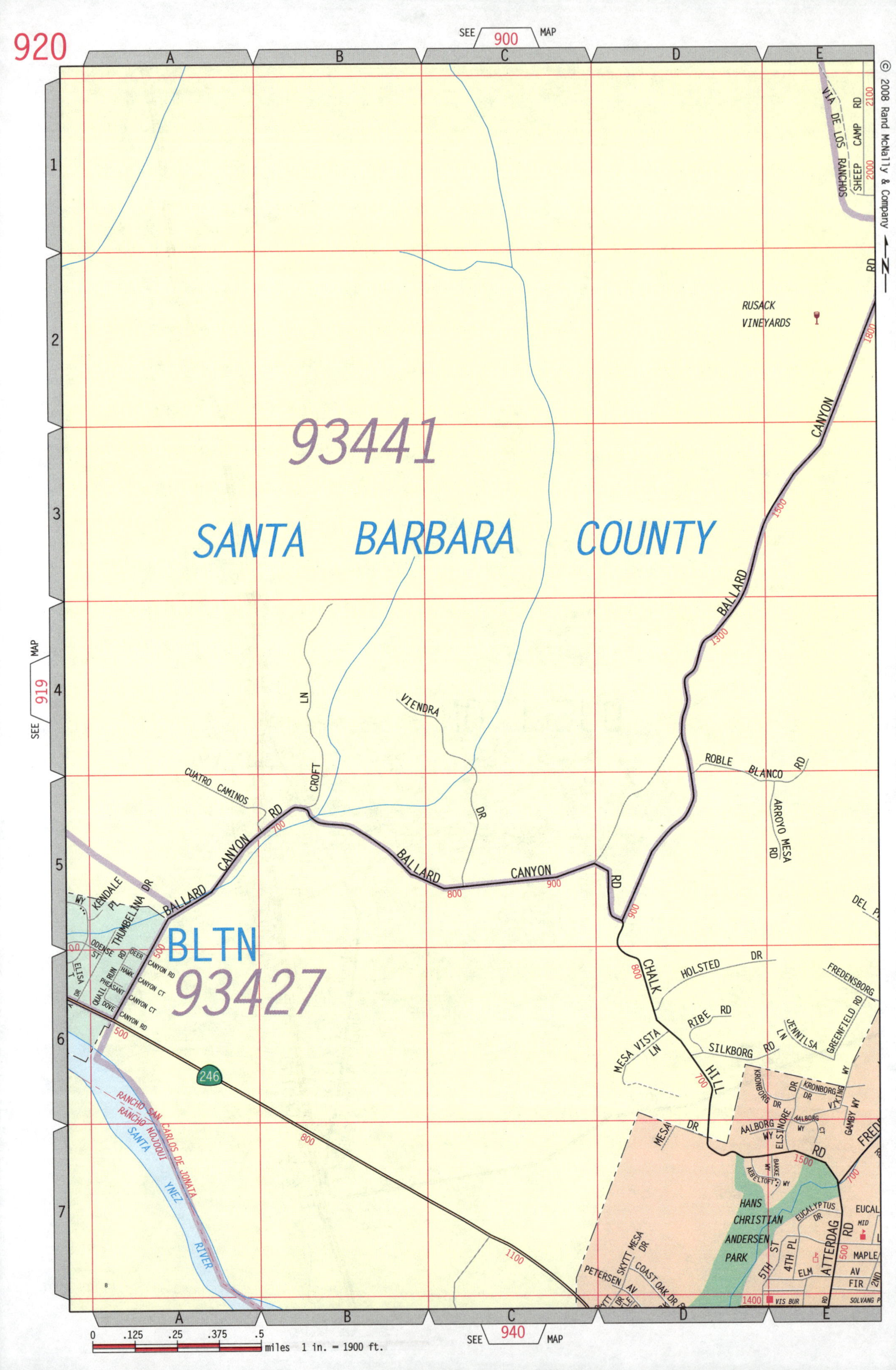

SEE 900 MAP
SEE 919 MAP
SEE 940 MAP
93441
SANTA BARBARA COUNTY
BLTN
93427
BALLARD CANYON RD
CHALK HILL RD
RUSACK VINEYARDS
ROBLE BLANCO RD
ARROYO MESA RD
VIENDRA DR
CROFT LN
CUATRO CAMINOS
HOLSTED DR
RIBE RD
SILKBORG RD
MESA VISTA LN
MESA DR
HANS CHRISTIAN ANDERSEN PARK
ATTERDAG RD
SANTA YNEZ RIVER
RANCHO SAN CARLOS DE JONATA
RANCHO NOJOQUI
246
VIA DE LOS RANCHOS
SHEEP CAMP RD
THUMBELINA DR
KENDALE PL
ODENSE ST
ELISA
QUAIL RUN RD
DEER CANYON RD
HAWK CANYON CT
PHEASANT CANYON CT
DOVE CANYON RD
FREDENSBORG
GREENFIELD RD
JENNILSA LN
KRONBORG DR
VIKING WY
AALBORG WY
ELSINORE RD
GAMBY WY
EUCALYPTUS DR
5TH ST
4TH PL
ELM
MAPLE AV
FIR
PETERSEN AV
SKYTT MESA DR
COAST OAK DR
VIS BUR
SOLVANG
0 .125 .25 .375 .5 miles 1 in. = 1900 ft.

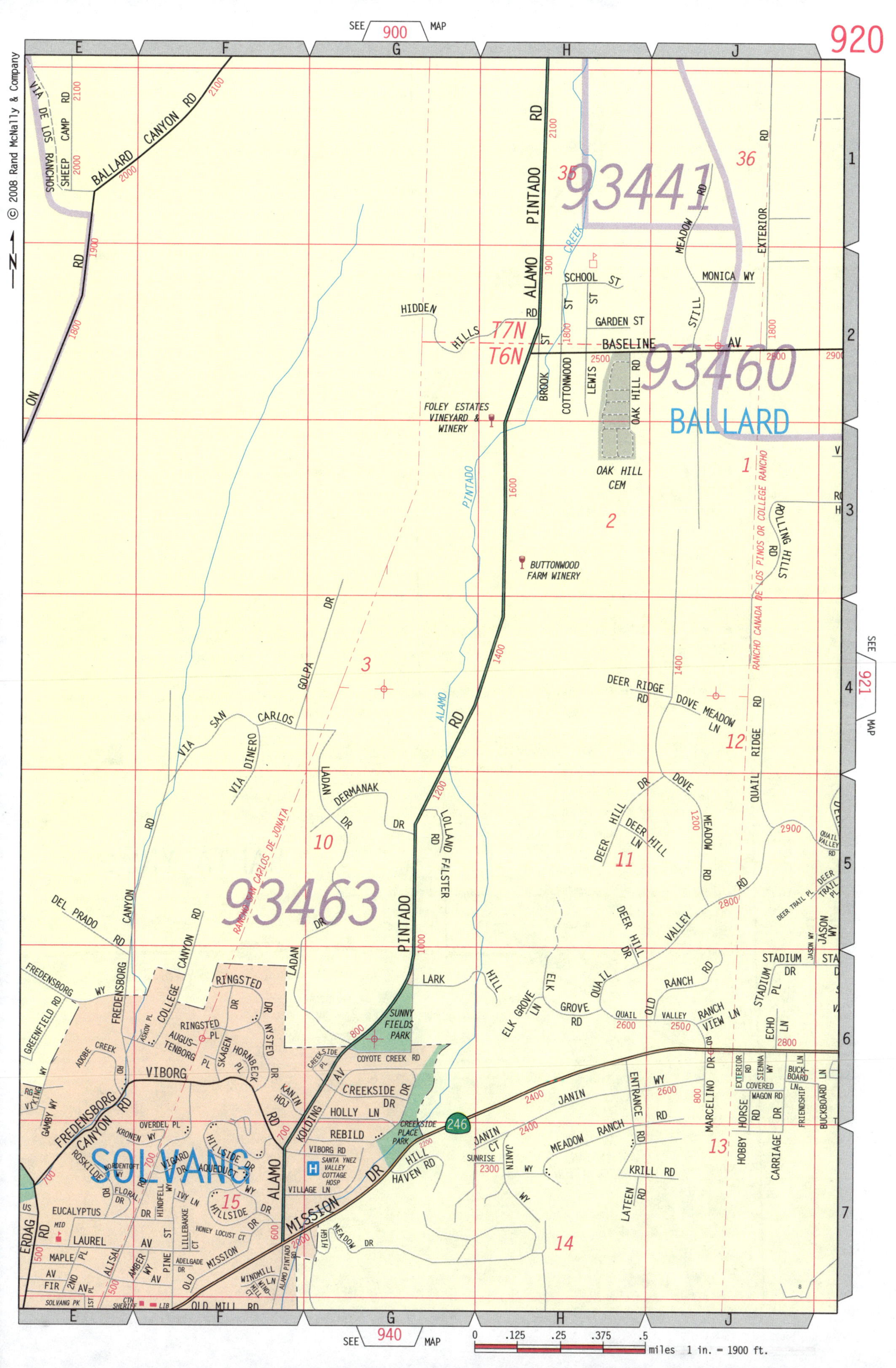
SEE 900 MAP
E F G H J
1 2 3 4 5 6 7
© 2008 Rand McNally & Company
BALLARD CANYON RD
VIA DE LOS RANCHOS
SHEEP CAMP RD
ALAMO PINTADO RD
93441
93460
93463
BALLARD
SOLVANG
T7N
T6N
SCHOOL ST
MONICA WY
MEADOW RD
STILL
EXTERIOR RD
HIDDEN HILLS RD
GARDEN ST
BASELINE AV
BROOK ST
COTTONWOOD ST
LEWIS ST
OAK HILL RD
FOLEY ESTATES VINEYARD & WINERY
OAK HILL CEM
BUTTONWOOD FARM WINERY
RANCHO CANADA DE LOS PINOS OR COLLEGE RANCHO
ROLLING HILLS RD
PINTADO CREEK
DEER RIDGE RD
DOVE MEADOW LN
QUAIL RIDGE RD
GOLPA DR
VIA SAN CARLOS
VIA DINERO
LADAN DR
DERMANAK DR
LOLLAND FALSTER RD
DEER HILL DR
DEER HILL LN
DOVE MEADOW RD
QUAIL VALLEY RD
DEER TRAIL PL
DEER TRAIL
DEER TRAIL PL
JASON WY
STADIUM DR
STADIUM PL
RANCHO SAN CARLOS DE JONATA
DEL PRADO RD
CANYON RD
COLLEGE CANYON RD
FREDENSBORG CANYON RD
FREDENSBORG WY
GREENFIELD RD
RINGSTED DR
RINGSTED PL
NYSTED DR
AUGUSTENBORG PL
SKAGEN DR
HORNBECK PL
LARK
HILL
ELK GROVE LN
ELK GROVE RD
QUAIL VALLEY
OLD VALLEY RANCH RD
RANCH VIEW LN
ECHO LN
SUNNY FIELDS PARK
COYOTE CREEK RD
CREEKSIDE PL
CREEKSIDE DR
ADOBE CREEK RD
VIBORG RD
VIKING WY
GAMBY WY
KANIN HOJ
KOLDING AV
HOLLY LN
REBILD DR
CREEKSIDE PLACE PARK
246
JANIN WY
ENTRANCE RD
MARCELINO DR
EXTERIOR RD
SIENNA WY
COVERED WAGON RD
HOBBY HORSE RD
BUCKBOARD LN
FRIENDSHIP LN
CARRIAGE DR
OVERDEL PL
KRONEN WY
HILLSIDE DR
AQUEDUCT WY
VIGARD DR
ROSKILDE RD
NORDENTOFT WY
FLORAL DR
SANTA YNEZ VALLEY COTTAGE HOSP
VILLAGE LN
HAVEN RD
HILL
MISSION DR
JANIN CT
SUNRISE WY
MEADOW RANCH RD
KRILL RD
LATEEN RD
EUCALYPTUS DR
HINDFELL WY
IVY LN
LILLEBAKKE CT
HONEY LOCUST CT
LAUREL AV
MAPLE PL
ALISAL RD
AMBER WY
PINE ST
ADELGADE DR
MISSION DR
FIR AV
2ND AV
OLD MILL RD
WINDMILL LN
HIGH MEADOW DR
SOLVANG PK
CTH SHERIFF LIB
ALAMO PINTADO RD
ERDAG RD
10 11 12 13 14 15
1 2 3 35 36
SEE 921 MAP
SEE 940 MAP
0 .125 .25 .375 .5 miles 1 in. = 1900 ft.

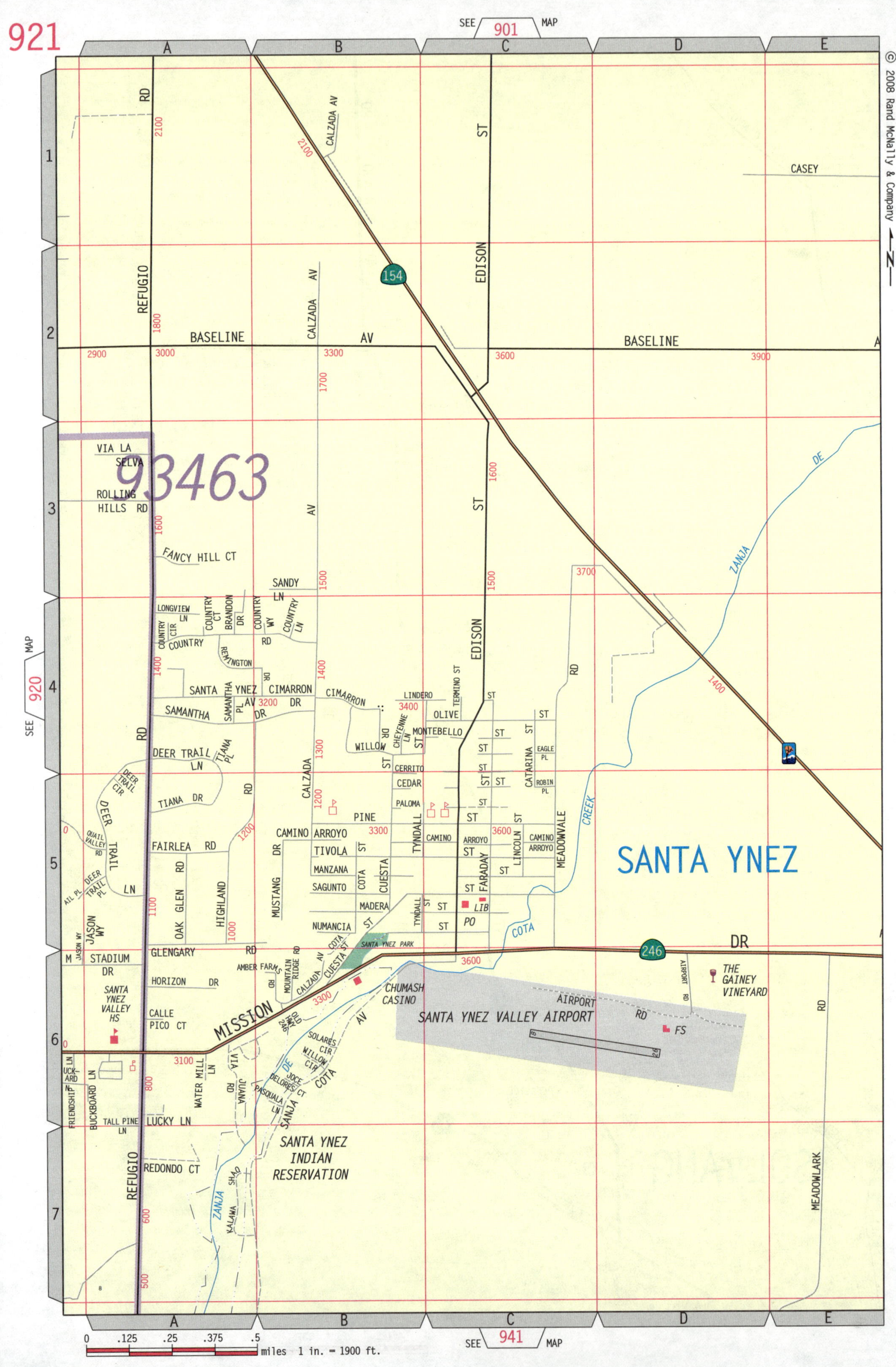
SEE 901 MAP
SEE 920 MAP
SEE 941 MAP
93463
SANTA YNEZ
REFUGIO RD
BASELINE AV
CALZADA AV
EDISON ST
154
246
MISSION DR
VIA LA SELVA
ROLLING HILLS RD
FANCY HILL CT
SANDY LN
LONGVIEW LN
COUNTRY CIR
COUNTRY CT
BRANDON DR
COUNTRY WY
COUNTRY LN
COUNTRY RD
REMINGTON DR
SANTA YNEZ AV
CIMARRON DR
SAMANTHA DR
SAMANTHA PL
DEER TRAIL LN
TIANA PL
TIANA DR
DEER TRAIL CIR
QUAIL VALLEY RD
FAIRLEA RD
OAK GLEN RD
HIGHLAND RD
MUSTANG DR
CAMINO ARROYO
TIVOLA ST
MANZANA
SAGUNTO
COTA ST
CUESTA ST
MADERA
NUMANCIA ST
PINE
CERRITO
CEDAR
PALOMA
TYNDALL ST
LINDERO
TERMINO ST
OLIVE ST
MONTEBELLO ST
WILLOW DR
CHEYENNE LN
CATARINA ST
EAGLE PL
ROBIN PL
LINCOLN ST
FARADAY ST
MEADOWVALE RD
LIB
PO
SANTA YNEZ PARK
ZANJA DE COTA CREEK
JASON WY
STADIUM DR
GLENGARY RD
HORIZON DR
AMBER FARMS RD
MOUNTAIN RIDGE RD
CALLE PICO CT
SANTA YNEZ VALLEY HS
CHUMASH CASINO
SANTA YNEZ VALLEY AIRPORT
AIRPORT RD
FS
THE GAINEY VINEYARD
OLD HWY 246
SOLARES CIR
WILLOW CIR
JOCE CT
DELORES CT
PASQUALA LN
SANJA COTA AV
VIA JUANA RD
WATER MILL LN
BUCKBOARD LN
FRIENDSHIP LN
TALL PINE LN
LUCKY LN
REDONDO CT
SANTA YNEZ INDIAN RESERVATION
SHAD
KALAWA
CASEY
MEADOWLARK RD
0 .125 .25 .375 .5 miles 1 in. = 1900 ft.

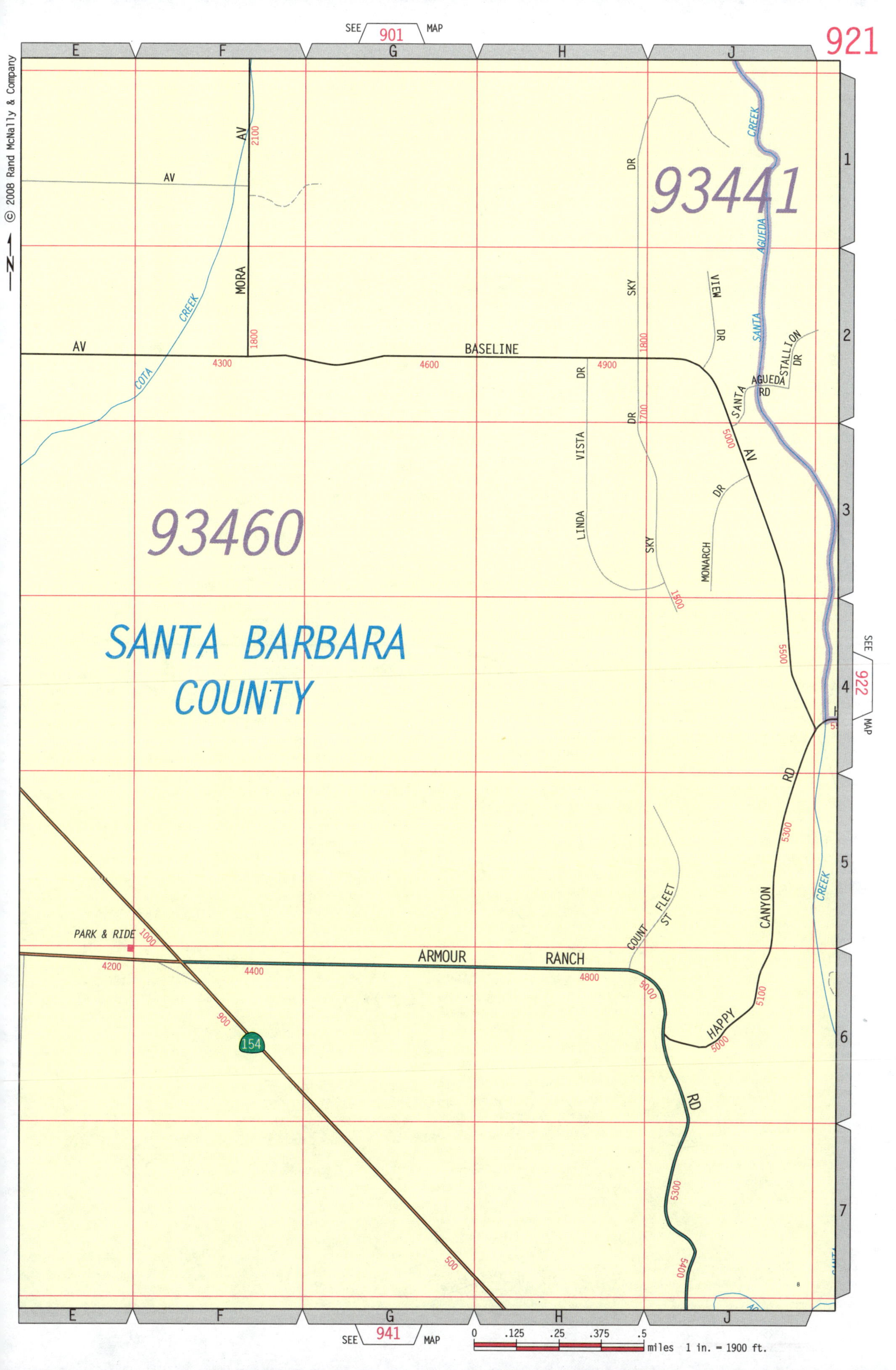

SEE 901 MAP
E
F
G
H
J
1
2
3
4
5
6
7
93441
93460
SANTA BARBARA
COUNTY
BASELINE
AV
MORA
AV
COTA
CREEK
SANTA AGUEDA CREEK
SKY DR
LINDA VISTA DR
VIEW DR
STALLION DR
AGUEDA RD
SANTA
MONARCH DR
ARMOUR RANCH
RD
HAPPY CANYON RD
COUNT FLEET ST
PARK & RIDE
154
SEE 922 MAP
SEE 941 MAP
0 .125 .25 .375 .5
miles 1 in. = 1900 ft.

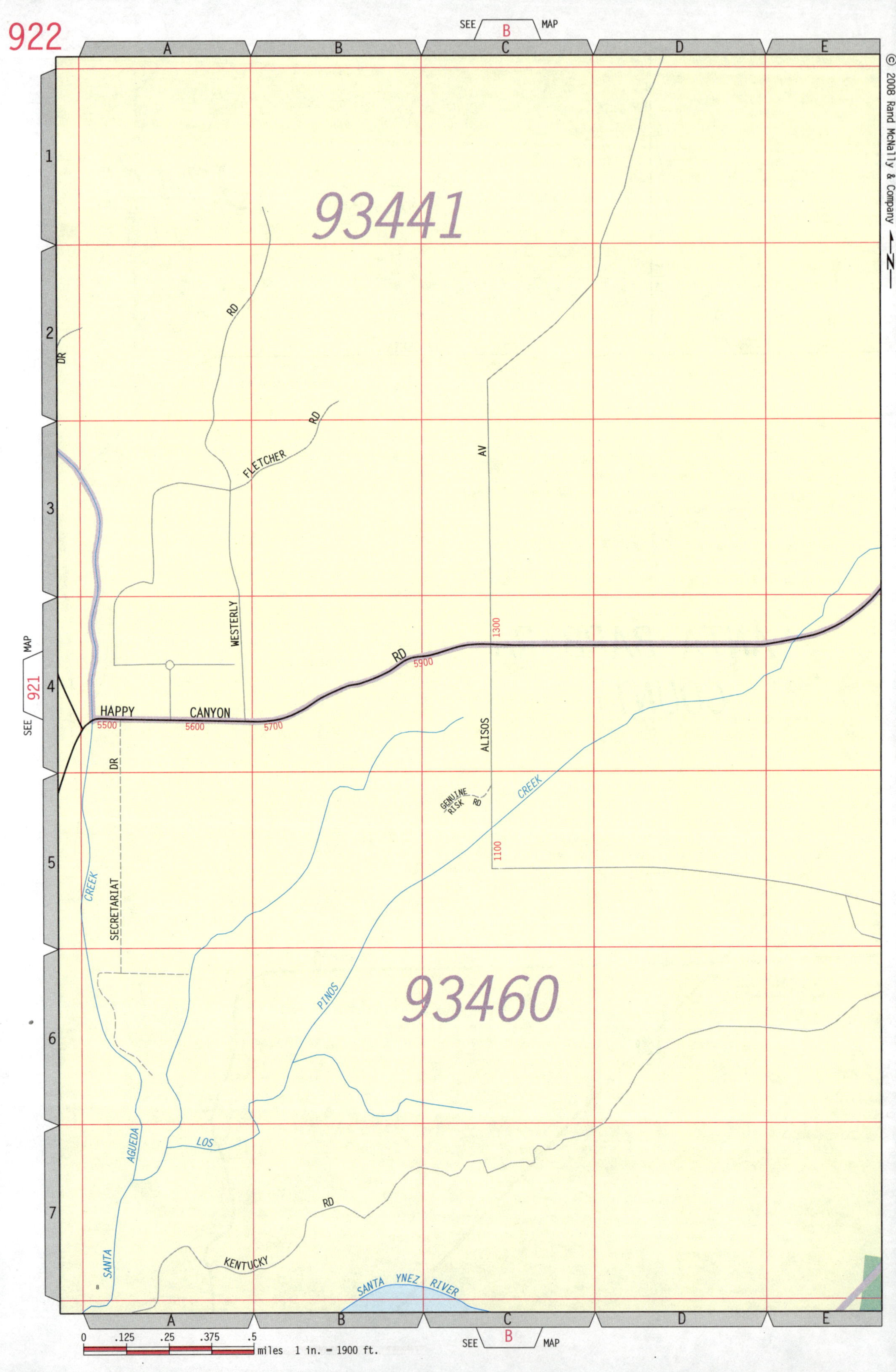

SEE B MAP
A
B
C
D
E
1
2
3
4
5
6
7
93441
93460
RD
DR
FLETCHER RD
WESTERLY RD
AV
ALISOS
1300
1100
HAPPY CANYON RD
5500
5600
5700
5900
SEE 921 MAP
SECRETARIAT DR
GENUINE RISK RD
CREEK
PINOS CREEK
LOS
AGUEDA
SANTA
KENTUCKY RD
SANTA YNEZ RIVER
0 .125 .25 .375 .5 miles 1 in. = 1900 ft.

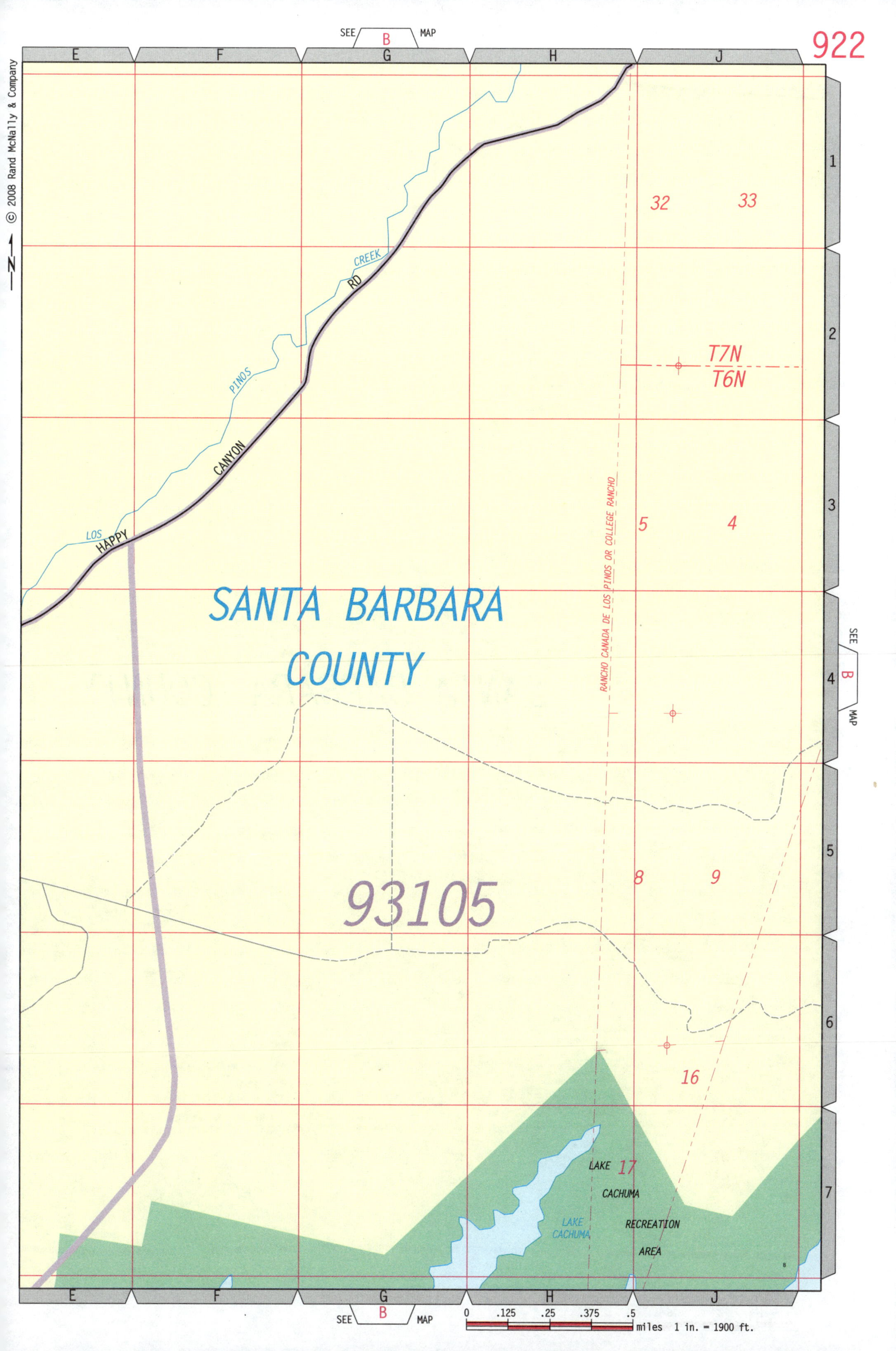
SEE B MAP
E
F
G
H
J
1
2
3
4
5
6
7
32
33
T7N
T6N
5
4
8
9
16
17
HAPPY CANYON RD
LOS PINOS CREEK
SANTA BARBARA COUNTY
RANCHO CANADA DE LOS PINOS OR COLLEGE RANCHO
93105
LAKE CACHUMA RECREATION AREA
LAKE CACHUMA
SEE B MAP
SEE B MAP
0 .125 .25 .375 .5 miles 1 in. = 1900 ft.

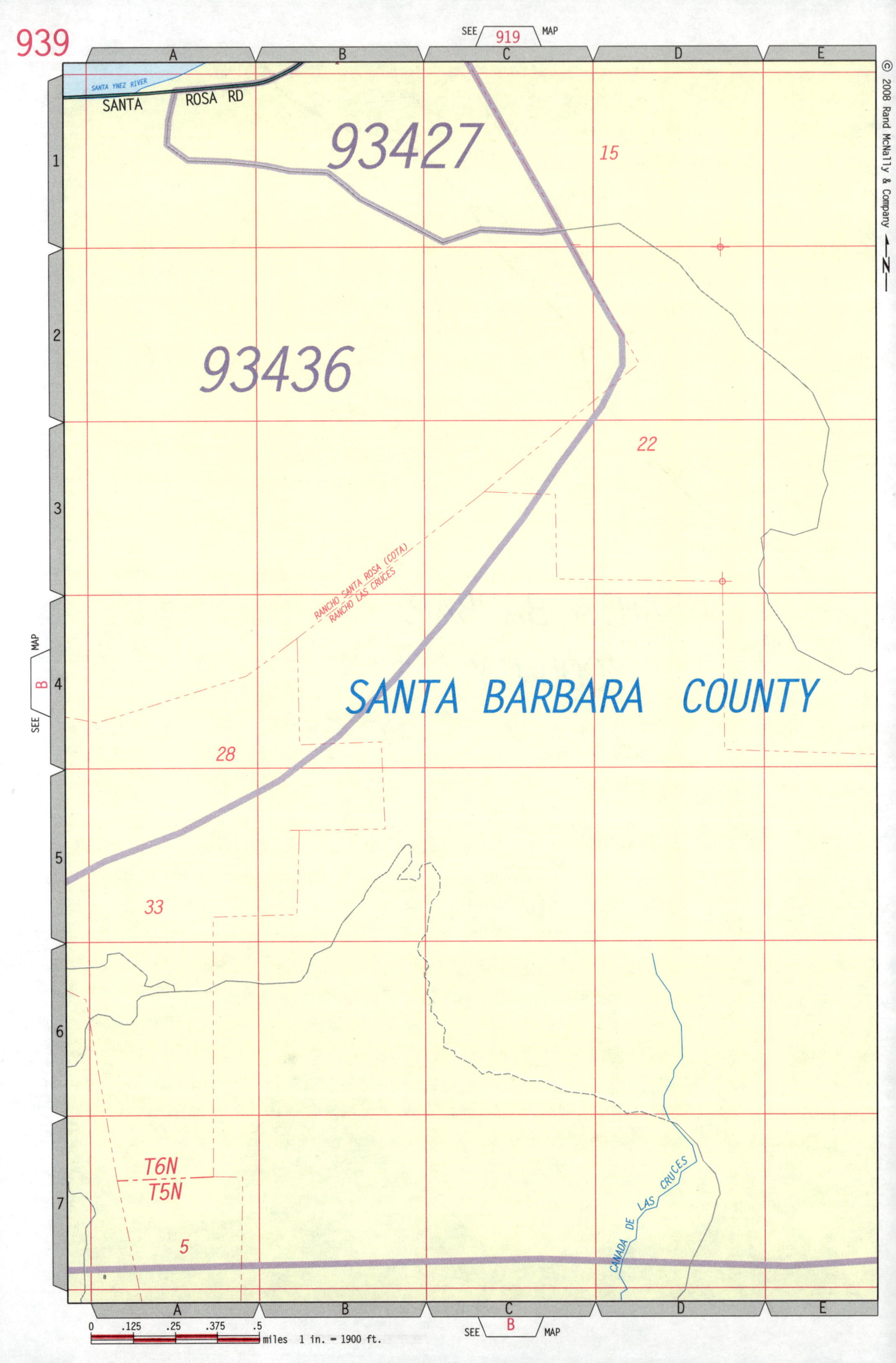
SEE 919 MAP
A
B
C
D
E
1
2
3
4
5
6
7
SANTA YNEZ RIVER
SANTA ROSA RD
93427
93436
15
22
28
33
5
RANCHO SANTA ROSA (COTA)
RANCHO LAS CRUCES
SANTA BARBARA COUNTY
T6N
T5N
CANADA DE LAS CRUCES
SEE B MAP
0 .125 .25 .375 .5
miles 1 in. = 1900 ft.

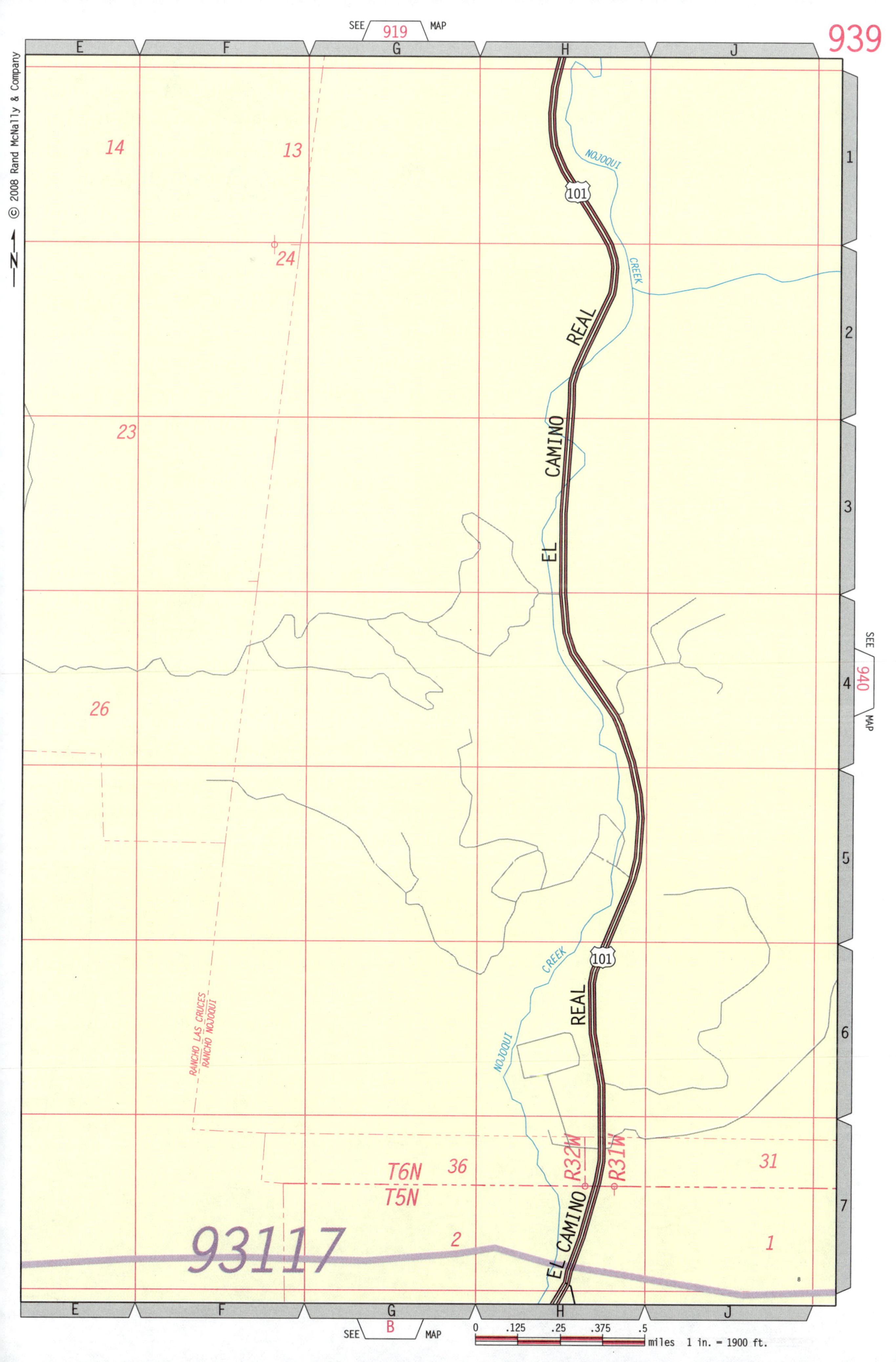
SEE 919 MAP
E
F
G
H
J
1
2
3
4
5
6
7
SEE 940 MAP
14
13
24
23
26
NOJOQUI
CREEK
101
EL CAMINO REAL
RANCHO LAS CRUCES
RANCHO NOJOQUI
R32W
R31W
T6N
T5N
36
31
2
1
93117
SEE B MAP
0 .125 .25 .375 .5
miles 1 in. = 1900 ft.

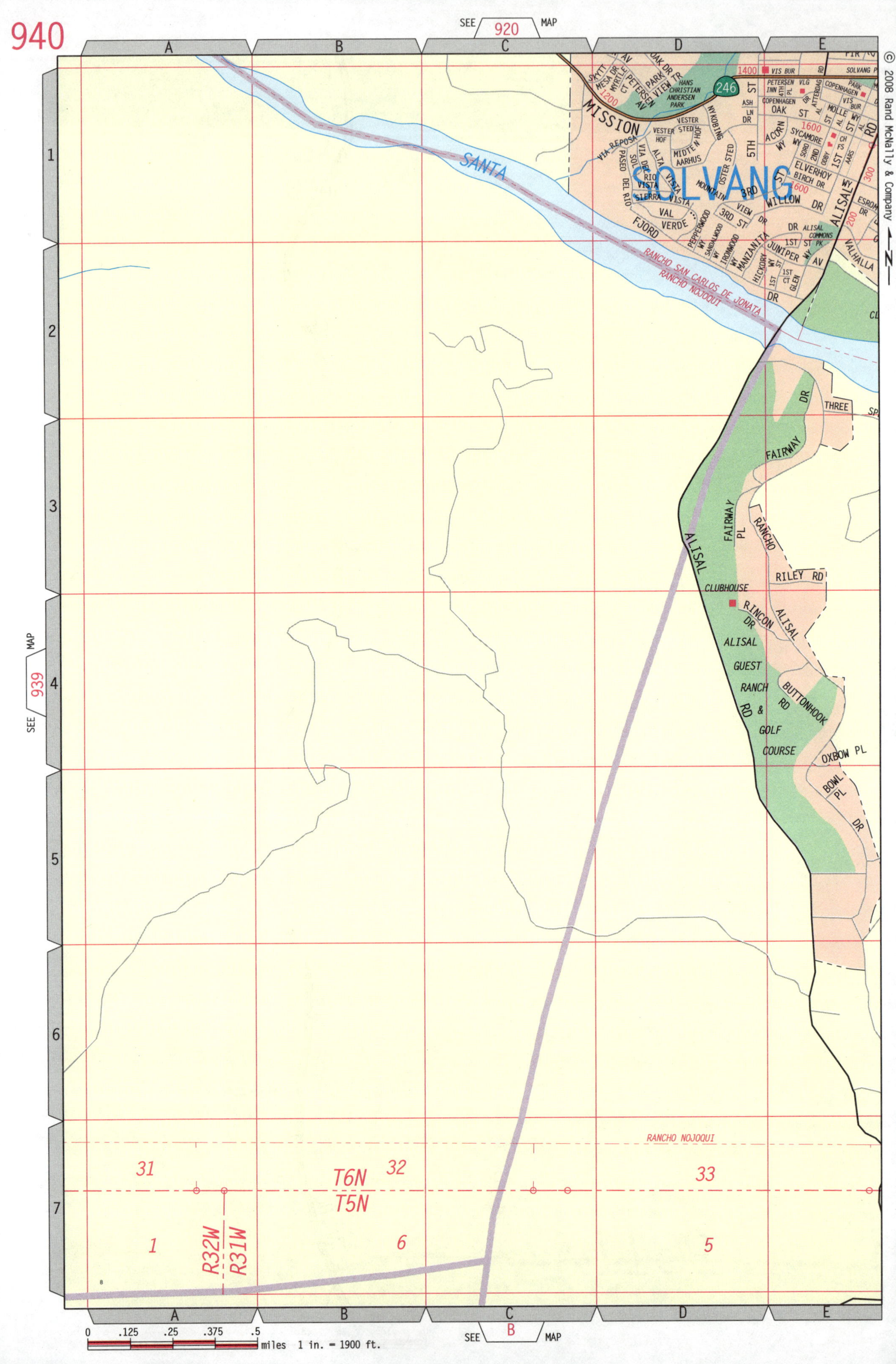
SEE 920 MAP
SEE 939 MAP
SEE B MAP
SOLVANG
SANTA
MISSION
246
HANS CHRISTIAN ANDERSEN PARK
RANCHO SAN CARLOS DE JONATA
RANCHO NOJOQUI
ALISAL RD
ALISAL GUEST RANCH & GOLF COURSE
CLUBHOUSE
FAIRWAY DR
FAIRWAY PL
RANCHO ALISAL
RILEY RD
RINCON DR
BUTTONHOOK RD
OXBOW PL
BOWL PL
DR
THREE
VALHALLA
T6N
T5N
R32W
R31W
31
32
33
1
6
5
0 .125 .25 .375 .5 miles 1 in. = 1900 ft.
© 2008 Rand McNally & Company

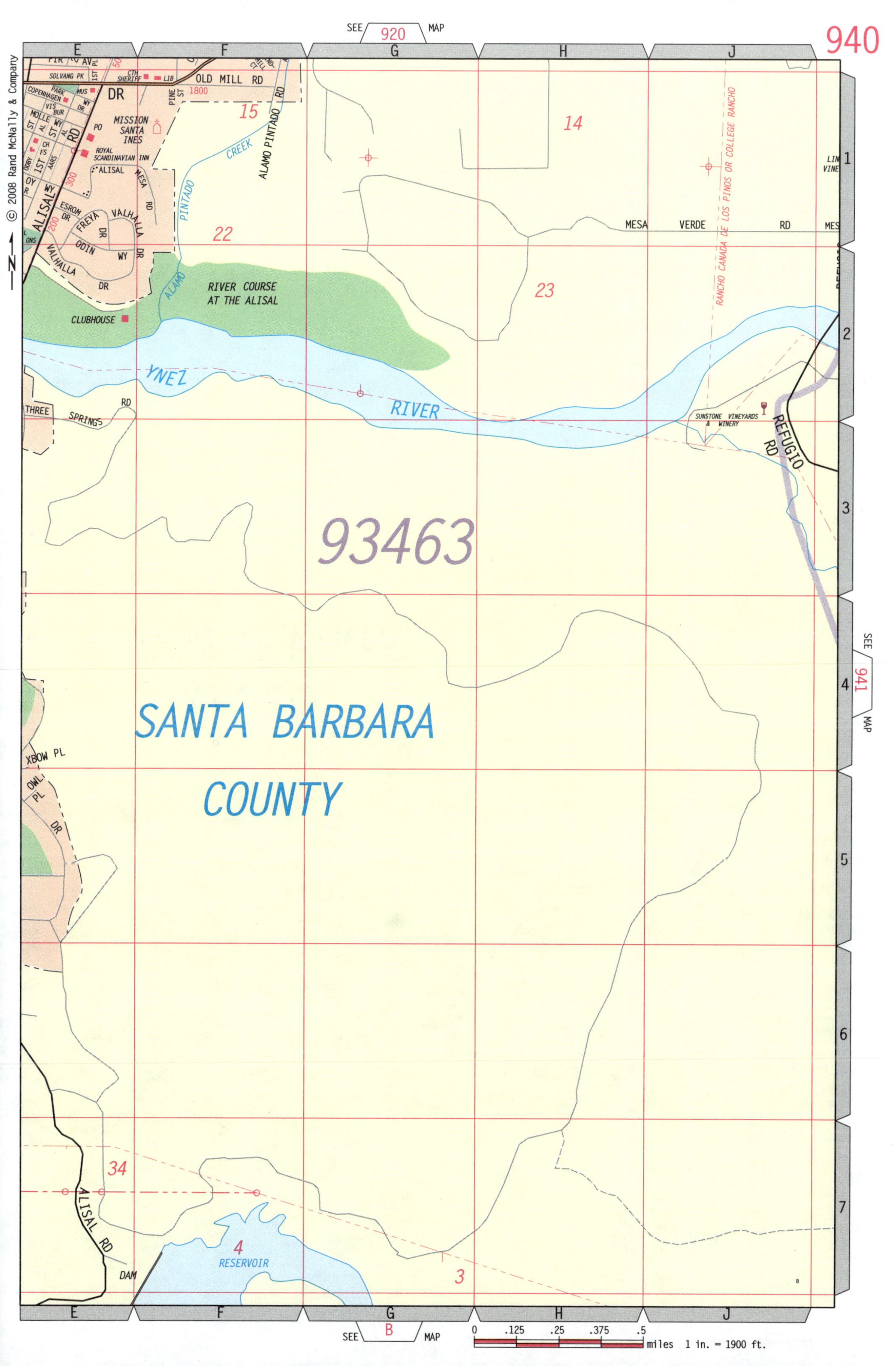
SEE 920 MAP
E
F
G
H
J
OLD MILL RD
MISSION SANTA INES
ROYAL SCANDINAVIAN INN
ALISAL
ALAMO PINTADO RD
PINTADO CREEK
MESA VERDE RD
RANCHO CANADA DE LOS PINOS OR COLLEGE RANCHO
VALHALLA DR
ODIN WY
FREYA DR
ESROM DR
RIVER COURSE AT THE ALISAL
CLUBHOUSE
YNEZ RIVER
THREE SPRINGS RD
SUNSTONE VINEYARDS & WINERY
REFUGIO RD
93463
SANTA BARBARA COUNTY
XBOW PL
OWL PL
DR
ALISAL RD
DAM
RESERVOIR
SEE 941 MAP
SEE B MAP
miles 1 in. = 1900 ft.

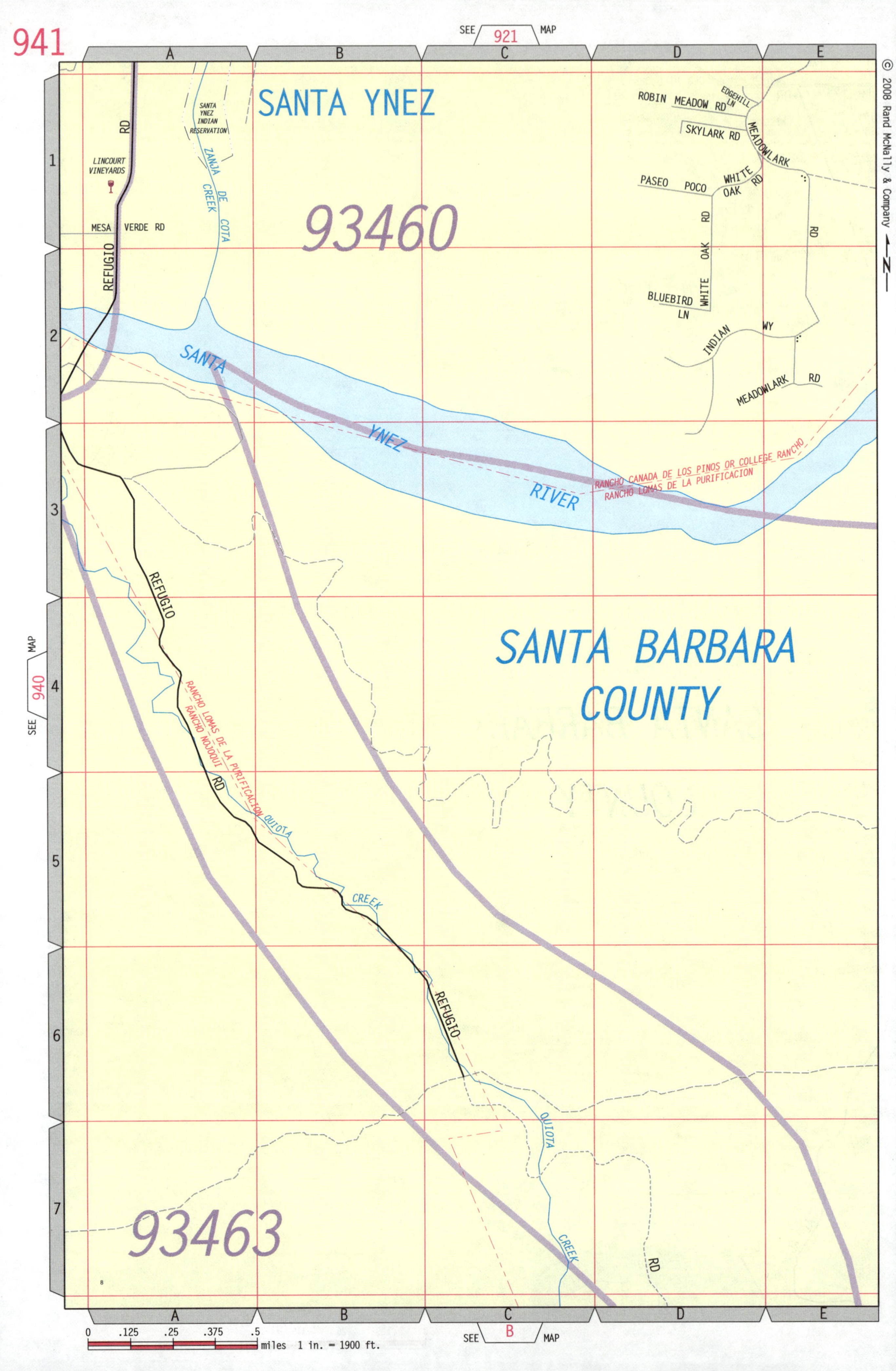
SEE 921 MAP
SANTA YNEZ
SANTA YNEZ INDIAN RESERVATION
LINCOURT VINEYARDS
REFUGIO RD
ZANJA DE COTA CREEK
MESA VERDE RD
93460
ROBIN MEADOW RD
EDGEHILL LN
SKYLARK RD
MEADOWLARK
PASEO POCO
WHITE OAK RD
BLUEBIRD LN
INDIAN WY
MEADOWLARK RD
SANTA YNEZ RIVER
RANCHO CANADA DE LOS PINOS OR COLLEGE RANCHO
RANCHO LOMAS DE LA PURIFICACION
REFUGIO RD
SANTA BARBARA COUNTY
RANCHO LOMAS DE LA PURIFICACION
RANCHO NOJOQUI
QUIOTA CREEK
REFUGIO
QUIOTA CREEK
RD
93463
SEE 940 MAP
0 .125 .25 .375 .5 miles 1 in. = 1900 ft.
SEE B MAP

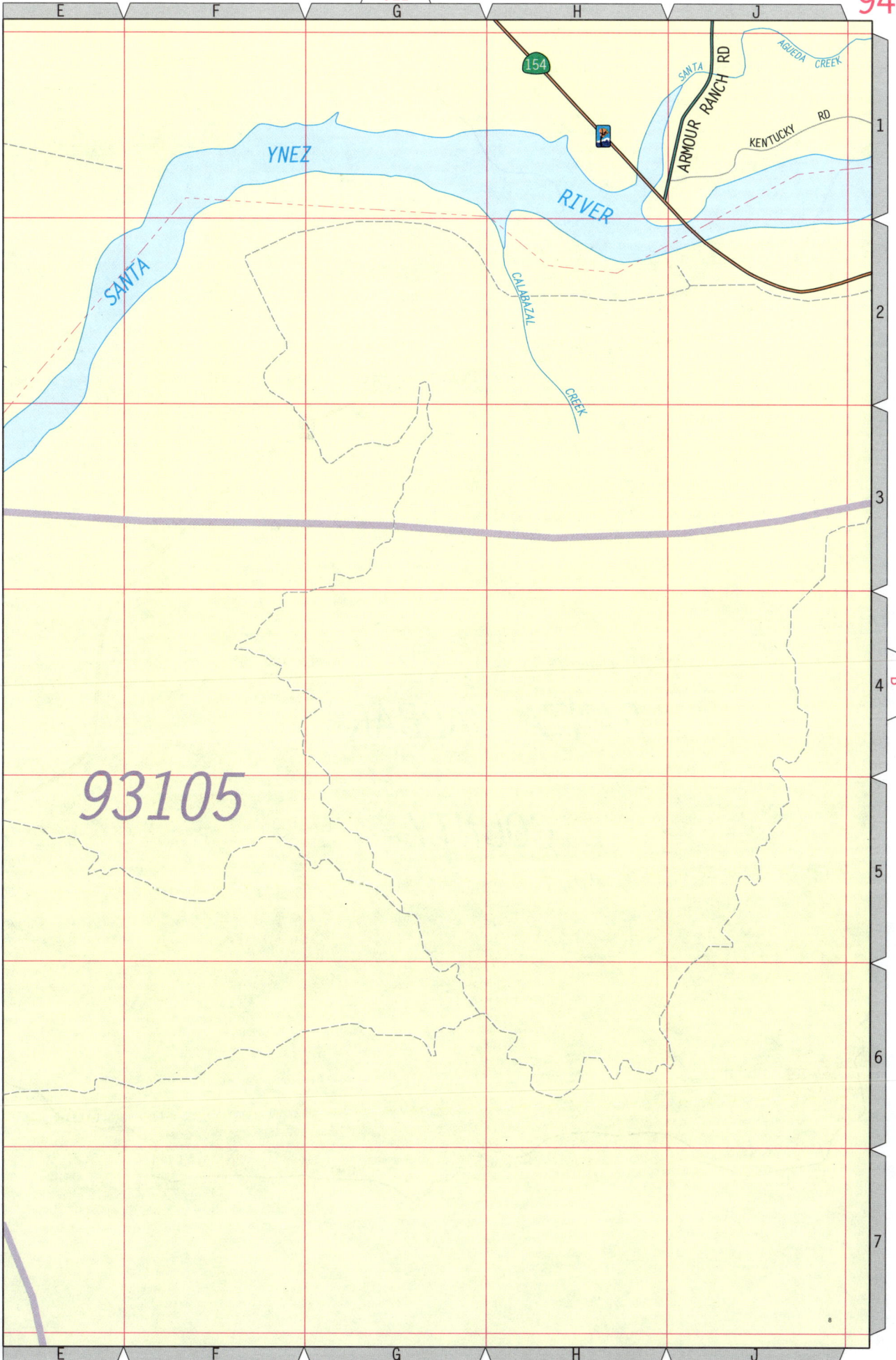

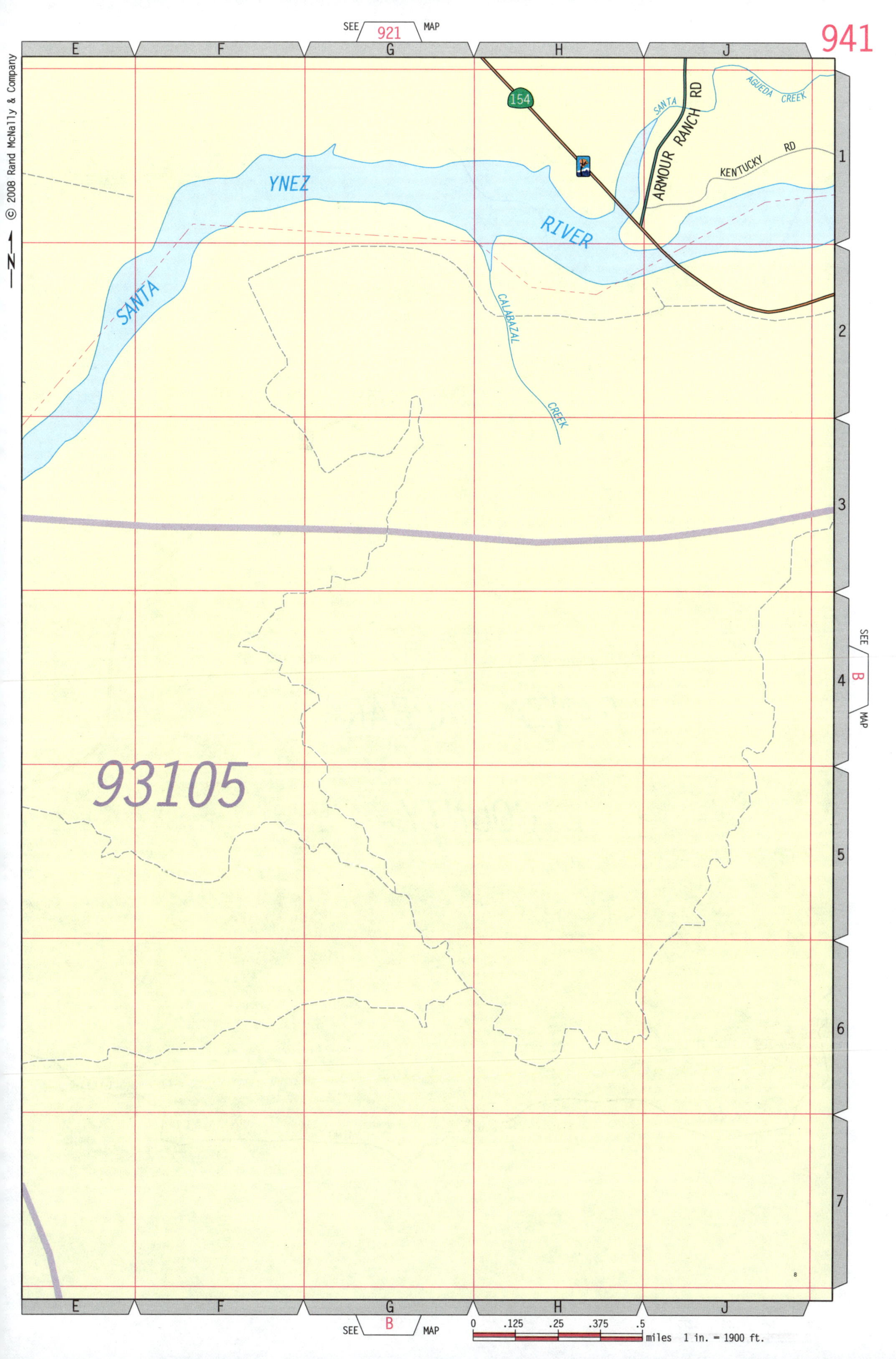
SEE 921 MAP
E
F
G
H
J
154
SANTA
AGUEDA CREEK
ARMOUR RANCH RD
KENTUCKY RD
SANTA
YNEZ
RIVER
CALABAZAL
CREEK
93105
1
2
3
4
5
6
7
SEE B MAP
SEE B MAP
0
.125
.25
.375
.5
miles 1 in. = 1900 ft.

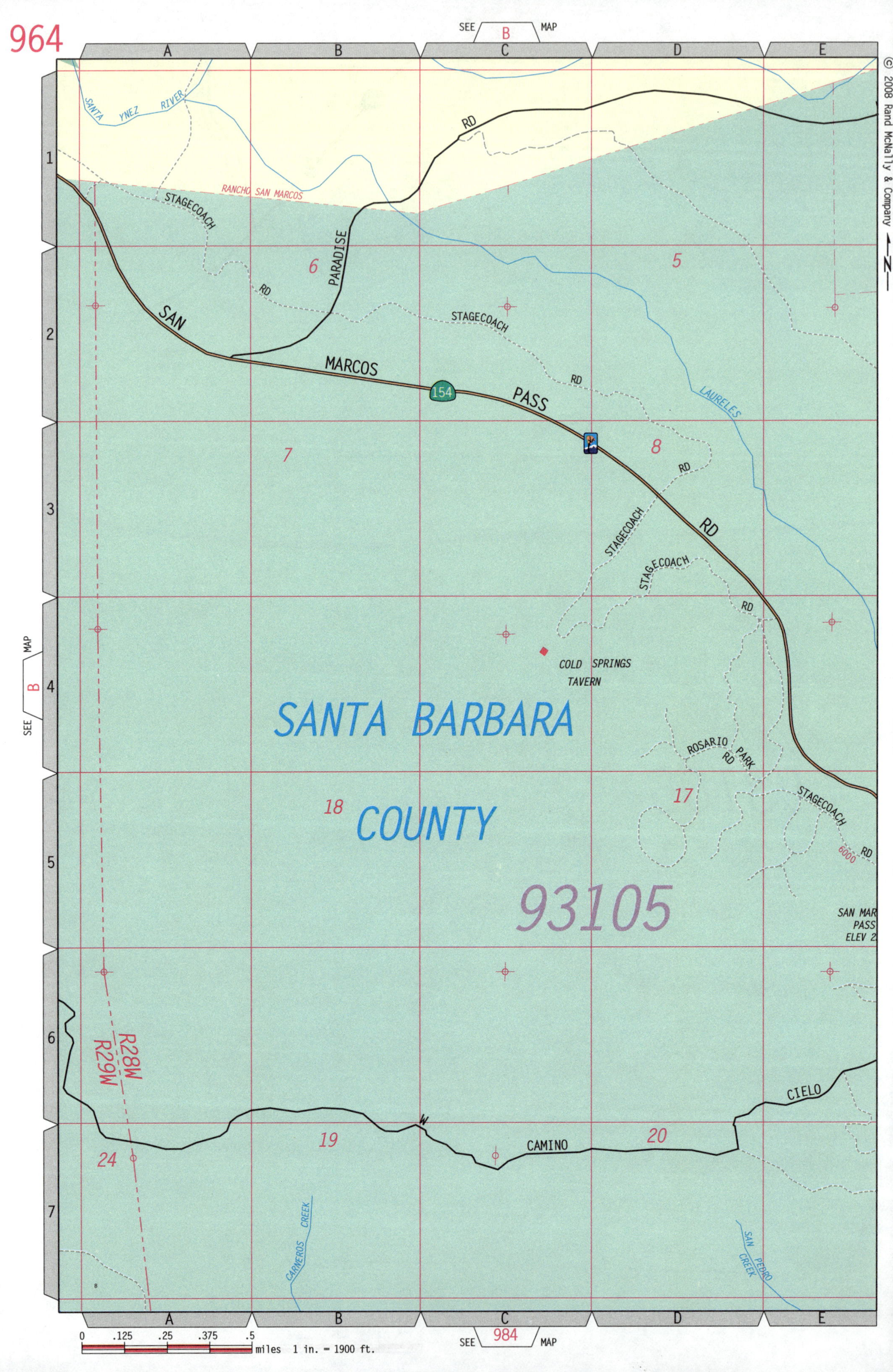
SEE B MAP
A
B
C
D
E
1
2
3
4
5
6
7
SANTA YNEZ RIVER
RD
RANCHO SAN MARCOS
STAGECOACH
PARADISE
6
5
RD
SAN
STAGECOACH
MARCOS
154
PASS
RD
LAURELES
7
8
RD
STAGECOACH
RD
STAGECOACH
RD
COLD SPRINGS TAVERN
SANTA BARBARA
ROSARIO PARK RD
18
COUNTY
17
STAGECOACH
6000
RD
93105
SAN MAR PASS ELEV 2
R28W
R29W
CIELO
W
19
CAMINO
20
24
CARNEROS CREEK
SAN PEDRO CREEK
SEE B MAP
SEE 984 MAP
0 .125 .25 .375 .5
miles 1 in. = 1900 ft.

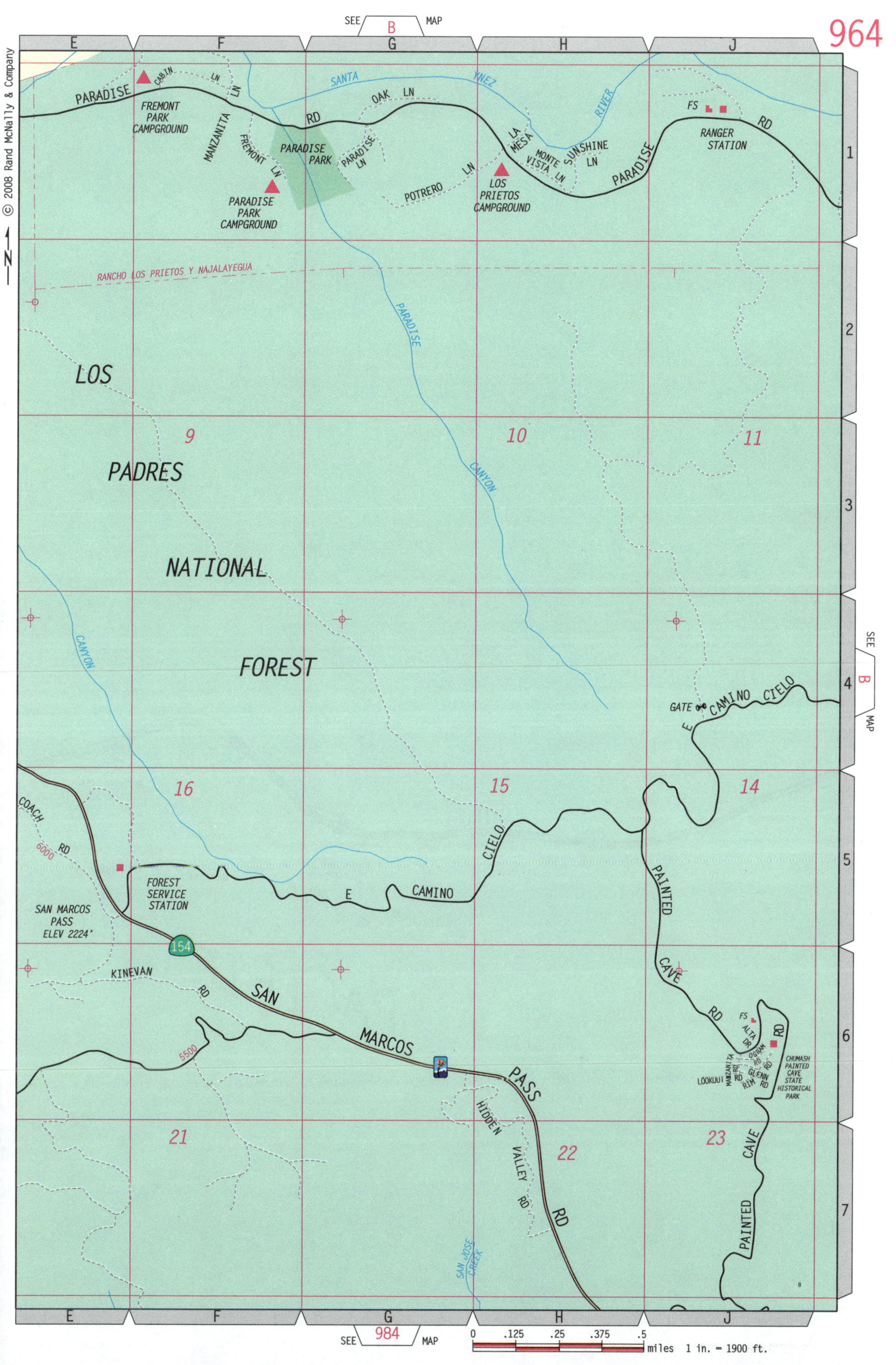
SEE B MAP
E
F
G
H
J
PARADISE
CABIN
LN
LN
FREMONT
PARK
CAMPGROUND
MANZANITA
FREMONT
LN
RD
PARADISE
PARK
PARADISE
LN
PARADISE
PARK
CAMPGROUND
SANTA
YNEZ
RIVER
OAK LN
POTRERO
LN
LA
MESA
MONTE
VISTA
LN
SUNSHINE
LN
LOS
PRIETOS
CAMPGROUND
PARADISE
RD
FS
RANGER
STATION
RANCHO LOS PRIETOS Y NAJALAYEGUA
PARADISE
CANYON
LOS
PADRES
NATIONAL
FOREST
CANYON
9
10
11
GATE
E CAMINO CIELO
16
15
14
COACH
RD
6000
FOREST
SERVICE
STATION
SAN MARCOS
PASS
ELEV 2224'
CIELO
E CAMINO
PAINTED
CAVE
RD
154
KINEVAN
RD
SAN
MARCOS
PASS
RD
5500
HIDDEN
VALLEY
RD
FS
ALTA
DR
OGRAM
RD
RD
GLENN
RD
RIM
RD
MANZANITA
LOOKOUT
CHUMASH
PAINTED
CAVE
STATE
HISTORICAL
PARK
21
22
23
CAVE
PAINTED
SAN JOSE
CREEK
1
2
3
4
5
6
7
SEE B MAP
SEE 984 MAP
0 .125 .25 .375 .5
miles 1 in. = 1900 ft.

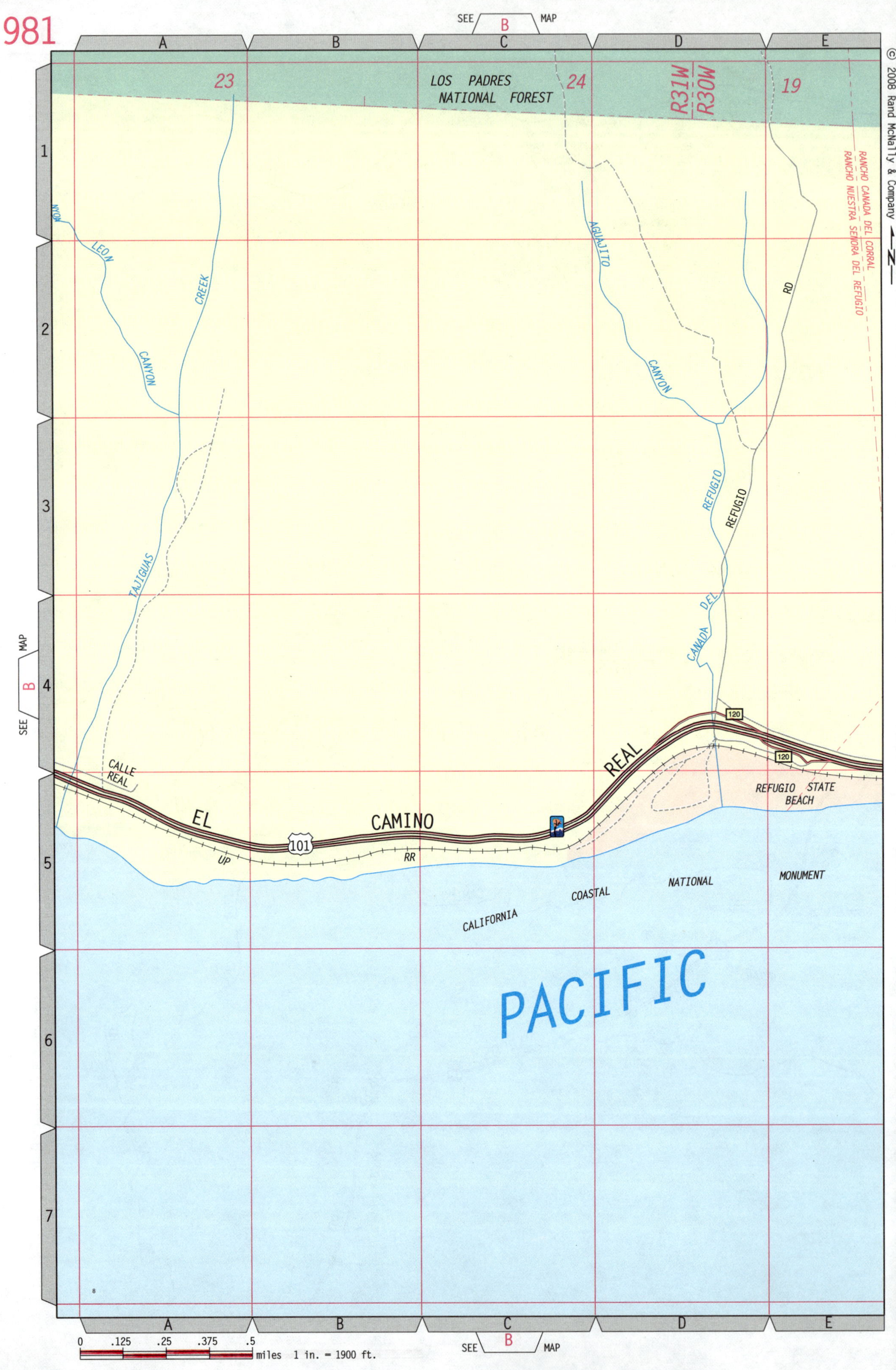
SEE B MAP
A
B
C
D
E
1
2
3
4
5
6
7
23
24
19
LOS PADRES
NATIONAL FOREST
R31W
R30W
RANCHO CANADA DEL CORRAL
RANCHO NUESTRA SENORA DEL REFUGIO
LEON
CANYON
CREEK
TAJIGUAS
AGUAJITO
CANYON
REFUGIO
CANADA DEL
REFUGIO
RD
120
CALLE
REAL
EL
CAMINO
REAL
101
UP
RR
REFUGIO STATE
BEACH
CALIFORNIA
COASTAL
NATIONAL
MONUMENT
PACIFIC
0 .125 .25 .375 .5
miles 1 in. = 1900 ft.

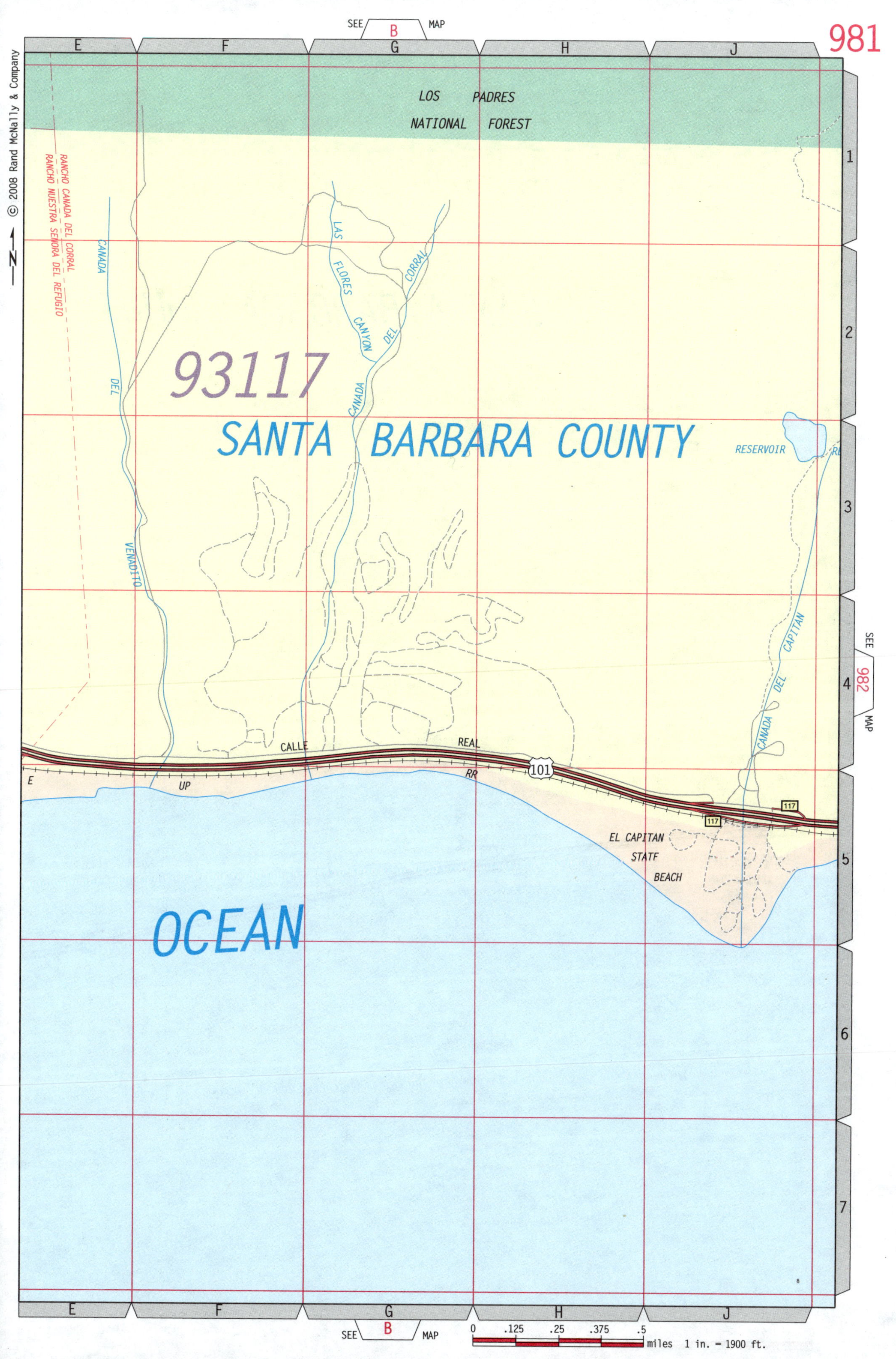
SEE B MAP
E
F
G
H
J
LOS PADRES
NATIONAL FOREST
RANCHO CANADA DEL CORRAL
RANCHO NUESTRA SEÑORA DEL REFUGIO
CANADA
DEL
VENADITO
LAS
FLORES
CANYON
CORRAL
DEL
CANADA
93117
SANTA BARBARA COUNTY
RESERVOIR
CANADA
DEL
CAPITAN
CALLE
REAL
101
E
UP
RR
117
117
EL CAPITAN
STATE
BEACH
OCEAN
1
2
3
4
5
6
7
SEE 982 MAP
SEE B MAP
0
.125
.25
.375
.5
miles 1 in. = 1900 ft.

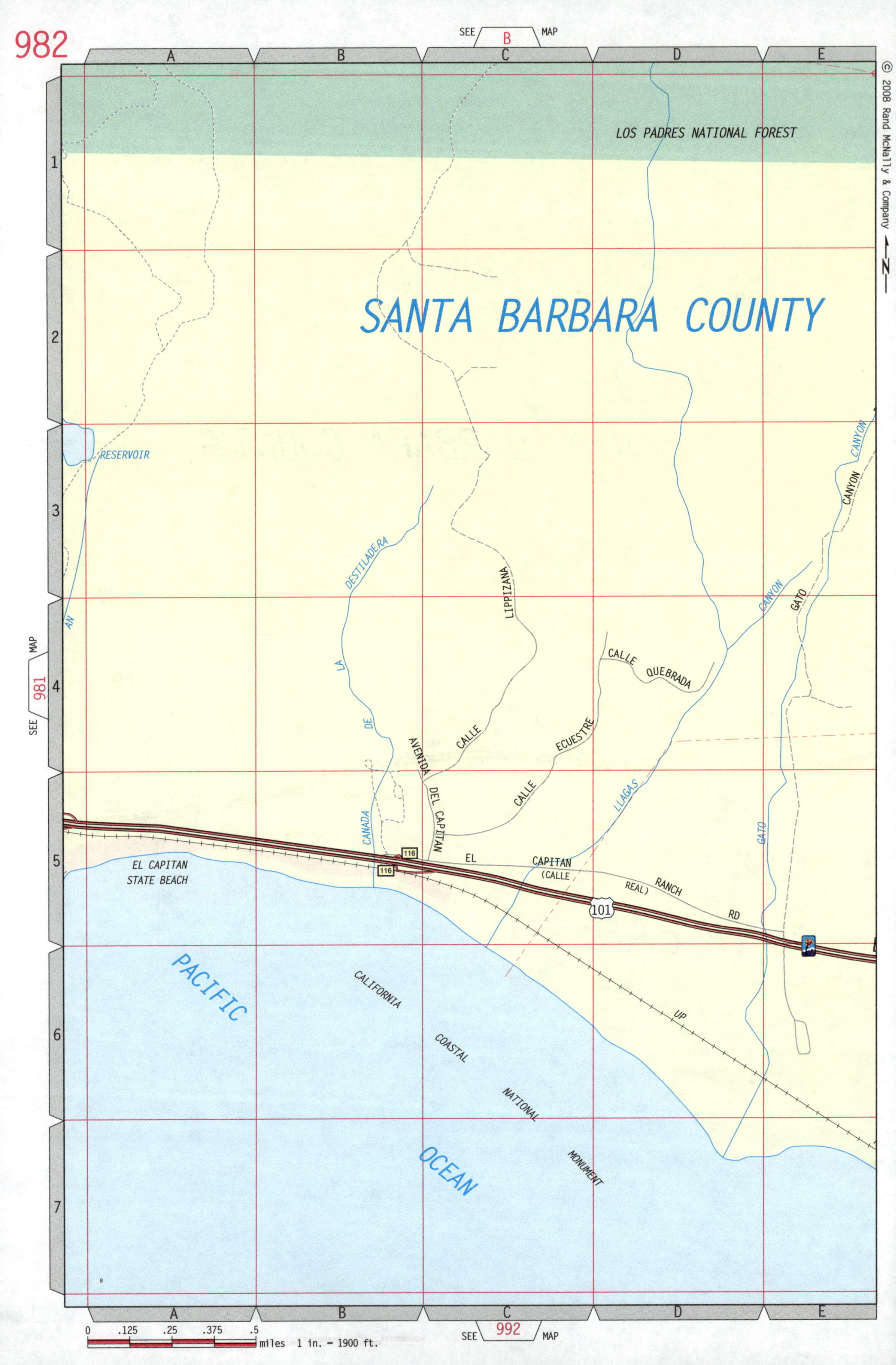
SEE B MAP
A
B
C
D
E
1
2
3
4
5
6
7
LOS PADRES NATIONAL FOREST
SANTA BARBARA COUNTY
RESERVOIR
LA DE DESTILADERA
LIPPIZANA
CANYON
CANYON
CANYON
GATO
CALLE QUEBRADA
AVENIDA DEL CAPITAN
CALLE
CALLE ECUESTRE
CALLE
LLAGAS
CANADA
GATO
116
116
EL CAPITAN (CALLE REAL) RANCH RD
101
EL CAPITAN STATE BEACH
PACIFIC OCEAN
CALIFORNIA COASTAL NATIONAL MONUMENT
UP
SEE 981 MAP
0 .125 .25 .375 .5
miles 1 in. = 1900 ft.
SEE 992 MAP

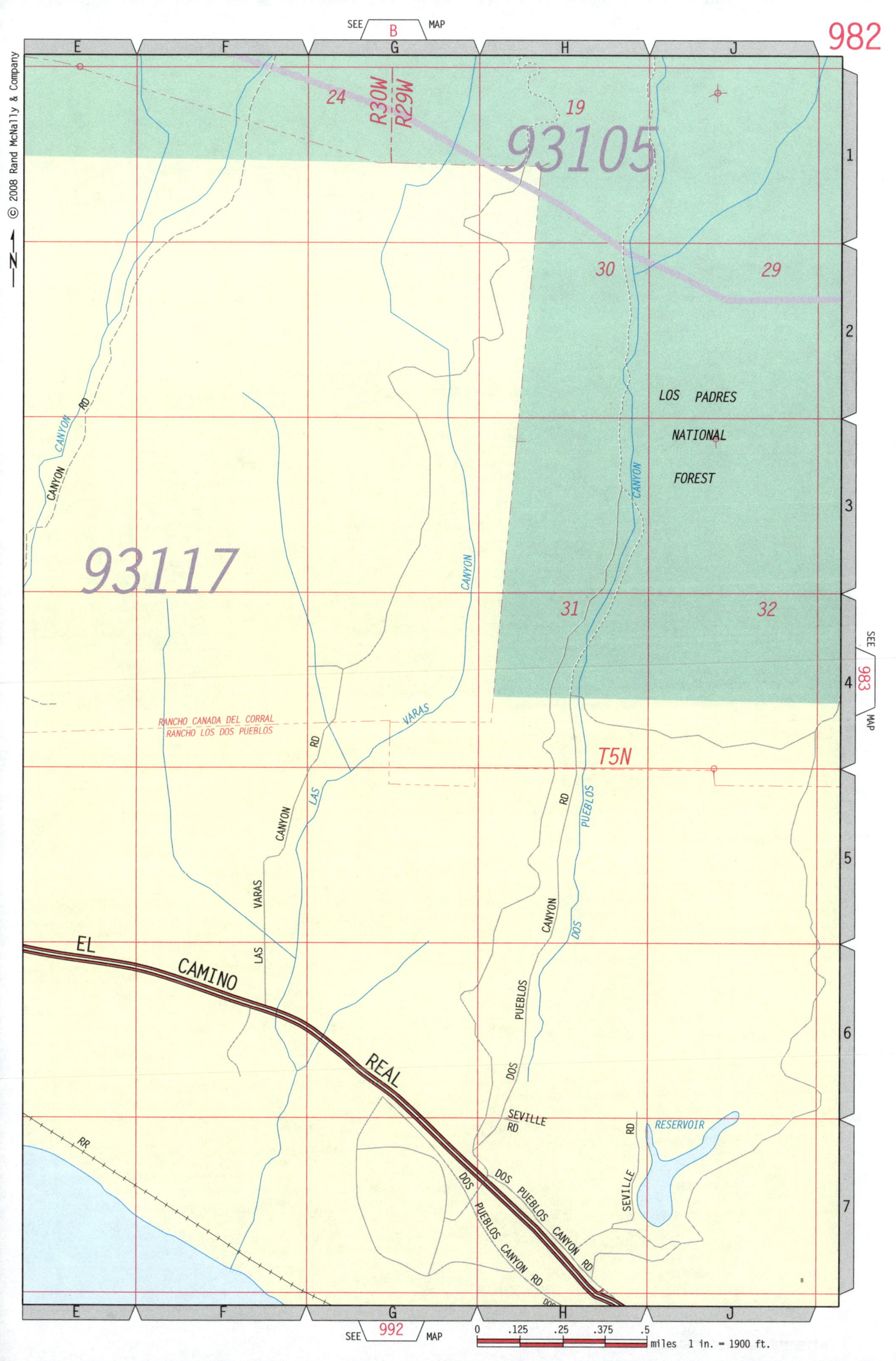

SEE B MAP
E
F
G
H
J
1
2
3
4
5
6
7
24
19
30
29
31
32
R30W
R29W
93105
93117
LOS PADRES
NATIONAL
FOREST
CANYON
CANYON RD
CANYON
CANYON
RANCHO CANADA DEL CORRAL
RANCHO LOS DOS PUEBLOS
VARAS
LAS
RD
CANYON
VARAS
LAS
T5N
RD
PUEBLOS
CANYON
DOS
PUEBLOS
DOS
EL
CAMINO
REAL
SEVILLE RD
RD
RESERVOIR
SEVILLE
DOS PUEBLOS CANYON RD
DOS PUEBLOS CANYON RD
RR
SEE 983 MAP
SEE 992 MAP
0
.125
.25
.375
.5
miles 1 in. = 1900 ft.

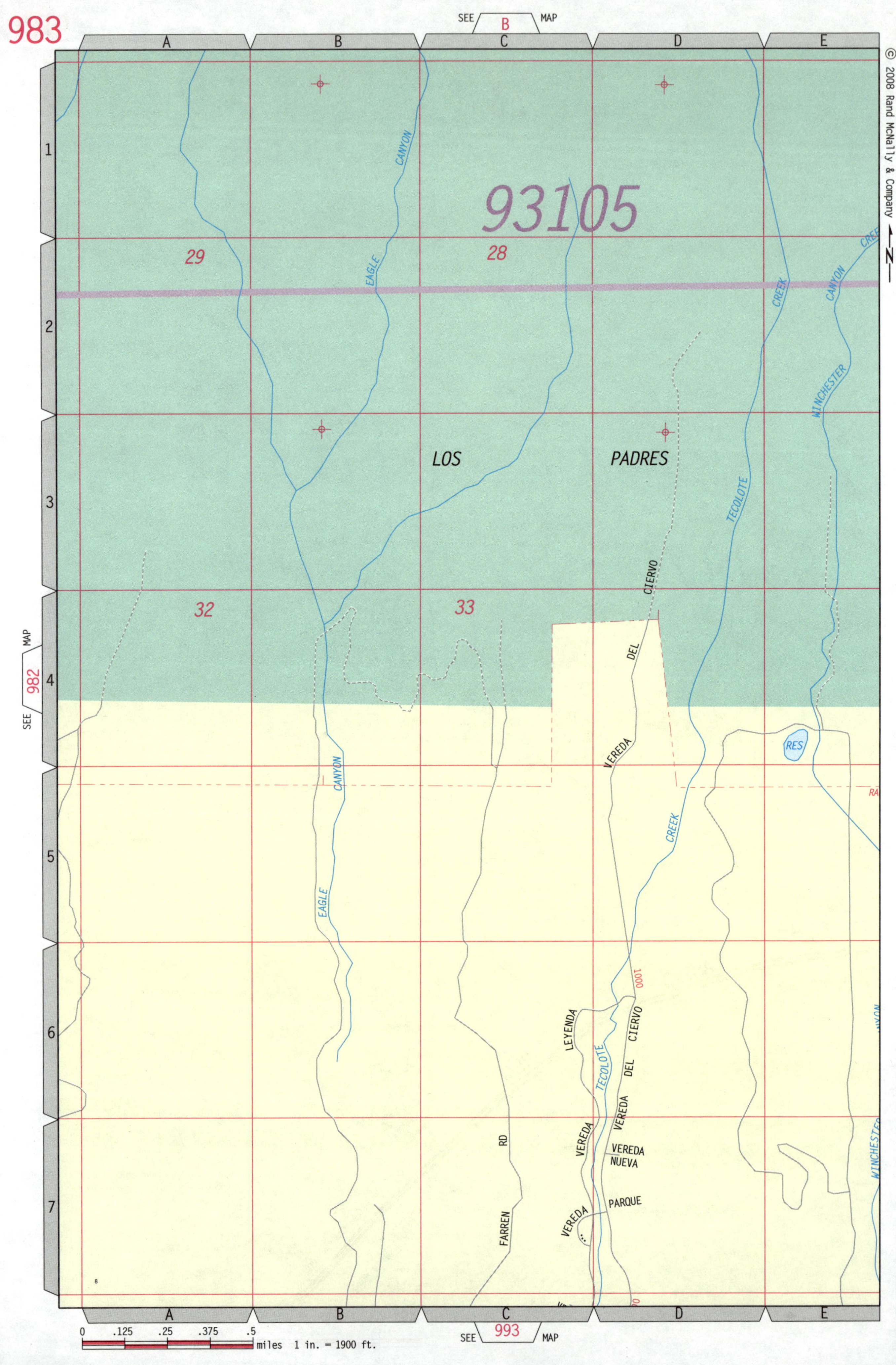
SEE B MAP
A
B
C
D
E
1
2
3
4
5
6
7
93105
29
28
32
33
EAGLE
CANYON
LOS
PADRES
CIERVO
DEL
VEREDA
TECOLOTE
CREEK
WINCHESTER
CANYON
RES
1000
LEYENDA
VEREDA
NUEVA
PARQUE
RD
FARREN
SEE 982 MAP
SEE 993 MAP
0 .125 .25 .375 .5
miles 1 in. = 1900 ft.

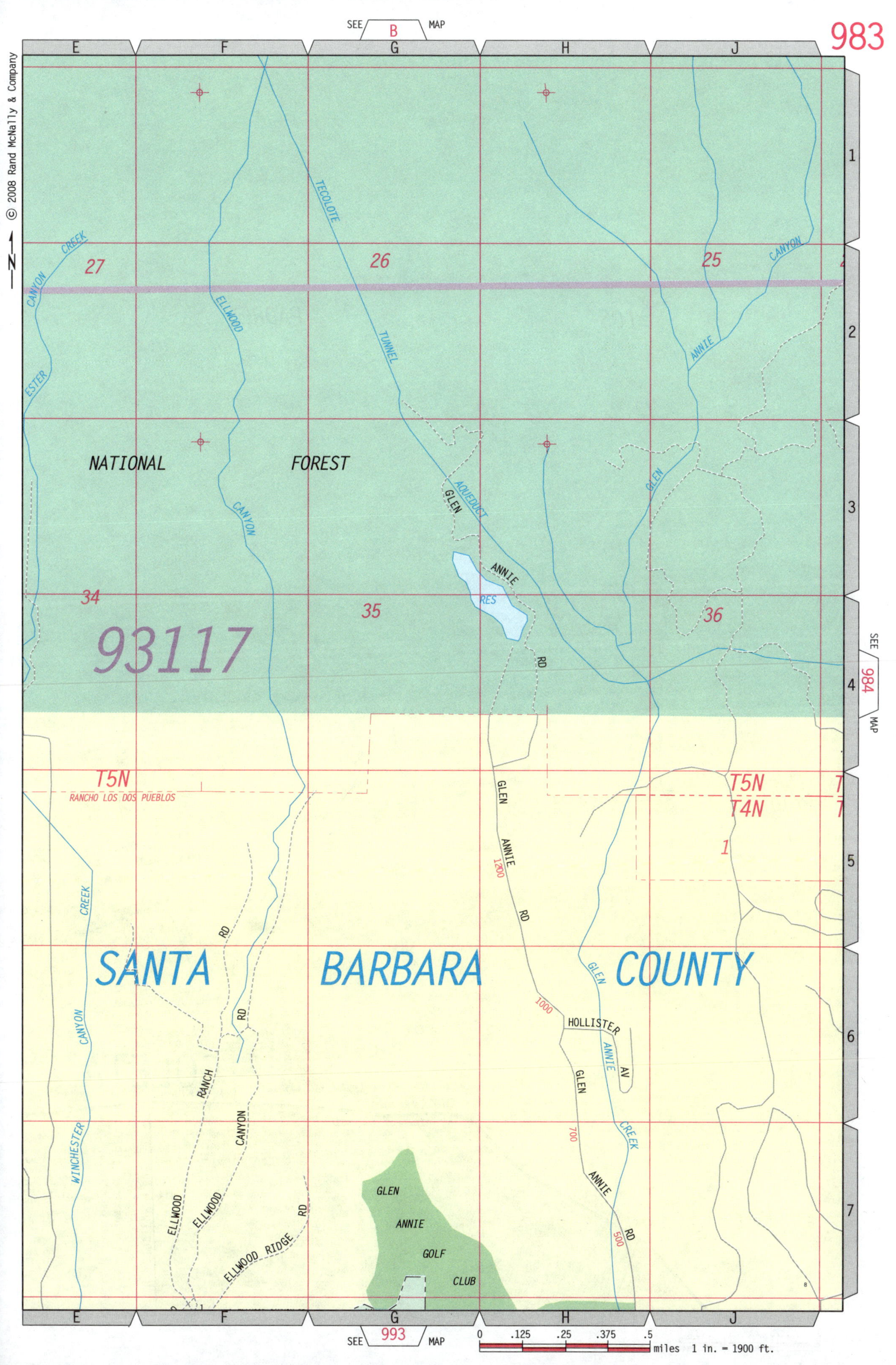
SEE B MAP
E
F
G
H
J
1
2
3
4
5
6
7
27
26
25
34
35
36
TECOLOTE
TUNNEL
AQUEDUCT
CREEK
CANYON
ESTER
ELLWOOD
CANYON
ANNIE
GLEN
NATIONAL
FOREST
GLEN
ANNIE
RES
RD
93117
SEE 984 MAP
T5N
RANCHO LOS DOS PUEBLOS
T5N
T4N
1
GLEN
ANNIE
1200
RD
CREEK
CANYON
WINCHESTER
SANTA
BARBARA
COUNTY
RD
RD
RANCH
CANYON
ELLWOOD
ELLWOOD
ELLWOOD RIDGE
RD
GLEN
1000
HOLLISTER
AV
ANNIE
GLEN
700
CREEK
ANNIE
RD
500
GLEN
ANNIE
GOLF
CLUB
SEE 993 MAP
0 .125 .25 .375 .5
miles 1 in. = 1900 ft.

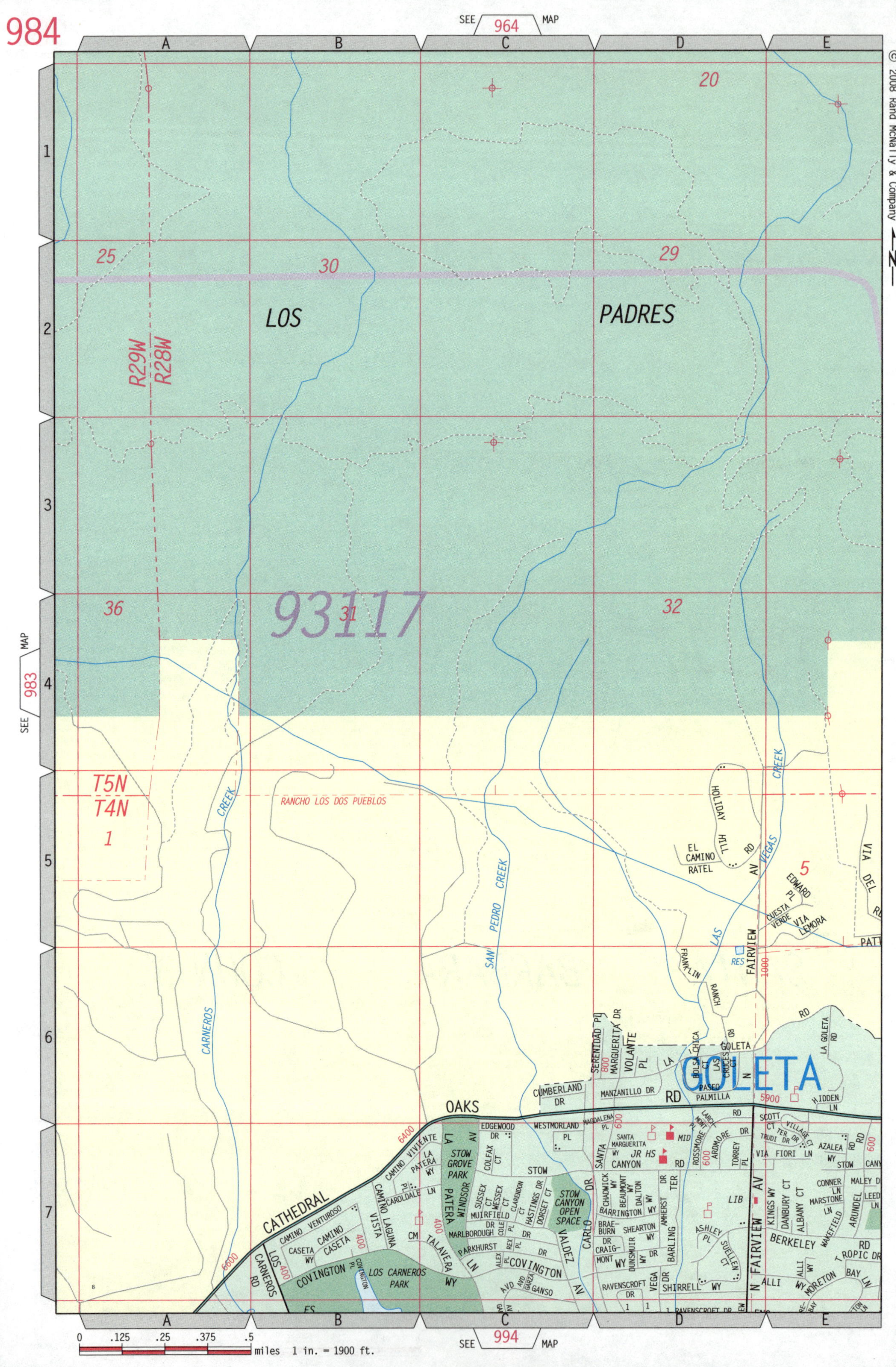
SEE 964 MAP
LOS
PADRES
93117
R29W
R28W
T5N
T4N
RANCHO LOS DOS PUEBLOS
CARNEROS CREEK
SAN PEDRO CREEK
LAS VEGAS CREEK
HOLIDAY HILL RD
EL CAMINO RATEL
FAIRVIEW AV
FRANKLIN RANCH RD
GOLETA
CATHEDRAL OAKS RD
STOW GROVE PARK
STOW CANYON OPEN SPACE
LOS CARNEROS PARK
SEE 983 MAP
SEE 994 MAP
miles 1 in. = 1900 ft.

SEE 964 MAP

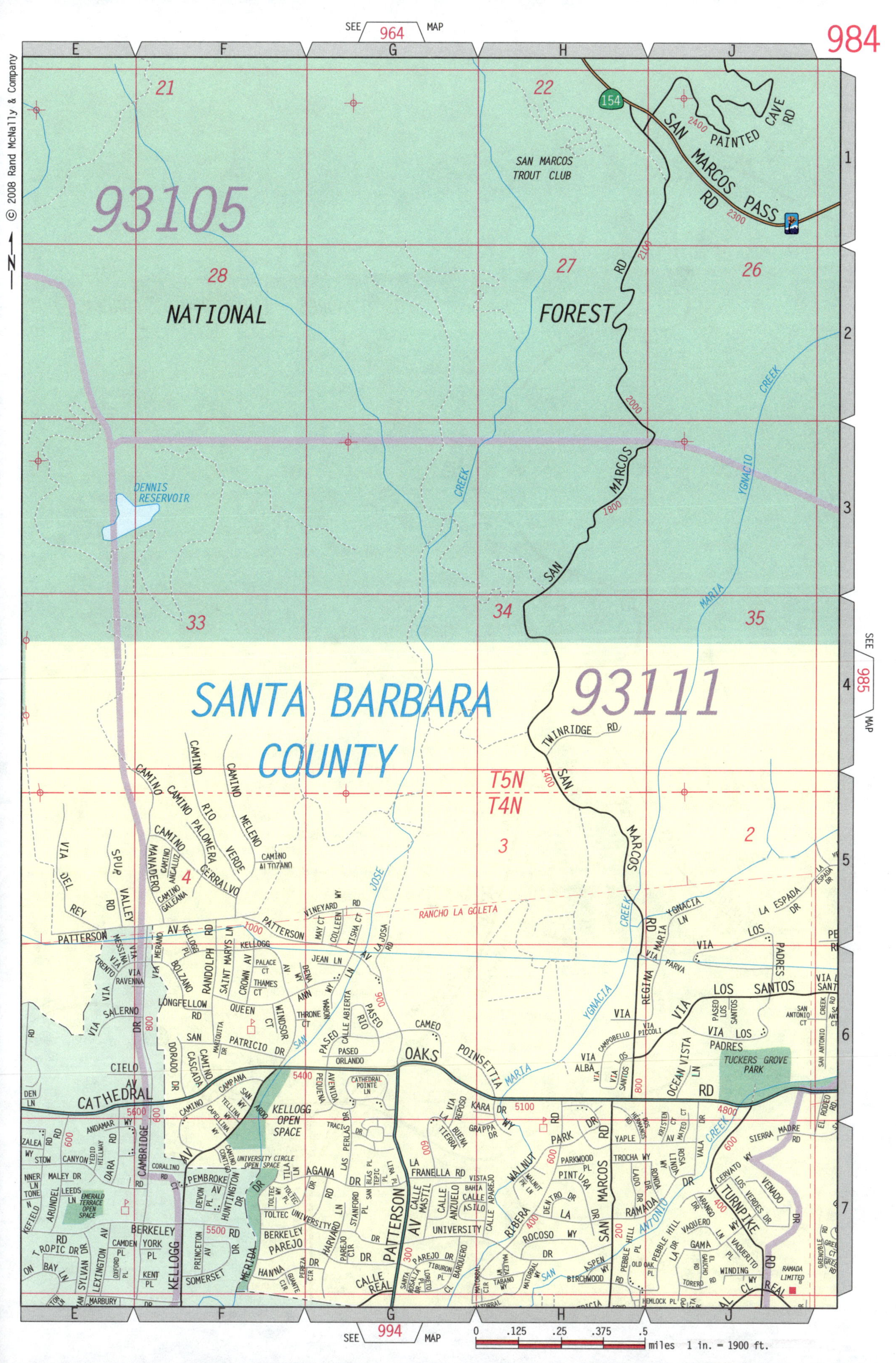
93105
93111
NATIONAL FOREST
SANTA BARBARA COUNTY
SAN MARCOS TROUT CLUB
DENNIS RESERVOIR
SAN MARCOS PASS RD
PAINTED CAVE RD
SAN MARCOS RD
TWINRIDGE RD
T5N
T4N
RANCHO LA GOLETA
PATTERSON AV
CATHEDRAL OAKS RD
KELLOGG OPEN SPACE
TUCKERS GROVE PARK
EMERALD TERRACE OPEN SPACE
UNIVERSITY CIRCLE OPEN SPACE
CALLE REAL
TURNPIKE RD
HOLLISTER AV
SAN JOSE CREEK
MARIA YGNACIO CREEK
SAN ANTONIO CREEK
RAMADA LIMITED

SEE 985 MAP

SEE 994 MAP

0 .125 .25 .375 .5 miles 1 in. = 1900 ft.

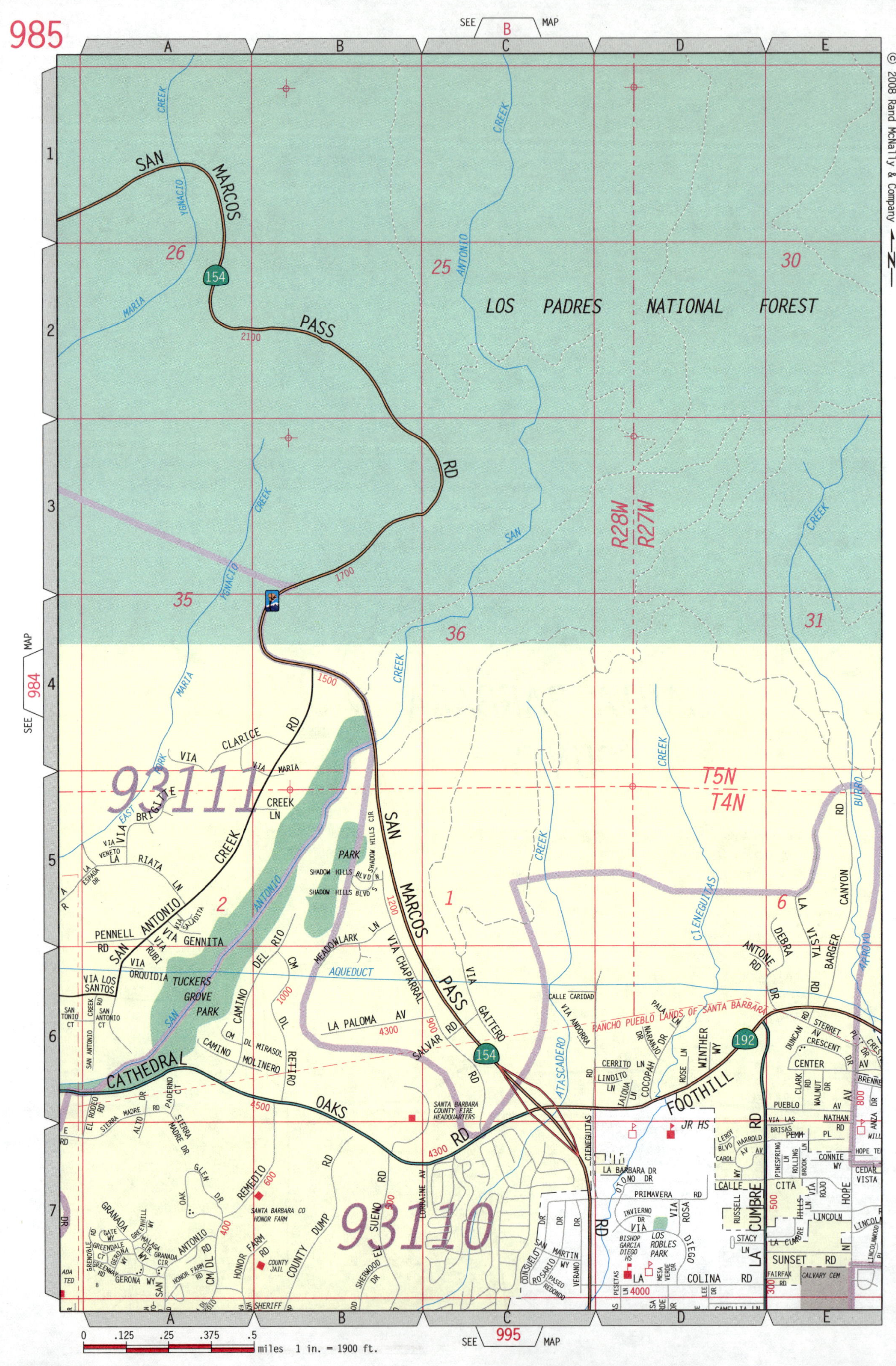

SEE B MAP
SEE 984 MAP
SEE 995 MAP
© 2008 Rand McNally & Company
LOS PADRES NATIONAL FOREST
SAN MARCOS PASS RD
154
192
YGNACIO CREEK
MARIA CREEK
SAN ANTONIO CREEK
EAST FORK
R28W
R27W
T5N
T4N
26
25
30
35
36
31
2
1
6
93111
93110
2100
1700
1500
1200
1000
900
600
500
400
300
800
4300
4500
4000
VIA CLARICE
VIA MARIA
BRIGITTE
CREEK LN
VIA VENETO
LA RIATA LN
LA ESPADA DR
SAN ANTONIO CREEK RD
PENNELL RD
VIA GENNITA
VIA RUBI
VIA ORQUIDIA
VIA LOS SANTOS
TUCKERS GROVE PARK
SHADOW HILLS PARK
SHADOW HILLS BLVD
SHADOW HILLS CIR
MEADOWLARK LN
VIA CHAPARRAL
CAMINO DEL RIO
CM DL MIRASOL
CAMINO MOLINERO
RETIRO
LA PALOMA AV
SALVAR RD
VIA GAITERO
AQUEDUCT
CATHEDRAL OAKS RD
EL RODEO RD
SIERRA MADRE
ALTO
PADERNO CT
SANTA BARBARA COUNTY FIRE HEADQUARTERS
REMEDIO
GLEN DR
OAK
GRANADA
GERONA WY
SAN ANTONIO RD
HONOR FARM RD
SANTA BARBARA CO HONOR FARM
COUNTY JAIL
COUNTY DUMP RD
SUENO RD
SHERWOOD DR
LORRAINE AV
SHERIFF
CALLE CARIDAD
VIA ANDORRA
RANCHO PUEBLO LANDS OF SANTA BARBARA
ATASCADERO CREEK
CIENEGUITAS CREEK
CIENEGUITAS RD
CERRITO LN
LINDITO LN
COCOPAH DR
NARANJO DR
PALA LN
ROSE LN
WINTHER WY
FOOTHILL RD
JR HS
LA BARBARA DR
OTONO DR
PRIMAVERA RD
VIA ROSA
INVIERNO DR
BISHOP GARCIA DIEGO HS
LOS ROBLES PARK
DIEGO
COLINA RD
SAN MARTIN WY
ROSARIO
PASEO REDONDO
VERANO
CONSUELO
LA CUMBRE RD
RUSSELL
STACY LN
CALLE
LEROY
HARROLD AV
CAROL AV
ANTONE RD
DEBRA
LA VISTA RD
BARGER
CANYON RD
BURRO
ARROYO
STERRET AV
CRESCENT DR
DUNCAN AV
CENTER AV
CLARK AV
WALNUT DR
PUEBLO AV
NATHAN
VIA LAS BRISAS
PEMM PL
PINESPRING LN
ROLLING
BROOK LN
CONNIE WY
CITA
HOPE AV
CEDAR VISTA
LINCOLN
SUNSET RD
FAIRFAX RD
CALVARY CEM
ANZA
BRENNER
0 .125 .25 .375 .5 miles 1 in. = 1900 ft.

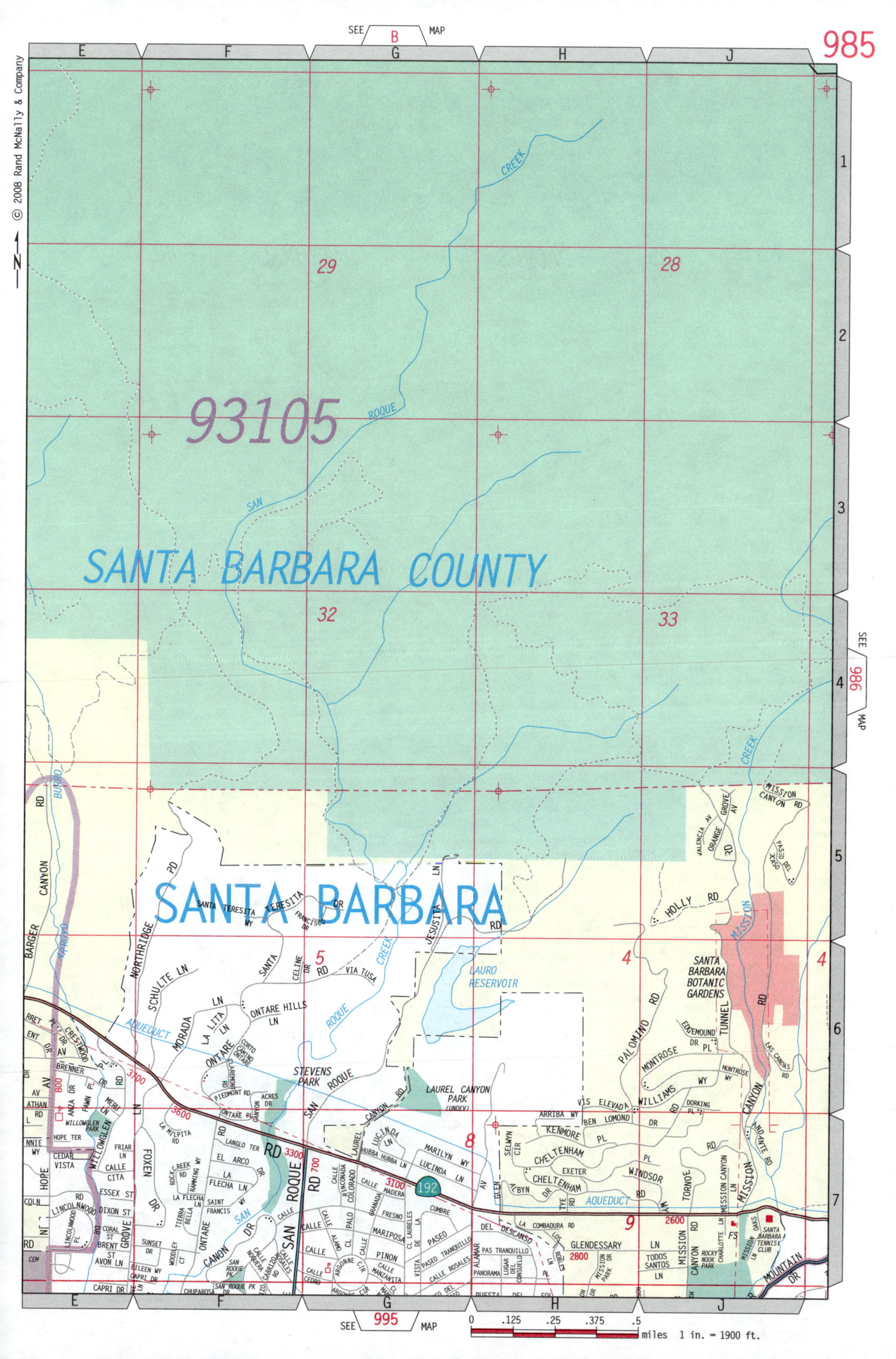
SEE B MAP
93105
SANTA BARBARA COUNTY
SANTA BARBARA
SAN ROQUE CREEK
LAURO RESERVOIR
SANTA BARBARA BOTANIC GARDENS
STEVENS PARK
LAUREL CANYON PARK (UNDEV)
SANTA BARBARA TENNIS CLUB
ROCKY NOOK PARK
AQUEDUCT
MISSION CANYON RD
MOUNTAIN DR
SEE 986 MAP
SEE 995 MAP
0 .125 .25 .375 .5 miles 1 in. = 1900 ft.

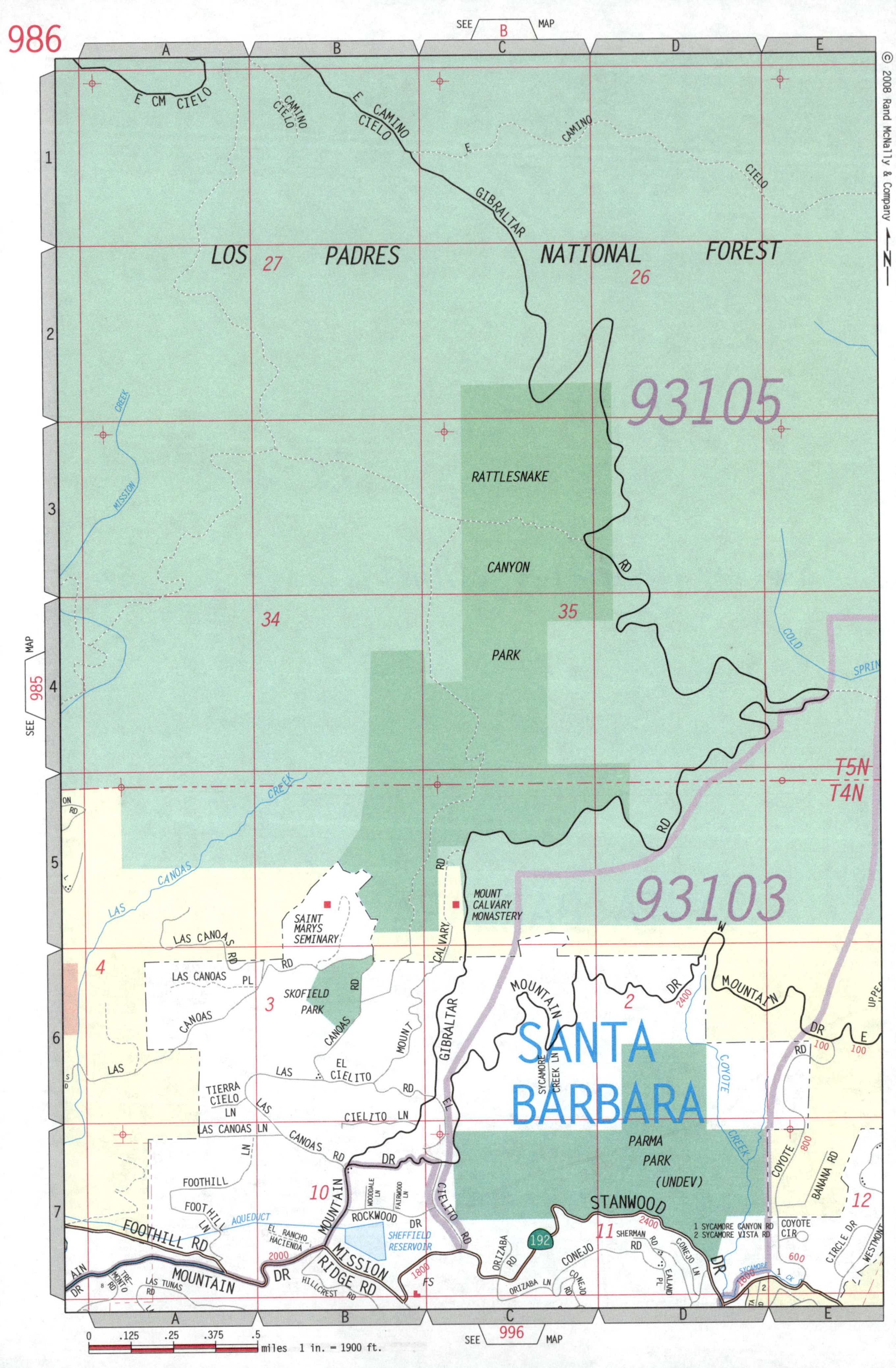

SEE B MAP
SEE 985 MAP
SEE 996 MAP
LOS PADRES NATIONAL FOREST
93105
93103
RATTLESNAKE CANYON PARK
MOUNT CALVARY MONASTERY
SAINT MARYS SEMINARY
SKOFIELD PARK
SANTA BARBARA
PARMA PARK (UNDEV)
SHEFFIELD RESERVOIR
E CM CIELO
CAMINO CIELO
E CAMINO CIELO
GIBRALTAR RD
MISSION CREEK
LAS CANOAS CREEK
COLD SPRING
T5N
T4N
LAS CANOAS RD
LAS CANOAS PL
CANOAS RD
MOUNT CALVARY RD
EL CIELITO RD
TIERRA CIELO LN
CIELITO LN
LAS CANOAS LN
MOUNTAIN DR
W MOUNTAIN DR
E MOUNTAIN DR
SYCAMORE CREEK LN
COYOTE CREEK
COYOTE RD
BANANA RD
COYOTE CIR
CIRCLE DR
WESTMONT
UPPER
FOOTHILL LN
FOOTHILL RD
AQUEDUCT
EL RANCHO HACIENDA
WOODDALE LN
FAIRWOOD LN
ROCKWOOD DR
MISSION RIDGE RD
HILLCREST RD
LAS TUNAS RD
TREMONTO RD
CIELITO RD
ORIZABA RD
ORIZABA LN
CONEJO RD
CONEJO LN
STANWOOD DR
SHERMAN RD
EALAND PL
SYCAMORE CK
192
FS
1 SYCAMORE CANYON RD
2 SYCAMORE VISTA RD
27
26
34
35
4
3
2
10
11
12
2400
2000
1800
800
600
100
miles 1 in. = 1900 ft.
0 .125 .25 .375 .5

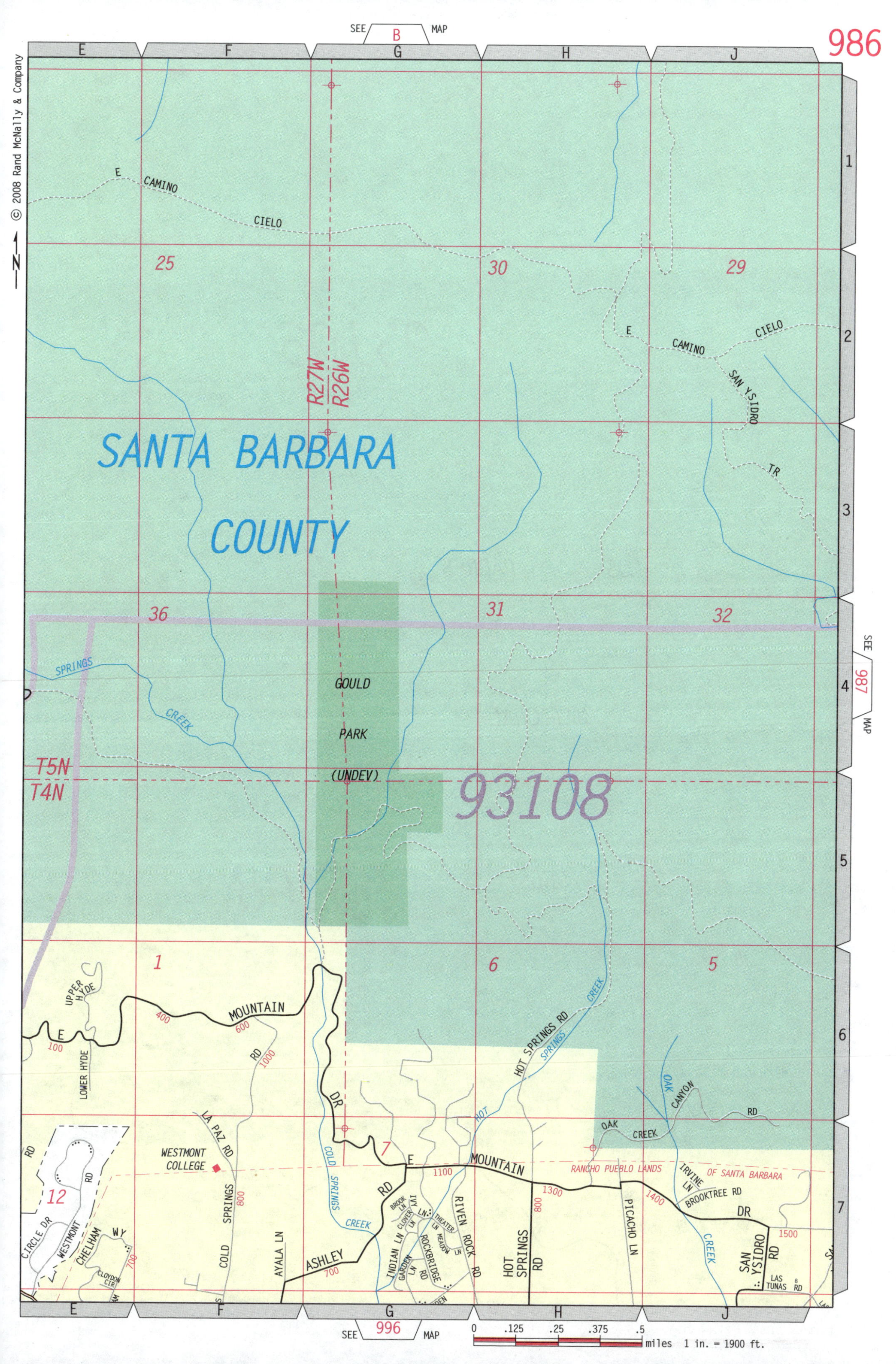
SEE B MAP
E
F
G
H
J
1
2
3
4
5
6
7
E CAMINO CIELO
25
30
29
R27W
R26W
SAN YSIDRO TR
SANTA BARBARA
COUNTY
36
31
32
SEE 987 MAP
SPRINGS CREEK
GOULD
PARK
(UNDEV)
T5N
T4N
93108
1
6
5
UPPER HYDE
E MOUNTAIN
400
600
100
LOWER HYDE
RD 1000
HOT SPRINGS RD
SPRINGS CREEK
OAK CANYON RD
OAK CREEK
DR
LA PAZ RD
WESTMONT COLLEGE
RD
12
CIRCLE DR
WESTMONT RD
CHELHAM WY
CLOYDON CIR
COLD SPRINGS
800
COLD SPRINGS CREEK
AYALA LN
ASHLEY RD
700
7
E MOUNTAIN
1100
HOT
RIVEN ROCK RD
RANCHO PUEBLO LANDS OF SANTA BARBARA
1300
PICACHO LN
1400
IRVINE LN
BROOKTREE RD
DR
1500
CREEK
SAN YSIDRO RD
LAS TUNAS RD
HOT SPRINGS RD
INDIAN LN
CLOVER LN
ROCKBRIDGE RD
GARDEN LN
THEATER LN
MEADOW LN
SEE 996 MAP
0 .125 .25 .375 .5 miles 1 in. = 1900 ft.

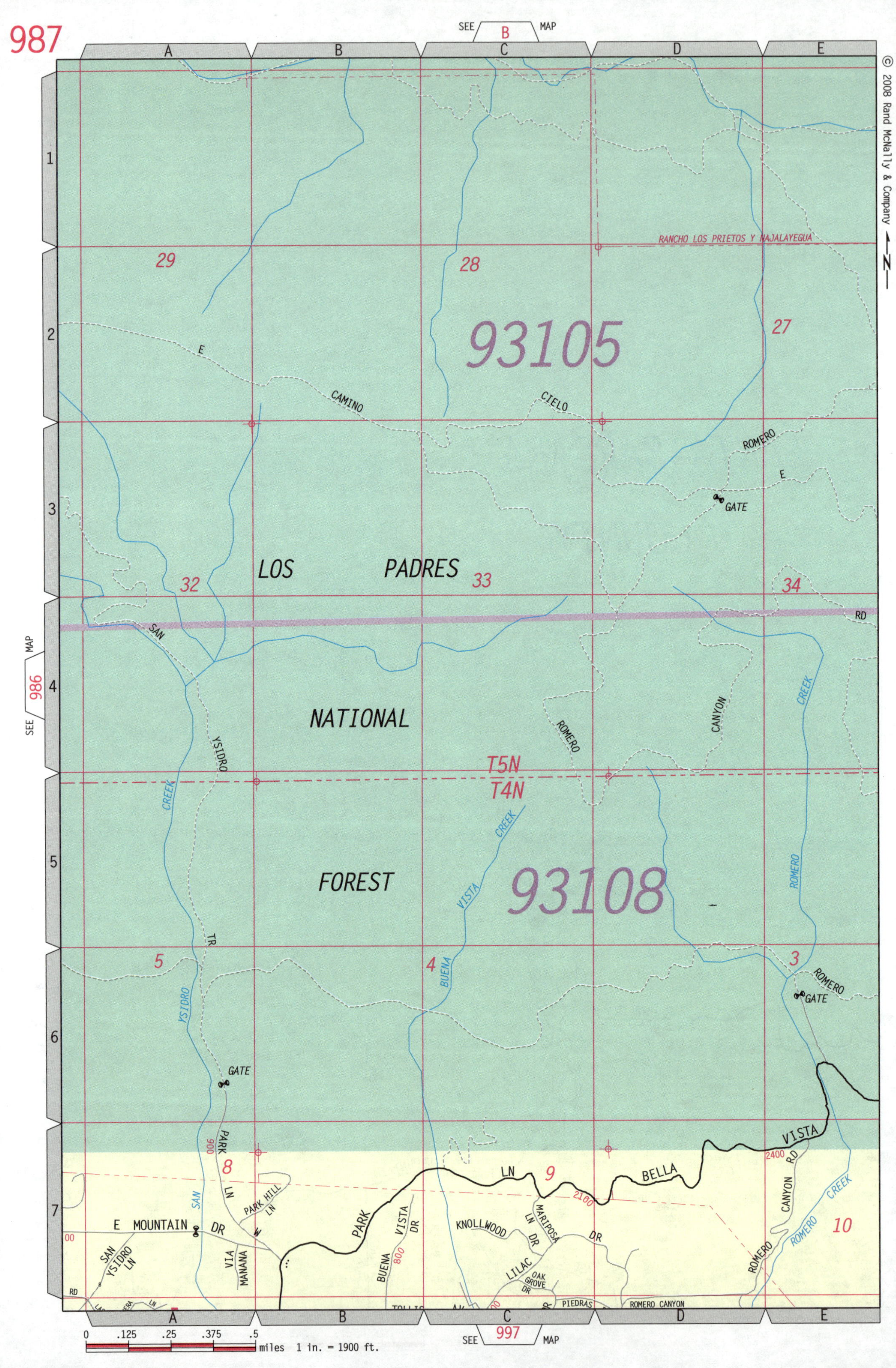
SEE B MAP
SEE 986 MAP
SEE 997 MAP
© 2008 Rand McNally & Company
RANCHO LOS PRIETOS Y NAJALAYEGUA
93105
93108
LOS PADRES NATIONAL FOREST
T5N
T4N
29
28
27
32
33
34
5
4
3
8
9
10
E CAMINO CIELO
ROMERO CANYON RD
GATE
SAN YSIDRO TR
SAN YSIDRO CREEK
BUENA VISTA CREEK
ROMERO CREEK
PARK LN
PARK HILL LN
E MOUNTAIN DR
SAN YSIDRO LN
VIA MANANA
BUENA VISTA DR
KNOLLWOOD DR
MARIPOSA LN
LILAC DR
OAK GROVE DR
PIEDRAS
ROMERO CANYON
BELLA VISTA
2400
2100
900
800
0 .125 .25 .375 .5 miles 1 in. = 1900 ft.

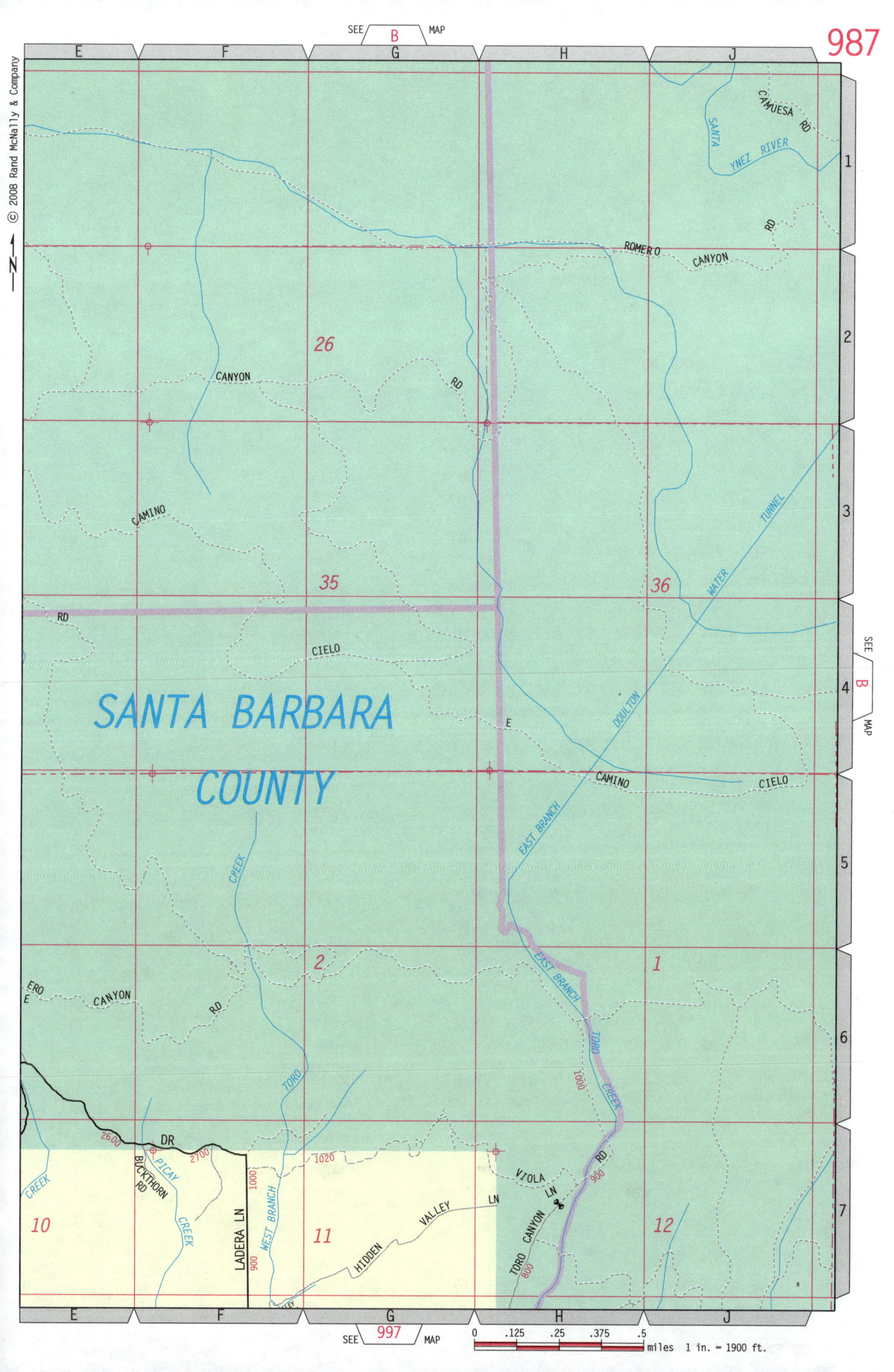
SEE B MAP
E
F
G
H
J
1
2
3
4
5
6
7
SEE B MAP
CAMUESA RD
SANTA YNEZ RIVER
RD
ROMERO CANYON
26
CANYON
RD
CAMINO
35
36
WATER TUNNEL
RD
CIELO
SANTA BARBARA COUNTY
DOULTON
E
CAMINO CIELO
EAST BRANCH
CREEK
2
1
EAST BRANCH
ERO
E
CANYON
RD
TORO CREEK
1000
TORO
2600
DR
2700
1020
VIOLA
RD
900
CREEK
PICAY
BUCKTHORN RD
CREEK
1000
LN
LN
10
LADERA LN
WEST BRANCH
900
11
HIDDEN VALLEY
TORO CANYON
800
12
E
F
G
H
J
SEE 997 MAP
0 .125 .25 .375 .5
miles 1 in. = 1900 ft.

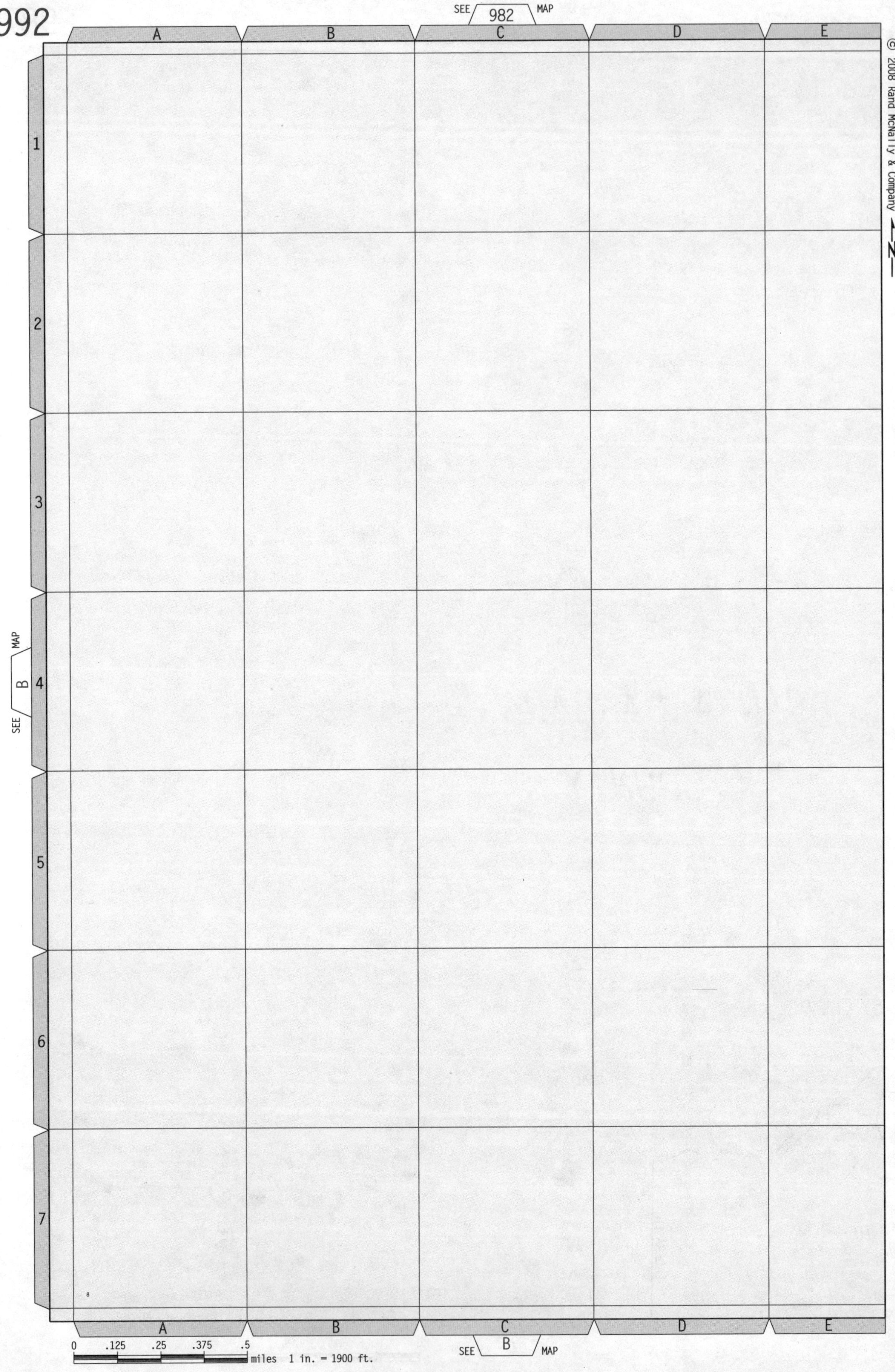

SEE 982 MAP
A
B
C
D
E
1
2
3
4
5
6
7
SEE B MAP
SEE B MAP
0 .125 .25 .375 .5
miles 1 in. = 1900 ft.

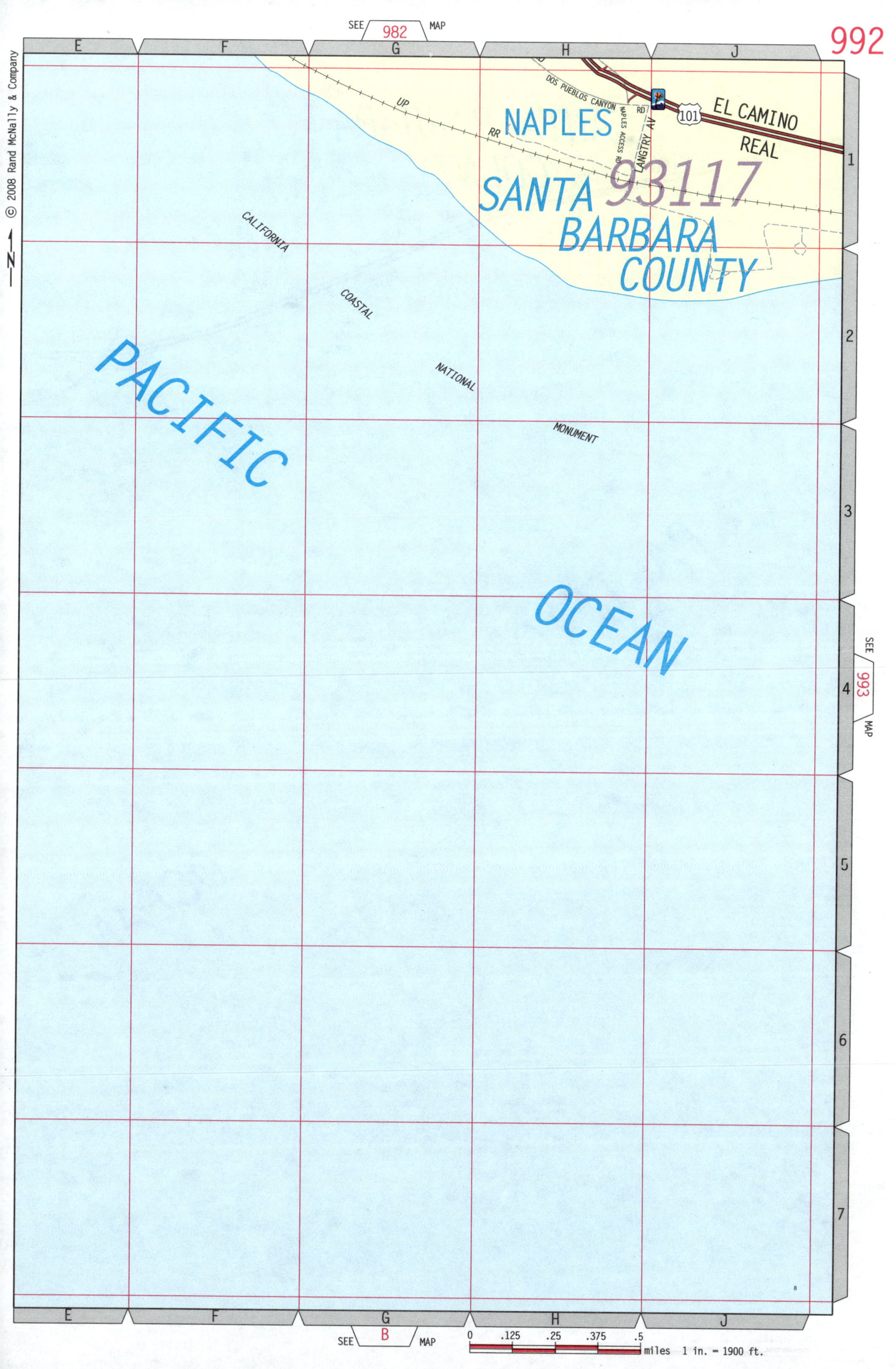
SEE 982 MAP
E
F
G
H
J
DOS PUEBLOS CANYON RD
UP RR
NAPLES
NAPLES ACCESS RD
LANGTRY AV
101
EL CAMINO REAL
SANTA BARBARA COUNTY
93117
CALIFORNIA COASTAL NATIONAL MONUMENT
PACIFIC OCEAN
1
2
3
4
5
6
7
SEE 993 MAP
SEE B MAP
0 .125 .25 .375 .5 miles 1 in. = 1900 ft.

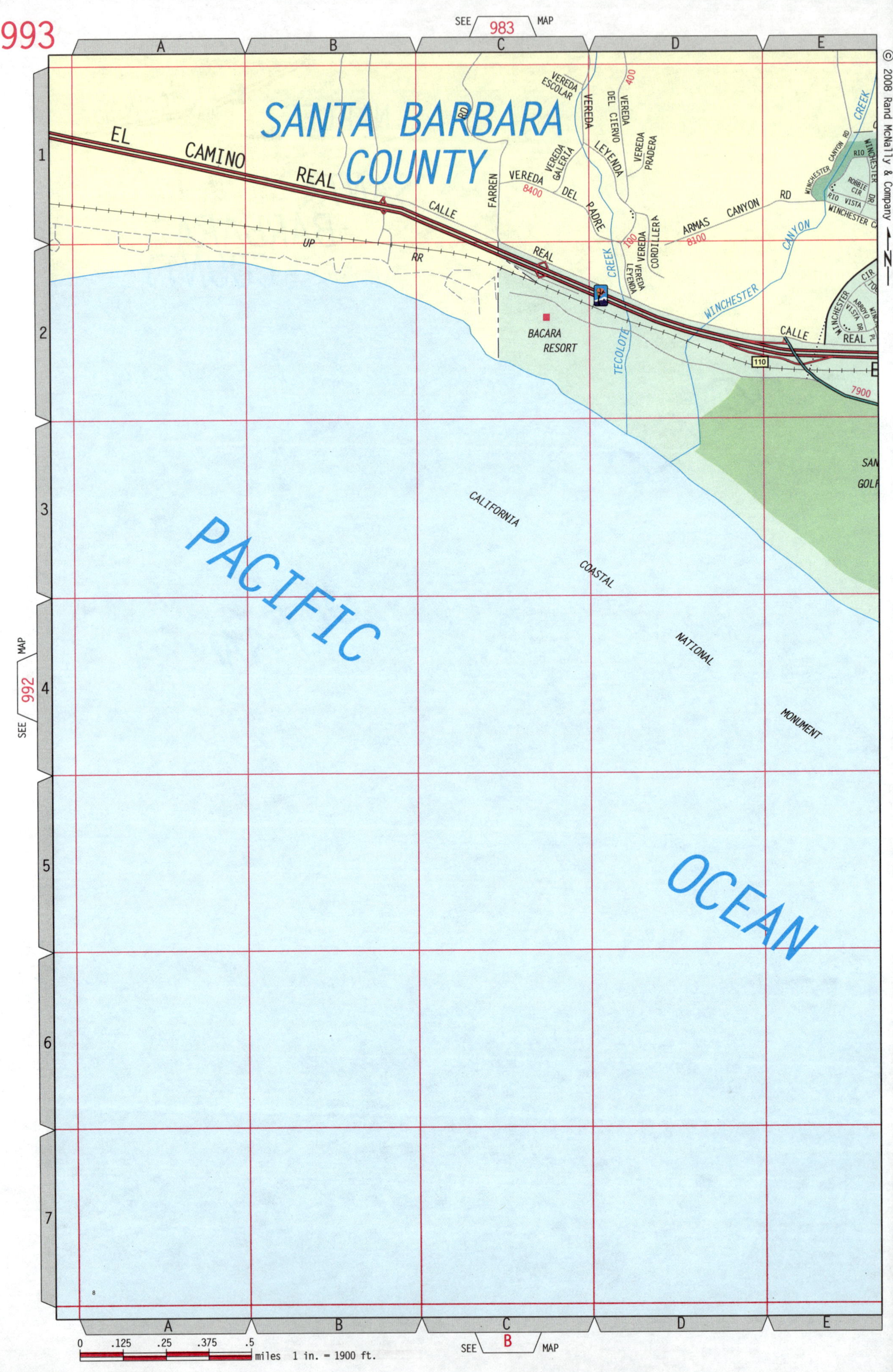

SEE 983 MAP
SANTA BARBARA COUNTY
EL CAMINO REAL
CALLE REAL
UP RR
VEREDA ESCOLAR
VEREDA
DEL CIERVO
VEREDA
VEREDA LEYENDA
VEREDA PRADERA
VEREDA GALERIA
VEREDA DEL PADRE
FARREN RD
8400
400
100
VEREDA CORDILLERA
VEREDA LEYENDA
ARMAS CANYON RD
8100
TECOLOTE CREEK
WINCHESTER CANYON
CREEK
WINCHESTER CANYON RD
RIO
ROBBIE CIR
RIO VISTA
WINCHESTER
BACARA RESORT
CALLE REAL
110
7900
PACIFIC
OCEAN
CALIFORNIA COASTAL NATIONAL MONUMENT
SEE 992 MAP
SEE B MAP
0 .125 .25 .375 .5 miles 1 in. = 1900 ft.

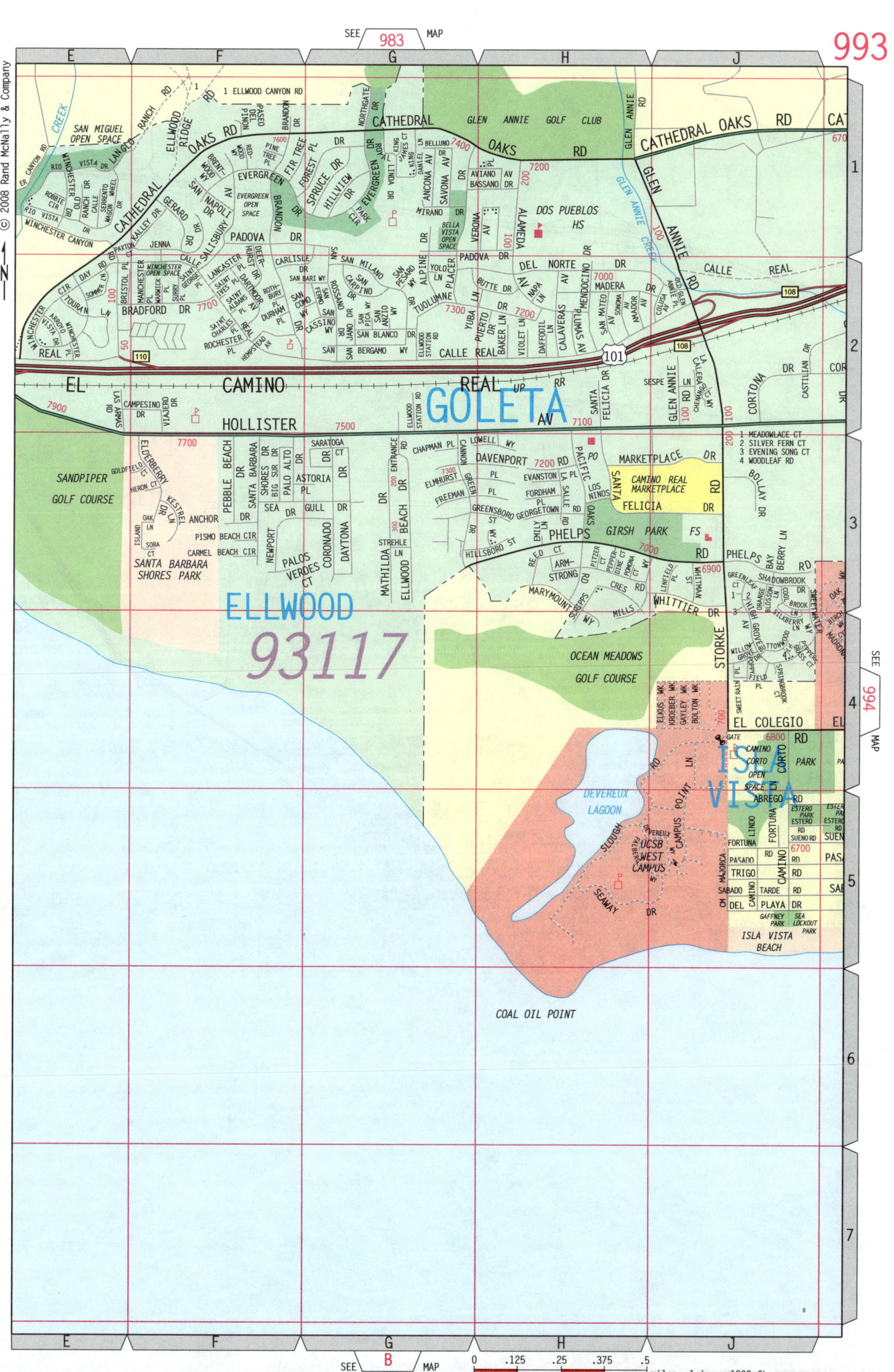
SEE 983 MAP
SEE 994 MAP
SEE B MAP
E
F
G
H
J
1
2
3
4
5
6
7
GOLETA
ELLWOOD
93117
ISLA VISTA
CATHEDRAL OAKS RD
GLEN ANNIE GOLF CLUB
SAN MIGUEL OPEN SPACE
DOS PUEBLOS HS
EVERGREEN OPEN SPACE
BELLA VISTA OPEN SPACE
WINCHESTER OPEN SPACE
CALLE REAL
EL CAMINO REAL
HOLLISTER AV
101
110
108
SANDPIPER GOLF COURSE
SANTA BARBARA SHORES PARK
CAMINO REAL MARKETPLACE
GIRSH PARK
OCEAN MEADOWS GOLF COURSE
DEVEREUX LAGOON
UCSB WEST CAMPUS
CAMINO CORTO OPEN SPACE
ISLA VISTA BEACH
COAL OIL POINT
STORKE RD
GLEN ANNIE RD
EL COLEGIO RD
PHELPS RD
WHITTIER DR
1 MEADOWLACE CT
2 SILVER FERN CT
3 EVENING SONG CT
4 WOODLEAF RD
1 ELLWOOD CANYON RD
0 .125 .25 .375 .5 miles 1 in. = 1900 ft.

SEE 984 MAP

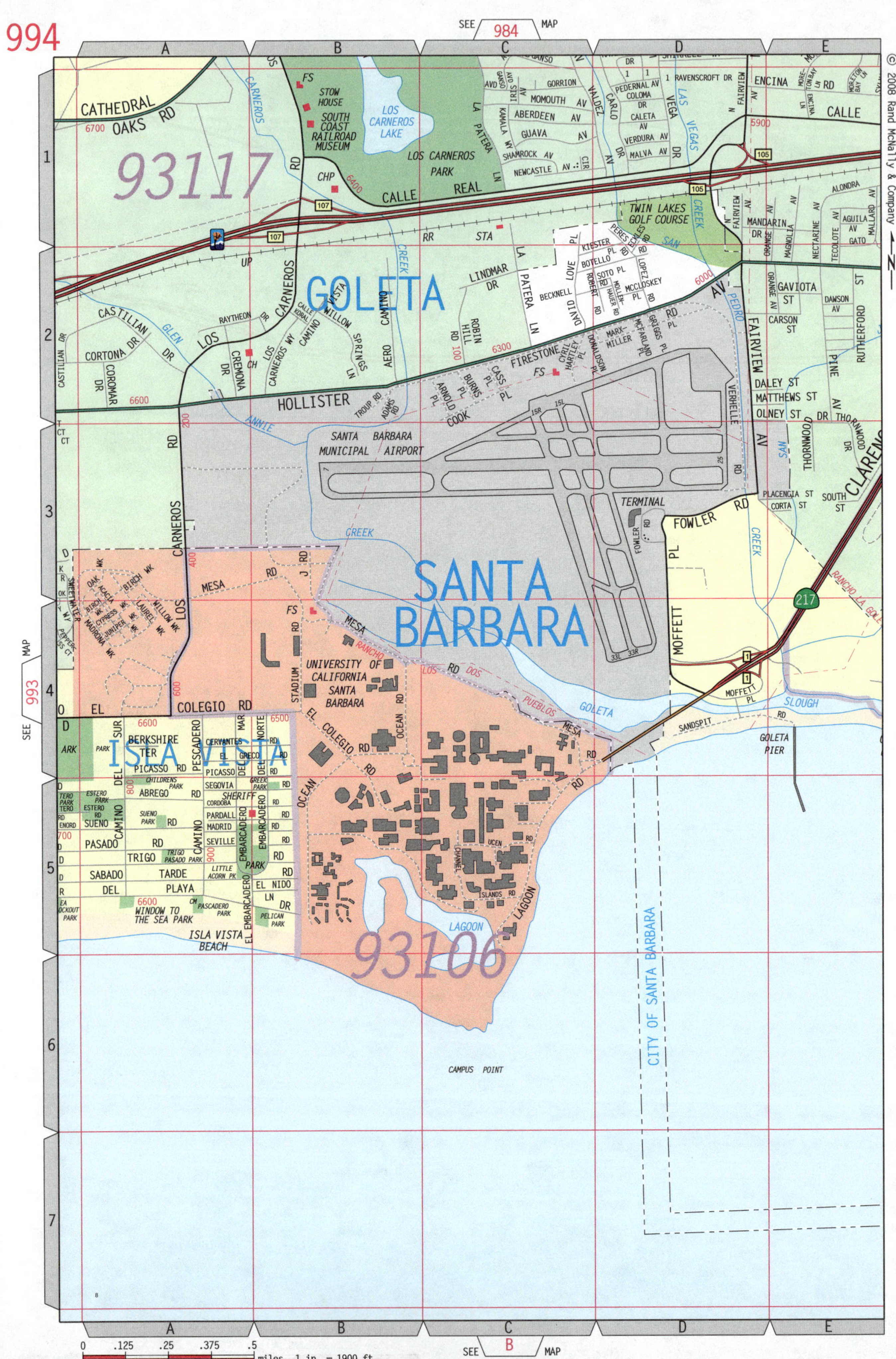
GOLETA
SANTA BARBARA
ISLA VISTA
93117
93106
SANTA BARBARA MUNICIPAL AIRPORT
UNIVERSITY OF CALIFORNIA SANTA BARBARA
LOS CARNEROS LAKE
LOS CARNEROS PARK
STOW HOUSE
SOUTH COAST RAILROAD MUSEUM
TWIN LAKES GOLF COURSE
TERMINAL
CAMPUS POINT
LAGOON
GOLETA PIER
ISLA VISTA BEACH
WINDOW TO THE SEA PARK
CITY OF SANTA BARBARA
CATHEDRAL OAKS RD
CALLE REAL
HOLLISTER
FAIRVIEW AV
LOS CARNEROS RD
EL COLEGIO RD
MESA RD
FOWLER RD
MOFFETT PL
SANDSPIT RD
GOLETA SLOUGH
ENCINA
CALLE
CLARENCE

SEE 993 MAP

0 .125 .25 .375 .5 miles 1 in. = 1900 ft.

SEE B MAP

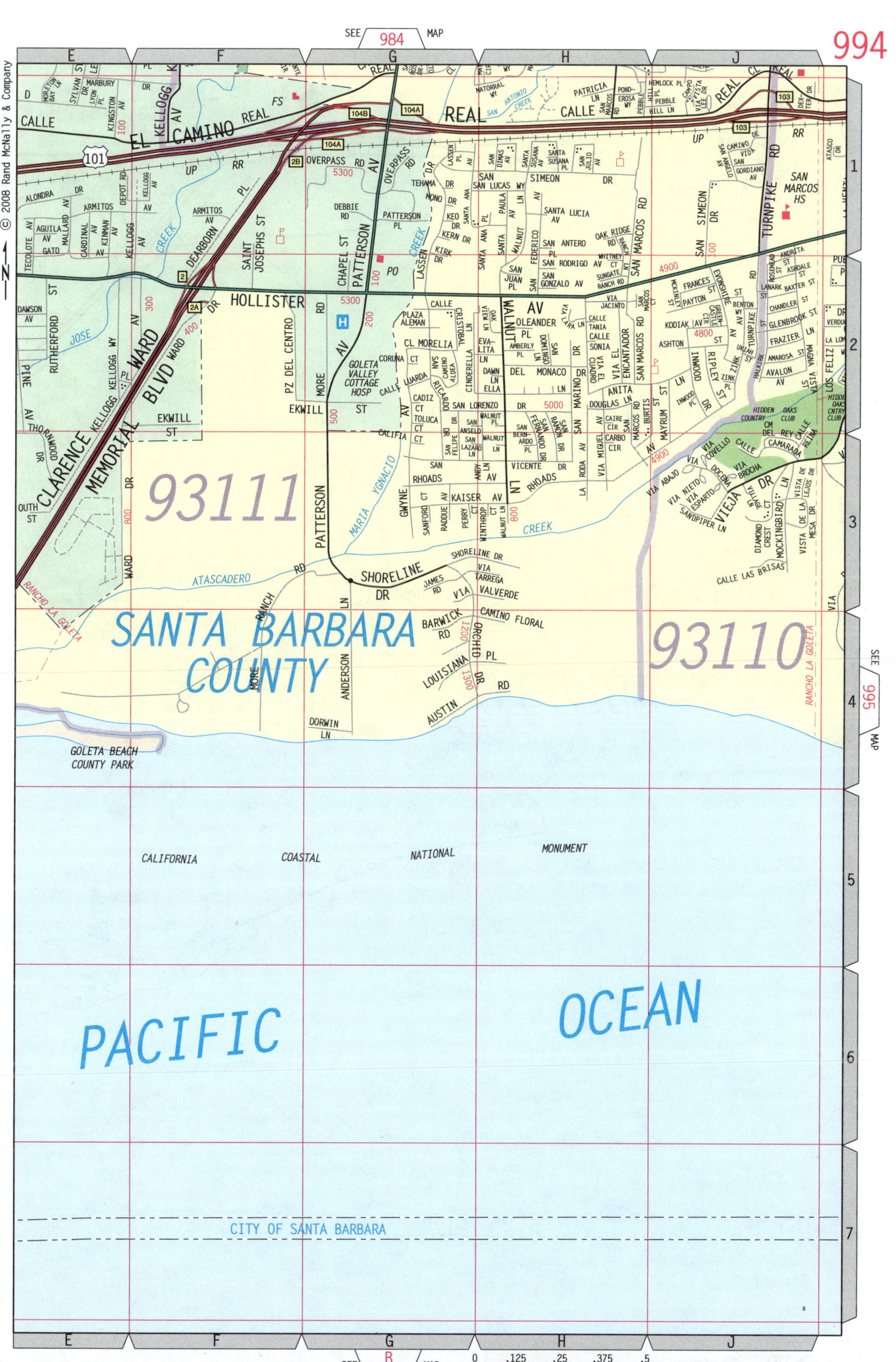
SEE 984 MAP
E
F
G
H
J
1
2
3
4
5
6
7
EL CAMINO REAL
CALLE REAL
101
104A
104B
103
2B
2A
2
UP RR
OVERPASS RD
HOLLISTER AV
WARD MEMORIAL BLVD
CLARENCE
KELLOGG AV
DEARBORN PL
SAINT JOSEPHS ST
CHAPEL ST
PATTERSON AV
PATTERSON RD
OVERPASS RD
PZ DEL CENTRO
MORE RD
EKWILL ST
GOLETA VALLEY COTTAGE HOSP
PO
FS
SAN SIMEON DR
SAN MARCOS RD
TURNPIKE RD
SAN MARCOS HS
WALNUT LN
SANTA ANA PL
OLEANDER PL
DEL MONACO DR
SAN LORENZO DR
RHOADS AV
KAISER AV
VICENTE DR
SHORELINE DR
ATASCADERO CREEK
SAN JOSE CREEK
SAN ANTONIO CREEK
MARIA YGNACIO CREEK
93111
93110
SANTA BARBARA COUNTY
MORE RANCH RD
ANDERSON LN
ORCHID DR
LOUISIANA PL
AUSTIN RD
DORWIN LN
BARWICK RD
CAMINO FLORAL
VIA VALVERDE
HIDDEN OAKS CNTRY CLUB
VIA ABAJO
VIEJA DR
CALLE LAS BRISAS
MOCKINGBIRD LN
VISTA DE LA MESA DR
RANCHO LA GOLETA
GOLETA BEACH COUNTY PARK
CALIFORNIA COASTAL NATIONAL MONUMENT
PACIFIC OCEAN
CITY OF SANTA BARBARA
SEE 995 MAP
SEE B MAP
0 .125 .25 .375 .5 miles 1 in. = 1900 ft.

SEE 985 MAP

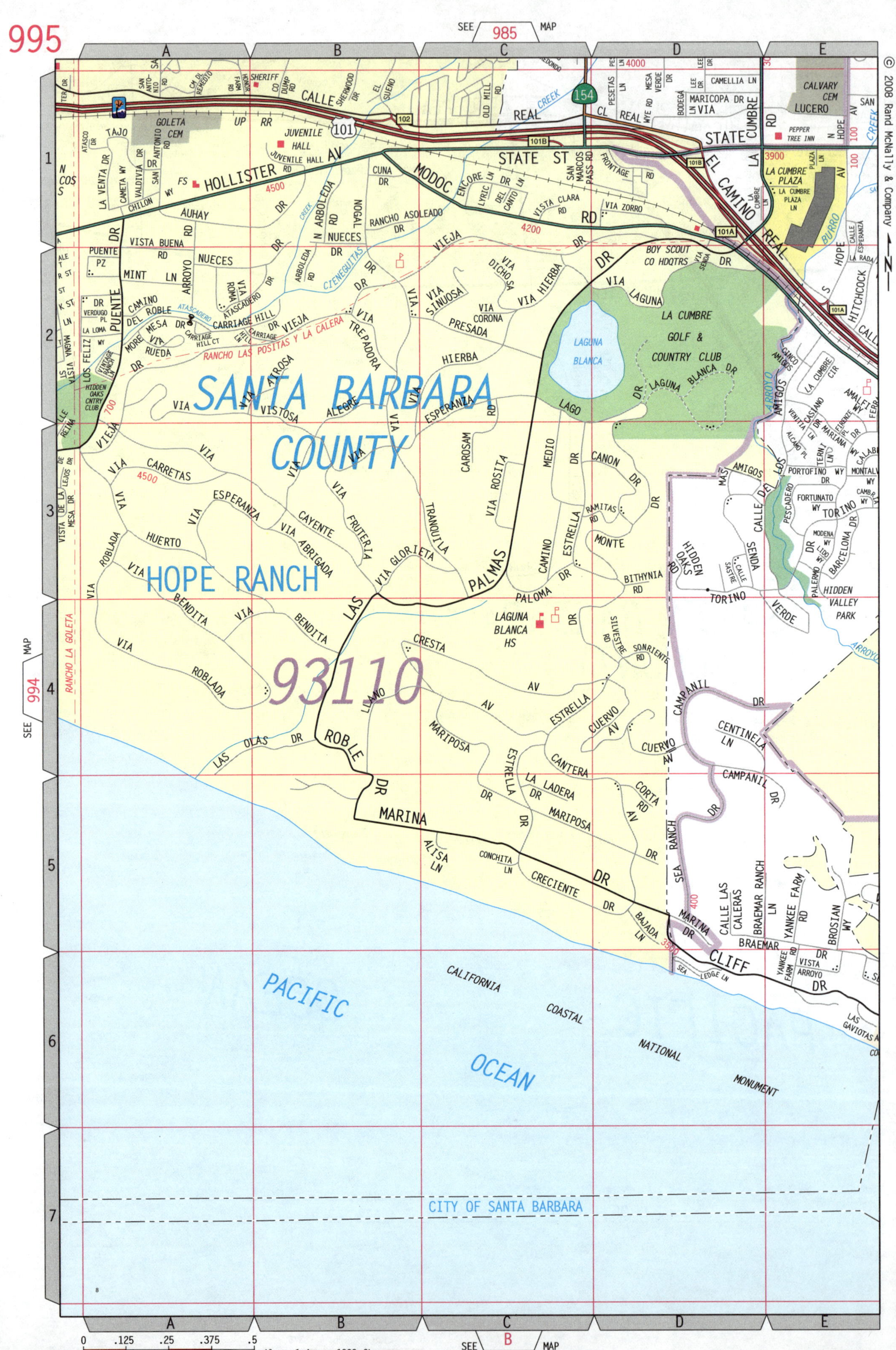
SANTA BARBARA
COUNTY
HOPE RANCH
93110
PACIFIC
OCEAN
CALIFORNIA COASTAL NATIONAL MONUMENT
CITY OF SANTA BARBARA
LAGUNA BLANCA
LA CUMBRE GOLF & COUNTRY CLUB
LAGUNA BLANCA HS
GOLETA CEM
CALVARY CEM
LA CUMBRE PLAZA
HIDDEN VALLEY PARK
JUVENILE HALL
SHERIFF
BOY SCOUT CO HDQTRS
HIDDEN OAKS CNTRY CLUB
PEPPER TREE INN
HOLLISTER AV
STATE ST
CALLE REAL
EL CAMINO REAL
MODOC RD
LAS PALMAS DR
MARINA DR
CLIFF DR
RANCHO LAS POSITAS Y LA CALERA
RANCHO LA GOLETA
101
154
© 2008 Rand McNally & Company

SEE 994 MAP

SEE B MAP

0 .125 .25 .375 .5 miles 1 in. = 1900 ft.

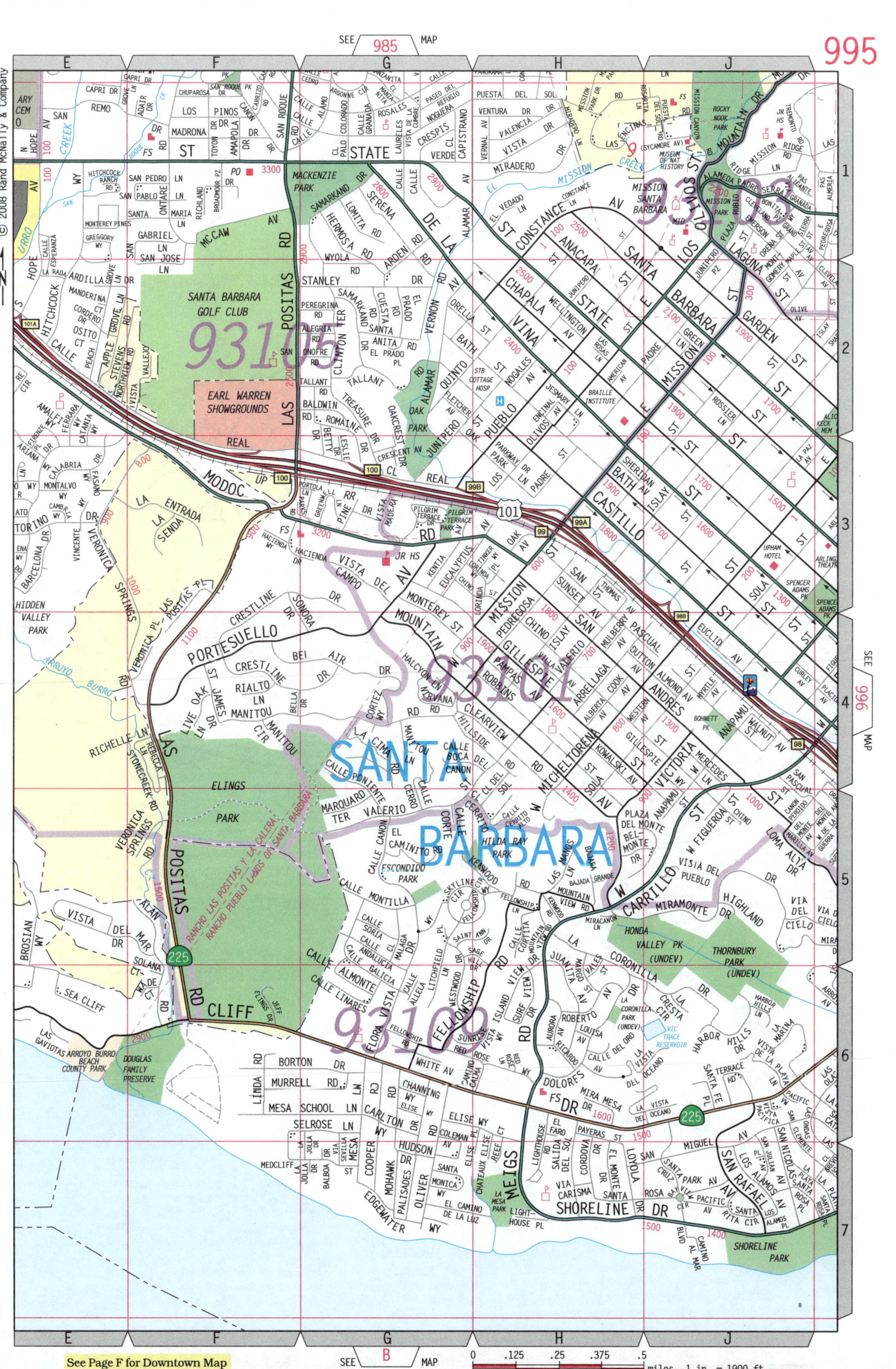
SEE 985 MAP
SEE B MAP
SEE 996 MAP
SANTA BARBARA
93105
93101
93109
SANTA BARBARA GOLF CLUB
EARL WARREN SHOWGROUNDS
MACKENZIE PARK
OAK PARK
ELINGS PARK
ESCONDIDO PARK
HILDA RAY PARK
HIDDEN VALLEY PARK
HONDA VALLEY PK (UNDEV)
THORNBURY PARK (UNDEV)
ARROYO BURRO BEACH COUNTY PARK
DOUGLAS FAMILY PRESERVE
LA MESA PARK
SHORELINE PARK
ROCKY NOOK PARK
MISSION SANTA BARBARA
MUSEUM OF NAT HISTORY
BRAILLE INSTITUTE
STB COTTAGE HOSP
UPHAM HOTEL
VIC TRACE RESERVOIR
STATE ST
CLIFF DR
SHORELINE DR
LAS POSITAS RD
MISSION ST
CARRILLO ST
MODOC RD
PORTESUELLO
MEIGS
FELLOWSHIP RD
101
225
0 .125 .25 .375 .5 miles 1 in. = 1900 ft.

See Page F for Downtown Map

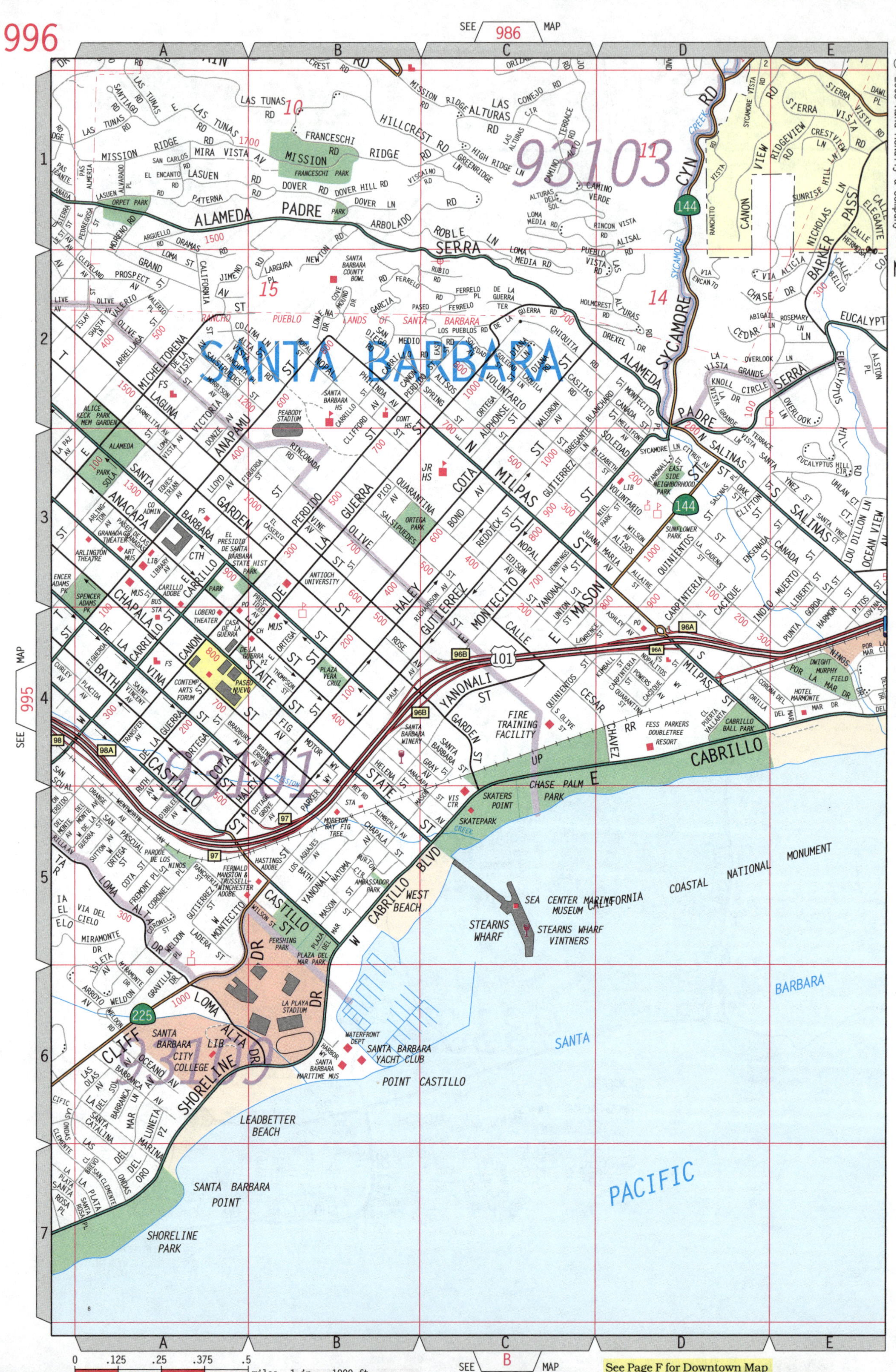

SEE 986 MAP
SANTA BARBARA
93103
93101
93109
MISSION
ALAMEDA PADRE SERRA
FRANCESCHI PARK
ORPET PARK
ALICE KECK PARK MEM GARDEN
ALAMEDA PARK
PEABODY STADIUM
SANTA BARBARA HS
SANTA BARBARA COUNTY BOWL
ORTEGA PARK
EAST SIDE NEIGHBORHOOD PARK
SUNFLOWER PARK
EL PRESIDIO DE SANTA BARBARA STATE HIST PARK
LOBERO THEATER
ARLINGTON THEATRE
SPENCER ADAMS PK
ANTIOCH UNIVERSITY
PASEO NUEVO
CONTEMP ARTS FORUM
PLAZA VERA CRUZ
FIRE TRAINING FACILITY
SANTA BARBARA WINERY
FESS PARKERS DOUBLETREE RESORT
CABRILLO BALL PARK
DWIGHT MURPHY FIELD
HOTEL MARMONTE
CHASE PALM PARK
SKATERS POINT
SKATEPARK
MORETON BAY FIG TREE
HASTINGS ADOBE
FERNALD MANSION & TRUSSELL-WINCHESTER ADOBE
AMBASSADOR PARK
WEST BEACH
SEA CENTER MARINE MUSEUM
STEARNS WHARF
STEARNS WHARF VINTNERS
CALIFORNIA COASTAL NATIONAL MONUMENT
PERSHING PARK
PLAZA DEL MAR PARK
LA PLAYA STADIUM
WATERFRONT DEPT
SANTA BARBARA YACHT CLUB
SANTA BARBARA MARITIME MUS
POINT CASTILLO
SANTA BARBARA CITY COLLEGE
LEADBETTER BEACH
SANTA BARBARA POINT
SHORELINE PARK
SANTA BARBARA
PACIFIC
CABRILLO
SHORELINE DR
CLIFF DR
MILPAS ST
STATE ST
SYCAMORE CYN RD
101
144
225
SEE 995 MAP
SEE B MAP
See Page F for Downtown Map
miles 1 in. = 1900 ft.
0 .125 .25 .375 .5

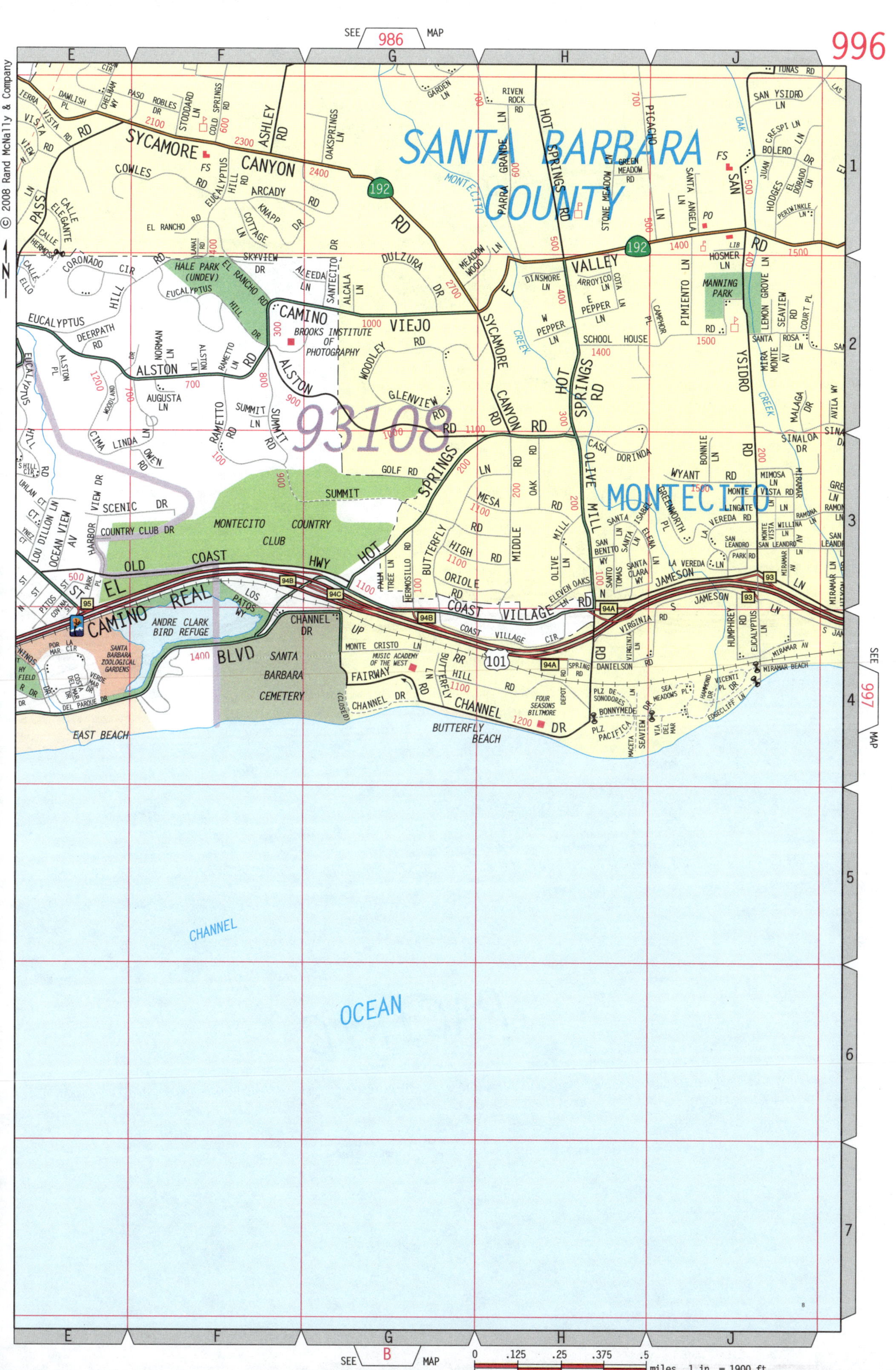
SEE 986 MAP
SANTA BARBARA COUNTY
MONTECITO
93108
SYCAMORE CANYON RD
ASHLEY RD
COWLES RD
EUCALYPTUS HILL RD
ARCADY RD
KNAPP DR
COTTAGE LN
EL RANCHO RD
PASS
CALLE ELEGANTE
CORONADO
HILL CIR
HALE PARK (UNDEV)
EL RANCHO RD
SKYVIEW DR
ALEEDA LN
SANTECITO DR
ALCALA LN
DULZURA DR
MEADOW WOOD LN
CAMINO VIEJO RD
BROOKS INSTITUTE OF PHOTOGRAPHY
WOODLEY RD
GLENVIEW RD
ALSTON RD
EUCALYPTUS
DEERPATH RD
ALSTON PL
NORMAN LN
RAMETTO LN
AUGUSTA LN
SUMMIT LN
SUMMIT RD
RAMETTO RD
CIMA LINDA LN
OWEN RD
SCENIC DR
COUNTRY CLUB DR
MONTECITO COUNTRY CLUB
SUMMIT
GOLF RD
HOT SPRINGS RD
OLD COAST HWY
EL CAMINO REAL
ANDRE CLARK BIRD REFUGE
SANTA BARBARA ZOOLOGICAL GARDENS
LOS PATOS WY
CHANNEL DR
SANTA BARBARA CEMETERY
EAST BEACH
CHANNEL DR
FAIRWAY RD
MONTE CRISTO LN
MUSIC ACADEMY OF THE WEST
BUTTERFLY LN
HILL RD
BUTTERFLY BEACH
FOUR SEASONS BILTMORE
COAST VILLAGE RD
COAST VILLAGE CIR
RIVEN ROCK RD
PARRA GRANDE LN
HOT SPRINGS RD
STONE MEADOW LN
GREEN MEADOW RD
PICACHO LN
SANTA ANGELA LN
SAN YSIDRO RD
SAN YSIDRO LN
CRESPI LN
BOLERO DR
EL DORADO LN
HODGES LN
PERIWINKLE LN
EAST VALLEY RD
DINSMORE LN
ARROYO COTA LN
E PEPPER LN
W PEPPER LN
SCHOOL HOUSE RD
CAMPHOR PL
PIMIENTO LN
MANNING PARK
HOSMER LN
LEMON GROVE LN
SEAVIEW RD
COURT PL
SANTA ROSA LN
MIRA MONTE AV
MALAGA DR
AVILA WY
SINALOA DR
CASA DORINDA
OLIVE MILL RD
BONNIE LN
WYANT RD
MESA RD
MIDDLE RD
OAK RD
HIGH RD
ORIOLE RD
BUTTERFLY LN
HERMOSILLO RD
PALM TREE LN
ELEVEN OAKS LN
SANTA ISABEL LN
GREENWORTH PL
LA VEREDA RD
SAN BENITO WY
SANTA ELENA LN
SANTA CLARA WY
JAMESON LN
S JAMESON LN
VIRGINIA RD
HUMPHREY RD
EUCALYPTUS LN
MIRAMAR AV
MIRAMAR BEACH
DANIELSON RD
SEA MEADOWS PL
HAMMOND DR
VICENTI PL
EDGECLIFF LN
BONNYMEDE DR
PLZ PACIFICA
SEAVIEW DR
CHANNEL DR
OCEAN
CHANNEL
SEE 997 MAP
SEE B MAP
0 .125 .25 .375 .5 miles 1 in. = 1900 ft.
© 2008 Rand McNally & Company

SEE 987 MAP

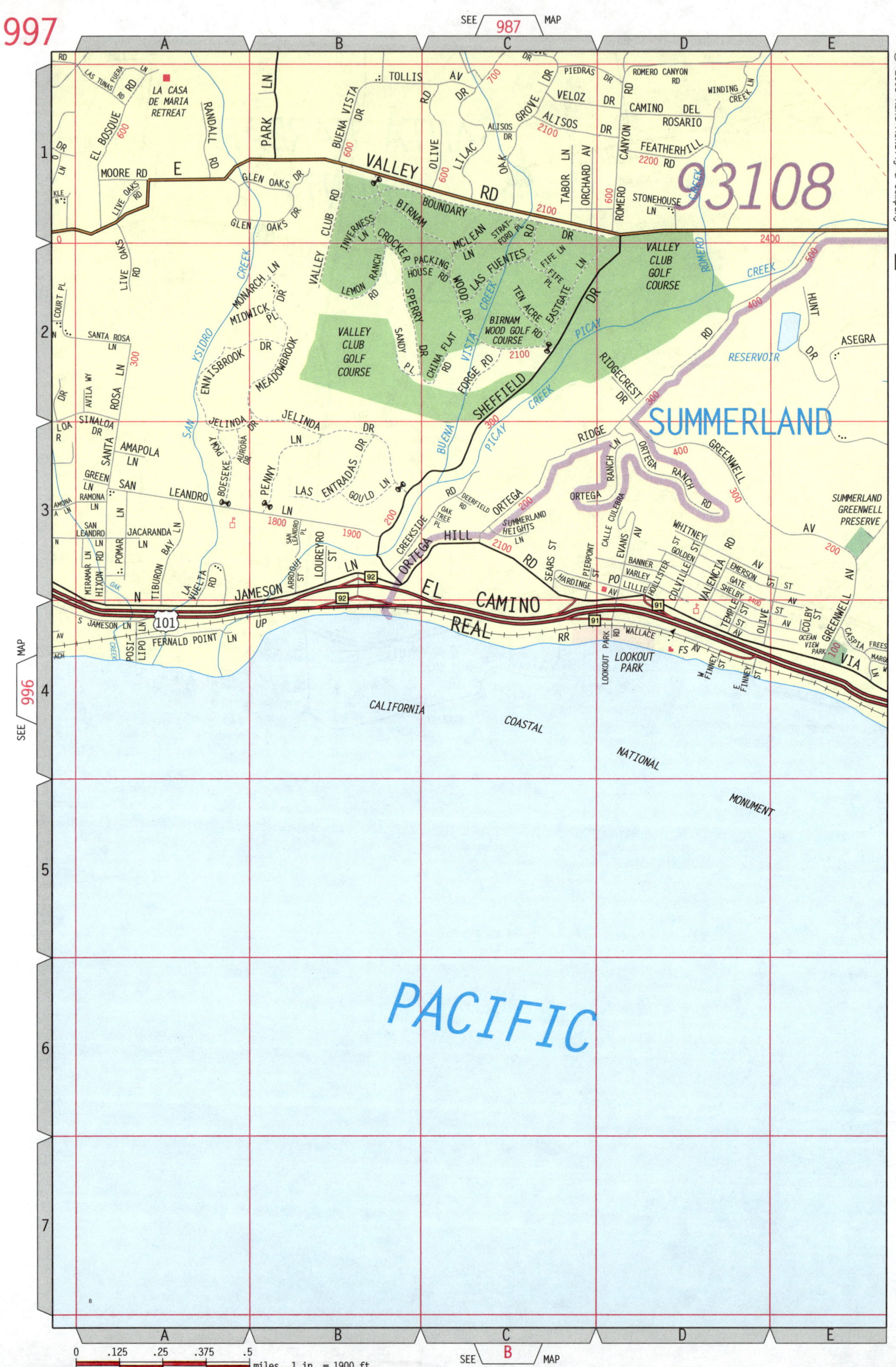

LA CASA DE MARIA RETREAT
VALLEY CLUB GOLF COURSE
BIRNAM WOOD GOLF COURSE
93108
SUMMERLAND
SUMMERLAND GREENWELL PRESERVE
LOOKOUT PARK
RESERVOIR
CALIFORNIA COASTAL NATIONAL MONUMENT
PACIFIC
EAST VALLEY RD
SHEFFIELD DR
ORTEGA HILL RD
EL CAMINO REAL
N JAMESON LN
S JAMESON LN
FERNALD POINT LN
SAN LEANDRO LN
SAN YSIDRO CREEK
PICAY CREEK
ROMERO CREEK
BUENA VISTA CREEK
RIDGECREST DR
GREENWELL AV
VIA REAL
LILLIE AV
WALLACE AV

SEE 996 MAP

SEE B MAP

0 .125 .25 .375 .5 miles 1 in. = 1900 ft.

SEE 987 MAP

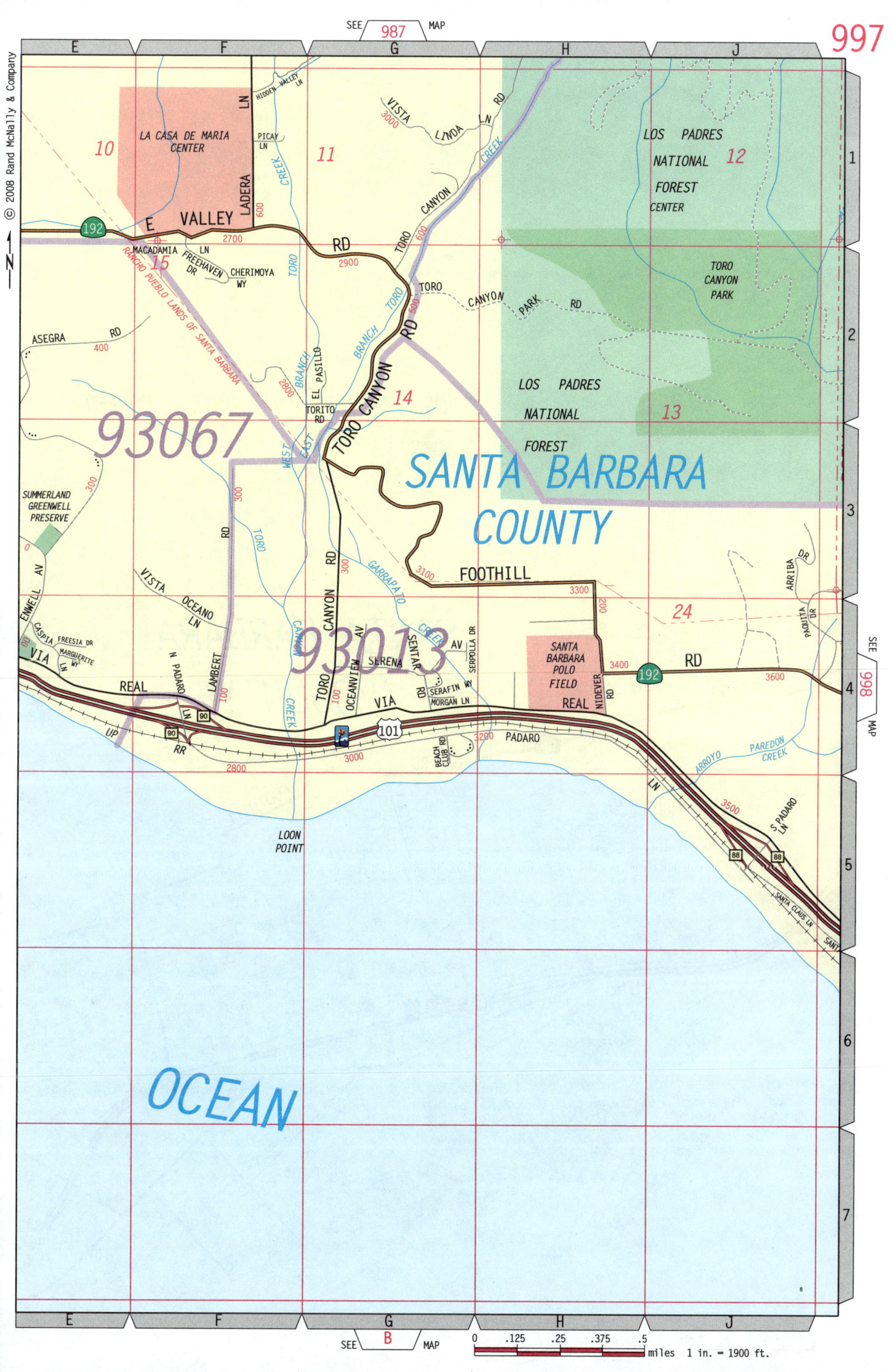

LA CASA DE MARIA CENTER
LOS PADRES NATIONAL FOREST CENTER
TORO CANYON PARK
LOS PADRES NATIONAL FOREST
SANTA BARBARA COUNTY
93067
93013
SUMMERLAND GREENWELL PRESERVE
SANTA BARBARA POLO FIELD
LOON POINT
OCEAN
E VALLEY RD
FOOTHILL RD
TORO CANYON RD
TORO CANYON PARK RD
VIA REAL
PADARO LN
RANCHO PUEBLO LANDS OF SANTA BARBARA
ASEGRA RD
VISTA OCEANO LN
VISTA LINDA LN RD
LADERA LN
HIDDEN VALLEY LN
PICAY LN
MACADAMIA LN
FREEHAVEN DR
CHERIMOYA WY
EL PASILLO
TORITO RD
LAMBERT RD
N PADARO LN
OCEANVIEW AV
SERENA
SENTAR RD
SERAFIN WY
MORGAN LN
SERPOLLA DR
NIDEVER RD
BEACH CLUB RD
CASPIA
FREESIA DR
MARGUERITE WY
ENWELL AV
S PADARO LN
SANTA CLAUS LN
ARRIBA DR
PAQUITA DR
UP RR
TORO CREEK
CANYON CREEK
GARRAPATO CREEK
ARROYO PAREDON CREEK
WEST EAST BRANCH
BRANCH TORO
192
101
90
88
© 2008 Rand McNally & Company

SEE 998 MAP

SEE B MAP

0 .125 .25 .375 .5 miles 1 in. = 1900 ft.

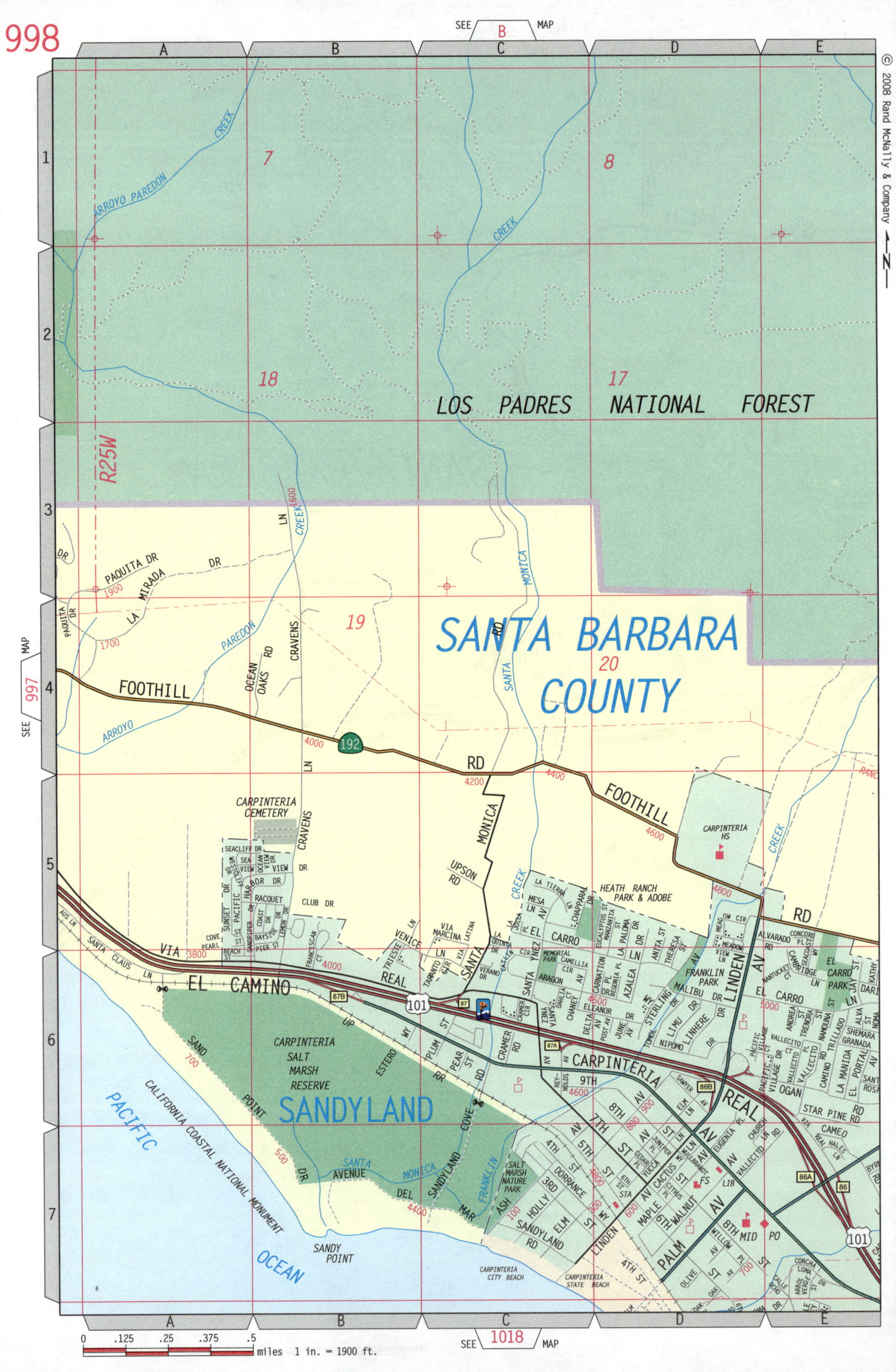
SEE B MAP
LOS PADRES NATIONAL FOREST
SANTA BARBARA COUNTY
SANDYLAND
PACIFIC OCEAN
CALIFORNIA COASTAL NATIONAL MONUMENT
CARPINTERIA SALT MARSH RESERVE
CARPINTERIA CEMETERY
CARPINTERIA HS
HEATH RANCH PARK & ADOBE
FRANKLIN PARK
MEMORIAL PARK
EL CARRO PARK
SALT MARSH NATURE PARK
CARPINTERIA CITY BEACH
CARPINTERIA STATE BEACH
SANDY POINT
ARROYO PAREDON CREEK
SANTA MONICA CREEK
FRANKLIN CREEK
FOOTHILL RD
EL CAMINO REAL
VIA REAL
CARPINTERIA AV
LINDEN AV
SANTA MONICA RD
CRAVENS LN
PAQUITA DR
LA MIRADA DR
OCEAN OAKS RD
UPSON RD
SANDYLAND RD
AVENUE DEL MAR
SAND POINT RD
R25W
SEE 997 MAP
SEE 1018 MAP
0 .125 .25 .375 .5 miles 1 in. = 1900 ft.

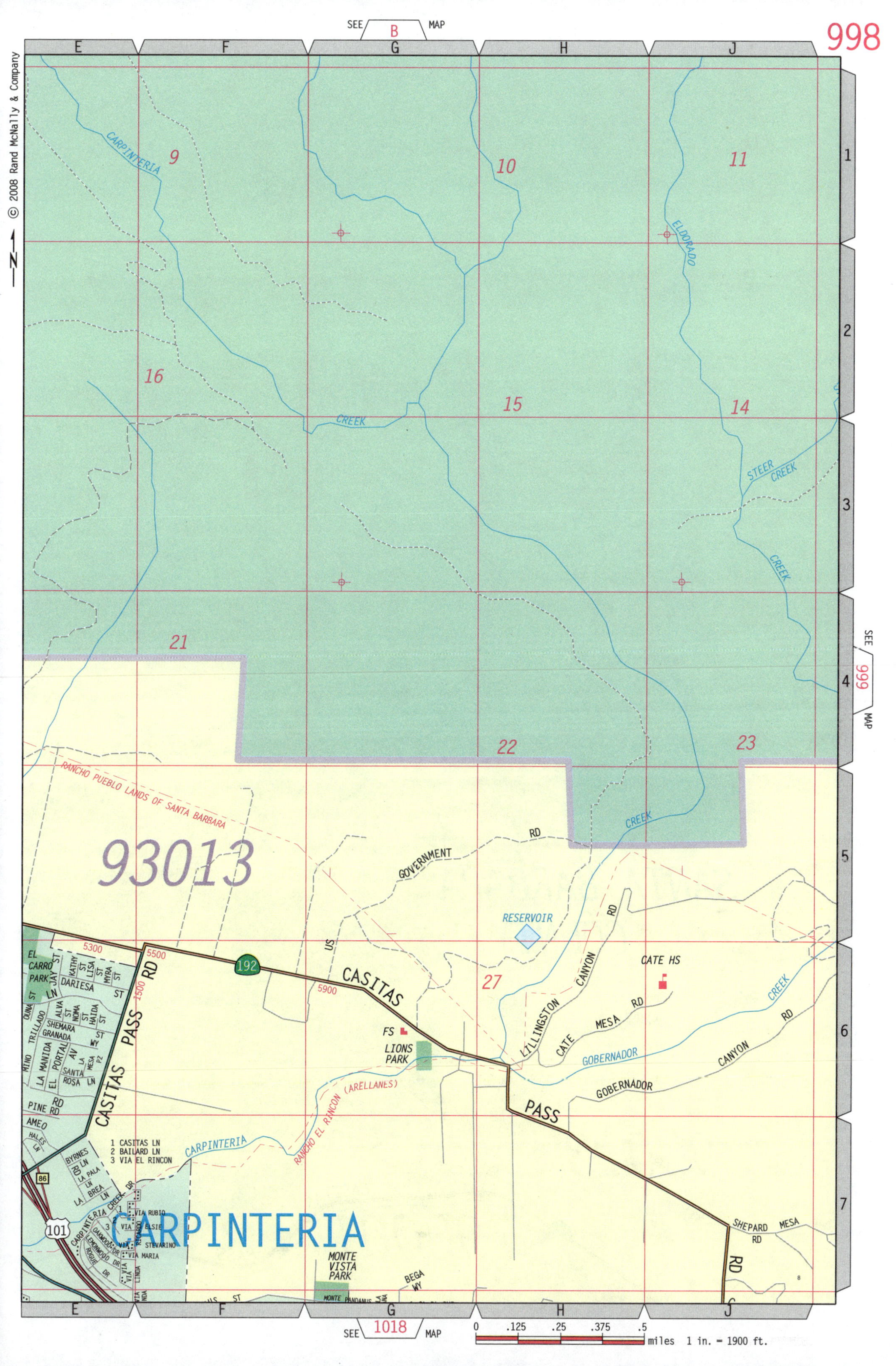
SEE B MAP
SEE 999 MAP
SEE 1018 MAP
© 2008 Rand McNally & Company
E
F
G
H
J
1
2
3
4
5
6
7
9
10
11
14
15
16
21
22
23
27
CARPINTERIA
ELDORADO
CREEK
STEER CREEK
RANCHO PUEBLO LANDS OF SANTA BARBARA
93013
GOVERNMENT RD
RESERVOIR
CATE HS
LILLINGSTON CANYON RD
CATE MESA RD
GOBERNADOR CREEK
GOBERNADOR CANYON RD
US 192
CASITAS PASS RD
5300
5500
5900
1500
FS
LIONS PARK
RANCHO EL RINCON (ARELLANES)
CARPINTERIA CREEK
SHEPARD MESA RD
EL CARRO PARK
JAY ST
KATHY ST
LISA ST
MYRA ST
DARIESA LN
ST
ALVA ST
NOMA AV
HAIDA ST
SHEMARA
GRANADA
LA MANIDA
EL PORTAL AV
SANTA ROSA LN
LA MESA
PINE RD
AMEO
HALES LN
1 CASITAS LN
2 BAILARD LN
3 VIA EL RINCON
BYRNES RD
LA PALA LN
LA BREA LN
VIA RUBIO
VIA ELSIE
VIA STEVARINO
VIA MARIA
VIA LINDA
86
101
CARPINTERIA
MONTE VISTA PARK
BEGA WY
0 .125 .25 .375 .5 miles 1 in. = 1900 ft.

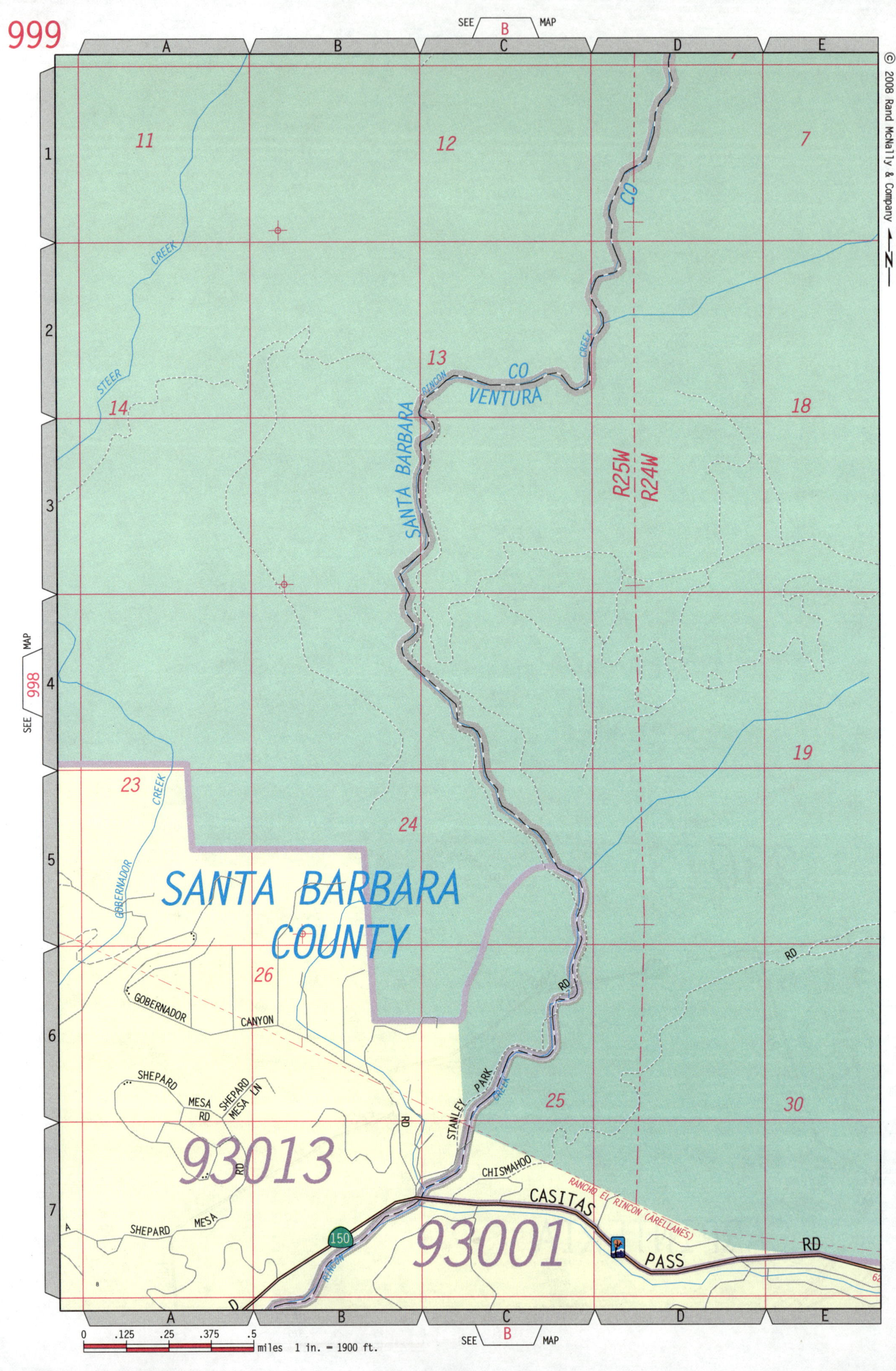

SEE B MAP
A
B
C
D
E
1
2
3
4
5
6
7
SEE 998 MAP
11
12
7
CO
CREEK
STEER
CREEK
13
RINCON
CO
VENTURA
14
18
SANTA BARBARA
R25W
R24W
23
CREEK
24
19
SANTA BARBARA
COUNTY
GOBERNADOR
26
RD
GOBERNADOR
CANYON
SHEPARD
MESA
SHEPARD
MESA LN
RD
STANLEY
PARK
CREEK
25
30
93013
RD
RD
CHISMAHOO
CASITAS
RANCHO EL RINCON (ARELLANES)
SHEPARD
MESA
150
93001
PASS
RD
RINCON
0
.125
.25
.375
.5
miles 1 in. = 1900 ft.
SEE B MAP

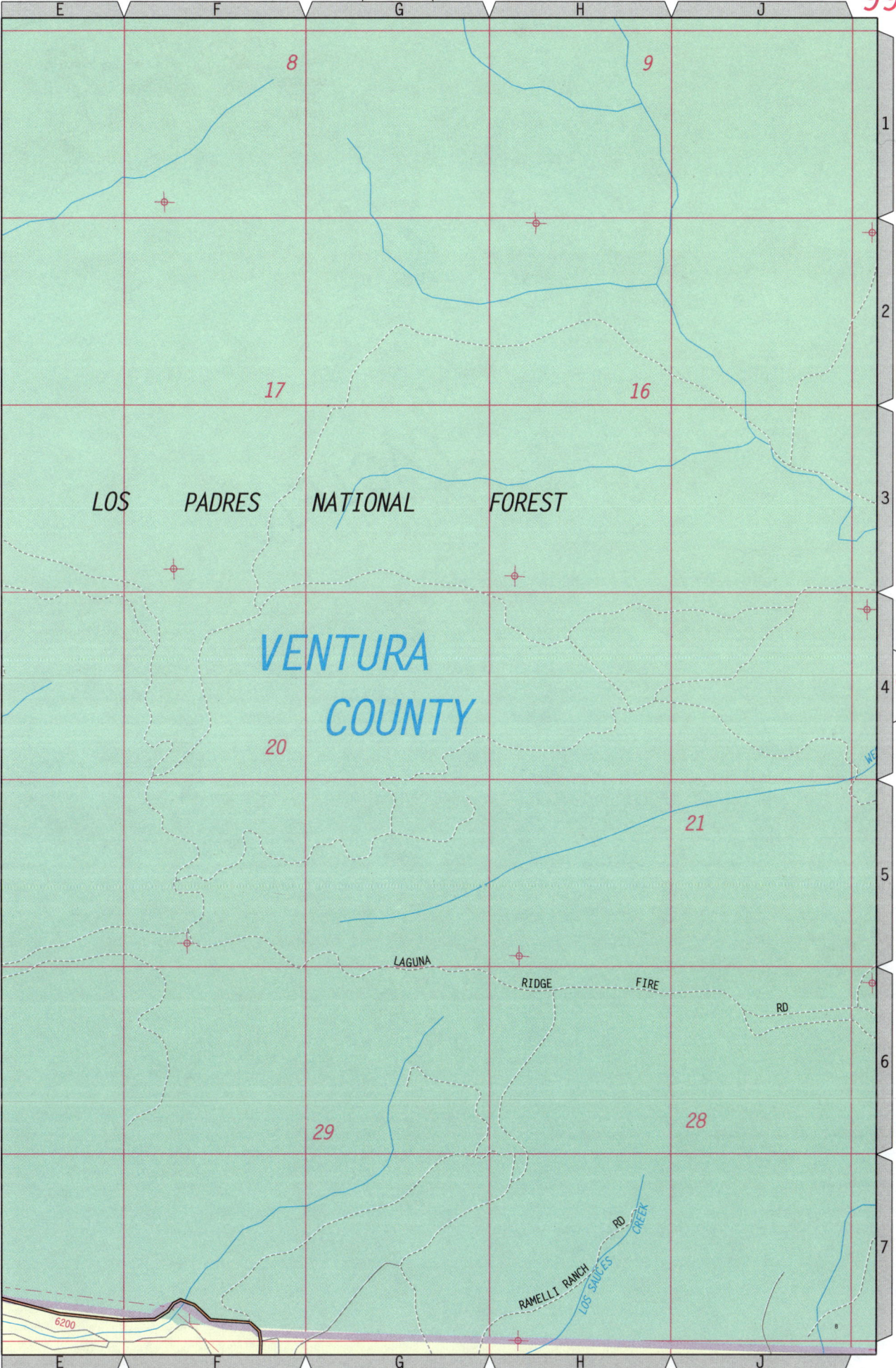

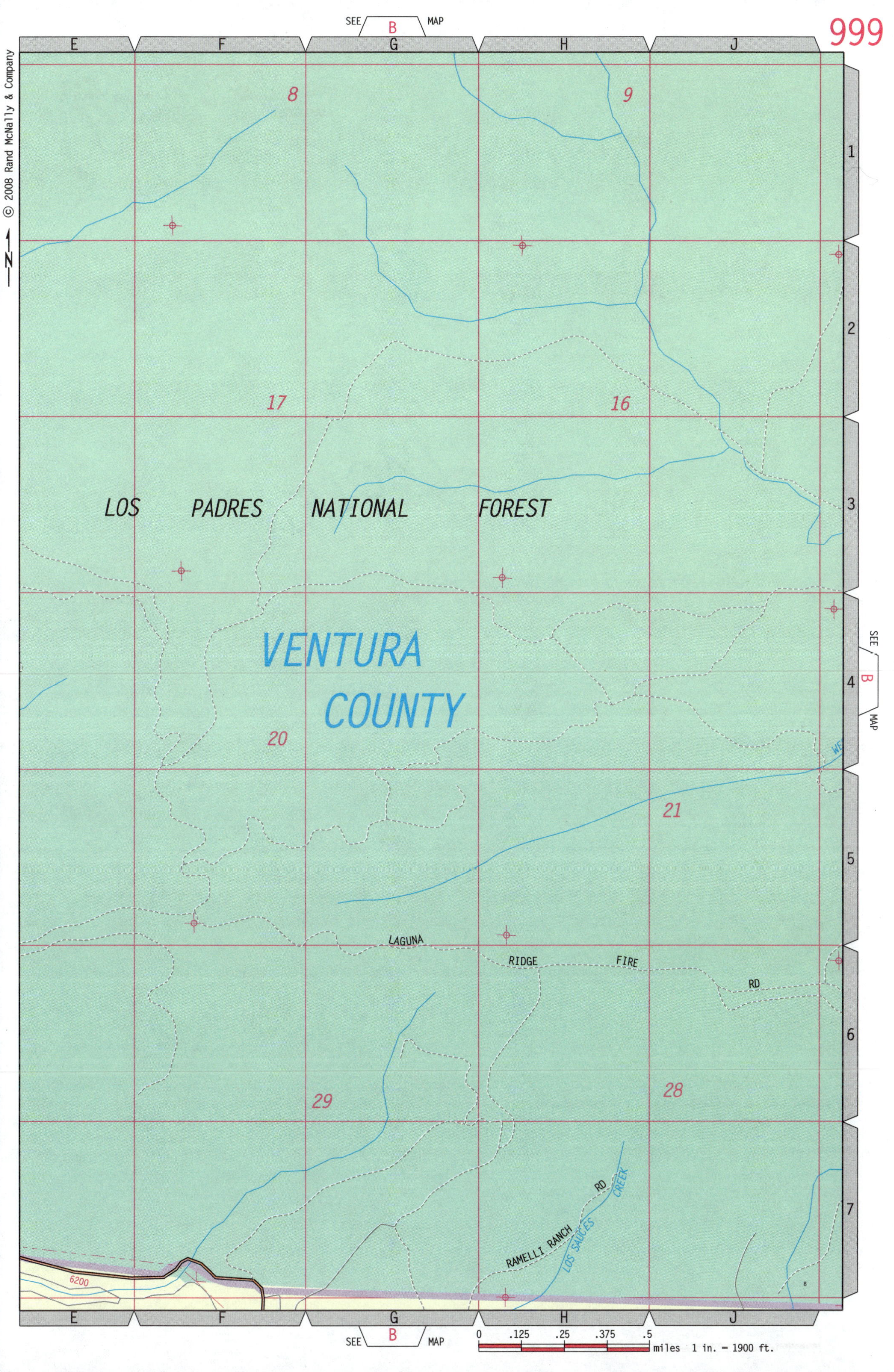
SEE B MAP
E
F
G
H
J
8
9
17
16
LOS PADRES NATIONAL FOREST
VENTURA
COUNTY
20
21
LAGUNA RIDGE FIRE RD
29
28
RAMELLI RANCH RD
LOS SAUCES CREEK
6200
1
2
3
4
5
6
7
SEE B MAP
0 .125 .25 .375 .5
miles 1 in. = 1900 ft.

SEE 998 MAP

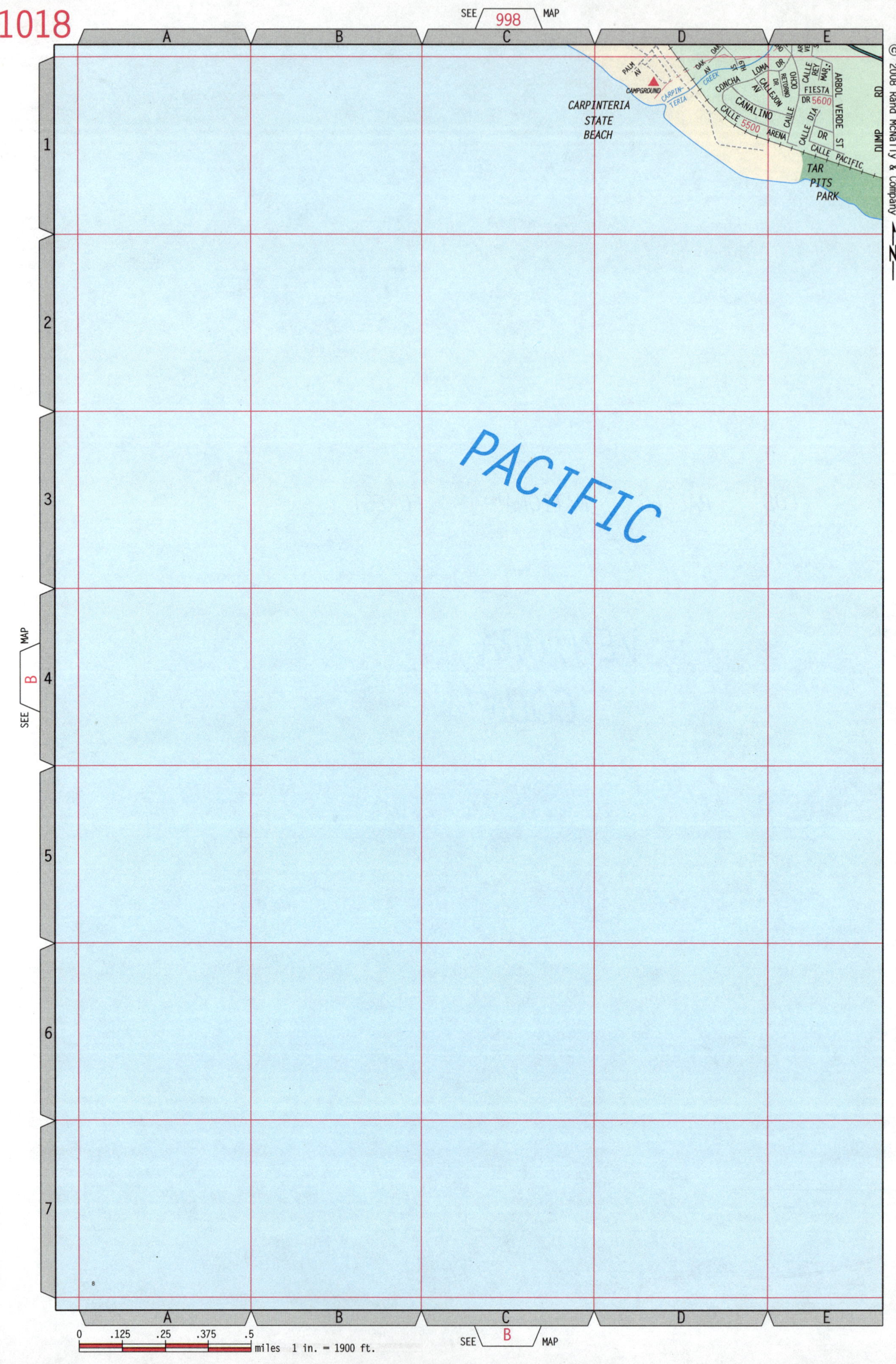
CARPINTERIA
STATE
BEACH
PALM AV
CAMPGROUND
CARPINTERIA CREEK
OAK AV
6TH ST
CONCHA
LOMA AV
CALLEJON
RETORNO DR
OCHO
CALLE REY
FIESTA DR
5600
CANALINO
CALLE 5500
ARENA
CALLE DIA DR
ARBOL VERDE ST
CALLE PACIFIC
DUMP RD
TAR
PITS
PARK
PACIFIC
0 .125 .25 .375 .5 miles 1 in. = 1900 ft.

SEE B MAP

SEE B MAP

SEE 998 MAP

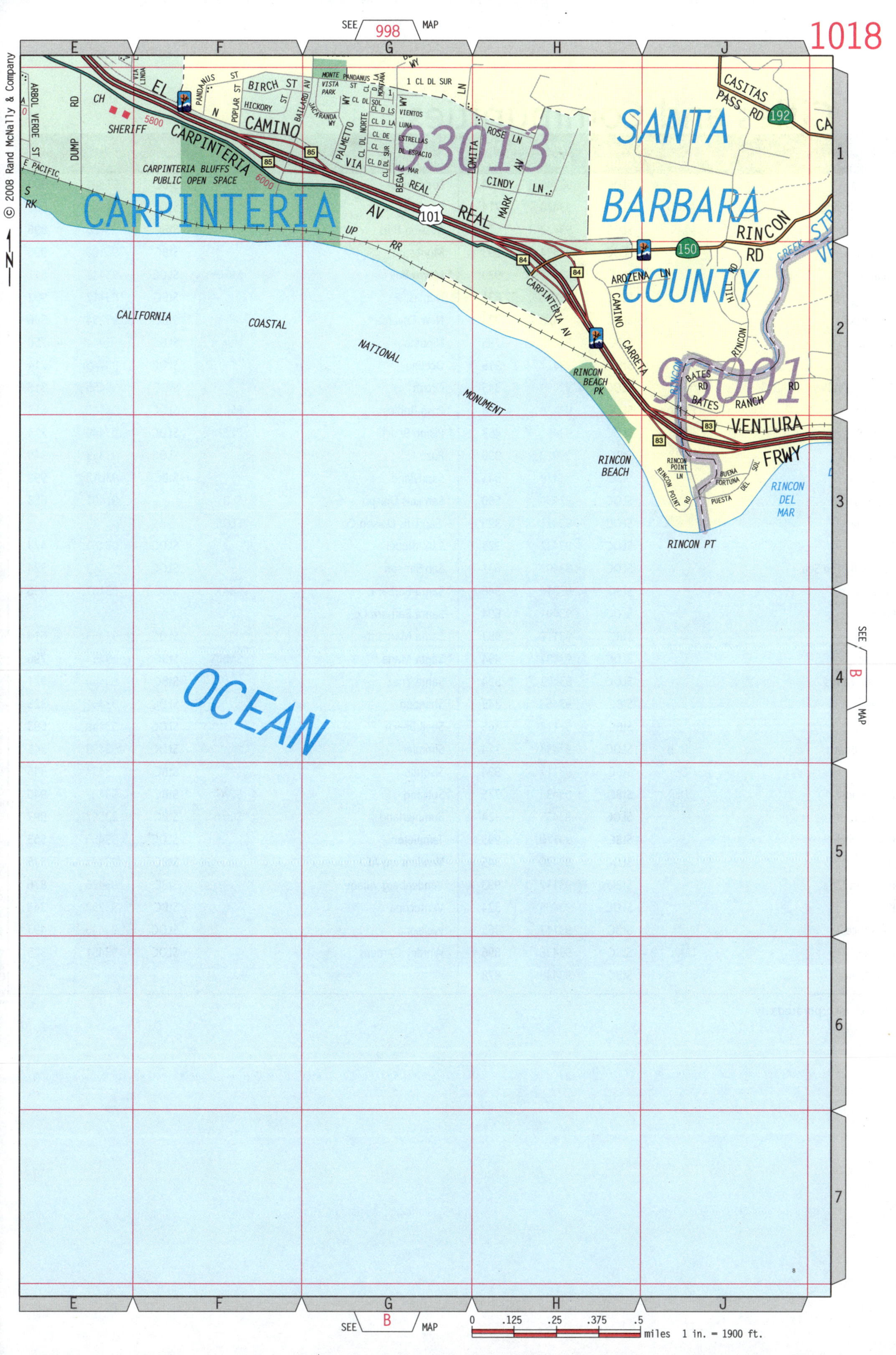

CARPINTERIA
CARPINTERIA BLUFFS PUBLIC OPEN SPACE
SANTA BARBARA COUNTY
93013
93001
EL CAMINO REAL
CARPINTERIA AV
VENTURA FRWY
RINCON RD
CASITAS PASS RD
RINCON BEACH PK
RINCON BEACH
RINCON PT
RINCON DEL MAR
SHERIFF
CALIFORNIA COASTAL NATIONAL MONUMENT
OCEAN
UP RR

SEE B MAP

SEE B MAP

0 .125 .25 .375 .5 miles 1 in. = 1900 ft.

Cities and Communities

Community Name	Abbr.	County	ZIP Code	Map Page
Adelaida		SLOC	93446	324
* Arroyo Grande	ARGD	SLOC	93420	714
* Atascadero	ATAS	SLOC	93422	573
Avila Beach		SLOC	93424	693
Ballard		StBC	93463	920
Baywood Park		SLOC	93402	631
Bee Rock		SLOC	93426	324
Betteravia		StBC	93455	795
* Buellton	BLTN	StBC	93427	919
California Valley		SLOC	93453	345
Cambria	Cmbr	SLOC	93428	528
Camp Roberts		SLOC	93451	453
* Carpinteria	CARP	StBC	93013	998
Casmalia		StBC	93429	345
Cayucos		SLOC	93430	590
Cholame		SLOC	93431	325
Creston		SLOC	93432	325
Cuesta By The Sea		SLOC	93402	631
Cuyama		StBC	93214	346
Edna		SLOC	93401	694
Ellwood		StBC	93117	993
Estrella		SLOC	93451	494
Garden Farms		SLOC	93422	594
Garey		StBC	93454	345
Gaviota		StBC	93117	365
* Grover Beach	GBCH	SLOC	93433	714
* Goleta	GOL	StBC	93117	994
* Guadalupe	GDLP	StBC	93434	775
Harmony		SLOC	93435	324
Hope Ranch		StBC	93110	995
Huasna		SLOC	93420	345
Isla Vista		StBC	93117	993
Klau		SLOC	93465	324
Las Cruces		StBC	93117	365
* Lompoc	LMPC	StBC	93436	896
Los Alamos		StBC	93440	878
Los Olivos		StBC	93441	900
Los Osos		SLOC	93402	631
Mission Hills		StBC	93436	896
Montecito		StBC	93108	996
* Morro Bay	MOBY	SLOC	93442	611
Naples		StBC	93117	992
New Cuyama		StBC	93254	806
Nipomo	Npmo	SLOC	93444	756
Oceano		SLOC	93445	714
Orcutt		StBC	93455	816
* Paso Robles	PSRS	SLOC	93446	513
* Pismo Beach	PBCH	SLOC	93449	714
Pozo		SLOC	93453	345
Sandyland		StBC	93013	998
* San Luis Obispo	SLO		93401	653
-- San Luis Obispo Co	SLOC			
San Miguel		SLOC	93451	473
San Simeon		SLOC	93452	324
* Santa Barbara	SBAR	StBC	93101	996
--Santa Barbara Co	StBC			
Santa Margarita		SLOC	93453	614
* Santa Maria	SMRA	StBC	93454	796
Santa Ynez		StBC	93460	921
Shandon		SLOC	93461	325
Shell Beach		SLOC	93449	693
Simmler		SLOC	93453	345
Sisquoc		StBC	93454	345
* Solvang	SLVG	StBC	93463	940
Summerland	Summ	StBC	93067	997
Templeton		SLOC	93465	553
Vandenberg AFB		StBC	93437	875
Vandenberg Village		StBC	93436	876
Ventucopa		StBC	93252	346
Wellsona		SLOC	93446	493
Whitley Gardens		SLOC	93451	325

*Indicates incorporated city

List of Abbreviations

PREFIXES AND SUFFIXES

AL	ALLEY
ARC	ARCADE
AV, AVE	AVENUE
AVCT	AVENUE COURT
AVD	AVENIDA
AVD D LA	AVENIDA DE LA
AVD D LOS	AVENIDA DE LOS
AVD DE	AVENIDA DE
AVD DE LAS	AVENIDA DE LAS
AVD DEL	AVENIDA DEL
AVDR	AVENUE DRIVE
AVEX	AVENUE EXTENSION
AV OF	AVENUE OF
AV OF THE	AVENUE OF THE
AVPL	AVENUE PLACE
BAY	BAY
BEND	BEND
BL, BLVD	BOULEVARD
BLCT	BOULEVARD COURT
BLEX	BOULEVARD EXTENSION
BRCH	BRANCH
BRDG	BRIDGE
BYPS	BYPASS
BYWY	BYWAY
CIDR	CIRCLE DRIVE
CIR	CIRCLE
CL	CALLE
CL DE	CALLE DE
CL DL	CALLE DEL
CL D LA	CALLE DE LA
CL D LAS	CALLE DE LAS
CL D LOS	CALLE DE LOS
CL EL	CALLE EL
CLJ	CALLEJON
CL LA	CALLE LA
CL LAS	CALLE LAS
CL LOS	CALLE LOS
CLTR	CLUSTER
CM	CAMINO
CM DE	CAMINO DE
CM DL	CAMINO DEL
CM D LA	CAMINO DE LA
CM D LAS	CAMINO DE LAS
CM D LOS	CAMINO DE LOS
CMTO	CAMINITO
CMTO DEL	CAMINITO DEL
CMTO D LA	CAMINITO DE LA
CMTO D LAS	CAMINITO DE LAS
CMTO D LOS	CAMINITO DE LOS
CNDR	CENTER DRIVE
COM	COMMON
COMS	COMMONS
CORR	CORRIDOR
CRES	CRESCENT
CRLO	CIRCULO
CRSG	CROSSING
CST	CIRCLE STREET
CSWY	CAUSEWAY
CT	COURT
CTAV	COURT AVENUE
CTE	CORTE
CTE D	CORTE DE
CTE DEL	CORTE DEL
CTE D LAS	CORTE DE LAS
CTO	CUT OFF
CTR	CENTER
CTST	COURT STREET
CUR	CURVE
CV	COVE
DE	DE
DIAG	DIAGONAL
DR	DRIVE
DRAV	DRIVE AVENUE
DRCT	DRIVE COURT
DRLP	DRIVE LOOP
DVDR	DIVISION DR
EXAV	EXTENSION AVENUE
EXBL	EXTENSION BOULEVARD
EXRD	EXTENSION ROAD
EXST	EXTENSION STREET
EXT	EXTENSION
EXWY	EXPRESSWAY
FOREST RT	FOREST ROUTE
FRWY	FREEWAY
FRY	FERRY
GDNS	GARDENS
GN, GLN	GLEN
GRN	GREEN
GRV	GROVE
HTS	HEIGHTS
HWY	HIGHWAY
ISL	ISLE
JCT	JUNCTION
LN	LANE
LNCR	LANE CIRCLE
LNDG	LANDING
LNDR	LAND DRIVE
LNLP	LANE LOOP
LP	LOOP
MNR	MANOR
MT	MOUNT
MTWY	MOTORWAY
MWCR	MEWS COURT
MWLN	MEWS LANE
NFD	NAT'L FOREST DEV
NK	NOOK
OH	OUTER HIGHWAY
OVL	OVAL
OVLK	OVERLOOK
OVPS	OVERPASS
PAS	PASEO
PAS DE	PASEO DE
PAS DE LA	PASEO DE LA
PAS DE LAS	PASEO DE LAS
PAS DE LOS	PASEO DE LOS
PAS DL	PASEO DEL
PASG	PASSAGE
PAS LA	PASEO LA
PAS LOS	PASEO LOS
PASS	PASS
PIKE	PIKE
PK	PARK
PKDR	PARK DRIVE
PKWY, PKY	PARKWAY
PL	PLACE
PLWY	PLACE WAY
PLZ, PZ	PLAZA
PT	POINT
PTAV	POINT AVENUE
PTH	PATH
PZ DE	PLAZA DE
PZ DEL	PLAZA DEL
PZ D LA	PLAZA DE LA
PZ D LAS	PLAZA DE LAS
PZWY	PLAZA WAY
RAMP	RAMP
RD	ROAD
RDAV	ROAD AVENUE
RDBP	ROAD BYPASS
RDCT	ROAD COURT
RDEX	ROAD EXTENSION
RDG	RIDGE
RDSP	ROAD SPUR
RDWY	ROAD WAY
RR	RAILROAD
RUE	RUE
RUE D	RUE D
RW	ROW
RY	RAILWAY
SKWY	SKYWAY
SQ	SQUARE
ST	STREET
STAV	STREET AVENUE
STCT	STREET COURT
STDR	STREET DRIVE
STEX	STREET EXTENSION
STLN	STREET LANE
STLP	STREET LOOP
ST OF	STREET OF
ST OF THE	STREET OF THE
STOV	STREET OVERPASS
STPL	STREET PLACE
STPM	STREET PROMENADE
STWY	STREET WAY
STXP	STREET EXPRESSWAY
TER	TERRACE
TFWY	TRAFFICWAY
THWY	THROUGHWAY
TKTR	TRUCK TRAIL
TPKE	TURNPIKE
TRC	TRACE
TRCT	TERRACE COURT
TR, TRL	TRAIL
TRWY	TRAIL WAY
TTSP	TRUCK TRAIL SPUR
TUN	TUNNEL
UNPS	UNDERPASS
VIA D	VIA DE
VIA DL	VIA DEL
VIA D LA	VIA DE LA
VIA D LAS	VIA DE LAS
VIA D LOS	VIA DE LOS
VIA LA	VIA LA
VW	VIEW
VWY	VIEW WAY
VIS	VISTA
VIS D	VISTA DE
VIS D L	VISTA DE LA
VIS D LAS	VISTA DE LAS
VIS DEL	VISTA DEL
WK	WALK
WY	WAY
WYCR	WAY CIRCLE
WYDR	WAY DRIVE
WYLN	WAY LANE
WYPL	WAY PLACE

DIRECTIONS

E	EAST
KPN	KEY PENINSULA NORTH
KPS	KEY PENINSULA SOUTH
N	NORTH
NE	NORTHEAST
NW	NORTHWEST
S	SOUTH
SE	SOUTHEAST
SW	SOUTHWEST
W	WEST

BUILDINGS

CH	CITY HALL
CHP	CALIFORNIA HIGHWAY PATROL
COMM CTR	COMMUNITY CENTER
CON CTR	CONVENTION CENTER
CONT HS	CONTINUATION HIGH SCHOOL
CTH	COURTHOUSE
FAA	FEDERAL AVIATION ADMIN
FS	FIRE STATION
HOSP	HOSPITAL
HS	HIGH SCHOOL
INT	INTERMEDIATE SCHOOL
JR HS	JUNIOR HIGH SCHOOL
LIB	LIBRARY
MID	MIDDLE SCHOOL
MUS	MUSEUM
PO	POST OFFICE
PS	POLICE STATION
SR CIT CTR	SENIOR CITIZENS CENTER
STA	STATION
THTR	THEATER
VIS BUR	VISITORS BUREAU

OTHER ABBREVIATIONS

BCH	BEACH
BLDG	BUILDING
CEM	CEMETERY
CK	CREEK
CO	COUNTY
COMM	COMMUNITY
CTR	CENTER
EST	ESTATE
HIST	HISTORIC
HTS	HEIGHTS
LK	LAKE
MDW	MEADOW
MED	MEDICAL
MEM	MEMORIAL
MT	MOUNT
MTN	MOUNTAIN
NATL	NATIONAL
PKG	PARKING
PLGD	PLAYGROUND
RCH	RANCH
RCHO	RANCHO
REC	RECREATION
RES	RESERVOIR
RIV	RIVER
RR	RAILROAD
SPG	SPRING
STA	SANTA
VLG	VILLAGE
VLY	VALLEY
VW	VIEW

City ZIP Pg-Grid

A
PBCH 93449 714-D3
MonC 93451 453-A3; SMRA 93455 796-D5; SMRA 93458 796-D4
LMPC 93436 896-F6; LMPC 93436 916-F1; StBC 93436 896-F5
LMPC 93436 916-F2
NK TR SLOC 93451 453-A6
RG CT SLVG 93463 920-E7
RG WY SLVG 93463 920-D7
S DR SLVG 93463 940-D1
RD PSRS 93446 514-C7; SLOC 93446 514-C7
L SLVG 93463 940-E1
RD StBC 93455 816-G4
' ST SLO 93401 654-A3
D SLOC 93465 553-E1
EN AV GOL 93117 994-C1
EN CT GBCH 93433 714-E6
O RD SLOC 93422 594-F5
L LN SBAR 93108 996-D2
SON RD SLOC 93465 553-D1
) RD StBC 93117 993-J5; StBC 93117 994-A5
SLO 93401 673-H1
AV SLOC 93430 591-C5; StBC 93437 855-G7; StBC 93437 875-G1
ST MOBY 93442 611-F7; SMRA 93458 776-G3
WK StBC 93117 994-A3
O RD StBC 93441 900-H4
PL SLOC 93420 715-B3
DR ARGD 93420 714-G3
LN SLOC 93446 469-G3
WY SLVG 93463 940-E1
V SLOC 93401 694-F1
DR SBAR 93105 995-F1
WY SMRA 93458 796-F2
S RD SBAR 93117 994-B2
S ST Cmbr 93428 548-H1
S WY LMPC 93436 896-C6
ST PBCH 93449 714-C3
IDA RD SLOC 93446 513-A2
ADE DR SLVG 93463 920-F7
NE LN SMRA 93454 796-H4
WY SLOC 93420 735-F6
WY Npmo 93444 756-C4
CT SMRA 93458 796-F4
RD PSRS 93446 494-B4; SLOC - 612-C7; SLOC 93405 612-C7; SLOC 93405 632-E1; SLOC 93446 494-B4
E CANYON RD SLOC 93432 574-C3
E CREEK RD SLVG 93463 920-E6
E FALLS RD StBC 93436 896-F3
EE SLOC 93430 591-C5
AV SMRA 93458 776-G4
TOFT WY SLVG 93463 920-D7
LN SLOC 93424 693-A1
DR SLO 93401 674-C2; SLOC 93401 674-C2
CAMINO GOL 93117 994-B2; SBAR 93117 994-B2
TECH CENTER WY PSRS 93446 494-F7
VISTA PL SLO 93401 674-B2
MED LN SLOC 93446 513-E3
A DR StBC 93111 984-G7
A WY StBC 93436 876-D6
LL DR SLOC 93465 553-C2
S AV SMRA 93454 776-G6; SMRA 93458 776-F6
CITA RD SLOC 93422 594-F5
MANANTIAL LN ATAS 93422 594-C2

STREET Name City ZIP Pg-Grid
AGUILA AV ATAS 93422 573-G4; GOL 93117 994-E1
AIRFIELD RD StBC 93437 875-B2
AIR PARK DR SLOC 93445 714-D7; SMRA 93455 796-E6; SMRA 93455 816-F1
AIRPARK DR SMRA 93455 816-G1
AIR PARK LN SMRA 93455 816-F1
E AIRPORT AV LMPC 93436 896-F7
W AIRPORT AV LMPC 93436 896-C7; StBC 93436 896-C7
AIRPORT DR SLO 93401 674-B2; SLOC 93401 674-B2
AIRPORT RD PSRS 93446 494-C7; PSRS 93446 514-C2; PSRS 93446 534-C1; SLOC 93446 494-C3; StBC 93460 921-C6
AJAY DR StBC 93455 816-H5
ALABAMA AV StBC 93437 875-D4
ALAMAR AV SBAR 93105 985-H7; SBAR 93105 995-G1
ALAMEDA AV GOL 93117 993-H1
ALAMEDA DR PSRS 93446 513-G2
ALAMEDA RD SLOC 93405 633-C5
ALAMEDA PADRE SERRA SBAR 93103 995-J1; SBAR 93103 996-A1; SBAR 93108 996-D2
ALAMO LMPC 93436 896-E4
ALAMO AV ATAS 93422 573-J1
ALAMO DR SLOC 93402 651-F1
ALAMO CREEK DR PSRS 93446 533-J1; PSRS 93446 534-A2
ALAMO PINTADO AV StBC 93441 900-G5; StBC 93463 900-G5
ALAMO PINTADO RD SLVG 93463 920-F7; SLVG 93463 940-E1; StBC 93463 900-H7; StBC 93463 920-H2; StBC 93463 940-F1
ALAN RD SBAR 93109 995-F5; StBC 93109 995-F5
ALASKA WY StBC 93437 875-D2
ALBA CT SMRA 93458 796-F4
ALBAN PL Cmbr 93428 548-G1
ALBANY CT GOL 93117 984-E7
ALBANY WY SLOC 93451 453-C6
ALBERT DR SLO 93405 654-A2
ALBERT ST SMRA 93458 796-G2
ALBERT WY SLOC 93420 735-C7; SLOC 93420 755-C2
ALBERTA AV SBAR 93101 995-H4
ALBIREO AV StBC 93436 876-C6
ALCALA DR SMRA 93454 777-B7
ALCALA LN StBC 93108 996-G2
ALCAMO PL SBAR 93105 995-E3
ALCANTARA AV ATAS 93422 573-J4
ALCAZAR DR SMRA 93455 796-H5
ALCO DR SMRA 93458 776-F3
ALCOR AV StBC 93436 876-D6
ALCOTAN LN ATAS 93422 594-D1
ALCOTT AV LMPC 93436 896-B6
ALDEBARAN AV StBC 93436 876-E5
ALDEN AV LMPC 93436 896-C6
ALDEN CT LMPC 93436 896-C6
ALDER AV MOBY 93442 611-E2
ALDER CT SLO 93401 674-D2
ALDER LN BLTN 93427 919-F4; SLO 93401 674-D2; SMRA 93455 796-J5
ALDER ST ARGD 93420 714-H6
ALDERBERRY DR StBC 93455 816-B1
ALDO WY SLOC 93451 473-F2
ALEEDA LN SBAR 93108 996-F2
ALEGRE AV ATAS 93422 574-A7; Npmo 93444 756-B4
ALEGRIA RD SBAR 93105 995-G2
ALEJANDRO WY SLOC 93420 755-A2
ALEX PL GOL 93117 984-C7
ALEXANDER AV LMPC 93436 896-B6; SLOC 93402 631-G7

ALHAMBRA AV SMRA 93458 796-E4
AL-HIL DR SLO 93405 653-G1
ALICE LN SLOC 93445 714-E7
ALICE PL SLOC 93446 533-E4
ALICITA CT SLO 93401 653-J7
ALINA LN Npmo 93444 756-A4
ALISA LN StBC 93110 995-C5
ALISAL AV SLO 93401 654-B3
ALISAL RD SBAR 93103 996-D1; SLVG - 940-D3; SLVG 93463 920-E7; SLVG 93463 940-E1; StBC - 940-E1; StBC 93463 940-E7
ALISAL MESA RD SLVG 93463 940-E1
ALISON AV SMRA 93458 776-F5
ALISOS AV StBC 93441 922-C4; StBC 93460 922-C4
ALISOS DR StBC 93108 997-C1
ALISOS RD SLOC 93420 695-H7; SLOC 93420 715-H1
ALISOS ST SBAR 93103 996-C2
ALLAIRE ST SBAR 93103 996-D3
ALLEGRO CT PSRS 93446 513-H4
ALLEMANDE LN ATAS 93422 573-G4
ALLEN CT SLOC 93465 553-B2
ALLEN RD SLOC 93446 469-J6; SLOC 93446 470-B5
ALLEN ST ARGD 93420 715-A5
ALLENE WY SLOC 93401 674-C3; SLOC 93405 633-A5
ALLESANDRO ST MOBY 93442 611-H6
ALLEY OOP WY SLOC 93420 754-J2
ALLI WY GOL 93117 984-D7
ALLIANCE WY SLOC 93405 693-D3
ALLISON CT SLOC 93420 755-C3
ALMA CT GBCH 93433 714-F4
ALMAGUER ST GDLP 93434 774-J6
ALMENDRA CT PSRS 93446 514-A4
ALMERIA AV SMRA 93458 796-E3
ALMIRA HTS SLOC 93446 533-F2
ALMIRA PARK WY SLOC 93446 533-E1
ALMOND AV LMPC 93436 896-F6; SBAR 93101 995-J4
ALMOND LN SMRA 93458 776-G4
ALMOND ST PSRS 93446 513-G5; SLO 93405 653-H3
ALMOND CREST CT PSRS 93446 513-E4
ALMOND SPRINGS DR PSRS 93446 513-E4
ALOHA PL SLOC 93445 714-D7
ALOMA WY SLOC 93420 735-B4
ALONDRA DR GOL 93117 994-E1
ALONDRA RD ATAS 93422 594-D2; SLOC 93422 594-D2
ALPHONSE ST SBAR 93103 996-C3
ALPHONSO ST SLO 93401 654-A6
ALPINE AV SLOC 93405 633-A5
ALPINE DR GOL 93117 993-G2
N ALPINE ST ARGD 93420 714-H5
S ALPINE ST ARGD 93420 714-H6
ALRITA CT SLO 93401 654-C5
ALRITA ST SLO 93401 654-C5; SLOC 93401 654-C5
ALSACE LN SLOC 93420 715-B3
AL SERENO LN SLOC 93402 631-H7; SLOC 93402 651-J1
ALSTON LN SBAR 93108 996-F2
ALSTON PL SBAR 93108 996-E2
ALSTON RD SBAR 93108 996-F2; StBC 93108 996-F2
ALTA CT MOBY 93442 611-G7
ALTA DR StBC 93105 964-J6
ALTA ST SLO 93401 654-B3; StBC 93441 900-H5
ALTADENA LN PSRS 93446 513-G2
ALTAIR AV StBC 93436 876-D6
ALTAIR PL StBC 93436 876-D6
ALTA MIRA LN SLOC 93401 674-D7

ALTA PRADERA LN ATAS 93422 573-E5
ALTA VISTA SLVG 93463 940-D1
ALTA VISTA AV ATAS 93422 573-H4
ALTA VISTA LN Npmo 93444 756-E7; Npmo 93444 776-E1
ALTA VISTA RD SBAR 93103 996-A2
ALTA VISTA WY SLOC 93420 715-A3
ALTO DR StBC 93110 985-A7
ALTON DR SMRA 93458 776-F5
ALTOS DE PIEDRA SLOC 93401 694-E1
ALTURAS RD ATAS 93422 553-C7; ATAS 93422 573-C1
ALTURAS DEL SOL SBAR 93103 996-C1
ALUFFO RD SLOC 93446 470-C7
ALVA ST CARP 93013 998-E6
ALVARADO PL SBAR 93103 996-A1
ALVARADO RD ATAS 93422 593-F2; CARP 93013 998-D5; SLOC 93422 593-F2
E ALVIN AV SMRA 93454 776-H6; SMRA 93454 777-A6
W ALVIN AV SMRA 93454 776-G6; SMRA 93458 776-G6
ALYDAR PL SLOC 93446 513-E3
ALYSSUM CIR Npmo 93444 755-J3; Npmo 93444 756-A3
ALYSSUM CT SLO 93401 674-C1
AMADO ST Npmo 93444 756-C3
AMADOR AV GOL 93117 993-H2; SLOC 93405 633-A5
AMADOR WY Npmo 93444 755-D5
AMALFI WY SBAR 93105 995-E2
AMANDA WY SLOC 93446 493-E6
AMAPOA AV ATAS 93422 573-J6
AMAPOLA DR SBAR 93105 995-F1
AMAPOLA LN StBC 93108 997-A3
AMARANTH LN Npmo 93444 756-A3
AMARGON RD ATAS 93422 573-G1
AMARILLO DR SLOC 93420 734-J5
AMARONE LN SMRA 93458 796-E4
AMAROSA ST StBC 93110 994-J2
AMBER CT SLOC 93446 533-E6
AMBER DR SLOC 93446 533-E6
AMBER LN SMRA 93454 796-H4
AMBER ST GDLP 93434 775-A6
AMBER WY Npmo 93444 755-H2; SLVG 93463 920-F7
AMBER FARMS RD StBC 93460 921-A6
AMBER GRAIN PL PSRS 93446 534-C1
AMBERLEY PL StBC 93455 816-F4
AMBERLY PL StBC 93111 994-H2
AMBROSIA CT SLO 93401 674-C2
AMBROSIA LN SLO 93401 674-C2
AMBUSH TRAIL PL SLOC 93446 533-E2
AMELIA WY Npmo 93444 756-B5
AMERICAN AV SBAR 93105 995-H2
AMERICAN WY Npmo 93444 755-E2
AMETHYST DR StBC 93455 816-J5; StBC 93455 817-A5
AMHERST DR GOL 93117 984-D7
AMHERST PL Cmbr 93428 548-F1; LMPC 93436 916-G2
AMIGO PL Npmo 93444 755-H4
AMOS PL ATAS 93422 593-C2; SLOC 93422 593-C2
AMY LN SMRA 93454 777-A5
ANA BAY RD SLOC 93424 693-A3
ANABELLE ST SMRA 93458 796-F3
ANACAPA CIR SLO 93405 653-F1
ANACAPA ST SBAR 93101 995-H1; SBAR 93101 996-A3; SBAR 93105 995-H1
ANAPAMU ST SBAR 93101 995-J5
E ANAPAMU ST SBAR 93101 996-B2; SBAR 93103 996-B2
W ANAPAMU ST SBAR 93101 995-J4; SBAR 93101 996-A3

ANCHOR CIR SLOC 93426 469-J1
ANCHOR DR GOL 93117 993-F3
ANCHOR ST MOBY 93442 611-F7
ANCHOR WY SLOC 93426 469-J1
ANCONA AV GOL 93117 993-G1
ANDAMAR WY GOL 93117 984-E7
ANDANTE RD StBC 93105 985-J7
ANDERSON LN StBC 93111 994-G4
ANDERSON RD SLOC 93446 533-A5
ANDORRA CT SMRA 93458 796-E4
ANDOVER PL Cmbr 93428 528-G7
ANDRE AV SLOC 93402 631-J7; SLOC 93402 632-A7
ANDRE DR ARGD 93420 714-H3
ANDREA CIR PSRS 93446 513-J6
ANDREA ST CARP 93013 998-E6
ANDREWS AV LMPC 93436 896-C6
ANDREWS ST SLO 93401 654-A3
ANDRITA RD ATAS 93422 573-G7
ANDRITA ST StBC 93110 994-J2
ANDROMEDA DR StBC 93436 896-D1
ANDROS ST MOBY 93442 611-E2
ANDY LN StBC 93111 994-H3
ANGELA AV PSRS 93446 513-F4
ANGELA CT StBC 93455 816-J5
ANGELES RD StBC 93455 816-H2
ANGELINA CT Npmo 93444 756-B5
ANGELLO TR GBCH 93433 714-E4
ANGIE LOU LN SLOC 93401 674-B3
ANGLERS WY SLOC 93446 469-G4
ANGUS ST PSRS 93446 533-H1
ANGUS RANCH WY SLOC 93446 470-E5
ANISE LN Npmo 93444 756-A2
ANITA AV GBCH 93433 714-F7
ANITA LN StBC 93111 994-H2
ANITA ST CARP 93013 998-D6
ANN CT SMRA 93454 777-A6
ANNA CIR SLOC 93420 755-B3
ANNE AV SLOC 93402 631-H7
ANNEFORD CIR SLOC 93401 674-E6
ANNIE WY SMRA 93455 796-J6
ANTARES AV StBC 93436 876-D6
ANTELOPE TR StBC 93455 816-G7
ANTHONY SLOC 93446 513-B1
ANTHONY PL SMRA 93458 796-F4
E ANTHONY WY LMPC 93436 896-E6
W ANTHONY WY LMPC 93436 896-D6
ANTLER DR SLOC 93420 695-C6
ANTLER RIDGE WY StBC 93455 816-G7
ANTONE LN SMRA 93454 777-B5
ANTONE RD StBC 93110 985-D6
ANZA DR SBAR 93105 985-E7
APACHE CT PSRS 93446 513-H6
APACHE TR SLOC 93420 735-F6
APION CT PSRS 93446 513-J3
APOLLO WY StBC 93436 876-D7
APPALOOSA DR PSRS 93446 513-H6
APPALOOSA TR StBC 93455 816-E5
APPALOOSA WY SLOC 93420 734-J4
W APPLE AV LMPC 93436 916-D1
APPLEGATE WY SLOC 93420 735-E6
APPLE GROVE LN SBAR 93105 995-E2; StBC 93105 995-E2
APPLE ORCHARD LN SLOC 93405 693-C2
APPY WY SLOC 93420 715-D2
W APRICOT AV LMPC 93436 916-C1
APRICOT ST Npmo 93444 756-A4
AQUARIUS RD StBC 93436 876-C5
AQUEDUCT WY SLVG 93463 920-F7
AQUINNAH LN StBC 93455 817-C7

ARABIAN CIR ARGD 93420 714-H2
ARABIAN LN PSRS 93446 513-H7
ARABIAN TR StBC 93455 816-E5
ARABIAN WY SLOC 93420 735-A2
ARAGON DR CARP 93013 998-C6
ARAGON RD ATAS 93422 574-C3
ARALIA CT SLO 93401 674-D1
ARANGO DR StBC 93111 984-J7
ARAUJO CT ATAS 93422 594-C1
ARBOLADO LN PSRS 93446 533-J2
ARBOLADO RD SBAR 93103 996-B1; SLOC 93446 533-J2
ARBOL DEL ROSAL WY ATAS 93422 594-C2
ARBOLEDA RD StBC 93110 995-B2
N ARBOLEDA RD StBC 93110 995-B1
ARBOLES WY SLOC 93420 734-H6; SMRA 93455 796-H5
ARBOLITOS CT SMRA 93458 796-D5
ARBOL VERDE ST CARP 93013 998-E7; CARP 93013 1018-E1
ARBOR DR StBC 93437 855-D6
ARBOR LN StBC 93455 796-H7
ARBOR RD SLOC 93446 533-D2
ARBOREA CT StBC 93455 816-J3
ARBORVIEW LN StBC 93436 896-F3
ARBUTUS AV MOBY 93442 611-G7
ARCADE RD ATAS 93422 574-A5
ARCADIA AV MOBY 93442 611-G7
ARCADIA DR ARGD 93420 715-A7
ARCADY RD StBC 93108 996-F1
ARCHBRIAR CT StBC 93436 896-E3
ARCHER CT LMPC 93436 896-C6
ARCHER ST LMPC 93436 896-C6; SLO 93401 653-J5
ARCHER WY Npmo 93444 756-A3
ARCIERO CT PSRS 93446 514-A3
ARCIERO WY PSRS 93446 513-J4; PSRS 93446 514-A4
ARCTIC AV SMRA 93454 796-H1
ARCTURUS AV StBC 93436 876-D5
ARDANA DR SLOC 93446 513-B3
ARDATH DR Cmbr 93428 548-G1
ARDEN AV BLTN 93427 919-G4
ARDEN RD SBAR 93105 995-G2
ARDEN WY BLTN 93427 919-G4; SLOC 93420 734-H5
ARDILLA AV ATAS 93422 573-G3
ARDILLA DR SBAR 93105 995-E2
ARDILLA RD ATAS 93422 573-E2
ARDMORE DR GOL 93117 984-D7
ARDMORE RD PSRS 93446 514-A4
ARENA AV ATAS 93422 553-H7; ATAS 93422 573-H1
ARENA RD ATAS 93422 553-G7
ARGONNE CIR SBAR 93105 985-G7; SBAR 93105 995-G1
ARGUELLO BLVD StBC 93437 895-A6
ARGUELLO RD SBAR 93103 996-A1
ARIBA RD SLOC 93446 533-E1
ARIES AV StBC 93436 876-D6
ARIZONA AV ATAS 93422 553-H7; ATAS 93422 573-H1; StBC 93437 875-C4
ARIZONA BLVD MonC 93451 453-A4; SLOC 93451 453-A4
ARLEEN AV PSRS 93446 513-F2
ARLINGTON AV SBAR 93101 996-A3
ARLINGTON ST Cmbr 93428 528-E6
ARLISS DR Cmbr 93428 548-H2
ARMAND AV SLOC 93451 473-F1
ARMAS CANYON RD StBC 93117 993-D1
ARMITOS AV GOL 93117 994-E1
ARMOUR RANCH RD StBC 93460 921-G6; StBC 93460 941-J1
ARMSTRONG AV SMRA 93454 776-J7

ARMSTRONG RD GOL 93117 993-H3
ARMSTRONG ST LMPC 93436 896-C6
ARNEB AV StBC 93436 876-D7
ARNOLD AV LMPC 93436 896-C6
ARNOLD CIR LMPC 93436 896-C6
ARNOLD PL SBAR 93117 994-C2
ARORA WY SMRA 93458 776-G3
AROZENA LN StBC 93013 1018-H2
ARRELLAGA ST SBAR 93101 995-H4; SBAR 93101 996-A2; SBAR 93103 996-A2
ARRIBA DR StBC 93013 997-J3
ARRIBA PL SLOC 93420 755-A2
ARRIBA WY SBAR 93105 985-H7; SMRA 93458 776-F4; StBC 93105 985-H7
ARROQUI ST StBC 93108 997-B3
ARROWHEAD DR StBC 93455 817-E5
ARROYICO LN StBC 93108 996-H2
ARROYO AV ARGD 93420 715-A6; ATAS 93422 573-J1; SBAR 93109 995-J6; SBAR 93109 996-A6
ARROYO CT StBC 93455 816-J6
ARROYO DR SLOC 93446 533-E5
ARROYO LN SLOC 93405 653-C5
ARROYO RD StBC 93110 995-A2
ARROYO WY StBC 93455 816-J6
ARROYO GRANDE SLO RD Rt#227 ARGD 93420 715-A3; SLOC 93420 715-A3
ARROYO MESA RD StBC 93463 920-E5
ARROYO VISTA DR GOL 93117 993-E2
ARROYO VISTA LN SLOC 93420 715-C2
ARTESIA AV StBC 93436 895-F6
ARTHUR LN SLOC 93422 594-F4; SMRA 93455 796-J6
ARTIGA LN ATAS 93422 573-E2
ARUNDEL RD GOL 93117 984-E7
ARVINE CT ATAS 93422 594-C2
ASCOT CT Cmbr 93428 528-G7; Cmbr 93428 548-G1
ASEGRA RD Summ 93067 997-E2
ASH AV CARP 93013 998-C7; Npmo 93444 756-C1; SLOC 93430 590-J1; SMRA 93454 777-A6
ASH LN SLVG 93463 940-D1
ASH ST ARGD 93420 714-G6; ATAS 93422 574-B7; GBCH 93433 714-G6; SLOC 93402 631-E6; StBC 93437 855-D6
ASHBROOK LN StBC 93455 817-B6
ASHBY LN Cmbr 93428 528-E5
ASHDALE ST StBC 93110 994-J2
ASHLAND LN Npmo 93444 756-C4
ASHLEY AV SBAR 93103 996-D4
ASHLEY LN SLOC 93465 553-C3
ASHLEY PL GOL 93117 984-D7; StBC 93455 816-G4
ASHLEY RD StBC 93108 986-G7; StBC 93108 996-F1
ASHMORE ST SLO 93401 674-D2
ASHTON AV SMRA 93458 776-F3
ASHTON ST StBC 93111 994-J2
ASHTON WY SLOC 93465 553-C3
ASHWOOD PL PSRS 93446 534-B2
ASILO ARGD 93420 714-H2
ASKOV PL SLVG 93463 920-F6
ASPEN CT Npmo 93444 756-A6
ASPEN LN SMRA 93454 777-A6
ASPEN ST ARGD 93420 714-G6; SLOC 93402 631-F6; StBC 93437 855-D6
ASPEN WY StBC 93111 984-H7
ASTER AV LMPC 93436 896-D6
ASTER LN LMPC 93436 896-D6
ASTER PL StBC 93455 816-H1
ASTER ST SLOC 93445 734-G1

STREET Name City ZIP Pg-Grid

ASTOR AV
Cmbr 93428 548-G2
ASTOR CT
LMPC 93436 896-C6
ASTORIA PL
GOL 93117 993-F3
ASUNCION RD
SLOC 93422 594-G4
ATAJO AV
ATAS 93422 573-G4
ATALAYA ST
ATAS 93422 553-E6
ATASCADERO AV
ATAS 93422 573-J4
ATAS 93422 574-A6
ATAS 93422 594-A1
SLOC 93422 594-A1
ATASCADERO DR
StBC 93110 995-A2
ATASCADERO MALL
ATAS 93422 573-H4
ATASCADERO RD
ATAS 93422 594-C3
MOBY 93442 611-E4
SLOC 93422 594-C3
ATASCADERO RD Rt#-41
MOBY 93442 611-G3
SLOC 93442 611-G3
SLOC 93442 612-A1
ATASCADERO ST
SLO 93405 653-F7
ATASCO DR
StBC 93110 995-A1
ATHERLY LN
StBC 93455 796-H7
ATLANTIC PL
SMRA 93458 776-F2
ATLANTIC CITY AV
GBCH 93433 714-D4
ATOLL ST
SLOC 93445 714-E7
ATTERDAG RD
SLVG 93463 920-E7
SLVG 93463 940-E1
ATWELL ST
Cmbr 93428 548-F2
AUBURN CT
SLOC 93446 471-C3
AUDUBON AV
LMPC 93436 896-B6
AUGUSTA CT
SLO 93401 654-B5
SMRA 93455 796-G6
AUGUSTA DR
Npmo 93444 755-F1
AUGUSTA LN
SBAR 93108 996-F2
AUGUSTA ST
SLO 93401 654-B5
StBC 93440 878-H2
AUGUSTENBORG PL
SLVG 93463 920-F6
AUHAY DR
StBC 93110 995-A1
AUKLET CT
SLOC 93420 735-A6
AURELIA LN
SLOC 93420 735-F6
AURIGA AV
StBC 93436 876-D5
AURORA AV
SBAR 93109 995-H6
AURORA DR
StBC 93108 997-A3
AURORA RD
ATAS 93422 574-C4
AURORA WY
SLOC 93465 553-C1
AUSTIN CT
PSRS 93446 513-J7
SLOC 93402 651-F1
AUSTIN RD
StBC 93111 994-G4
AUTO PARK DR
SMRA 93455 816-G1
StBC 93455 816-G1
AUTO PARK WY
SLO 93405 673-G1
AUTO PLAZA DR
SMRA 93455 796-J4
AUTO PLAZA LN
SMRA 93454 796-J5
SMRA 93455 796-J5
AUTUMN PL
SLOC 93420 754-H1
AUTUMN WOODS PL
SMRA 93454 777-A6
AVALON AV
StBC 93110 994-J2
AVALON ST
LMPC 93436 916-B3
MOBY 93442 611-F3
SLO 93405 653-F6
StBC 93436 916-B3
AVENAL AV
ATAS 93422 573-J7
AVENIDA CABALLO
StBC 93460 901-A5
AVENIDA DE AMIGOS
Npmo 93444 756-C3
AVENIDA DE DIAMANTE
ARGD 93420 714-J4
AVENIDA DEL CAPITAN
StBC 93117 982-C5
AVENIDA DEL SOL
ATAS 93422 553-H7
PSRS 93446 513-H5
AVENIDA DE SOCIOS
Npmo 93444 756-C4
AVENIDA GANSO
GOL 93117 984-C7
GOL 93117 994-C1
AVENIDA GARZA
GOL 93117 984-C7
AVENIDA GORRION
GOL 93117 994-C1
AVENIDA MANZANA
ATAS 93422 553-E7
AVENIDA MARIA
ATAS 93422 594-C1
AVENIDA MONTECITO VERDE
Npmo 93444 756-C4
AVENIDA PELICANOS
SLOC 93445 714-F7
AVENIDA PEQUENA
StBC 93111 984-G6
AVENIDA REDONDO
SMRA 93458 776-F4
AVENIDA RIVIERA
SMRA 93458 776-F4
AVENUE 1
SLOC 93451 453-B5
AVENUE 2
SLOC 93451 453-B5
AVENUE 3
SLOC 93451 453-B4
AVENUE 6
SLOC 93451 453-A4
AVENUE 7
SLOC 93451 453-A4
AVENUE 8
MonC 93451 453-B4
SLOC 93451 453-A4
AVENUE 9
MonC 93451 453-A3
SLOC 93451 453-A4
AVENUE 10
MonC 93451 453-A3
SLOC 93451 453-A4
AVENUE 11
MonC 93451 453-A3
SLOC 93451 453-A4
AVENUE 12
MonC 93451 453-A3
SLOC 93451 453-A4
AVENUE 13
MonC 93451 453-A3
AVENUE 14
MonC 93451 453-A3
AVENUE 15
MonC 93451 453-A3
AVENUE 50
MonC 93451 453-A1
AVENUE 51
MonC 93451 453-A1
AVENUE 52
MonC 93451 453-A1
AVENUE DEL MAR
StBC 93013 998-B7
AVENUE OF FLAGS
StBC - 919-H6
BLTN 93427 919-H5
StBC 93427 919-H6
AVIANO AV
GOL 93117 993-G1
AVIANO PL
GOL 93117 993-H1
AVIATION DR
LMPC 93436 896-C5
SMRA 93455 796-F6
AVILA WY
StBC 93108 997-A2
AVILA BEACH DR
SLOC 93405 693-C3
SLOC 93424 693-C3
SLOC 93449 693-C3
AVILA VALLEY DR
SLOC 93405 693-C2
AVION RD
ATAS 93422 594-D1
AVIS ST
SLOC 93420 735-E4
AVOCADO AV
Npmo 93444 756-C1
AVOCADO CT
Npmo 93444 756-C2
AVOCADO LN
SLOC 93401 674-G3
AVOCET CIR
GDLP 93434 774-H6
AVOCET WY
SLOC 93420 735-A5
AVOLA AV
SMRA 93458 796-E3
AVON AV
Cmbr 93428 548-G2
AVON LN
SBAR 93105 985-E7
AWAKEN PL
SLOC 93446 494-G5
AYALA LN
StBC 93108 986-F7
AZALEA CT
Npmo 93444 755-J5
SLO 93401 674-C1
AZALEA DR
CARP 93013 998-D6
AZALEA LN
StBC 93437 875-H3
AZALEA WY
GOL 93117 984-E7
AZOR LN
ATAS 93422 594-D1
AZUCENA AV
ATAS 93422 573-J6
AZURE ST
MOBY 93442 611-E2

B

B CT
LMPC 93436 896-F5
B ST
SLOC 93430 590-J1
SLOC 93451 453-B4
N B ST
LMPC 93436 896-F6
LMPC 93436 916-F1
S B ST
LMPC 93436 916-F2
BADEN AV
GBCH 93433 714-E6
BADGER RD
StBC 93460 901-C3
BADGER CANYON LN
SLOC 93420 695-B7
SLOC 93420 715-B1
BAHIA CT
SLO 93401 654-C5
BAILARD AV
CARP 93013 1018-F1
BAILARD LN
CARP 93013 998-E7
BAILEY AV
LMPC 93436 896-B7
StBC 93436 896-B7
StBC 93436 916-B2
BAJADA
SBAR 93109 995-H5
BAJADA AV
ATAS 93422 573-H2
BAJADA LN
StBC 93110 995-D5
BAJADA GRANDE
SBAR 93109 995-H5
BAKEMAN NE
ARGD 93420 714-G6
BAKEMAN NW
ARGD 93420 714-G6
BAKEMAN LN
ARGD 93420 714-G6
BAKER AV
PBCH 93449 693-G7
BAKER LN
GOL 93117 993-H2
BAKERSFIELD AV
SLOC 93430 590-J1
SLOC 93430 591-A1
BAKERSFIELD ST
PBCH 93449 714-C1
BAKKE WY
SLVG 93463 920-E7
BALBOA CT
LMPC 93436 916-B2
BALBOA DR
SBAR 93109 995-G7
SMRA 93454 776-J5
SMRA 93454 777-A5
BALBOA RD
ATAS 93422 573-C1
BALBOA ST
GBCH 93433 714-F4
MOBY 93442 611-G6
SLO 93405 653-F6
BALDWIN RD
SBAR 93105 995-G2
BALDWIN WY
SMRA 93458 776-F3
BALI ST
MOBY 93442 611-E2
BALLARD ST
Npmo 93444 756-C2
BALLARD CANYON RD
BLTN 93427 920-A5
StBC 93427 920-A5
StBC 93441 900-F7
StBC 93441 920-D4
StBC 93463 900-F7
StBC 93463 920-E1
BALLESTRAL AV
SMRA 93455 796-G6
BALM RIDGE CT
SLOC 93401 673-G6
BALM RIDGE RD
SLOC 93401 673-G7
BAMBI CT
ARGD 93420 714-J7
BANANA RD
StBC 93108 986-E7
BANBURY RD
Cmbr 93428 548-H1
BANDEROLA CT
SLO 93401 653-J6
BANK ST
Npmo 93444 756-C3
BANNEKER PL
Npmo 93444 755-D4
BANNER AV
Summ 93067 997-D3
BANYAN PL
Npmo 93444 756-C4
BANYAN WY
SMRA 93455 796-G6
BANYON ST
StBC 93437 855-F7
BARBADOS ST
SLOC 93445 734-H1
BARBARA CT
Npmo 93444 755-C4
SLOC 93420 755-C4
BARBARA ST
SMRA 93458 776-G6
SMRA 93458 796-G3
BARBERRY CT
StBC 93436 896-F3
BARBERRY WY
Npmo 93444 755-E1
BARCA ST
GBCH 93433 714-E6
BARCELLUS AV
SMRA 93454 796-H2
BARCELONA
PBCH 93449 693-G6
BARCELONA DR
SBAR 93105 995-E3
BARD CT
SLOC 93401 673-G6
BARDMORE CT
SMRA 93455 796-G6
BARGER CANYON RD
StBC 93110 985-E6
BAR-K LN
Npmo 93444 756-C3
BARKER PASS RD
SBAR 93108 996-E2
StBC 93108 996-E2
BARLEY GRAIN RD
SLOC 93446 533-J3
SLOC 93446 534-A3
BARLING TER
GOL 93117 984-D7
BARLOW LN
MOBY 93442 611-G7
BARN RD
SLOC 93446 471-C5
N BARNES RD
SLOC 93446 473-E5
S BARNES RD
SLOC 93446 473-D7
SLOC 93446 493-E1
BARNETTE RD
StBC 93455 817-A5
BAROLO PL
SMRA 93458 796-E4
BARON CANYON RANCH RD
SLOC 93401 673-F7
BARRANCA AV
SBAR 93109 996-A6
BARRANCA CT
SLO 93401 654-D6
BARRANCA LN
SBAR 93109 996-A6
BARRANCO HTS
ATAS 93422 573-F7
BARRANCO RD
ATAS 93422 573-F7
BARRENDA AV
ATAS 93422 573-J2
BARRETT ST
SMRA 93458 796-F1
BARRINGTON CT
LMPC 93436 916-G2
BARRINGTON DR
SMRA 93458 776-G5
BARRINGTON PL
LMPC 93436 916-G2
BARRINGTON WY
GOL 93117 984-D7
BARTON AV
LMPC 93436 896-C5
E BARTON AV
LMPC 93436 896-E6
W BARTON AV
LMPC 93436 896-C6
BARWICK RD
StBC 93111 994-G4
BASELINE AV
StBC 93460 920-H2
StBC 93460 921-A2
StBC 93460 922-A4
StBC 93463 920-H2
BASIN ST
SLOC 93445 714-G7
BASQUE DR
StBC 93455 816-J5
StBC 93455 817-A5
BASSANO DR
GOL 93117 993-G1
BASSI DR
SLOC 93401 693-D1
SLOC 93405 693-D1
BASS POINT RD
SLOC 93426 469-J2
BASSWOOD ST
StBC 93437 855-G7
BATES RD
StBC 93013 1018-J2
VeCo 93001 1018-J2
BATES RANCH RD
VeCo 93001 1018-J2
BATH ST
SBAR 93101 995-H3
SBAR 93101 996-A4
SBAR 93105 995-G2
BATHURST DR
StBC 93455 817-B4
BATTERING ROCK RD
SLOC 93446 533-H4
BATTLES RD
SMRA 93458 796-E3
E BATTLES RD
SMRA 93454 796-H3
SMRA 93454 797-A3
StBC 93454 797-A3
W BATTLES RD
SMRA 93454 796-G3
SMRA 93458 796-G3
BAUER AV
StBC 93455 817-A5
BAXTER LN
PBCH 93449 714-B1
BAXTER ST
StBC 93110 994-J2
BAY AV
MOBY 93442 611-G6
SMRA 93454 777-A5
BAY ST
PBCH 93449 714-B1
BAY ABI LN
SLOC 93420 695-C5
BAYBERRY LN
GOL 93117 993-J3
BAYCLIFF DR
PBCH 93449 693-J7
BAYFRONT DR
PBCH 93449 693-J7
BAY LAUREL PL
SLOC 93424 693-C2
BAYLOR LN
SMRA 93454 776-J5
BAY OAKS DR
SLOC 93402 631-H7
BAYSHORE DR
MOBY 93442 611-G7
MOBY 93442 631-G1
BAYSIDE DR
CARP 93013 998-B5
BAYSIDE PL
SLOC 93420 734-J5
BAYVIEW
PBCH 93449 693-F6
BAYVIEW AV
MOBY 93442 611-F4
BAY VIEW CIR
SBAR 93109 995-J7
BAYVIEW DR
SMRA 93454 777-A5
BAYVIEW LN
PBCH 93449 714-D3
SLOC 93420 734-H3
BAYVIEW HEIGHTS DR
SLOC 93402 631-H7
SLOC 93402 651-J1
SLOC 93402 652-A1
BAY VISTA LN
SLOC 93402 631-H7
BAYWOOD ST
StBC 93437 855-E6
BAYWOOD WY
SLOC 93402 631-G4
BEA CT
SLOC 93420 755-C2
BEACH
PBCH 93449 714-C3
BEACH BLVD
StBC 93437 875-A7
StBC 93437 894-H1
E BEACH CIR
SLOC 93426 470-A3
BEACH ST
CARP 93013 998-A6
MOBY 93442 611-F6
SLO 93401 653-J5
SLOC 93445 734-E1
BEACH CLUB RD
StBC 93013 997-G4
BEACHCOMBER DR
MOBY 93442 611-D1
PBCH 93449 693-E5
BEACHCOMBER DR N
PBCH 93449 693-E5
BEACHCOMBER DR S
PBCH 93449 693-E5
BEACHWOOD CT
SLOC 93446 533-E6
BEACON RD
PSRS 93446 494-F6
SLOC 93446 494-F6
BEAR CANYON LN
SLOC 93420 715-B2
BEAR CREEK DR
BLTN 93427 919-H6
BEATTIE DR
LMPC 93436 916-F2
BEAUMONT WY
GOL 93117 984-D7
BEAVER CREEK LN
SLOC 93446 533-H2
BECK RD
StBC 93436 896-G3
BECKETT PL
GBCH 93433 714-D4
BECKNELL RD
SBAR 93117 994-C2
BEDFORD CT
SLO 93401 654-C6
BEDFORD PL
StBC 93455 816-J1
BEDLOE LN
ARGD 93420 715-A5
BEE ST
Npmo 93444 756-C2
BEEBEE ST
SLO 93401 653-J6
BEE CANYON RD
SLOC 93420 695-B7
BEECH CT
BLTN 93427 919-F4
BEECH ST
ARGD 93420 714-H6
SLO 93401 673-H1
StBC 93437 855-D6
N BEECHNUT AV
Npmo 93444 756-C1
S BEECHNUT AV
Npmo 93444 756-D2
BEECHWOOD DR
PSRS 93446 534-A1
BEE ROCK RD
SLOC 93426 470-F1
SLOC 93451 473-A1
BEE TREE RD
SLOC 93451 473-D5
BEGA WY
CARP 93013 1018-G1
StBC 93013 998-G7
StBC 93013 1018-G1
BEGONIA PL
CARP 93013 998-D6
BEGONIA ST
SLOC 93445 734-G1
BEL AIR DR
SBAR 93105 995-F4
BEL AIR PL
PSRS 93446 533-J1
PSRS 93446 534-A1
BELANGER DR
Npmo 93444 756-C4
BELGIAN PL
SLOC 93420 735-A2
BELGIAN WOODS RD
SLOC 93465 553-B6
BELL AV
LMPC 93436 896-E6
BELL RD
StBC 93254 806-F3
BELL ST
ARGD 93420 714-H5
StBC 93440 878-F1
BELL ST Rt#-135
StBC 93440 878-G1
BELLA DR
SBAR 93105 995-F4
BELLAGIO CT
StBC 93455 816-J2
BELLA TERRA CT
SLOC 93449 694-C5
BELLA TIERRA PL
SLOC 93446 493-A5
BELLA VISTA CT
PSRS 93446 513-J3
PSRS 93446 514-A3
BELLA VISTA DR
MOBY 93442 611-H6
StBC 93108 987-D7
BELLA VISTA RD
ATAS 93422 573-G5
BELLEVUE ORCHARD LN
SLOC 93405 693-C2
BELLFLOWER LN
LMPC 93436 896-D6
BELLO RD
SMRA 93455 796-J6
SMRA 93455 797-A6
BELLO ST
PBCH 93449 714-B2
BELLUNO DR
GOL 93117 993-G1
BELMONT CT
SMRA 93458 796-F4
BELMONTE DR
SBAR 93101 995-H5
BELRIDGE ST
SLOC 93445 714-E7
BENCHMARK RD
PSRS 93446 514-A3
BENEDICT ST
SLOC 93451 473-F1
BENIAMINO WY
SLOC 93405 632-F3
BENICIA LN
PSRS 93446 513-G2
BENJI LN
StBC 93455 816-H5
BEN LOMOND DR
StBC 93105 985-H7
W BENNET ST
Npmo 93444 756-C2
BENNETT AV
ARGD 93420 714-H5
E BENNETT ST
Npmo 93444 756-D2
BENNETT WY
SLOC 93465 553-C1
BENNETTA DR
SMRA 93458 776-H3
BENSON AV
Cmbr 93428 548-F2
BENTLEY AV
SMRA 93458 776-F3
BENTON RD
SLOC 93446 493-F3
BENTON WY
SLO 93405 653-H3
StBC 93111 994-J2
BENT TREE DR
StBC 93455 816-J1
N BENT TREE DR
StBC 93455 816-G2
S BENT TREE DR
StBC 93455 816-G2
BENWILEY AV
SMRA 93458 776-G5
BERKELEY DR
LMPC 93436 916-G2
BERKELEY RD
GOL 93111 984-F7
GOL 93117 984-E7
StBC 93111 984-F7
BERKELEY WY
SMRA 93454 776-J4
BERKSHIRE LN
StBC 93455 816-F4
BERKSHIRE TER
StBC 93117 994-A4
BERMUDA PL
Npmo 93444 756-C4
BERNARDO AV
MOBY 93442 611-G7
BERNITA PL
Npmo 93444 756-A4
BERRY LN
SMRA 93455 796-D5
BERRYESSA LN
StBC 93455 817-E5
BERRY PATCH LN
SLOC 93446 534-B5
SLOC 93465 534-B5
BERRYWOOD DR
StBC 93455 816-J3
BERWICK DR
Cmbr 93428 548-F2
MOBY 93442 611-F5
BERWYN DR
StBC 93455 817-A2
BETA CT
ARGD 93420 714-G5
BETH CT
SMRA 93454 776-J6
BETHANY DR
StBC 93455 816-H6
BETHEL LN
SMRA 93458 796-D4
N BETHEL RD
SLOC 93446 533-C6
SLOC 93465 533-C6
SLOC 93465 553-B1
S BETHEL RD
SLOC 93465 553-B2
E BETTERAVIA RD
SMRA 93454 796-H5
SMRA 93454 797-B4
StBC 93454 796-H5
StBC 93454 797-B4
W BETTERAVIA RD
SMRA 93454 796-B5
SMRA 93455 796-B5
StBC 93455 795-C2
StBC 93455 796-B5
BETTIGA WY
PBCH 93449 714-C2
BETTY DR
SBAR 93105 995-G2
BEVERLY AV
PSRS 93446 513-F3
BEVERLY CT
StBC 93455 816-E4
BEVERLY DR
Npmo 93444 756-B5
StBC 93455 816-E4
BEV ROSE PL
SMRA 93458 796-F4
BIANCHI LN
SLO 93401 653-H5
BICKNELL AV
SMRA 93458 776-G3
BIDDLE RANCH RD
SLOC 93401 674-F6
BIENVENIDA CT
ATAS 93422 574-B7
BIG BEAR CIR
SLOC 93446 471-C7
BIG BUCK LN
SLOC 93446 471-D6
BIG CANYON CT
SLOC 93420 715-C3
BIG HORN WY
Npmo 93444 756-C3
BIG PINE DR
SMRA 93454 776-J5
SMRA 93454 777-A5
BIG SUR DR
GOL 93117 993-F3
BILBAO DR
SMRA 93454 777-B7
BILLIE CT
StBC 93455 816-G5
BILLS WY
ARGD 93420 714-G2
ARGD 93449 714-G2
SLOC 93420 714-G2
SLOC 93449 714-G2
BINNS CT
SLO 93401 654-B5
BINSCARTH RD
SLOC 93402 631-F6
BIRCH
SLO 93401 673-H1
BIRCH AV
MOBY 93442 611-E2
SLOC 93430 590-J1
StBC 93437 855-G7
E BIRCH AV
LMPC 93436 896-E6
BIRCH DR
SLVG 93463 940-E1
BIRCH LN
BLTN 93427 919-G5
BIRCH ST
ATAS 93422 574-B7
CARP 93013 1018-F1
GDLP 93434 775-A6
SMRA 93458 776-G4
BIRCH WK
StBC 93117 994-A3
BIRCHWOOD CT
SLOC 93446 533-E6
BIRCHWOOD RD
StBC 93111 984-H7
StBC 93111 994-H1
BIRDIE CT
PSRS 93446 513-J7
BIRDIE LN
SLOC 93420 735-A4
BIRKDALE LN
SLOC 93401 674-E6
BIRNAM WOOD DR
StBC 93108 997-B1
BISCAYNE ST
SMRA 93458
BISHOP ST
SLO 93401
BISON LN
StBC 93463
BITHYNIA RD
StBC 93110
BITTERN ST
SLOC 93420
BIVOUAC RD
SLOC 93451
BIXBY RD
Cmbr 93428
BLACK RD
SMRA 93455
SMRA 93458
StBC 93429
StBC 93455
StBC 93455
StBC 93458
StBC 93458
BLACKBERRY AV
ARGD 93420
BLACKBURN ST
PSRS 93446
SLOC 93465
BLACK HAWK WY
Npmo 93444
BLACK HORSE LN
SLOC 93446
BLACK LAKE CIR
Npmo 93444
BLACKLAKE CANYON
Npmo 93444
Npmo 93444
SLOC 93420
BLACK MOUNTAIN RD
MOBY 93442
MOBY 93442
BLACK OAK DR
StBC 93455
BLACKOAK DR
PSRS 93446
BLACK OAK LN
Npmo 93444
BLACK RIDGE LN
Npmo 93444
BLACK SAGE CIR
Npmo 93444
BLACKSTONE CT
StBC 93455
BLACKWOOD CT
StBC 93455
BLAISDEL LN
StBC 93436
BLAKE ST
StBC 93455
BLANCA ST
MOBY 93442
SLOC -
BLANCHARD ST
SBAR 93103
BLANCHE CT
SMRA 93458
BLANKER PL
StBC 93455
BLARNEY LN
SLOC 93405
BLISS ST
ATAS 93422
BLOSSER RD
SMRA 93455
SMRA 93455
SMRA 93458
StBC 93455
N BLOSSER RD
SMRA 93458
StBC 93458
BLOSSOM CT
PSRS 93446
BLOSSOM DR
StBC 93455
BLUEBELL WY
SLO 93401
BLUEBERRY AV
ARGD 93420
BLUEBERRY LN
SLOC 93401
BLUEBIRD LN
SLOC 93446
StBC 93460
BLUEBIRD ST
SMRA 93454
BLUEBIRD GLEN RD
StBC 93427
BLUE BLOSSOM WY
BLTN 93427
BLUE FOX RD
SLOC 93420
BLUEGILL DR
SLOC 93446
BLUE GRANITE LN
SLOC 93405
BLUE GUM LN
Npmo 93444
BLUE HEAVEN LN
PSRS 93446
BLUE HERON CIR
GDLP 93434
BLUE HERON DR
SLOC 93424
BLUE HERON LN
GDLP 93434
SLOC 93446
BLUE HERON VIEW LN
SLOC 93402
BLUE JAY
PSRS 93446
BLUEJAY DR
StBC 93455
StBC 93455
BLUE LAKE LN
SMRA 93454
SMRA 93454
BLUE LUPINE LN
SLOC 93446
BLUE OAK WY
PSRS 93446
BLUE RIDGE DR
SMRA 93455
BLUERIDGE LN
StBC 93437
BLUEROCK CT
SLO 93401
BLUEROCK DR
SLO 93401
BLUE ROCK RD
SLOC 93446

City ZIP Pg-Grid

AGE RD
SLOC 93446 493-C6
KY DR
SLOC 93420 695-E6
PRINGS LN
Npmo 93444 756-C2
AV
LMPC 93436 916-F2
T
SLOC 93426 469-H2
ST
Npmo 93444 756-B3
PL
Cmbr 93428 528-G7
Cmbr 93428 548-G1
WALK LN
StBC 93455 817-A4
OOK RD
SLOC 93426 470-A1
LN
SLOC 93446 470-B4
SPRINGS RD
StBC 93427 919-G2
ITE
PSRS 93446 514-B7
ITE DR
SLOC 93424 693-B3
ATAS 93422 594-C1
A CT
GBCH 93433 714-E7
A LN
SBAR 93110 995-D1
R RD
LMPC 93436 916-C3
StBC 93436 916-C3
R AV
PBCH 93449 693-H7
E PKWY
StBC 93108 997-A3
PL
SLOC 93420 735-A4
LN
PSRS 93446 513-J7
DR
PSRS 93446 513-H5
D DR
StBC 93108 996-J1
S CT
GBCH 93433 714-D4
Y DR
GOL 93117 993-J3
RD
ATAS 93422 573-B3
CHICA CT
GOL 93117 984-D6
N DR
MOBY 93442 611-F5
N WK
StBC 93117 993-J4
ZA LN
SLOC 93446 471-B5
AV
SBAR 93103 996-C3
ST
SLO 93405 653-J2
SLO 93405 654-A2
TI DR
SLO 93401 673-J1
AV
PSRS 93446 513-F2
SLOC 93430 591-C5
A PL
SLOC 93451 473-F2
A PZ
SBAR 93103 995-J1
A ST
MOBY 93442 611-E3
PBCH 93449 693-E4
SMRA 93454 776-J7
SMRA 93454 796-J1
A LATERAL RD
StBC 93458 775-H6
StBC 93458 776-A6
A SCHOOL RD
Npmo 93444 755-G7
Npmo 93444 775-G1
StBC 93458 775-H4
E LN
StBC 93108 996-J3
E JEAN LN
SLOC 93420 735-A3
MEDE DR
StBC 93108 996-H4
ST
SMRA 93454 796-H1
SMRA 93454 797-A1
SMRA 93458 796-E1
AUX PL
SLOC 93420 715-B2
A LN
Npmo 93444 756-E6
S DR
SMRA 93454 776-J4
IDA ST
SLO 93405 653-F7
N DR
SBAR 93109 995-F6
E CT
SMRA 93454 797-A1
N WY
SLOC 93451 453-C6
LO RD
SBAR 93117 994-C2
NWOOD
SLOC 93401 674-B3
AINVILLEA ST
SLO 93401 674-C1
VARD DEL CAMPO
SLO 93401 654-B6
DARY DR
StBC 93108 997-C1
DARY OAKS CT
SMRA 93455 796-F6
DR
SLOC 93402 651-F1
PL
SLVG 93463 940-E5
LN
SMRA 93455 796-J5
ANYON RD
StBC 93460 901-C5
AR PL
SMRA 93458 776-F3
OOD CT
SLO 93401 674-D1
OOD ST
SMRA 93458 776-G3

STREET Name City ZIP Pg-Grid

BOYSEN AV
SLO 93405 653-H2
BOYSENBERRY ST
ARGD 93420 714-G6
BRACKEN LN
Npmo 93444 756-A3
BRADBURY AV
SBAR 93101 996-A4
BRADFORD AV
Cmbr 93428 548-H2
BRADFORD CIR
Cmbr 93428 548-H2
BRADFORD DR
GOL 93117 993-E2
BRADFORD RD
Cmbr 93428 548-H2
BRADLEY AV
MOBY 93442 611-G7
MOBY 93442 631-G1
BRADLEY RD
SMRA 93454 776-J5
SMRA 93454 777-A7
SMRA 93454 796-J2
SMRA 93454 797-A2
SMRA 93455 796-J5
SMRA 93455 797-A4
StBC 93454 796-J4
StBC 93454 797-A4
StBC 93455 816-J1
StBC 93455 817-A3
BRADY LN
SLOC 93420 715-C7
BRAEBURN DR
GOL 93117 984-D7
BRAEMAR DR
SBAR 93109 995-D5
StBC 93109 995-D5
BRAEMAR RANCH LN
SBAR 93109 995-D5
BRAHMA ST
PSRS 93446 533-H1
BRAMADERO RD
StBC 93441 900-J5
BRAMBLE RD
SLOC 93420 695-C5
BRAMBLES CT
SLOC 93465 533-C7
BRANCH ST
SLO 93401 653-J5
SLO 93401 654-A5
E BRANCH ST
Npmo 93444 756-C1
E BRANCH ST Rt#-227
ARGD 93420 715-A5
W BRANCH ST
ARGD 93420 714-H4
Npmo 93444 756-C2
W BRANCH ST Rt#-227
ARGD 93420 714-J5
ARGD 93420 715-A5
BRANCH CREEK CIR
PSRS 93446 534-A1
BRANCH MILL RD
ARGD 93420 715-C4
SLOC 93420 695-F7
SLOC 93420 715-F2
BRAND PL
Cmbr 93428 548-F2
BRANDON CT
StBC 93455 816-F5
BRANDON DR
GOL 93117 993-F1
StBC 93460 921-A4
BRANDY CT
SMRA 93454 776-J4
BRANT ST
SLOC 93420 734-J5
SLOC 93420 735-A6
BRASS BUTTON CT
SLOC 93424 693-B1
BREAKER ST
SLOC 93445 734-E1
BRECK ST
SLO 93401 654-A4
BREEZY GLEN DR
StBC 93455 817-A3
BREGANTE LN
SBAR 93103 996-C3
BRENNER DR
SBAR 93105 985-E6
BRENT ST
SBAR 93105 985-E7
BRENTWOOD CIR
SLOC 93420 734-H5
BRENTWOOD LN
StBC 93455 816-J4
BRENTWOOD WY
GOL 93117 993-F1
BRESSI PL
SLO 93405 653-H3
BREWER ST
SLOC 93465 553-E1
BRIAN AV
SMRA 93454 777-B6
BRIAN ST
SMRA 93454 777-B7
BRIARCLIFF DR
StBC 93455 816-F4
BRIAR ROSE LN
Npmo 93444 756-A5
BRIARWOOD DR
SLO 93401 654-C7
BRIARWOOD LN
Npmo 93444 756-A1
BRIARWOOD PL
SLOC 93465 553-A2
BRIARWOOD RD
StBC 93455 796-A7
StBC 93455 816-B1
BRIDEGEPORT LN
StBC 93437 855-F7
BRIDGE ST
ARGD 93420 715-A5
Cmbr 93428 528-F5
SLO 93401 653-H6
BRIDGE CANYON WY
SLOC 93451 473-C6
BRIDGE CREEK RD
SLOC 93401 674-H2
BRIDGEGATE LN
PSRS 93446 533-G1
BRIDGEPORT RD
StBC 93455 817-A3
BRIDLE RIDGE TR
SLOC 93405 633-F7
BRIDLE TRAIL LN
SLOC 93446 471-C5
BRIDLE TRAILS LN
StBC 93454 797-D6

STREET Name City ZIP Pg-Grid

BRIGHTON AV
ARGD 93420 714-D4
ARGD 93433 714-D4
GBCH 93433 714-D4
BRIGHTON LN
Cmbr 93428 528-D5
BRIGHTON PL
StBC 93455 816-G5
BRINKERHOFF AV
SBAR 93101 996-B4
StBC 93441 901-F5
StBC 93460 901-F5
BRISA CT
PBCH 93449 693-E5
BRISA BLANDA DR
SLOC 93420 734-J4
BRISA DEL MAR
LMPC 93436 896-E4
BRISCO RD
ARGD 93420 714-G5
BRISTLECONE LN
Npmo 93444 756-B4
BRISTOL CT
StBC 93455 816-E4
BRISTOL DR
StBC 93437 855-F7
BRISTOL PL
GOL 93117 993-E2
BRISTOL ST
Cmbr 93428 528-E6
BRITTANY AV
ARGD 93420 714-G6
BRITTANY CIR
SLO 93405 653-F1
BRITTNEY CT
StBC 93455 817-B6
BRITTNEY LN
StBC 93455 817-B6
BRIZZOLARA ST
SLO 93401 653-H4
BROAD ST
SLO 93401 653-J4
SLO 93401 654-A5
SLO 93405 653-H3
BROAD ST Rt#-227
SLO 93401 654-A6
SLO 93401 674-B1
SLOC 93401 654-A6
SLOC 93401 674-B1
BROADMOOR DR
ARGD 93420 715-A7
BROADMOOR PZ
SBAR 93105 995-F1
BROADWAY
StBC 93455 816-F6
N BROADWAY Rt#-135
SMRA 93454 776-H6
S BROADWAY Rt#-135
SMRA 93454 776-H7
SMRA 93454 796-H1
SMRA 93455 796-H5
BRODERSON AV
SLOC 93402 631-G6
BROKEN ARROW RD
Npmo 93444 735-H4
BROKEN SPUR PL
SLOC 93446 514-G7
SLOC 93446 534-G1
BROOK CT
LMPC 93436 896-D6
BROOK LN
SLOC 93446 471-D6
StBC 93108 986-G7
BROOK ST
SLO 93401 653-H6
StBC 93463 920-H2
BROOKHILL DR
PSRS 93446 514-B7
PSRS 93446 534-B1
BROOKLINE LN
SLOC 93401 674-D7
BROOKPINE DR
SLO 93401 674-D1
SLOC 93401 674-D1
BROOKSIDE AV
StBC 93455 816-J3
BROOKSIDE DR
LMPC 93436 896-D6
BROOKSIDE PL
StBC 93455 816-J3
BROOKTREE RD
StBC 93108 986-J7
BROSIAN WY
SBAR 93109 995-E5
StBC 93109 995-E5
BROWN RD
StBC 93434 795-A3
StBC 93455 795-E2
StBC 93458 795-E2
BROWNSTONE LN
SMRA 93454 777-A7
BRUNSWICK DR
SMRA 93455 796-H6
BRYAN PL
Cmbr 93428 528-E7
BRYCE PL
StBC 93455 816-H2
BUCHON ST
SLO 93401 653-J5
SLO 93401 654-A4
BUCKBOARD LN
StBC 93463 920-J6
StBC 93463 921-A6
BUCKBRUSH DR
SLOC 93420 695-B6
BUCK CANYON RD
StBC 93460 901-C4
BUCKEYE CT
SLO 93401 674-E1
BUCKEYE ST
StBC 93437 855-G7
BUCKHORN DR
SLOC 93446 469-H4
BUCKHORN RD
Npmo 93444 756-A4
BUCKINGHAM PL
Cmbr 93428 548-G1
BUCKLEY DR
Cmbr 93428 528-E4
BUCKLEY RD
SLOC 93401 673-H3
SLOC 93401 674-A3
BUCK RIDGE LN
SLOC 93420 695-A7
SLOC 93420 715-A1
BUCKSKIN DR
SLOC 93402 632-A7
SMRA 93454 777-A6

STREET Name City ZIP Pg-Grid

BUCKTAIL LN
SLOC 93446 471-D6
BUCKTHORN LN
StBC 93436 896-F3
BUCKTHORN RD
StBC 93108 987-F7
BUELLTON DR
StBC 93437 875-D1
BUELLTON PKWY
BLTN 93427 919-H6
StBC - 919-H6
StBC 93427 919-H6
BUELLTON LOMPOC RD Rt#-246
StBC 93436 896-H7
StBC 93436 916-H1
BUENA AV
ATAS 93422 573-J1
BUENA FORTUNA
StBC 93013 1018-J3
VeCo 93001 1018-J3
BUENA FORTUNA CIR
ATAS 93422 574-C7
ATAS 93422 594-C1
BUENA VISTA AV
SLO 93401 654-B3
SLO 93405 654-B2
BUENA VISTA DR
PSRS 93446 494-B6
PSRS 93446 513-J2
SLOC 93446 493-J7
SLOC 93446 494-A6
SLOC 93446 513-J2
StBC 93108 987-B7
StBC 93108 997-B1
BUGGYWHIP LN
SLOC 93446 471-E6
BULL CANYON RD
SLOC 93454 777-B5
SMRA 93454 777-B5
BULLOCK LN
SLO 93401 654-B7
SLO 93401 674-C1
SLOC 93401 654-B7
SLOC 93401 674-C1
BUMBLE BEE LN
SLOC 93465 553-B5
BUNCH CT
SMRA 93458 796-E4
BUNDY CIR
BLTN 93427 919-H6
BUNFILL DR
SMRA 93455 796-J7
BUNGALOW DR
SMRA 93458 796-G4
BUNKHOUSE CT
SLOC 93446 533-J5
BUNNY AV
SMRA 93454 776-H6
SMRA 93458 776-F6
BUR CLOVER WY
SLOC 93453 695-E3
BURGANDY CT
SMRA 93458 796-F4
BURGANDY LN
SLOC 93446 514-J1
BURKET PL
PSRS 93446 513-E4
BURKHILL LN
SLOC 93420 694-H7
BURLINGTON DR
StBC 93455 816-F4
BURLWOOD LN
SLOC 93465 553-B2
BURNHAM DR
StBC 93436 876-E7
BURNING HILLS LN
SLOC 93465 553-B2
BURNING TREE WY
StBC 93436 876-E5
BURNS PL
SBAR 93117 994-C2
BURNT ROCK WY
SLOC 93446 533-H5
BURRO VERDE
PSRS 93446 513-J5
BURTIS ST
StBC 93111 994-H2
BURTON CIR
Cmbr 93428 528-G7
Cmbr 93428 548-G1
SBAR 93101 996-B5
BURTON DR
Cmbr 93428 528-G7
Cmbr 93428 548-G1
N BURTON ST
Npmo 93444 756-B1
S BURTON ST
Npmo 93444 756-C2
BURTON MESA BLVD
StBC 93436 876-D7
StBC 93436 896-F1
E BUSH AV
LMPC 93436 896-F6
BUSH CT
LMPC 93436 896-E6
BUSH DR
SLOC 93402 631-H6
BUSH LN
StBC 93455 816-E4
BUSHNELL ST
SLO 93401 654-A5
BUTT RD
StBC 93429 855-E3
BUTTE AV
MOBY 93442 611-G6
SLOC 93405 632-J5
BUTTE DR
GOL 93117 993-H2
SLOC 93402 631-E6
BUTTER CUP LN
SLOC 93424 693-A1
BUTTERCUP LN
PSRS 93446 514-A6
BUTTERFLY CT
SMRA 93455 796-J7
SMRA 93455 797-A7
BUTTERFLY LN
Npmo 93444 756-B3
SBAR 93108 996-G3
SLOC 93402 631-E7
StBC 93108 996-G3
BUTTONHOOK RD
SLVG 93463 940-E4
BUTTON SAGE WY
SLOC 93453 695-E3
BUTTONWILLOW PL
Npmo 93444 756-A3

STREET Name City ZIP Pg-Grid

BUTTONWOOD LN
GOL 93117 993-J4
BYRNES LN
CARP 93013 998-E7
BYRON LN
Npmo 93444 735-E7

C

C CT
LMPC 93436 896-F5
C ST
SLOC 93451 453-B5
N C ST
LMPC 93436 896-F6
LMPC 93436 916-F1
S C ST
LMPC 93436 916-F2
CABALLERO LN
SMRA 93455 796-H5
CABALLEROS AV
SLOC 93401 674-C5
CABALLO LN
StBC 93460 901-B4
CABALLO PL
PSRS 93446 513-E2
SLOC 93446 513-E2
CABALLO RD
StBC 93460 901-F5
CABALLO WY
SMRA 93458 776-F4
CABAZON RD
ATAS 93422 573-B6
CABIN LN
StBC 93105 964-F1
CABOOSE AV
SMRA 93458 776-F3
CABO SAN JOSE
SMRA 93455 796-H5
CABO SAN LUCAS
SMRA 93455 796-H5
CABO SAN LUCAS CIR
SMRA 93455 796-J5
CABRILLO AV
ATAS 93422 573-J2
ATAS 93422 574-A2
SLOC 93430 591-A2
E CABRILLO BLVD
SBAR 93101 996-D4
SBAR 93103 996-D4
SBAR 93108 996-D4
StBC 93108 996-D4
W CABRILLO BLVD
SBAR 93101 996-B5
CABRILLO CT
GBCH 93433 714-F4
StBC 93437 855-F7
CABRILLO HWY
SLOC 93420 734-H7
SLOC 93420 755-B1
CABRILLO HWY Rt#-1
Cmbr 93428 528-B2
Cmbr 93428 548-J1
GBCH 93433 714-C4
GBCH 93449 714-C4
GDLP 93434 775-A3
LMPC 93436 916-H1
MOBY - 591-C6
MOBY 93430 591-C6
MOBY 93442 591-C6
MOBY 93442 611-E4
MOBY 93442 612-A6
Npmo 93444 755-B2
Npmo 93444 775-A3
PBCH 93449 714-C4
SLO 93405 633-F6
SLO 93405 653-H1
SLOC - 591-C6
SLOC - 612-A6
SLOC 93405 612-A6
SLOC 93405 632-F1
SLOC 93405 633-B4
SLOC 93405 653-H1
SLOC 93420 734-H1
SLOC 93420 754-H1
SLOC 93420 755-A1
SLOC 93430 590-E1
SLOC 93430 591-C6
SLOC 93433 714-C4
SLOC 93442 591-C6
SLOC 93442 611-G6
SLOC 93442 612-A6
SLOC 93445 714-C4
SLOC 93445 734-H1
SLOC 93445 755-B6
SLOC 93445 775-A3
SLOC 93452 528-B2
StBC 93429 816-B4
StBC 93429 855-G6
StBC 93434 775-A7
StBC 93434 795-A2
StBC 93436 916-H1
StBC 93437 855-G6
StBC 93455 795-C5
StBC 93455 816-B4
CABRILLO LN
SLOC 93401 674-C5
CABRILLO PL
MOBY 93442 611-G7
CACHUMA DR
SLO 93401 653-J7
CACIQUE ST
SBAR 93103 996-D4
CACTUS LN
CARP 93013 998-D7
CADDIE LN
PSRS 93446 513-J7
CADET PL
SLOC 93446 534-J2
CADIZ CT
StBC 93111 994-G2
CAGNEY WY
LMPC 93436 896-F5
CAIN DR
StBC 93455 816-G5
CAIRE CIR
StBC 93111 994-H2
CALA CT
ATAS 93422 594-C2
CALABAZA WY
SLOC 93446 494-F4
CALABRIA DR
SBAR 93105 995-E3
CALAVERAS AV
GOL 93117 993-H2
SLOC 93405 633-B5
CALDERON DR
SMRA 93455 796-J5

STREET Name City ZIP Pg-Grid

CALETA AV
GOL 93117 994-D1
CALETA LN
ATAS 93422 574-A7
CALF CANYON HWY Rt#-58
SLOC 93422 614-G3
SLOC 93453 614-G3
CALICO CT
Npmo 93444 755-J5
CALICO LN
StBC 93455 816-G7
CALIENTE AV
StBC 93254 806-B1
CALIFIA CT
StBC 93111 994-G3
CALIFORNIA BLVD
MonC 93451 453-A3
SLO 93401 654-A3
SLO 93405 653-J1
SLO 93405 654-A3
SLOC 93405 653-J1
SLOC 93407 653-J1
SMRA 93455 816-F4
StBC 93437 855-F7
StBC 93437 875-D3
StBC 93455 816-F4
CALIFORNIA LN
PSRS 93446 514-C7
CALIFORNIA ST
ARGD 93420 714-J5
ARGD 93420 715-A6
SBAR 93103 996-A2
CALIMESA WY
SLOC 93420 735-D7
CALIMEX PL
Npmo 93444 755-J2
CALKINS RD
StBC 93441 900-H4
CALLE ABIERTA
StBC 93111 984-G6
CALLE ALAMO
SBAR 93105 985-G7
SBAR 93105 995-G1
CALLE ALLELA
SBAR 93109 995-G6
CALLE ALMONTE
SBAR 93109 995-G6
CALLE ALTO
PSRS 93446 513-E2
CALLE ANDALUCIA
SBAR 93109 995-G5
CALLE ANZUELO
StBC 93111 984-G7
CALLE APAREJO
StBC 93111 984-H7
CALLE ARENA
CARP 93013 1018-E1
CALLE ASILO
StBC 93111 984-G7
CALLE BARQUERO
StBC 93111 984-G7
CALLE BELLO
SBAR 93108 996-E2
CALLE BENDITA
SLOC 93420 754-J2
CALLE BOCA DEL CANON
SBAR 93101 995-G4
CALLE BONITA
SMRA 93455 796-J5
StBC 93441 901-A4
StBC 93460 901-A5
CALLE BREVO
SBAR 93109 996-A7
CALLE CABALLO
SLOC 93422 594-C4
CALLE CAMARADA
StBC 93110 994-J3
CALLE CANON
SBAR 93101 995-G5
SBAR 93109 995-G5
CALLE CAPISTRANO
SBAR 93105 995-G1
CALLE CARIDAD
StBC 93110 985-C6
CALLE CARMAN
ARGD 93420 714-H4
CALLE CEDRO
SBAR 93105 985-G7
CALLE CERRITO
SBAR 93101 995-G5
CALLE CERRITO ALTO
SBAR 93101 995-H5
CALLE CERRO
SBAR 93101 995-G5
CALLE CESAR CHAVEZ
SBAR 93103 996-C4
CALLE CESAR E CHAVEZ ST
GDLP 93434 774-H6
CALLE CHORRO
PSRS 93446 513-E2
CALLE CIELO
Npmo 93444 755-H6
CALLE CINCO
StBC 93436 896-H1
CALLE CITA
SBAR 93105 985-E7
SBAR 93110 985-E7
StBC 93110 985-E7
CALLE CONSUETTA
PBCH 93449 693-G6
CALLE CORDONIZ
SLOC 93402 631-H7
SLOC 93402 651-J1
CALLE CORDOVA
PBCH 93449 693-G6
CALLE COREA
PBCH 93449 693-G6
CALLE CORTE
SBAR 93101 995-G5
CALLE CORTITA
SBAR 93109 995-H5
CALLE CORTO
SMRA 93454 777-C7
CALLE CRESPIS
SBAR 93105 995-G1
CALLE CRISTOBAL
StBC 93111 994-G2
CALLE CROTALO
SLOC 93401 654-D7
CALLE CUERVO
ARGD 93420 714-H3
CALLE CULEBRA
Summ 93067 997-D3
CALLE CYNTHIA
ATAS 93422 594-C1

STREET Name City ZIP Pg-Grid

CALLE DEBRON
SLOC 93420 735-E4
CALLE DE CAMPO
SMRA 93454 777-A7
CALLE DE ESTRELLAS
CARP 93013 1018-G1
CALLE DE FRANCISCO
SLOC 93446 513-B1
CALLE DE LA LUNA
CARP 93013 1018-G1
CALLE DE LA MAR
CARP 93013 1018-G1
CALLE DE LA MONTANA
CARP 93013 1018-G1
CALLE DEL CAMINOS
SLO 93401 674-C2
SLOC 93401 674-C2
CALLE DEL ESPACIO
CARP 93013 1018-G1
CALLE DEL NORTE
CARP 93013 1018-G1
CALLE DEL ORO
SBAR 93109 995-H6
CALLE DE LOS AMIGOS
SBAR 93105 995-E3
StBC 93105 995-E3
CALLE DE LOS DESCA
SLOC 93420 714-J7
CALLE DE LOS SUEI
SLOC 93420 714-H7
CALLE DE LOS VIENTOS
CARP 93013 1018-G1
CALLE DEL SOL
CARP 93013 1018-G1
Npmo 93444 755-H6
SBAR 93101 995-H5
CALLE DEL SUR
CARP 93013 1018-G1
CALLE DE TOPO
Npmo 93444 755-J2
CALLE DIA
CARP 93013 1018-E1
CALLE DIEZ
StBC 93436 876-H7
CALLE DOS
SLOC 93445 734-G1
CALLE DUENDE
SLOC 93420 735-E4
CALLE ECUESTRE
StBC 93117 982-C4
CALLE ELEGANTE
StBC 93108 996-E1
CALLE ESPERANZA
SBAR 93105 995-E2
CALLE FRESA
Npmo 93444 755-F3
CALLE FRESNO
SBAR 93105 985-G7
CALLE GALICIA
SBAR 93109 995-G6
CALLE GRANADA
PBCH 93449 693-G6
SBAR 93105 985-G7
SBAR 93105 995-G1
CALLE GRANDE CIR
SMRA 93455 796-H5
CALLE HERMOSA
SLOC 93401 693-F2
StBC 93108 996-E1
CALLE JAZMIN
SLO 93401 653-J7
CALLE JOAQUIN
SLO 93401 673-G1
SLO 93405 673-G2
SLOC 93405 673-G2
CALLEJON AV
CARP 93013 1018-D1
CALLE KORAL
GOL 93117 994-B2
CALLE LAGUNA
SLOC 93420 735-C6
CALLE LA PALTA
SLOC - 611-J1
SLOC 93442 611-J1
CALLE LAS BRISAS
StBC 93110 994-J3
CALLE LAS CALERAS
SBAR 93109 995-D5
CALLE LAURELES
SBAR 93105 985-G7
SBAR 93105 995-G1
SMRA 93458 796-E4
CALLE LINARES
SBAR 93109 995-G6
CALLE LINDERO
StBC 93436 876-H7
CALLE LIPPIZANA
StBC 93117 982-C4
CALLE LORA
StBC 93436 896-H2
CALLE LOS CHARROS
SLOC 93446 533-J4
SLOC 93446 534-A4
CALLE LUARDA
StBC 93111 994-G2
CALLE LUPITA
SLO 93401 653-J7
CALLE MADERA
SBAR 93105 985-G7
CALLE MALAGA
SBAR 93109 995-G5
CALLE MALVA
SLO 93401 653-J7
CALLE MANZANITA
SBAR 93105 985-G7
SBAR 93105 995-G1
CALLE MARANA
StBC 93436 876-H7
CALLE MARGARITA
SMRA 93458 796-E4
CALLE MARIPOSA
SBAR 93105 985-G7
CALLE MASTIL
StBC 93111 984-G7
CALLE MILANO
ATAS 93422 594-D1
CALLE MIRASOL
SMRA 93458 796-E4
CALLE MIRO
StBC 93436 896-H2
CALLE MONTILLA
SBAR 93109 995-G5
CALLE MORELIA
StBC 93111 994-G2
CALLENDER RD
Npmo 93444 735-B7
SLOC 93420 734-H7
SLOC 93420 735-A7

STREET Name	City	ZIP	Pg-Grid
CALLE NETO	StBC	93436	876-H7
CALLE NOGUERA	SBAR	93105	985-F7
	SBAR	93105	995-G1
CALLE NUEVE	StBC	93436	876-J7
CALLE OCHO	CARP	93013	998-E7
	CARP	93013	1018-E1
CALLE PACIFIC	CARP	93013	1018-E1
CALLE PALO COLORADO	SBAR	93105	985-G7
	SBAR	93105	995-G1
CALLE PASADO	StBC	93436	896-G1
CALLE PATTITO	SLOC	93446	534-A4
CALLE PEQUENO	SMRA	93454	777-C7
CALLE PICO CT	StBC	93460	921-A6
CALLE PINON	SBAR	93105	985-G7
CALLE PONIENTE	SBAR	93101	995-G4
CALLE PORTOS	StBC	93436	896-H2
CALLE PRIMERA	StBC	93436	896-H2
CALLE PROPANO	SLOC	93446	533-F4
CALLE PUERTA VALLARTA	SBAR	93103	996-D4
CALLE QUARTA	StBC	93436	896-G2
CALLE QUATRO	SLOC	93445	734-G1
CALLE QUEBRADA	StBC	93117	982-D4
CALLE REAL	GOL	93111	994-F1
	GOL	93117	993-E2
	GOL	93117	994-C1
	SBAR	93105	995-G3
	SBAR	93110	995-C1
	StBC	93105	995-F3
	StBC	93110	984-J7
	StBC	93110	994-J1
	StBC	93110	995-C1
	StBC	93111	984-G7
	StBC	93111	994-J1
	StBC	93117	981-G4
	StBC	93117	982-C5
	StBC	93117	993-C2
CALLE REAL Rt#-154	SBAR	93110	995-D1
	StBC	93110	995-D1
CALLE REFUGIO	ATAS	93422	574-A6
CALLE REINA	StBC	93110	994-J3
CALLE REY MAR	CARP	93013	1018-E1
CALLE RINCONADA	SBAR	93105	985-G7
CALLE ROSALES	SBAR	93105	985-F7
	SBAR	93105	995-G1
CALLE SASTRE	SBAR	93105	995-D3
CALLE SEGUNDA	StBC	93436	896-G2
CALLE SEIS	StBC	93436	896-H1
CALLE SERENA	SMRA	93455	796-H5
CALLE SERENO	ATAS	93422	553-J7
CALLE SERRENTO	GOL	93117	993-E1
CALLE SIETE	StBC	93436	876-H7
CALLE SONIA	StBC	93111	994-H2
CALLE SORIA	SBAR	93109	995-G5
CALLE TANIA	StBC	93111	994-H2
CALLE TERCERA	StBC	93436	896-G2
CALLE TIO	Npmo	93444	755-G2
CALLE TRES	SLOC	93445	734-G1
CALLE UNO	SLOC	93445	734-G1
CALLE VALENCIA	PBCH	93449	693-G6
CALLIE CT	ARGD	93420	715-B4
CALLISTO LN	Npmo	93444	756-A5
CALOR DR	BLTN	93427	919-G5
CALVERT AV	LMPC	93436	896-F5
CALVIN CT	GBCH	93433	714-E6
CALZADA AV	StBC	93460	901-B5
	StBC	93460	921-B1
CAMAROSA ST	SMRA	93458	796-F4
CAMBORNE PL	Cmbr	93428	548-G1
CAMBRIA	SLO	93401	653-J7
CAMBRIA AV	StBC	93455	816-J2
CAMBRIA RD	Cmbr	93428	528-F6
CAMBRIA WY	SBAR	93105	995-E3
CAMBRIA PINES RD	Cmbr	93428	528-D5
CAMBRIDGE CT	StBC	93455	816-G4
CAMBRIDGE DR	GOL	93111	984-F7
	GOL	93117	984-F7
	GOL	93117	994-F1
	LMPC	93436	916-E3
CAMBRIDGE LN	CARP	93013	998-E6
CAMBRIDGE ST	Cmbr	93428	528-E6
CAMBRIDGE WY	StBC	93454	797-C7
CAMDEN CT	SLO	93401	654-B6
CAMDEN PL	GOL	93117	984-E7
CAMDEN ST	LMPC	93436	916-G2
CAMELLIA CIR	CARP	93013	998-C6
CAMELLIA CT	LMPC	93436	896-D6
	SLO	93401	653-J7
CAMELLIA LN	SBAR	93110	995-D1
	SLOC	93446	533-B1
CAMELOT DR	StBC	93455	816-F4
CAMEO DR	StBC	93455	817-B5
CAMEO PL	StBC	93455	816-G5
CAMEO RD	CARP	93013	998-E7
CAMEO WY	SLOC	93420	734-J4
CAMERON AV	SMRA	93455	796-G6
CAMERON CT	ARGD	93420	714-H6
CAMERON DR	StBC	93437	855-E7
CAMETA WY	StBC	93110	995-A1
CAMILLIA DR	Npmo	93444	756-A5
CAMINO ALDEA	StBC	93111	994-G2
CAMINO AL MAR AL	SBAR	93109	995-J7
CAMINO ALTO	SBAR	93103	996-C1
CAMINO ALTOZANO	StBC	93111	984-F5
CAMINO ANDALUZ	StBC	93111	984-F5
CAMINO ARROYO	StBC	93460	921-B5
CAMINO CABALLO	Npmo	93444	755-E3
	Npmo	93444	756-A2
CAMINO CALMA	SBAR	93109	995-H6
CAMINO CAMPANA	StBC	93111	984-F6
CAMINO CARRETA	StBC	93013	1018-H2
CAMINO CASCADA	StBC	93111	984-F6
CAMINO CASETA	GOL	93117	984-B7
CAMINO CERRALVO	StBC	93111	984-F5
CAMINO CIELO	StBC	93105	986-B1
E CAMINO CIELO	StBC	-	987-J5
	StBC	93105	964-J4
	StBC	93105	986-A1
	StBC	93105	987-C2
	StBC	93108	987-G4
W CAMINO CIELO	StBC	93105	964-E6
CAMINO CODORNIZ	Npmo	93444	755-H3
CAMINO COLEGIO	SMRA	93458	796-F2
E CAMINO COLEGIO	SMRA	93454	796-J2
W CAMINO COLEGIO	SMRA	93454	796-G2
	SMRA	93458	796-G2
CAMINO CONTENTO	SLOC	93420	734-J4
CAMINO CONTIGO	StBC	93111	984-F7
CAMINO CORTO	StBC	93117	993-J4
CAMINO DE ARBOLES	SLOC	93420	755-A2
CAMINO DEL MIRASOL	StBC	93110	985-B6
CAMINO DEL ORO	Npmo	93444	755-H5
CAMINO DEL REMEDIO	StBC	93110	985-A7
	StBC	93110	995-A1
CAMINO DEL RETIRO	StBC	93110	985-B6
CAMINO DEL REY	SLOC	93420	734-J4
	StBC	93110	994-J3
CAMINO DEL RIO	StBC	93110	985-B5
CAMINO DEL ROBLE	StBC	93110	995-A2
CAMINO DEL ROBLES	ATAS	93422	553-E6
CAMINO DEL ROSARIO	StBC	93108	997-D1
CAMINO DEL SOL	SLOC	93451	473-F2
CAMINO DEL SUR	StBC	93117	994-A4
CAMINO DE PLAZA	ARGD	93420	714-G4
CAMINO DE UNOS	SLOC	93420	734-J4
CAMINO DE VIDA	StBC	93111	994-J1
CAMINO EDNA	SLOC	93401	694-J2
CAMINO ENCANTO	Npmo	93444	735-J4
	Npmo	93444	736-A4
CAMINO ESCONDIDO	SLOC	93420	735-C4
CAMINO FLORAL	StBC	93111	994-H4
CAMINO GALEANA	StBC	93111	984-F5
CAMINO LAGUNA VISTA	GOL	93117	984-B7
CAMINO LINDO	StBC	93117	993-J5
CAMINO LOBO	PSRS	93446	514-A7
	PSRS	93446	534-A1
CAMINO MAJORCA	StBC	93117	993-J5
CAMINO MANADERO	StBC	93111	984-F5
CAMINO MARIPOSA	Npmo	93444	755-F5
CAMINO MEDIO	StBC	93110	995-C3
CAMINO MELENO	StBC	93111	984-F5
CAMINO MERCADO	ARGD	93420	714-H4
CAMINO MOLINERO	StBC	93110	985-A6
CAMINO PALOMERA	StBC	93111	984-F5
CAMINO PERRILLO	SLOC	93420	735-D6
CAMINO PESCADERO	GOL	93117	994-A4
CAMINO RIO VERDE	StBC	93111	984-F5
CAMINO ROBLE	Npmo	93444	755-J3
CAMINO SAN CARLOS	StBC	93427	919-H2
CAMINO TALAVERA	GOL	93117	984-C7
CAMINO TRILLADO	CARP	93013	998-E6
CAMINO VENTUROSO	GOL	93117	984-B7
CAMINO VERDE	SBAR	93103	996-C1
CAMINO VIEJO	SBAR	93108	996-G2
	StBC	93108	996-G2
CAMINO VISTA	GOL	93117	994-B2
CAMINO VIVIENTE	GOL	93117	984-B7
CAMLIN CT	StBC	93455	816-F5
CAMP LN	GDLP	93434	774-J6
CAMP WY	SLOC	93451	453-C6
CAMPANA PL	ARGD	93420	715-B3
CAMPANIL DR	SBAR	93105	995-D4
	SBAR	93109	995-D5
	SBAR	93110	995-D4
CAMPBELL DR	SLOC	93402	652-C3
CAMPBELL LN	ATAS	93422	573-G1
CAMPESINO DR	GOL	93117	993-E2
CAMPHOR CT	StBC	93437	875-J1
CAMPHOR PL	StBC	93108	996-J2
CAMPHOR ST	StBC	93437	875-H1
CAMPINA CT	ATAS	93422	594-C2
CAMPO RD	ATAS	93422	573-E1
CAMPONDONICO AV	GDLP	93434	775-A6
CAMPO VISTA DR	StBC	93111	994-J1
CAMPUS WY	SLOC	93405	653-J2
W CAMPUS POINT LN	StBC	93117	993-J5
CAMUESA RD	StBC	-	987-J1
CANADA ST	SBAR	93103	996-D2
CANADA ESTE RD	StBC	93460	901-B5
CANAL ST	SMRA	93458	776-F4
CANALINO DR	CARP	93013	1018-D1
CANARY LN	SLOC	93446	470-B4
CANDELABRA PL	SLOC	93401	674-D5
CANDELEROS	SMRA	93455	796-H5
CANDICE CT	SLOC	93420	715-B7
CANDLEWOOD CT	PSRS	93446	533-J1
CANET RD	SLOC	93405	632-D1
CANFIELD AV	LMPC	93436	896-F5
CANFIELD CT	LMPC	93436	896-E5
	StBC	93436	896-E5
CANFIELD DR	LMPC	93436	896-F5
	StBC	93436	896-F5
CANFIELD LN	LMPC	93436	896-E5
	SMRA	93454	796-H3
CANNON GREEN DR	GOL	93117	993-G3
CANON DR	SBAR	93105	985-F7
	SBAR	93105	995-F1
	StBC	93110	995-D3
CANON PERDIDO ST	SBAR	93101	995-J5
	SBAR	93101	996-A4
	SBAR	93103	996-B2
	SBAR	93109	995-J5
CANON VIEW RD	StBC	93108	986-E7
	StBC	93108	996-D1
CANOPY DR	SMRA	93458	796-G4
CANTATA CT	StBC	93437	855-F7
CANTATA LN	StBC	93455	817-C7
CANTEBURY CT	StBC	93437	855-E7
CANTERA AV	StBC	93110	995-C4
CANTERBERRY	SLO	93401	673-H1
CANTERBURY LN	Cmbr	93428	528-E5
CANVASBACK PL	StBC	93424	693-B2
CANYON DR	SMRA	93454	777-A5
CANYON WY	ARGD	93420	715-A3
CANYON ACRES DR	SBAR	93105	985-F7
CANYON CREEK RD	StBC	93455	817-B6
CANYON CREST LN	PSRS	93446	513-G7
	PSRS	93446	533-G1
CANYON VISTA DR	SLOC	93446	533-B1
CAPANNA CT	PBCH	93449	714-D2
CAPANNA ST	PBCH	93449	714-D3
CAPELLA DR	StBC	93436	876-C7
CAPELLINA WY	StBC	93111	984-F6
CAPISTRANO AV	ATAS	93422	573-J3
	ATAS	93422	574-A2
	PBCH	93449	693-H7
CAPISTRANO CT	GBCH	93433	714-E6
	SLO	93405	653-D6
CAPISTRANO LN	SMRA	93455	796-H6
CAPITOL DR	SMRA	93454	776-J7
	SMRA	93454	796-J1
CAPITOLA ST	GBCH	93433	714-F7
	SMRA	93458	796-F4
CAPITOL HILL	PSRS	93446	513-H5
CAPITOLIO WY	SLO	93401	654-B7
CAPRI DR	SBAR	93105	985-E7
	SBAR	93105	995-E1
CAPRI ST	MOBY	93442	611-E2
CAPRICORN CT	StBC	93436	876-C6
CAPSTAN CIR	SLOC	93426	469-J2
CAPTAINS CIR	SLOC	93426	469-J1
CAPTAINS WK	SLOC	93426	469-J1
CARAWAY CT	StBC	93455	817-C6
CARBO CIR	StBC	93111	994-H3
CARBO RD	SLOC	93422	594-D6
CARBON CANYON TR	SLOC	93465	553-B5
CARDELINA LN	ATAS	93422	594-C2
CARDIFF DR	Cmbr	93428	548-G2
CARDIFF LN	StBC	93455	817-A2
CARDINAL AV	GOL	93117	994-E1
CARDINAL CT	ARGD	93420	714-G3
CARDINAL WY	PSRS	93446	534-A2
CARDO WY	Npmo	93444	755-D5
CARIBOU WY	StBC	93455	816-G7
CARILLO ST	Npmo	93444	756-C2
CARINA DR	StBC	93436	876-C7
	StBC	93436	896-C1
CARINO CT	PSRS	93446	513-J3
CARISSA CT	SLO	93401	673-H2
	StBC	93455	816-H4
CARISSA LN	StBC	93437	875-J3
CARLA CT	SLO	93401	654-C6
	SMRA	93454	776-J6
CARLIN DR	GDLP	93434	774-J6
CARLISLE DR	GOL	93117	993-F2
CARLO DR	GOL	93117	984-C7
	GOL	93117	994-D1
CARLOTTI DR	SMRA	93454	776-J4
CARLSON ST	StBC	93455	816-G5
CARLTON WY	SBAR	93109	995-G6
CARMEL CT	GBCH	93433	714-E7
	MOBY	93442	611-G7
CARMEL LN	SMRA	93454	776-J5
CARMEL RD	SLOC	93422	594-E2
CARMEL ST	MOBY	93442	611-G7
	SLO	93401	653-J5
CARMEL BEACH CIR	GOL	93117	993-F3
CARMELDE LN	GBCH	93433	714-D4
CARMELIA LN	SMRA	93458	796-E4
CARMELITA AV	ATAS	93422	573-H5
	ATAS	93422	593-F1
	SBAR	93101	996-A2
CARMELLA DR	ARGD	93420	714-G6
CARMEN LN	SMRA	93454	796-G4
	SMRA	93458	796-D4
CARMENITA CT	SMRA	93458	796-G4
CARNATION PL	CARP	93013	998-D6
CARNER CT	PSRS	93446	513-J7
CAROB ST	StBC	93437	875-J1
CAROL AV	StBC	93110	985-D7
CAROL PL	ARGD	93420	714-G6
CAROLDALE LN	GOL	93117	984-B7
CAROLDALE PL	GOL	93117	984-B7
CAROLYN CT	Npmo	93444	756-C4
CAROLYN DR	SLO	93405	653-E7
CAROLYNE WY	StBC	93455	817-A4
CAROSAM RD	StBC	93110	995-C3
CARPENTER ST	SLO	93405	653-J2
CARPENTER CANYON RD Rt#-227	SLOC	93401	694-G1
	SLOC	93420	694-G3
	SLOC	93420	695-A6
	SLOC	93420	715-A1
CARPINTERIA AV	CARP	93013	998-C6
	CARP	93013	1018-F1
CARPINTERIA ST	SBAR	93103	996-D4
CARPINTERIA CREEK DR	CARP	93013	998-E7
	CARP	93013	1018-E1
CARRIAGE DR	StBC	93463	920-J7
CARRIAGE LN	SLOC	93420	695-C6
CARRIAGE HILL CT	StBC	93110	995-A2
CARRIAGE HILL DR	StBC	93110	995-A2
CARRIAGE HILL LN	StBC	93110	995-A2
CARRILLO RD	SBAR	93103	996-B2
CARRILLO ST	SBAR	93101	996-B2
	SBAR	93103	996-B2
E CARRILLO ST	SBAR	93101	996-A3
W CARRILLO ST	SBAR	93101	995-H5
	SBAR	93101	996-A4
	SBAR	93109	995-H5
CARRINGTON PL	ARGD	93420	714-G6
CARRIZO	LMPC	93436	896-E3
CARRIZO RD	ATAS	93422	553-E6
	SBAR	93105	985-F7
	SBAR	93105	995-F1
CARSON LN	SLOC	93445	714-E7
CARSON ST	GOL	93117	994-E2
CASA PL	SLOC	93445	734-G1
CASA ST	SLO	93405	653-J2
CASA BELLA CT	ATAS	93422	574-B6
CASA BLANCA CT	PSRS	93446	513-F3
CASA DORINDA	StBC	93108	996-H3
CASALS DR	PSRS	93446	513-J7
CASANOVA AV	ATAS	93422	573-F7
CASA REAL PL	Npmo	93444	755-H6
CASCABEL RD	ATAS	93422	573-F4
CASCADA LN	Npmo	93444	755-H3
CASCADA RD	ATAS	93422	574-A6
	SLOC	93422	593-F3
CASCADE LN	Npmo	93444	756-B6
	SLOC	93446	471-B5
CASELLI WY	SMRA	93455	796-J7
CASERO CT	ATAS	93422	594-C2
CASETA WY	GOL	93117	984-B7
CASEY AV	StBC	93460	921-E1
CASHIN ST	ATAS	93422	594-D2
CASIANO DR	SBAR	93105	995-E3
CASITAS AV	ATAS	93422	573-G7
	MOBY	93442	611-F3
CASITAS CT	SLO	93405	653-D6
CASITAS LN	CARP	93013	998-E7
CASITAS RD	SBAR	93103	996-C2
CASITAS ST	SLOC	93445	734-G1
CASITAS PASS RD	CARP	93013	998-E7
	StBC	93013	998-E7
CASITAS PASS RD Rt#-150	StBC	93013	999-C7
	VeCo	-	999-C7
	VeCo	93001	999-C7
CASITAS PASS RD Rt#-192	StBC	93013	998-G6
	StBC	93013	1018-J1
CASMALIA RD	StBC	93429	816-C5
	StBC	93455	816-C5
CASON AV	ATAS	93422	574-A6
CASPER CT	PSRS	93446	533-J1
CASPER RD	SLOC	93465	553-C2
CASPIA LN	Summ	93067	997-E4
CASS AV	SLOC	93430	591-A2
CASS PL	SBAR	93117	994-C2
CASTAIC	SLO	93401	653-J7
CASTAIC AV	PBCH	93449	693-H7
CASTANO AV	ATAS	93422	574-B3
CASTEEL LN	SLOC	93465	553-B3
CASTENADA LN	ATAS	93422	593-G1
CASTILIAN DR	GOL	93117	993-J2
	GOL	93117	994-A2
CASTILLO CT	ARGD	93420	714-H2
	SLO	93405	653-D6
CASTILLO RD	SLOC	93401	673-D5
	SLOC	93405	673-D5
CASTILLO ST	SBAR	93101	995-H3
	SBAR	93101	996-A4
	SBAR	93105	995-H3
CASTILLO ST Rt#-225	SBAR	93101	996-B5
CASTILLO DEL MAR	ARGD	93420	715-A6
CASTLE LN	SMRA	93454	776-J7
CASTLE ST	Cmbr	93428	548-F2
CASTLEROCK LN	SMRA	93455	796-G6
CAT LN	SMRA	93454	777-B5
CATALINA DR	SLO	93405	653-G3
CATALINA PL	SLOC	93446	471-C3
CATALPA CT	ATAS	93422	574-B7
CATALPA ST	ATAS	93422	574-B7
	StBC	93437	855-G7
CATANIA WY	SBAR	93105	995-E3
CATARINA ST	StBC	93460	921-C5
CAT CANYON RD	SLOC	93420	737-F2
CATE MESA RD	StBC	93013	998-H6
CATHEDRAL LN	SLOC	93420	715-A7
CATHEDRAL CANYON CT	PSRS	93446	533-J2
CATHEDRAL OAKS RD	GOL	93111	984-E6
	GOL	93117	984-E6
	GOL	93117	993-E1
	GOL	93117	994-A1
	StBC	93110	984-E6
	StBC	93110	985-A6
	StBC	93111	984-E6
	StBC	93111	985-A6
	StBC	93117	984-B7
	StBC	93117	993-G1
	StBC	93117	994-A1
CATHEDRAL OAKS RD Rt#-192	StBC	93110	985-C6
CATHEDRAL POINTE LN	StBC	93111	984-G6
CATLIN CIR	CARP	93013	998-C6
CATRINA WY	SMRA	93458	776-G6
CATTAIL RD	SLOC	93465	533-E7
	SLOC	93465	553-E1
CATTLEMAN WY	PSRS	93446	534-A2
CATTLE RUN LN	SLOC	93420	695-D5
CAUDILL ST	SLO	93401	654-A6
CAVALIER LN	SLO	93405	653-F7
CAVE LANDING RD	PBCH	93449	693-B3
	SLOC	93424	693-B3
	SLOC	93449	693-B3
CAYMUS CT	PSRS	93446	534-A2
CAYUCOS AV	ATAS	93422	573-G2
	SLOC	93465	553-D1
CAYUCOS DR	SLO	93405	653-G7
	SLO	93405	673-F1
	SLOC	93430	590-J1
	SLOC	93430	591-A1
CAYUCOS RD	SLOC	93430	590-J1
	SLOC	93430	591-A1
CAYUCOS CREEK RD	SLOC	93430	590-J1
CAZADERO ST	SLO	93401	654-B3
CEBADA PL	SLOC	93451	473-E4
CEBADA RD	ATAS	93422	573-D2
CEBRIAN AV	StBC	93254	806-B1
CECCHETTI RD	SLOC	93420	715-F1
CECELIA CT	SLO	93401	654-B5
CECELIA DR	SMRA	93454	796-J3
CECIL CT	PSRS	93446	513-H5
CEDAR	SLO	93401	673-H1
CEDAR AV	MOBY	93442	611-E2
CEDAR CT	SLO	93401	654-C6
CEDAR LN	BLTN	93427	919-G4
	SBAR	93108	996-D2
CEDAR PL	CARP	93013	9
CEDAR RD	SMRA	93458	7
CEDAR ST	ARGD	93420	7
	GDLP	93434	7
	StBC	93437	8
	StBC	93460	9
CEDAR GREEN CT	Npmo	93444	7
CEDARHURST DR	StBC	93455	8
CEDAR VISTA	SBAR	93105	9
	SBAR	93110	9
N CEDARWOOD AV	Npmo	93444	7
S CEDARWOOD AV	Npmo	93444	7
CEDARWOOD DR	PSRS	93446	5
CELESTIAL WY	SLOC	93465	5
	StBC	93436	8
CELINE DR	SBAR	93105	9
CEMETERY RD	ATAS	93422	5
	SLOC	93451	4
CENCERO RD	ATAS	93422	5
	SLOC	93422	5
CENEGAL RD	ATAS	93422	5
CENTAUR AV	StBC	93436	8
CENTENNIAL ST	SMRA	93454	7
	StBC	93440	8
CENTER AV	StBC	93105	9
	StBC	93110	9
CENTER CT	MOBY	93442	6
CENTER LN	SLO	93401	6
CENTER ST	Cmbr	93428	5
	SLO	93405	6
S CENTERPOINTE PKWY	SMRA	93454	7
	SMRA	93455	7
CENTINELA LN	SBAR	93109	9
CENTRA RD	SLOC	93446	4
CENTRAL AV	BLTN	93427	9
	SMRA	93454	7
E CENTRAL AV	LMPC	93436	8
W CENTRAL AV	LMPC	93436	8
	StBC	93436	8
	StBC	93436	8
CENTRAL PARK DR	SMRA	93458	77
CENTRE POINT PL	Npmo	93444	75
CENTURY LN	SLOC	93420	71
CENTURY ST	SMRA	93455	79
CERCIS LN	StBC	93437	87
CERRITO LN	StBC	93110	98
CERRITO PL	MOBY	93442	61
CERRITO ST	StBC	93460	92
CERRO CT	SLO	93405	65
CERRO ALTO RD	SLOC	-	59
CERRO GORDO AV	SLOC	93430	59
CERRO ROBLES	SLOC	93401	69
CERRO ROMAULDO AV	SLO	93405	65
CERRO VISTA CIR	ARGD	93420	71
	SLOC	93405	65
CERRO VISTA DR	PBCH	93449	71
CERRO VISTA LN	ARGD	93420	71
CERVANTES RD	StBC	93117	99
CERVATO WY	StBC	93111	98
CESAR E CHAVEZ DR	SMRA	93458	77
CETONA LN	SMRA	93458	79
CHABOW LN	SLOC	93420	69
CHADWELL DR	SMRA	93454	77
CHADWICK WY	GOL	93117	98
CHALFONTE CT	SMRA	93454	797
CHALK HILL RD	SLVG	93463	92
	StBC	93463	92
CHAMISAL LN	SLOC	93420	73
CHAMISO DR	StBC	93440	87
CHAMPAGNE LN	SLOC	93446	49
CHAMPIONS LN	Npmo	93444	755
CHANCELLOR ST	StBC	93455	817
CHANDLER LN	ATAS	93422	593
CHANDLER RD	StBC	93436	896
CHANDLER ST	SLO	93401	654
	StBC	93110	994
CHANEY AV	CARP	93013	998
	SLOC	93430	591

City ZIP Pg-Grid
IEL DR
SBAR 93108 996-F4
SMRA 93458 776-G4
StBC 93108 996-F4
IEL ISLANDS RD
StBC 93106 994-C5
IING LN
LMPC 93436 896-E5
IING WY
SBAR 93109 995-G6
ALA ST
SBAR 93101 995-H2
SBAR 93101 996-A3
SBAR 93105 995-H2
ARRAL CIR
SLO 93401 674-D1
ARRAL DR
StBC 93437 855-E7
ARRAL LN
ARGD 93420 714-J3
Npmo 93444 756-A2
SLOC 93446 471-C6
ARRAL RD
SLOC 93402 631-J7
SLOC 93446 534-G3
ARRAL ST
SMRA 93454 796-H2
EL ST
GOL 93111 994-G2
SMRA 93454 776-J7
SMRA 93454 777-A7
SMRA 93458 776-F7
LIN CIR
LMPC 93436 896-E5
LIN LN
SLO 93405 654-A2
MAN DR
GDLP 93434 774-J6
MAN PL
GOL 93117 993-G3
PARAL DR
CARP 93013 998-C5
AN WY
SLOC 93420 715-E1
ING LN
Cmbr 93428 528-E5
LES DR
SLOC 93401 674-E7
LES ST
GBCH 93433 714-E4
LIE LN
SMRA 93454 777-B5
LOTTE DR
SMRA 93454 776-J6
LOTTE LN
StBC 93105 985-J7
OLAIS RD
PSRS 93446 533-G1
PSRS 93446 534-A2
SLOC 93446 533-G1
SLOC 93446 534-A2
RO WY
Npmo 93444 755-H4
TER CT
StBC 93455 817-A4
E DR
SBAR 93108 996-D2
A ST
Npmo 93444 756-A4
EAUX ELISE
SBAR 93109 995-H7
HAM LN
Cmbr 93428 528-D6
HAM WY
StBC 93455 817-A2
PLIN AV
ATAS 93422 573-G4
KERSPOT DR
SLOC 93426 470-A2
HAM WY
StBC 93108 986-E7
StBC 93108 996-E1
SEA CT
ARGD 93420 714-G5
SEA LN
Cmbr 93428 528-D5
TENHAM RD
StBC 93105 985-H7
IANGO CT
GOL 93117 993-J2
IMOYA WY
StBC 93108 997-F2
ISH LN
SLOC 93465 553-E1
OKEE CT
PSRS 93446 513-H6
OKEE PL
Npmo 93444 735-J7
Npmo 93444 755-H1
RY AV
StBC 93455 816-J5
ERRY AV
ARGD 93420 715-C4
LMPC 93436 896-E7
IERRY AV
ARGD 93420 715-A6
LMPC 93436 896-C7
RRY ST
PSRS 93446 513-F6
StBC 93437 855-D6
RRY BLOSSOM PL
Npmo 93444 756-E7
RY HILL DR
StBC 93455 817-A2
RRY HILL RD
StBC 93455 817-A2
RRY WOOD
BLTN 93427 919-G5
SAPEAKE PL
SLOC 93420 735-C6
STER LN
Cmbr 93428 548-F2
STNUT AV
SLOC 93422 594-G6
ESTNUT AV
LMPC 93436 916-E1
HESTNUT AV
LMPC 93436 916-B1
ESTNUT CT
LMPC 93436 916-G1
STNUT LN
SMRA 93458 776-G4
STNUT ST
PSRS 93446 513-F4
StBC 93437 855-G7
IESTNUT ST
Npmo 93444 756-C2
HESTNUT ST
Npmo 93444 756-C2

STREET Name City ZIP Pg-Grid
CHEYENNE CT
Npmo 93444 755-F3
CHEYENNE DR
PSRS 93446 513-H6
CHEYENNE LN
StBC 93460 921-B4
CHIA PL
SLOC 93422 594-F2
CHIANINA PL
SLOC 93422 594-E2
CHIANTI CT
SLOC 93465 553-C3
CHIANTI LN
SMRA 93458 796-E4
CHICA DR
SLOC 93420 734-H5
CHICAGO WY
SLOC 93451 453-C6
CHICO AV
SLOC 93405 633-E5
CHICO RD
ATAS 93422 553-G7
CHICORY LN
PSRS 93446 514-A6
CHILMARK LN
StBC 93455 817-B7
CHILON WY
StBC 93110 995-A1
CHILTON ST
ARGD 93420 714-G4
CHINA FLAT RD
StBC 93108 997-C2
CHINO ST
SBAR 93101 995-G3
CHIPMUNK RD
SLOC 93446 469-H4
CHIQUITA RD
SBAR 93103 996-C2
CHISMAHOO RD
VeCo - 999-C7
VeCo 93001 999-C7
CHISPA RD
SLOC 93422 594-G3
CHISWICK WY
Cmbr 93428 528-D5
CHOLARE RD
ATAS 93422 573-B6
SLOC 93422 573-B7
CHORRO ST
SLO 93401 653-J4
SLO 93401 654-A5
SLO 93405 653-H2
N CHORRO ST
SLO 93405 653-H2
CHORRO CREEK RD
SLOC - 612-A7
SLOC 93442 612-A7
CHORRO VALLEY RD
SLOC 93405 632-J4
SLOC 93405 633-A5
CHRISTINA CT
PSRS 93446 513-H4
CHRISTINA ST
SMRA 93454 776-H6
CHRISTINA WY
PBCH 93449 714-F3
SLO 93405 653-G2
CHRISTINE PL
SLOC 93420 695-C6
CHRISTMAS TREE PL
SLOC 93445 734-G1
CHRISTOPHER DR
StBC 93436 896-G2
CHRISTOPHER LN
SMRA 93454 777-B7
CHUKAR ST
SLOC 93420 734-J6
CHUMASH CT
PSRS 93446 513-H6
CHUMASH DR
SLO 93401 653-J7
CHUMASH LN
SLOC 93402 651-J1
CHUMASH SPRING RD
SLOC 93422 573-A7
SLOC 93422 593-A1
CHUPAROSA CT
ATAS 93422 594-C1
CHUPAROSA DR
SBAR 93105 995-F1
CHUPARROSA DR
SLO 93401 673-G2
CHURCH LN
CARP 93013 998-D7
CHURCH ST
SLO 93401 653-J5
SLO 93401 654-A5
E CHURCH ST
SMRA 93454 776-H7
SMRA 93454 777-A7
W CHURCH ST
SMRA 93458 776-F7
CIDER LN
SLOC 93402 673-A5
CIELITO LN
SBAR 93105 986-B6
CIELO AV
GOL 93111 984-E6
GOL 93117 984-E6
CIELO CT
PSRS 93446 513-J3
CIELO LN
Npmo 93444 756-B6
CIELO GRANDE
ATAS 93422 553-H6
CIELO LINDO
PBCH 93449 693-H7
CIELO VISTA
SLOC 93446 513-C3
CIENAGA ST Rt#-1
SLOC 93420 734-H1
SLOC 93445 734-H1
CIENEGUITAS RD
SBAR 93110 985-C7
StBC 93110 985-C7
CIMA CT
SLO 93401 653-J6
CIMA LINDA LN
SBAR 93108 996-E3
CIMARRON DR
StBC 93460 921-B4
CIMARRON WY
Npmo 93444 735-H4
SLOC 93402 632-B7
SLOC 93402 652-B1
SLOC 93420 735-H4
CINCO AMIGOS
SBAR 93105 995-E2

STREET Name City ZIP Pg-Grid
CINDERELLA LN
StBC 93111 994-G2
CINDY LN
CARP 93013 1018-H1
CINDY WY
ARGD 93420 715-B4
CINNABAR CT
StBC 93455 816-J5
StBC 93455 817-A5
CIRCLE DR
SBAR 93108 986-E7
SLOC 93405 653-J1
SLOC 93430 591-B3
StBC 93437 855-D6
CIRCLE LN
SLOC 93430 591-B3
CIRCLE B RD
PSRS 93446 514-A1
SLOC 93446 513-J1
SLOC 93446 514-A1
CIRCLE OAK DR
ATAS 93422 574-B7
ATAS 93422 594-B1
SLOC 93426 469-H2
CIRRUS WY
PSRS 93446 494-E7
CITATION CT
SMRA 93455 816-E2
CITRUS AV
SBAR 93103 996-D3
CITRUS CT
SMRA 93458 796-G4
CITRUS LN
Npmo 93444 756-B4
CITRUS PL
CARP 93013 998-D7
CIVIC CENTER PZ
LMPC 93436 916-E2
CLAIRE DR
SLO 93405 653-E7
CLAMATH CT
SLOC 93446 471-D6
CLAMSHELL MOUNTAIN WY
Npmo 93444 736-D6
CLARABELLE DR
MOBY 93442 611-F5
CLAREMONT CT
StBC 93437 855-E6
CLAREMONT PL
SMRA 93458 796-G3
CLAREMONT RD
SBAR 93105 985-F6
CLARENCE AV
ARGD 93420 715-B4
CLARENCE CT
SMRA 93458 796-F4
CLARENCE WARD MEM BLVD Rt#217
GOL 93111 994-E3
GOL 93117 994-E3
SBAR 93117 994-E3
StBC 93106 994-E3
StBC 93111 994-E3
StBC 93117 994-E3
CLARENDON CT
GOL 93117 984-C7
CLARINTA AV
SLOC 93402 631-H7
CLARION CT
SLOC 93401 674-B2
E CLARK AV
StBC 93454 817-F5
StBC 93455 816-H6
StBC 93455 817-F5
W CLARK AV
StBC 93455 816-F6
CLARK RD
StBC 93110 985-E6
CLARK ST
StBC 93437 895-B5
CLARKIE WY
SLOC 93420 735-B3
CLARK VALLEY RD
SLOC 93402 652-B2
CLASSEN RANCH LN
SLOC 93446 533-D5
CLAYBROOK CT
StBC 93455 816-H5
CLEAR LAKE DR
StBC 93455 817-E4
CLEARVIEW LN
SLO 93405 653-D6
CLEARVIEW RD
SBAR 93101 995-G4
CLEARWATER LN
Npmo 93444 756-C2
CLELLAND AV
SLOC 93402 631-F7
CLEMENS WY
LMPC 93436 916-F2
CLEVELAND AV
SBAR 93103 995-J1
SBAR 93103 996-A2
CLEVELAND ST
Npmo 93444 756-A5
CLEVENGER DR
ARGD 93420 714-G3
CLIFF AV
PBCH 93449 693-J7
CLIFF DR
SBAR 93109 995-D6
StBC 93105 995-D6
StBC 93109 995-D6
StBC 93110 995-D6
CLIFF DR Rt#-225
SBAR 93101 996-A6
SBAR 93109 995-F6
SBAR 93109 996-A6
StBC 93105 995-F6
StBC 93109 995-F6
CLIFFORD AV
SBAR 93103 996-B3
CLIFFROSE LN
BLTN 93427 919-G4
CLIFFSIDE DR
SLOC 93446 469-G4
CLIFTON ST
SBAR 93103 996-D3
CLIMBING TREE LN
SLOC 93465 534-C6
CLINTON CT
ARGD 93420 714-H3
SMRA 93454 777-A6
CLINTON TER
SBAR 93105 995-G2
CLOUD WY
PSRS 93446 494-D7

STREET Name City ZIP Pg-Grid
CLOVER DR
SLO 93405 653-G1
CLOVER LN
StBC 93108 986-G7
StBC 93441 901-E2
CLOVER RIDGE LN
SLOC 93401 673-F5
CLOYDON CIR
StBC 93108 986-E7
CLUBHOUSE CIR
ARGD 93420 714-G3
CLUBHOUSE DR
PSRS 93446 513-G2
StBC 93455 816-F4
CLUBHOUSE LN
SMRA 93454 776-J7
CLUB HOUSE RD
StBC 93436 876-E6
CLUB MOSS LN
SLOC 93424 693-A1
CLUB VIEW DR
SLOC 93401 674-E6
CLYDELL WY
PBCH 93449 714-D2
CLYDESDALE CIR
PSRS 93446 513-H6
COACH RD
ARGD 93420 715-C4
COACHMAN WY
StBC 93455 816-G4
COACHWHIP LN
SLOC 93426 470-A3
COAST DR
CARP 93013 998-B5
COAST RD
StBC 93454 797-B4
COAST OAK DR
SLVG 93463 920-D7
SLVG 93463 940-D1
COAST VIEW DR
SLOC 93420 715-B7
COAST VILLAGE CIR
SBAR 93108 996-G4
StBC 93108 996-G4
COAST VILLAGE RD
SBAR 93108 996-G4
StBC 93108 996-G4
COBBLE DR
SMRA 93458 796-G4
COBBLE CREEK WY
SLOC 93465 533-C6
COBBLESTONE LN
SMRA 93454 777-C7
StBC 93437 855-F7
COBBLESTONE WY
SLOC 93420 695-C4
COBRE PL
ARGD 93420 715-B3
COBURN LN
PBCH 93449 693-G6
COCOPAH DR
StBC 93110 985-D6
CODY AV
SLOC 93430 591-C5
COFFEE LN
SLOC 93420 715-A1
COFFEEBERRY CT
SLOC 93424 693-B2
COINER CT
StBC 93440 878-H2
COINER ST
StBC 93440 878-H2
COLBERT DR
LMPC 93436 896-E5
COLBY ST
Summ 93067 997-E4
COLD SPRINGS RD
StBC 93108 986-F7
StBC 93108 996-F1
COLE CT
ATAS 93422 574-A6
COLE PL
GOL 93117 984-C7
COLEBROOK DR
SMRA 93458 776-F4
COLEMAN AV
SBAR 93109 995-G6
COLEMAN DR
LMPC 93436 896-E5
MOBY 93442 611-D6
COLEMAN LN
LMPC 93436 896-E5
COLFAX CT
GOL 93117 984-C7
COLIMA CT
ATAS 93422 573-G1
COLIMA RD
ATAS 93422 553-F7
ATAS 93422 573-G1
COLINA CT
SLO 93401 654-C6
COLINA LN
SBAR 93103 996-A2
COLINA ST
ARGD 93420 715-A4
COLLADO CTE
ARGD 93420 714-J3
COLLEEN AV
SMRA 93458 776-F6
COLLEEN WY
StBC 93111 984-G5
COLLEGE AV
SLOC 93405 653-J1
E COLLEGE AV
LMPC 93436 896-F7
W COLLEGE AV
LMPC 93436 896-C7
COLLEGE DR
SMRA 93454 776-J7
SMRA 93454 796-J4
SMRA 93455 796-J5
StBC 93454 796-J4
StBC 93455 796-J7
StBC 93455 816-J1
COLLEGE CANYON RD
SLVG 93463 920-F6
StBC 93463 920-F6
COLLI WY
SLOC 93420 715-E1
COLOMA DR
GOL 93117 994-D1
COLOMA LN
Npmo 93444 755-E2
COLONIAL PL
Npmo 93444 735-F7
Npmo 93444 755-E1
COLONY DR
SLOC 93405 633-E6

STREET Name City ZIP Pg-Grid
COLORADO AV
StBC 93437 855-D7
COLORADO RD
ATAS 93422 594-B1
COLORADO ST
SMRA 93454 796-H4
COLT LN
Npmo 93444 756-C3
COLUMBIA DR
SMRA 93454 796-J3
SMRA 93454 797-A3
COLUMBINE CT
SLO 93401 674-B1
COLUMBUS DR
SMRA 93454 776-J5
SMRA 93454 777-A5
COLUSA AV
GOL 93117 993-J2
SLOC 93405 632-J5
SLOC 93405 633-A5
COLVILLE ST
Summ 93067 997-D3
COMANCHE AV
StBC 93455 816-J5
COMBINE ST
PSRS 93446 514-B3
COMET LN
SLOC 93420 734-J3
COMMANCHE WY
SLOC 93446 471-D7
COMMERCE CT
LMPC 93436 896-D5
COMMERCE DR
BLTN 93427 919-J4
COMMERCE WY
PSRS 93446 514-B7
PSRS 93446 534-B1
COMMUNITY LP
StBC 93437 875-D2
CONCEPCION AV
Npmo 93444 756-C3
SMRA 93454 776-J6
SMRA 93454 796-J1
CONCEPCION CT
StBC 93437 855-D7
CONCHA LOMA DR
CARP 93013 998-E7
CARP 93013 1018-D1
CONCHITA AV
SMRA 93458 796-E4
CONCHITA LN
StBC 93110 995-C5
CONCHO WY
SLOC 93446 533-H6
SLOC 93465 533-H6
CONCORD AV
SMRA 93454 777-A5
CONCORD PL
CARP 93013 998-E5
CONCRETE CT
SLOC 93446 533-F5
CONDADO VISTA CT
SLOC 93420 695-B4
CONDICT BLVD
PSRS 93446 514-C7
CONDOR LN
SLOC 93465 553-B1
CONDOR ST
SMRA 93454 796-H3
CONEJO AV
MOBY 93442 611-F3
SLO 93401 654-B3
CONEJO CT
SLOC 93402 631-J7
CONEJO LN
SBAR 93103 986-D7
SBAR 93103 996-D1
CONEJO RD
ATAS 93422 553-F7
ATAS 93422 573-E1
SBAR 93103 986-C7
SBAR 93103 996-C1
CONESTOGA LN
Npmo 93444 755-E2
CONGRESS AV
SLOC 93420 735-D4
CONIFER PL
SLOC 93465 533-H6
CONNER LN
GOL 93117 984-E7
CONNIE WY
SBAR 93110 985-E7
CONOVER LN
SLOC 93465 533-C7
SLOC 93465 553-C1
CONSTANCE AV
SBAR 93105 995-H1
CONSTANCE LN
SBAR 93105 995-H1
CONSTANCIA
ATAS 93422 574-A5
CONSTELLATION RD
StBC 93436 876-D6
StBC 93436 896-C1
CONSTELLATION WY
StBC 93436 876-D7
CONSUELO DR
SBAR 93110 985-C7
CONTENTA CT
SLO 93401 673-G2
CONTRA COSTA AV
SLOC 93405 633-A5
COOK AV
SBAR 93101 995-H4
COOK CT
SLOC 93465 534-C7
COOK PL
SBAR 93117 994-C3
COOK ST
SMRA 93454 796-J1
SMRA 93458 796-F1
COOL BROOK LN
GOL 93117 993-J3
COOLEY LN
SMRA 93455 796-G5
COOLIDGE DR
SLOC 93445 714-D6
COOL VALLEY RD
PSRS 93446 534-A2
COOPER DR
LMPC 93436 896-F5
COOPER RD
SBAR 93109 995-G7
COPADO WY
ATAS 93422 553-E6
COPENHAGEN DR
SLVG 93463 940-E1
CORAL AV
MOBY 93442 611-E2

STREET Name City ZIP Pg-Grid
CORAL CIR
PBCH 93449 714-D3
CORAL CT
PBCH 93449 714-D2
CORAL DR
SMRA 93454 777-B7
CORAL ST
SBAR 93105 985-E7
SLO 93405 653-F7
CORALINO RD
GOL 93111 984-F7
CORBEROSA DR
SLOC 93420 715-B1
CORBETT CANYON RD
ARGD 93420 715-C2
SLOC 93401 694-H2
SLOC 93401 695-A3
SLOC 93420 694-H2
SLOC 93420 695-A3
SLOC 93420 715-C2
CORBETT CANYON RD Rt#-227
ARGD 93420 715-A4
CORBETT HIGHLANDS PL
SLOC 93420 695-B4
CORBINA DR
SMRA 93458 796-E4
CORDERO DR
SBAR 93105 995-E2
StBC 93105 995-E2
CORDIAL CT
SMRA 93458 776-G3
CORDOBA AV
LMPC 93436 896-D5
CORDOBA RD
StBC 93117 994-A5
CORDOBAN LN
SMRA 93455 796-H5
CORDOVA DR
SBAR 93109 995-H7
SLO 93405 653-D6
CORMORANT WY
SLOC 93424 693-B3
CORNELL CT
SMRA 93454 776-J4
CORNERSTONE LN
SLOC 93420 715-A7
CORNUS CT
SLO 93401 674-D2
CORNUTA WY
Npmo 93444 756-C1
CORNWALL AV
ARGD 93420 714-H5
CORNWALL ST
Cmbr 93428 528-E6
COROMAR AV
ATAS 93422 574-A5
COROMAR DR
GOL 93117 994-A2
CORONA CT
PSRS 93446 513-H6
SLO 93401 654-B5
CORONA RD
ATAS 93422 573-B2
CORONA DEL MAR
SBAR 93103 996-D4
CORONA DEL TERRA
ARGD 93420 714-G5
CORONADO AV
SLOC 93430 591-C5
CORONADO CIR
SBAR 93108 996-E2
CORONADO CT
GBCH 93433 714-F4
CORONADO DR
GOL 93117 993-G3
LMPC 93436 916-B2
CORONADO WY
LMPC 93436 916-B2
CORONEL PL
SBAR 93101 996-A5
CORONEL ST
SBAR 93101 996-A5
SBAR 93109 996-A5
CORRAL AV
PSRS 93446 534-A1
CORRAL PL
ARGD 93420 715-B3
CORRAL RD
StBC 93437 855-F6
CORRAL DE PIEDRA RD
SLOC 93401 694-E1
CORRAL DE QUATI RD
StBC 93441 900-J5
CORRALITOS
PBCH 93449 693-H7
CORRALITOS AV
SLO 93401 654-B3
CORRALITOS RD
SLOC 93420 695-E6
SLOC 93420 715-E1
CORRIDA DR
SLO 93401 653-J6
SLO 93401 654-A6
CORRIENTE RD
ATAS 93422 573-C2
CORRIETTA CT
SLOC 93465 553-D2
CORRINE CT
SMRA 93454 777-A7
CORSAIR CIR
SMRA 93455 816-F1
CORSICA DR
StBC 93455 817-B5
CORSICA PL
SLOC 93420 715-A2
CORTA AV
ATAS 93422 573-H4
CORTA RD
StBC 93110 995-D5
CORTA ST
GOL 93117 994-E3
CORTA BELLA WY
StBC 93455 816-J2
CORTE DE MAYO
SLOC 93420 734-H3
CORTEZ AV
ATAS 93422 574-B3
CORTEZ CT
SLO 93405 653-E6
CORTEZ DR
SMRA 93454 776-J5
SMRA 93454 777-A5
CORTEZ WY
SBAR 93101 995-G4
CORTINA AV
ATAS 93422 574-B4

STREET Name City ZIP Pg-Grid
CORTO WY
PBCH 93449 714-D3
CORTO CAMINO ONTARE
SBAR 93105 985-F6
CORTONA DR
GOL 93117 993-J2
GOL 93117 994-A2
CORUNA CT
StBC 93111 994-G2
CORY CT
ATAS 93422 594-C2
StBC 93455 816-H6
CORY WY
Npmo 93444 755-J2
Npmo 93444 756-A2
COSIMA LN
StBC 93455 817-A6
COSSA CT
SMRA 93454 777-B6
COSTA PL
SMRA 93455 796-G6
COSTA AZUL DR
SLOC 93402 631-E7
COSTA BRAVA
PBCH 93449 693-G6
COSTA DEL MAR DR
SBAR 93103 996-E4
COSTA DEL SOL
PBCH 93449 693-G6
COSTA RICA
PBCH 93449 693-H7
COTA LN
StBC 93108 996-H2
COTA ST
SBAR 93101 996-A4
SBAR 93103 996-C3
StBC 93460 921-B5
COTTAGE LN
PSRS 93446 513-H2
SMRA 93455 796-J5
StBC 93108 996-F1
COTTAGE GROVE AV
SBAR 93101 996-B5
COTTONTAIL
SLOC 93446 470-C4
COTTONTAIL LN
SLOC 93402 651-J1
COTTONWOOD CIR
PSRS 93446 534-A1
COTTONWOOD DR
PSRS 93446 534-A1
COTTONWOOD LN
SLOC 93405 653-D4
COTTONWOOD ST
StBC 93437 855-G7
StBC 93463 920-H2
COUGAR CREEK WY
SLOC 93420 695-B7
COUGAR RIDGE RD
StBC 93427 919-G2
COUGAR RIDGE WY
SLOC 93420 737-C4
COUGHLIN WY
StBC 93455 816-J5
COUNT FLEET ST
StBC 93460 921-H5
COUNTRY CIR
StBC 93460 921-A4
COUNTRY CT
StBC 93460 921-A4
COUNTRY LN
SLOC 93401 674-A4
SMRA 93455 796-G5
StBC 93460 921-B4
COUNTRY RD
StBC 93460 921-A4
StBC 93463 921-A4
COUNTRY WY
StBC 93460 921-B4
COUNTRY BROOK LN
SLOC 93446 533-D5
COUNTRY CLUB DR
ATAS 93422 573-J3
PSRS 93446 513-J7
SBAR 93103 996-E3
SBAR 93108 996-E3
SLOC 93401 674-D7
SLOC 93401 694-D1
SLOC 93424 693-B2
COUNTRY CLUB LN
SMRA 93455 796-G7
COUNTRY CLUB VILLAGE DR
SMRA 93455 796-G5
COUNTRY HILL RD
Npmo 93444 756-A6
StBC 93455 816-J4
StBC 93455 817-A4
COUNTRY HILLS LN
SLOC 93420 715-C3
COUNTRY OAK WY
SLOC 93420 715-D2
COUNTRYSIDE LN
SLOC 93401 674-D7
COUNTRY VIEW LN
PSRS 93446 513-E4
COUNTRYWOOD CT
LMPC 93436 896-E6
StBC 93437 855-F7
StBC 93455 816-F4
COUNTRYWOOD DR
LMPC 93436 896-E6
StBC 93455 816-F4
COUNTRY WOOD LN
SLOC 93420 755-C1
COUNTY DUMP RD
StBC 93110 985-B7
StBC 93110 995-B1
COUNTY KERRY LN
SLOC 93422 593-C2
COUPER DR
SLO 93405 653-H1
COURT PL
StBC 93108 996-J2
N COURT ST
SLOC 93402 631-F6
S COURT ST
SLOC 93402 631-F6
N COURTLAND ST
ARGD 93420 714-F5
ARGD 93433 714-F5
GBCH 93433 714-F5
S COURTLAND ST
ARGD 93420 714-F6
COURTNEY DR
StBC 93436 896-F2
StBC 93455 796-H7
COURTYARD LN
SMRA 93455 796-G5

STREET Name City ZIP Pg-Grid

COVE CT
SLOC 93445 714-E7
COVE LN
SLOC 93426 470-A2
COVE ST
CARP 93013 998-A5
COVE MOUND DR
SBAR 93103 996-B2
COVENTRY CT
StBC 93455 816-G4
COVENTRY LN
Cmbr 93428 528-E6
COVERED WAGON RD
StBC 93463 920-J6
COVEY LN
SLOC 93402 651-J1
StBC 93455 816-J1
COVINA ST
SBAR 93103 996-E4
COVINGTON DR
ARGD 93420 715-A7
COVINGTON PL
GOL 93117 984-B7
COVINGTON WY
GOL 93117 984-B7
COWLES RD
StBC 93108 996-E1
COW MEADOW PL
SLOC 93446 533-F6
SLOC 93465 533-F6
COWPER ST
Cmbr 93428 548-G1
COX LN
SMRA 93454 776-H5
SMRA 93454 777-A5
SMRA 93458 776-F5
W COX LN
SMRA 93458 776-G5
COYOTE CIR
SBAR 93108 986-E7
COYOTE DR
SLOC 93420 734-H4
COYOTE RD
SBAR 93108 986-E7
StBC 93108 986-E7
COYOTE CANYON RD
SLOC 93401 674-J2
COYOTE CREEK RD
SLVG 93463 920-G6
COYOTE SPRINGS RD
SLOC - 737-D6
SLOC 93420 737-D6
CRAIG DR
SMRA 93458 796-E2
StBC 93436 896-F2
CRAIG WY
SLO 93405 653-G2
SLOC 93420 714-J1
CRAIGMONT DR
GOL 93117 984-D7
CRAMER CIR
CARP 93013 998-C6
CRAMER RD
CARP 93013 998-C6
CRANBERRY ST
ARGD 93420 714-F6
CRANDALL WY
SLO 93405 653-J2
SLOC 93405 653-J2
CRANESBILL PL
SLOC 93424 693-B2
CRAVENS LN
CARP 93013 998-B5
StBC - 998-B4
StBC 93013 998-B4
CRAWFORD AV
SLOC 93430 591-C5
CRAZY HORSE CT
PSRS 93446 513-H6
CRAZY HORSE DR
PSRS 93446 513-H6
CRECIENTE DR
StBC 93110 995-C5
CREEK LN
StBC 93111 985-B5
CREEK RD
SLOC 93445 734-F1
W CREEK RD
SLOC 93405 633-H7
SLOC 93405 653-H1
CREEKSAND LN
PSRS 93446 533-G1
CREEKSIDE
SLO 93401 673-G1
CREEKSIDE CT
PSRS 93446 534-B1
CREEKSIDE DR
ARGD 93420 714-H6
SLVG 93463 920-G6
CREEKSIDE LN
SLOC 93446 471-A5
StBC 93437 855-F7
CREEKSIDE PL
SLVG 93463 920-G6
CREEKSIDE RD
StBC 93108 997-B3
CREEKSIDE RANCH RD
SLOC 93465 533-F7
CREMONA DR
GOL 93117 994-A2
CRENSHAW CT
PSRS 93446 513-J7
CRESCENT AV
SBAR 93105 995-G3
StBC 93455 816-H6
CRESCENT DR
StBC 93110 985-E6
CRESCENT LN
SLOC 93420 695-D7
CRESCENT OAKS WY
PSRS 93446 514-B6
CREST AV
SLOC 93402 631-H7
CREST DR
PBCH 93449 714-F3
CREST ST
MOBY 93442 611-F4
SLOC 93445 714-E7
CRESTA AV
StBC 93110 995-B4
CRESTLINE DR
PSRS 93446 513-F3
SBAR 93105 995-F4
CRESTMONT CT
StBC 93455 816-J2
CRESTMONT DR
SLOC 93401 674-D5
StBC 93455 816-J2

CRESTON RD
PSRS 93446 513-H5
PSRS 93446 514-A7
PSRS 93446 534-A2
SLOC 93446 534-F5
SLOC 93465 534-F5
CRESTON ST
SMRA 93454 776-H5
SMRA 93454 777-A5
SMRA 93458 776-F5
CRESTON EUREKA RD
SLOC 93432 574-B2
SLOC 93465 574-B2
CRESTON EUREKA RD Rt#-41
ATAS 93422 574-E1
SLOC 93422 574-E1
SLOC 93432 574-E1
SLOC 93465 574-E1
CRESTON RIDGE LN
SLOC 93446 534-G6
CRESTVIEW CIR
SLO 93401 654-D6
CRESTVIEW LN
StBC 93108 996-E1
CRESTVIEW PL
Npmo 93444 755-D3
CREST VIEW WY
SLOC 93451 473-C4
CRESTWOOD CT
StBC 93455 816-H5
CRESTWOOD DR
StBC 93105 985-E6
StBC 93455 816-H5
CRESTWOOD PL
StBC 93105 985-E6
CREW LN
StBC 93455 816-E4
CRILENE CT
StBC 93455 816-J2
CRILENE LN
StBC 93455 816-J2
CRIMEA CT
SMRA 93458 796-E4
CRIMSON CT
StBC 93455 816-F5
CRISPIN AV
SLOC 93451 473-F1
CRISTOBAL AV
ATAS 93422 573-J5
ATAS 93422 574-A5
CROCKER ST
SLOC 93465 553-D2
CROCKER SPERRY DR
StBC 93108 997-B1
CROCKET CIR
SLOC 93402 631-F7
SLOC 93402 651-F1
CROFT LN
StBC 93441 920-B5
CROSBY DR
LMPC 93436 896-E5
CROSBY WY
Npmo 93444 756-A3
CROSS RD
StBC 93437 855-A6
CROSS ST
ARGD 93420 715-A5
SLO 93401 673-H2
CROSS CANYONS RD
SLOC 93451 473-H1
CROSS CREEK WY
SLOC 93401 674-H6
CROSSROAD LN
SMRA 93455 796-J5
CROWLEY WY
StBC 93455 817-E5
CROWN AV
StBC 93111 984-F6
CROWN CT
SMRA 93454 776-J7
CROWN TER
ARGD 93420 715-A4
CROWN WY
PSRS 93446 514-A4
CROWN HILL ST
ARGD 93420 715-A4
CROWS NEST LP
SLOC 93426 469-J2
CROYDEN LN
Cmbr 93428 528-E6
CRUISE CIR
SLOC 93446 471-B5
CRUM RD
SLOC 93465 553-D2
CRYSTAL CIR
LMPC 93436 896-E5
CRYSTAL DR
StBC 93455 817-E5
CRYSTAL LN
Npmo 93444 756-C4
CRYSTAL CANYON CT
PSRS 93446 533-J2
CRYSTAL SPRINGS RD
SLOC - 737-D7
CUATRO CAMINOS
StBC 93441 920-A5
CUCARACHA CT
SLO 93405 653-E7
CUERDA CORTE CIR
ARGD 93420 714-J3
CUERNO LARGO WY
SLOC 93446 533-E1
CUERVO AV
SBAR 93110 995-D4
StBC 93110 995-D4
CUERVO WY
ATAS 93422 594-C1
CUESTA AV
MOBY 93442 611-F3
SLOC 93405 653-J1
SLOC 93407 653-J1
CUESTA CT
ATAS 93422 574-B7
CUESTA DR
SLO 93405 653-G1
CUESTA PL
ARGD 93420 715-A4
CUESTA RD
SBAR 93105 995-G2
SLOC 93422 573-A7
CUESTA ST
StBC 93460 921-B5
CUESTA COLLEGE RD
SLOC 93405 632-J4
CUESTA VERDE
StBC 93117 984-E5
CUMBERLAND DR
GOL 93117 984-C6

CUMBRE CT
ATAS 93422 594-C2
SLO 93401 653-J6
CUMBRE RD
PSRS 93446 533-J2
SLOC 93446 533-J2
SLOC 93446 534-A3
CUNA DR
StBC 93110 995-B1
CURBARIL AV
ATAS 93422 573-H5
ATAS 93422 574-A4
SLOC 93422 574-A4
SLOC 93432 574-A4
CURLEW CT
SLOC 93420 734-J6
CURLEY AV
SBAR 93101 995-J4
SBAR 93101 996-A4
CURLY RD
StBC 93429 855-E1
CURRENT LN
PSRS 93446 513-G7
PSRS 93446 533-G1
CURRYER ST
SMRA 93458 776-G5
SMRA 93458 796-G1
CURTIS CT
SMRA 93455 797-A5
CURTIS PL
SLOC 93420 735-C4
CURVADO CIR
ATAS 93422 573-H1
CUTTER RD
SLOC 93426 469-H2
CUTTLEBON CT
StBC 93455 816-G4
CUYAMA AV
PBCH 93449 693-G7
CUYAMA DR
SLO 93401 653-J7
CUYAMA HWY Rt#-166
Npmo 93444 776-H1
SLOC 93454 776-H1
SLOC 93454 777-C1
CYCLAMEN CT
SLO 93401 674-C1
CYCLONE ST
Npmo 93444 756-A4
CYNBALARIA CT
StBC 93455 816-H4
CYNDIE LN
StBC 93455 816-E4
CYNTHIA DR
StBC 93436 896-F3
CYNTHIA LN
SLOC 93465 553-C2
CYPRESS AV
MOBY 93442 611-F7
SLOC 93430 590-J1
E CYPRESS AV
LMPC 93436 916-F2
W CYPRESS AV
LMPC 93436 916-C2
CYPRESS CT
StBC 93436 876-F5
CYPRESS LN
BLTN 93427 919-G5
CYPRESS ST
PBCH 93449 714-B2
SLO 93401 653-J5
SMRA 93454 796-J1
SMRA 93454 797-A1
SMRA 93458 776-F7
SMRA 93458 796-F1
StBC 93437 855-H7
CYPRESS WK
StBC 93117 994-A4
CYPRESS WY
SMRA 93454 797-A1
StBC 93436 876-F5
CYPRESS GLEN CT
SLOC 93430 590-H1
CYPRESS HOLLOW RD
SLOC - 591-G1
SLOC 93430 591-G1
CYPRESS RIDGE PKWY
SLOC 93420 734-J3
SLOC 93420 735-A5
CYRIL HARTLEY PL
SBAR 93117 994-C2

D

D ST
SLOC 93430 590-J1
SLOC 93451 453-B5
N D ST
LMPC 93436 896-E5
LMPC 93436 916-E1
S D ST
LMPC 93436 916-E2
DAFFODIL AV
Npmo 93444 755-J3
Npmo 93444 756-A3
DAFFODIL LN
GOL 93117 993-H2
DAGO LN
SLOC 93446 470-B7
DAHLIA CT
CARP 93013 998-C6
S DAHLIA CT
LMPC 93436 916-D2
DAHLIA LN
SLO 93401 674-B1
DAHLIA PL
StBC 93455 816-H2
DAHLIA ST
Npmo 93444 756-C1
N DAHLIA ST
LMPC 93436 916-D1
DAIRY LN
SLOC 93420 695-A4
DAIRY WY
BLTN 93427 919-F5
DAIRY CREEK RD
SLOC 93405 633-A4
DAIRYLAND RD
BLTN 93427 919-G5
DAISY ST
SLOC 93445 734-H1
N DAISY ST
LMPC 93436 896-G6
LMPC 93436 916-G1
DAKOTA DR
StBC 93455 816-H1
DAKOTA LN
SLOC 93420 736-E2

DALE AV
SLOC 93420 735-F5
DALE WY
StBC 93455 816-H5
DALEY ST
GOL 93117 994-D2
DALIDIO DR
SLO 93405 653-G7
DALLONS DR
PSRS 93446 513-J2
PSRS 93446 514-A2
DAL PORTO LN
SMRA 93454 796-G5
SMRA 93458 796-G5
DALTON WY
GOL 93117 984-D7
DALY AV
SLO 93405 653-G1
DAMAR ST
MOBY 93442 611-E2
DAMASK CT
SMRA 93458 796-F4
DAMASSA ST
BLTN 93427 919-J4
DAN CT
SMRA 93454 797-A1
DANA ST
SLO 93401 653-J4
E DANA ST
Npmo 93444 756-C2
W DANA ST
Npmo 93444 756-C2
DANA WY
MOBY 93442 611-G7
MOBY 93442 631-G1
N DANA FOOTHILL RD
Npmo 93444 735-H3
Npmo 93444 736-A4
S DANA FOOTHILL RD
Npmo 93444 736-E7
Npmo 93444 756-F2
DANBURY CT
GOL 93117 984-E7
DANCER AV
StBC 93455 816-H4
DANDELION LN
SLOC 93465 553-C1
DANE CREST
SLOC 93420 695-B6
DANFORD CANYON RD
Npmo 93444 737-B7
DANIA AV
BLTN 93427 919-J5
DANIEL DR
SMRA 93454 796-H4
DANIELSON RD
StBC 93108 996-H4
DANIJAY WY
SMRA 93454 776-J5
DANLEY CT
PSRS 93446 514-A2
DANNY LN
Npmo 93444 756-A3
DANTE DR
SMRA 93458 796-F4
DARA RD
GOL 93117 984-E7
DARBETON AV
SMRA 93458 776-F3
DARBY LN
Npmo 93444 756-C3
DARIEN CT
SLOC 93445 714-G7
DARIESA ST
CARP 93013 998-E6
DARLENE LN
StBC 93455 816-H5
DARRELLONA AV
SLOC 93451 473-H3
DARTMOOR AV
GOL 93117 993-F2
DARTMOOR LN
SMRA 93455 796-H6
DARTMOUTH DR
SLO 93405 653-H2
DARTMOUTH LN
StBC 93455 816-H3
W DATE AV
LMPC 93436 896-D7
DATE CT
LMPC 93436 896-C7
DAUPHIN ST
SMRA 93455 796-H7
StBC 93455 796-H7
DAVENPORT RD
GOL 93117 993-H3
DAVENPORT CREEK RD
SLOC 93401 674-B5
DAVID CT
SLOC 93401 673-E7
SLOC 93405 673-E7
DAVID RD
StBC 93455 816-J5
StBC 93455 817-A5
DAVID LOVE PL
SBAR 93117 994-C2
DAVID SANCHEZ CT
SMRA 93454 776-J5
DAVIES AV
SLOC 93430 591-C5
DAVIS CANYON RD
SLOC 93402 673-A5
DAWLISH PL
StBC 93108 996-E1
DAWN DR
BLTN 93427 919-H5
DAWN LN
StBC 93111 994-H2
DAWN RD
Npmo 93444 755-D2
DAWSON AV
GOL 93117 994-E2
DAWSON ST
MOBY 93442 591-E7
DAY
SLOC 93430 591-C5
DAY RD
GOL 93117 993-E2
DAY ST
Npmo 93444 756-B1
DAY BREAK LN
SLOC 93465 553-B6
DAYTONA DR
GOL 93117 993-G3
DE ANZA CT
ATAS 93422 553-E5
SLO 93405 653-D6
DEARBORN PL
GOL 93117 994-F2

DE ARMOND PL
SMRA 93454 796-H2
DEBBIE RD
GOL 93111 994-G1
DEBRA DR
StBC 93110 985-E5
DEER RD
SLOC 93405 654-A1
SLOC 93446 469-H4
DEER CANYON RD
BLTN 93427 920-A6
SLOC 93420 695-A6
DEER CREEK RD
SLOC 93420 737-F1
DEER CREEK WY
SLOC 93446 494-H7
SLOC 93446 514-H1
DEERFIELD LN
PSRS 93446 534-B1
DEERFIELD RD
StBC 93108 997-C3
DEER HILL DR
StBC 93463 920-H5
DEER HILL LN
StBC 93463 920-H5
DEERHURST DR
GOL 93117 993-F1
DEERPATH RD
SBAR 93108 996-E2
DEER RIDGE RD
StBC 93463 920-H4
DEER RUN LN
StBC 93455 816-G7
DEER RUN RD
StBC 93455 816-H7
DEER SPRINGS DR
PSRS 93446 534-B2
DEER TRAIL CIR
ARGD 93420 714-G2
StBC 93463 921-A5
DEER TRAIL CT
SLOC 93426 469-H2
DEER TRAIL LN
StBC 93460 921-A4
StBC 93463 921-A5
DEER TRAIL PL
StBC 93463 920-J5
StBC 93463 921-A5
DEER VIEW LN
SLOC 93465 534-C6
DEERWEED LN
SLOC 93426 470-B2
DE GAMMA DR
SMRA 93454 776-J5
SMRA 93454 777-A5
DEGASPARIS ST
GDLP 93434 774-J6
DEIGRATIA PL
SLOC 93420 694-J6
DEJOY CT
SMRA 93458 776-F5
DEJOY ST
SMRA 93458 776-F5
DEL CT
PBCH 93449 714-C2
DE LA GUERRA RD
SBAR 93103 996-C2
E DE LA GUERRA ST
SBAR 93101 996-B3
SBAR 93103 996-B3
W DE LA GUERRA ST
SBAR 93101 995-J5
SBAR 93101 996-A4
DE LA GUERRA TER
SBAR 93103 996-C2
DELANEY PL
SLOC 93446 471-C3
DELANO ST
PBCH 93449 714-C1
DE LA VINA ST
SBAR 93101 995-G1
SBAR 93101 996-A4
SBAR 93105 995-G1
DE LA VISTA AV
SBAR 93103 996-A2
DEL CANTO LN
StBC 93110 995-C1
DEL CIELO CT
StBC 93437 855-E6
DELKENER CT
StBC 93455 817-B5
DELLA DR
SMRA 93458 796-F4
DEL LAGO DR
StBC 93455 816-J2
DEL MAR AV
GBCH 93433 714-E7
SBAR 93109 996-A7
SLOC 93430 591-C5
DEL MAR CT
SLO 93405 653-G2
DEL MAR DR
SLOC 93402 631-H7
DEL MAR RD
SLOC 93422 572-H5
DEL MONACO DR
StBC 93111 994-H2
DEL MONTE AV
SBAR 93101 995-J5
SBAR 93101 996-A5
DEL NORTE
SMRA 93455 796-J5
DEL NORTE DR
GOL 93117 993-H2
DEL NORTE ST
SLOC 93402 631-F7
DEL NORTE WY
SLO 93405 653-G2
StBC 93455 816-J6
DEL ORO
SBAR 93109 996-A7
DEL ORO CT
SLO 93401 673-G2
DEL PARQUE DR
SBAR 93103 996-E4
DEL PLAYA DR
StBC 93106 994-A5
StBC 93117 993-J5
StBC 93117 994-A5
DEL PRADO RD
StBC 93463 920-E5
DEL REY
PBCH 93449 714-C3
DEL REY LN
SMRA 93454 776-J3
DEL RIO AV
SLO 93405 653-D6
DEL RIO RD
ATAS 93422 553-C7

DEL RIO RD
ATAS 93422 573-B1
DEL SOL AV
SBAR 93109 996-A6
DEL SOL CT
SLO 93401 673-H2
DEL SOL PL
SLOC 93446 533-E4
DEL SOL ST
ARGD 93420 714-G6
DEL SUR
SMRA 93455 796-J5
DEL SUR WY
SLO 93405 653-G2
DELTA AV
CARP 93013 998-C6
DELTA ST
SLOC 93445 714-E7
SLOC 93445 734-E1
DEN ST
StBC 93440 878-G1
DENA WY
SMRA 93454 776-H6
SMRA 93454 777-A6
StBC 93111 984-F6
DENEB PL
StBC 93436 876-D6
DENNIS LN
SLOC 93420 714-G1
SLOC 93449 714-G1
DENTRO DR
StBC 93111 984-H7
DENVER WY
SLOC 93451 453-C6
DEPOT AV
SLOC 93401 674-E7
SLOC 93401 694-E1
DEPOT DR
SMRA 93458 776-G6
DEPOT RD
GOL 93117 994-E1
StBC 93108 996-H4
DEPOT ST
SMRA 93455 796-G5
SMRA 93458 776-G5
SMRA 93458 796-G2
DERBY LN
Cmbr 93428 528-E5
PSRS 93446 513-E6
DEREK CT
Npmo 93444 756-A3
DERMANAK DR
StBC 93463 920-G5
DESCANSO ST
SLO 93405 653-E6
DE SOTO DR
SMRA 93454 776-J5
SMRA 93454 777-A5
DEVAUL RANCH DR
SLO 93405 653-E7
SLO 93405 673-E1
DEVAULT PL
Cmbr 93428 528-D7
DEVEREUX WY
StBC 93117 993-H5
DEVON CT
ATAS 93422 573-H5
DEVON PL
GOL 93111 984-F7
DEVONSHIRE DR
ARGD 93420 715-A7
DEVONSHIRE PL
StBC 93455 817-A3
DEWEY DR
SLOC 93445 714-E7
DE WOLFF AV
StBC 93436 895-G6
DEXTER DR
StBC 93110 994-J1
DIABLO DR
SLO 93405 653-D6
SLOC 93405 653-D6
DIABLO CANYON RD
SLOC 93402 651-A7
DIAMENTE ST
SMRA 93458 796-F4
DIAMOND CIR
ARGD 93420 714-J7
DIAMOND DR
StBC 93455 816-J5
StBC 93455 817-A5
DIAMOND CREST CT
StBC 93110 994-J3
DIAN DR
SMRA 93455 796-J7
DIANA LN
SBAR 93103 996-C2
DIANA PL
ARGD 93420 714-H6
DIANA RD
SBAR 93103 996-C2
DIBBLEE AV
SBAR 93101 996-A5
DICKINSON ST
StBC 93455 817-B4
DICKSON DR
StBC 93455 796-H7
StBC 93455 816-H1
DIEGO RIVERA LN
SLOC 93420 734-J7
SLOC 93420 754-J1
DIESEL AV
SMRA 93458 776-F3
DINSMORE LN
StBC 93108 996-H2
DIVIDE WY
SMRA 93458 776-F3
DIVISION ST
Npmo 93444 755-F7
Npmo 93444 756-B5
Npmo 93444 775-B2
DIXIE LN
SLOC 93420 694-J5
DIXIELEE ST
StBC 93455 816-H2
DIXON ST
SBAR 93105 985-E7
DIXSON ST
ARGD 93420 714-F6
DOANE AV
SMRA 93454 796-J1
SMRA 93454 797-A1
DODDS WY
SLOC 93432 574-J3
DODSON WY
ARGD 93420 714-H6
DOE LN
SLOC 93446 469-D2

DOESKIN PL
SLOC 93465 5
DOESKIN TR
StBC 93455 8
DOGWOOD AV
MOBY 93442 6
DOGWOOD CT
StBC 93455 8
DOGWOOD DR
BLTN 93427 9
DOGWOOD ST
StBC 93437 8
DOLCETTO LN
SMRA 93458 7
DOLLIVER ST Rt#-1
GBCH 93433 7
GBCH 93449 7
PBCH 93449 7
DOLORES AV
ATAS 93422 5
DOLORES CT
SMRA 93455 7
DOLORES DR
SBAR 93109 9
DOLORES LN
SLOC 93465 5
DOLPHIN AV
SLOC 93445 7
DOMINCA CT
SMRA 93454 7
DOMINGUES ST
SMRA 93454 7
DOMINION RD
StBC 93454 7
StBC 93454 8
DOMINO AV
StBC 93455 8
StBC 93455 8
DON AV
SLOC 93402 63
DONALD WY
StBC 93455 8
DONALDSON PL
SBAR 93117 99
DONEGAL DR
SLOC 93405 65
DONELSON PL
SLOC 93465 55
DONNA AV
SLOC 93402 63
DONNA WY
SLO 93405 65
DONNER CT
SMRA 93454 77
E DONOVAN RD
SMRA 93454 77
SMRA 93454 77
W DONOVAN RD
SMRA 93454 77
SMRA 93458 77
StBC 93458 77
DON PABLO DR
StBC 93455 81
DON RICARDO PL
StBC 93455 81
DONZE AV
SBAR 93101 99
DOOLITTLE WY
Npmo 93444 75
DORADO DR
StBC 93111 98
DORAL CT
SLOC 93401 67
DORAL DR
StBC 93436 87
DORIS AV
SLOC 93402 63
DORIS LN
SLOC 93420 71
DORKING AV
Cmbr 93428 54
DORKING PL
StBC 93105 98
DOROPHY AV
SLOC 93453 61
DOROTHY CT
PSRS 93446 51
PSRS 93446 51
DOROTHY ST
PSRS 93446 51
DORRANCE WY
CARP 93013 99
DORSET CT
GOL 93117 98
DORSET ST
Cmbr 93428 52
DORSEY CT
PSRS 93446 53
DORTHY LN
SLOC 93420 73
DORWIN LN
StBC 93111 99
DOS CANADAS RD
Npmo 93444 73
Npmo 93444 73
DOS CERROS
ARGD 93420 71
DOS HERMANOS RD
StBC 93111 98
DOS PUEBLOS CANYON RD
StBC 93117 98
StBC 93117 99
DOTY DR
SLOC 93420 73
DOUBLE POINT WY
SLOC 93446 47
DOUGLAS LN
StBC 93111 99
DOUGLAS WY
SMRA 93454 79
DOUGLASS AV
StBC 93436 89
DOVE
PSRS 93446 51
DOVE CT
SLOC 93420 71
DOVE LN
LMPC 93436 91
DOVE RD
SLOC 93446 46
DOVE CANYON RD
BLTN 93427 92
DOVEDALE AV
Cmbr 93428 54
DOVE MEADOW LN
StBC 93463 92
DOVE MEADOW RD
StBC 93463 92

STREET Name City ZIP Pg-Grid

R CT
GBCH 93433 714-F5
R LN
Cmbr 93428 528-E5
SBAR 93103 996-B1
R RD
SBAR 93103 996-B1
R HILL RD
SBAR 93103 996-B1
RLEE DR
StBC 93455 816-G5
R AV
SLOC 93420 714-H7
EY CIR
BLTN 93427 919-H5
ING AV
Cmbr 93428 548-G2
MOBY 93442 611-G5
ING CT
StBC 93437 855-E7
StBC 93437 875-E1
ING LN
StBC 93455 796-H7
O DR
StBC 93436 876-C7
E CIR
SLO 93405 653-F6
E DR
StBC 93455 796-H7
StBC 93455 816-J1
E ST
Cmbr 93428 548-F2
ER RANCH PL
SLOC 93446 534-H2
EL DR
SBAR 93103 996-D2
OON AV
Cmbr 93428 548-G2
WOOD
PBCH 93449 714-D3
WOOD CT
PSRS 93446 534-B1
WOOD DR
PSRS 93446 534-B1
StBC 93455 816-A1
WOOD ST
GBCH 93433 714-F7
MOBY 93442 611-F6
I CANYON RD
StBC 93436 878-G7
StBC 93440 878-G3
IM LN
Npmo 93444 756-C5
IMER CIR
StBC 93455 816-H5
CREEK RD
PSRS 93446 494-C7
PSRS 93446 514-F1
SLOC 93446 494-B7
SLOC 93446 514-F1
WELL PL
PSRS 93446 534-B2
IN CT
StBC 93455 816-F4
AN DR
PBCH 93449 714-F3
E DR
SMRA 93454 776-J5
StBC 93455 816-H6
URA AV
ATAS 93422 573-H2
URA DR
StBC 93108 996-G2
P RD
CARP 93013 1018-E1
BAR ST
MOBY 93442 611-F5
CAN RD
SLO 93401 654-B7
SLOC 93465 553-D1
StBC 93110 985-E6
ES
PBCH 93449 714-C3
ES ST
MOBY 93442 611-F6
LIN ST
SLOC 93420 735-A6
SMUIR WY
GOL 93117 984-D7
TOV DR
SLOC 93420 735-D6
ANGO RD
SLOC 93422 594-E2
HAM PL
GOL 93117 993-F2
TY PL
SLOC 93446 494-G6
ARD RD
StBC 93455 816-A2
TON AV
SBAR 93101 995-H4
ALI DR
SMRA 93458 796-E4
NA CT
PSRS 93446 513-H3
R ST
StBC 93455 816-G6

E

CT
LMPC 93436 896-E6
PL
LMPC 93436 896-E6

SLOC 93430 590-J2
SLOC 93451 453-A4
SMRA 93455 796-C4
SMRA 93455 816-C2
SMRA 93458 796-C2
StBC 93455 816-C2
ST
LMPC 93436 896-E5
LMPC 93436 916-E1
ST
LMPC 93436 916-E2
LE CT
PSRS 93446 513-J7
SMRA 93454 796-H3
LE PL
StBC 93460 921-C4
LE ST
SMRA 93454 796-H3
LE CREEK CT
ATAS 93422 594-C3
LE NEST CT
SLOC 93424 693-A1
LE POINT LN
SLOC 93446 471-B5

EAGLE RANCH RD
SLOC - 593-H6
SLOC 93422 593-H6
EAGLETON AV
SMRA 93458 776-E3
EAGLE VISTA WY
SLOC 93422 594-C4
EALAND PL
SBAR 93103 986-D7
EARL LN
StBC 93455 816-J5
EAST AV
SMRA 93454 776-J5
SMRA 93454 796-J1
EAST MALL
ATAS 93422 573-J3
EAST ST
SBAR 93103 996-C2
EASTBOURNE TER
StBC 93455 816-G4
EASTBROOK DR
LMPC 93436 896-D6
EASTBURY WY
SMRA 93455 796-G5
EASTER ST
MOBY 93442 611-E2
EASTGATE
BLTN 93427 919-G5
EASTGATE LN
StBC 93108 997-C2
EASTMAN ST
SLOC 93420 735-D4
EASTON RD
StBC 93441 900-H6
EASTVIEW PL
Npmo 93444 755-D3
PSRS 93446 534-C1
EASTVIEW WY
SLOC 93420 734-H5
EASTWOOD DR
StBC 93455 816-J4
EASY LN
Npmo 93444 755-H4
EASY ST
ARGD 93420 714-J2
BLTN 93427 919-J4
SMRA 93458 776-F3
EATON DR
ARGD 93420 715-A7
EBB TIDE WY
PBCH 93449 693-F6
EBONY DR
PSRS 93446 534-A1
EBONY ST
SMRA 93458 776-G3
StBC 93437 855-H7
ECHO CT
PSRS 93446 514-A6
ECHO LN
StBC 93463 920-J6
ECHO CANYON CT
SLOC 93420 715-C3
ECKLES RD
SBAR 93117 994-D1
EDDY ST
SLOC 93465 553-D2
EDENBURY RD
StBC 93455 816-F4
EDGECLIFF LN
StBC 93108 996-J4
EDGEHILL LN
StBC 93460 941-D1
EDGEMOUND DR
StBC 93105 985-J6
EDGEVIEW LN
SLOC 93420 734-J5
EDGEWATER LN
PSRS 93446 513-G7
EDGEWATER WY
SBAR 93109 995-G7
EDGEWOOD AV
StBC 93455 816-J2
EDGEWOOD CT
SLOC 93446 471-C3
EDGEWOOD DR
GOL 93117 984-C7
SLO 93401 654-D6
EDIE CT
SMRA 93454 777-A7
EDISON AV
SBAR 93103 996-C3
EDISON ST
StBC 93460 901-C7
StBC 93460 921-C2
EDITH DR
StBC 93455 817-B5
EDMANDS AV
ARGD 93420 715-B4
EDNA RD Rt#-227
SLOC 93401 674-D4
SLOC 93401 694-F1
EDNA RANCH CIR
SLOC 93401 695-A1
EDNA VALLEY LN
SLOC 93420 694-H5
EDUCATION DR
SLOC 93405 632-J3
EDWARD PL
StBC 93117 984-E5
EDWARD ST
SMRA 93458 796-G2
EDWARDS PL
LMPC 93436 896-E6
EFFIE WY
PBCH 93449 714-F3
EGRET LN
GDLP 93434 774-J6
SLOC 93446 471-D6
EILEEN LN
StBC 93455 816-H5
EILEEN WY
SBAR 93105 985-E7
EKWILL ST
GOL 93111 994-F2
StBC 93111 994-F2
EL ACEBO
SMRA 93455 796-J5
ELAINE AV
SMRA 93458 796-F4
ELAINE ST
PSRS 93446 514-A6
ELAINE WY
PBCH 93449 714-F3
EL ARCO DR
SBAR 93105 985-F7
EL BORDO AV
ATAS 93422 574-B7
EL BOSQUE RD
StBC 93108 997-A1

EL CALLE JON
SMRA 93454 777-A7
EL CAMINITO RD
SBAR 93109 995-G5
EL CAMINO ST
SMRA 93454 776-H7
SMRA 93458 776-F6
EL CAMINO DE LA LUZ
SBAR 93109 995-G7
EL CAMINO RATEL
StBC 93117 984-D5
EL CAMINO REAL
ATAS 93422 553-E6
ATAS 93422 573-G2
ATAS 93422 574-A5
ATAS 93422 594-C1
SLOC 93422 594-G7
SLOC 93422 614-G2
SLOC 93453 614-G2
EL CAMINO REAL Rt#-58
SLOC 93453 614-F3
EL CAMINO REAL U.S.-101
ARGD - 714-J5
ARGD - 715-B6
ATAS - 553-D3
BLTN - 919-H7
CARP - 998-A6
CARP - 1018-F1
GBCH - 714-F3
GOL - 993-A1
GOL - 994-E1
MonC - 453-B3
Npmo - 735-H6
Npmo - 736-A7
Npmo - 756-D4
Npmo - 776-H4
PBCH - 693-E3
PBCH - 714-F3
PSRS - 513-F2
PSRS - 533-F3
SBAR - 995-D1
SBAR - 996-E3
SLO - 653-H5
SLO - 654-B2
SLO - 673-F4
SLOC - 453-B3
SLOC - 473-E5
SLOC - 493-F3
SLOC - 513-F2
SLOC - 533-F3
SLOC - 553-D3
SLOC - 594-C3
SLOC - 614-C6
SLOC - 653-H5
SLOC - 654-B2
SLOC - 673-F4
SLOC - 693-E3
SLOC - 714-A1
SLOC - 715-B6
SLOC - 735-E2
SLOC - 776-H4
SMRA - 776-H4
SMRA - 777-A6
SMRA - 797-A7
StBC - 797-A7
StBC - 817-B4
StBC - 878-H1
StBC - 900-C1
StBC - 919-H7
StBC - 939-H3
StBC - 981-A5
StBC - 982-E6
StBC - 992-J1
StBC - 993-A1
StBC - 994-E1
StBC - 995-D1
StBC - 996-E3
StBC - 997-C3
StBC - 998-A6
StBC - 1018-F1
Summ - 997-C3
VeCo - 1018-F1
E EL CAMPO RD
SLOC 93420 715-B7
SLOC 93420 735-C1
W EL CAMPO RD
SLOC 93420 734-J5
SLOC 93420 735-B3
EL CAPITAN WY
SLO 93401 674-C2
EL CAPTITAN RANCH RD
StBC 93117 982-C5
EL CARRO LN
CARP 93013 998-C5
EL CASERIO
SBAR 93101 996-B3
EL CASERIO CT
SLO 93401 654-C6
EL CAZADOR WY
Npmo 93444 737-B4
EL CENTRO RD
ATAS 93422 574-A5
EL CENTRO WY
SLO 93401 654-B3
EL CERRITO
SLO 93401 654-C5
StBC 93455 816-H6
EL CERRITO CT
SLO 93401 654-C5
StBC 93437 855-E6
EL CERRITO DR
Npmo 93444 755-J6
EL CIELITO RD
SBAR 93103 986-C6
SBAR 93105 986-B6
EL COLEGIO RD
StBC 93106 994-B4
StBC 93117 993-J4
StBC 93117 994-A4
EL CORRAL ST
SLOC 93446 533-E1
EL CORTE RD
ATAS 93422 574-B5
ELDER
StBC 93437 855-E6
ELDERBERRY DR
GOL 93117 993-F3
ELDERBERRY LN
SLOC 93424 693-A1
EL DESCANSO AV
ATAS 93422 573-H5
EL DORADO AV
SLOC 93405 633-B5
EL DORADO CT
PSRS 93446 513-H4

EL DORADO DR
SLOC 93420 734-J5
EL DORADO LN
StBC 93108 996-J1
EL DORADO RD
ATAS 93422 574-B5
StBC 93436 876-D6
EL DORADO ST
SLOC 93402 631-E7
EL DORADO WY
PBCH 93449 693-E5
ELEANOR DR
CARP 93013 998-C6
EL EMBARCADERO
StBC 93117 994-A5
ELENA ST
MOBY 93442 611-E3
EL ENCANTO RD
SBAR 93103 996-A1
ELEVEN OAKS LN
StBC 93108 996-H3
EL FARO
SBAR 93109 995-H6
EL GAUCHO RD
StBC 93111 984-J7
EL GRECO RD
StBC 93117 994-A4
ELIANO ST
ATAS 93422 594-D2
ELISA CT
BLTN 93427 919-J6
ELISE PL
SBAR 93109 995-G7
ELISE WY
SBAR 93109 995-G6
ELIZA DR
SMRA 93458 796-E4
ELIZABETH CT
SLOC 93465 553-C2
ELIZABETH ST
SBAR 93103 996-C3
SMRA 93454 776-J6
SMRA 93454 796-H1
ELK PT
SLOC 93446 471-C3
ELK GROVE LN
StBC 93463 920-H6
ELK GROVE RD
StBC 93463 920-H6
ELKHORN LN
StBC 93455 816-G7
ELKS LN
SLO 93401 653-H6
SMRA 93454 776-J6
ELKUS WK
StBC 93117 993-J4
ELLA LN
StBC 93111 994-H2
ELLA ST
SLO 93401 654-A5
ELLEN LN
SMRA 93455 796-J5
ELLEN WY
SLO 93405 653-J3
ELLIOT ST
SMRA 93455 796-J5
ELLIS AV
Cmbr 93428 548-H2
ELLWOOD BEACH DR
GOL 93117 993-G3
ELLWOOD CANYON RD
StBC 93117 983-F7
StBC 93117 993-F1
ELLWOOD RANCH RD
StBC 93117 983-F7
StBC 93117 993-F1
ELLWOOD RIDGE RD
GOL 93117 993-F1
StBC 93117 993-F1
ELLWOOD STATION RD
GOL 93117 993-G2
ELM
SLO 93401 673-H1
ELM AV
CARP 93013 998-C7
MOBY 93442 611-E2
SLVG 93463 920-E7
SMRA 93458 776-G5
ELM CT
PSRS 93446 513-H5
SLO 93405 653-H2
ELM LN
CARP 93013 998-D6
LMPC 93436 895-J2
LMPC 93436 896-A2
ELM ST
GDLP 93434 775-A6
StBC 93437 855-D7
N ELM ST
ARGD 93420 714-G5
S ELM ST
ARGD 93420 714-G6
SLOC 93420 714-G6
SLOC 93445 714-G6
SLOC 93445 734-G1
EL MEDIO DR
SMRA 93458 796-E4
EL MERCADO
SLO 93405 653-G6
ELMHURST PL
GOL 93117 993-G3
EL MIRADOR CT
SLO 93401 673-G3
EL MIRLO
SMRA 93455 796-J5
EL MONTE DR
SBAR 93109 995-H7
EL MONTE RD
ATAS 93422 572-J3
ATAS 93422 573-A2
SLOC 93422 572-J3
EL MORRO AV
SLOC 93402 631-H5
SLOC 93402 632-A5
ELMWOOD DR
StBC 93455 816-B1
EL NIDO CT
SMRA 93455 796-H5
EL NIDO LN
StBC 93117 994-B5
EL NIDO ST
SMRA 93455 796-H5
EL PARQUE AV
ATAS 93422 573-H7
EL PASEO
SLO 93401 654-C5
EL PASILLO
StBC 93108 997-G2

EL PASO WY
SLOC 93451 453-D6
EL POMAR DR
SLOC 93465 533-J7
SLOC 93465 534-A7
SLOC 93465 553-G1
S EL POMAR RD
SLOC 93465 534-G7
EL PORTAL AV
CARP 93013 998-E6
EL PORTAL DR
PBCH 93449 693-D4
EL PORTAL ST
StBC 93455 816-J6
EL PRADO PL
SBAR 93105 995-G2
EL PRADO RD
SBAR 93105 995-G2
EL RANCHO LN
SLOC 93420 715-G2
EL RANCHO RD
SBAR 93108 996-F2
StBC 93108 996-F1
StBC 93429 855-B2
StBC 93437 855-A4
EL RANCHO HACIENDA
SBAR 93105 986-B7
EL RANCHO OESTE RD
StBC 93429 855-A1
EL RANCHO RD LATERAL
StBC 93429 855-A3
EL RETIRO AV
ATAS 93422 573-H4
EL RODEO RD
StBC 93110 984-J7
StBC 93110 985-A7
EL SERENO AV
SLOC 93430 591-C5
ELSINORE DR
SLVG 93463 920-E7
EL SUENO RD
StBC 93110 985-B7
StBC 93110 995-B1
EL SUENO WY
SLOC 93420 715-C2
EL TIGRE CT
SLO 93405 653-F7
EL VEDADO LN
SBAR 93105 995-H1
EL VERANO AV
ATAS 93422 573-H1
ELVERHOY WY
SLVG 93463 940-E1
EL VIENTO
PBCH 93449 714-E2
ELVIRA WY
Npmo 93444 756-A3
ELWELL AV
SLOC 93420 735-G6
EMAN CT
ARGD 93420 714-J5
EMBARCADERO
MOBY 93442 611-E4
EMBARCADERO DEL MAR
StBC 93106 994-A5
StBC 93117 994-A5
EMBARCADERO DEL NORTE
StBC 93106 994-B5
StBC 93117 994-B5
EMBASSY AV
SMRA 93458 776-G3
EMERALD CIR
MOBY 93442 611-E3
EMERALD CT
StBC 93455 816-J3
EMERALD DR
SMRA 93454 777-A7
EMERALD WY
PBCH 93449 693-H7
PBCH 93449 714-D3
EMERALD BAY DR
ARGD 93420 714-J4
EMERSON AV
SBAR 93103 995-J1
EMERSON RD
Cmbr 93428 548-G1
EMERSON ST
Summ 93067 997-D3
EMILY LN
GOL 93117 993-H3
EMILY ST
SLO 93401 654-A5
EMMONS RD
Cmbr 93428 548-F2
EMPIRE DR
SMRA 93458 776-G3
EMPIRE ST
SLOC 93401 694-F1
EMPLEO ST
SLO 93401 673-H1
EMPRESA DR
SLO 93401 673-J1
EMPRESS CIR
SMRA 93454 776-J7
ENCANTO
LMPC 93436 896-E3
ENCANTO AV
PBCH 93449 693-D5
ENCANTO CT
PSRS 93446 513-G5
ENCANTO LN
SLO 93401 673-G2
ENCHANTO RD
ATAS 93422 573-C2
ENCINA AV
SLOC 93453 614-G3
ENCINA CT
ATAS 93422 573-H2
ENCINA LN
GOL 93117 994-E1
ENCINA RD
GOL 93117 994-D1
ENCINAL AV
ATAS 93422 574-A4
ENCINAL ST
SLOC 93446 513-F7
SLOC 93446 533-F1
ENCINITAS CT
GBCH 93433 714-F6
ENCINO AV
ATAS 93422 573-G4
ENCINO CT
SLO 93401 654-C5
ENCINO LN
Npmo 93444 756-A2
ENCORE DR
StBC 93110 995-C1

ENNISBROOK DR
StBC 93108 997-A2
ENOS DR
SMRA 93454 796-J3
SMRA 93458 796-G3
ENSENADA AV
ATAS 93422 573-J2
ATAS 93422 574-A2
ENSENADA ST
SBAR 93103 996-D3
ENTERPRISE AV
StBC 93436 896-D1
ENTRADA W
PBCH 93449 714-D3
ENTRADA AV
ATAS 93422 573-J3
ENTRADA CT
StBC 93437 855-F7
ENTRADA DR
PBCH 93449 714-D3
ENTRADA WY
SMRA 93458 796-G2
ENTRANCE RD
GOL 93117 993-G3
PSRS 93446 514-C7
StBC 93463 920-H6
EQUESTRIAN AV
SBAR 93101 996-A3
EQUESTRIAN RD
SLOC 93446 471-C5
EQUESTRIAN WY
ARGD 93420 714-G3
ERHART RD
SLOC 93449 694-F7
SLOC 93449 714-G1
ERIC LN
SLOC 93465 553-B2
ERICA CT
SLOC 93445 734-H1
ERICA PL
StBC 93436 896-G2
ERIE WY
StBC 93455 817-E5
ERMINIA WY
SMRA 93458 796-F4
ERNA WY
PBCH 93449 714-F3
ERNEST PL
Cmbr 93428 548-H1
ERROL ST
MOBY 93442 611-F4
ESCABROSO CT
ATAS 93422 573-A6
ESCABROSO RD
SLOC 93422 572-J6
SLOC 93422 573-A6
ESCALANTE ST
GDLP 93434 775-B5
ESCALERAS RD
SLOC 93422 572-J3
ESCALON PL
ATAS 93422 573-J1
ESCARPA AV
ATAS 93422 574-A3
ESCONDIDO RD
ATAS 93422 573-E6
ESCUELA CT
SLO 93405 653-E6
ESCUELA ST
StBC 93254 806-C1
ESPALIER DR
SMRA 93455 796-G6
ESPARTO AV
PBCH 93449 693-H7
ESPERANZA LN
SLOC 93401 673-J3
ESPLANADA AV
StBC 93455 816-J6
ESROM DR
SLVG 93463 940-E1
ESSEX CT
SMRA 93458 776-G3
ESSEX ST
SBAR 93105 985-E7
ESTATE WY
Npmo 93444 755-E4
ESTELITA CT
SLO 93401 653-J7
ESTERO AV
MOBY 93442 611-G7
ESTERO RD
StBC 93117 993-J5
StBC 93117 994-A5
ESTERO WY
CARP 93013 998-B6
ESTES DR
SMRA 93454 797-A1
ESTRADA AV
ATAS 93422 553-H7
ATAS 93422 573-H1
ESTRADA AV Rt#-58
SLOC 93453 614-G3
ESTRADA PL
SMRA 93455 796-G6
ESTRELLA CIR
SLOC 93446 494-G2
ESTRELLA CT
SLOC 93405 653-D7
ESTRELLA DR
StBC 93110 995-C3
ESTRELLA RD
SLOC 93422 594-C6
SLOC 93446 494-E1
SLOC 93451 473-H4
SLOC 93451 494-E1
ESTRELLA DEL MAR CT
SLOC 93424 693-B3
ESTRIGA CT
SMRA 93458 796-E4
ESTUARY WY
GBCH 93433 714-D4
ETO CIR
SLO 93405 653-E7
ETO LN
SLOC 93402 632-A7
ETO RD
SLOC 93402 632-A6
ETON RD
Cmbr 93428 528-H7
Cmbr 93428 548-H1
EUCALYPTUS AV
SBAR 93101 995-G3
EUCALYPTUS DR
SLVG 93463 920-E7
EUCALYPTUS LN
SLOC 93465 534-J7
StBC 93108 996-J4
StBC 93455 816-H3

EUCALYPTUS RD
Npmo 93444 755-C4
SLOC 93405 654-A1
SLOC 93420 755-C3
EUCALYPTUS ST
CARP 93013 998-D5
EUCALYPTUS HILL CIR
SBAR 93103 996-E3
EUCALYPTUS HILL DR
SBAR 93108 996-F2
EUCALYPTUS HILL RD
SBAR 93103 996-E2
SBAR 93108 996-E2
StBC 93108 996-F1
EUCLID AV
SBAR 93101 995-J4
EUGENIA PL
CARP 93013 998-D7
EUREKA LN
SLOC 93465 553-H5
EUREKA ST
SLOC 93405 633-E5
EUROPA AV
StBC 93436 896-C1
EVALITA LN
StBC 93111 994-H2
EVANS AV
Summ 93067 997-D3
EVANS RD
SLOC 93401 674-B4
EVANSTON PL
GOL 93117 993-H3
EVE ST
Npmo 93444 756-B1
EVELYN CT
Cmbr 93428 528-E5
SMRA 93454 776-J4
EVENING SONG CT
GOL 93117 993-J3
EVENSONG WY
Cmbr 93428 528-H7
Cmbr 93428 548-H1
EVERGLADE LN
SLOC 93420 715-J3
EVERGREEN
BLTN 93427 919-G5
EVERGREEN AV
SMRA 93454 776-H6
SMRA 93458 776-F6
EVERGREEN DR
GOL 93117 993-F1
EVERGREEN WY
Npmo 93444 755-G3
EVERSDEN DR
StBC 93437 855-E7
EVERSDEN LN
StBC 93454 797-D7
EVERT CT
PSRS 93446 513-J7
EVONSHIRE AV
StBC 93111 994-J2
EVY LN
SLOC 93420 715-A1
EWING AV
SLOC 93420 735-F5
EWING LN
SLOC 93420 735-G5
EXCEL WY
SLOC 93420 715-F1
EXETER LN
Cmbr 93428 528-D5
EXETER PL
StBC 93105 985-H7
EXLINE RD
SLOC 93446 493-D5
S EXLINE RD
SLOC 93446 493-D5
EXOTIC GARDEN DR
Cmbr 93428 528-C3
EXPERIMENTAL STATION RD
PSRS 93446 513-H3
EXPOSITION CT
SLO 93401 653-J6
EXPOSITION DR
SLO 93401 653-J6
EXTERIOR RD
StBC 93460 900-J7
StBC 93460 920-J2
StBC 93463 920-J6

F

F ST
SLOC 93430 590-J2
SLOC 93453 614-F3
StBC 93455 796-B5
N F ST
LMPC 93436 896-E5
LMPC 93436 916-E1
S F ST
LMPC 93436 916-E2
FAEH AV
ARGD 93420 714-H5
FAIRCHILD LN
StBC 93440 878-H2
FAIRCHILD WY
SLOC 93402 631-J7
FAIRFAX RD
StBC 93110 985-E7
FAIRLANE DR
StBC 93437 855-F7
StBC 93437 875-E1
FAIRLANE PL
StBC 93455 796-H7
FAIRLEA RD
StBC 93460 921-A5
StBC 93463 921-A5
FAIRMONT AV
StBC 93455 816-H2
FAIRMONT CT
StBC 93437 855-D6
FAIR OAKS AV
ARGD 93420 714-J5
ARGD 93420 715-A5
FAIR OAKS DR
StBC 93455 796-H7
StBC 93455 816-J1
FAIR RIDGE DR
StBC 93455 817-B6
FAIRVIEW AV
GOL 93117 994-D2
MOBY 93442 611-H7
SBAR 93117 994-D2
StBC 93117 994-D2
N FAIRVIEW AV
GOL 93117 984-D7
GOL 93117 994-D1
SBAR 93117 994-D1

STREET Name City ZIP Pg-Grid

N FAIRVIEW AV StBC 93117 984-D6
FAIR VIEW DR ARGD 93420 714-G5
FAIRVIEW LN PBCH 93449 714-D3; PSRS 93446 513-E3
FAIRVIEW RD SLO 93401 654-C5; SLOC 93401 654-C5
FAIRVIEW ST SLO 93401 654-A4
FAIRWAY DR PSRS 93446 513-J7; PSRS 93446 514-A7; SLO 93405 653-E7; SLVG 93463 940-E3; SMRA 93455 796-E6
FAIRWAY PL SLVG 93463 940-D3
FAIRWAY RD StBC 93108 996-G4
FAIRWAY VISTA DR SMRA 93455 796-F5
FAIRWOOD LN SBAR 93103 986-B7
FAITH PL Npmo 93444 756-D7
FALBERG WY StBC 93117 993-H5
FALCON DR PSRS 93446 534-A2; StBC 93436 876-D5
FALCON RD ATAS 93422 593-D2
FALCON CREST DR SLOC 93420 715-B7; SLOC 93420 735-A1
FALCON RIDGE RD SLOC 93402 652-B1
FALDA RD ATAS 93422 553-G7; ATAS 93422 573-G1
FALLBROOK CT PSRS 93446 533-J1; PSRS 93446 534-A1
FALLBROOK ST Cmbr 93428 548-F2
FALLEN LEAF LN ATAS 93422 553-E6
FALLEN LEAF RD StBC 93455 817-E4
FALLING STAR LN SLOC - 572-B5
FAN CT SLOC 93426 469-J1
FANCY HILL CT StBC 93460 921-A3
FARADAY ST StBC 93460 921-C5
FARM LN SLOC 93422 594-F6
FARM RD LMPC 93436 895-H3; LMPC 93436 896-A4
FARM HOUSE LN SLOC 93401 674-C3
FARMHOUSE PL ARGD 93420 715-B5
FARMLAND DR BLTN 93427 919-F4
FARNEL RD SMRA 93458 796-E1
FARNSWORTH DR ARGD 93420 715-A7
FA-ROUSSE WY SLOC 93446 494-H6; SLOC 93446 514-H1
FARRELL DR SMRA 93454 797-A1
FARREN RD StBC 93117 983-C7; StBC 93117 993-C1
FARRIER CT SLO 93405 673-F1
FARROLL AV ARGD 93420 714-G6
FARROLL RD GBCH 93433 714-D6
FASANO WY SBAR 93105 995-E3
FAVA CT SLOC 93465 553-A3
FAWN LN SLOC 93446 469-D2
FAWN PL SBAR 93105 985-E7
FAWN CANYON RD StBC 93460 901-C4
FEARN AV SLOC 93402 631-F6
FEATHERHILL RD StBC 93108 997-D1
FEED MILL RD SLOC 93405 653-J1; SLOC 93405 654-A1
FEIJOA PL Npmo 93444 755-G1
FEIN AV PSRS 93446 513-F2
FELICIA DR SMRA 93455 796-G6
FELICIA WY SLO 93401 674-C1
FELICITY WY Npmo 93444 756-C4
FELLOWSHIP CIR SBAR 93109 995-G5
FELLOWSHIP LN SBAR 93109 995-H5
FELLOWSHIP RD SBAR 93109 995-G6
FEL MAR DR SLO 93405 653-G2
FELTON WY SLO 93405 653-H2
FERN DR Cmbr 93428 548-G1
FERN LN StBC 93437 875-H3; StBC 93455 816-J2
FERN ST SLOC 93445 734-G1
FERNALD POINT LN StBC 93108 997-A4
FERNANDEZ RD SLO 93405 653-H5
FERN CANYON LN SLOC 93401 693-F3
FERNDALE DR StBC 93455 816-H1
FERNDALE RD SLOC 93420 735-B4
FERNVIEW ST StBC 93455 816-J3
FERNWOOD DR SLO 93401 654-C6
FERRARA WY SBAR 93105 995-E2
FERRASCI RD Cmbr 93428 528-J6
FERRELL AV SLOC 93402 631-G6
FERRELO PL SBAR 93103 996-C2
FERRELO RD SBAR 93103 996-B2
FERRINI RD SLO 93405 653-H2; SLOC 93405 653-H2
FERRO LN PSRS 93446 513-H5
FERRO CARRIL RD ATAS 93422 553-G7
FERROCARRIL RD ATAS 93422 553-F5
N FERROCARRIL RD ATAS 93422 553-E5
FESLER ST SMRA 93454 776-F7; SMRA 93458 776-F7
E FESLER ST SMRA 93454 776-H7; SMRA 93454 777-A7
FIDDLENECK LN SLOC 93424 693-B2
FIELDSTONE CIR PSRS 93446 534-B1
FIELDSTONE LN SMRA 93454 777-A7
FIELDVIEW PL ARGD 93420 715-B5
FIERO LN SLOC 93401 674-B2
FIESTA DR CARP 93013 1018-E1
FIESTA WY SMRA 93458 776-F4
FIFE LN StBC 93108 997-C2
FIFE PL StBC 93108 997-C2
FIFTH AVDR SMRA 93458 776-G3
FIG AV SBAR 93101 996-B4
FIG ST MOBY 93442 611-F7
FIGUEROA ST SBAR 93101 995-J4; SBAR 93101 996-A3
W FIGUEROA ST SBAR 93101 995-J5
FIGUEROA MOUNTAIN RD StBC 93441 900-H3
FILAMINA ST SMRA 93454 777-A6
FILAREE WY SLOC 93453 695-E2
FILBERT ST PSRS 93446 513-E5
FINCH ST SLOC 93465 553-D2
FINNEY RD Cmbr 93428 548-J2
E FINNEY ST Summ 93067 997-D4
W FINNEY ST Summ 93067 997-D4
FINNIANS WY Npmo 93444 756-A3
FIR AV LMPC 93436 916-C2; MOBY 93442 611-E2; SLVG 93463 920-E7
E FIR AV LMPC 93436 916-F3
W FIR AV LMPC 93436 916-C3
FIR PL Npmo 93444 756-B4
FIR ST GDLP 93434 775-A6; StBC 93437 855-E6
FIREFIGHTER RD StBC 93429 855-H5; StBC 93437 855-G5
FIREFOX DR SMRA 93455 796-J7
FIREHOUSE CANYON RD SLOC 93424 693-B2
FIRENZE PL SBAR 93105 995-E3
FIRE ROCK LP SLOC 93446 533-H3
FIRESTONE CT SMRA 93455 796-G6
FIRESTONE RD SBAR 93117 994-C2
FIRESTONE WY StBC 93436 876-F5
FIRETHORN LN PSRS 93446 514-A6; StBC 93437 875-J3
FIR TREE PL GOL 93117 993-F1
FIRTREE WY SLOC 93446 533-E6
FISHER CT SLOC 93465 553-E1
FISHERMANS CT SLOC 93446 471-A6
FIVE CITIES DR PBCH 93449 714-D3
FIXLINI ST SLO 93401 654-B4
FJORD DR SLVG 93463 940-D1
FLAG WY PSRS 93446 534-A1
FLAGSTONE CIR StBC 93437 855-F7
FLAGSTONE DR StBC 93455 816-F5
FLEMING LN StBC 93455 796-H7
FLETCHER AV SBAR 93105 995-G2; SLO 93401 654-B5
FLETCHER RD StBC 93441 922-A3
FLORA RD ARGD 93420 715-C4
FLORA ST SLO 93401 654-B5
FLORA WY SMRA 93458 796-G4
FLORADALE AV StBC 93436 896-A6; StBC 93436 916-A1
FLORAL DR SLVG 93463 920-E7
FLORA VISTA DR SBAR 93109 995-G6
FLORENCE AV SLO 93401 654-A5
FLORENCE ST SLOC 93465 553-D2
FLORES AV SLOC 93430 591-B5
FLORES RD ATAS 93422 573-G4
FLORETTE DR StBC 93455 817-B4
FLORIN ST PBCH 93449 693-E5
FLOWER AV GDLP 93434 775-B6; StBC 93434 775-B6
FLOWER ST StBC 93455 816-H1
FLOYD CT SMRA 93454 777-B5
FLYING ARROW WY SLOC 93446 470-A4
FLYROD DR SLOC 93446 471-D2
FONTANA SLO 93401 653-H7
FONTANA RD PSRS 93446 514-B7
E FOOTHILL BLVD SLO 93405 653-H2
W FOOTHILL BLVD SLO 93405 653-E3; SLOC 93405 653-E3
FOOTHILL LN SBAR 93105 986-A7
FOOTHILL RD PBCH 93449 693-J7; StBC 93254 806-B7
FOOTHILL RD Rt#-192 CARP 93013 998-D5; SBAR 93105 985-D6; SBAR 93105 986-A7; SBAR 93110 985-D6; StBC 93013 997-G3; StBC 93013 998-A4; StBC 93105 985-D6; StBC 93105 986-A7; StBC 93110 985-D6
FORBES PL SMRA 93455 796-J6
FORDHAM PL GOL 93117 993-H3
FOREMAN CT SLO 93405 653-F7
FOREMASTER LN GBCH 93433 714-E4
FOREST AV SLOC 93465 553-D1
FOREST CIR StBC 93455 816-J4
FOREST DR GOL 93117 993-G1
FOREST GLEN DR ARGD 93420 714-H6
FORGE RD StBC 93108 997-C2
FORMOSA ST MOBY 93442 611-E2
FORTINI PL PSRS 93446 533-E4; SLOC 93446 533-E4
FORTUNA CT ARGD 93420 715-B4; SLO 93405 653-D7
FORTUNA LN StBC 93117 993-J5
FORTUNA RD StBC 93117 993-J5
FORTUNATO WY SBAR 93105 995-E3
E FOSTER RD StBC 93455 816-J3; StBC 93455 817-A3
W FOSTER RD SMRA 93455 816-F3
FOUNDERS AV StBC 93455 817-A2
FOUNTAIN AV SLOC 93445 714-E7; SLOC 93445 734-E1
FOUNTAIN DR StBC 93455 817-A3
FOUR PAWS WY SLOC 93446 534-G6
FOWLER LN SLOC 93420 734-H5
FOWLER RD SBAR 93117 994-D3; StBC 93117 994-D3
FOXBURROW CT StBC 93455 816-G4
FOX CANYON LN SLOC 93420 695-B7
FOXEN CT StBC 93455 816-F4
FOXEN DR SBAR 93105 985-F7
FOXEN LN StBC 93440 878-H2
FOXEN BLUFF LN SLOC 93420 735-A2
FOXEN CANYON LN SLOC 93424 693-B1
FOXEN CANYON RD StBC 93441 900-F2; StBC 93454 797-J6; StBC 93463 900-F2
FOXENWOOD CIR SMRA 93455 816-G4
FOXENWOOD DR StBC 93455 816-E4
FOXENWOOD LN SMRA 93455 816-G3; StBC 93455 816-G4
FOX HILLS RD SLOC 93446 513-C3
FOX HOLLOW RD SLOC 93401 654-C2
FOXTAIL LN SLOC 93465 533-C7; SLOC 93465 553-C1
FRADY LN PBCH 93449 714-C2
FRAMBUESA DR SLO 93405 653-D6
FRANCES ST PSRS 93446 514-A6; StBC 93111 994-J2
FRANCES WY PBCH 93449 714-F3
FRANCESCHI RD SBAR 93103 996-B1
FRANCIA ST SLOC 93420 714-H7
FRANCINE LN StBC 93455 816-J2
FRANCIS AV SLO 93401 654-A6
FRANCIS LN SMRA 93455 796-J5
FRANCIS WY Npmo 93444 756-F2
FRANCISCAN CT CARP 93013 998-B6
FRANCISCO DR SBAR 93105 985-F5
FRANK CT Npmo 93444 756-A4
FRANK LN SMRA 93458 776-F6
FRANKIE LN SLOC 93420 735-C5; SLOC 93465 553-E1
FRANKLIN DR PBCH 93449 714-B1
FRANKLIN RD StBC 93455 817-A4
FRANKLIN RANCH RD GOL 93117 984-D6; StBC 93117 984-D6
FRAZIER LN StBC 93110 994-J2
FREDENSBORG WY SLVG 93463 920-E6; StBC 93463 920-E6
FREDENSBORG CANYON RD SLVG 93463 920-E6; StBC 93463 920-E6
FREDERICK AV SLO 93401 654-A6
FREDERICK ST SMRA 93455 796-J6; SMRA 93455 797-A6
FREDERICKS ST SLO 93405 653-J2; SLO 93405 654-A2
FREDRICH DR StBC 93436 896-G2
FREEAR DR BLTN 93427 919-J5
FREEDOM PL BLTN 93427 919-H6
FREEHAVEN DR StBC 93108 997-F2
FREEMAN LN SLOC 93402 632-A6
FREEMAN PL GOL 93117 993-G3
FREESIA DR Summ 93067 997-E4
FRWY U.S.-101 ATAS - 553-E5; ATAS - 573-F1; ATAS - 574-A4; ATAS - 594-B1; SLOC - 553-E5; SLOC - 594-C3
FREMONT LN StBC 93105 964-F1
FREMONT PL SBAR 93101 996-A5
FREMONT ST SMRA 93454 777-B5
FRESNO AV ATAS 93422 573-H2; MOBY 93442 611-G7; SLOC 93405 632-J5; SLOC 93430 590-J1; SLOC 93430 591-A2
FRESNO ST PBCH 93449 714-C1; PSRS 93446 513-E6; SLOC 93402 631-E6
FRESNO WY SLOC 93451 453-D6
FREYA DR SLVG 93463 940-E1
FRIAR LN SBAR 93105 985-E7
FRIENDSHIP LN StBC 93463 920-J7
FRISCO WY SLOC 93420 735-G5
FROG HOLLOW DR SLOC 93422 593-B1
FROG POND PL SLOC 93422 593-B1
E FRONT RD ATAS 93422 574-B7
W FRONT RD ATAS 93422 574-A6
FRONT ST GBCH 93433 714-D4; MOBY 93442 611-F5; SLOC 93424 693-A4; SLOC 93445 734-F1
FRONT ST Rt#-1 SLOC 93445 714-E7; SLOC 93445 734-E1
FRONTAGE RD StBC 93110 995-D1; StBC 93455 817-A2
N FRONTAGE RD Npmo 93444 735-J7; Npmo 93444 756-B2; SLOC 93420 735-H5
S FRONTAGE RD Npmo 93444 756-B3
FRONTIER WY SLOC 93465 533-C7; SLOC 93465 553-C1
FROSTY WY SMRA 93455 796-J7
FUENTE PL SLOC 93422 594-E4
FUENTE DEL ORO ATAS 93422 553-H6
FUERA LN StBC 93108 997-A1
FULLER RD SLO 93401 674-C2; SLOC 93401 674-C2; SLOC 93446 469-H4
FUNSTON AV SLO 93401 654-A6
FURUKAWA WY SMRA 93458 796-E2
FUTURA LN SLOC 93420 735-G6

G

G ST SLOC 93430 590-J2; SLOC 93430 591-A2
G ST Rt#-58 SLOC 93453 614-F3
N G ST LMPC 93436 896-E6; LMPC 93436 916-E1
S G ST LMPC 93436 916-E2
GABLE LN SMRA 93458 796-G4
GAGE IRVING RD SLOC 93446 469-G4
GAHAN PL PSRS 93446 533-E4; SLOC 93446 533-E4
GAIL PL SLO 93401 654-A6
GAINE ST Cmbr 93428 548-F2
GAIT WY SLOC 93420 735-A2
GALAXY ST Npmo 93444 756-A6
GALAXY WY StBC 93436 876-D5
GALLANT PL SLOC 93401 674-E6
GALLEON WY SLO 93405 653-F7
GALLINA CT ATAS 93422 573-D5
GAMBLE LN PSRS 93446 513-H2
GAMBY WY SLVG 93463 920-E7; StBC 93427 919-H1
GANADOR CT SLO 93401 653-J6
GANCHO AV ATAS 93422 573-J2
GARBADA RD ATAS 93422 574-B3
GARCERO RD ATAS 93422 573-A1
GARCIA SLOC 93430 591-B5
GARCIA AV SLOC 93430 591-C5
GARCIA DR SLO 93405 653-F7; SLO 93405 673-F1
GARCIA RD ATAS 93422 553-D6; SBAR 93103 996-B2; SLOC 93422 553-D6
GARDEN AL SLO 93401 653-J4
GARDEN CT StBC 93437 855-E7
GARDEN DR SMRA 93458 776-H4
GARDEN LN StBC 93108 986-G7; StBC 93108 996-G1
GARDEN ST ARGD 93420 715-A5; SBAR 93101 995-J2; SBAR 93101 996-A3; SBAR 93105 995-J2; SLO 93401 653-J4; SLO 93401 654-A5; SLOC 93402 631-F5; StBC 93463 920-H2
GARDENGATE LN StBC 93436 896-E3
GARDENIA AV LMPC 93436 896-F7
GARDENIA CIR PSRS 93446 513-H7
GARDENIA CT PSRS 93446 513-H7
GARDENIA ST LMPC 93436 896-F5
GARDENIA WY Npmo 93444 756-A3
GARFIELD PL ARGD 93420 714-G7
GARFIELD ST SLO 93401 654-A3
GARIBALDI AV SLO 93401 654-B6
GARNET WY SMRA 93454 777-A7
GARNETTE DR SLO 93405 653-E7
GARRETT LN SLOC 93420 754-J2
GARRETT ST GDLP 93434 774-J6; StBC 93455 816-G6
GARY PL SLOC 93401 674-E6
GARY WY SLOC 93451 453-D6
GARZA CT ATAS 93422 594-C2
GASOLINE ALLEY PL SLOC 93420 754-J2; SLOC 93420 755-A2
GATE WY StBC 93110 985-A7
GATES CT PSRS 93446 513-H6
GATEWAY DR SLOC 93446 471-D6
GATEWOOD WY SMRA 93454 777-B7
GATHE DR SLO 93405 653-E7
GATO AV GOL 93117 994-E2
GATO CANYON RD StBC 93105 982-E4; StBC 93117 982-E4
GAUCHO CT SLOC 93465 553-E1
GAUCHO WY SMRA 93458 776-F4
GAVANZA RD ATAS 93422 593-E3; SLOC 93422 593-E3
GAVILAN RD SLOC 93422 593-F3
GAVIOTA ST GOL 93117 994-E2; StBC 93441 900-G5; StBC 93463 900-G5
GAY DR BLTN 93427 919-J5
GAYLENE DR SMRA 93458 776-F4
GAYLEY WK StBC 93117 993-J4
GAYNFAIR TER ARGD 93420 714-H7
GAZELLE WY StBC 93455 816-G7
GEM CT SMRA 93454 777-A7
GEMINI AV StBC 93436 876-D5
GENOA WY StBC 93455 817-B4
GENTLE BREEZE WY SLOC 93420 734-H7
GENUINE RISK RD StBC 93460 922-C5
GEORGE DR StBC 93455 817-A5
GEORGE LN StBC 93455 816-H6
GEORGE ST SLO 93401 654-A5
GEORGE WY Npmo 93444 755-G3
GEORGE MILLER DR LMPC 93436 896-D5
GEORGETOWN RD GOL 93117 993-H3
GEORGIA AV SLOC 93405 633-A5
GERARD DR GOL 93117 993-F1
GERDA ST SLO 93401 654-B5
GERMAINE WY PSRS 93446 514-B2
GERONA WY StBC 93110 985-A7
GERTIE PL Npmo 93444 756-A4
GIBRALTAR RD SBAR 93105 986-C6; StBC 93103 986-C6; StBC 93105 986-C1
GIBSON LN SMRA 93454 796-H2
GIBSON RD SLOC 93465 553-E1
GILARDI RD SLOC 93405 632-G2
GILBERT AV SLOC 93430 591-C5
GILBERT ST MOBY 93442 611-E2
GILEA CT SMRA 93455 796-H5
GILEAD LN PSRS 93446 514-A4
GILLESPIE ST SBAR 93101 995-H4
GILLESPIE WY SBAR 93101 995-H4
GINA CT PSRS 93446 513-J4
GINGER LN PSRS 93446 514-A7
GINGKO CT SMRA 93458 776-G3
GIUSEPPE WY SLOC 93420 734-G5
GLACIER LN StBC 93455 817-E5
GLADE AV SLOC 93445 714-E7; SLOC 93445 734-E1
GLEASON ST Cmbr 93428 548-J2
GLEN AV StBC 93455 816-H1
GLEN CT PSRS 93446 513-E5
GLEN WY SLVG 93463 940-E2
GLEN ALBYN DR StBC 93105 985-H7
GLEN ANNIE RD GOL 93117 993-H1; StBC 93117 983-G3; StBC 93117 993-H1
GLENBROOK PL SLOC 93446 471-C3
GLENBROOK ST StBC 93110 994-J2; StBC 93111 994-J2
GLEN CAIRON DR StBC 93455 816-J5
GLENCREST LN PSRS 93446 513-F3
GLENDESSARY LN SBAR 93105 985-H7; StBC 93105 985-H7
GLEN EAGLES DR StBC 93455 816-J5
GLEN ELLEN CT LMPC 93436 896-C6
GLEN ELLEN LN LMPC 93436 896-C6; StBC 93455 817-A2
GLENGARY RD StBC 93460 921-A6; StBC 93463 921-A6
GLENHAVEN PL Npmo 93444
GLENN AV SLOC 93405
GLENN RD StBC 93105
GLENN ST SLOC 93402
GLENNHEIN CT SLOC 93401
GLENNORA WY BLTN 93427
GLENOAK DR ARGD 93420
GLEN OAKS CT StBC 93455
GLEN OAKS DR StBC 93108
GLENRIDGE LN StBC 93455
GLENVIEW CT StBC 93437
GLENVIEW DR StBC 93455
GLENVIEW LN SLOC 93401
GLENVIEW RD StBC 93108
GLENWOOD DR StBC 93455
GLINES AV StBC 93455
GLORIA CIR LMPC 93436
GLORY ST Npmo 93444
GOBBLER HILL RD SLOC 93446
GOBERNADOR CANYON RD StBC 93013; StBC 93013
GODDARD DR StBC 93436
GODELL ST SLOC 93465
GOLD CREST DR Npmo 93444
GOLDEN DR SMRA 93458
GOLDENEYE LN SLOC 93424
GOLDEN GATE AV Summ 93067
GOLDEN GROVE CT SLOC 93420
GOLDEN HAWK LN SLOC 93420
GOLDEN HILL RD PSRS 93446; SLOC 93446
GOLDEN LEAF LN Npmo 93444
GOLDEN LEAF ST Npmo 93444
GOLDEN MEADOW DR SLOC 93446
GOLDEN OAK LN SLOC 93420
GOLDENROD LN SLO 93401
GOLDEN WEST PL ARGD 93420
GOLDFIELD CT GOL 93117
GOLD RUSH LN SLOC 93446
GOLDSMITH CT SMRA 93454
GOLF PL PSRS 93446
GOLF RD SBAR 93108; StBC 93108
GOLF BALL RD Npmo 93444
GOLF COURSE LN Npmo 93444
GOLONDRINA CT ATAS 93422
GOLPA DR StBC 93463
GONZALES DR StBC 93440
GONZALES LN StBC 93440
GOODCHILD LN SMRA 93455
GOODLAND ST StBC 93455
GOODMAN CT PSRS 93446
GOODWIN RD StBC 93455
GOOSEBERRY CIR SLOC 93426
GOOSEFOOT CT SLOC 93424
GOPHER GLEN WY SLOC 93402
GORRION WY ATAS 93422
GOSHAWK LN SLOC 93420
GOSSIP ROCK RD Npmo 93444
GOUGH AV SLOC 93465
GOULD LN StBC 93108
GRACE LN ARGD 93420; Npmo 93444
GRACIA WY SLOC 93420
GRACIOSA RD StBC 93455
GRADE MOUNTAIN WY Npmo 93444
GRANA PL SLOC 93451
GRANACHE WY SLOC 93465
GRANADA CIR StBC 93110
GRANADA DR SLO 93401
GRANADA ST SMRA 93458

City ZIP Pg-Grid
DA WY
CARP 93013 998-E6
StBC 93110 985-A7
AV
SBAR 93103 995-J1
SBAR 93103 996-A2
SLO 93401 654-A2
SLO 93405 654-A2
SLOC 93405 654-A2
StBC 93441 900-H6
D AV
ARGD 93420 714-H5
ARGD 93433 714-H5
GBCH 93433 714-H5
D AV Rt#-227
ARGD 93420 714-J5
ND AV
GBCH 93433 714-D5
CT
StBC 93455 816-J6
CANYON DR
PSRS 93446 514-A6
E AV
Npmo 93444 756-A4
VIEW DR
GBCH 93433 714-E4
E RD
SLOC 93465 533-F7
AV
SLOC 93420 735-D4
RD
StBC 93429 855-H1
ST
SMRA 93454 776-H5
SMRA 93458 776-G5
VINE RD
SMRA 93454 777-A6
VINE WY
SLOC 93465 553-B3
A DR
StBC 93111 984-G7
VALLEY WY
SMRA 93454 777-B6
Y HOLLOW WY
PSRS 93446 514-A6
S AV
SLO 93401 654-A3
SLO 93405 654-A2
S CREEK RD
ATAS 93422 573-E4
LLA DR
SBAR 93109 996-A6
AV
SBAR 93101 996-C4
ST
StBC 93455 816-G6
FOX LN
SLOC 93446 471-B5
CT
PSRS 93446 534-A1
LN
SBAR 93105 995-J2
StBC 93108 997-A3
PL
SLOC 93420 734-J3
SLOC 93420 735-A3
ST
Cmbr 93428 548-H1
ACRE DR
StBC 93455 816-J1
BRIAR CT
StBC 93455 816-J2
BRIAR LN
SLOC 93446 471-D6
BRIER PL
SLOC 93401 674-J5
BRIER RD
StBC 93436 876-E5
BROOK LN
SLOC 93446 471-D6
CASTLE CIR
StBC 93111 994-J2
DALE CT
StBC 93110 985-A7
FIELD AV
SLOC 93420 734-H7
SLOC 93420 754-H1
FIELD RD
StBC 93463 920-E6
GATE RD
SLOC 93401 694-G1
HEART CIR
SLOC 93420 735-B7
HILL WY
StBC 93110 985-A7
LEAF CT
GOL 93117 993-J3
LEAF LN
Npmo 93444 756-A4
MEADOW RD
StBC 93108 996-H1
OAKS DR
SLOC 93402 631-H7
PINE LN
SLOC 93446 471-B6
RIDGE CT
StBC 93455 816-F4
RIDGE LN
SBAR 93103 996-C1
SBORO LN
SLOC 93401 674-D6
SBORO ST
GOL 93117 993-G3
STONE LN
SMRA 93454 777-C7
TREE LN
StBC 93455 816-J4
WAY RD
StBC 93110 985-A7
WELL AV
StBC 93108 997-D3
Summ 93067 997-D3
WELL LN
SBAR 93105 995-G3
WOOD AV
MOBY 93442 611-E2
WOOD DR
ARGD 93420 715-C4
PSRS 93446 513-E5
WOOD RD
StBC 93455 816-B1
WORTH PL
StBC 93108 996-J3
GORY WY
SBAR 93105 995-E1
ORY AV
PSRS 93446 513-G4
ORY CT
SLO 93401 654-C6

STREET Name City ZIP Pg-Grid
GREGORY CT
SMRA 93454 777-A6
GRELL LN
SLOC 93445 714-G7
SLOC 93445 734-G1
GRENOBLE RD
StBC 93110 985-A7
GRETA PL
SLO 93401 654-B6
GREYSTONE CT
StBC 93455 816-G4
GREYSTONE PL
SLOC 93401 674-D6
GREYSTONE WY
Cmbr 93428 528-F6
GRIEB DR
ARGD 93420 714-G3
GRIFFIN ST
GBCH 93433 714-E6
GRIGGS PL
SBAR 93117 994-D2
GROVE CT
ARGD 93420 715-B5
GROVE LN
SBAR 93105 985-E7
SBAR 93105 995-E1
GROVE ST
Cmbr 93428 528-F6
Npmo 93444 756-C3
PSRS 93446 513-E6
SLO 93401 654-A3
SLOC 93402 631-F6
GUADALUPE AV
StBC 93437 855-D7
StBC 93437 875-D1
GUADALUPE RD
SLOC 93420 735-B7
SLOC 93420 755-B1
GUADALUPE RD Rt#-1
SLOC 93420 755-B2
GUADALUPE ST Rt#-1
GDLP 93434 775-A6
GUAM AV
StBC 93437 875-E3
GUANTE CIR
StBC 93111 984-F7
GUAVA AV
GOL 93117 994-C1
E GUAVA AV
LMPC 93436 916-G1
W GUAVA AV
LMPC 93436 916-C1
GUERNSEY CT
PSRS 93446 533-H1
GUERRA LN
SLOC 93405 653-D3
GUILDFORD DR
Cmbr 93428 528-E6
GULARTE LN
GDLP 93434 775-B5
GULARTE RD
ARGD 93420 715-B3
GULF ST
SLO 93405 653-F6
GUNDERSON LN
SMRA 93458 776-G5
GUNNER ST
SMRA 93458 776-F6
GUS WY
SLOC 93420 735-C3
GUSTA RD
ATAS 93422 574-B6
GUTIERREZ ST
SBAR 93101 996-C4
SBAR 93103 996-C3
GWEN PL
SLOC 93445 714-G7
GWYNE AV
StBC 93111 994-G3

H

H ST
SLOC 93430 591-A2
SLOC 93453 614-F3
N H ST Rt#-1
LMPC 93436 896-E5
LMPC 93436 916-E1
StBC 93436 896-E5
S H ST
LMPC 93436 916-E2
HACIENDA AV
SLOC 93401 674-C5
HACIENDA CIR
PSRS 93446 514-A5
HACIENDA DR
ARGD 93420 715-A7
SBAR 93105 995-F3
SLOC 93430 591-C4
HACIENDA LN
SLOC 93446 469-J6
HACIENDA WY
SBAR 93105 995-F3
SMRA 93458 776-F4
HACKBERRY LN
StBC 93437 855-H7
HACKNEY WY
SLOC 93446 471-D5
HADDON DR
Cmbr 93428 548-G1
HADLEY WY
StBC 93455 816-H1
HAGER LN
StBC 93427 919-H2
HAGERMAN DR
SMRA 93455 796-F7
SMRA 93455 816-F1
HAGGERTY WY
Npmo 93444 756-C1
HAIDA ST
CARP 93013 998-E6
HAINES AV
SLOC 93430 591-C5
HAL ST
SMRA 93454 777-A6
HALCON RD
ATAS 93422 574-D7
ATAS 93422 594-D1
ATAS 93432 574-D7
SLOC 93432 574-D7
HALCYON LN
SBAR 93101 995-G4
HALCYON RD
SLOC 93420 714-H7
SLOC 93420 734-H1
SLOC 93420 735-A5
N HALCYON RD
ARGD 93420 714-H5
S HALCYON RD
ARGD 93420 714-H6
SLOC 93420 714-H6
HALE CREEK RD
SLOC - 593-E5
SLOC 93422 593-E5
SLOC 93453 614-A3
HALES LN
CARP 93013 998-E7
HALEY ST
SBAR 93101 996-B4
SBAR 93103 996-B4
HALKIRK ST
StBC 93110 994-J2
HAMILTON LN
StBC 93455 817-C7
HAMMOND DR
StBC 93108 996-J4
HAMPSHIRE LN
StBC 93455 817-A2
HAMPSHIRE PL
StBC 93455 816-F4
HAMPTON CT
SLOC 93422 594-D2
HAMPTON DR
StBC 93455 796-H7
HAMPTON LN
SLOC 93446 493-A7
SLOC 93446 513-A1
HAMPTON PL
ARGD 93420 714-G6
HANA LN
Npmo 93444 755-H2
HANCOCK AV
SMRA 93454 796-J3
SMRA 93454 797-A3
HANCOCK DR
LMPC 93436 896-D3
StBC 93436 896-D3
HANFORD ST
PBCH 93449 714-B1
HANGAR ST
SMRA 93455 796-E7
HANGING TREE LN
SLOC 93446 533-J5
SLOC 93446 534-A6
SLOC 93465 534-A6
HANKS PL
SLOC 93446 494-F2
HANNA DR
StBC 93111 984-F7
HANOVER PL
SLOC 93401 674-D6
HANOVER WY
SMRA 93458 776-G3
HANS PL
Npmo 93444 736-B7
HANSEN LN
SLOC 93401 654-D7
SLOC 93401 674-D1
HANSON RD
PSRS 93446 514-D7
PSRS 93446 534-D2
SLOC 93446 514-D7
SLOC 93446 534-D2
HANSON WY
SMRA 93458 776-E7
SMRA 93458 796-E2
StBC 93458 776-E7
StBC 93458 796-E2
HANSON HILL RD
SLOC 93420 715-C1
HAPPY CANYON RD
StBC 93105 922-E3
StBC 93441 922-E3
StBC 93460 921-J6
StBC 93460 922-E3
HAPPY HUNTING CIR
SLOC 93446 471-C7
HARBOR CIR
SLOC 93446 471-A5
HARBOR DR
CARP 93013 998-A5
HARBOR ST
MOBY 93442 611-F6
HARBOR WY
SBAR 93109 996-B6
HARBOR HILLS DR
SBAR 93109 995-J6
HARBOR HILLS LN
SBAR 93109 995-J6
HARBOR LIGHTS LN
SLOC 93424 693-A3
HARBOR VIEW DR
SBAR 93103 996-E3
SBAR 93108 996-E3
HARBOR VIEW ST
PBCH 93449 714-B2
HARDEN ST
ARGD 93420 715-A4
HARDING AV
SMRA 93454 776-H5
SMRA 93454 777-A5
W HARDING AV
SMRA 93454 776-G5
SMRA 93458 776-F5
HARDING DR
SLOC 93445 714-D7
HARDINGE AV
Summ 93067 997-C3
HARFORD CANYON RD
SLOC 93424 693-A3
HARLEY DR
SLOC 93465 553-E1
HARLOE AV
PBCH 93449 714-B2
HARMON ST
SBAR 93103 996-E4
HARMONY LN
SLOC 93420 715-D1
StBC 93455 817-B4
HARMONY WY
SLOC 93401 654-D6
HARNESS CT
SLOC 93465 553-E1
HARP RD
StBC 93455 817-A6
HARPER CT
SMRA 93454 776-J5
HARRIER LN
Npmo 93444 756-B4
HARRIS DR
StBC 93436 896-G2
HARRIS ST
SLO 93401 653-J5
HARRIS GRADE RD
StBC 93436 876-G3
StBC 93436 896-E3
StBC 93455 876-G3
HARRISON DR
SMRA 93454 777-B6
HARRISON ST
ARGD 93420 715-A4
HARROLD AV
StBC 93110 985-D7
HARSIN LN
StBC 93455 816-H2
HART DR
SMRA 93454 776-J7
SMRA 93454 796-J1
HART LN
ARGD 93420 714-J5
ARGD 93420 715-A5
HARTFORD ST
Cmbr 93428 528-F6
HARTLEY PL
SMRA 93455 796-J4
SMRA 93455 797-A6
HARTNELL RD
StBC 93455 816-F5
StBC 93455 816-G5
HARTZELL CT
SLOC 93422 593-B1
HARVARD LN
StBC 93111 984-G7
StBC 93111 994-G1
HARVEST PL
Npmo 93444 756-A3
HARVEST WY
SLOC 93422 594-E6
HARVEST MEADOW PL
PSRS 93446 534-B2
HARVEST RIDGE WY
SLOC 93446 534-G1
HARVEY ST
Cmbr 93428 548-F2
HASKIN ST
SLO 93401 654-A5
HASLAM DR
SMRA 93454 796-H2
HASS LN
SLOC 93445 714-G7
HASSET CT
StBC 93455 816-H1
HASTINGS DR
GOL 93117 984-C7
HASTINGS ST
Cmbr 93428 528-E6
HATHWAY AV
SLO 93405 653-J2
SLO 93405 654-A2
HATTERAS ST
MOBY 93442 611-D2
HAVENCREST DR
StBC 93455 817-B6
HAVEN HILL WY
SLOC 93420 736-B1
HAWK CANYON CT
BLTN 93427 920-A6
HAWKINS CT
ARGD 93420 715-A5
HAWKINS WY
SMRA 93455 796-J6
HAWK VIEW CT
SLOC 93420 715-A7
SLOC 93420 735-B1
HAWLEY ST
SLOC 93465 553-D2
HAWTHORN ST
SMRA 93458 776-G3
StBC 93437 855-H7
HAWTHORNE LN
Npmo 93444 735-H5
HAWTHORNE ST
LMPC 93436 916-F2
HAY BARN LN
SLOC 93405 653-C3
HAYS ST
SLO 93405 654-A2
HAZEL DR
SLO 93405 653-E7
HAZEL LN
Npmo 93444 756-A5
HAZELNUT ST
StBC 93437 855-H7
HEADWATERS RD
SLOC 93465 533-E7
SLOC 93465 553-E1
HEARST CT
SMRA 93454 777-B6
HEARTHSTONE DR
SMRA 93454 777-C7
HEARTS PL
SLOC 93446 493-F2
HEATH LN
Cmbr 93428 528-E6
HEATH ST
StBC 93437 855-H7
StBC 93437 875-H1
HEATHER CIR
StBC 93455 817-A4
HEATHER CT
Npmo 93444 756-B4
SLOC 93465 553-C1
HEATHER LN
StBC 93437 875-H3
HEATHERWOOD LN
StBC 93455 817-B6
HEDLEY DR
SLO 93405 653-E7
HEIDI CT
PSRS 93446 513-H4
SMRA 93454 777-B6
HEIDI PL
SLOC 93420 735-B3
HEIDI WY
SLOC 93446 493-E6
HELEN ST
PSRS 93446 513-J6
HELEN WY
Npmo 93444 756-G6
HELENA AV
SBAR 93101 996-B4
SLOC 93453 614-F3
HELENA ST
SLO 93401 654-B5
SLOC 93420 714-H7
StBC 93440 878-G2
HELGREN CT
SLOC 93465 553-B1
HELROY RD
SLOC 93420 735-E6
HEMI RD
SLOC 93420 735-F3
HEMINGWAY LN
SLOC 93465 553-B3
HEMLOCK AV
MOBY 93442 611-F2
HEMLOCK PL
StBC 93111 994-J1
HEMLOCK ST
StBC 93437 855-E7
HEMLOCK WY
StBC 93455 816-H4
E HEMLOCK WY
StBC 93455 816-H4
W HEMLOCK WY
StBC 93455 816-H4
HEMPSTEAD AV
GOL 93117 993-F2
HENDERSON LN
SLOC 93445 734-G1
HENDERSON ST
SLO 93401 654-B3
SLO 93405 654-B2
HENDRICKS RANCH RD
SLOC 93446 469-G5
HENNING DR
StBC 93441 900-H5
HENRIETTA AV
SLOC 93402 631-F6
HENRY AV
SMRA 93455 796-J5
SMRA 93455 797-A5
HENRY CT
StBC 93440 878-G1
HENRY ST
SLO 93401 654-A5
HERADO AV
StBC 93437 875-D1
HERCULES AV
StBC 93436 876-D5
HERDSMAN WY
SLOC 93465 533-C5
HEREDIA ST
SMRA 93455 796-J6
HEREFORD LN
SLOC 93446 533-H2
HERENCIA CT
ATAS 93422 594-C2
HERITAGE LN
SLOC 93420 714-J1
StBC 93440 878-J2
HERITAGE RD
SLOC 93446 471-A4
HERITAGE LOOP RD
SLOC 93446 471-B3
HERMOSA AV
ATAS 93422 573-H5
HERMOSA CT
GBCH 93433 714-F6
LMPC 93436 916-B2
StBC 93437 855-E6
HERMOSA DR
PBCH 93449 693-E5
SMRA 93458 776-F6
HERMOSA RD
SBAR 93105 995-G1
HERMOSA ST
SMRA 93454 776-H6
SMRA 93458 776-G6
HERMOSA WY
SLO 93405 653-G3
HERMOSA VISTA WY
SLOC 93420 734-H4
HERMOSILLA AV
ATAS 93422 573-G2
HERMOSILLO RD
SBAR 93108 996-G3
StBC 93108 996-G3
HERNANDEZ DR
GDLP 93434 774-J6
HERON CT
GOL 93117 993-F3
HERON LN
SLOC 93446 469-F2
HERON POINT DR
SLOC 93446 469-G3
HESPERIAN LN
Cmbr 93428 528-G7
HETRICK AV
Npmo 93444 735-G6
Npmo 93444 755-H1
SLOC 93420 735-G5
HIAWATHA LN
SLOC 93420 714-H7
HIBISCUS CT
Npmo 93444 755-J3
Npmo 93444 756-A3
StBC 93455 817-A3
HIBISCUS LN
StBC 93437 875-J3
HIBISCUS ST
SLOC 93445 734-G1
E HICKORY AV
LMPC 93436 916-E2
W HICKORY AV
LMPC 93436 916-C2
HICKORY LN
SLOC 93446 513-D7
HICKORY ST
CARP 93013 1018-F1
StBC 93437 855-E6
HICKORY WY
SLVG 93463 940-D2
HIDALGO AV
ATAS 93422 573-J1
HIDALGO ST
SLOC 93430 591-B4
HIDDEN LN
GOL 93117 984-E6
HIDDEN CREEK CANYON DR
SLOC 93405 693-C2
HIDDEN HILLS RD
SLOC 93420 735-F6
StBC 93463 920-G2
HIDDEN OAK RD
ARGD 93420 714-J3
HIDDEN OAKS RD
SBAR 93105 995-D3
HIDDEN PINE LN
SLOC 93420 715-A1
HIDDEN PINES WY
SMRA 93458 776-G3
HIDDEN RANCH WY
SLOC 93420 735-E7
HIDDEN SPRINGS RD
SLOC 93401 674-C5
HIDDEN VALLEY LN
StBC 93108 987-G7
StBC 93108 997-F1
HIDDEN VALLEY RD
StBC 93105 964-H6
HIGH RD
StBC 93108 996-G3
HIGH ST
SLO 93401 653-J5
SLO 93401 654-A5
HIGHCASTLE LN
StBC 93455 816-G4
HIGH GROVE AV
GOL 93117 993-J3
HIGHLAND DR
PBCH 93449 714-D3
SBAR 93109 995-J5
SLO 93405 653-F1
SLOC 93402 631-F7
SLOC 93405 653-H2
StBC 93455 816-H6
HIGHLAND RD
StBC 93460 921-A5
HIGHLAND WY
GBCH 93433 714-E6
HIGHLAND HILLS RD
Npmo 93444 736-A5
HIGHLAND PARK DR
PSRS 93446 513-E4
HIGH MEADOW DR
Npmo 93444 756-A6
SLVG 93463 920-G7
StBC 93463 920-G7
HIGH MEADOW RD
SLOC 93446 470-B4
HIGH RIDGE LN
SBAR 93103 996-C1
HIGH RIDGE RD
SLOC 93446 534-H4
HIGH SCHOOL HILL RD
ATAS 93422 573-H4
HIGH VIEW DR
SLOC 93420 715-A1
HIGHWAY Rt#-46
PSRS 93446 513-J3
PSRS 93446 514-F1
PSRS 93446 533-F3
SLOC 93446 514-J1
SLOC 93446 533-E3
SLOC 93465 533-C5
HIGHWAY Rt#-135
StBC 93440 878-D1
HIGHWAY Rt#-150
CARP 93013 1018-H2
StBC 93013 1018-J1
HIGHWAY Rt#-154
StBC 93440 900-C2
StBC 93441 900-C2
StBC 93460 900-J5
StBC 93460 901-A6
StBC 93460 921-B1
StBC 93460 941-H1
HIGHWAY Rt#-166
StBC 93254 806-A1
HIGHWAY Rt#-246
BLTN - 919-H5
BLTN - 920-A6
BLTN 93427 919-F4
BLTN 93427 920-A6
StBC 93427 919-E4
StBC 93436 919-B4
StBC 93463 920-A6
HIGOS WY
Npmo 93444 756-B4
HIGUERA ST
SLO 93401 653-J4
SLO 93401 654-A3
SLO 93401 673-H1
HIGUERA ST Rt#-227
SLO 93401 653-H6
S HIGUERA ST
SLO 93401 653-H7
SLO 93401 673-G3
SLOC 93401 673-G3
SLOC 93405 673-G3
HILL CT
StBC 93455 817-A4
HILL RD
StBC 93108 996-G4
HILL ST
MOBY 93442 611-F4
Npmo 93444 756-B3
SLO 93405 653-H3
StBC 93440 878-G2
HILLCREST DR
ARGD 93420 714-G4
Cmbr 93428 528-F6
MOBY 93442 611-F5
PSRS 93446 513-E5
HILLCREST PL
SLO 93401 654-A3
HILLCREST RD
SBAR 93103 986-B7
SBAR 93103 996-B1
StBC 93460 901-D3
HILL HAVEN RD
StBC 93463 920-G7
HILLSBORO DR
SMRA 93454 777-B6
HILLSBORO ST
GOL 93117 993-G3
HILLSBORO WY
GOL 93117 993-H3
HILLSIDE CIR
StBC 93437 855-F7
HILLSIDE CT
ARGD 93420 715-B5
HILLSIDE DR
SLVG 93463 920-F7
HILLSIDE LN
SLOC 93420 694-J7
SLOC 93420 714-J1
HILLSIDE RD
SBAR 93101 995-G4
HILLTOP DR
PSRS 93446 513-E6
HILLTOP LN
SLOC 93451 473-C4
HILLTOP RD
StBC 93455 817-A3
HILLTOP WY
SLOC 93424 693-B2
HILLVIEW DR
GOL 93117 993-G1
HILLVIEW PL
SLOC 93420 755-A2
HILLVIEW RD
StBC 93455 816-J1
HILLVIEW ST
MOBY 93442 611-F4
HIND LN
SLO 93401 673-H1
HINDFELL WY
SLVG 93463 920-F7
HINDS AV
PBCH 93449 714-B3
HINDS PL
SMRA 93455 796-J6
HINES LN
SMRA 93454 796-H4
HISCHIER LN
SLOC 93420 695-C7
SLOC 93420 715-D1
HITCHCOCK WY
SBAR 93105 995-E2
HITCHCOCK RANCH RD
SBAR 93105 995-E1
HIXON RD
StBC 93108 997-A3
HOBBS LN
StBC 93455 816-H5
HOBBY HORSE RD
StBC 93463 920-J7
HODGES LN
StBC 93108 996-J1
StBC 93108 997-A1
HODGES RD
ARGD 93420 714-G3
HOGAN CT
Npmo 93444 735-D7
HOGAN PL
PSRS 93446 513-H7
PSRS 93446 533-J1
HOG CANYON RD
SLOC 93446 494-H2
SLOC 93451 494-H2
HOLDEN AV
SLOC 93445 714-F7
HOLDEN PL
Cmbr 93428 548-H2
HOLDER PARK LN
Npmo 93444 756-E7
Npmo 93444 776-D1
HOLIDAY HILL
SLOC 93446 469-H4
HOLIDAY HILL RD
StBC 93117 984-D5
HOLLEY
SLO 93401 673-H1
HOLLISTER AV
GOL 93111 994-F2
GOL 93117 993-F2
GOL 93117 994-B2
PBCH 93449 714-B2
SBAR 93117 994-B2
SLOC 93405 633-A4
StBC 93110 994-F2
StBC 93110 995-A1
StBC 93111 994-F2
StBC 93117 983-H6
HOLLISTER LN
SLOC 93402 631-J6
SLOC 93402 632-A6
HOLLISTER ST
StBC 93441 900-H5
StBC 93463 900-G5
Summ 93067 997-D3
W HOLLOW DR
SLOC 93446 513-D1
HOLLY AV
CARP 93013 998-C7
HOLLY DR
SLOC 93446 471-C3
HOLLY LN
SLVG 93463 920-G6
HOLLY RD
StBC 93105 985-J5
HOLLY ST
GDLP 93434 775-A6
HOLLY WY
PBCH 93449 714-F3
HOLLYHOCK LN
SLOC 93465 534-B6
HOLLYHOCK WY
SLO 93401 674-C1
HOLLY OAK LN
StBC 93455 796-H7
HOLLYSPRINGS LN
StBC 93455 817-A6
HOLMCREST RD
SBAR 93103 996-C2
HOLSTED DR
StBC 93463 920-D6
HOLSTEIN DR
PSRS 93446 533-H1
HONDA AV
ATAS 93422 573-J2
HONDO CT
PSRS 93446 534-B1
HONDONADA RD
SLOC 93420 715-D1
HONEY WY
SLOC 93465 553-D1
HONEY GROVE LN
Npmo 93444 756-C5
HONEY LOCUST CT
SLVG 93463 920-F7
HONEYSUCKLE LN
PSRS 93446 514-A6
SLOC 93420 694-J7
SLOC 93420 695-A7
HONEYSUCKLE WY
LMPC 93436 896-D6
HONOLULU AV
SLOC 93445 714-D7
HONOR FARM RD
StBC 93110 985-A7
StBC 93110 995-A1
N HOPE AV
SBAR 93105 985-E7
SBAR 93105 995-E1
SBAR 93110 985-E7
SBAR 93110 995-E1
StBC 93105 985-E7
StBC 93110 985-E7
S HOPE AV
SBAR 93105 995-E2
HOPE ST
SLO 93405 654-A2
HOPE TER
SBAR 93105 985-E7
HOPE WY
Npmo 93444 756-A3
HOPE TERRACE CT
StBC 93455 816-H5
HOPKINS ST
SLOC 93465 553-A2
HORIZON CT
PSRS 93446 494-C6
HORIZON DR
SLOC 93460 921-A6
StBC 93463 921-A6
HORIZON LN
SLOC 93401 673-J2
SLOC 93465 553-A5

STREET Name City ZIP Pg-Grid

HORNBECK PL — SLVG 93463 920-F6
HORSEMAN CT — SMRA 93454 777-B6
HORSESHOE WY — SLOC 93446 534-J3
HORSTMAN ST — SLOC 93465 553-E1
HOSMER LN — StBC 93108 996-J2
HOSPITAL DR — ATAS 93422 573-J3
HOT SPRINGS RD — SBAR 93108 996-G3; StBC 93108 986-H6; StBC 93108 996-H1
HOURIHAN RANCH RD — Npmo 93444 756-G6
HOUSTON DR — SLOC 93402 651-F1
HOUSTON WY — PBCH 93449 714-F3
HOWARD AV — SLOC 93402 631-E6
HOWARD ST — SLO 93401 653-J3
HUASNA DR — SLO 93405 653-F7; SLO 93405 673-G1
HUASNA RD — ARGD 93420 715-B4; SLOC 93420 715-D3
HUASNA RIVER RD — SLOC - 737-F2; SLOC 93420 737-F2
HUASNA TOWNSITE RD — SLOC 93420 737-E1
HUBBA HUBBA LN — SBAR 93105 985-G7; StBC 93105 985-G7
HUBBARD AV — StBC 93254 806-C2
HUBER ST — GBCH 93433 714-E6
HUCKLEBERRY AV — ARGD 93420 714-F5
HUCKLEBERRY LN — SLO 93401 674-E1
HUDSON AV — Cmbr 93428 548-H2
HUDSON DR — SBAR 93109 995-G7
HUEBNER LN — ARGD 93420 715-B5
HUERO RD — SLOC 93422 594-D6
HUERTO WY — ATAS 93422 594-C1
HUMBERT AV — SLO 93401 654-A6
HUMBOLDT AV — SLOC 93405 633-A4
HUMBOLDT DR — Npmo 93444 756-B6; SMRA 93458 796-E4
HUMBOLDT ST — SLOC 93402 631-E6
HUMMEL DR — StBC 93455 816-H3
HUMMINGBIRD — PSRS 93446 514-A7; SLOC 93446 470-C4
HUMMINGBIRD LN — StBC 93455 816-J1
HUMPHREY RD — StBC 93108 996-J4
HUNT DR — Summ 93067 997-E2
HUNTER PL — SLOC 93446 493-E4
HUNTER RIDGE LN — Npmo 93444 755-G3
HUNTERS KNOLL — SLOC 93446 469-G4
HUNTINGTON AV — GBCH 93433 714-F6
HUNTINGTON DR — GOL 93111 984-F7
HUNTINGTON PL — LMPC 93436 916-G2
HUNTINGTON RD — Cmbr 93428 528-E7
HUNTINGTON WY — StBC 93455 817-E5
HURON WY — StBC 93455 817-E5
HUSTON ST — GBCH 93433 714-E6
HUTTON RD — Npmo 93444 756-F7; Npmo 93444 776-G1
HUTTON ST — SLO 93401 653-J5

I

I ST — LMPC 93436 896-E7; SLOC 93430 591-A2; SLOC 93453 614-F3
N I ST — LMPC 93436 896-E7; LMPC 93436 916-E1
S I ST — LMPC 93436 916-E2
IAIQUA LN — StBC 93110 985-D6
IBIS CIR — GDLP 93434 774-H6
IBIS LN — SLOC 93446 471-D6
ICELAND AV — StBC 93437 875-E2
IDA PL — Npmo 93444 756-A4
IDE ST — ARGD 93420 715-A5
IDYLLWILD PL — SLOC 93420 754-J1; SLOC 93420 755-A1
IGLOO RD — StBC 93437 875-E6
IKEDA WY — ARGD 93420 715-C4
ILENE DR — SLO 93405 653-E7
ILIFF LN — SMRA 93458 776-G4
ILLINOIS WY — Npmo 93444 755-E6
IL TRENO PL — SLOC 93446 494-A6
IMPALA TR — StBC 93455 816-G7
IMPERIAL AV — SLOC 93405 633-E5
IMPERIAL WY — StBC 93455 816-J6
INDEPENDENCE CT — StBC 93455 816-H5
INDIAN LN — StBC 93108 986-G7
INDIAN WY — StBC 93460 941-D2
INDIANA WY — Npmo 93444 755-F6
INDIAN HILLS WY — SLOC 93420 735-A1
INDIAN KNOB RD — SLOC 93401 693-F2
INDIAN VALLEY RD — MonC - 453-D3; MonC 93451 453-D3; SLOC 93451 453-D4; SLOC 93451 473-G1
INDIGO CIR — MOBY 93442 611-E3
INDIO DR — PBCH 93449 693-E5
INDIO MUERTO ST — SBAR 93103 996-D4
INDUSTRIAL — SLOC 93451 453-C5
INDUSTRIAL PKWY — SMRA 93455 796-F7
INDUSTRIAL WY — BLTN 93427 919-G5; LMPC 93436 916-G1; SLO 93401 674-B1; SLOC 93401 674-B1
INDUSTRIAL TAXI WY — PSRS 93446 494-C6
INGA RD — Npmo 93444 755-J3; Npmo 93444 756-A2
INGALLS CT — PSRS 93446 513-G2
INGER DR — SMRA 93454 796-H4
INNESLEY DR — ARGD 93420 715-A7
INVERNESS AV — StBC 93436 876-E6
INVERNESS DR — PSRS 93446 533-J1
INVERNESS LN — StBC 93108 997-B2
INVERNESS PL — SLOC 93401 674-D6
INVIERNO DR — SBAR 93110 985-D7
INWOOD DR — StBC 93111 994-J2
INWOOD PL — StBC 93111 994-J2
INYO AV — SLOC 93405 633-A5
INYO ST — SLOC 93402 631-E6
IRELANE DR — BLTN 93427 919-H5
IRIS AV — GOL 93117 994-C1
IRIS CT — LMPC 93436 896-D6
IRIS LN — SMRA 93455 796-J5
IRIS ST — SLO 93401 654-B4; SLOC 93445 734-H1
IRISH WY — PBCH 93449 714-E3
IRISH HILLS — SLOC 93402 652-A1
IRONBARK ST — SLO 93401 674-D1
IRONRIDGE CT — SMRA 93455 796-F6
IRON STONE LP — SLOC 93446 533-H4
IRONWOOD AV — MOBY 93442 611-E2
IRONWOOD CT — MOBY 93442 611-F3
IRONWOOD DR — SMRA 93455 816-B1; StBC 93455 816-B1
IRONWOOD PL — SLOC 93465 553-A1
IRONWOOD ST — StBC 93437 855-D7
IRONWOOD WY — SLVG 93463 940-D2
IRVINE LN — StBC 93108 986-J7
IRVINE STOVALL MEM HWY Rt-166 — Npmo 93444 776-H1; SLOC 93454 776-H1; SLOC 93454 777-B1
ISABELLA WY — SLO 93405 653-D7
ISLAND CT — SLOC 93445 714-F7
ISLAND ST — MOBY 93442 611-E2
ISLAND OAK LN — GOL 93117 993-F3
ISLAND VIEW DR — SBAR 93109 995-H6
ISLAY ST — SBAR 93101 995-J3; SBAR 93101 996-A2; SBAR 93103 996-A2; SLO 93401 653-J5; SLO 93401 654-A4
ISLETA AV — SBAR 93109 996-A6
IVA CT — Cmbr 93428 528-F6
IVAR ST — Cmbr 93428 548-F2
IVORY DR — StBC 93455 817-B4
IVY LN — PSRS 93446 513-J5; SLVG 93463 920-F7; StBC 93108 986-G7

J

J RD — StBC 93106 994-B3
J ST — SLOC 93430 591-A2; SLOC 93453 614-G3
N J ST — LMPC 93436 916-E1
S J ST — LMPC 93436 916-E2
JACANA CT — SLOC 93420 735-A6
JACARANDA CT — SMRA 93458 796-D5
JACARANDA LN — SLOC 93402 652-D2; StBC 93108 997-A3
JACARANDA ST — StBC 93437 855-F7
JACARANDA WY — CARP 93013 1018-G1
JACKIE LN — SMRA 93454 797-A1
JACK RABBIT RD — SLOC 93420 736-E2
JACKS WY — SLOC 93446 469-G4
JACKSON DR — PSRS 93446 513-H5
JACOB RD — Npmo 93444 737-B7
JACOB ST — SMRA 93455 796-J5
JACOB WY — SLOC 93465 553-C3
JACQUELINE PL — Npmo 93444 755-C3
JADE CT — StBC 93455 817-C5
JADE CANYON WY — SLOC 93432 574-J4
JALA CT — SMRA 93454 776-H5
JALAMA CT — GBCH 93433 714-F6
JALISCO CT — SLO 93405 653-D6
JAMAICA ST — MOBY 93442 611-E1
JAMES RD — StBC 93111 994-G3
JAMES ST — PSRS 93446 513-F6; SLOC 93465 553-D2
JAMES WY — ARGD 93420 714-H3; ARGD 93420 715-A3; PBCH 93449 714-D3
JAMESON CT — SLOC 93420 754-J1
N JAMESON LN — StBC 93108 996-J3; StBC 93108 997-A3; Summ 93067 997-A3
S JAMESON LN — StBC 93108 996-J3; StBC 93108 997-A4
JAMIE LP — SMRA 93454 797-A1
JAMI LEE CT — SLO 93401 654-D6
JANE DR — SLO 93405 653-E7
JANE ST — SMRA 93458 796-G3
JANELLE LN — SMRA 93458 796-F3
JANET AV — GBCH 93433 714-F7
JANET DR — PBCH 93449 714-F3; StBC 93455 817-B5
JANICE DR — SLO 93405 653-E7
JANICE ST — PSRS 93446 514-A6
JANIN CT — StBC 93463 920-H7
JANIN WY — StBC 93463 920-H6
JANUARY ST — Npmo 93444 756-B4
JAQUIMA RD — ATAS 93422 573-B2
JARDINE RD — SLOC 93446 494-G4; SLOC 93446 514-G1
JARED LN — StBC 93441 901-E1
JASMINE LN — StBC 93455 816-H2
JASMINE PL — ARGD 93420 714-F6
JASMINE ST — LMPC 93436 896-F6
JASMINE WY — Npmo 93444 756-A3
JASON CT — SLOC 93420 755-C3
JASON DR — LMPC 93436 896-C6
JASON WY — SMRA 93455 796-E5; StBC 93463 920-J6; StBC 93463 921-A5
JASPER WY — Npmo 93444 756-A4
JAVA ST — MOBY 93442 611-E1
JAY CT — Npmo 93444 756-B3
JAY ST — CARP 93013 998-E6
JAYCEE DR — SLO 93405 653-G2
JAYE CT — SMRA 93458 796-F4
JAYTON AV — SMRA 93458 776-F3
JEAN DR — SLO 93405 653-E7
JEAN LN — StBC 93111 984-G6
JEAN ST — Cmbr 93428 548-F2
JEANETTE LN — Npmo 93444 756-B5
JEANNE WY — PSRS 93446 514-A6
JEFF ELINGS DR — StBC 93109 995-F6
JEFFERSON CT — StBC 93455 817-A4
JEFFREY CT — SMRA 93454 797-A1
JEFFREY DR — SLO 93405 653-G2
JELINDA DR — StBC 93108 997-B2
JENA CT — PSRS 93446 513-J2
JENNA DR — GOL 93117 993-F1
JENNER WY — SLOC 93420 735-A4
JENNIE LN — Npmo 93444 755-H2
JENNIFER CT — GBCH 93433 714-F7; SMRA 93454 776-J6
JENNIFER ST — SLO 93401 654-A5
JENNILSA LN — StBC 93463 920-E6
JENNINGS AV — SBAR 93103 996-C3
JENNINGS DR — ARGD 93420 715-A7
JENNY PL — ARGD 93420 714-H3
JENSEN RANCH RD — StBC 93455 817-B6
JERRY LN — SMRA 93454 777-A6
JERSEY CT — PSRS 93446 533-H1; SLOC 93422 594-D3
JESMARY LN — SBAR 93105 995-H2
JESPERSEN RD — SLOC 93401 673-J4
JESPERSON RD — SLOC 93401 673-J5; SLOC 93401 674-A6
JESSELLE CT — SMRA 93454 776-J5
JESSICA PL — Npmo 93444 756-B5
JESSIE CT — SMRA 93454 777-A6
JESUSITA LN — SBAR 93105 985-G6; StBC 93105 985-G6
JETTY AV — SLOC 93445 714-E7
JEWEL ST — SMRA 93454 776-H5; SMRA 93454 777-A5; SMRA 93458 776-F5
JILL AV — SMRA 93458 796-E2
JIMENO RD — SBAR 93103 996-A2
JOAN PL — SLOC 93401 674-D7
JOANNE DR — StBC 93455 796-H7
JOCE DELORES CT — StBC 93460 921-B6
JODI CT — SMRA 93454 797-A1
JODI DR — LMPC 93436 896-C6
JOHE LN — SLOC 93405 653-D3
JOHNSON AV — SLO 93401 654-A3; SLOC 93401 654-B4
JOHNSON DR — SMRA 93458 776-H3
JOLON RD — ATAS 93422 573-F7
JONATA ST — StBC 93441 900-H5
JONATA PARK RD — BLTN 93427 919-H4; StBC 93427 919-H4; StBC 93440 900-A5
JONATHAN PL — SMRA 93454 777-A7
JONES LN — Npmo 93444 735-D7
JONES ST — SMRA 93454 796-J1; SMRA 93454 797-A1; SMRA 93458 796-G1; StBC 93454 797-B1
JORDAN CT — SLOC 93420 755-C3
JORDAN LN — SLOC 93465 553-B2
JORDAN RD — Cmbr 93428 528-D4
JORNADA LN — ATAS 93422 574-C7; ATAS 93422 594-C1
JOSEPH ST — SMRA 93454 777-B6
JOSHUA ST — Npmo 93444 756-E7
JOVITA PL — Npmo 93444 735-J5
JOY WY — SMRA 93458 776-F3
JOYCE CT — SLO 93401 654-B5
JOYCE WY — PBCH 93449 714-F3
JUANA MARIA AV — SBAR 93103 996-C3
JUAN CRESPI LN — StBC 93108 996-J1
JUANITA AV — SBAR 93109 995-H5; SLOC 93445 714-D7
JUAREZ AV — ATAS 93422 573-J2
JUBILEE CT — SMRA 93458 776-G3
JUDGE AV — SLOC 93420 714-H7
JULESTON DR — SMRA 93458 776-F3
JULIA DR — GDLP 93434 774-J7
JULIE LN — SLOC 93465 553-D1
JULLIEN DR — StBC 93455 816-H6
JUNE AV — CARP 93013 998-D6
JUNIPER AV — SLVG 93463 940-E2
JUNIPER PL — CARP 93013 998-D7
JUNIPER ST — ARGD 93420 714-G5; MOBY 93442 611-F2; Npmo 93444 756-A3; StBC 93437 855-D7
JUNIPER WK — StBC 93117 994-A4
JUNIPERO AV — ATAS 93422 574-A5
JUNIPERO PZ — SBAR 93105 995-J2
JUNIPERO ST — SBAR 93105 995-H2
JUNO CT — Npmo 93444 756-C4
JUPITER AV — StBC 93436 896-D1
JUPITER DR — Npmo 93444 756-A5
JUVENILE HALL RD — StBC 93110 995-B1

K

K ST — SLOC 93451 473-F2; SLOC 93453 614-G3
N K ST — LMPC 93436 896-D7; LMPC 93436 916-D1
S K ST — LMPC 93436 916-D2
KAHN WY — StBC 93440 878-G1
KAISER AV — StBC 93111 994-G3
KALAWA SHAQ — StBC 93460 921-A7
KALLE LN — StBC 93455 816-H5
KALLEY DR — GOL 93117 993-F1
KAMALA WY — GOL 93117 994-C1
KAMEO ST — SMRA 93458 796-E2
KANIN HOJ — SLVG 93463 920-F6
KANSAS AV — SLOC 93405 633-B5; SLOC 93451 453-A4; StBC 93437 875-E1
KAPALUA DR — StBC 93455 816-D4
KAPAREIL LN — PSRS 93446 514-A4
KARA DR — StBC 93111 984-G6
KAREN CT — PBCH 93449 714-F3
KAREN DR — SLO 93405 653-E7
KAREN PL — BLTN 93427 919-H5
KAREN WY — PBCH 93449 714-F3
KARI LN — StBC 93455 816-E4
KARINA WY — SLOC 93420 715-A1
KARL CT — Npmo 93444 755-J3
KARNES RD — StBC 93455 817-B5
KATE CT — SMRA 93454 776-J6
KATHERINE CT — PSRS 93446 514-A7
KATHERINE DR — PSRS 93446 514-A7
KATHLEEN CT — SMRA 93458 776-E7
KATHRYAN CT — Npmo 93444 735-E7; SLOC 93420 735-E7
KATHRYN DR — Cmbr 93428 528-E4
KATHRYN WY — SMRA 93454 777-A5
KATHY CT — SLOC 93401 674-E7
KATHY ST — CARP 93013 998-E6
KATSURA AV — StBC 93437 855-H7; StBC 93437 875-H1
KATY CANYON WY — SLOC 93420 694-G6; SLOC 93449 694-G6
KAY ST — Cmbr 93428 548-H2
KAYLA CT — PSRS 93446 513-H4
KEENAN RD — StBC 93463 900-G5
KELLOGG AV — GOL 93111 984-F7; GOL 93111 994-F1; GOL 93117 994-F1; StBC 93111 984-F6
KELLOGG PL — GOL 93117 994-E2; StBC 93111 984-F5
KELLOGG WY — GOL 93117 994-E2
KELSEY CT — SMRA 93454 776-J4
KEN AV — StBC 93455 817-A6
KENAI CT — StBC 93455 816-H4
KENDAL LN — Cmbr 93428 528-D5
KENDALE PL — BLTN 93427 919-J5; BLTN 93427 920-A5
KENDALE RD — BLTN 93427 919-J6
KENDALL RD — SLOC 93401 674-D3
KENDRA CT — SLO 93401 654-B5
KENMORE PL — StBC 93105 985-H7
KENNEDY LN — SLOC 93451 473-G3
KENNETH AV — StBC 93455 817-B5
KENNETH DR — Cmbr 93428 548-F2
KENNINGTON DR — StBC 93455 816-F5
KENSINGTON AV — SMRA 93454 777-A5
KENSINGTON WY — SMRA 93454 777-A6
KENT CT — SMRA 93458 776-F4
KENT PL — GOL 93117 984-F7
KENT ST — Cmbr 93428 528-E6; Npmo 93444 756-B2
KENTIA AV — SBAR 93101 995-G3
KENTON CT — PSRS 93446 533-H1
KENTUCKY AV — SLOC 93430 591-A1
KENTUCKY RD — StBC 93460 922-A7; StBC 93460 941-J1
KENTUCKY ST — SLO 93405 653-J2; SLO 93405 654-A2
KENTWOOD DR — SLO 93401 654-C6
KENWOOD RD — SBAR 93109 995-G5
KEO DR — StBC 93111 994-G1
KERN AV — MOBY 93442 611-G7; MOBY 93442 631-G1; SLOC 93405 633-A5
KERN DR — StBC 93111 994-G1
KERRY AV — Cmbr 93428 548-H1
KERRY DR — SLO 93405 653-E7
KERWIN ST — Cmbr 93428 548-F2
KESTREL LN — GOL 93117 993-F3; SLOC 93405 693-C2; SLOC 93424 693-C2
KESTREL WY — Npmo 93444 756-B4
KEYSTONE LN — SMRA 93454 777-A7
KIESTER PL — SBAR 93117 994-C2
KILARNEY CT — SLOC 93405 653-D6
KILER CANYON RD — SLOC 93446 513-A7; SLOC 93446 533-B1
KILER CREEK PL — SLOC 93446 533-A1
KIMBALL ST — SBAR 93103 996-D4
KIMBERLY AV — SBAR 93101 996-B5
KIMBERLY DR — PSRS 93446 534-B1
KIM SUE LN — BLTN 93427 919-H5
KINEVAN RD — StBC 93105 964-E6
KING CT — SLO 93401 653-J6
KING ST — SLO 93401 653-J5
KING ARTHURS CT — StBC 93455 816-G5
KING DANIEL LN — GOL 93117 993-G1
KINGFISHER LN — SLOC 93424 693-B1
KING JAMES CT — GOL 93117 993-G1
KINGS AV — MOBY 93442 611-H7
KINGS DR — PSRS 93446 534-B1
KINGS LN — SMRA 93454 776-J7; SMRA 93454 777-A7
KINGS WY — GOL 93117 984-E7
KINGSBURY DR — ARGD 93420 715-A7
KINGSBURY RD — SLOC 93432 574-G1
KINGSTON AV — GOL 93117 994-E1
KINGSTON DR — Npmo 93444 755-C4; SMRA 93458 776-F5
KINMAN AV — GOL 93117 994-E1
KIP LN — SLOC 93420 734-H5
KIRBY WY — Npmo 93444 756-A6
KIRK DR — StBC 93111 994-G1
KIT WY — StBC 93455 817-A4
KITTIWAKE ST — SLOC 93420 735-A6
KIWI LN — Npmo 93444 755-F4
KLAMATH RD — SLOC 93405 654-A1
KLECK RD — PSRS 93446 513-H3
KLEIN BLVD — LMPC 93436 895-J3
KNAPP DR — StBC 93108 996-F1
KNIGHT CT — PSRS 93446 513-J5
KNIGHTBRIDGE DR — SMRA 93455
KNIGHTS LN — SMRA 93454
W KNOLL CIR — SLOC 93446
KNOLL DR — SLO 93401
E KNOLL LN — SLOC 93446
KNOLL CIRCLE DR — SBAR 93103
KNOLLGLEN CT — PSRS 93446
KNOLLWOOD DR — Cmbr 93428; StBC 93108
E KNOTTS ST — Npmo 93444
KNUDSEN WY — SMRA 93458
KOA AV — MOBY 93442
KODIAK AV — StBC 93111
KODIAK LN — SLOC 93420
KODIAK ST — MOBY 93442
KOLDING AV — SLVG 93463
KONA WY — StBC 93455
KORINA AV — StBC 93437
KOVAL LN — SMRA 93455
KOWALSKI AV — SBAR 93101
KRILL RD — StBC 93463
KRIS DR — StBC 93455
KRISTEN CT — StBC 93111
KRISTY CT — SLO 93401
KROEBER WK — StBC 93117
KRONBORG DR — SLVG 93463
KRONEN WY — SLVG 93463
KYLE CT — SLOC 93420

L

L ST — SLOC 93451; StBC 93437
N L ST — LMPC 93436; LMPC 93436
S L ST — LMPC 93436
LA BARBARA DR — SBAR 93110; StBC 93110
LABRADOR LN — SLOC 93420
LA BREA AV — SMRA 93458
LA BREA CT — SLOC 93445; StBC 93437
LA BREA LN — CARP 93013
LA BUENA TIERRA — StBC 93111
LA CADENA ST — SBAR 93103
LA CALERA WY — GOL 93117
LA CAMARILLA PL — Npmo 93444; Npmo 93444
LA CANADA — ARGD 93420
LA CANADA DR — SLO 93405
LA CANADA LN — ATAS 93422
LA CIMA RD — SBAR 93101; SBAR 93105
LA CITA CT — SLO 93401
LA COLIMA — PBCH 93449
LA COLINA RD — SBAR 93110
LA COMBADURA RD — StBC 93105
LA CORONILLA DR — SBAR 93109
LA COSTA CT — ATAS 93422; SLOC 93445
LA COSTA DR — SMRA 93455
LA COSTA LN — StBC 93436
LA CRESCENTA WY — SLOC 93422
LA CRESTA CIR — SBAR 93109
LA CRESTA DR — ARGD 93420
LA CRUZ WY — SLOC 93446
LA CUMBRE CIR — SBAR 93105
LA CUMBRE LN — Npmo 93444; SBAR 93105
LA CUMBRE RD — SBAR 93105; SBAR 93110; SBAR 93110; StBC 93105; StBC 93110
LA CUMBRE HILLS LN — SBAR 93110; StBC 93110
LA CUMBRE PLAZA LN — SBAR 93105
LADAN DR — StBC 93463

N — SMRA 93455 796-G7
LN — SLOC 93446 493-F2
A — LMPC 93436 896-E4
A CT — SLO 93401 654-A6
A LN — PSRS 93446 533-J2; SLOC 93446 533-J2; SLOC 93446 534-A2; StBC 93108 987-F7; StBC 93108 997-F1
A PL — ARGD 93420 715-A4
A ST — SBAR 93101 996-A5
R — StBC 93111 984-H7
LOS WY — SLOC 93451 473-F1
ST — SLOC 93420 714-H7
RADA — SBAR 93105 995-F3; StBC 93105 995-F3
RADA AV — SLO 93405 653-G2
RADA LN — SLOC 93445 734-G1
ADA DR — StBC 93111 984-J5; StBC 93111 985-A5
UELA CT — ATAS 93422 574-B5
A VINEYARD — SLOC 93420 735-E2
A CT — SLOC 93420 695-B4
CHA LN — SBAR 93105 985-F7
RICITA — PBCH 93449 714-E2
NELLA RD — StBC 93111 984-G7
IA WY — StBC 93111 984-J7; StBC 93111 994-J1
RZA — PBCH 93449 714-D2
VIOTA — PBCH 93449 714-E2
V — ATAS 93422 573-J6
DR — StBC 93110 995-C2
ETA RD — GOL 93117 984-D6; StBC 93117 984-D6
N RD — StBC 93106 994-C5
ACIA — SMRA 93455 796-J5
ARDIA LN — GDLP 93434 775-B5
A AV — SMRA 93454 796-J2
A CT — GBCH 93433 714-F4
A DR — SLOC 93445 714-D7; SLOC 93445 734-D1
A LN — SLO 93405 653-E6
A PL — SLOC 93446 533-E5
A ST — SBAR 93101 995-J1; SBAR 93101 996-A2; SBAR 93103 995-J1; SBAR 93105 995-J1
A WY — SLOC 93446 533-E5
A BLANCA DR — StBC 93110 995-D2
A DEL CAMPO — SLOC 93446 533-J3; SLOC 93446 534-A3
A NEGRA LN — SLOC 93420 735-A7
A RIDGE FIRE — VeCo - 999-G5
N — SMRA 93454 777-A5
LA CT — GBCH 93433 714-E7
LA DR — SBAR 93109 995-G7
LA PL — CARP 93013 998-C5
LA ST — MOBY 93442 611-E3
A RD — StBC 93111 984-G6
A DR — Npmo 93444 755-J6
ST — SLOC 93445 714-E7
CANYON RD — StBC 93437 855-F7; StBC 93437 875-F1
CHORRO RD — SLOC 93405 633-E4
MARIE DR — StBC 93455 817-E5
IDE AV — SLOC 93445 714-D7
IDE PKWY — SMRA 93455 796-H4
IDE VILLAGE DR — SLOC 93446 471-C3
IEW CT — StBC 93455 816-H1
VIEW DR — ATAS 93422 573-J6
IEW DR — SLOC 93426 469-F1; SLOC 93426 470-A1
IEW RD — SLOC 93426 469-E1; StBC 93455 816-H1
IEW ST — SLO 93405 653-F7
YSABEL RD — SLOC 93446 533-H4

LAKOTA WY — SLOC 93422 594-D4
LALA LN — SLOC 93422 593-B1
LA LADERA DR — StBC 93110 995-C5
LA LATA DR — BLTN 93427 919-G5
LA LATA PL — BLTN 93427 919-G4
LA LINIA AV — ATAS 93422 574-A6
LA LITA LN — SBAR 93105 985-F6
LA LOMA AV — MOBY 93442 611-H6
LA LOMA CT — SLO 93405 653-F2
LA LOMA DR — Npmo 93444 755-J6; Npmo 93444 756-A5
LA LOMA WY — StBC 93110 995-A2
LA LOMITA WY — SLOC 93401 674-E2
LA LUNA CT — SLO 93405 653-D6
LA LUZ RD — ATAS 93422 553-G7
LA MANIDA — CARP 93013 998-E6
LA MARINA — SBAR 93109 995-J6; SBAR 93109 996-A6
LAMBERT RD — StBC 93013 997-F4; Summ 93067 997-F4
LA MESA — StBC 93105 964-H1
LA MESA PZ — CARP 93013 998-E6
LA MILPITA RD — SBAR 93105 985-F7
LA MIRADA DR — Npmo 93444 755-J6; StBC 93013 997-J4; StBC 93013 998-A4
LA MIRADA LN — SLOC 93402 651-J1
LAMPLIGHTER LN — SLOC 93420 715-C3; SLOC 93455 816-G5
LAMPTON ST — Cmbr 93428 548-F2
LANA LN — LMPC 93436 896-C6
LANA ST — PSRS 93446 513-J6; PSRS 93446 514-A6
LANAI RD — SBAR 93108 996-F1; StBC 93108 996-F1
LANARK ST — StBC 93110 994-J2; StBC 93111 994-J2
LANCASTER DR — ARGD 93420 714-G7; StBC 93455 796-H7; StBC 93455 816-H1
LANCASTER PL — GOL 93117 993-F2
LANCASTER ST — Cmbr 93428 528-E7
LANCER DR — StBC 93455 816-J6
LANDFILL RD — StBC 93437 875-F4
LANDLUBBER LN — SLOC 93426 469-H2
LANDS END RD — SLOC 93426 469-J2
LANGLO TER — SBAR 93105 985-F7
LANGLO RANCH RD — GOL 93117 993-E1; StBC 93117 983-F7; StBC 93117 993-E1
LANGTON ST — Cmbr 93428 548-G1
LANGTRY AV — StBC 93117 992-H1
LA NORIA — SMRA 93455 796-J5
LANTANA CT — StBC 93455 817-A3
LANTANA ST — Npmo 93444 755-H4
LANTANA WY — Npmo 93444 755-E1
LA PALA LN — CARP 93013 998-E7
LA PALOMA — PBCH 93449 693-E5
LA PALOMA AV — StBC 93105 985-B6
LA PALOMA CT — ATAS 93422 594-C1
LA PALOMA DR — CARP 93013 998-D6
LA PATERA LN — GOL 93117 984-C7; GOL 93117 994-C1; SBAR 93117 994-C2
LA PATERA WY — GOL 93117 984-C7
LA PAZ AV — SBAR 93101 995-J3; SBAR 93101 996-A3
LA PAZ CIR — ARGD 93420 715-B4; SMRA 93455 796-J5
LA PAZ LN — ATAS 93422 594-B2
LA PAZ RD — StBC 93108 986-F7
LA PITA PL — BLTN 93427 919-H4
LA PLATA — SBAR 93109 995-J7; SBAR 93109 996-A7
LA POSADA — SLO 93401 674-C2
LA PRADERA RD — SLOC 93422 594-F5
LA PRADERO RD — SLOC 93422 594-E6
LA PUESTA DEL SOL — PBCH 93449 714-E3

LA PURISIMA AV — SMRA 93455 796-J6
LA PURISIMA CT — SLOC 93451 473-F1
LA PURISIMA ST — GDLP 93434 774-H6
LAQUILA LN — SBAR 93103 996-C2
LA QUINTA DR — CARP 93013 998-C5; Npmo 93444 755-J6
LA QUINTA RD — ATAS 93422 574-B6
LA QUINTA WY — StBC 93436 876-D5
LARA LN — SLOC 93445 734-G1
LARABLE CT — PSRS 93446 534-B1
LA RADA — SBAR 93105 995-E2
LA RAMADA DR — StBC 93111 984-H7
LARAMIE DR — SLOC 93420 734-H5
LARCH AV — StBC 93455 816-J2; StBC 93455 817-A2
LARCHMONT CT — StBC 93455 816-J2
LARCHMONT DR — ARGD 93420 714-J5
LARCHMONT PL — GOL 93117 984-D6
LAREDO DR — SLOC 93420 734-H4
LARGA AV — ATAS 93422 573-H5
LARGURA PL — SBAR 93103 996-B2
LARIAT DR — SLOC 93402 632-A7
LARIAT LP — SLOC 93426 470-A1
LA RIATA LN — StBC 93111 985-A5
LARK — PSRS 93446 514-A7
LARK CT — SMRA 93454 796-H3
LARK ST — SMRA 93454 796-H3
LARK ELLEN DR — PSRS 93446 534-B1
LARKFIELD PL — PSRS 93446 534-B1
LARK HILL — SLVG 93463 920-G6; SLOC 93463 920-G6
LARKIN DR — StBC 93455 817-A5
LARKSPUR DR — SMRA 93455 796-G6
LARKSPUR LN — PSRS 93446 514-B6
LARKSPUR ST — SLO 93401 674-C2
N LARKSPUR ST — LMPC 93436 896-F7
LA RODA AV — StBC 93111 994-H3
LARRABEE ST — SMRA 93455 796-J6; SMRA 93455 797-A6
LARRYTON AV — SMRA 93458 776-F3
LA SALLE DR — SMRA 93454 776-J5
LA SALLE RD — GOL 93117 993-H3
LASALLE CANYON RD — StBC 93436 895-G7
LAS ALTURAS CIR — SBAR 93103 996-C1
LAS ALTURAS RD — SBAR 93103 996-C1
LAS ARMAS RD — GOL 93117 993-E2
LAS BRISAS DR — PSRS 93446 513-G5
LAS CANOAS LN — SBAR 93105 986-A7
LAS CANOAS PL — SBAR 93105 986-A6
LAS CANOAS RD — SBAR 93105 986-A6; SBAR 93105 985-J6; StBC 93105 986-A5
LAS CASITAS — ATAS 93422 594-C1
LAS CRUCES CT — GOL 93117 984-D6
LA SELVA AV — GBCH 93433 714-E6
LAS ENCINAS DR — SLOC 93402 631-J7; SLOC 93402 651-J1
LAS ENCINAS RD — SBAR 93105 995-H1; StBC 93105 995-H1
LA SENDA — StBC 93105 995-F3
LAS ENTRADAS DR — StBC 93108 997-B3
LA SERENA PL — SMRA 93455 796-G7
LA SERENA WY — Npmo 93444 755-J4
LA SERENATA WY — Npmo 93444 755-H3
LA SERENTA CT — StBC 93455 816-J2
LAS FLORES — SLOC 93420 714-H7
N LAS FLORES DR — Npmo 93444 755-H5
S LAS FLORES DR — Npmo 93444 755-J6; Npmo 93444 756-A6
LAS FLORES PL — SMRA 93454 796-H2
LAS FLORES WY — SMRA 93454 796-H2; SMRA 93458 796-F2
LAS FUENTES RD — StBC 93108 997-C2
LAS GAVIOTAS — SBAR 93109 995-E6

LAS LOMAS AV — ATAS 93422 574-B6
LAS LOMAS DR — SLOC 93420 694-J7
LAS MANOS LN — SBAR 93109 995-H5
LAS OLAS AV — SBAR 93109 996-A6
LAS OLAS DR — StBC 93110 995-A4
LAS ONDAS — SBAR 93109 995-J6; SBAR 93109 996-A6
LAS PALMAS DR — StBC 93105 995-B4; StBC 93110 995-B4
LAS PERLAS DR — StBC 93111 984-G7
LAS POSAS AV — SMRA 93458 796-E4
LAS POSITAS PL — SBAR 93105 995-F3
LAS POSITAS RD — SBAR 93105 995-F2; StBC 93105 995-F2
LAS POSITAS RD Rt#-225 — SBAR 93105 995-F4; StBC 93105 995-F4
LAS PRADERAS DR — SLO 93401 673-G2
LAS ROSAS LN — SBAR 93105 995-H2
LASSEN AV — SLOC 93405 633-A5
LASSEN CT — PSRS 93446 514-B7
LASSEN DR — Npmo 93444 756-A6; SMRA 93458 796-E4; StBC 93111 994-G2
LASSEN PL — StBC 93111 994-G1
LAS TABLAS RD — SLOC 93465 553-B1
LAST CHANCE RD — SLOC 93451 453-A6
LAS TUNAS RD — SBAR 93103 986-A7; SBAR 93103 995-J1; SBAR 93103 996-A1; StBC 93108 986-J7; StBC 93108 987-A7; StBC 93108 997-A1
E LAS TUNAS RD — SBAR 93103 996-A1
LAS TUNAS ST — MOBY 93442 611-G6
LASUEN RD — SBAR 93103 996-A1
LAS VARAS CANYON RD — StBC 93117 982-F6
LAS VEGAS ST — MOBY 93442 611-E3
LA TAPADERA LN — Npmo 93444 735-J3
LATEEN RD — StBC 93463 920-H7
LA TEENA PL — SLOC 93420 714-J1; SLOC 93420 715-A1
LATHAM PL — Cmbr 93428 528-G7; Cmbr 93428 548-G1
LA TIERRA LN — CARP 93013 998-C5
LATIGO CT — PSRS 93446 534-B1
LATIGO DR — StBC 93463 900-F5
LA TIJERA CT — SLOC 93445 734-G1
LAUGHLIN LN — StBC 93440 878-H2
LAUNA LN — ARGD 93420 715-A5
LAUNDRY AV — StBC 93437 875-F3
LAURA CT — SLOC 93465 553-B2
LAURA WY — PSRS 93446 513-J6
LAUREATE LN — SLOC 93405 653-D3
LAUREL AV — MOBY 93442 611-F3; SLVG 93463 920-E7
E LAUREL AV — LMPC 93436 916-E1
W LAUREL AV — LMPC 93436 916-B1
LAUREL CT — StBC 93455 816-J2
LAUREL LN — SLO 93401 654-C6
LAUREL PL — Cmbr 93428 548-F2
LAUREL RD — ATAS 93422 573-E7
LAUREL ST — SLOC 93424 693-A4; StBC 93437 855-E6
LAUREL WK — StBC 93117 994-A4
LAUREL CANYON RD — SBAR 93105 985-G7; StBC 93105 985-G7
LAURELWOOD DR — PSRS 93446 534-B1; StBC 93455 816-J5
LAUREN LN — SMRA 93454 777-A5
LAURIE WY — SLOC 93420 734-H7
LA UVA LN — ATAS 93422 573-F1
LAVELLE CT — StBC 93455 816-J5
LAVENDER LN — SLOC 93465 553-D1
LA VENTA DR — StBC 93110 995-A1
LA VEREDA LN — StBC 93108 996-J3
LA VEREDA RD — StBC 93108 996-J3
LA VERNE AV — StBC 93455 816-H5

LA VERNE ST — SLOC 93445 714-F7
LA VIDA LN — SLOC 93420 715-A2
LA VIGNA LN — SMRA 93458 796-E4
LA VINEDA — SLO 93401 654-B5
LA VIRADA WY — SLO 93405 653-E6
LA VISTA CT — ARGD 93420 714-G7
LA VISTA RD — StBC 93105 985-E5; StBC 93110 985-E5
LA VISTA DEL OCEANO — SBAR 93109 995-H6
LA VISTA GRANDE — SBAR 93103 996-D2; SBAR 93108 996-D2
LAVONNE DR — SMRA 93454 776-J6
LA VUELTA RD — StBC 93108 997-A3
LAWNWOOD CT — SLO 93401 654-C7
LAWNWOOD DR — SLO 93401 654-C7
LAWRENCE DR — SLO 93401 654-A6
LAWRENCE LN — LMPC 93436 896-C6
LAWRENCE PL — Npmo 93444 756-G6
LAWRENCE ST — SBAR 93103 996-C4
LAWSON PL — Cmbr 93428 548-H2
LAWTON AV — SLO 93401 654-A6
LAWTON LN — SLOC 93465 553-B3
LAZO WY — SMRA 93458 776-F4
LAZY LN — SLOC 93445 714-F7
LEAF ST — Npmo 93444 756-C1
LEAH WY — PSRS 93446 513-J4
LEANNA DR — ARGD 93420 714-J7
LEDO PL — ARGD 93420 714-G5
LEE — SLOC 93430 591-C5
LEE DR — SBAR 93110 985-D7; SBAR 93110 995-D1; SMRA 93454 776-H5; SMRA 93454 777-A5; SMRA 93458 776-F5
LEE RD — StBC 93429 855-H1
LEE ANN CT — SLO 93401 654-D6
LEEDS LN — GOL 93117 984-E7
LEEWARD AV — PBCH 93449 693-H7
LEFF ST — SLO 93401 653-J5; SLO 93401 654-A5
LEFT LN — SLOC 93420 715-E1
LEGADO — ATAS 93422 573-G3
LEGGE AV — StBC 93436 895-J6
LEIF LN — SLOC 93420 714-H1
LEIGH ST — SMRA 93455 796-J6
LEIGHTON ST — Cmbr 93428 528-E7
LEISURE DR — ARGD 93420 714-G3
LELA LN — SMRA 93454 796-H2
LELAND ST — PSRS 93446 513-E6
LEMA DR — Npmo 93444 756-A3
E LEMON AV — LMPC 93436 896-E7
W LEMON AV — LMPC 93436 896-C7
LEMON DR — CARP 93013 998-B5
W LEMON PL — LMPC 93436 896-B7
LEMON ST — SLO 93405 653-J3; SMRA 93458 796-F1
LEMON GROVE LN — StBC 93108 996-J2
LEMON RANCH RD — StBC 93108 997-B2
LEMONWOOD DR — CARP 93013 998-E7
LEMOORE ST — PBCH 93449 714-C1
LENOSA LN — ATAS 93422 553-A7
LENOX CT — PSRS 93446 513-H2
LEON ST — StBC 93455 817-A5
LEONA AV — SLO 93401 654-B6
LEONA DR — Cmbr 93428 548-G1
LEONA ST — SMRA 93454 777-B6
LEONARD PL — Cmbr 93428 548-H3
LEONI DR — GBCH 93433 714-D6
LEOPOLDO CT — SMRA 93454 776-H5
LE POINT ST — ARGD 93420 715-A4
LE POINT TER — ARGD 93420 715-A4
LE RIDA AV — SMRA 93458 796-E4
LEROY BLVD — StBC 93110 985-D7

LEROY CT — SLO 93405 654-A2
LE SAGE DR — GBCH 93433 714-C5
LESLEY CT — SMRA 93454 777-A6
LESLIE DR — SBAR 93105 995-G3
LESLIE ST — StBC 93440 878-G1
LES MAISONS DR — StBC 93455 816-J1; StBC 93455 817-A2
LE VALLEY RD — StBC 93436 896-F3
LEWIS AV — ATAS 93422 573-J3
LEWIS DR — StBC 93436 896-F3
LEWIS LN — SLOC 93401 674-D7
LEWIS PL — StBC 93436 896-G3
LEWIS RD — SMRA 93455 796-J5
LEWIS ST — StBC 93463 920-H2
LEXINGTON AV — GOL 93117 984-E7; GOL 93117 994-E1; SMRA 93458 776-G3
LEXINGTON CT — SLO 93401 654-B6
LIBERATOR CT — SMRA 93455 796-F7
LIBERATOR ST — SMRA 93455 796-F7
LIBERTY ST — SBAR 93103 996-E3; SMRA 93454 796-G2; SMRA 93458 796-F2
LIBRA DR — StBC 93436 876-C5
LIBRARY AV — SBAR 93101 996-A3
LICHEN PL — SLOC 93465 534-A7
LIDO WY — SBAR 93105 995-E3
LIERLY LN — ARGD 93420 715-B5
LIGA RD — ATAS 93422 553-G7; ATAS 93422 573-G1
LIGHTHOUSE PL — SBAR 93109 995-H7
LIGHTHOUSE RD — SBAR 93109 995-H7
LIGHTNING ST — SMRA 93455 796-F7; SMRA 93455 816-F1
LILAC DR — SLOC 93402 631-F7; StBC 93108 987-C7; StBC 93108 997-C1
LILAC ST — LMPC 93436 896-F7; SLOC 93445 734-G1; SMRA 93458 776-G3
LILLEBAKKE CT — SLVG 93463 920-F7
LILLIE AV — Summ 93067 997-D3
LILLINGSTON CANYON RD — StBC 93013 998-H6
LILLY CT — SLOC 93420 755-C2
LILY LN — SLO 93401 674-C2; SMRA 93455 796-J5
LIMA DR — SLO 93405 653-F7
W LIME AV — LMPC 93436 916-C2
LIMERICK LN — PBCH 93449 714-E2
LIMESTONE WY — SLOC 93446 533-F5
LIMOUSIN LN — SLOC 93422 594-E2
LIMU DR — CARP 93013 998-D6
LINCOLN AV — SLOC 93420 735-D4; SLOC 93465 553-C2
LINCOLN RD — SBAR 93110 985-E7
LINCOLN ST — SLO 93405 653-H3; SMRA 93458 776-H5; SMRA 93458 796-G1; StBC 93460 921-C5
LINCOLNWOOD DR — SBAR 93105 985-E7; SBAR 93110 985-E7
LINCOLNWOOD PL — SBAR 93110 985-E7
LINDA CIR — PSRS 93446 513-J6; PSRS 93446 514-A6
LINDA DR — ARGD 93420 714-G5; SMRA 93454 776-J7; SMRA 93454 796-J1
LINDA LN — SLO 93401 673-H2
LINDA RD — SBAR 93109 995-F6
LINDA LEE ST — StBC 93455 816-H2
LINDA VISTA AV — ATAS 93422 573-H5
LINDA VISTA DR — LMPC 93436 896-F6; StBC 93460 921-H3
LINDEMAN LN — SMRA 93454 796-H4
LINDEN AV — CARP 93013 998-D6; SLOC 93422 594-G7
LINDEN CT — Cmbr 93428 548-J2
LINDERO ST — StBC 93460 921-B4
LINDITO LN — StBC 93110 985-D6
LINDMAR DR — GOL 93117 994-C2

LINDON LN — Npmo 93444 756-A2
LINDY DR — GDLP 93434 774-J6
LINETTA DR — SMRA 93454 777-B7
LINFIELD PL — GOL 93117 993-J3
LINGATE LN — StBC 93108 996-J3
LINHERE DR — CARP 93013 998-D6
LINKS DR — Npmo 93444 735-F7; Npmo 93444 755-F1
LINNE RD — PSRS 93446 514-B7; SLOC 93446 514-D7; SLOC 93446 534-F1
LINNET LN — Npmo 93444 756-B3
LINWOOD LN — StBC 93455 816-H1
LION LN — SLOC 93446 469-G4
LIPPIZAN LN — PSRS 93446 513-H7
LIRA PL — StBC 93111 984-G7
LIRIO CT — SLO 93401 653-J7
LISA LN — Npmo 93444 756-A5
LISA ST — CARP 93013 998-E6
LISA WY — StBC 93455 816-H2
LISTOWEL LN — SLOC 93422 593-C2
LITAHNI LN — SLOC 93420 736-E1
LITCHFIELD LN — SBAR 93109 995-G6
LITCHFIELD PL — SBAR 93109 995-G5
LITTLE CT — SLOC 93449 694-F6
LITTLE COUNTRY RD — SLOC 93422 594-D2
LITTLE CREEK LN — SLOC 93446 471-B5; SLOC 93463 900-H7
LITTLE FAWN PL — SLOC 93446 534-J2
LITTLE MORRO CREEK RD — MOBY 93442 611-F4; SLOC - 611-G4; SLOC - 612-B3
LITTLE OAK CT — StBC 93455 816-G7
LITTLE QUAIL PL — PSRS 93446 534-C2
LIVE OAK DR — BLTN 93427 919-G5; SLOC 93446 469-G4
LIVE OAK LN — SBAR 93105 995-F4; SLO 93401 693-F3
LIVE OAK RD — SLOC 93446 533-B3; StBC 93441 901-E4; StBC 93460 901-E4
LIVE OAK RIDGE RD — Npmo 93444 755-G1
LIVE OAKS RD — StBC 93108 997-A1
LIZZIE CT — SLO 93401 654-B4
LIZZIE ST — SLO 93401 654-B4
LLANO AV — StBC 93110 995-B4
LLANO RD — ATAS 93422 573-B3
LLOYD AV — SBAR 93101 996-A3
LLOYD PL — LMPC 93436 896-C6
LOBELIA LN — SLO 93401 674-C1
LOBO LN — StBC 93455 816-H2
LOBOS AV — ATAS 93422 573-G2
LOCH LOMOND DR — StBC 93455 816-J3
LOCKFORD CT — StBC 93437 875-E1
LOCKFORD ST — StBC 93455 816-J3
LOCKWOOD LN — StBC 93455 816-B1
E LOCUST AV — LMPC 93436 916-E2
W LOCUST AV — LMPC 93436 916-C2
LOCUST ST — PSRS 93446 513-E4; SMRA 93458 776-G3
LOGAN CT — SLOC 93420 755-C3
LOGAN WY — SMRA 93455 796-J6
LOGANBERRY AV — ARGD 93420 714-F5
LOGANBERRY LN — SLOC 93424 693-A1
LOIRE LN — SLOC 93420 715-A2
LOIS LN — Npmo 93444 756-B4
LOLITA LN — SMRA 93458 796-G4
LOLITA ST — ATAS 93422 573-J1
LOLLAND FALSTER RD — StBC 93463 920-G5
LOMA LN — SLOC 93446 533-E5
LOMA ST — SBAR 93103 996-A2; SLOC 93402 631-G6
LOMA WY — StBC 93455 816-J5
LOMA ALTA DR — SBAR 93109 995-J5; SBAR 93109 996-A5

STREET Name City ZIP Pg-Grid

LOMA BONITA SLO 93401 653-J6
LOMA MEDIA RD SBAR 93103 996-C1
LOMA VISTA AV SBAR 93101 996-A3
LOMA VISTA LN Npmo 93444 756-C3
LOMBARDDO CT PSRS 93446 513-H7
LOMITA LN CARP 93013 1018-H1; StBC 93013 1018-H1
LOMITA RD SBAR 93105 995-G1
LOMITAS RD ATAS 93422 573-B3
LOMPOC SLO 93401 653-J7
LOMPOC CASMALIA RD StBC 93429 855-D2; StBC 93437 855-F6
LOMPOC CASMALIA RD Rt#-1 LMPC 93436 896-D1; StBC 93436 876-A4; StBC 93436 896-D1; StBC 93437 855-G7; StBC 93437 875-G1; StBC 93437 876-A4
LONDON LN Cmbr 93428 548-J2
LONDONDERRY LN Cmbr 93428 548-H1
LONE OAK WY SLOC 93465 553-C1
LONE PALM DR Cmbr 93428 528-B1; SLOC 93452 528-B1
LONG ST SLO 93401 673-H2
LONG TER SMRA 93455 796-J6
LONGBRANCH AV GBCH 93433 714-E5
LONG CANYON RD StBC 93441 901-D4; StBC 93460 901-D4
LONGDEN CT ARGD 93420 715-A7
LONGDEN DR ARGD 93420 715-A7
LONGDRIVE LN SMRA 93455 796-F6
LONGFELLOW RD StBC 93111 984-F6
LONG HILL PL SLOC 93446 534-J1
LONGHORN CT PSRS 93446 533-H1
LONGHORN LN SLOC 93420 715-A2; SLOC 93446 471-D6
LONG VALLEY RD StBC 93441 901-E1; StBC 93460 901-E5
LONGVIEW AV PBCH 93449 694-C7; PBCH 93449 714-C1
LONGVIEW LN SLO 93405 654-A2; SLOC 93405 654-A2; SLOC 93446 471-B5
LONGVIEW RD StBC 93460 921-A4; StBC 93463 921-A4
LOOKOUT LP SLOC 93426 469-J2
LOOKOUT RD StBC 93105 964-J6
LOOKOUT PARK RD Summ 93067 997-D4
LOOMIS ST SLO 93401 654-B2; SLO 93405 654-A2; SLOC 93405 654-B2
LOOP RD SLOC 93446 469-H4
LOPEZ DR SLOC 93420 695-F7; SLOC 93420 715-D2; SLOC 93453 695-G4
LOPEZ RD SBAR 93117 994-D2
LOQUAT AV LMPC 93436 916-B2
W LOQUAT AV LMPC 93436 916-C2
W LOQUAT CT LMPC 93436 916-D2
LORENA ST ATAS 93422 573-J1
LORENCITA DR SMRA 93455 796-G7
LORENZ CT Npmo 93444 776-G1
LORETO CT GBCH 93433 714-F6
LORETO PL StBC 93111 984-G7
LORIENDA CT SLOC 93420 715-A2
LORINDA PL SBAR 93101 995-H3
LORINDA WY SBAR 93101 995-G3
LORRAINE AV StBC 93110 985-C7; StBC 93455 816-J6
LORRAINE WY SLOC 93446 513-F2
LOS AGUAJES AV SBAR 93101 996-B5
LOS ALAMOS SLO 93401 653-J7
LOS ALAMOS AV SBAR 93109 995-J7; StBC 93437 855-D7; StBC 93437 875-D1
LOS ALAMOS PL SBAR 93109 995-J7
LOS ALTOS RD ATAS 93422 573-D7; ATAS 93422 593-C1
LOS ANGELES AV SLOC 93405 633-E5
LOS ARBOLES SLOC 93402 631-F7
LOS ARBOLES AV ATAS 93422 573-J4
LOS BERROS RD ARGD 93420 714-J7; SLOC 93420 714-J7; SLOC 93420 715-A7; SLOC 93420 735-B1
LOS CARNEROS RD GOL 93117 984-B7; GOL 93117 994-A2; SBAR 93117 994-A2; StBC 93106 994-A2; StBC 93117 994-A4
LOS CARNEROS WY GOL 93117 994-B2
LOS CERRITOS AV ATAS 93422 573-H4
LOS CERROS DR SLO 93405 653-F2
LOS CIERVOS ARGD 93420 714-H2
LOS FELIZ SLO 93401 653-J7
LOS FELIZ DR StBC 93110 995-A2
LOS GALLOS CT Npmo 93444 756-B5
LOS GATOS RD ATAS 93422 573-G5
LOS NINOS GOL 93117 993-H3
LOS OLIVOS AV SLOC 93402 631-H6
LOS OLIVOS LN ARGD 93420 715-A5
LOS OLIVOS ST SBAR 93105 995-H3
E LOS OLIVOS ST SBAR 93103 995-J2; SBAR 93105 995-J2
LOS OLIVOS MEADOWS RD StBC 93463 900-G5
LOS OSOS RD ATAS 93422 593-G1; SLOC 93422 593-G1
LOS OSOS VALLEY RD SLO 93401 673-F1; SLO 93405 653-D6; SLO 93405 673-F1; SLOC 93402 631-F6; SLOC 93402 632-A7; SLOC 93402 652-C1; SLOC 93405 652-C1; SLOC 93405 653-A3; SLOC 93405 673-F1
LOS PADRES CT SLOC 93402 631-F7
LOS PADRES RD Npmo 93444 756-A6; StBC 93455 816-H2
LOS PADRES WY BLTN 93427 919-J3
LOS PALMAS WY SLOC 93401 674-D7
LOS PALOS DR SLO 93401 673-G2
LOS PALOS RD ATAS 93422 594-E1; SLOC 93422 594-E1
LOS PATOS WY SBAR 93103 996-F3; SBAR 93108 996-F3
LOS PINOS DR SBAR 93105 995-F1
LOS PUEBLOS ATAS 93422 594-C1
LOS PUEBLOS RD SBAR 93103 996-C2
LOS RANCHOS RD SLOC 93401 674-E5
LOS REYES WY SLOC 93420 755-A2
LOS ROBLES SLO 93405 653-G1
LOS ROBLES LN SBAR 93105 985-H7
LOS ROBLES RD SLOC 93465 533-A7; SLOC 93465 553-A1
LOST OAK DR SLOC 93402 631-J6
LOST SPRINGS LN SLOC 93446 513-E2
LOS VERDES DR SLO 93401 673-G2; StBC 93111 984-J7
LOS VINEROS RD SLOC 93420 715-F1
LOTHAR LN SLOC 93446 534-A5
LOU DILLON CT SBAR 93103 996-E3
LOU DILLON LN SBAR 93103 996-E3
LOUISA AV SBAR 93109 995-H6
LOUISA TER SMRA 93455 796-J6
LOUISIANA PL StBC 93111 994-G4
LOUREYRO ST StBC 93108 997-B3
LOWELL WY GOL 93117 993-G3
LOWENA DR SBAR 93103 996-B2
LOWER HYDE StBC 93108 986-E6
LOYOLA DR SBAR 93109 995-H7
L P RANCH RD SLOC 93465 534-C7
LUBOVA WY SLOC 93451 473-F3
LUCAS DR SMRA 93454 776-J6; SMRA 93454 796-J1
LUCAS LN SLOC 93424 693-B4
LUCCA AV StBC 93441 900-H5
LUCERNE RD SLOC 93430 590-H2
LUCIA CT SMRA 93454 777-A6
LUCILLE AV Cmbr 93428 548-H1
LUCINDA CT StBC 93455 816-J3
LUCINDA LN ATAS 93422 573-F7; SBAR 93105 985-G7
LUCKY LN StBC 93460 921-A6
LUDLOW AV Cmbr 93428 548-G1
LUGAR DEL CONSUELO SBAR 93105 985-H7; SBAR 93105 995-H1
LUISITA ST MOBY 93442 611-G7
LUKE WY SLOC 93420 754-H1
LUNAR CIR StBC 93436 896-D1
LUNETA DR SLO 93405 653-G3
LUNETA PZ SBAR 93109 996-A6
LUPIN LN StBC 93455 816-H2
LUPINE LN SLOC 93465 534-B7; SLOC 93465 553-J4
LUPINE ST SLOC 93402 631-F5
N LUPINE ST LMPC 93436 896-F6; LMPC 93436 916-F1
LUPINE CANYON RD SLOC 93405 693-B2; SLOC 93424 693-B1
LUZON ST MOBY 93442 611-E1
LYDIA LN StBC 93455 816-J5
LYLE AV Cmbr 93428 548-H2
LYLE LN PSRS 93446 513-J4
LYMAN ST SLOC 93420 735-D4
LYN RD SLOC 93420 735-C5
LYNCH CANYON DR SLOC 93426 469-F1
LYNHURST CIR StBC 93455 816-J4
LYNN DR SLO 93405 653-E7
LYNN ST GBCH 93433 714-F7
LYNNE DR SMRA 93454 776-J5
LYON PL GOL 93117 994-E1
LYRIC LN StBC 93110 995-C1
LYSANDRA CT SLOC 93465 553-C2

M

M PL LMPC 93436 896-D7
N M ST LMPC 93436 896-D7; LMPC 93436 916-D1
S M ST LMPC 93436 916-D2
MABLE CT StBC 93455 816-J2
MACADAMIA LN StBC 93108 997-F2
MACAW CT Npmo 93444 756-B3
MACETA LN StBC 93108 996-H4
MACHADO AV SMRA 93455 796-G7
MACHADO LN SLOC 93401 674-D5
MACLEOD WY Cmbr 93428 548-H1
MACON CT StBC 93455 816-E4
MACON DR StBC 93437 855-F7
MADBURY CT SLOC 93401 674-D7
MADERA AV MOBY 93442 611-G7; SLOC 93405 632-J5; SLOC 93405 633-A5
MADERA DR GOL 93117 993-H2
MADERA PL ATAS 93422 553-F7
MADERA ST SLOC 93402 631-E7; StBC 93460 921-B5
MADERO CT SLOC 93420 735-B3
MADISON DR SLOC 93453 614-F3
MADISON ST Cmbr 93428 548-F2
MADONNA RD SLO 93405 653-F7; SLOC 93405 653-F7
MADONNA RD Rt#-227 SLO 93401 653-G6; SLO 93405 653-G6
MADRESELVA LN ATAS 93422 594-C2
MADRID CT ATAS 93422 594-C1; SLO 93401 653-J6
MADRID RD SLOC 93422 594-E2; StBC 93117 994-A5
MADRONA DR SBAR 93105 995-F1
MADRONA WK StBC 93117 994-A4
MADRONE CT StBC 93455 816-B1
MADRONE LN SLO 93401 674-D2
MADRONE RD ATAS 93422 573-B5
MADRONE ST SLOC 93446 533-F1
MADURO ATAS 93422 594-C1
MAGDALENA AV ATAS 93422 574-A2
MAGDALENA DR SLOC 93451 473-J3
MAGDALENA PL GOL 93117 984-C7
MAGELLAN DR SMRA 93454 777-A5
MAGGIE LN StBC 93455 816-G1
MAGNA VISTA ST StBC 93110 994-J2
MAGNOLIA SLO 93401 673-H1
MAGNOLIA AV ATAS 93422 573-J3; ATAS 93422 574-A2; GOL 93117 994-E2
MAGNOLIA DR ARGD 93420 714-H7
MAGNOLIA ST StBC 93437 855-E7; StBC 93437 875-E1
MAGPIE LN SLOC 93446 470-B5
MAHONEY LN GDLP 93434 774-J6
MAHONEY RD SLOC 93446 493-A2; SMRA 93455 796-B6; StBC 93455 796-B6
MAHONEY CANYON RD SLOC 93451 453-J7; SLOC 93451 473-H1
MAIL POUCH LN SLOC 93405 633-F7
MAIN AV PBCH 93449 714-C2
MAIN ST Cmbr 93428 528-F6; Cmbr 93428 548-H1; MOBY 93442 611-E2; PBCH 93449 714-B2; StBC 93440 878-G1
E MAIN ST SMRA 93454 777-C7; SMRA 93454 797-E1; StBC 93454 777-C7; StBC 93454 797-E1
E MAIN ST Rt#-166 SMRA 93454 776-H7; SMRA 93454 777-A7
N MAIN ST SLOC 93446 533-E7; SLOC 93465 533-E7; SLOC 93465 553-E1
S MAIN ST SLOC 93465 553-D2
W MAIN ST GDLP 93434 774-G6; GDLP 93434 775-B6; StBC 93434 774-E6; StBC 93434 775-B6
W MAIN ST Rt#-166 GDLP 93434 775-G6; SMRA 93454 776-G7; SMRA 93458 776-G7; StBC 93434 775-G6; StBC 93458 775-G6; StBC 93458 776-C7
MAININI RANCH RD SLOC 93405 633-D6
MAJESTIC DR StBC 93455 816-H1
MALAGA CIR StBC 93110 985-A7
MALAGA DR StBC 93108 996-J2
MALEY DR GOL 93117 984-E7
MALEZA AV ATAS 93422 574-B3
MALEZA WY StBC 93111 984-H7
MALIBU CT GBCH 93433 714-F5
MALIBU DR CARP 93013 998-D6; SLO 93401 653-J7
MALIBU WY LMPC 93436 916-B2
MALIK LN SLOC 93401 674-F7
N MALLAGH ST Npmo 93444 756-B1
S MALLAGH ST Npmo 93444 756-C2
MALLARD PSRS 93446 514-B6
MALLARD AV GOL 93117 994-E1
MALLARD CT SLOC 93446 471-C6
MALLARD WY SLOC 93401 674-H3
MALVA AV GOL 93117 994-D1
MALVASIA CT SLOC 93465 553-A3
MALVERN ST Cmbr 93428 548-H1
MAMMOTH DR SMRA 93454 777-B6
MAMMOTH LN SLOC 93446 471-B5
MANANITA AV ATAS 93422 573-H1
MANCHESTER CT StBC 93437 875-E1; StBC 93455 816-F4
MANCHESTER PL GOL 93117 993-F2
MANDA CT StBC 93455 816-J1
MANDA DR StBC 93455 816-J1
MANDARIN DR GOL 93117 994-D1
MANDARIN LN SLOC 93420 694-H4
MANDERINA CT SBAR 93105 995-E2
MANDEVILLE CT StBC 93455 817-B5
MANDI CT Npmo 93444 755-G3
E MANGO AV LMPC 93436 916-F2
MANHATTAN AV GBCH 93433 714-E5
MANITOU CIR SBAR 93105 995-F4
MANITOU LN SBAR 93101 995-G4
MANITOU RD SBAR 93101 995-F4; SBAR 93105 995-F4
MANKINS CT ATAS 93422 594-C2
MANLEY DR StBC 93436 896-F2
MANNIX AV SLOC 93430 591-C5
MANOR LN SMRA 93455 796-G5
MANOR WY Cmbr 93428 528-F6
MANUELA WY SLOC 93420 695-F7
MANZANA ST StBC 93460 921-B5
MANZANILLO DR GOL 93117 984-D6
MANZANITA DR SLOC 93402 631-F7; SLVG 93463 940-D2
MANZANITA LN SMRA 93454 777-A6; StBC 93105 964-F1
MANZANITA RD StBC 93105 964-J6; StBC 93436 876-F5
MANZANITA ST CARP 93013 998-D5
MANZANITA WY SLO 93401 674-D1
MAPLE SLO 93401 673-H1
MAPLE AV CARP 93013 998-D7; MOBY 93442 611-F2; SLOC 93402 631-F6; SLVG 93463 920-E7
E MAPLE AV LMPC 93436 916-F1
W MAPLE AV LMPC 93436 916-B1
MAPLE CT SMRA 93454 796-J4
MAPLE ST ARGD 93420 714-G6; ATAS 93422 574-B7; PSRS 93446 513-F6; SBAR 93103 995-J2; StBC 93437 855-D6
MAPLEWOOD CT PSRS 93446 513-E6
MARAVILLA LMPC 93436 896-E3
MARBELLA CT GBCH 93433 714-F6
MARBELLA LN SLOC 93465 553-B1
MARBELLA WY SMRA 93454 777-B7
MARBURY DR GOL 93111 994-E1; GOL 93117 994-E1
MARCELINO DR StBC 93463 920-J7
MARCELLA LN SLOC 93420 695-C7
MARCHANT AV ATAS 93422 573-J4; ATAS 93422 574-A5
MARCHANT WY ATAS 93422 573-J6
MARCIA WY SMRA 93458 776-F6
MARCO LN ATAS 93422 573-G1
MARCUM ST StBC 93455 816-F6
MARCUS WY SLOC 93420 735-C4
MARENGO DR MOBY 93442 611-H6
MARGARITA AV GBCH 93433 714-E4; SLO 93401 653-J7; SLOC 93453 614-G3
MARGATE AV Cmbr 93428 528-G7; Cmbr 93428 548-G1
MARGETTS AV SLOC 93465 553-B2
MARGIE AV StBC 93455 816-J2
MARGIE PL Npmo 93444 756-C4
MARGO ST SBAR 93109 995-H5
MARGO WY PBCH 93449 714-F3
MARGUERITE WY Summ 93067 997-E4
MARIA AV SLOC 93453 614-F3
MARIAH DR SMRA 93454 776-J4
MARIAH LN PSRS 93446 513-H4
MARIAN DR SMRA 93454 797-A1
MARIAN WY PBCH 93449 714-F3
MARIANA WY SBAR 93105 995-E3
MARIANELA ST SLOC 93402 631-E7
MARIA YGNACIA LN StBC 93111 984-J6
MARICOPA DR SBAR 93110 995-D1
MARICOPA RD ATAS 93422 573-F2
MARIE CT SMRA 93454 777-A5
MARIE DR SLOC 93420 735-A2
MARIE LN SLOC 93420 694-H7
MARIGOLD CT SLO 93401 674-C1
MARIGOLD LN PSRS 93446 534-C1
MARIGOLD WY LMPC 93436 896-C6
MARILLA AV SBAR 93101 995-J5
MARILYN WY SBAR 93105 985-G7; SMRA 93454 797-A1
MARIN AV SLOC 93405 633-A4
MARINA DR SBAR 93110 995-D5; StBC 93110 995-B5
MARINA ST MOBY 93442 611-F6
MARINERS CV SLO 93405 653-F6
MARION AV PSRS 93446 513-F2
MARION CT StBC 93436 876-E6
MARIOTT RD SMRA 93454 796-H4
MARIPOSA CIR ARGD 93420 715-B4
MARIPOSA DR SLO 93401 673-G2; StBC 93110 995-C4
MARIPOSA LN StBC 93108 987-C7
MARIPOSA WY SMRA 93454 796-H2; SMRA 93458 796-F2
MARIQUITA AV ATAS 93422 573-H3
MARIQUITA DR StBC 93111 984-F6
MARITIME DR StBC 93455 817-B4
MARJORIE PL Cmbr 93428 548-H1
MARK AV CARP 93013 1018-H1
MARKET AV MOBY 93442 611-F6
MARKETPLACE DR GOL 93117 993-H3
MARLBERRY ST SMRA 93455 796-G6
MARLBOROUGH DR GOL 93117 984-C7
MARLBOROUGH LN Cmbr 93428 548-F2
MARLEE LN SLOC 93446 513-D6
MARLENE DR SLO 93405 653-G1; StBC 93455 816-J5
MARLOMA LN SLOC 93420 715-G3
MARQUARD TER SBAR 93101 995-G5
MARQUIS PL SMRA 93454 776-J7
MARQUITA AV SLOC 93446 533-F5
MARS AV StBC 93436 896-D1
MARS CT Npmo 93444 756-A5
MARSALA AV SMRA 93458 796-E4
MARSALA DR GBCH 93433 714-E6
MARSEILLE CT GBCH 93433 714-F6
MARSH RD SLOC - 572-A5; SLOC 93430 572-A5
MARSH ST SLO 93401 653-J5; SLO 93401 654-A4; SLO 93405 653-J5
MARSHA CT SMRA 93454 777-B6
MARSHA DR SLO 93405 653-E7
MARSHALL DR SLOC 93401 673-G6
MARSHALL LN StBC 93436 896-F2
MARSHALL WY SLOC 93401 674-D6
MARSTONE LN GOL 93117 984-E7
MARTHA LN Npmo 93444 756-A4
MARTIN AV StBC 93455 816-H5
MARTIN RD SLOC 93465 553-D1
MARTIN WY MOBY 93442 611-F4
MARTINDALE RD Cmbr 93428 528-G7
MARTINEZ DR SLOC 93451 473-G3
MARTINGALE AV SLOC 93402 632-A7
MARTINIQUE DR SLOC 93445 734-G1
MARTITA PL Npmo 93444 756-C4
MARVIN AV StBC 93455 816-H1
MAR VISTA DR SLOC 93402 631-F7
MAR VISTA PL SLOC 93424 693-B3
MARXMILLER PL SBAR 93117 994-D2
MARY AV Npmo 93444 756-B2
MARY DR SMRA 93458 776-F5
MARY ANNE CT PSRS 93446 513-H3
MARY AUSTIN LN SLOC 93422 593-B1
MARYKNOLL DR GDLP 93434 774-J6
MARYMOUNT WY GOL 93117 993-H3; StBC 93117 993-H3
MAS AMIGOS SBAR 93105 995-D3
MASATANI CT GDLP 93434 774-J7
MASON ST SBAR 93101 996-B5
MASON ST SBAR 93103
E MASON ST Rt#-144 SBAR 93103
S MASON ST ARGD 93420
MASON WY SLO 93401
MASTERS CIR Npmo 93444
MATEO CT StBC 93111
MATHILDA DR GOL 93117
MATILIJA LN SLOC 93420; SLOC 93420
MATORRAL CIR StBC 93111; StBC 93111
MATORRAL WY StBC 93111; StBC 93111
MATTEI RD StBC 93460
MATTHEW WY ARGD 93420
MATTHEWS ST GOL 93117
MATTIE RD PBCH 93449; PBCH 93449; SLOC 93449
MAUD AV SLOC 93453
MAUI CIR SLOC 93445
MAXWELLTON ST SLOC 93401
MAY CT StBC 93111
MAY ST ARGD 93420
MAYA LN ATAS 93422
MAYBELLE CT SLOC 93445
MAYER AV SLOC 93430
MAYFIELD ST StBC 93455
MAYRUM ST StBC 93111
MAYTEN ST SMRA 93458
MAYWOOD CT SLOC 93420
MCCABE DR Cmbr 93428
MCCARTHY AV SLOC 93445
MCCAW AV SBAR 93105
MCCLELLAND ST SMRA 93454; SMRA 93454
MCCLOSKEY PL SBAR 93117
MCCLOUD ST SMRA 93455
MCCOLLUM ST SLO 93405
MCCOY LN SMRA 93454; SMRA 93455; SMRA 93455
MCELHANY AV SMRA 93454; SMRA 93454; SMRA 93458
MCFARLAND PL SBAR 93117
MCKINLEY ST ARGD 93420; StBC 93111
MCLAUGHLIN RD LMPC 93436; StBC 93436
MCLEAN LN StBC 93108
MCMILLAN AV SLO 93401
MCMURRAY RD BLTN -; BLTN 93427; StBC -; StBC 93427
MCNEIL AV SMRA 93454; SMRA 93454
MEAD LN StBC 93455
MEADOW CIR CARP 93013
MEADOW DR StBC 93455
MEADOW LN StBC 93108
MEADOW RD BLTN 93427
MEADOW ST SLO 93405
MEADOW VW SLOC 93424
MEADOW WY ARGD 93420
MEADOWBROOK CT StBC 93437
MEADOW BROOK DR StBC 93455
MEADOWBROOK DR StBC 93108
MEADOWBROOK LN SLOC 93402
MEADOWGATE DR SMRA 93458
MEADOWLACE CT GOL 93117
MEADOWLARK DR ARGD 93420; ARGD 93449
MEADOW LARK LN SLOC 93446
MEADOWLARK LN SLOC 93446; StBC 93105
MEADOWLARK RD PSRS 93446; SLOC 93446

STREET Name City ZIP Pg-Grid

WLARK RD
StBC 93454 797-E6
StBC 93460 921-E7
StBC 93460 941-D1
W OAK DR
SLOC 93420 735-B5
WOOD PL
SLOC 93420 735-F7
W RANCH RD
StBC 93463 920-H7
WVALE RD
StBC 93460 921-C5
W VIEW DR
BLTN 93427 919-F5
StBC 93455 796-J7
StBC 93455 797-A7
StBC 93455 816-J1
StBC 93455 817-A1
W VIEW LN
CARP 93013 998-D5
SLOC 93465 553-A3
W WOOD LN
StBC 93108 996-G2
FF ST
SBAR 93109 995-F7
AH LN
StBC 93436 876-E5
RD
SBAR 93103 996-B2
CT
SLOC 93465 553-C2
HAU RD
Npmo 93444 736-B7
RD
SBAR 93109 995-H7
KE AV
SLO 93405 653-H2
ER LN
SLO 93401 673-H1
SLOC 93401 673-H1
E CT
SMRA 93454 776-J4
E LN
Npmo 93444 756-B4
A CT
SMRA 93455 796-J7
ONT AV
SBAR 93103 996-D2
LN
SLOC 93401 674-B3
Y DR
PSRS 93446 513-J6
PSRS 93446 514-A6
Y LN
SLOC 93445 734-H1
SE AV
Cmbr 93428 548-G2
LE WY
LMPC 93436 916-F3
Y LN
SLOC 93449 694-G7
L DR
SLOC 93445 714-D7
CINO AV
SLOC 93405 633-A5
CINO DR
GOL 93117 993-H2
SHA LN
StBC 93455 817-B7
DR
BLTN 93427 919-G5
NE AV
GBCH 93433 714-D6
A CT
SMRA 93458 796-F3
O AV
SLOC 93405 632-J6
O ST
PBCH 93449 714-C1
DES AV
ATAS 93422 574-A2
DES AV Rt#-41
ATAS 93422 573-J3
ATAS 93422 574-A3
DES LN
ARGD 93420 714-J4
SBAR 93101 995-J4
R CT
StBC 93455 817-B5
RY AV
StBC 93436 896-D1
RY CT
Npmo 93444 756-A6
RY DR
Npmo 93444 756-A5
SMRA 93455 816-G1
TH AV
Npmo 93444 756-C4
TH LN
SMRA 93455 796-F5
A DR
StBC 93111 984-F7
AN CT
SMRA 93455 796-G6
I CT
SLOC 93424 693-A1
T LN
SLOC 93446 494-J7
N AV
Cmbr 93428 548-H2
OOCK CT
StBC 93455 816-H5
EE WY
StBC 93455 816-H6
HILL RD
PSRS 93446 513-E6
SLOC 93446 513-E6
.N
SBAR 93105 985-E6
DR
ARGD 93420 714-J7
ARGD 93420 715-A7
SLVG 93463 920-D7
.N
CARP 93013 998-C5
SBAR 93109 995-G7
RD
PSRS 93446 513-J3
PSRS 93446 514-A3
SBAR 93106 994-B4
SBAR 93117 994-B4
SLOC 93422 594-E4
StBC 93106 994-A3
StBC 93108 996-H3
StBC 93117 994-B4
A RD
Npmo 93444 755-D4
Npmo 93444 756-A4

S MESA RD
Npmo 93444 756-A4
MESA ST
MOBY 93442 611-G6
MESA ALTA LN
SLOC 93420 734-H4
MESA CIRCLE DR
StBC 93436 876-C7
MESA GRANDE DR
SLOC 93420 734-H4
MESA OAKS LN
StBC 93436 896-G3
MESA PINES WY
SLOC 93420 755-B2
MESA RANCH RD
SLOC 93420 735-B2
MESA SANDS WY
Npmo 93444 756-B4
MESA SCHOOL LN
SBAR 93109 995-F6
MESA VERDE DR
SBAR 93110 985-D7
SBAR 93110 995-D1
MESA VERDE LN
Npmo 93444 755-J5
MESA VERDE RD
StBC 93463 940-H1
StBC 93463 941-A1
MESA VIEW DR Rt#-1
SLOC 93420 734-H5
MESA VIEW LN
SMRA 93454 777-A5
MESA VISTA CT
PSRS 93446 513-J3
MESA VISTA LN
StBC 93463 920-D6
MESETA PL
SLOC 93420 714-J7
MESQUITE LN
ARGD 93420 714-J3
ARGD 93420 715-A3
StBC 93436 896-F3
MESSINA CT
GBCH 93433 714-E6
MICHAEL CT
LMPC 93436 896-C6
MICHAEL LN
SLOC 93420 735-B2
MICHAEL ST
StBC 93455 817-B6
MICHELE CT
SLOC 93420 755-C3
MICHELLE DR
StBC 93455 816-H3
E MICHELTORENA ST
SBAR 93101 995-J3
SBAR 93101 996-A2
SBAR 93103 996-A2
W MICHELTORENA ST
SBAR 93101 995-H4
MICHIGAN AV
SLOC 93451 453-A5
MICHIGAN WY
Npmo 93444 755-D5
MIDDLE RD
SBAR 93108 996-H3
StBC 93108 996-H3
MIDDLE RIDGE PL
Npmo 93444 755-F1
MIDDLETREE LN
ATAS 93422 594-C2
SLOC 93422 594-C2
MIDTEN HOF
SLVG 93463 940-D1
MIDWAY AV
StBC 93437 875-E3
MIDWICK PL
StBC 93108 997-A2
MIGUEL CT
SLOC 93420 755-C3
MIGUELITO CT
SLO 93401 654-B7
MILES AV
StBC 93455 816-H1
MILES OAK LN
Npmo 93444 755-J2
MILKY WY
StBC 93436 876-C7
StBC 93436 896-C1
MILL RD
PSRS 93446 514-E3
SLOC 93446 514-H3
MILL ST
SLO 93401 653-J4
SLO 93401 654-A3
SLOC 93420 735-C5
SMRA 93454 776-J7
SMRA 93458 776-G7
MILLER CIR
ARGD 93420 715-A4
MILLER CT
PSRS 93446 513-H7
PSRS 93446 533-H1
MILLER ST
SMRA 93454 776-H6
SMRA 93454 796-H3
SMRA 93455 796-H6
N MILLER ST
SMRA 93454 776-H5
MILLER WY
ARGD 93420 714-J4
ARGD 93420 715-A4
MILLS LN
GDLP 93434 774-J6
MILLS ST
Cmbr 93428 548-H1
MILLS WY
GOL 93117 993-H4
MILLSTONE AV
StBC 93455 816-J3
MILPAS ST
SBAR 93103 996-B2
N MILPAS ST
SBAR 93103 996-C3
N MILPAS ST Rt#-144
SBAR 93103 996-D3
S MILPAS ST
SBAR 93103 996-D4
S MILPAS ST Rt#-144
SBAR 93103 996-D4
MILTON ST
SLOC 93420 735-C4
MIMOSA CT
Npmo 93444 755-J4
MIMOSA LN
StBC 93108 996-J3
MIMOSA ST
MOBY 93442 611-F4

MINDORO ST
MOBY 93442 611-D1
MINDORO WY
MOBY 93442 611-D1
MINT LN
StBC 93110 995-A2
MIOSSI RD
SLO 93405 654-C2
SLOC 93401 654-C2
SLOC 93405 654-C2
MIRABELLA LN
SLOC 93420 734-J4
MIRACANON LN
SBAR 93109 995-H5
MIRA CIELO DR
SLOC 93401 674-F7
MIRADA DR
SLO 93405 653-E6
MIRADA LN
ATAS 93422 574-A6
MIRADERO DR
SBAR 93105 995-H1
MIRA FLORES AV
ATAS 93422 573-H4
MIRA FLORES DR
StBC 93455 817-A7
MIRALESTE LN
SLOC 93401 674-D6
MIRA LOMA DR
StBC 93455 816-J2
StBC 93455 817-A2
MIRA LOMA WY
SLOC 93446 513-E2
MIRAMAR AV
StBC 93108 996-J3
MIRA MAR CT
GBCH 93433 714-F4
MIRAMAR LN
PBCH 93449 693-D5
StBC 93108 997-A3
MIRAMAR BEACH
StBC 93108 996-J4
MIRA MESA DR
SBAR 93109 995-H6
MIRAMON AV
ATAS 93422 573-J1
MIRA MONTE AV
StBC 93108 996-J2
MIRAMONTE DR
SBAR 93101 995-J5
SBAR 93109 995-J5
SBAR 93109 996-A5
MIRANDA CT
SMRA 93458 776-H3
MIRANO DR
GOL 93117 993-G1
MIRASOL CT
SMRA 93458 796-D4
MIRA SOL DR
SLO 93405 653-G1
MIRASOL WY
ATAS 93422 553-F6
S MIRASOL WY
ATAS 93422 553-F7
MIRA VISTA AV
SBAR 93103 996-A1
MIRA VISTA WY
SLOC 93446 513-E1
MIRLO CT
ATAS 93422 594-C1
MISSION DR
SLOC 93451 473-H3
MISSION DR Rt#-246
SLVG 93463 920-F7
SLVG 93463 940-C1
StBC 93460 921-A6
StBC 93463 920-F7
StBC 93463 921-A6
MISSION LN
SLO 93405 653-H3
MISSION ST
SBAR 93101 995-H4
SLO 93405 653-H3
SLOC 93451 453-E7
SLOC 93451 473-F2
E MISSION ST
SBAR 93101 995-J2
SBAR 93105 995-J2
W MISSION ST
SBAR 93101 995-J2
SBAR 93105 995-J2
MISSION CANYON LN
StBC 93105 985-J7
MISSION CANYON RD
SBAR 93105 995-J1
SBAR 93105 985-J5
StBC 93105 986-A5
StBC 93105 995-J1
MISSION GATE RD
StBC 93436 896-J5
MISSION OAKS LN
StBC 93105 985-J7
MISSION PARK DR
StBC 93105 985-H7
StBC 93105 995-H1
MISSION RIDGE RD
SBAR 93103 995-J1
SBAR 93103 996-A1
MISSION RIDGE RD Rt#-192
SBAR 93103 986-B7
SBAR 93103 996-B1
MISSION SPRINGS RD
SLOC 93420 695-E5
MISSION VALLEY WY
SLOC 93451 473-D2
MISTLETOE LN
SLOC 93446 469-G3
MISTY CANYON WY
SLOC 93432 574-F2
MISTY ELM CT
StBC 93455 816-J3
MISTY GLEN PL
Npmo 93444 755-F1
MISTY VIEW WY
Npmo 93444 735-D7
MITCHELL DR
SLO 93401 654-A6
SLOC 93402 631-F5
MITCHELL LN
SLOC 93420 734-H7
MITCHELL ST
SMRA 93455 816-F3
MI TIERRA LN
StBC 93455 816-H4
MIZAR PL
StBC 93436 876-D6
MOCCASIN LN
SLOC 93446 471-B5

MOCHUELO CT
ATAS 93422 574-C7
MOCKERNUT
StBC 93437 875-H1
MOCKINGBIRD LN
SLOC 93465 553-B1
StBC 93110 994-J3
MODELLO AV
SLOC 93401 654-C2
SMRA 93458 796-E4
MODENA WY
SBAR 93105 995-E3
MODOC AV
SLOC 93405 632-J5
MODOC RD
SBAR 93101 995-F3
SBAR 93105 995-F3
StBC 93105 995-F3
StBC 93110 995-C1
MOFFETT PL
SBAR 93117 994-D4
StBC 93117 994-D4
MOGUL AV
SMRA 93458 776-F3
MOHAWK CT
PSRS 93446 513-H7
MOHAWK RD
SBAR 93109 995-G7
MOJAVE LN
SLOC 93446 533-H2
MOLERA DR
SMRA 93458 796-E4
MOLLE WY
SLVG 93463 940-E1
MOLLENHAUER RD
SBAR 93117 994-D2
MOMOUTH AV
GOL 93117 994-C1
MONA WY
PSRS 93446 513-J6
MONACO CT
GBCH 93433 714-F6
StBC 93455 817-B4
MONADELLA ST
SLOC 93420 734-H7
SLOC 93420 754-H1
MONA LEI CT
SLOC 93445 714-G7
MONARCH DR
StBC 93460 921-J3
MONARCH LN
Npmo 93444 756-B5
SLOC 93402 631-E6
SMRA 93454 776-J7
StBC 93108 997-A2
MON CHERE LN
SMRA 93458 776-G3
MONICA CT
SMRA 93454 777-A7
MONICA WY
StBC 93460 920-J2
StBC 93463 920-J2
MONITA RD
ATAS 93422 573-G7
MONO AV
SLOC 93405 632-J5
MONO CT
GBCH 93433 714-F4
MONO DR
StBC 93111 994-G1
MONO PL
StBC 93455 816-H2
MONROE DR
SLOC 93445 714-D7
MONROE ST
SMRA 93454 776-H5
SMRA 93458 776-G5
MONTALBAN ST
SLO 93405 653-J3
MONTALVO WY
SBAR 93105 995-E3
MONTANA AV
StBC 93437 855-E7
MONTANA BLVD
MonC 93451 453-A3
SLOC 93451 453-A3
MONTANA WY
SLOC 93402 631-F7
MONTANO DR
StBC 93455 796-H7
MONTCLAIR PL
SLOC 93420 734-J5
MONTE DR
StBC 93110 995-D3
MONTE RD
SLOC 93401 673-E7
SLOC 93401 693-E1
SLOC 93449 693-E4
MONTE ST
PSRS 93446 533-F1
SLOC 93446 533-F1
MONTEBELLO ST
StBC 93460 921-B4
MONTEBELLO OAKS DR
PSRS 93446 513-H4
PSRS 93446 514-A4
MONTE CARLO CT
StBC 93455 817-B4
MONTECIELO DR
StBC 93460 901-D6
MONTECITO AV
ATAS 93422 574-B7
PBCH 93449 693-H7
MONTECITO DR
SLO 93401 673-H1
MONTECITO PL
SBAR 93103 996-D2
MONTECITO RD
SLOC 93430 591-D3
E MONTECITO ST
SBAR 93101 996-C4
SBAR 93103 996-C4
W MONTECITO ST
SBAR 93101 996-A5
W MONTECITO ST Rt#-225
SBAR 93101 996-B5
SBAR 93109 996-A5
MONTECITO RIDGE DR
SLOC 93420 695-A7
MONTE CRISTO LN
StBC 93108 996-G4
MONTEGO ST
ARGD 93420 714-G4
MONTEREY AV
MOBY 93442 611-F7
MONTEREY CT
ATAS 93422 573-G2
MONTEREY RD
ATAS 93422 553-E7

MONTEREY RD
ATAS 93422 573-E1
SLOC 93446 473-F3
SLOC 93446 493-F2
SLOC 93451 473-F3
SMRA 93455 796-H6
MONTEREY ST
SBAR 93101 995-G3
SLO 93401 653-J4
SLOC 93401 654-A4
MONTEREY PINES
SBAR 93105 995-E1
MONTE VERDE DR
ATAS 93422 594-E1
SMRA 93455 796-G7
MONTE VISTA
SLO 93405 653-J2
MONTE VISTA LN
StBC 93105 964-H1
StBC 93108 996-J3
MONTE VISTA RD
StBC 93108 996-J3
MONTEZ CT
GDLP 93434 774-J7
MONTGOMERY ST
SBAR 93103 995-J2
MONTROSE DR
SLO 93405 653-G1
MONTROSE PL
StBC 93105 985-J6
MONTROSE WY
StBC 93105 985-J6
MONTURA LN
ATAS 93422 574-A6
MOODY CT
PSRS 93446 513-J7
MOON RDG
SLOC 93424 693-B1
MOONCREST LN
StBC 93455 816-H4
MOON DANCE DR
StBC 93455 816-G1
MOONGLOW RD
LMPC 93436 896-C1
StBC 93436 896-C1
MOONLITE DR
SMRA 93455 796-J7
MOON RIDGE RD
SLOC 93446 469-J5
MOON SHADOW
SLOC 93446 469-H4
MOONSTONE BEACH DR
Cmbr 93428 528-C4
MOORE LN
SLOC 93420 694-H7
SLOC 93420 714-G1
MOORE RD
StBC 93108 997-A1
MOPACIETO PL
Npmo 93444 756-F6
MORA AV
StBC 93460 901-F7
StBC 93460 921-F2
MORABITO PL
SLOC 93401 674-D3
MORADA LN
SBAR 93105 985-F6
MORALES ST
StBC 93254 806-B1
MORAN CT
PSRS 93446 513-J7
MORE RD
GOL 93111 994-G2
MORE MESA DR
StBC 93110 995-A2
MORENO RD
SBAR 93103 996-A1
MORE RANCH RD
StBC 93111 994-F4
MORETON BAY LN
GOL 93117 984-E7
GOL 93117 994-E1
MORGAN DR
PBCH 93449 714-E2
MORGAN LN
PSRS 93446 513-H7
StBC 93013 997-G4
MORGAN TR
StBC 93455 816-E5
MORNING GLORY WY
SLO 93401 674-C1
MORNING RIDGE RD
StBC 93455 817-A3
MORNING RISE LN
ARGD 93420 714-G6
MORNINGSIDE DR
StBC 93455 817-B3
MORNINGSIDE RD
SLOC 93422 594-C4
MORNING STAR WY
SLOC 93401 674-A4
MORRETTI CANYON RD
SLOC 93401 674-J6
MORRISON AV
SBAR 93103 996-A2
SMRA 93454 796-G2
SMRA 93458 796-F2
MORRISON ST
SLO 93401 654-B6
MORRO AV
MOBY 93442 611-F6
PBCH 93449 693-H7
MORRO DR
SMRA 93454 777-A6
MORRO RD Rt#-41
ATAS 93422 573-H7
ATAS 93422 593-D1
SLOC - 572-J7
SLOC 93422 572-J7
SLOC 93422 573-A7
SLOC 93422 593-D1
MORRO ST
SLO 93401 653-J3
SLO 93401 654-A4
SLO 93405 653-J3
MORRO BAY BLVD
MOBY 93442 611-F6
MORRO COVE RD
MOBY 93442 611-F7
MOSS AV
PSRS 93446 513-H5
MOSS CT
SMRA 93454 776-J6
MOSS LN
Npmo 93444 756-G7
Npmo 93444 776-G1
SLOC 93465 553-H2
MOSS BEACH CT
GBCH 93433 714-F4

MOTLEY
SLO 93405 654-A2
MOTOR WY
SBAR 93101 996-B4
MOUNTAIN AV
SBAR 93101 995-G4
MOUNTAIN DR
SBAR 93103 985-J7
SBAR 93103 986-C6
SBAR 93103 995-J1
SBAR 93105 985-J7
SBAR 93105 986-B7
SBAR 93105 995-J1
StBC 93105 995-J1
MOUNTAIN DR Rt#-192
SBAR 93103 986-B7
SBAR 93105 986-B7
E MOUNTAIN DR
StBC 93108 986-F6
StBC 93108 987-A7
W MOUNTAIN DR
SBAR 93103 986-D6
StBC 93103 986-D6
StBC 93108 986-D6
MOUNTAIN LN
SLOC 93405 654-A1
MOUNTAIN QUAIL LN
SLOC 93424 693-B2
MOUNTAIN RANCH RD
SLOC 93446 470-A6
MOUNTAIN RIDGE RD
StBC 93460 921-B6
MOUNTAIN SPRINGS RD
PSRS 93446 513-E3
SLOC 93446 513-B3
MOUNTAIN VIEW BLVD
StBC 93437 855-G7
StBC 93437 875-H1
MOUNTAIN VIEW DR
ATAS 93422 573-J6
ATAS 93422 574-A7
SLOC 93402 631-J6
SLVG 93463 940-D1
StBC 93455 816-H6
MOUNTAIN VIEW RD
Npmo 93444 755-D4
SBAR 93109 995-H5
SLOC 93420 734-H3
MOUNTAIN VIEW ST
SLO 93405 653-H3
MOUNT BISHOP RD
SLOC 93405 633-H7
SLOC 93405 653-J1
MOUNT CALVARY RD
SBAR 93105 986-C6
StBC 93105 986-C6
MOUNT LOWE RD
SLOC 93401 654-H2
SLOC 93453 654-H2
MOUNT VERNON DR
SMRA 93454 777-B6
MOUNT WHITNEY WY
SMRA 93454 777-B6
MOURNING DOVE LN
SLOC 93424 693-B1
MUGU LN
SLO 93401 653-J7
MUIRFIELD
SLO 93401 673-H1
MUIRFIELD CT
SMRA 93455 796-G6
MUIRFIELD DR
ARGD 93420 714-J7
GOL 93117 984-C7
MUIRFIELD PL
StBC 93436 876-E6
MULBERRY AV
SBAR 93101 995-H4
MULBERRY DR
StBC 93437 875-H1
MULBERRY LN
ARGD 93420 714-H7
MULLIGAN LN
SLOC 93420 735-A5
MURL DR
SLO 93405 653-E7
MURPHY AV
SLOC 93453 614-F3
MURRAY DR
SMRA 93454 776-J4
MURRAY PL
Cmbr 93428 528-E7
MURRAY ST
SLO 93405 653-J3
MURRELL RD
SBAR 93109 995-F6
MUSCAT CT
SLOC 93465 553-A3
MUSSELMAN DR
ATAS 93422 574-C7
MUSTANG CIR
ARGD 93420 714-H3
MUSTANG CT
StBC 93455 816-E4
MUSTANG DR
SLO 93405 653-J2
SLOC 93420 734-J5
SLOC 93420 735-A5
StBC 93460 921-B5
MUSTANG SPRINGS RD
SLOC 93446 513-D2
MUSTARD CREEK RD
SLOC 93446 493-B5
MUTSUHITO AV
SLO 93401 654-A6
MYRA ST
CARP 93013 998-E6
MYRTLE AV
SBAR 93101 995-J4
MYRTLE CT
SLVG 93463 940-D1
MYRTLE DR
SLO 93405 653-E7
MYRTLE ST
ARGD 93420 715-B5
MYRTLEWOOD DR
PSRS 93446 534-A1
MYRTLEWOOD RD
StBC 93455 816-B1

N

N PL
LMPC 93436 896-D7
N ST
MonC 93451 453-A1
SLOC 93451 473-F2
StBC 93437 875-E1

N N ST
LMPC 93436 896-D7
LMPC 93436 916-D1
S N ST
LMPC 93436 916-D2
NABAL CT
SLOC 93445 714-G7
NACIMIENTO AV
ATAS 93422 573-H4
GBCH 93433 714-E4
NACIMIENTO LAKE DR
PSRS 93446 513-C2
SLOC 93446 513-C2
NACIMIENTO LAKE DR Rt#-G14
PSRS 93446 513-E3
SLOC 93446 471-C1
SLOC 93446 493-A5
SLOC 93446 513-B1
NACIMIENTO SHORES RD
SLOC 93426 470-C2
NAGANO RD
SLOC - 611-G4
NAMOUNA ST
CARP 93013 998-E6
NAN CT
SMRA 93454 776-H6
NANCY AV
SLOC 93402 631-F6
NANCY DR
SLO 93405 653-E7
NANDINA LN
Npmo 93444 756-C1
NANETTE LN
PSRS 93446 513-J6
PSRS 93446 514-A6
NANTUCKET CT
CARP 93013 998-E6
NAOMI AV
PBCH 93449 693-G7
NAPA AV
MOBY 93442 611-F7
SLOC 93405 633-C5
NAPA LN
GOL 93117 993-H2
NAPLES ST
GBCH 93433 714-F6
NAPLES ACCESS RD
StBC 93117 982-H7
StBC 93117 992-H1
NARANJO DR
StBC 93110 985-D6
NARLENE WY
PBCH 93449 714-F3
NARROW CT
SLOC 93405 653-D3
NARROW GAUGE WY
SLOC 93420 695-B4
NARTATEZ CT
SMRA 93458 796-F4
NASELLA LN
SLOC 93405 653-D5
NASSAU ST
MOBY 93442 611-E1
NATHAN RD
StBC 93110 985-E6
NATHAN WY
SLOC 93420 755-B2
NATOMA AV
SBAR 93101 996-B5
NAULT AV
Cmbr 93428 548-G2
NAVAJO AV
PSRS 93446 513-H5
NAVAJO PL
StBC 93455 817-A7
NAVAJOA AV
ATAS 93422 573-J5
NAVARETTE AV
ATAS 93422 573-G4
NAVARRA WY
SMRA 93454 777-B7
NAVIDAD RD
ATAS 93422 573-H1
NAZARIO CT
Npmo 93444 756-B5
NEAL SPRINGS RD
SLOC 93446 534-C5
SLOC 93465 533-J7
SLOC 93465 534-A6
NEBRASKA AV
StBC 93437 855-D7
StBC 93437 875-D1
NECTARINE AV
GOL 93117 994-E2
E NECTARINE AV
LMPC 93436 896-G7
W NECTARINE AV
LMPC 93436 896-C7
NEGRANTI RD
SLOC - 591-H4
NELSON DR
GDLP 93434 774-J7
NELSON ST
ARGD 93420 715-A5
NELSON WY
Npmo 93444 756-C6
NEPTUNE AV
StBC 93436 896-D1
NEPTUNE DR
Npmo 93444 756-A5
NEVA CT
SMRA 93454 776-H4
NEVADA AV
MonC 93451 453-A3
SLOC 93405 633-A5
StBC 93437 875-E3
NEVADA CT
SLOC 93402 631-E6
NEVADA ST
ARGD 93420 715-A5
NEVIS ST
MOBY 93442 611-E1
SLOC - 611-E1
NEW BEACH RD
StBC 93436 894-J1
StBC 93437 894-J1
NEWCASTLE AV
GOL 93117 994-C1
NEWCASTLE CIR
GOL 93117 994-C1
StBC 93455 816-G5
NEWCASTLE CT
StBC 93437 855-D6
NEWHALL AV
Cmbr 93428 548-G2
NEWLOVE DR
SMRA 93454 796-H3

STREET Name City ZIP Pg-Grid
NEWLOVE DR
SMRA 93458 796-G3
NEWMAN DR
ARGD 93420 714-J6
NEW MEXICO AV
StBC 93437 875-E2
StBC 93437 895-B1
NEWPORT AV
ARGD 93420 714-F4
Cmbr 93428 548-G1
GBCH 93420 714-F4
GBCH 93433 714-E4
NEWPORT DR
GOL 93117 993-F3
LMPC 93436 916-B2
NEWPORT ST
SLO 93405 653-F7
W NEWPORT ST
SLO 93405 653-F7
NEWSOME ST
StBC 93254 806-C1
NEWSOM SPRINGS RD
SLOC 93420 715-C5
NEW SOUTH RD
StBC 93429 855-A1
NEWTON DR
Cmbr 93428 528-F7
Cmbr 93428 548-G1
NEWTON RD
SBAR 93103 996-B2
NEW WINE PL
SLOC 93465 553-B2
NIBLICK RD
PSRS 93446 513-G7
PSRS 93446 514-A7
NICE AV
GBCH 93433 714-E6
NICHOLAS LN
SBAR 93108 996-E1
StBC 93108 996-E1
NICHOLSON AV
SMRA 93454 777-A7
SMRA 93454 797-A3
StBC 93454 797-A3
NICKERSON DR
PSRS 93446 513-H6
NICKLAUS DR
SMRA 93455 796-F6
NICKLAUS ST
PSRS 93446 513-H7
PSRS 93446 533-J1
NICOLA RANCH RD
SLOC - 612-E7
NIDEVER RD
StBC 93013 997-H4
NIEL PARK ST
SBAR 93103 996-D3
NIGHTHAWK DR
PSRS 93446 534-A1
NIGHT HAWK WY
SLOC 93424 693-A2
NIGHTINGALE
PSRS 93446 514-A6
NIGHTSHADE LN
SMRA 93455 796-H5
NIGHTSHADE PL
SLOC 93453 695-D3
NILES CT
SMRA 93454 777-B6
NINA PL
BLTN 93427 919-H5
NINOS DR
SBAR 93103 996-E4
NIPOMO AV
SLOC 93402 631-H6
SLOC 93402 632-A6
NIPOMO DR
CARP 93013 998-D6
NIPOMO ST
SLO 93401 653-J4
SLOC 93445 734-F1
NIRVANA RD
SBAR 93101 995-G4
NITA ST
SMRA 93454 776-J6
NIVERTH PL
SMRA 93455 796-J6
SMRA 93455 797-A6
NOB HILL RD
SLOC 93446 469-H4
NOBLE DR
StBC 93437 855-E7
NOBLE WY
SMRA 93454 776-J5
NODDY CT
SLOC 93420 735-A6
NOEL ST
ARGD 93420 714-F6
NOGAL
LMPC 93436 896-E3
NOGAL DR
StBC 93110 995-B1
NOGALES AV
ATAS 93422 573-H1
SBAR 93105 995-H2
NOGUERA PL
ARGD 93420 715-B5
NOJOQUI
SLO 93401 653-J7
NOJOQUI AV
StBC 93441 900-H5
NOKOMIS CT
SLOC 93402 651-E1
NOMA ST
CARP 93013 998-E6
NOPAL ST
SBAR 93103 996-B2
NOPAL WY
Npmo 93444 756-B4
NOPALITOS WY
SBAR 93103 996-D4
NORDENTOFT WY
SLVG 93463 920-E7
NORFOLK ST
Cmbr 93428 528-D6
NORMA DR
PBCH 93449 714-F3
NORMA LN
GBCH 93433 714-F4
NORMA WY
StBC 93111 984-G6
NORMAN LN
SBAR 93108 996-F2
NORMANDEL LN
ATAS 93422 553-E6
NOROESTE AV
SMRA 93458 796-E4
NORRIS ST
StBC 93455 816-G6
NORSWING DR
SLOC 93445 714-D6
NORTE RD
SLOC 93422 594-F6
NORTH AV
StBC 93455 816-F5
E NORTH AV
LMPC 93436 896-F7
W NORTH AV
LMPC 93436 896-C6
NORTH RD
LMPC 93436 895-J3
LMPC 93436 896-A3
NORTH ST
SMRA 93458 796-G5
StBC 93441 900-H4
NORTHAMPTON ST
Cmbr 93428 528-F6
NORTHBROOK DR
LMPC 93436 896-D6
NORTH CENTER CT
StBC 93455 816-H3
NORTHFORK PL
SLOC 93446 471-D6
NORTH FORTY RD
SLOC 93422 594-F6
NORTHGATE DR
GOL 93117 993-G1
StBC 93117 993-G1
NORTHOAKS DR
StBC 93436 876-C5
NORTH POINT CIR
StBC 93455 816-H3
NORTHPOINT PL
LMPC 93436 896-D6
NORTHRIDGE RD
SBAR 93105 985-F6
StBC 93105 985-F6
NORTH STAR LN
SLOC 93446 493-F3
NORTHVIEW AV
SLOC 93420 734-H4
NORTHVIEW PL
PSRS 93446 534-C1
NORTHVIEW RD
SBAR 93105 995-E2
StBC 93105 995-E2
NORTHWOOD RD
Npmo 93444 755-C2
SLOC 93420 755-C2
NORTON LN
Cmbr 93428 548-H3
NORWICH AV
Cmbr 93428 548-G2
MOBY 93442 611-F5
NORWOOD ST
SLOC 93420 735-D4
NOTTINGHAM DR
Cmbr 93428 528-D7
StBC 93455 816-F4
NOVA DR
SMRA 93454 776-J6
NOYES RD
ARGD 93420 714-G2
SLOC 93420 694-J7
SLOC 93420 714-G2
NUDOSO RD
ATAS 93422 573-C4
NUECES DR
StBC 93110 995-B1
NUEVA AV
SMRA 93458 796-E3
NUMANCIA ST
StBC 93460 921-B5
NURSERY WY
SLOC 93405 693-C2
NUTHATCH LN
SLOC 93426 470-A3
NUTMEG AV
MOBY 93442 611-F3
NUTMEG LN
SMRA 93455 796-J5
NUTWOOD CIR
PSRS 93446 533-E5
SLOC 93446 533-E5
NYGREN RD
SLOC 93446 473-E5
SLOC 93451 473-D4
NYKOBING
SLVG 93463 940-D1
NYSTED DR
SLVG 93463 920-F6

O

S O PL
LMPC 93436 916-D2
O ST
MonC 93451 453-A1
N O ST
LMPC 93436 896-D5
LMPC 93436 916-D1
S O ST
LMPC 93436 916-D2
OAHU ST
MOBY 93442 611-E1
OAK AV
CARP 93013 998-D7
CARP 93013 1018-D1
MOBY 93442 611-F7
SBAR 93101 995-H3
SLOC 93422 594-F6
E OAK AV
LMPC 93436 896-F7
W OAK AV
LMPC 93436 896-C7
OAK DR
SLOC 93451 473-G3
OAK LN
SLOC 93446 533-G1
StBC 93105 964-G1
W OAK PL
LMPC 93436 896-C7
OAK RD
StBC 93108 996-H3
OAK ST
ARGD 93420 714-J5
PSRS 93446 513-F2
SBAR 93103 996-D3
SLO 93405 653-J3
SLVG 93463 940-E1
SMRA 93454 796-H1
StBC 93455 816-H6
OAK WK
StBC 93117 994-A3
OAK WY
SLOC 93420 695-C7
OAK BLUFFS DR
StBC 93455 817-B7
OAKBROOK DR
StBC 93437 855-E7
OAKBROOK LN
StBC 93455 817-C6
OAK CREEK CANYON RD
StBC 93108 986-H7
OAK CREST DR
SLOC 93424 693-B1
OAKCREST DR
SBAR 93105 995-G2
OAK CREST LN
StBC 93441 900-J6
StBC 93460 900-J6
OAK CREST WY
SMRA 93454 777-A5
OAK FLAT RD
SLOC 93446 493-A6
N OAKGLEN AV
Npmo 93444 756-A1
S OAKGLEN AV
Npmo 93444 756-C3
OAK GLEN DR
StBC 93110 985-A7
OAK GLEN RD
StBC 93460 921-A5
OAK GROVE CT
PSRS 93446 513-H6
OAK GROVE DR
StBC 93108 987-C7
StBC 93108 997-C1
OAK GROVE LN
SLOC 93420 735-H5
OAK HAVEN LN
SLOC 93420 695-D6
OAKHILL CT
StBC 93455 816-G7
OAK HILL DR
StBC 93436 876-E5
OAKHILL DR
StBC 93455 816-G7
OAK HILL RD
ARGD 93420 715-B4
PSRS 93446 513-H7
SLOC 93420 715-C1
StBC 93463 920-H2
OAK HILL TER
StBC 93436 876-F6
OAKHURST CT
StBC 93455 816-H7
OAKHURST DR
Cmbr 93428 528-F6
OAK KNOLL DR
SLOC 93446 533-E6
OAK KNOLL RD
StBC 93455 817-B5
OAK LEAF CIR
ARGD 93420 714-G3
OAKLEY AV
SMRA 93455 796-F5
SMRA 93458 776-F5
SMRA 93458 796-F1
OAKLEY CT
SMRA 93458 796-F2
OAK MEADOW LN
PSRS 93446 514-A6
OAKMONT AV
StBC 93436 876-E6
OAKMONT PL
Npmo 93444 735-F7
SLOC 93420 735-F7
OAK PARK BLVD
ARGD 93420 714-G3
ARGD 93433 714-F5
ARGD 93449 714-G3
GBCH 93420 714-F5
GBCH 93433 714-F5
PBCH 93420 714-G3
PBCH 93449 714-G3
SLOC 93420 714-G3
SLOC 93449 714-G3
OAK PARK LN
SBAR 93105 995-G3
OAK POINTE DR
StBC 93436 896-G3
OAKRIDGE DR
SLO 93405 653-F1
SLOC 93402 631-J7
OAK RIDGE RD
StBC 93111 994-H1
OAKRIDGE RD
LMPC 93436 895-J3
LMPC 93436 896-A2
OAK RIDGE WY
PSRS 93446 514-B6
OAKRIDGE PARK RD
StBC 93455 817-B6
OAK SHORES DR
SLOC 93426 469-H2
OAKSPRINGS LN
StBC 93108 996-G1
OAK TRAIL RD
StBC 93441 901-C3
StBC 93460 901-C3
W OAK TRAIL RD
StBC 93441 901-B2
OAK TREE PL
StBC 93108 997-C3
OAK TREE WY
BLTN 93427 919-G4
OAK TREE VALLEY PL
SLOC 93446 494-G5
OAK VALLEY CT
StBC 93455 816-G7
OAK VIEW CT
SLOC 93424 693-B2
OAKVIEW DR
SLOC 93446 470-C4
OAK VIEW LN
StBC 93111 994-H2
OAK VIEW RD
StBC 93441 901-B2
OAKWOOD CIR
StBC 93436 876-E6
OAKWOOD CT
ARGD 93420 715-B4
SLO 93401 654-C6
StBC 93436 876-E6
OAK WOOD DR
PBCH 93449 714-E2
OAKWOOD DR
CARP 93013 998-E7
SMRA 93454 796-H2
OAKWOOD RD
StBC 93436 876-E6
OAKWOOD ST
PSRS 93446 514-A3
OBISPO AV
SLOC 93430 591-B4
OBISPO RD
ATAS 93422 553-F7
OBISPO ST
GDLP 93434 775-A6
OBISPO PACIFIC TR
SLOC 93420 694-J6
OCEAN
PBCH 93449 714-C3
E OCEAN AV Rt#-1
LMPC 93436 916-F1
E OCEAN AV Rt#-246
LMPC 93436 916-H1
StBC 93436 916-H1
N OCEAN AV
SLOC 93430 590-H1
S OCEAN AV
SLOC 93430 590-J2
SLOC 93430 591-A2
W OCEAN AV
LMPC 93436 916-C2
StBC 93436 894-G2
StBC 93436 895-A3
StBC 93436 916-A1
StBC 93437 895-D6
OCEAN BLVD
PBCH 93449 693-G7
SLOC 93430 591-B4
OCEAN RD
StBC 93106 994-B4
OCEAN ST
SLOC 93445 734-E1
OCEAN WY
PBCH 93449 714-B1
W OCEAN WY
LMPC 93436 916-C1
OCEANAIRE CT
SLO 93405 653-G7
OCEANAIRE DR
SLO 93405 653-F6
OCEAN FRONT LN
SLOC 93430 590-J2
OCEANO AV
SBAR 93109 996-A6
OCEAN OAKS RD
StBC 93013 998-B4
OCEAN PARK RD
StBC 93436 894-G2
OCEAN VIEW AV
GBCH 93433 714-D4
PBCH 93449 714-C2
SBAR 93103 996-E3
OCEANVIEW AV
StBC 93013 997-G4
OCEAN VIEW BLVD
StBC 93437 855-E6
StBC 93437 875-C1
OCEAN VIEW CT
SLOC 93430 591-B5
OCEAN VIEW DR
CARP 93013 998-B5
OCEAN VIEW PL
SLOC 93402 631-H7
OCEAN VISTA LN
StBC 93111 984-J6
OCONNOR WY
SLOC 93405 633-A6
SLOC 93405 653-B1
OCOTILLO AV
SMRA 93455 796-G6
ODBY AL
SLVG 93463 940-E1
ODENSE ST
BLTN 93427 919-J6
BLTN 93427 920-A5
ODIE LN
StBC 93455 816-H3
ODIN WY
SLVG 93463 940-E2
ODYSSEY CT
StBC 93436 876-C6
OGAN RD
CARP 93013 998-E6
OGDEN DR
Cmbr 93428 548-F2
OGRAM RD
StBC 93105 964-J6
OHIO WY
Npmo 93444 755-E5
OJAI
PBCH 93449 714-C3
OJAI DR
SLO 93401 653-J7
OKLAHOMA AV
SLOC 93405 633-C5
OLD LP
SLOC 93451 473-G2
OLD 246 HWY
StBC 93460 921-B6
OLD ADOBE WY
SLOC 93432 574-G4
OLD CALZADA RD
StBC 93441 901-B6
StBC 93460 901-B6
OLD COAST HWY
SBAR 93103 996-E3
SBAR 93108 996-E3
StBC 93117 939-H7
OLD COUNTY RD
SLOC 93465 553-E1
OLD CREEK RD
SLOC 93430 591-C3
OLD DAIRY RD
BLTN 93427 919-G5
OLD GLEN ANNIE PL
GOL 93117 993-J2
OLD GROVE LN
SLOC 93446 534-J6
OLD MILL CT
StBC 93455 816-G4
OLD MILL LN
StBC 93455 816-F5
OLD MILL RD
SLVG 93463 940-F1
StBC 93110 985-C7
StBC 93110 995-C1
OLD MISSION DR
SLVG 93463 920-F7
OLD MORRO RD
ATAS 93422 593-D1
SLOC 93422 593-D1
OLD MORRO RD E
ATAS 93422 573-H7
ATAS 93422 593-G1
OLD MORRO RD W
SLOC 93422 572-J7
SLOC 93422 573-A7
OLD OAK PL
StBC 93111 984-H7
OLD OAK RD
SMRA 93454 776-J6
SMRA 93454 777-A6
OLD OAK PARK RD
ARGD 93420 714-G2
ARGD 93449 714-G2
SLOC 93420 694-G7
SLOC 93420 714-G2
SLOC 93449 694-G7
SLOC 93449 714-G2
OLD PEACHY CANYON RD
SLOC 93446 513-D6
OLD PRICE CANYON RD
SLOC 93401 694-F1
OLD RANCH DR
GOL 93117 993-E1
OLD RANCH LN
Npmo 93444 755-E2
OLD RANCH RD
ARGD 93420 714-J5
StBC 93463 920-J6
OLD SANTA ROSA RD
ATAS 93422 574-B7
OLD SETTLER RD
SLOC 93446 513-C6
OLD SUMMIT RD
SLOC 93420 735-H5
OLD TISBURY LN
StBC 93455 817-B7
OLD WEST WY
SLOC 93426 469-J1
OLD WILLOW RD
SLOC 93420 694-H7
OLD WINDMILL LN
Npmo 93444 756-D5
OLD WINDMILL WY
SLO 93401 673-J2
SLOC 93401 673-J2
OLD WRANGLER LN
SLOC 93446 471-B6
OLEA CT
SLO 93401 674-D1
OLEANDER LN
PSRS 93446 514-A6
OLEANDER PL
LMPC 93436 896-D7
StBC 93111 994-H2
OLEARY CANYON WY
SLOC 93420 737-C4
OLIVE AV
CARP 93013 998-D7
SBAR 93101 995-J2
SBAR 93101 996-A2
SBAR 93103 995-J2
SBAR 93103 996-A2
E OLIVE AV
LMPC 93436 916-F2
W OLIVE AV
LMPC 93436 916-C2
StBC 93436 916-C2
OLIVE CT
PSRS 93446 513-F6
OLIVE DR
PSRS 93446 513-F6
SMRA 93454 796-H4
OLIVE RD
StBC 93108 997-C1
OLIVE ST
ARGD 93420 714-H6
MOBY 93442 611-F7
PSRS 93446 513-F4
SBAR 93101 996-A2
SBAR 93103 996-A2
SLO 93405 653-J3
SLOC 93446 513-F7
StBC 93460 921-C4
Summ 93067 997-D4
S OLIVE ST
SBAR 93103 996-C4
OLIVE HILL RD
StBC 93455 817-B6
OLIVE MILL LN
StBC 93108 996-H3
OLIVE MILL RD
SBAR 93108 996-H3
StBC 93108 996-H3
OLIVER RD
SBAR 93109 995-G7
OLIVERA AV
SLOC 93420 755-A2
OLIVERA ST
GDLP 93434 775-A5
OLIVET AV
StBC 93441 900-G5
StBC 93463 900-G5
OLIVEWOOD RD
StBC 93455 816-B1
OLIVIA CT
PSRS 93446 513-J6
OLIVOS LN
Npmo 93444 756-A2
OLMEDA AV
ATAS 93422 573-H2
OLNEY ST
GOL 93117 994-D2
SBAR 93117 994-D2
OLYMPIA DR
SMRA 93458 796-F4
OLYMPIC WY
Npmo 93444 755-H3
ONSTOTT RD
StBC 93436 896-F2
ONTARE PL
SBAR 93105 985-F7
ONTARE RD
SBAR 93105 985-F6
SBAR 93105 995-F1
ONTARE HILLS LN
SBAR 93105 985-F6
ONTARIO RD
SLOC 93401 673-E6
SLOC 93401 693-E1
SLOC 93405 673-E6
SLOC 93405 693-D3
ONTARIO WY
StBC 93455 817-E5
ONTIVEROS RD
StBC 93460 900-J7
StBC 93460 901-A7
ONYX CT
StBC 93455 817-B5
OOP CT
SLOC 93420 754-J2
OPAL CIR
ARGD 93420 714-J7
OPAL CT
SMRA 93454 776-H4
ORAMAS RD
SBAR 93103 996-A1
ORANGE AV
GOL 93117 994-E2
SBAR 93101 996-A5
ORANGE DR
SLO 93405 653-J2
ORANGE ST
SMRA 93454 796-J1
SMRA 93454 797-A1
SMRA 93458 796-F1
ORANGE BLOSSOM LN
GOL 93117 993-J3
ORANGE GROVE AV
StBC 93105 985-J5
ORCAS ST
MOBY 93442 611-D1
ORCAS WY
MOBY 93442 611-E1
ORCHARD AV
ARGD 93420 715-A5
StBC 93108 997-C1
ORCHARD DR
PSRS 93446 513-J5
ORCHARD RD
Npmo 93444 756-A4
SLOC 93465 553-A4
ORCHARD ST
SMRA 93454 776-H5
SMRA 93458 776-F5
ORCHID DR
StBC 93111 994-G4
ORCHID LN
ARGD 93420 715-B6
SMRA 93455 796-J5
ORCHID ST
LMPC 93436 896-F5
ORCUTT AV
StBC 93437 875-D1
ORCUTT EXWY Rt#-135
SMRA 93455 796-H7
SMRA 93455 816-F7
StBC 93455 796-H7
StBC 93455 816-F7
ORCUTT RD
SLO 93401 654-B7
SLO 93401 674-D1
SLOC 93401 654-B7
SLOC 93401 674-D1
SLOC 93401 695-A1
SLOC 93420 695-A1
SLOC 93453 695-D3
SMRA 93455 796-H7
StBC 93455 796-H7
StBC 93455 816-H5
ORCUTT FRONTAGE RD
SMRA 93455 816-G1
StBC 93455 796-H7
StBC 93455 816-G1
ORCUTT-GAREY RD
StBC 93454 817-J3
ORCUTT VIEW CT
StBC 93455 816-G6
OREGON AV
MonC 93451 453-A3
SLOC 93451 453-A3
StBC 93437 875-E1
ORELLA ST
SBAR 93105 995-G2
ORENA ST
SBAR 93103 995-J1
ORIE CT
SMRA 93454 777-B7
ORILLA DEL MAR DR
SBAR 93103 996-D4
ORILLAS CT
ATAS 93422 553-H7
ORILLAS WY
ATAS 93422 553-H7
ORIN
Cmbr 93428 548-H1
ORINDA CT
ATAS 93422 553-H7
ORIOLE RD
StBC 93108 996-G3
ORIOLE WY
PSRS 93446 534-B2
ORION AV
StBC 93436 876-C6
ORIZABA LN
SBAR 93103 986-C7
SBAR 93103 996-C1
ORIZABA RD
SBAR 93103 986-C7
ORLANDO DR
Cmbr 93428 548-F2
ORLEN LN
SLOC 93465 553-A1
ORME PL
Cmbr 93428 528-G7
Cmbr 93428 548-G1
ORMONDE RD
SLOC 93420 694-F4
SLOC 93449 694-F4
E ORMONDE RD
SLOC 93420 694-H6
ORO DR
ARGD 93420 715-B4
ORR RD
StBC 93429 855-H1
ORTEGA RD
ATAS 93422 594-A3
SLOC 93422 593-J3
SLOC 93422 594-A3
E ORTEGA ST
SBAR 93101 996-B4
SBAR 93103 996-C2
W ORTEGA ST
SBAR 93101 996-A4
ORTEGA HILL RD
Summ 93067 997-B3
ORTEGA RANCH LN
StBC 93108 997-C3
ORTEGA RANCH RD
StBC 93108 997-D3
ORTEGA RIDGE RD
StBC 93108 997-C3
Summ 93067 997-C3
ORTON ST
MOBY 93442 611-F5
ORVILLE AV
Cmbr 93428 548-H2
SLOC 93430 591-B4
ORVILLE PL
Cmbr 93428 548-H2
OSAGE ST
Npmo 93444 755-H5
OSITO CT
SBAR 93105 995-E2
OSO FLACO LAKE RD
Npmo 93444
SLOC 93445
SLOC 93445
OSO GRANDE CIR
SMRA 93458
OSOS CT
SLOC 93402
OSOS ST
SLO 93401
SLO 93401
OSOS WY
PSRS 93446
PSRS 93446
OSPREY CT
SLOC 93465
OSTER STED
SLVG 93463
OSWEGO WY
StBC 93455
OTERO LN
PSRS 93446
SLOC 93446
OTERO RD
ATAS 93422
OTONO DR
SBAR 93110
OTONO PL
Npmo 93444
OUR PL
SLOC 93446
OUR HILL LN
SLOC 93446
OUTLAND CT
ARGD 93420
OVERDEL PL
SLVG 93463
OVERLOOK LN
SBAR 93103
SBAR 93108
OVERPASS RD
GOL 93111
OWEN CT
GBCH 93433
OWEN RD
SBAR 93108
OXBOW PL
SLVG 93463
OXEN CT
PSRS 93446
OXEN ST
PSRS 93446
OXFORD AV
Cmbr 93428
SMRA 93454
OXFORD DR
LMPC 93436
OXFORD PL
GOL 93117
OXFORD ST
SMRA 93454

P

P ST
MonC 93451
N P ST
LMPC 93436
S P ST
LMPC 93436
PABLO LN
Npmo 93444
PABST LN
StBC 93455
PACHECO ST
GDLP 93434
PACHECO WY
SLOC 93405
PACIFIC AV
PSRS 93446
SBAR 93109
SLOC 93430
SLOC 93430
PACIFIC BLVD Rt#-1
GBCH 93433
SLOC 93433
SLOC 93445
PACIFIC DR
PBCH 93449
PACIFIC ST
MOBY 93442
SLO 93401
SLO 93401
StBC 93455
PACIFIC VW
SBAR 93109
PACIFICA DR
GBCH 93433
PACIFIC COAST RAILWAY PL
ARGD 93420
PACIFIC DUNES CIR
GDLP 93434
PACIFIC DUNES WY
GDLP 93434
PACIFIC GROVE PL
SMRA 93454
PACIFIC OAKS RD
GOL 93117
PACIFIC PINE DR
SLOC 93449
PACIFIC POINTE WY
ARGD 93420
PACIFIC VIEW DR
CARP 93013
PACIFIC VILLAGE CT
CARP 93013
PACIFIC VILLAGE DR
CARP 93013
PACKING HOUSE RD
StBC 93108
PADARO LN
StBC 93013
N PADARO LN
StBC 93013
Summ 93067
S PADARO LN
StBC 93013
PADDOCK AV
PBCH 93449
PADEN ST
SMRA 93454
SMRA 93454
PADERNO CT
StBC 93110
PADOVA DR
GOL 93117
PADRE CT
StBC 93455

STREET Name City ZIP Pg-Grid

LN
Npmo 93444 755-D1
ST
SBAR 93103 995-J2
SBAR 93105 995-J2
NG DR
GDLP 93434 774-J6
D CAVE RD
StBC 93105 964-J5
StBC 93105 984-J1
D SKY WY
SLOC 93420 735-B2
HORSE PL
SLOC 93446 533-D3
HORSE TR
StBC 93455 816-E5
LN
ATAS 93422 574-A6
Npmo 93444 755-H5
ST
SMRA 93458 796-F4
N
StBC 93110 985-D6
AV
SLOC 93445 714-E7
CT
StBC 93111 984-F6
MISSION WY
SLOC 93451 473-F1
MO DR
SBAR 93105 995-E3
DE AV
PBCH 93449 693-H7
DE DR
SMRA 93454 777-A7
SMRA 93454 797-A1
SADE DR
SMRA 93454 777-A6
DES AV
SLOC 93402 631-G6
DES DR
SBAR 93109 995-G7
AV
CARP 93013 998-D7
CARP 93013 1018-D1
MOBY 93442 611-F7
SBAR 93101 996-B4
T
ARGD 93420 714-G6
PSRS 93446 513-H5
R
LMPC 93436 896-E6
T
SLO 93401 653-J4
SLO 93401 654-A3
WY
BLTN 93427 919-H5
AV
ATAS 93422 573-H2
COURT DR
SMRA 93454 796-H2
DESERT CT
PSRS 93446 533-J1
R ST
Npmo 93444 756-A3
TTO AV
LMPC 93436 916-G2
TTO DR
SMRA 93455 796-G6
TTO WY
CARP 93013 1018-G1
TREE LN
StBC 93108 996-G3
LTO CT
PSRS 93446 513-G3
LTO DR
GOL 93117 993-F3
IA DR
SLOC 93446 533-E5
StBC 93110 995-C4
IA PL
SLOC 93420 715-C2
IA ST
Npmo 93444 755-J5
Npmo 93444 756-A5
StBC 93460 921-B5
IAR AV
ATAS 93422 574-B4
PBCH 93449 693-H7
SLO 93405 653-H2
INO
PBCH 93449 714-D3
INO CIR
PSRS 93446 513-H7
SLOC 93420 734-H5
INO DR
SLOC 93402 632-A7
INO LN
PSRS 93446 513-H7
INO RD
StBC 93105 985-H6
SECOS
ARGD 93420 714-H3
VERDES
SLOC 93446 469-D2
VERDES CT
GOL 93117 993-F3
VERDE RD
ATAS 93422 593-D1
SLOC 93422 593-D1
T
SMRA 93454 797-A1
A CT
PSRS 93446 513-J6
SLOC 93465 553-B1
A DR
PBCH 93449 714-F3
AS AV
SBAR 93101 995-H4
AS PL
SLOC 93420 695-C5
ONA WY
ATAS 93422 594-C1
ST
MOBY 93442 611-D1
ITA PL
SBAR 93103 996-A2
ANUS ST
CARP 93013 1018-G1
StBC 93013 1018-F1
RAMA DR
MOBY 93442 591-D7
MOBY 93442 611-E1
PBCH 93449 714-F3
PSRS 93446 513-F3
SLOC - 591-D7
SLOC - 611-E1
SLOC 93442 591-D7
SLOC 93442 611-E1

PANORAMA PL
SBAR 93105 985-H7
PAQUITA DR
StBC 93013 997-J4
StBC 93013 998-A3
PAR AV
PSRS 93446 513-J7
PARADISE DR
SLOC 93420 715-F2
PARADISE LN
SLOC 93402 652-C2
StBC 93105 964-G1
PARADISE RD
StBC 93105 964-E1
PARADISE MEADOWS LN
SLOC 93465 553-A3
PARAISO
ARGD 93420 714-H2
PARAISO DR
SMRA 93458 796-F4
PARDALL RD
StBC 93117 994-A5
PAREJO CIR
StBC 93111 984-G7
PAREJO DR
StBC 93111 984-F7
PARK AV
PBCH 93449 714-C3
SLO 93401 654-A3
SLOC 93430 591-A2
SMRA 93454 796-H1
SMRA 93458 796-G1
StBC 93455 816-F5
PARK CIR
BLTN 93427 919-G5
GOL 93117 993-G1
PARK LN
GBCH 93433 714-D4
StBC 93108 987-B7
StBC 93108 997-B1
PARK LN W
StBC 93108 987-A7
PARK PL
PBCH 93449 693-G7
SBAR 93103 996-E3
PARK ST
BLTN 93427 919-H5
MOBY 93442 611-E4
PSRS 93446 513-F2
StBC 93441 900-H6
PARK WY
ARGD 93420 714-H5
SLVG 93463 940-E1
PARKDALE LN
StBC 93455 817-A4
PARKER ST
SLO 93401 653-H5
PARKER WY
SBAR 93101 996-B5
PARK HILL LN
StBC 93108 987-A7
PARKHURST DR
GOL 93117 984-C7
PARKLAND DR
StBC 93455 817-A3
PARKLAND TER
SLO 93401 654-B5
PARKS RD
SBAR 93105 995-F3
PARKSIDE CT
StBC 93437 855-F7
PARKSIDE WY
LMPC 93436 896-D6
PARKVIEW N
StBC 93455 816-H3
PARKVIEW S
StBC 93455 816-H4
PARK VIEW AV
GBCH 93433 714-D4
PARKVIEW AV
SMRA 93458 796-G2
PARK VIEW DR
MOBY 93442 631-G1
PARK VIEW LN
Npmo 93444 756-A3
PARKVIEW LN
PSRS 93446 534-C1
PARKVIEW RD
BLTN 93427 919-F5
PARK VIEW ST
StBC 93440 878-H2
PARKVIEW ST
StBC 93437 855-F7
PARK VIEW TR
SLVG 93463 940-D1
PARKWAY DR
SBAR 93105 995-H3
PARKWAY CIRCLE DR
SLOC 93446 471-E4
PARKWOOD PL
StBC 93111 984-H7
PARRA GRANDE LN
StBC 93108 996-H1
PARRIZA CT
ATAS 93422 573-F3
ATAS 93422 574-A4
PARTNER RD
SLOC 93405 653-C3
PARTRIDGE
PSRS 93446 514-A6
PARTRIDGE DR
SLO 93405 653-E7
PARTRIDGE LN
SLOC 93446 471-B5
PAR VIEW LN
SLOC 93420 735-A4
PASADENA DR
SLOC 93402 631-G4
PASADENA LN
PSRS 93446 513-G2
PASADENA RD
SLOC 93422 594-D5
PASADO RD
StBC 93117 993-J5
StBC 93117 994-A5
PASATIEMPO DR
SLO 93405 653-G1
PASEO
PBCH 93449 714-C3
PASEO ST
ARGD 93420 715-A4
PASEO ALICANTE
SBAR 93103 995-J1
PASEO ALMERIA
SBAR 93103 996-A1
PASEO CAMEO
StBC 93111 984-G6
PASEO CIELO
SMRA 93455 796-H5

PASEO DE CABALLO
ATAS 93422 574-B5
SLOC 93405 633-F7
PASEO DE LAS GRANADAS
SBAR 93101 996-A3
PASEO DEL DESCANSO
SBAR 93105 985-H7
SBAR 93105 995-H1
PASEO DEL LAGO
ATAS 93422 553-J7
PASEO DEL OCASO
StBC 93105 985-J5
PASEO DEL PINON
GOL 93117 993-F1
PASEO DEL REFUGIO
SBAR 93105 985-G7
SBAR 93105 995-G1
PASEO DEL RIO
SLVG 93463 940-D1
PASEO DE VACA
ATAS 93422 574-B5
PASEO DE YACA
SLOC 93401 673-F5
PASEO EXSELSUS
SLOC 93465 553-A3
PASEO FERRELO
SBAR 93103 996-C2
PASEO JACARANDA
SMRA 93458 796-E5
PASEO LADERA
PBCH 93449 714-E3
PASEO LADERA LN
SLOC 93449 694-F7
SLOC 93449 714-F1
PASEO LOS SANTOS
StBC 93111 984-J6
PASEO ORLANDO
StBC 93111 984-G6
PASEO PACIFICO
ATAS 93422 553-C6
PASEO PALMILLA
GOL 93117 984-D6
SMRA 93458 796-E4
PASEO POCO
SLOC 93451 473-C1
StBC 93460 941-D1
PASEO REDONDO
SBAR 93110 985-C7
PASEO RIO
StBC 93111 984-G6
PASEO TRANQUILLO
SBAR 93105 985-G7
PASEO VINEDO
SLOC 93401 695-B1
PASO ROBLES AV
SLOC 93402 631-H5
PASO ROBLES BLVD
PSRS 93446 514-B3
PASO ROBLES DR
SLO 93405 654-B2
StBC 93108 996-E1
PASO ROBLES ST
PSRS 93446 513-G5
SLOC 93445 714-F7
SLOC 93445 734-F1
PASO VERDE CT
ATAS 93422 573-B6
PASQUALA LN
StBC 93460 921-B6
PASTORIA AV
SMRA 93458 796-E4
PATCHETT RD
SLOC 93420 694-H4
PATERNA RD
SBAR 93103 996-A1
PATO AV
StBC 93254 806-B1
PATO LN
SLOC 93402 631-E7
SLOC 93402 651-B3
PATRIA CIR
ATAS 93422 594-C1
PATRIA CT
PSRS 93446 514-A3
PATRICIA CT
SLO 93405 653-G1
SMRA 93455 796-J7
PATRICIA DR
SLO 93405 653-G1
PATRICIA LN
PSRS 93446 513-J7
PSRS 93446 514-A7
StBC 93111 994-H1
PATRICIO LN
Npmo 93444 755-F3
PATRICK WY
SMRA 93455 796-J6
PATTERSON AV
GOL 93111 984-F5
GOL 93111 994-G2
GOL 93117 984-E5
StBC 93111 984-F5
StBC 93111 994-G3
StBC 93117 984-E5
PATTERSON PL
Cmbr 93428 528-G7
Cmbr 93428 548-H1
GOL 93111 994-G1
PATTERSON RD
StBC 93455 816-H5
StBC 93455 817-A5
PATTI LN
SMRA 93458 776-F6
PATTY KAY CT
Npmo 93444 755-G3
PAUL PL
ARGD 93420 714-G7
PAULA ST
MOBY 93442 611-F3
PAULA RAY LN
BLTN 93427 919-H4
PAULDING CIR
ARGD 93420 715-A4
PAULINE CT
StBC 93455 816-J2
PAULINE WY
SLO 93401 654-A5
PAWNEE CT
PSRS 93446 513-H6
PAXTON CT
GOL 93117 993-E1
PAYERAS ST
SBAR 93109 995-H6
PAYTON ST
StBC 93111 994-J2
PAYTON WY
Npmo 93444 755-C3
SLOC 93420 755-C3
SMRA 93455 797-A6

P C LAKE RD
StBC 93437 875-H5
PEACE LN
SLOC 93449 714-G1
PEACEFUL POINT LN
SLOC 93420 735-A1
PEACH AV
LMPC 93436 916-F2
PEACH ST
SLO 93401 653-J4
SLO 93401 654-A3
PEACH GROVE LN
SBAR 93105 995-E2
PEACHTREE CT
PSRS 93446 513-E6
PEACHTREE LN
PSRS 93446 513-F6
PEACHY CT
PSRS 93446 513-F6
PEACHY CANYON RD
PSRS 93446 513-E6
SLOC 93446 513-A6
PEACOCK CT
SLOC 93465 553-B1
PEACOCK LN
StBC 93455 796-H7
PEACOCK PL
SLOC 93445 734-G1
PEACOCK WY
Npmo 93444 756-C4
PEANUT WY
SLOC 93420 734-H7
W PEAR AV
LMPC 93436 916-C1
PEAR ST
CARP 93013 998-C6
PEARL DR
ARGD 93420 714-J7
PEARL ST
CARP 93013 998-A5
PBCH 93449 693-H7
PEARLIE LN
Npmo 93444 756-C4
PEAR VALLEY WY
SLOC 93451 473-C1
PEARWOOD AV
ARGD 93420 715-C3
SLOC 93420 715-C3
PEBBLE ST
GBCH 93433 714-F6
PEBBLE BEACH CT
PSRS 93446 533-J1
PEBBLE BEACH DR
GOL 93117 993-F3
PEBBLE BEACH PL
SMRA 93454 776-J2
PEBBLEBEACH WY
SLOC 93401 674-E6
PEBBLE HILL DR
StBC 93111 984-J7
PEBBLE HILL LN
StBC 93111 994-J1
PEBBLE HILL PL
StBC 93111 984-H7
StBC 93111 994-H1
PECAN CT
StBC 93437 875-J1
PECAN PL
ARGD 93420 714-H6
PECAN ST
ARGD 93420 714-H6
StBC 93437 875-J1
PECHO RD
SLOC 93402 631-F6
PECHO ST
MOBY 93442 611-G7
PECHO VALLEY RD
SLOC 93402 631-E7
SLOC 93402 651-B3
PECOS CT
ATAS 93422 573-B5
PEDERNAL AV
GOL 93117 994-D1
PEDREGOSA ST
SBAR 93101 995-H4
SBAR 93103 995-H4
SBAR 93103 996-A1
E PEDREGOSA ST
SBAR 93103 996-A1
PEGASUS AV
StBC 93436 876-C6
PEGGY LEE CT
Npmo 93444 755-G2
PELICAN LN
GDLP 93434 774-H6
PELICAN PL
MOBY 93442 611-F6
PELLHAM DR
StBC 93436 896-F2
PEMBROKE AV
GOL 93111 984-F7
PEMBROKE CT
GOL 93111 984-F7
PEMBROOK DR
Cmbr 93428 528-D6
LMPC 93436 916-G2
PEMM PL
SBAR 93110 985-E7
StBC 93110 985-E7
PENDLETON LN
SLOC 93465 553-B1
PENMAN WY
SLO 93405 653-H3
PENMAN SPRINGS RD
SLOC 93446 514-F7
SLOC 93446 534-F1
PENNELL RD
StBC 93111 985-A5
PENNINGTON CREEK RD
SLOC 93405 632-J3
SLOC 93405 633-A3
PENNSYLVANIA ST
SMRA 93454 796-H4
PENNY LN
SLO 93401 654-A4
StBC 93108 997-B3
E PEPPER LN
StBC 93108 996-H2
W PEPPER LN
StBC 93108 996-H2
PEPPER ST
SLO 93401 654-A3
PEPPERDINE CT
GOL 93117 993-H3
PEPPERGRASS CT
GOL 93117 993-J4
PEPPER TREE LN
StBC 93455 816-H1

PEPPER TREE RANCH RD
StBC 93460 901-C6
PEPPERWOOD PL
SMRA 93454 777-A5
PEPPERWOOD WY
SLVG 93463 940-D2
PEQUENIA AV
ATAS 93422 573-H5
PERALTA ST
GDLP 93434 775-B5
PERCH LN
SLOC 93446 471-D3
PEREGRINA RD
SBAR 93105 995-G2
PEREGRINE LN
Npmo 93444 756-A4
PEREIRA DR
SLO 93405 653-F7
PERES RD
SBAR 93117 994-D1
PEREZA CIR
StBC 93111 984-F7
PERGOLA ST
SMRA 93458 796-G4
PERIMETER RD
SLOC 93451 471-H1
E PERIMETER RD
SLOC 93451 453-A7
SLOC 93451 473-B1
N PERIMETER RD
SLOC 93405 653-J1
SLOC 93405 654-A1
SLOC 93407 653-J1
S PERIMETER RD
SLOC 93405 653-J2
SLOC 93405 654-A1
PERIWINKLE LN
StBC 93108 996-J1
PERKINS LN
SLO 93401 654-A6
PERKINS RD
StBC 93254 806-B3
PERKINS ST
StBC 93440 878-G1
PERLA LN
SLO 93401 673-G2
PERRY CT
StBC 93111 994-G3
PERSHING DR
SLOC 93445 714-D7
PERSHING ST
SMRA 93454 796-G2
SMRA 93458 796-F2
PERSIMMON PL
SLOC 93446 471-D3
PERUVIAN WY
SLOC 93446 471-C5
PESCADERO DR
SBAR 93105 995-E3
PESCADO CT
ATAS 93422 573-H4
PESETAS LN
SBAR 93110 985-D7
SBAR 93110 995-D1
PETALUMA ST
SLOC 93405 633-E5
PETERS PL
SLOC 93401 674-E7
PETERSEN AV
SLVG 93463 920-C7
SLVG 93463 940-D1
PETERSEN RANCH RD
SLOC 93465 553-C1
PHEASANT
PSRS 93446 514-B7
PHEASANT LN
SLOC 93446 471-B5
PHEASANT CANYON CT
BLTN 93427 920-A6
PHEASANT VIEW DR
StBC 93455 816-J1
PHELAN RANCH WY
SLOC 93420 735-C3
PHELPS RD
GOL 93117 993-H3
StBC 93117 993-H3
PHILBRIC RD
SMRA 93454 797-F2
StBC 93454 797-F2
PHILINDA AV
SBAR 93103 996-B2
PHILLIPS LN
SLO 93401 653-J3
SLO 93401 654-A3
PHILLIPS RD
SLOC 93420 715-A1
SLOC 93465 533-E7
PHOEBE CT
Npmo 93444 756-B4
PHOEBE ST
Npmo 93444 756-B4
PHULLAHARI RD
SLOC - 572-A5
SLOC 93430 572-A5
PHYLLIS RAE CT
Npmo 93444 735-J4
PICACHO LN
StBC 93108 986-H7
StBC 93108 996-H1
PICASSO RD
StBC 93117 994-A4
PICAY LN
StBC 93108 997-F1
PICKWICK LN
Cmbr 93428 548-H2
PICO AV
SBAR 93103 996-B3
PICO CT
SLO 93405 653-F7
PICO ST
MOBY 93442 611-E3
PIEDMONT PL
PSRS 93446 513-E5
PIEDMONT RD
SBAR 93105 985-F6
PIEDRA CT
SLOC 93401 674-F7
PIEDRAS DR
StBC 93108 997-C1
PIEDRAS ALTOS
ATAS 93422 573-H5
PIEDRA SPRINGS RD
SLOC 93420 695-E5
PIER AV
PBCH 93449 693-H7
SLOC 93445 714-D7
PIER ST
CARP 93013 998-B6

PIERCE AV
Cmbr 93428 548-H1
PIERCE DR
SMRA 93454 777-B6
PIERPONT ST
Summ 93067 997-C3
PIKE LN
SLOC 93445 714-E7
PILGRIM WY
ARGD 93420 715-A6
PILGRIM TERRACE DR
SBAR 93101 995-G3
PIMIENTO LN
StBC 93108 996-J2
PINAL AV
ATAS 93422 574-A3
SLOC 93453 614-G2
StBC 93455 816-G6
PINA SELVA PL
SLOC 93465 533-H6
PINE
SLO 93401 673-H1
PINE AV
GOL 93117 994-E2
SLOC 93402 631-G6
SLOC 93422 594-G6
E PINE AV
LMPC 93436 896-E7
W PINE AV
LMPC 93436 896-C7
PINE CT
Cmbr 93428 528-G7
PINE DR
SBAR 93105 995-G3
PINE LN
LMPC 93436 895-J2
LMPC 93436 896-A2
PINE ST
ARGD 93420 714-G5
PSRS 93446 513-F2
SLVG 93463 920-F7
SLVG 93463 940-F1
SMRA 93458 776-G5
SMRA 93458 796-G2
StBC 93460 921-B5
PINE BRANCH RD
SLOC 93426 470-A2
PINECONE WY
SLOC 93420 734-J4
PINECOVE DR
SLOC 93405 653-G7
PINE CREEK CT
StBC 93455 817-B6
PINECREST PL
Npmo 93444 756-B4
PINEDORADO RD
ATAS 93422 573-J7
ATAS 93422 574-A6
PINEHURST DR
StBC 93436 876-F6
PINEHURST WY
SLOC 93401 674-D6
PINEKNOLLS DR
Cmbr 93428 528-F6
PINELAKE ST
StBC 93455 816-J3
PINERIDGE DR
Cmbr 93428 548-H1
PINE RIDGE LN
SLOC 93420 735-B5
PINE RIDGE RD
SLOC 93426 470-A2
PINESPRING LN
SBAR 93110 985-E7
PINETREE LN
SLOC 93449 714-G1
PINE TREE PL
GOL 93117 993-F1
PINE VIEW DR
SLOC 93420 715-A2
PINEWOOD CT
ATAS 93422 574-B7
PINEWOOD DR
Cmbr 93428 528-F6
SMRA 93455 816-B1
StBC 93455 816-B1
PINEY LN
MOBY 93442 611-G7
PINEY WY
Cmbr 93428 528-G7
MOBY 93442 611-G6
PINION PT
SLOC 93446 469-G4
PINNACLE CT
PSRS 93446 514-A4
PINNACLE DR
SMRA 93458 796-E4
PINO WY
PSRS 93446 513-J5
PIN OAK LN
SLOC 93446 533-J4
PINO SOLO AV
ATAS 93422 574-B6
PINO SOLO CT
Npmo 93444 756-A3
PINO SOLO DR
StBC 93455 817-A7
PINTA RD
StBC 93437 895-E1
PINTAIL AV
SLOC 93446 471-D6
PINTO
PBCH 93449 714-D3
PINTO CIR
SLOC 93420 734-J5
PINTO LN
SLOC 93446 471-C6
PINTURA DR
StBC 93111 984-H7
PINZON CT
ATAS 93422 594-C2
PIONA LN
ATAS 93422 594-C1
PIONEER AV
Npmo 93444 756-B2
PIONEER CT
SMRA 93454 777-B7
PIONEER DR
SMRA 93454 777-B6
PIONEER ST
GDLP 93434 774-J6
GDLP 93434 775-A5
StBC 93434 775-A5
PIONEER TRAIL RD
PSRS 93446 534-C1
PIPPIN LN
SLOC 93402 673-C7
PIRA RD
StBC 93437 875-E7

PIRA RD
StBC 93437 895-E1
PIRITA RD
StBC 93437 875-E7
PISMO AV
ATAS 93422 573-H6
PBCH 93449 714-B2
SLOC 93402 631-J5
SLOC 93402 632-A5
PISMO ST
SLO 93401 653-J5
SLO 93401 654-A4
PISMO BEACH CIR
GOL 93117 993-F3
PITOS ST
SBAR 93103 996-E4
PITT PL
Cmbr 93428 548-G2
PITZER CT
GOL 93117 993-H3
PLACENCIA ST
GOL 93117 994-E3
SBAR 93117 994-E3
PLACENTIA AV
PBCH 93449 693-H7
PLACER AV
SLOC 93405 633-A5
PLACER DR
GOL 93117 993-G2
PLACIDA AV
SBAR 93101 996-A4
PLANCHA WY
SLOC 93420 715-B3
PLATA LN
ATAS 93422 574-A6
PLATA RD
ARGD 93420 715-B4
PLATINO LN
ARGD 93420 715-B4
PLAYA PL
PBCH 93449 693-E5
PLAYA BLANCA CT
SMRA 93455 796-H5
PLAYA BLANCA ST
SMRA 93455 796-H6
PLAYA DEL SOL
PBCH 93449 693-H7
PLAYA VISTA PL
SLOC 93424 693-A3
PLAYER LN
PSRS 93446 513-J7
PSRS 93446 533-J1
PLAZA
PBCH 93449 714-C3
PLAZA DR
SMRA 93454 796-H2
PLAZA LN
SBAR 93105 995-E1
PLAZA ALEMAN
StBC 93111 994-G2
PLAZA DEL CENTRO
GOL 93111 994-F2
StBC 93111 994-F2
PLAZA DEL MAR
SBAR 93101 996-B5
PLAZA DEL MONTE
SBAR 93101 995-H5
PLAZA DE SONODORES
StBC 93108 996-H4
PLAZA PACIFICA
StBC 93108 996-H4
PLAZA RUBIO
SBAR 93103 995-J1
PLEASANT LN
SLOC 93420 715-B7
PLEASANT PL
StBC 93455 817-B5
PLEMAN PL
SMRA 93458 776-G5
PLOMO CT
ARGD 93420 715-B3
PLOVER CT
SLOC 93420 735-A5
PLUM ST
CARP 93013 998-C6
PLUMA CT
ATAS 93422 594-C1
PLUMAS AV
GOL 93117 993-H2
SLOC 93405 632-J5
PLUMAS CT
PSRS 93446 514-B7
PSRS 93446 534-B1
PLUMERIA CT
StBC 93455 817-A3
PLUMM ORCHARD LN
SLOC 93465 553-B4
PLUTO AV
StBC 93436 896-C2
PLUTO ST
Npmo 93444 756-A5
PLYMOUTH ST
Cmbr 93428 528-E6
PLYMOUTH HILL ST
SLOC 93446 513-F2
POA PL
SLOC 93405 653-D6
POAGUE RD
Npmo 93444 756-F5
POCAHONTAS CT
PSRS 93446 513-H6
POCO RD
SLOC 93465 574-G1
POINSETTIA ST
SLO 93401 674-C2
POINSETTIA WY
StBC 93111 984-G6
POINT LOBO LN
SMRA 93454 776-J5
POINT SAL DUNES CIR
GDLP 93434 774-J6
POINT SAL DUNES WY
GDLP 93434 774-J6
POLARIS AV
StBC 93436 876-C6
POLARIS DR
Npmo 93444 756-A5
POLK ST
SMRA 93458 776-G4
POLY CANYON RD
SLOC 93405 654-A1
N POLY VUE DR
SLOC 93405 653-J1
S POLY VUE DR
SLOC 93405 653-J1
SLOC 93405 654-A1
POMAR LN
StBC 93108 997-A3

STREET Name City ZIP Pg-Grid

POMAR RD
SLOC 93422 593-F3
POMEROY AV
PBCH 93449 714-B2
POMEROY RD
Npmo 93444 735-F7
Npmo 93444 755-G2
Npmo 93444 756-A3
SLOC 93420 735-E4
POMMEL DR
StBC 93463 900-F6
POMONA CT
GOL 93117 993-H3
POND RD
SLOC 93445 734-F1
PONDEROSA LN
PSRS 93446 534-B1
PONDEROSA PL
Npmo 93444 756-A4
PONDEROSA ST
MOBY 93442 611-F4
PONDEROSA WY
StBC 93111 994-H1
PONTIAC LN
StBC 93455 817-E5
POOLE ST
ARGD 93420 715-A5
POOPOUT HILL RD
SLOC 93451 473-A1
POPLAR AV
SLOC 93422 594-F7
POPLAR ST
ARGD 93420 714-G5
CARP 93013 1018-F1
SMRA 93458 776-G2
StBC 93013 1018-F1
POPPINGA WY
StBC 93455 816-G4
POPPY LN
PSRS 93446 514-C7
PSRS 93446 534-C1
SLO 93401 674-C1
SLOC 93420 735-F5
StBC 93455 816-H2
N POPPY ST
LMPC 93436 896-G6
LMPC 93436 916-G1
POPPY FIELD PL
GOL 93117 993-J4
POPPY VALLEY RD
StBC 93427 919-G1
POPULUS AV
SLO 93401 674-E1
POQUITA LN
SLOC 93451 473-F2
POQUITO PL
SLOC 93420 734-H4
POR LA MAR CIR
SBAR 93103 996-E4
POR LA MAR DR
SBAR 93103 996-E4
PORTAL RD
ATAS 93422 573-E5
PORTER ST
PBCH 93449 714-B2
PORTERVILLE ST
PBCH 93449 714-C2
PORTESUELLO AV
SBAR 93101 995-F4
SBAR 93105 995-F4
PORTLAND DR
SMRA 93458 776-H3
PORTOFINO WY
SBAR 93105 995-E3
PORTOLA LN
SBAR 93105 995-F3
PORTOLA RD
ATAS 93422 573-G3
ATAS 93422 574-A6
PORTOLA ST
SLO 93405 653-D6
PORTOLA WY
ATAS 93422 573-G3
POSADA LN
SLOC 93465 553-C1
POSILIPO LN
StBC 93108 997-A4
POST AV
CARP 93013 998-D6
POTE RD
StBC 93437 875-E7
StBC 93437 895-E1
POTRERO LN
StBC 93105 964-G1
POTRERO RD
ATAS 93422 553-F7
POWER RD
SLOC 93451 473-G2
POWERLINE RD
SLOC 93422 594-D5
POWERS AV
SBAR 93103 996-D4
PRADERA CT
ARGD 93420 715-C4
PRADERA PL
Npmo 93444 756-A3
PRADO LN
ATAS 93422 593-H1
PRADO PL
SLOC 93451 473-F2
PRADO RD
SLO 93401 653-H7
SLO 93401 673-J1
SLO 93401 674-A1
SLOC 93401 673-J1
SLOC 93401 674-A1
PRAIRIE LN
SMRA 93458 796-G4
PRAIRIE RD
SLOC 93446 494-G7
SLOC 93446 514-G1
PREFUMO CANYON RD
SLO 93405 653-D6
SLOC 93405 652-F7
SLOC 93405 653-A6
PREISKER LN
SMRA 93454 776-H4
SMRA 93458 776-H3
PRELL RD
SMRA 93454 797-B5
StBC 93454 797-B5
PREMIER CT
SMRA 93454 777-B7
PRESCOTT DR
MOBY 93442 611-F5
PRESCOTT LN
StBC 93455 816-G1
PRESIDIO AV
SBAR 93101 996-B3
PRESIDIO WY
SMRA 93458 776-G3
PRESTON LN
MOBY 93442 611-F4
PRESTON ST
Cmbr 93428 548-H2
PRETTY DOE LN
SLOC 93446 471-D6
PRICE ST
PBCH 93449 693-J7
PBCH 93449 714-A1
SLO 93401 653-J5
E PRICE ST
Npmo 93444 756-D2
W PRICE ST
Npmo 93444 756-C2
PRICE CANYON RD
PBCH 93449 714-C2
SLOC 93401 694-E3
SLOC 93420 694-E3
SLOC 93449 694-E3
SLOC 93449 714-C2
PRICE RANCH RD
StBC 93440 878-J1
PRICKLY PEAR WY
SLOC 93453 695-E4
PRIMAVERA LN
Npmo 93444 756-B6
PRIMAVERA RD
SBAR 93110 985-D7
PRIMERO ST
StBC 93254 806-B1
PRIMROSE CT
LMPC 93436 896-D6
PRIMROSE LN
Npmo 93444 756-A3
PSRS 93446 514-A6
StBC 93437 875-J3
StBC 93455 816-H2
PRINCESS CT
Npmo 93444 756-C4
PRINCETON AV
GOL 93111 984-F7
PRINCETON DR
StBC 93455 816-H6
PRINCETON PL
LMPC 93436 916-G2
SLO 93405 653-G1
PRINCIPAL AV
ATAS 93422 574-B6
PRINTZ RD
ARGD 93420 714-J1
ARGD 93420 715-A2
SLOC 93420 714-J1
SLOC 93420 715-A2
PRISCILLA LN
ARGD 93420 714-G5
PRIVATE DR
SLOC 93401 693-E3
PRODUCE PL
SLOC 93420 734-H2
SLOC 93445 734-H2
PROFESSIONAL PKWY
Npmo 93444 755-C4
SLOC 93420 755-C4
PROMONTORY PL
PSRS 93446 514-A4
PRONGHORN CT
SLOC 93426 469-H2
PROPELLER DR
PSRS 93446 494-C6
PROSPECT AV
PSRS 93446 514-A3
SBAR 93103 995-J2
SBAR 93103 996-A2
PROSPECT ST
SLOC 93401 674-D3
PROSPERITY WY
Npmo 93444 756-A3
PROVANCE AV
SMRA 93458 796-F4
PROVENCE DR
SLOC 93420 715-A2
E PRUNE AV
LMPC 93436 896-E7
W PRUNE AV
LMPC 93436 896-C7
PUEBLO AV
ATAS 93422 574-A4
StBC 93110 985-E6
PUEBLO ST
SBAR 93105 995-H3
PUEBLO VISTA RD
SBAR 93103 996-C2
PUENTE DR
StBC 93110 994-J3
StBC 93110 995-A2
PUENTE PZ
StBC 93110 995-A2
PUENTE RD
ATAS 93422 573-C5
PUERTO DR
GOL 93117 993-H2
PUESTA DEL SOL
ARGD 93420 714-H2
StBC 93013 1018-J3
VeCo 93001 1018-J3
PUESTA DEL SOL RD
SBAR 93105 995-H1
StBC 93105 995-J1
PUFFIN WY
SLOC 93465 553-B2
PULLMAN AV
SMRA 93458 776-F3
PUMA CT
SLOC 93401 673-F7
PUMP HANDLE LN
SLOC 93446 533-G2
PUNTA GORDA ST
SBAR 93103 996-E4
PURISIMA RD
LMPC 93436 896-F3
StBC 93436 896-F3
PURPLE SAGE LN
SLO 93401 674-D2
PUTTER AV
PSRS 93446 513-J7
PSRS 93446 514-A7
PYRACANTHA LN
StBC 93437 875-J3

Q

N Q ST
LMPC 93436 896-D7
LMPC 93436 916-D1
S Q ST
LMPC 93436 916-D2
QUAIL CIR
LMPC 93436 916-F1
SLO 93405 653-E7
QUAIL CT
ARGD 93420 714-G3
StBC 93455 816-G7
QUAIL DR
SLO 93405 653-E7
QUAIL LN
SLOC 93402 651-J1
QUAIL RUN
PSRS 93446 514-B7
QUAIL WY
SLOC 93424 693-C2
QUAIL CANYON RD
StBC 93455 817-E6
QUAIL CROSSING LN
SLOC 93446 470-B4
QUAILHILL LN
SLOC 93420 714-H1
QUAIL MEADOWS CT
StBC 93455 816-J1
QUAIL MEADOWS DR
StBC 93455 796-J7
StBC 93455 816-J1
QUAIL OAKS LN
Npmo 93444 755-J3
QUAIL RIDGE CT
ARGD 93420 714-J3
QUAIL RIDGE DR
ATAS 93422 573-J4
StBC 93455 816-F4
QUAIL RIDGE RD
StBC 93463 920-J5
QUAIL RUN RD
BLTN 93427 920-A6
QUAIL SUMMIT
PSRS 93446 514-A6
QUAIL VALLEY RD
StBC 93463 920-H6
StBC 93463 921-A5
QUAILWOOD LN
SLOC 93420 735-F4
QUAN AV
SLOC 93420 714-H7
QUARANTINA ST
SBAR 93103 996-B3
QUARTERHORSE LN
PSRS 93446 513-H7
QUARTERHORSE TR
StBC 93455 816-E5
QUARTERHORSE WY
SLOC 93420 735-A2
SLOC 93446 471-C4
QUEBRADA LN
SLOC 93420 715-A2
QUEEN ANN LN
StBC 93111 984-F6
QUEENANNE RD
PSRS 93446 534-B1
QUEENS CT
SMRA 93454 776-J7
QUICK DRAW LN
SLOC 93426 470-A1
QUICKSILVER WY
SLOC 93465 553-B3
QUIET OAKS DR
SLOC 93420 735-E4
QUINIENTOS ST
SBAR 93103 996-D3
QUINTA CT
SLOC 93446 533-E5
QUINTANA PL
MOBY 93442 611-F5
QUINTANA RD
MOBY 93442 611-F5
MOBY 93442 612-A7
SLOC - 612-A7
SLOC 93442 611-J7
SLOC 93442 612-A7
QUINTO ST
SBAR 93105 995-G2
QUITO ST
Npmo 93444 756-C4

R

R ST
MonC 93451 453-A1
N R ST
LMPC 93436 896-C7
LMPC 93436 916-C1
S R ST
LMPC 93436 916-C2
RAABERG WY
SMRA 93458 776-F6
RACCOON LN
SLOC 93446 470-B4
RACCOON RD
SLOC 93446 469-H4
RACHEL CT
SLO 93401 654-A5
RACHEL DR
SMRA 93454 777-A5
RACHEL LN
PSRS 93446 513-J6
RACHEL ST
SLO 93401 654-A5
RACQUET CLUB DR
CARP 93013 998-B5
RADCLIFF AV
Cmbr 93428 548-G2
RADCLIFF LN
StBC 93455 816-G4
RADCLIFFE ST
MOBY 93442 611-F5
RADDUE AV
StBC 93111 994-G3
RAFAEL WY
SLO 93405 653-G3
RAFTER WY
SLOC 93446 513-J2
RAIL CT
SLOC 93420 735-A5
RAILROAD AV
SLO 93401 654-A5
SMRA 93458 776-G3
SMRA 93458 796-G1
RAILROAD ST
PSRS 93446 513-G5
SLOC 93445 714-E7
SLOC 93445 734-E1
RAILWAY AV
StBC 93441 900-H5
RAINBOW CT
PSRS 93446 513-H6
SLOC 93465 553-C1
RAINBOW DR
SMRA 93455 796-J7
RAINBOWS END WY
SLOC 93422 593-C1
RAINEY DR
StBC 93455 816-J6
RAINIER WY
SMRA 93458 776-G3
RAIN TREE CT
SMRA 93455 796-J6
RAIN TREE DR
SMRA 93455 796-J6
RALCOA WY
SLOC 93420 754-J2
RALPH ST
SMRA 93458 796-F4
RAMADA DR
PSRS 93446 533-F3
SLOC 93446 533-F4
SLOC 93465 533-E6
RAMAGE AV
ATAS 93422 573-G3
RAMAL LN
Npmo 93444 736-A3
RAMBLIN ROSE WY
SLOC 93420 695-A7
SLOC 93420 715-A1
RAMBOUILLET RD
PSRS 93446 513-J7
PSRS 93446 533-J1
RAMELLI RANCH RD
VeCo - 999-H7
VeCo 93001 999-H7
RAMETTO LN
SBAR 93108 996-F2
RAMETTO RD
SBAR 93108 996-F3
RAMITAS RD
StBC 93110 995-C3
RAMMING WY
SBAR 93105 985-F7
RAMONA AV
GBCH 93433 714-D5
SLOC 93402 631-G5
RAMONA DR
SLO 93405 653-G2
RAMONA LN
StBC 93108 996-J3
StBC 93108 997-A3
RAMONA RD
ATAS 93422 553-E7
ATAS 93422 573-F1
RAMOS LN
SMRA 93454 796-H3
RAMSEY ST
Cmbr 93428 528-F7
Cmbr 93428 548-F1
RANADA CIR
ATAS 93422 594-D1
RANCH LN
StBC 93111 994-H1
RANCH RD
BLTN 93427 919-G5
RANCH ST
SMRA 93454 776-J7
SMRA 93454 796-J1
RANCH CLUB DR
BLTN 93427 919-G5
RANCHERIA ST
SBAR 93101 996-A5
RANCHITA CANYON RD
SLOC 93451 494-F1
RANCHITO LN
SLOC 93401 674-D5
RANCHITO VISTA RD
SBAR 93108 996-D1
StBC 93108 996-D1
RANCHO DR
SLO 93405 653-G1
RANCHO PKWY
ARGD 93420 714-H4
RANCHO RD
Npmo 93444 756-D3
RANCHO ALISAL DR
SLVG - 940-D3
SLVG 93463 940-D3
StBC 93463 940-D3
RANCHO ASOLEADO DR
StBC 93110 995-B1
SBAR 93109 995-H7
RANCHO CARO RD
SLOC 93446 534-A4
RANCHO OAK DR
SLOC 93401 674-B5
RANCHO PASO DR
SLOC 93446 533-E5
RANCHO VERDE
SMRA 93458 776-F4
RANCHO VIEJO
ATAS 93422 553-J7
RANCH VIEW LN
StBC 93463 920-J6
RANDALL DR
Cmbr 93428 548-G2
RANDALL RD
StBC 93108 997-A1
RANDOLPH RD
StBC 93111 984-F6
RANDOM OAKS DR
SLOC 93422 594-E4
RANDY LN
SLOC 93420 734-G6
RANGE PL
Npmo 93444 756-D5
RANGE RD
SLOC 93405 633-E2
RANGE ST
Npmo 93444 756-C6
RANUNCULO CT
ATAS 93422 594-C2
RAPF AV
SLOC 93430 591-C5
RAPTOR ST
SLOC 93420 734-H7
SLOC 93420 754-H1
RASPBERRY AV
ARGD 93420 714-F6
RAVEN CT
SMRA 93454 796-J3
RAVENNA AV
SLOC 93402 631-G7
RAVENSCROFT DR
GOL 93117 984-D7
GOL 93117 994-D1
RAWHIDE PL
PSRS 93446 513-J4
RAY RD
SMRA 93458 775-J7
SMRA 93458 795-H2
StBC 93455 795-G4
StBC 93458 775-J7
StBC 93458 795-H2
RAYAR RD
ATAS 93422 573-C3
RAYMOND AV
StBC 93455 816-H1
RAYTHEON DR
GOL 93117 994-A2
RAYVILLE LN
StBC 93455 796-C5
READY RD
SLOC 93426 470-A1
REALITO AV
ATAS 93422 573-E7
REATA WY
ATAS 93422 574-B5
REBA ST
SLO 93401 654-B5
REBECCA LN
StBC 93105 995-F4
REBECCA ST
GBCH 93433 714-F7
REBILD DR
SLVG 93463 920-G7
RED BARK RD
SMRA 93454 776-J6
SMRA 93454 777-A6
REDBERRY PL
Npmo 93444 735-F7
Npmo 93444 755-E1
REDBIRD CT
StBC 93455 816-J1
RED BROME PL
SLOC 93453 695-E2
RED CLOUD RD
PSRS 93446 513-H6
REDDICK ST
SBAR 93103 996-C3
RED GUM LN
Npmo 93444 755-H3
RED OAK LN
SLOC 93446 469-G3
RED OAK WY
SLOC 93420 735-D5
REDONDO CT
GBCH 93433 714-F6
StBC 93460 921-A7
REDONDO LN
SLOC 93465 534-D7
SLOC 93465 553-H1
REDONDO RD
SLOC 93422 593-G4
RED RIVER DR
PSRS 93446 514-A6
RED ROBIN LN
PSRS 93446 514-C7
RED ROCK RD
SLOC 93420 714-J1
RED ROSE LN
SBAR 93109 995-H6
RED ROSE WY
SBAR 93109 995-G6
RED TAIL HAWK LN
SLOC 93446 493-F3
RED TAIL MEADOW LN
SLOC 93420 734-J4
REDWILLOW DR
StBC 93455 816-H6
RED WINGS ST
Npmo 93444 756-B6
REDWOOD
BLTN 93427 919-G5
SLO 93401 673-H1
REDWOOD AV
StBC 93455 816-J2
REDWOOD CT
PSRS 93446 534-B1
SLOC 93402 631-J7
REDWOOD DR
PSRS 93446 534-B1
REDWOOD WY
GOL 93117 993-F1
REE ST
SMRA 93455 796-J6
REED CT
GOL 93117 993-H3
REEF CT
PBCH 93449 714-D2
REFLECTION PL
SLOC 93465 533-E7
N REFUGIO AV
StBC 93460 901-A7
REFUGIO PL
ARGD 93420 714-H3
REFUGIO RD
StBC 93117 981-D3
StBC 93460 901-A7
StBC 93460 921-A2
StBC 93460 940-J3
StBC 93460 941-A3
StBC 93463 921-A7
StBC 93463 940-J3
StBC 93463 941-A2
N REFUGIO RD
StBC 93460 901-A6
REFUGIO ST
GBCH 93433 714-F6
REGAL DR
SMRA 93454 776-J7
REGENT CT
SMRA 93454 776-J7
REGENT ST
LMPC 93436 916-G2
REGINA CT
SMRA 93458 796-E4
REGIO PL
ATAS 93422 553-E6
REGIS
Cmbr 93428 548-G1
REGULUS AV
StBC 93436 876-D6
REINA CT
SLO 93405 653-D7
REMINGTON CT
SLOC 93446 514-A2
REMINGTON DR
StBC 93460 921-A4
N RENA ST
ARGD 93420 714-H5
S RENA ST
ARGD 93420 714-H6
RENATE WY
PSRS 93446 513-J4
RENEE CT
StBC 93455 817-A4
RENNEL ST
MOBY 93442 611-D1
RENO CT
MOBY 93442 611-E3
RENWICK AV
StBC 93436 895-C4
StBC 93437 895-C4
RESERVOIR RD
ARGD 93420 714-J5
SLOC 93446 471-E4
SLOC 93451 471-E4
RESERVOIR CANYON RD
SLOC 93401 654-D2
SLOC 93453 654-H4
RETORNO DR
CARP 93013 1018-E1
REVERE ST
StBC 93455 817-B5
REX PL
GOL 93117 984-C7
REY RD
SBAR 93101 996-B5
REYNOLDS AV
CARP 93013 998-C6
RHINESTONE CT
StBC 93455 817-B5
RHOADS AV
StBC 93111 994-G3
RIALTO LN
SBAR 93105 995-F4
RIATA CT
PSRS 93446 534-B1
RIATA LN
Npmo 93444 735-J4
Npmo 93444 736-A3
RIBE RD
StBC 93463 920-D6
RIBERA RD
StBC 93111 984-H7
StBC 93111 994-G1
RICARDO AV
SBAR 93109 995-H6
RICARDO CT
SLO 93401 654-B7
RICE CT
ARGD 93420 714-G6
RICE ST
SLOC 93445 714-E7
E RICE RANCH RD
StBC 93455 816-H7
StBC 93455 817-A7
W RICE RANCH RD
StBC 93455 816-G6
RICH CT
SLO 93401 654-B5
RICHARD AV
Cmbr 93428 548-H2
SLOC 93430 591-B4
RICHARD DR
SMRA 93458 796-G3
RICHARD ST
SLO 93401 654-C6
SMRA 93458 796-G3
RICHARDSON AV
SBAR 93103 996-B4
RICHELLE LN
SBAR 93105 995-E4
StBC 93105 995-E4
RICHLAND DR
SBAR 93105 995-F1
RICHMIND CT
SMRA 93455 796-H7
RICHMOND RD
StBC 93429 855-F2
RICK RD
StBC 93455 816-E4
RIDDERING ST
SMRA 93455 796-J5
RIDGE LN
SBAR 93103 995-J1
RIDGE RD
Npmo 93444 755-H2
PBCH 93449 714-F3
SLOC 93465 553-B4
StBC 93460 901-C4
RIDGECREST DR
StBC 93108 997-D2
RIDGECREST PL
Npmo 93444 736-B3
RIDGECREST ST
StBC 93455 816-J3
RIDGEMARK DR
SMRA 93455 796-F6
RIDGEMONT WY
SLOC 93420 734-J5
RIDGE RIDER RD
SLOC 93426 469-J1
RIDGERUNNER RD
SLOC 93420 695-D7
SLOC 93420 715-D1
RIDGEVIEW CT
PSRS 93446 513-E5
RIDGEVIEW DR
PSRS 93446 513-E5
N RIDGE VIEW DR
StBC 93455 796-J7
S RIDGE VIEW DR
StBC 93455 816-G2
RIDGEVIEW RD
StBC 93108 996-E1
RIDGEVIEW WY
ARGD 93420 715-A3
SLOC 93420 715-A3
RIDGEWAY CT
ATAS 93422 573-H3
RIDGEWAY ST
MOBY 93442 611-G7
RIDGEWOOD CT
StBC 93437 855-E6
RIDGEWOOD ST
StBC 93437 855-D6
RIESLING LN
SLOC 93465 553-A3
RIGEL AV
StBC 93436 876-C5
RIGHETTI RD
SLOC 93401 654-J7
SLOC 93401 674-J2
RILEY RD
SLVG 93463 940-E3
RIM RD
StBC 93105 964-J6
RIMES CT
SMRA 93458 796-F4
RIMROCK LN
SLOC 93401 674-D7
SLOC 93401 694-D1
RIM ROCK RD
Npmo 93444 735-H4
RINCON CT
GBCH 93433 714-F6
RINCON DR
SLVG 93463 940-D4
RINCON RD
SLOC 93422
RINCON RD Rt#-150
StBC 93013
RINCONADA RD
SBAR 93101
SBAR 93103
RINCONCITO
LMPC 93436
RINCON HILL RD
StBC 93013
RINCON POINT LN
StBC 93013
RINCON POINT RD
StBC 93013
RINCON VISTA RD
SBAR 93103
RINGSTED DR
SLVG 93463
RINGSTED PL
SLVG 93463
RIO RD
SLOC 93420
SLOC 93420
RIO BLANCO CT
ATAS 93422
RIO LADO
ATAS 93422
RIO RITA RD
ATAS 93422
RIOS CT
SMRA 93454
RIO VISTA
SLVG 93463
RIO VISTA DR
GOL 93117
RIO VISTA LN
SLOC 93432
SMRA 93454
RIO VISTA PL
SLOC 93451
RIO VISTA RD
Npmo 93444
RIPARIAN WY
SLOC 93446
RIPLEY ST
StBC 93111
RITA LN
StBC 93455
RITCHIE CT
GBCH 93433
RITCHIE RD
GBCH 93433
RIVEN ROCK RD
StBC 93108
StBC 93108
RIVER AV
SLOC 93445
RIVER RD
SLOC 93446
SLOC 93451
N RIVER RD
MonC 93451
PSRS 93446
SLOC 93446
SLOC 93446
SLOC 93446
SLOC 93451
S RIVER RD
PSRS 93446
PSRS 93446
SLOC 93446
SLOC 93446
RIVER VW
SLOC 93424
RIVERA
ATAS 93422
RIVERBANK LN
PSRS 93446
RIVER BIRCH CT
SMRA 93454
RIVERGLEN DR
PSRS 93446
RIVER OAKS DR
PSRS 93446
RIVER PARK RD
StBC 93436
StBC 93436
RIVER ROCK CT
SMRA 93454
RIVER RUN RD
SLOC 93465
RIVERSIDE AV
PSRS 93446
RIVERSIDE CT
SMRA 93458
RIVERSIDE DR
LMPC 93436
RIVERSIDE RD
Npmo 93444
Npmo 93444
Npmo 93444
RIVERSIDE ST
SLOC 93405
RIVERTON DR
SMRA 93458
RIVERVIEW DR
BLTN 93427
RIVER VIEW LN
SLOC 93432
RIVERVIEW TER
LMPC 93436
RIVIERA CIR
Npmo 93444
Npmo 93444
RIVIERA LN
SMRA 93455
RIZAL AV
SLOC 93420
ROAD C
StBC 93460
ROADRUNNER DR
StBC 93455
ROAD RUNNER LN
SLOC 93432
ROADRUNNER LN
SLOC 93420
ROBBIE CIR
GOL 93117
ROBBINS ST
SBAR 93101
ROBERT CT
Npmo 93444
ROBERT LN
SMRA 93458
ROBERT RD
SBAR 93117
ROBERTA DR
SLOC 93420

STREET
Name City ZIP Pg-Grid
T EMMET WY
SLOC 93422 593-C2
TO AV
SBAR 93109 995-H6
TO CT
SLO 93401 654-B7
CT
PSRS 93446 513-G2
PSRS 93446 514-A7
CIR
ARGD 93420 714-G3
ARGD 93449 714-G3
CT
StBC 93455 816-H7
PL
StBC 93460 921-C5
HILL RD
GOL 93117 994-C2
MEADOW RD
StBC 93460 941-D1
AR AV
StBC 93441 900-H7
StBC 93460 900-H7
StBC 93460 901-A7
DR
StBC 93110 995-B4
LN
SBAR 93103 996-C1
ST
SMRA 93454 796-H2
BLANCO RD
StBC 93463 920-D4
S AV
ATAS 93422 574-A4
S PL
ARGD 93420 714-G4
S RD
ARGD 93420 714-G4
S ST
SLOC 93446 533-F1
S PERDIDO DR
SLOC 93402 631-J6
ELLE WY
SLOC 93445 734-G1
ESTER PL
GOL 93117 993-F2
AWAY AV
GBCH 93433 714-D5
BRIDGE RD
StBC 93108 986-G7
CREEK RD
SBAR 93105 985-F7
DOVE CT
SLOC 93424 693-A1
ROSE LN
LMPC 93436 896-C6
SLOC 93424 693-B1
TERRACE WY
SLOC 93432 574-J4
VIEW PL
SLO 93401 654-A7
SLOC 93401 654-A7
VIEW ST
MOBY 93442 611-F4
WOOD DR
SBAR 93103 986-B7
SBAR 93105 986-B7
WREN LN
SLOC 93424 693-A1
Y PL
SLOC 93420 735-E5
Y CANYON RD
SLOC 93432 574-B2
SLOC 93465 574-B2
Y CREEK LN
SLOC 93401 673-G6
Y OAK LN
SLOC 93420 736-F2
Y POINT LN
SLOC 93422 593-C1
SO WY
StBC 93111 984-H7
DR
SMRA 93455 796-H7
O DR
ARGD 93420 714-J3
O WY
SLOC 93446 534-J4
O GROUNDS RD
Cmbr 93428 528-G7
MAN AV
Cmbr 93428 548-G1
MAN DR
SLOC 93402 631-F7
SLOC 93402 651-E1
RD
SLOC 93420 735-C5
IER CT
SMRA 93454 776-H4
IER PL
SMRA 93454 776-H4
IER WY
SMRA 93454 776-H4
RS CT
ARGD 93420 714-G7
RS DR
Cmbr 93428 528-G7
E DR
CARP 93013 998-E7
CT
ATAS 93422 573-B6
E LN
SLOC 93465 553-B2
E GATES DR
PSRS 93446 494-C6
ING BROOK LN
SBAR 93110 985-E7
ING GREEN DR
SMRA 93455 796-F6
ING HILL DR
StBC 93437 855-F7
ING HILLS RD
PSRS 93446 513-J6
PSRS 93446 514-A5
StBC 93463 920-J3
StBC 93463 921-A3
ING OAKS DR
SLOC 93420 735-F7
AINE DR
SBAR 93105 995-G2
AULDO RD
SLOC 93405 632-J4
SLOC 93405 633-A4
ERO CANYON RD
StBC - 987-H2
StBC 93105 987-D3
StBC 93108 987-C4
StBC 93108 997-D1

STREET
Name City ZIP Pg-Grid
ROMNEY DR
Cmbr 93428 548-G1
RONALD PL
SMRA 93458 796-G2
RONDA DR
StBC 93111 984-J7
ROOKER RANCH WY
SLOC 93420 714-J2
ROPA CT
ATAS 93422 553-D6
ROPER WY
StBC 93455 817-A4
ROSALES CT
StBC 93455 816-B1
ROSALIE DR
StBC 93455 817-B5
ROSALIND DR
SMRA 93458 776-G6
ROSA LINDA WY
StBC 93111 984-J7
ROSANA PL
Npmo 93444 756-B5
ROSARIO AV
ATAS 93422 573-H3
ROSARIO DR
SBAR 93110 985-C7
ROSARIO PARK RD
StBC 93105 964-D4
ROSARITA LN
StBC 93105 995-H1
ROSCHELLE LN
SMRA 93458 796-G3
ROSCOE PL
Cmbr 93428 548-H2
ROSE AL
SLO 93401 653-J4
ROSE AV
SBAR 93101 996-B4
SLO 93401 654-C6
SMRA 93454 776-H6
SMRA 93454 777-A6
SMRA 93458 776-G6
ROSE CT
GBCH 93433 714-F6
ROSE DR
Npmo 93444 755-J5
Npmo 93444 756-A5
ROSE LN
CARP 93013 1018-H1
PSRS 93446 513-H6
StBC 93110 985-D6
ROSE PL
SMRA 93454 776-J6
ROSE ST
SLOC 93445 734-H2
N ROSE ST
LMPC 93436 896-B7
S ROSE ST
LMPC 93436 916-C2
ROSEBAY WY
SLOC 93465 553-C1
ROSEMARY CT
ARGD 93420 714-H2
SLO 93401 674-D2
ROSEMARY DR
PSRS 93446 514-A7
ROSEMARY LN
ARGD 93420 714-J3
SBAR 93108 996-E2
ROSEMARY RD
StBC 93454 797-C2
ROSEMEAD ST
StBC 93110 994-J2
ROSEVINE LN
SLOC 93420 714-H1
ROSEWOOD DR
SMRA 93458 776-F7
ROSEWOOD LN
ARGD 93420 715-C4
ROSINA DR
SLOC 93402 631-F6
ROSITA AV
ATAS 93422 573-G1
SMRA 93458 796-D4
ROSITA ST
SLO 93405 653-G2
ROSKILDE RD
SLVG 93463 920-E7
ROSS LN
SLOC 93420 714-H7
StBC 93455 816-H4
ROSS RD
Cmbr 93428 548-H2
SLOC 93405 632-D1
ROSSI RD
SLOC 93465 553-C3
ROSSIER LN
SBAR 93101 995-J2
ROSSMORE RD
GOL 93117 984-D7
ROTHBURY PL
GOL 93117 993-F2
ROUGEOT PL
SLO 93405 653-H2
ROUGH RD
SLOC 93426 470-A1
ROUNDHOUSE AV
SLO 93401 654-A5
ROUND MOUNTAIN HTS
SLOC 93422 593-C1
SLOC 93422 594-F5
ROUND UP PL
SLOC 93420 715-D2
ROUNDUP RD
StBC 93441 901-E4
StBC 93460 901-E4
ROWAN RD
StBC 93437 855-H7
StBC 93437 875-H1
ROWLAND DR
SMRA 93454 777-B7
ROXY AV
StBC 93455 817-A6
ROYA AV
SLOC 93465 553-B1
ROYAL CT
PSRS 93446 513-F3
SLO 93405 653-E7
ROYAL PL
SMRA 93454 776-J7
SMRA 93454 777-A7
ROYAL TER
StBC 93455 816-J5
ROYAL WY
SLO 93405 653-E7
ROYAL LINDA DR
GOL 93117 993-G1
ROYAL OAK PL
SLOC 93420 715-B2

STREET
Name City ZIP Pg-Grid
ROYAL OAK RD
StBC 93455 817-A5
RUBEL WY
SMRA 93455 796-J5
RUBIO
GDLP 93434 775-A5
RUBIO LN
SLO 93405 653-E7
RUBIO RD
SBAR 93103 996-C2
RUBY CT
PBCH 93449 693-G6
SMRA 93454 777-A6
RUBY LN
Npmo 93444 756-A5
RUBY CREST CT
StBC 93455 816-H5
RUCKER RD
StBC 93436 876-G7
StBC 93436 896-G2
RUNNING BEAR CT
SLOC 93446 471-D7
RUNNING RABBIT CIR
SLOC 93446 471-C7
RUNNING STAG WY
PSRS 93446 534-B2
RUSS CT
ARGD 93420 714-G7
RUSSELL AV
SMRA 93458 776-F7
SMRA 93458 796-F2
N RUSSELL AV
SMRA 93458 776-F5
RUSSELL WY
StBC 93110 985-D7
RUSTIC WY
SLOC 93401 674-A3
RUTGERS DR
StBC 93455 816-H3
RUTH AV
SBAR 93101 996-A5
RUTH ST
SLO 93401 654-A5
RUTH WY
SLOC 93446 533-F6
RUTH ANN WY
ARGD 93420 714-G5
RUTH ELLEN WY
Npmo 93444 755-C4
SLOC 93420 755-C4
RUTHERFORD ST
GOL 93117 994-E2

S

N S ST
LMPC 93436 896-C7
LMPC 93436 916-C1
SABADO TARDE RD
StBC 93106 994-A5
StBC 93117 993-J5
StBC 93117 994-A5
SABRINA CT
SMRA 93458 796-E4
SACAGAWEA CT
PSRS 93446 513-H6
SACRAMENTO DR
SLO 93401 654-B7
SLO 93401 674-C1
SADDLE WY
SLOC 93426 469-H2
SADDLE BACK LN
SLOC 93446 471-C6
SADIE WY
SMRA 93455 796-J6
SAFETY E
SLOC 93405 653-J1
SAFETY W
SLOC 93405 653-J1
SAGAN CIR
StBC 93436 896-C2
SAGAN CT
StBC 93436 896-C2
SAGE AV
SLOC 93402 631-J6
SLOC 93402 632-A5
SAGE CT
LMPC 93436 896-C7
StBC 93437 875-H1
SAGE LN
SLOC 93446 471-B5
SAGE ST
ARGD 93420 714-G5
LMPC 93436 916-C2
StBC 93437 875-H1
SAGE HILL DR
SBAR 93109 995-G5
SAGEWOOD DR
SMRA 93454 776-J6
SAGUNTO ST
StBC 93460 921-B5
SAINT ALBANS PL
GOL 93117 993-F2
SAINT ANDREWS CIR
PSRS 93446 533-J1
SLOC 93446 533-J1
SAINT ANDREWS CT
StBC 93436 876-E6
SAINT ANDREWS WY
Npmo 93444 755-F1
SMRA 93455 796-H6
StBC 93436 876-F5
SAINT ANN DR
PSRS 93446 533-J1
SBAR 93109 995-G5
SAINT ANNES PL
StBC 93436 876-E6
SAINT CHARLES PL
GOL 93117 993-F2
SAINT FRANCIS WY
SBAR 93105 985-F7
SLOC 93451 473-F1
SAINT GEORGE PL
GOL 93117 993-F2
SAINT IVES CT
StBC 93455 816-G4
SAINT IVES PL
GOL 93117 993-F2
SAINT JAMES DR
SBAR 93105 995-F4
SAINT JAMES RD
Cmbr 93428 548-G2
SAINT JOHN CIR
GBCH 93433 714-F6
SAINT JOSEPH ST
StBC 93440 878-G2
SAINT JOSEPHS ST
GOL 93111 994-F2

STREET
Name City ZIP Pg-Grid
SAINT MARY AV
SLOC 93430 590-J2
SLOC 93430 591-A2
SAINT MARYS CT
StBC 93455 816-H3
SAINT MARYS LN
StBC 93111 984-F6
SAINT NICKS PL
SLOC 93445 734-G1
SAINT THOMAS AV
Cmbr 93428 548-F2
SAINT VINCENT AV
SBAR 93101 996-A4
SALIDA DEL SOL
ARGD 93420 714-J3
SBAR 93109 995-H7
SALINAS AV
SLOC 93465 553-D2
SALINAS PL
SBAR 93103 996-D3
SALINAS RD
SLOC 93422 594-F2
SALINAS ST
SLOC 93405 633-D5
N SALINAS ST
SBAR 93103 996-E3
N SALINAS ST
Rt#-144
SBAR 93103 996-D3
S SALINAS ST
SBAR 93103 996-D3
SALISBURY AV
GOL 93117 993-F2
SALISBURY LN
SLOC 93401 674-D6
SMRA 93454 776-J7
SALSIPUEDES ST
SBAR 93103 996-A2
SALVAR RD
StBC 93105 985-B6
SALVIA LN
ATAS 93422 594-C2
SAMANTHA DR
PSRS 93446 513-J7
SMRA 93458 776-G4
StBC 93460 921-A4
StBC 93463 921-A4
SAMANTHA PL
StBC 93460 921-A4
SAMARKAND DR
SBAR 93105 995-G1
SAN ADRIANO CT
SLO 93405 653-E6
SAN ADRIANO ST
SLO 93405 653-E6
SAN ANDRES AV
ATAS 93422 573-H4
ATAS 93422 574-A4
SAN ANDRES ST
SBAR 93101 995-H4
SAN ANGELO AV
StBC 93111 994-J1
SAN ANSELMO RD
ATAS 93422 553-H7
ATAS 93422 573-G2
SAN ANSELO
StBC 93111 994-G2
SAN ANTERO PL
StBC 93111 994-H1
SAN ANTONIO CT
StBC 93111 984-J6
StBC 93111 985-A6
SAN ANTONIO DR
SMRA 93455 796-H6
SAN ANTONIO LN
Npmo 93444 756-B2
SAN ANTONIO RD
ATAS 93422 594-C3
SLOC 93422 594-D4
StBC 93110 985-A7
StBC 93110 995-A1
SAN ANTONIO RD W
StBC 93429 855-E3
SAN ANTONIO ST
SLOC 93424 693-A4
SAN ANTONIO CREEK
RD
StBC 93111 985-A6
SAN ANZIO WY
GOL 93117 993-G2
SAN ARDO AV
ATAS 93422 573-H1
SAN ARDO WY
StBC 93111 984-F6
SAN AUGUSTIN DR
PSRS 93446 514-A7
PSRS 93446 534-A1
SAN BARI WY
GOL 93117 993-F2
SAN BENITO RD
ATAS 93422 553-F7
ATAS 93422 573-F1
SLOC 93405 633-D4
SAN BENITO WY
StBC 93108 996-H3
SAN BERGAMO WY
GOL 93117 993-G2
SAN BERNARDINO AV
SLOC 93405 633-D4
SAN BERNARDO PL
StBC 93111 994-H2
SAN BERNARDO CREEK
RD
SLOC - 612-F3
SAN BLANCO DR
GOL 93117 993-G2
SAN BLAS PL
StBC 93111 984-G7
SAN BUENAVENTURA WY
SLOC 93451 473-F1
SAN CARLOS DR
PSRS 93446 514-A7
PSRS 93446 534-A1
SLO 93401 654-A5
SAN CARLOS RD
ATAS 93422 593-J1
SBAR 93103 996-A1
SLOC 93422 593-J1
SAN CARPINO DR
GOL 93117 993-G2
SAN CASSINO WY
GOL 93117 993-G2
SAN CAYETANO RD
ATAS 93422 573-C5
SLOC 93422 572-J4
SLOC 93422 573-A4
SANCHEZ DR
GDLP 93434 774-J6

STREET
Name City ZIP Pg-Grid
SAN CLEMENTE
SBAR 93109 995-J6
SBAR 93109 996-A7
SAN CLEMENTE AV
ATAS 93422 573-H5
SAN COMO WY
GOL 93117 993-F2
SANDALWOOD AV
ARGD 93420 714-H6
MOBY 93442 611-E2
SANDALWOOD DR
StBC 93455 816-B1
SANDALWOOD LN
SLOC 93465 553-A2
SANDALWOOD WY
SLVG 93463 940-D2
SANDBAR CT
PSRS 93446 533-G1
SAND CANYON CT
SLOC 93420 715-C3
SAND CASTLE CT
GBCH 93433 714-E4
SANDCOVE LN
PSRS 93446 533-G1
SAND DOLLAR AV
SLOC 93445 734-E1
SANDERCOCK ST
SLO 93401 653-H5
SLO 93401 654-A5
SANDERLING CT
SLOC 93420 735-A5
SAND HARBOR CT
SLOC 93446 471-C3
SAND HILL LN
StBC 93454 797-D7
SAN DIEGO AV
SLOC 93405 633-C5
SAN DIEGO LP
GBCH 93433 714-F4
SAN DIEGO RD
ATAS 93422 593-G2
ATAS 93422 594-B2
SBAR 93103 996-B2
SLOC 93422 593-H2
SLOC 93422 594-A2
SAN DIEGO ST
SMRA 93455 796-H6
SAN DIEGO WY
ATAS 93422 594-C1
SAN DIMAS AV
StBC 93111 994-H1
SAN DIMAS CT
ATAS 93422 593-H1
SAN DIMAS RD
ATAS 93422 593-G2
SLOC 93422 593-G2
SAN DOMINGO LN
StBC 93111 994-H2
SAN DOMINICO AV
SLOC 93402 631-F7
SANDOVAL RD
SLOC 93422 594-F3
SANDOWN PL
Cmbr 93428 548-G1
SANDPIPER CIR
MOBY 93442 631-G1
SANDPIPER DR
CARP 93013 998-B5
SMRA 93455 796-F6
SANDPIPER LN
GDLP 93434 774-H6
MOBY 93442 611-G7
MOBY 93442 631-G1
SLOC 93445 714-D7
SLOC 93446 471-C6
StBC 93110 994-J3
SAND POINT DR
StBC 93013 998-A6
SANDRA CT
Npmo 93444 755-J3
SANDSPIT RD
StBC 93117 994-D4
SANDSTONE LN
SMRA 93454 777-A7
SANDWORT LN
SLOC 93420 734-J7
SANDY CT
StBC 93455 816-H3
SANDY LN
StBC 93460 921-B3
SANDY PL
StBC 93108 997-B2
SANDY WY
SLOC 93420 735-D6
SANDYDALE DR
Npmo 93444 755-J2
Npmo 93444 756-A2
SANDYION AV
SMRA 93458 776-F3
SANDYLAND RD
CARP 93013 998-C7
SANDYLAND COVE RD
CARP 93013 998-C7
StBC 93013 998-C7
SANDY OAKS LN
Npmo 93444 755-J2
SAN FEDERICO AV
StBC 93111 994-H2
SAN FELIPE CT
ATAS 93422 573-A6
SAN FELIPE DR
StBC 93111 994-G3
SAN FELIPE RD
SLOC 93422 572-J5
SLOC 93422 573-A6
SAN FERMO
GOL 93117 993-G2
SAN FERNANDO DR
PSRS 93446 514-A7
PSRS 93446 534-A1
StBC 93111 994-H2
SAN FERNANDO RD
ATAS 93422 553-D7
ATAS 93422 573-D1
SANFORD CT
StBC 93111 994-G3
SAN FRANCISCO AV
ATAS 93422 573-J6
SLOC 93405 633-E5
SAN FRANCISCO ST
SLOC 93424 693-A4
SAN GABRIEL LN
SBAR 93105 995-F1
SAN GABRIEL RD
ATAS 93422 573-E4
ATAS 93422 574-A7
ATAS 93422 593-J1
ATAS 93422 594-A1

STREET
Name City ZIP Pg-Grid
SAN GERONIMO RD
SLOC 93430 590-F1
SAN GONZALO AV
StBC 93111 994-H2
SAN GORDIANO AV
StBC 93111 994-J1
SAN GREGORIO DR
StBC 93455 817-A7
SAN GREGORIO RD
ATAS 93422 553-D6
ATAS 93422 573-B1
SAN GUILLERMO LN
ATAS 93422 594-A1
SANITARY FILL RD
SLOC 93451 453-B6
SAN JACINTO AV
ATAS 93422 573-H2
SAN JACINTO DR
SLOC 93402 651-F1
SAN JACINTO ST
MOBY 93442 611-E2
SANJA COTA AV
StBC 93460 921-B7
SAN JANO DR
GOL 93117 993-G2
SAN JOAQUIN AV
SLOC 93405 633-A4
SAN JOAQUIN ST
MOBY 93442 611-E2
SAN JOSE CT
SLO 93405 653-G3
SAN JOSE LN
SBAR 93105 995-F2
SAN JUAN AV
MOBY 93442 611-F3
SAN JUAN PL
StBC 93111 994-H2
SAN JUAN RD
SLOC 93422 594-A3
SAN JUAN ST
SLOC 93424 693-A4
SAN JUAN BAUTISTA
ST
SLOC 93451 473-F1
SAN JUANICO
SMRA 93455 796-H5
SAN JULIAN AV
SBAR 93109 995-J6
SAN JULIAN PL
SBAR 93109 995-J7
SAN JULIAN RD
LMPC 93436 916-G1
SAN JULIO AV
StBC 93111 994-H1
SAN LAZARO LN
StBC 93111 994-G3
SAN LEANDRO CT
SLOC 93402 631-F7
SAN LEANDRO LN
StBC 93108 996-J3
StBC 93108 997-A3
SAN LEANDRO PL
StBC 93108 997-B3
SAN LEANDRO PARK RD
StBC 93108 996-J3
SAN LINO CT
SMRA 93455 796-H6
SAN LORENZO DR
StBC 93111 994-G2
SAN LUCAS
ATAS 93422 573-A3
SAN LUCAS WY
StBC 93111 994-G1
SAN LUIS AV
ATAS 93422 574-A5
PBCH 93449 714-B2
SLOC 93402 631-H6
SAN LUIS DR
SLO 93401 654-A3
SMRA 93455 796-H6
SAN LUIS ST
SLOC 93424 693-A4
SAN LUIS BAY DR
SLOC 93401 693-C2
SLOC 93405 693-C2
SLOC 93424 693-C2
SAN LUISITO CREEK
RD
SLOC - 612-H5
SLOC 93405 612-H5
SLOC 93405 632-E1
SAN LUIS OBISPO RD
SLOC 93451 473-F3
SAN LUIS ST PKWY
SLOC 93424 693-A4
SAN MARCOS AV
StBC 93441 900-H6
SAN MARCOS CT
ATAS 93422 573-A5
SLO 93401 654-B6
StBC 93111 994-H2
SAN MARCOS RD
ATAS 93422 573-B5
ATAS 93422 593-D1
SLOC 93422 572-J5
SLOC 93422 573-A5
SLOC 93446 473-E7
SLOC 93446 493-D2
StBC 93105 984-H3
StBC 93111 984-H3
StBC 93111 994-H1
SAN MARCOS PASS RD
SBAR 93110 995-C1
StBC 93110 995-C1
SAN MARCOS PASS RD
Rt#-154
SBAR 93110 985-B5
SBAR 93110 995-C1
StBC 93105 964-A2
StBC 93105 984-J1
StBC 93105 985-A1
StBC 93110 985-B5
StBC 93111 985-B5
SAN MARINO DR
StBC 93111 994-H2
SAN MARTIN WY
SBAR 93110 985-C7
SAN MATEO AV
GOL 93117 993-H2
SAN MATEO DR
SLO 93401 654-B5
SAN MIGUEL AV
SBAR 93109 995-J7
SLO 93405 654-B2
SLOC 93451 453-B5
SAN MIGUEL CT
GDLP 93434 774-H6
SAN MIGUEL RD
SLOC 93422 573-B7

STREET
Name City ZIP Pg-Grid
SAN MIGUEL RD
SLOC 93422 593-A1
SAN MIGUEL ST
SLOC 93424 693-A4
SMRA 93455 796-H5
SAN MIGUELITO RD
LMPC 93436 916-D5
StBC 93436 916-D5
SAN MILANO DR
GOL 93117 993-G2
SAN NAPOLI DR
GOL 93117 993-F1
SAN NICOLAS AV
SBAR 93109 995-J6
SAN NICOLAS ST
SMRA 93455 796-H6
SAN ONOFRE RD
SBAR 93105 995-F2
SAN PABLO DR
SLOC 93451 473-H3
SAN PABLO LN
SBAR 93103 995-E1
SAN PALO RD
ATAS 93422 573-G2
SAN PAREDES RD
SLOC 93422 572-J5
SAN PASCUAL ST
SBAR 93101 995-H3
SBAR 93101 996-A5
SAN PASQUAL AV
StBC 93436 916-A4
SAN PATRICIO DR
StBC 93111 984-F6
SAN PEDRO AV
ATAS 93422 573-J1
SAN PEDRO LN
SBAR 93105 995-F1
SAN PESARO WY
GOL 93117 993-G2
SAN PICA WY
GOL 93117 993-G2
SAN RAFAEL AV
SBAR 93109 995-J7
SAN RAFAEL CT
ATAS 93422 574-B7
SAN RAFAEL DR
PSRS 93446 514-A7
SAN RAFAEL RD
ATAS 93422 573-H7
ATAS 93422 574-B7
ATAS 93422 593-H1
ATAS 93422 594-A1
SLOC 93422 593-H1
SAN RAFAEL ST
SLOC 93424 693-A4
SAN RAMON DR
StBC 93111 994-H2
SAN RAMON RD
ATAS 93422 553-E6
ATAS 93422 573-E1
SLOC 93422 553-E6
SAN REMO DR
SBAR 93105 995-E1
SAN RICARDO DR
StBC 93111 994-G2
SAN RICARDO LN
SLOC 93402 631-E7
SAN RODRIGO AV
StBC 93111 994-H2
SAN ROQUE RD
SBAR 93105 985-F7
SBAR 93105 995-F1
StBC 93105 985-G7
SAN ROSSANO DR
GOL 93117 993-G1
SAN SEBASTIAN CT
GBCH 93433 714-F6
SAN SEBASTIAN LN
SLOC 93402 631-F7
SAN SIMEON AV
SMRA 93455 796-H6
SAN SIMEON DR
SLO 93401 673-H1
StBC 93111 994-H1
SAN SIMEON CREEK RD
Cmbr 93428 528-G1
SLOC 93452 528-C2
SAN SORRENTO CT
GBCH 93433 714-F7
SANTA AGUEDA RD
StBC 93441 921-J2
StBC 93460 921-J2
SANTA ANA AV
StBC 93111 994-G1
SANTA ANA PL
StBC 93111 994-H2
SANTA ANA RD
ATAS 93422 573-A1
SANTA ANGELA LN
StBC 93108 996-J1
SANTA ANITA RD
SBAR 93105 995-G2
SANTA ANITA ST
SMRA 93455 796-H5
SANTA BARBARA AV
SLO 93401 654-A5
SLOC 93430 591-B4
StBC 93437 875-C4
StBC 93441 900-H6
StBC 93463 900-H6
SANTA BARBARA DR
SMRA 93455 796-H6
SANTA BARBARA RD
ATAS 93422 594-C2
SLOC 93422 593-J4
SLOC 93422 594-A4
SANTA BARBARA ST
GDLP 93434 774-H6
SBAR 93101 995-H1
SBAR 93101 996-A3
SBAR 93105 995-H1
SANTA BARBARA
SHORES DR
GOL 93117 993-F3
SANTA BELLA AV
PSRS 93446 514-A7
SANTA CATALINA
SBAR 93109 995-J6
SBAR 93109 996-A6
SANTA CLARA AV
SLOC 93405 633-D4
SANTA CLARA DR
LMPC 93436 916-E3
SANTA CLARA RD
SLOC 93422 594-D3
SANTA CLARA ST
SLO 93401 654-B6
SANTA CLARA WY
StBC 93108 996-H3

STREET Name City ZIP Pg-Grid

SANTA CLAUS LN
StBC 93013 997-J5
StBC 93013 998-A5
SANTA CRUZ AV
PSRS 93446 514-A7
SANTA CRUZ BLVD
SBAR 93109 995-J7
SANTA CRUZ CT
SMRA 93455 796-J5
SANTA CRUZ RD
ATAS 93422 553-E5
ATAS 93422 573-A1
SLOC 93405 633-C5
SANTA DOMINGO RD
SLOC 93420 715-J3
SANTA ELENA LN
StBC 93108 996-H3
SANTA FE AV
PBCH 93449 693-H7
PSRS 93446 514-A7
SANTA FE PL
SBAR 93109 995-J6
SANTA FE RD
ATAS 93422 574-B5
SLOC 93401 674-B3
SLOC 93422 593-J4
SLOC 93422 594-A5
SANTA FELICIA DR
GOL 93117 993-H2
SANTA INES ST
GDLP 93434 774-H6
SANTA INEZ AV
StBC 93437 875-E1
SANTA ISABEL
SLOC 93430 591-A2
SANTA ISABEL LN
StBC 93108 996-H3
SANTA LUCIA AV
SLOC 93402 631-G4
StBC 93111 994-H1
SANTA LUCIA DR
SLO 93405 653-G2
SANTA LUCIA RD
ATAS 93422 573-A2
SLOC 93422 573-B4
SANTA LUCIA CANYON RD
LMPC 93436 895-J1
LMPC 93436 896-A3
StBC 93436 895-J1
StBC 93436 896-A3
StBC 93437 875-J7
StBC 93437 876-A6
StBC 93437 895-J1
SANTA MARGARITA RD
SLOC 93422 594-C5
N SANTA MARGARITA RD
SLOC 93422 594-D4
SANTA MARGUERITA DR
GOL 93117 984-D7
SANTA MARGUERITA WY
GOL 93117 984-D7
SANTA MARIA AV
SLO 93405 654-B2
SLOC 93402 631-G4
StBC 93437 855-D7
StBC 93437 875-D1
SANTA MARIA LN
SBAR 93105 995-F1
SANTA MARIA WY
SMRA 93455 796-H6
StBC 93455 796-H6
StBC 93455 816-J1
SANTA MARIA VISTA
Npmo 93444 756-E7
Npmo 93444 776-F1
SANTA MONICA RD
CARP 93013 998-C6
StBC - 998-C6
StBC 93013 998-C6
SANTA MONICA WY
SBAR 93109 995-G7
SANTA PAULA AV
SLOC 93402 631-H4
StBC 93111 994-H1
SANTA RITA CIR
SBAR 93109 995-J7
SANTA RITA RD
SLOC - 572-A5
SLOC 93422 572-C1
SLOC 93430 572-A5
SLOC 93465 553-B3
SLOC 93465 572-C1
StBC 93436 878-E5
StBC 93440 878-D2
SANTA ROSA AV
SBAR 93109 995-H7
SANTA ROSA CT
StBC 93437 855-F7
SANTA ROSA LN
CARP 93013 998-E6
StBC 93108 996-J2
StBC 93108 997-A2
SANTA ROSA PL
SBAR 93109 995-J7
SBAR 93109 996-A7
SANTA ROSA RD
ATAS 93422 573-J7
ATAS 93422 574-A7
StBC - 919-E6
StBC 93427 919-E6
StBC 93427 939-A1
StBC 93436 916-H4
StBC 93436 919-B7
StBC 93436 939-A1
SANTA ROSA ST
SLO 93401 653-J3
SLO 93401 654-A4
SMRA 93455 796-H6
SANTA ROSA ST Rt#-1
SLO 93401 653-H2
SLO 93405 653-H2
SLOC 93405 653-H2
SANTA ROSA CREEK RD
Cmbr 93428 528-H6
SANTA ROSALIA WY
StBC 93111 984-G7
SANTA SUSANA AV
StBC 93111 994-H1
SANTA SUSANA PL
StBC 93111 994-H1
SANTA TERESITA DR
SBAR 93105 985-F6
SANTA TERESITA WY
SBAR 93105 985-F5
SANTA YNEZ AV
ATAS 93422 573-J5
CARP 93013 998-C6
PSRS 93446 534-A1
SLO 93405 654-B2
SLOC 93402 631-H6
StBC 93460 921-A4
StBC 93463 921-A4
SANTA YNEZ CT
SBAR 93103 996-E3
SANTA YNEZ ST
SBAR 93103 996-D3
StBC 93441 900-H6
StBC 93460 900-H6
StBC 93460 901-A6
SANTA YNEZ RIDGE RD
StBC 93437 895-B5
SANTA YSABEL AV
ATAS 93422 573-J4
ATAS 93422 574-A4
PSRS 93446 514-A7
SLOC 93402 631-G4
SLOC 93402 632-A4
SANTA YSABEL AV Rt#-41
ATAS 93422 573-J4
SANTA YSABEL DR
SLOC 93430 591-A2
SANTA YSABEL RD
SLOC 93446 533-G2
SANTECITO DR
SBAR 93108 996-G2
SAN TELMO
SMRA 93455 796-H5
SANTIAGO RD
SBAR 93103 996-A1
SANTILLAN AV
SMRA 93458 796-E4
SANTO THOMAS CT
GBCH 93433 714-E4
SANTO TOMAS LN
StBC 93108 996-H3
SAN VICENTE AV
ATAS 93422 573-H1
SAN VICENTE DR
StBC 93111 994-G3
SAN YSIDRO LN
Npmo 93444 755-G2
StBC 93108 987-A7
StBC 93108 996-J1
StBC 93108 997-A1
SAN YSIDRO RD
StBC 93108 986-J7
StBC 93108 996-J1
SAN YSIDRO ST
SMRA 93455 796-H6
SAN YSIDRO TR
StBC 93105 986-J2
StBC 93105 987-A4
StBC 93108 987-A4
SAPPHIRE DR
SMRA 93454 777-A6
SARA CT
StBC 93455 816-H3
SARA ST
SLOC 93465 553-B1
SARATOGA AV
GBCH 93433 714-D4
SARATOGA CT
GOL 93117 993-G3
SARAZEN CT
Npmo 93444 735-D7
SASHA WY
SMRA 93454 777-A5
SATINWOOD RD
StBC 93455 816-B1
SATURN AV
StBC 93436 876-D7
StBC 93436 896-D1
SATURN CT
Npmo 93444 756-A5
SAUSILITO RD
ATAS 93422 573-C2
SAVAGE ST
Npmo 93444 756-C2
SAVANNA DR
StBC 93440 878-G1
SAVANNAH CIR
SLOC 93420 715-A1
SAVANNAH DR
GBCH 93433 714-F6
SAVONA AV
GOL 93117 993-G1
SAVONA LN
SMRA 93458 796-E4
SAVOY DR
SMRA 93455 796-H6
SAWLEAF CT
SLO 93401 674-D2
SAWLEAF ST
SLO 93401 674-D1
SAWYER AV
CARP 93013 998-D6
SCANDI LN
SLOC 93420 715-H2
SCANDIA DR
BLTN 93427 919-J5
SCANDIA WY
BLTN 93427 919-J5
SCENIC CIR
ARGD 93420 714-H3
SCENIC DR
SBAR 93103 996-E3
SCENIC WY
SLOC 93402 631-J4
SCENIC VIEW WY
Npmo 93444 755-G6
SW SCHOLLS FERRY RD
StBC 93463 920-J6
SCHOOL RD
SLOC 93420 715-F2
SCHOOL ST
SMRA 93454 776-H5
SMRA 93454 796-H1
StBC 93463 920-H2
SCHOOLHOUSE CIR
PSRS 93446 513-H2
SCHOOLHOUSE LN
Cmbr 93428 528-H7
SCHOOL HOUSE RD
StBC 93108 996-H2
SCHULTE LN
SBAR 93105 985-F6
SCHUMAN PL
SMRA 93458 776-F3
SCOLARI LN
StBC 93440 878-H2
SCORPIO RD
StBC 93436 876-C5
SCOTT AV
MOBY 93442 611-F6
SCOTT CT
GOL 93117 984-D6
SCOTT DR
SMRA 93454 776-J6
SMRA 93454 777-A7
SMRA 93454 796-J1
SCOTT ST
PSRS 93446 534-A1
SCOTT LEE DR
SLOC 93445 714-G7
SCRIPPS CRES
GOL 93117 993-H4
SEA ST
Npmo 93444 756-B2
SEA VW
CARP 93013 998-A5
SEA BREEZE
PBCH 93449 714-D3
SEABREEZE WY
LMPC 93436 896-D6
SEABRIGHT AV
ARGD 93420 714-D5
GBCH 93420 714-D5
GBCH 93433 714-D5
SEA CLIFF
SBAR 93109 995-E6
SEACLIFF DR
CARP 93013 998-A5
PBCH 93449 693-F6
SEACOAST WY
CARP 93013 998-E6
SEA GULL DR
GOL 93117 993-F3
SEA HORSE LN
SLOC 93402 631-F7
SEA LEDGE LN
SBAR 93109 995-D6
SEA MEADOWS PL
StBC 93108 996-J4
SEA OAK LN
SLOC 93420 735-B5
SEA PINES PL
Npmo 93444 755-D1
SEAPORT DR
PBCH 93449 693-J7
SEA RANCH DR
SBAR 93109 995-D5
SBAR 93110 995-D5
SEARIDGE CT
PBCH 93449 693-E5
SEARS ST
Summ 93067 997-C3
SEASCAPE PL
SLOC 93402 631-E7
SEASIDE DR
SMRA 93454 776-J5
SEA VIEW AV
PBCH 93449 693-H7
SEAVIEW AV
MOBY 93442 611-F4
SEAVIEW CIR
PBCH 93449 714-C3
SEAVIEW DR
StBC 93108 996-H4
SEAVIEW LN
PBCH 93449 714-D3
SEAVIEW RD
StBC 93108 996-J2
SEAWARD DR
SMRA 93454 776-J4
SMRA 93454 777-A4
SEAWARD ST
SLO 93405 653-G7
SEAWAY DR
StBC 93117 993-H5
SEA WIND WY
SLOC 93402 631-E7
SEBASTIAN CT
SLOC 93451 473-F1
SEBASTIAN WY
Npmo 93444 756-B5
SECOND WIND WY
PSRS 93446 494-E7
SECRETARIAT DR
StBC 93441 922-A5
StBC 93460 922-A5
SECURITY CT
SLOC 93445 714-D7
SEE CANYON RD
SLOC 93402 673-A4
SLOC 93402 693-C2
SLOC 93405 693-C2
SLOC 93424 693-C2
SEGOVIA RD
StBC 93117 994-A5
SELBY ST
MOBY 93442 611-F5
SELMA ST
PBCH 93449 714-C2
SELROSE LN
SBAR 93109 995-F6
SELWYN CIR
StBC 93105 985-H7
SEMILLON LN
SLOC 93465 553-A3
SENDA VERDE
SBAR 93105 995-D3
SENDERO AV
ATAS 93422 574-A4
SENDERO ST
SLO 93401 653-J6
SENECA ST
SMRA 93454 777-B6
SENTAR RD
StBC 93013 997-G4
SENTIMENTAL LN
PSRS 93446 514-C7
SEPERADO AV
ATAS 93422 553-H7
ATAS 93422 573-J1
SEQUOIA CT
MOBY 93442 611-F2
PSRS 93446 514-B7
SEQUOIA DR
SLOC 93401 654-D7
SMRA 93454 796-H4
SEQUOIA LN
Npmo 93444 756-A5
SEQUOIA RD
StBC 93437 875-H1
SEQUOIA ST
MOBY 93442 611-E2
SLO 93401 654-D6
SERAFIN WY
StBC 93013 997-G4
SERENA AV
StBC 93013 997-G4
SERENA CT
ATAS 93422 573-J3
ATAS 93422 574-A3
SERENA RD
SBAR 93105 995-G1
SERENADE DR
PSRS 93446 513-H7
PSRS 93446 533-H1
SERENIDAD PL
GOL 93117 984-D6
SERENITY LN
SLOC 93420 734-J3
SERPA RANCH RD
SLOC 93401 674-B5
SERPENTINE LN
SLOC 93405 652-G7
SERPOLLA DR
StBC 93013 997-G4
SERRA AV
ATAS 93422 573-J4
SERRANO CIR
SLO 93405 653-H3
SERRANO DR
SLO 93405 653-H3
SERRANO HTS
SLO 93405 653-H3
SESPE LN
GOL 93117 993-H2
SEVADA LN
SLOC 93420 735-A1
SEVILLE LN
ATAS 93422 594-C1
SEVILLE RD
StBC 93117 982-H6
StBC 93117 994-A5
SHADOW LN
SLOC 93420 734-H7
SHADOWBROOK DR
GOL 93117 993-J3
SHADOWBROOK LN
SLOC 93402 673-B4
SHADOW CREEK LN
PSRS 93446 533-G1
SHADOW CREEK RD
PSRS 93446 533-J2
PSRS 93446 534-A2
SHADOWCREST DR
StBC 93455 817-A3
SHADOW HILLS BLVD N
StBC 93105 985-B5
SHADOW HILLS BLVD S
StBC 93105 985-B5
SHADOW HILLS CIR
StBC 93105 985-B5
SHADOW MEADOW WY
PSRS 93446 514-A6
SHADOW MOUNTAIN DR
BLTN 93427 919-G6
SHADY LN
StBC 93455 816-H3
SHADY CREEK DR
SLOC 93446 471-A5
SHADY GLADE DR
StBC 93455 816-J3
SHADY GLEN CT
StBC 93455 817-A4
SHADY GLEN DR
StBC 93455 817-A4
SHAFFER LN
PBCH 93449 714-B1
SHAMROCK AV
GOL 93117 994-C1
SHAMROCK LN
PBCH 93449 714-E3
SHANE LN
SLOC 93465 553-C3
SHANKLIN PL
StBC 93436 896-F3
SHANNA PL
GBCH 93433 714-F7
SHANNON LN
SLOC 93420 715-A1
SHANNON HILL DR
PSRS 93446 513-H5
SHANON CT
SMRA 93454 797-A1
SHARON LN
GBCH 93433 714-E4
SHARON PL
BLTN 93427 919-H4
SHARRY LN
StBC 93455 816-H5
SHASTA AV
MOBY 93442 611-G7
SHASTA LN
Npmo 93444 735-H4
SBAR 93101 996-A2
SLOC 93446 471-B5
SHASTA WY
StBC 93455 817-E5
SHAW ST
StBC 93440 878-H2
SHAY AV
SMRA 93458 776-F3
SHAYNA LN
SLOC 93422 594-D2
SHEARER AV
SLOC 93430 591-C5
SHEARTON WY
GOL 93117 984-D7
SHEARWATER CT
SLOC 93424 693-B3
SHEEHY RD
Npmo 93444 735-J5
Npmo 93444 736-A4
SHEEP CAMP RD
StBC 93463 900-E6
StBC 93463 920-E1
SHEERIN CT
ATAS 93422 594-C2
SHEFFIELD DR
LMPC 93436 916-G2
StBC 93108 997-C2
Summ 93067 997-C2
SHEFFIELD ST
Cmbr 93428 528-F6
SHEFIELD DR
SLO 93401 673-H1
SHEILA LN
SMRA 93458 796-G4
SHELBY ST
Summ 93067 997-D3
SHELBY WY
SLOC 93420 715-D2
SHELL BEACH RD
PBCH 93449 693-F6
SLOC 93449 693-E4
SHELLIE CT
StBC 93455 816-H3
SHELTER RIDGE PL
Npmo 93444 755-F1
SHEMARA ST
CARP 93013 998-E6
SHEPARD DR
SMRA 93454 796-J3
SHEPARD MESA LN
StBC 93013 999-A6
SHEPARD MESA RD
StBC 93013 998-J7
StBC 93013 999-A6
SHEPHERD DR
PSRS 93446 534-B1
StBC 93436 896-F2
SHERIDAN AV
SBAR 93101 995-H3
SHERIDAN RD
SLOC 93420 735-A7
SLOC 93420 755-A2
SHERMAN RD
SBAR 93103 986-D7
SHERMAN ST
SLOC 93420 735-D4
SHERRY PL
LMPC 93436 896-C6
SHERWOOD DR
Cmbr 93428 548-F2
StBC 93110 985-B7
StBC 93110 995-B1
StBC 93455 816-B1
SHERWOOD RD
PSRS 93446 514-A7
SHETLAND CT
StBC 93455 817-A4
SHETLAND PL
SLOC 93420 735-A2
SHETLAND WY
SLOC 93446 471-C4
SHIFFRAR LN
Npmo 93444 756-A6
SHILO CT
StBC 93455 816-G7
SHILOH PL
SLOC 93465 553-B1
SHIRLEY LN
StBC 93455 816-H3
SHIRRELL WY
GOL 93117 984-D7
SHOOTING STAR LN
SLOC 93424 693-A1
S SHORE DR
SLOC 93446 469-E2
SHORELINE DR
PBCH 93449 693-G7
SBAR 93101 996-A6
SBAR 93109 995-H7
SBAR 93109 996-A6
StBC 93111 994-G3
SHORT LN
SLOC 93446 469-D2
SHORT RD
StBC 93460 901-G3
SHORT ST
ARGD 93420 715-A5
SLO 93401 673-H2
SHORTHORN CT
PSRS 93446 533-H1
SHOSHONE DR
PSRS 93446 513-H6
SICILY ST
MOBY 93442 611-D1
SIENA LN
SMRA 93458 796-E4
SIENNA ST
MOBY 93442 611-E2
SIENNA WY
StBC 93463 920-J6
SIERRA CT
MOBY 93442 611-G7
SIERRA DR
ARGD 93420 714-G4
SIERRA LN
PSRS 93446 514-C7
PSRS 93446 534-C1
SIERRA RD
Npmo 93444 756-B6
SIERRA ST
SBAR 93103 995-J1
SIERRA WY
SLO 93401 654-B5
SIERRA MADRE AV
SMRA 93454 796-H2
SMRA 93454 797-A2
SIERRA MADRE DR
StBC 93110 985-A6
SIERRA MADRE RD
StBC 93110 984-J7
StBC 93110 985-A7
StBC 93111 984-J7
SIERRA MEADOWS LN
SLOC 93465 553-A4
SIERRA VISTA
SLVG 93463 940-D1
SMRA 93458 776-G4
SIERRA VISTA RD
ATAS 93422 573-G6
StBC 93108 996-E1
SIGNAL AV
SMRA 93458 776-G3
SIGNORA ROSA CT
PSRS 93446 514-A3
SILER LN
StBC 93455 816-H2
SILKBERRY LN
GOL 93117 993-J3
SILKBORG RD
StBC 93463 920-D6
SILLA RD
ATAS 93422 573-F1
SILVA PL
Npmo 93444 756-A6
SILVER WY
SLOC 93420 735-A1
SILVERADO AV
SMRA 93455 796-G6
SILVER CHARM DR
SLOC 93420 755-A1
SILVER DOLLAR LN
Npmo 93444 755-H3
SILVER FERN CT
GOL 93117 993-J3
SILVER LEAF CT
Npmo 93444 756-B5
SILVER LEAF DR
StBC 93455 816-H2
SILVER OAK DR
PSRS 93446 534-A2
SILVER OAK LN
SLOC 93424 693-B1
SILVER SADDLE LN
SLOC 93446 471-B6
SILVER SAGE LN
StBC 93436 896-F3
N SILVER SHOALS DR
PBCH 93449 693-F5
SILVER SPUR PL
SLOC 93445 734-F1
SILVERWOOD WY
PSRS 93446 534-A2
SILVERY MOON LN
PSRS 93446 514-C7
SILVESTRE RD
StBC 93110 995-D4
SIMAS ST
StBC 93434 775-C7
StBC 93455 795-C1
StBC 93458 775-C7
StBC 93458 795-C1
SIMMENTAL RD
SLOC 93422 594-E2
SIMMONS LN
Npmo 93444 756-A5
SIMS AV
PSRS 93446 513-F2
SINALOA AV
ATAS 93422 574-A4
SINALOA DR
StBC 93108 996-J3
StBC 93108 997-A3
SINGLETON CT
SLO 93405 673-F1
SINGLETON DR
SMRA 93455 796-J5
SINNARD LN
ATAS 93422 594-C2
SINSONTE CT
ATAS 93422 594-C1
SINTON RD
StBC 93455 795-H5
StBC 93458 795-H5
SIRIUS AV
StBC 93436 876-C6
SISQUOC
SLO 93401 653-J7
SISQUOC ST
StBC 93254 806-B1
SIX FLAGS CIR
BLTN 93427 919-H5
SKAGEN DR
SLVG 93463 920-F6
SKIPJACK LN
SLOC 93446 471-B5
SKY DR
StBC 93460 921-H2
SKYE ST
Cmbr 93428 528-F7
SKYLARK CT
SMRA 93455 796-J7
SMRA 93455 797-A7
SKYLARK LN
Npmo 93444 756-C3
SLO 93401 654-B4
SKYLARK RD
StBC 93460 941-D1
SKYLINE CIR
SBAR 93109 995-G5
SKYLINE DR
PBCH 93449 714-F3
SLO 93405 653-G1
SLOC 93402 631-F6
SKYLINE WY
SBAR 93109 995-G5
SKYLINK LN
SLOC 93446 471-B5
SKYLINKS DR
SMRA 93455 796-F6
SKY RIDGE DR
SLOC 93446 513-D1
SKYTT MESA DR
SLVG 93463 920-D7
SLVG 93463 940-C1
SKY VIEW DR
LMPC 93436 916-F2
SKYVIEW DR
PSRS 93446 513-H3
SBAR 93108 996-F2
StBC 93108 996-F2
SKYVIEW TR
SLOC 93402 673-B7
SLOC 93402 693-B1
SKYWAY DR
SMRA 93455 796-E6
SMRA 93455 816-G1
StBC 93455 816-G1
SLACK ST
SLO 93405 654-A2
SLOC 93405 654-A2
SLATE RANCH RD
SLOC 93446 513-C3
SLEEPY HOLLOW LN
SMRA 93454 777-A6
SLEEPY HOLLOW RD
PSRS 93446 533-J2
SLENDER ROCK PL
SLOC 93405 653-D5
SLOAN TER
SMRA 93455 796-J6
SLOUGH RD
StBC 93117 993-H5
SMALLWOOD CT
StBC 93455 817-A4
SMILEY PL
SLOC 93422 593-B1
SMITH AV
SLOC 93445 714-D7
SMITH CT
Cmbr 93428 548-H1
SMITH DR
SMRA 93458 776-G5
SMITH ST
SLO 93401 654-B5
SMRA 93458 776-G7
SMRA 93458 796-G2
SMITH POINT RD
SLOC 93426 469-J3
SLOC 93426 470-A3
SMOKE TREE LN
SMRA 93454 777-A6
SMUGGLERS POINT LN
SLOC 93446 471-B6
SNAPDRAGON WY
SLO 93401 674-D2
SNEAD LN
Npmo 93444 735-D7
SNEAD ST
PSRS 93446 533-H1
SNOW LN
Npmo 93444 736-A4
SNOWBERRY CT
SLOC 93424
SNOWBERRY LN
SMRA 93454
SNOWCONE PL
SLOC 93420
SNOWHILL CT
StBC 93455
SNOWY EGRET LN
SLOC 93402
SNOWY PLOVER LN
GDLP 93434
SOARES AV
StBC 93455
SOARES DR
Npmo 93444
SODA RD
SLOC 93446
SOFTCHESS PL
SLOC 93453
SOLA CT
SLO 93405
SOLA ST
SBAR 93101
SBAR 93101
SBAR 93103
SOLANA CT
GBCH 93433
SBAR 93109
SOLANO AV
SLOC 93405
SOLANO RD
ATAS 93422
PBCH 93449
SLOC 93422
SOLANO ST
SLOC 93402
SOLANO WY
SLOC 93446
SOLAR WY
PBCH 93449
StBC 93436
SOLARES CIR
StBC 93460
SOLEDAD AV
SBAR 93103
SOLEDAD CT
SMRA 93455
SOLEDAD RD
ATAS 93422
SLOC 93422
SOLEDAD ST
SBAR 93103
SOLIDA DEL SOL
PSRS 93446
SOLOMON RD
StBC 93455
SOLOMON VIEW RD
StBC 93455
SOLVANG ST
SLOC 93405
SOMBRERO DR
SLOC 93402
SOMBRERO WY
SMRA 93458
SOMBRILLA AV
ATAS 93422
ATAS 93422
SOMBRILLA CT
ATAS 93422
SOMBRILLO
ARGD 93420
SOMERSET CT
LMPC 93436
SOMERSET DR
GOL 93111
SOMERSET PL
LMPC 93436
SOMERSET WY
Cmbr 93428
SOMMER LN
GOL 93117
SONGBIRD ST
SLOC 93424
SONOMA AV
GOL 93117
SLOC 93405
SONORA AV
ATAS 93422
SONORA DR
SBAR 93105
SONRIENTE RD
StBC 93110
SONRISA CT
SLO 93405
SONYA LN
SMRA 93458
SOPHIE CT
SLOC 93420
SORA CT
GOL 93117
SORO AL
SLVG 93463
SORREL LN
SLOC 93446
SORRENTO LN
SMRA 93458
SOTO PL
SBAR 93117
SOUTH ST
GOL 93117
MOBY 93442
SLO 93401
SLO 93401
SOUTH ST Rt#-227
SLO 93401
SLO 93401
SOUTH BAY BLVD
MOBY 93402
MOBY 93405
MOBY 93442
MOBY 93442
SLOC -
SLOC 93402
SLOC 93405
SLOC 93442
SLOC 93442
SOUTHBROOK DR
LMPC 93436
SOUTHCREEK CT
StBC 93455
SOUTH DAKOTA AV
SLOC 93451
StBC 93437
SOUTHFORK PL
SLOC 93446
SOUTHLAND ST
Npmo 93444

STREET Name City ZIP Pg-Grid

ILAND WOODS LN
Npmo 93444 756-C4
ILYN PL
StBC 93455 817-A2
IPOINT CT
StBC 93455 816-H6
IRIDGE LN
Npmo 93444 755-F1
ISIDE PKWY
SMRA 93455 796-J5
IVIEW AV
SLOC 93420 734-H5
IVIEW CIR
PSRS 93446 534-C1
IWOOD DR
SLO 93401 654-B6
SLOC 93401 654-C6
A ST
Npmo 93444 756-B3
SH TR
SLOC 93420 734-J4
SLOC 93420 735-A4
SH CAMP RD
SLOC 93446 533-H2
SH MOSS LN
ARGD 93420 714-J3
SH OAKS DR
SLO 93401 674-D2
SH SPRINGS DR
SLOC 93449 694-B5
S ST
Npmo 93444 756-C2
OW ST
SLOC 93405 693-C2
OW HAWK LN
SLOC 93446 471-C6
ST
SMRA 93454 796-H2
ER DR
StBC 93455 816-J5
ER ST
Cmbr 93428 548-H2
WY
StBC 93436 876-D6
CT
SLOC 93426 469-H2
LER WY
SLOC 93446 469-J5
RE LN
SLO 93401 674-C2
SLOC 93401 674-C2
NBILL CT
SLOC 93424 693-B3
NER DR
SLO 93405 653-F7
SLO 93405 673-F1
T COMPLEX RD
SLOC 93405 633-H7
ED BASS LN
SLOC 93446 471-D3
ED WOOD LN
SLOC 93424 693-B3
G CT
SLO 93401 654-C6
G RD
SLOC 93446 469-J4
StBC 93108 996-H4
G ST
PSRS 93446 513-F3
SBAR 93103 996-C2
SLOC 93446 513-F3
GBROOK CT
GOL 93117 993-J4
G CANYON LN
Npmo 93444 735-J2
Npmo 93444 736-A2
G CANYON RD
SLOC 93460 901-D5
G MEADOW LN
SLOC 93422 593-C1
CE DR
GOL 93117 993-G1
SMRA 93454 777-B7
CE LN
Npmo 93444 756-B4
CE ST
ARGD 93420 714-G6
CEWOOD CT
SLOC 93446 533-E6
DR
StBC 93455 817-B5
VALLEY RD
StBC 93117 984-E5
LASS AV
SMRA 93455 796-G5
LASS CT
PSRS 93446 533-J1
LASS DR
PBCH 93449 693-F6
SMRA 93455 796-G5
LASS LN
SLOC 93446 471-B5
E CT
SLOC 93401 693-G1
RE CANYON RD
SLOC 93401 693-F2
RE KNOLL DR
SLOC 93401 693-F1
Y LN
SBAR 93110 985-D7
Y ANN TER
SMRA 93455 796-J6
SMRA 93455 797-A6
UM DR
StBC 93463 920-J6
StBC 93463 921-A6
UM PL
StBC 93463 920-J6
UM RD
StBC 93106 994-B4
ORD ST
Cmbr 93428 528-D6
SLO 93405 653-J2
SLO 93405 654-A2
CANYON RD
SLOC 93460 901-D6
E COACH RD
SLOC 93446 534-J7
SLOC 93465 534-J7
ECOACH RD
ARGD 93420 715-B4
SLOC 93420 715-C3
SLOC 93446 534-J4
StBC 93105 964-A1
LCUP LN
StBC 93436 896-G3
ION DR
StBC 93441 921-J2
StBC 93441 922-A2

STALLION WY
SLOC 93446 534-J4
STANFORD CIR
StBC 93436 876-E5
STANFORD DR
SLO 93405 653-G1
StBC 93455 816-J6
STANFORD PL
StBC 93111 984-G7
STANFORD RD
SMRA 93454 776-J4
STANISLAUS AV
SLOC 93405 633-D5
STANLEY AV
ARGD 93420 715-B4
STANLEY DR
SBAR 93105 995-G2
STANLEY PARK RD
StBC - 999-C7
StBC 93013 999-C7
VeCo - 999-C7
STANSBURY DR
StBC 93455 816-G5
STANTON ST
SLOC 93420 735-D4
STANWOOD DR Rt#-192
SBAR 93103 986-D7
SBAR 93103 996-D1
SBAR 93105 986-D7
SBAR 93108 996-D1
STARDUST CT
SMRA 93455 796-J7
StBC 93437 855-E6
STARDUST DR
SMRA 93455 796-J6
STARDUST LN
PSRS 93446 514-C7
STARDUST RD
StBC 93436 896-C1
STARFIRE ST
SMRA 93455 796-J7
STARLIGHT LN
ARGD 93420 714-H6
STARLING CT
PSRS 93446 534-A1
STARLING DR
PSRS 93446 534-A2
STARLITE CT
SMRA 93455 796-J6
STARLITE DR
Npmo 93444 756-A5
STAR PINE RD
CARP 93013 998-E6
STARR CT
SLOC 93402 651-J1
STATE ST
SBAR 93101 995-J3
SBAR 93101 996-A4
SBAR 93105 995-F1
SBAR 93110 995-D1
StBC 93105 995-D1
StBC 93110 995-C1
STATE PARK RD
MOBY 93442 611-G7
MOBY 93442 631-G1
STATION WY
ARGD 93420 714-J5
ARGD 93420 715-A5
STEELE ST
StBC 93441 900-G5
StBC 93463 900-G5
STEELHEAD RD
SLOC 93446 471-D3
STELLA CT
PSRS 93446 514-A3
STEMWOOD DR
SMRA 93458 776-G3
STENNER ST
SLO 93405 653-J2
STENNER CREEK RD
SLOC 93405 633-G6
STEPHANIE DR
SLO 93405 653-E6
STEPHEN PL
SMRA 93455 796-J6
STEPLEGATE LN
StBC 93455 817-B6
STERLING AV
CARP 93013 998-D6
STERLING LN
SLO 93405 653-D7
STERLING WY
CARP 93013 998-D6
STERN DECK RD
SLOC 93426 469-J1
STERRET AV
StBC 93110 985-E6
STEVENS RD
SBAR 93105 995-E2
StBC 93105 995-E2
STEVENSON DR
ARGD 93420 714-H3
STILL MEADOW RD
StBC 93441 920-J2
StBC 93463 920-J2
STILLWATER CT
PSRS 93446 533-G1
STILLWELL RD
StBC 93455 817-B5
STIMSON AV
PBCH 93449 714-C2
STINSON CT
GBCH 93433 714-F5
STOCKDALE RD
SLOC 93446 493-F4
STOCKTON ST
StBC 93455 817-B5
STODDARD LN
StBC 93108 996-F1
STOKES AV
SMRA 93454 776-J6
SMRA 93454 777-A6
STONEBRIDGE DR
SMRA 93454 777-C7
STONEBRIDGE LN
PSRS 93446 533-G1
StBC 93437 855-E7
STONEBROOK CIR
PSRS 93446 513-H2
STONEBROOK DR
LMPC 93436 896-D6
STONE BROOK RD
StBC 93455 816-G4
STONECREEK RD
StBC 93105 995-F4
STONEHOUSE LN
StBC 93108 997-D1
STONE MEADOW LN
StBC 93108 996-H1

STONERIDGE DR
SLO 93401 654-A6
STONEWOOD CT
StBC 93455 817-A4
STONEY PL
SLOC 93446 514-J7
SLOC 93446 534-J1
STONEY CREEK DR
PSRS 93446 533-J1
PSRS 93446 534-A1
STONEY PARK LN
SMRA 93458 776-G3
STORAGE RD
StBC 93437 875-F1
STORKE RD
GOL 93117 993-J4
StBC 93117 993-J4
STORMY WY
PSRS 93446 513-H4
STORY ST
Npmo 93444 756-C4
SLO 93401 654-A5
STOW ST
StBC 93441 900-H6
STOW CANYON RD
GOL 93117 984-C7
E STOWELL RD
SMRA 93454 796-H2
SMRA 93454 797-B2
StBC 93454 797-B2
W STOWELL RD
SMRA 93454 796-F2
SMRA 93458 796-F2
StBC 93458 796-C2
STRAND WY
SLOC 93445 714-D7
SLOC 93445 734-D1
STRATFORD AV
SMRA 93454 777-A5
SMRA 93454 797-A1
STRATFORD DR
StBC 93437 855-E7
STRATFORD PL
StBC 93108 997-C1
STRATFORD ST
PBCH 93449 714-C1
StBC 93455 816-J3
STRAWBERRY AV
ARGD 93420 714-F5
STREET 1
StBC 93455 795-H5
STREET 5
StBC 93455 795-G5
STREHLE LN
GOL 93117 993-G3
STUART
SLOC 93430 591-B4
STUART AV
SLOC 93430 591-C4
STUART DR
StBC 93455 817-A5
STUART ST
Cmbr 93428 548-H2
STUBBLEFIELD RD
StBC 93455 817-A7
STUBBS LN
StBC 93455 796-G7
STUB END CIR
SLOC 93426 469-J2
STUDIO DR
SLOC 93430 591-B4
STUPID RULE LN
SLOC 93446 493-H7
SUBURBAN RD
SLO 93401 673-H2
SLOC 93401 673-H2
SLOC 93401 674-A2
SUELDO ST
SLO 93401 673-J1
SUELLEN CT
GOL 93117 984-D7
SUENO RD
StBC 93117 993-J5
StBC 93117 994-A5
SUEY RD
SMRA 93454 777-B5
SMRA 93454 797-B1
StBC 93454 777-B7
StBC 93454 797-B1
SUEY CREEK RD
Npmo 93444 737-D7
SLOC - 737-D7
SLOC 93420 737-A4
SUEY CROSSING RD
SMRA 93454 777-B6
SUFFOLK ST
Cmbr 93428 528-F6
SUGAR ST
SMRA 93454 797-F2
StBC 93454 797-F2
SUGAR BUSH DR
SMRA 93454 777-A6
SULIVAN CT
ATAS 93422 594-C2
SULPHUR SPRINGS DR
PSRS 93446 513-G2
SUMAC CT
SLO 93401 674-D2
SUMAC ST
StBC 93437 875-H1
SUMMER LN
Npmo 93444 755-E3
SUMMER CREEK LN
PSRS 93446 513-G7
PSRS 93446 533-G1
SUMMER FALLOW PL
PSRS 93446 534-C1
SUMMERHILL DR
SMRA 93454 777-B7
SUMMERLAND HEIGHTS LN
StBC 93108 997-C3
Summ 93067 997-C3
SUMMERSILL AV
StBC 93437 855-E7
SUMMERWOOD LN
LMPC 93436 896-D6
SUMMIT DR
PBCH 93449 714-F3
PSRS 93446 514-A4
SUMMIT LN
SBAR 93108 996-F2
SUMMIT RD
SBAR 93108 996-F2
StBC 93108 996-G3
SUMMIT STATION RD
SLOC 93420 735-G6
SUMNER PL
StBC 93455 817-A3

SUNBEAM RD
StBC 93436 876-C7
StBC 93436 896-C1
SUNBURY AV
Cmbr 93428 528-E6
SUNCREST DR
SLOC 93465 553-B1
SUN DALE WY
Npmo 93444 755-E3
SUNDANCE LN
PSRS 93446 513-H4
SUNDAY DR
Npmo 93444 755-F1
SUNDOWN LN
SLOC 93420 715-H3
SUNFISH CIR
SLOC 93446 471-E3
SUNFLOWER CT
SMRA 93455 796-J6
SUNFLOWER WY
SLO 93401 674-C2
SUNGATE RANCH RD
StBC 93111 994-H2
SUNKIST LN
SLOC 93420 735-F5
SUNNYBROOK CT
LMPC 93436 896-D6
SUNNY HILL AV
SLOC 93402 631-F6
SUNNY OAKS LN
SLOC 93402 631-J7
SUNNY RIDGE PL
SLOC 93446 534-H1
SUNNYSIDE AV
StBC 93455 816-J3
SUNNYSIDE WY
SLOC 93465 553-C1
SUNNYSLOPE LN
Npmo 93444 756-C3
StBC 93455 817-A3
SUNRAY PL
SLOC 93420 714-H1
SUNRIDGE LN
Npmo 93444 755-J5
SUNRISE CT
PSRS 93446 533-J1
PSRS 93446 534-A1
SUNRISE DR
SMRA 93455 796-H6
SMRA 93455 797-A6
SUNRISE TER
ARGD 93420 714-J7
ARGD 93420 715-A7
SUNRISE TR
SLOC 93424 693-C2
SUNRISE WY
StBC 93463 920-G7
SUNRISE HILL LN
SBAR 93108 996-E1
StBC 93108 996-E1
SUNRISE RIDGE RD
SLOC 93446 469-H4
SUNRISE VISTA WY
SBAR 93109 995-G6
SUNROSE CT
SLO 93401 674-C1
SUNROSE LN
SLO 93401 674-C1
SUNSET AV
MOBY 93442 611-F4
SBAR 93101 995-H3
SMRA 93454 776-H6
SMRA 93454 777-A6
SMRA 93458 776-F6
SUNSET CT
MOBY 93442 611-F4
SUNSET DR
ARGD 93420 714-G5
CARP 93013 998-A5
PSRS 93446 513-F3
SBAR 93105 985-F7
SLO 93401 654-C5
SLOC 93402 631-H7
StBC 93437 855-F7
SUNSET LN
SLOC 93445 714-D7
SUNSET RD
StBC 93110 985-E7
SUNSHINE CT
SMRA 93455 796-J7
SUNSHINE LN
StBC 93105 964-H1
SUNVIEW DR
StBC 93455 816-H4
SUPERIOR ST
SMRA 93458 776-F7
SMRA 93458 796-F1
SURF
PBCH 93449 714-C3
SURF AV
SLOC 93445 714-D7
SURF ST
MOBY 93442 611-F5
PBCH 93449 714-D2
SURFBIRD CT
GDLP 93434 774-J6
SURFBIRD LN
GDLP 93434 774-H6
SURF VIEW DR
SBAR 93109 995-H6
SURREY WY
SMRA 93454 777-A5
SURRY PL
GOL 93117 993-F2
SUSAN PL
SMRA 93455 796-J4
SMRA 93455 797-A6
SUSANNAH LN
PSRS 93446 513-H4
SUSSEX CT
GOL 93117 984-C7
SUTLIFF RD
SLOC 93451 473-B5
SUTTER AV
SLOC 93405 632-J5
SLOC 93405 633-A5
SUTTER ST
SMRA 93454 777-B6
SUTTON AV
SBAR 93101 996-A5
SWALLOW CT
SMRA 93454 796-H3
SWALLOW LN
Npmo 93444 756-E4
SWALLOW ST
SMRA 93454 796-H3
SWAMP JOHN RD
SLOC 93446 469-G4

SWAN LN
SLOC 93446 471-D5
SWAZEY ST
SLO 93401 654-A5
SWEENEY LN
SLO 93401 654-A7
SWEENEY RD
StBC 93436 916-J1
SWEETBAY LN
SLO 93401 674-D2
SWEETBRIAR CT
StBC 93455 817-A5
SWEET DONNA PL
Npmo 93444 755-H3
SWEET GUM LN
Npmo 93444 755-H3
SWEETHEART LN
PSRS 93446 514-C7
SWEET RAIN PL
GOL 93117 993-J4
SWEETSAGE CT
StBC 93436 896-E3
SWEET SPRINGS LN
SLOC 93420 715-D1
SWEETWATER WY
GOL 93117 993-J3
StBC 93117 993-J3
SWIFT RD
Npmo 93444 756-E3
SWORD CT
SMRA 93454 797-B1
SYCAMORE CT
ARGD 93420 714-H7
SYCAMORE DR
ARGD 93420 714-H7
BLTN 93427 919-G4
SLO 93401 654-C6
SYCAMORE LN
SBAR 93103 996-D3
SYCAMORE RD
ATAS 93422 573-J1
ATAS 93422 574-A2
SYCAMORE ST
SMRA 93458 776-G4
SYCAMORE WY
SLVG 93463 940-E1
SYCAMORE CANYON DR
PSRS 93446 534-B1
SLOC 93405 652-H5
SLOC 93405 653-A5
SYCAMORE CANYON RD
PSRS 93446 534-B1
StBC 93108 996-H2
SYCAMORE CANYON RD Rt#-144
SBAR 93108 996-D2
SYCAMORE CANYON RD Rt#-192
SBAR 93108 986-D7
SBAR 93108 996-F1
StBC 93108 986-D7
StBC 93108 996-F1
SYCAMORE CREEK CT
StBC 93455 817-B6
SYCAMORE CREEK LN
Npmo 93444 735-H3
SBAR 93103 986-C6
SYCAMORE VISTA RD
StBC 93108 986-D7
StBC 93108 996-D1
SYDNEY ST
SLO 93401 654-B5
SYLVAN CT
StBC 93455 816-J3
SYLVAN DR
GOL 93117 984-E7
GOL 93117 994-E1
SYLVAN RIDGE RD
SLOC 93420 715-A1
SYLVESTER WY
SLOC 93446 494-A6
SYLVIA CIR
PSRS 93446 513-J6
SYLVIA CT
SLO 93401 654-B5
SYRAH CT
SLOC 93465 553-A3

T

N T ST
LMPC 93436 896-C7
LMPC 93436 916-C1
S T ST
LMPC 93436 916-C2
TABANO WY
StBC 93111 984-H7
TABITHA LN
SMRA 93454 776-J4
TABOR LN
StBC 93108 997-C1
TADPOLE CT
SLOC 93465 553-F1
TAFT AV
SLOC 93430 590-J1
SLOC 93430 591-A1
TAFT PL
Cmbr 93428 548-H1
TAFT ST
PBCH 93449 714-C1
SLO 93405 653-J3
SLO 93405 654-A3
SMRA 93454 776-H4
SMRA 93458 776-G4
TAG CT
SLOC 93420 755-C2
TAHITI ST
MOBY 93442 611-D1
TAHOE RD
SLOC 93405 654-A1
TAJO DR
StBC 93110 995-A1
TALLANT RD
SBAR 93105 995-G2
TALLEY FARMS RD
SLOC 93420 695-F5
TALL PINE LN
StBC 93463 921-A6
TALL TREE DR
Npmo 93444 755-H3
TALLYHO PL
StBC 93455 816-G5
TALLY HO RD
ARGD 93420 715-A4
TALLYHO RD
StBC 93455 816-G5
TALMADGE RD
StBC 93455 817-A5

TAMA LN
SMRA 93455 796-F5
TAMARA CT
StBC 93455 816-H5
TAMARA LN
SLOC 93432 574-F1
SLOC 93465 574-F1
TAMARACK CT
StBC 93436 876-F5
TAMARACK WY
SLOC 93465 553-E1
TAMARIND LN
BLTN 93427 919-G4
TAMARISK DR
StBC 93436 896-F3
TAMARISK WY
SLO 93401 674-D5
TAMERA DR
SLOC 93445 714-G7
TAMPICO RD
ATAS 93422 574-B4
TAMSEN ST
Cmbr 93428 528-F7
TANAGER CT
SLOC 93465 553-B1
TANBARK CT
SLOC 93424 693-A1
TANGAIR RD
StBC 93437 875-A4
E TANGERINE AV
LMPC 93436 896-F6
TANGLEWOOD CT
PSRS 93446 534-B1
SLO 93401 654-C6
TANGLEWOOD DR
PSRS 93446 534-A1
SLO 93401 654-C6
StBC 93455 816-B1
TANIS PL
Npmo 93444 756-A4
TANK FARM RD
SLO 93401 673-H2
SLO 93401 674-C1
SLOC 93401 673-H2
SLOC 93401 674-A2
TANNER DR
PSRS 93446 513-H5
TANNER LN
ARGD 93420 715-C4
TANYA CT
SMRA 93454 777-A5
TANYA DR
PSRS 93446 513-J7
TAPADERO DR
StBC 93463 900-F6
TAPIDERO AV
SLOC 93402 632-B7
TARAN CT
SMRA 93455 796-J6
TARANTO CIR
StBC 93013 998-C6
TARENTAISE ST
SLOC 93422 594-E2
TARRAGON CT
LMPC 93436 896-C7
TARSUS CIR
PSRS 93446 494-F7
N TASSAJARA DR
SLO 93405 653-G2
S TASSAJARA DR
SLO 93405 653-G2
TASSAJARA CREEK RD
SLOC - 614-A5
SLOC 93453 614-A5
TATTERSALL CT
StBC 93455 817-A4
TATTLER ST
SLOC 93420 735-A6
TATUM CT
StBC 93455 817-B4
TAUNTON DR
SMRA 93455 796-G5
TAURUS RD
StBC 93429 855-A2
StBC 93436 876-C5
TAYLOR PL
ARGD 93420 714-J5
TAYLOR ST
SMRA 93454 776-H4
SMRA 93458 776-F4
TEAK DR
PSRS 93446 534-A1
TEAKWOOD DR
StBC 93455 816-B1
TEAL
PSRS 93446 514-A7
TECOLOTE AV
GOL 93117 994-E2
TECOLOTE RD
ATAS 93422 573-E5
TECORIDA AV
ATAS 93422 573-J5
TEDDY BEAR LN
GBCH 93433 714-E4
TEE CT
Npmo 93444 735-E7
PSRS 93446 513-J7
TEELYNN AV
SMRA 93458 776-F3
E TEFFT ST
Npmo 93444 736-E7
Npmo 93444 756-D1
W TEFFT ST
Npmo 93444 755-J5
Npmo 93444 756-B3
TEHAMA AV
SLOC 93405 632-J5
TEHAMA DR
StBC 93111 994-G1
TEHAS CANYON RD
StBC 93441 900-J4
N TEJAS PL
Npmo 93444 755-H4
Npmo 93444 756-A4
S TEJAS PL
Npmo 93444 756-A4
TELEPHONE RD
StBC 93454 797-E6
StBC 93454 817-E4
StBC 93455 817-E4
TELFORD RD
SLOC 93446 469-J4
SLOC 93446 470-A4
TELLINA WY
StBC 93111 984-F6
TEMETATTE RIDGE LN
Npmo 93444 736-B3
TEMETTATE DR
Npmo 93444 737-B4

TEMPLE ST
SLOC 93420 714-H7
Summ 93067 997-D4
TEMPLETON RD
SLOC 93465 553-D3
SLOC 93465 574-A1
TEMPLETON CEMETERY RD
SLOC 93465 533-E6
TEMPLETON HILLS RD
SLOC 93465 553-B2
TEMPUS CIR
ARGD 93420 715-B4
TEN ACRE RD
StBC 93108 997-C2
TENBROOK ST
SLO 93401 654-A6
TENNESSEE WALKER WY
SLOC 93446 471-C5
TEN OAKS WY
Npmo 93444 755-H2
TEPIC PL
StBC 93111 984-G7
TEREBINTH LN
SLOC 93465 553-C1
TERESA DR
MOBY 93442 611-J6
TERESA ST
ATAS 93422 573-J1
TERI SUE LN
BLTN 93427 919-H4
TERMINAL DR
SMRA 93455 796-F7
SMRA 93455 816-F1
TERMINO ST
StBC 93460 921-C4
TERN ST
SLOC 93420 735-A5
TERNI LN
SBAR 93105 995-E3
TERRA RD
StBC 93437 895-B2
TERRA ST
MOBY 93442 611-E2
TERRA WY
StBC 93436 876-D7
StBC 93436 896-D1
TERRABELLA CT
PSRS 93446 514-A3
TERRACE AV
PBCH 93449 693-G7
StBC 93455 816-J2
TERRACE CT
BLTN 93427 919-G4
StBC 93437 855-E7
TERRACE DR
SMRA 93455 796-G6
TERRACE RD
SBAR 93103 996-C1
SBAR 93109 995-J6
TERRACE ST
Npmo 93444 756-C3
TERRACE HILL DR
PSRS 93446 513-E5
TERRACE VISTA LN
SBAR 93103 996-D3
TERRAZZO WY
StBC 93455 816-F5
TERRY CT
PBCH 93449 714-F3
StBC 93455 816-J1
TERRY DR
PBCH 93449 714-F3
TESSA CT
SLOC 93465 553-C3
TEXAS RD
SLOC 93446 473-A7
SLOC 93446 493-A1
SLOC 93451 473-A7
THALBERG AV
SLOC 93430 591-C5
THAMES CT
StBC 93111 984-F6
THEATER DR
PSRS 93446 533-F5
SLOC 93446 533-E6
SLOC 93465 533-E7
THEATER LN
StBC 93108 986-G7
THE ESPLANADE
PSRS 93446 513-G2
THELMA DR
SLO 93405 653-E7
THEODORA ST
Npmo 93444 756-A4
THE PIKE
ARGD 93420 714-G7
ARGD 93445 714-G7
GBCH 93433 714-E7
SLOC 93420 714-G7
SLOC 93445 714-E7
THERESA ST
CARP 93013 998-D6
THOMAS AV
SBAR 93101 995-H3
THOMAS CT
SLOC 93465 553-E1
THOMAS RD
BLTN 93427 919-J4
THOMAS HILL RD
SLOC 93420 715-D2
N THOMPSON AV
Npmo 93444 735-H5
Npmo 93444 736-A7
Npmo 93444 756-B1
SLOC 93420 735-H5
S THOMPSON AV
Npmo 93444 756-D3
Npmo 93444 776-H1
THOMPSON ST
SBAR 93101 996-B4
THOMPSON WY
SMRA 93455 796-E5
THORNBERRY RD
SLOC 93445 774-H4
SLOC 93445 775-A3
THORNBURG ST
SMRA 93455 796-G5
SMRA 93458 776-G7
SMRA 93458 796-G1
THORNTON CT
SLOC 93422 593-B1
THORNWOOD DR
GOL 93117 994-E3
THOROUGHBRED PL
SLOC 93420 735-A2
THREAD LN
SLOC 93401 674-C3

STREET Name	City	ZIP	Pg-Grid
THREE SISTERS DR	SLOC	93401	674-B4
THREE SPRINGS RD	SLVG	93463	940-E2
	StBC	93463	940-E2
THRONE CT	StBC	93111	984-F6
THUMBELINA DR	BLTN	93427	919-J6
	BLTN	93427	920-A5
THUNDER GULCH DR	SLOC	93420	755-A1
TIANA DR	StBC	93460	921-A5
	StBC	93463	921-A5
TIANA PL	StBC	93460	921-A4
TIBURON CIR	ATAS	93422	574-B7
TIBURON PL	StBC	93111	984-G7
TIBURON WY	SLOC	93401	654-D7
TIBURON BAY LN	StBC	93108	997-A4
TICIHO PL	SLOC	93405	632-G3
TIDE AV	MOBY	93442	611-E1
TIELO ST	SLOC	93451	473-F1
TIENDA PL	SLOC	93420	734-H6
TIERRA DR	SLOC	93402	631-J7
TIERRA RD	Npmo	93444	756-B6
	SLOC	93422	594-E5
TIERRA ST	ARGD	93420	714-G7
TIERRA BELLA	SBAR	93105	985-F7
TIERRA BRISAS DR	StBC	93455	816-J2
TIERRA CIELO LN	SBAR	93105	986-A6
TIERRA DEL PAJARO	SLOC	93405	693-D2
TIERRA MESA	ATAS	93422	553-H6
TIERRA NUEVA LN	SLOC	93445	714-G7
	SLOC	93445	734-H1
TIERRA REDONDA RD	SLOC	93426	470-B1
TIERRA VISTA RD	SLOC	93446	513-E2
TIFFANY DR	SMRA	93454	777-A6
TIFFANY PARK CIR	StBC	93455	817-B5
TIFFANY PARK CT	StBC	93455	817-C5
TIFFANY RANCH RD	SLOC	93420	695-A4
	SLOC	93453	695-A4
TIGER TAIL DR	ARGD	93420	714-J7
	ARGD	93420	715-A7
TILA LN	StBC	93111	984-F7
TILBURY CT	StBC	93455	817-A5
TILIA ST	StBC	93455	816-J3
TIMBER LN	SMRA	93458	796-G4
	StBC	93437	855-H7
	StBC	93437	875-G1
TIMBERLINE DR	SLOC	93446	471-C3
TIMOTHY CT	LMPC	93436	896-C6
TIMS RD	StBC	93441	901-D1
TIMSBURY WY	SMRA	93455	796-G5
TINKER WY	SBAR	93101	995-H3
TIPTON ST	Cmbr	93428	548-F1
TISHA CT	StBC	93111	984-G5
TISHLINI LN	SLOC	93465	553-B3
TITAN AV	StBC	93436	876-C5
TITAN ST	StBC	93455	817-B5
TIVOLA ST	StBC	93460	921-B5
TOBAGO ST	SLOC	93445	734-H1
TODD LN	ARGD	93420	714-H6
TODO SANTOS CT	SLOC	93445	734-G1
TODOS SANTOS LN	StBC	93105	985-J7
TOGNAZZINI AV	GDLP	93434	774-J6
	GDLP	93434	775-A6
TOLBERT PL	SLOC	93420	735-A2
TOLLIS AV	StBC	93108	997-B1
TOLOSA PL	SLOC	93420	694-G3
TOLOSA WY	SLO	93405	653-G2
TOLOSO RD	ATAS	93422	593-G1
TOLTEC DR	StBC	93111	984-F7
TOLTEC PL	StBC	93111	984-F7
TOLTEC WY	StBC	93111	984-F7
TOLUCA CT	StBC	93111	994-G2
TOMASINI RD	SLOC	93405	632-E1
TOMOL DR	CARP	93013	998-D6
TONINI DR	SLO	93405	653-F7
	SLO	93405	673-F1
TONYA LN	StBC	93455	816-J5
TOPAZ	PBCH	93449	714-D3
TOPAZ ST	PBCH	93449	693-E5
TOPAZ WY	SMRA	93454	777-A6
TORERO RD	StBC	93111	984-J7
TORINO DR	SBAR	93105	995-E3
TORITO RD	StBC	93108	997-G2
TORNOE RD	StBC	93105	985-J7
TORO LN	MOBY	93442	611-D1
TORO ST	SLO	93401	653-J3
	SLO	93401	654-A4
TORO CANYON RD	StBC	-	987-H7
	StBC	93013	997-G4
	StBC	93108	987-H7
	StBC	93108	997-G2
TORO CANYON RD Rt#-192	StBC	93013	997-G3
	StBC	93108	997-G3
TORO CANYON PARK RD	StBC	-	997-G2
	StBC	93108	997-G2
TORO CREEK RD	MOBY	93430	591-D6
	SLOC	-	572-F7
	SLOC	-	591-G4
	SLOC	93430	591-D6
TORREON RD	SLOC	93422	594-E2
TORREY PL	GOL	93117	984-D7
TORREY PINE PL	SLOC	93420	714-H1
TORREY PINES DR	PSRS	93446	533-J1
TOUCAN CT	Npmo	93444	756-B3
TOUCHSTONE LN	SMRA	93454	777-A7
TOULUMNE AV	SLOC	93405	633-E5
TOURAN LN	GOL	93117	993-E2
TOURNEY HILL LN	Npmo	93444	755-E1
TOWER RD	PSRS	93446	494-D4
	SLOC	93446	494-D4
	SLOC	93451	471-J1
TOWN CENTER DR	SMRA	93454	776-H7
TOWN CREEK LN	SLOC	93446	470-A5
TOWNHOUSE TER	PSRS	93446	513-F5
TOWNSEND LN	StBC	93455	816-H2
TOYON CT	ARGD	93420	715-B4
TOYON DR	SBAR	93105	995-F1
TOYON PL	SLOC	93424	693-B2
TRACI DR	StBC	93111	984-G7
TRACK WY	SLOC	93451	453-D6
TRACTOR ST	PSRS	93446	514-A2
TRADITIONS LP	PSRS	93446	513-G2
TRAFFIC WY	ARGD	93420	714-J5
	ARGD	93420	715-A5
	ATAS	93422	553-F6
	ATAS	93422	573-J3
S TRAFFIC WAY EXT	ARGD	93420	715-B6
TRAGER CANYON RD	SLOC	93446	513-C3
TRAILBLAZER LN	SLOC	93446	493-E3
TRAIL VIEW PL	Npmo	93444	755-C3
TRANQUIL HILLS CT	PSRS	93446	513-J5
TRANQUILLA AV	ATAS	93422	573-G1
TRANSFER AV	SBAR	93101	996-A4
TRAVIS DR	SLOC	93402	631-F7
	SLOC	93402	651-F1
TREASURE DR	SBAR	93105	995-G2
TREE LN	SLOC	93420	735-F5
TREE LINE DR	SMRA	93458	776-G3
TREE TRAP RD	SLOC	93426	469-J2
TREMONTO RD	SBAR	93103	986-A7
	SBAR	93103	995-J1
	SBAR	93103	996-A1
TRENORA ST	CARP	93013	998-E6
TRENTON AV	Cmbr	93428	548-G1
TRES CASA LN	Npmo	93444	755-J6
TREVINO CT	PSRS	93446	513-J7
	PSRS	93446	533-J1
TREVINO DR	Npmo	93444	756-A3
TREVOR WY	SLO	93401	654-A5
TRIESTE LN	CARP	93013	998-B6
	StBC	93013	998-B6
TRIFONE WY	Npmo	93444	735-J5
TRIGO CT	ATAS	93422	594-C2
TRIGO LN	PSRS	93446	513-H5
N TRIGO LN	PSRS	93446	513-J5
TRIGO RD	StBC	93117	993-J5
	StBC	93117	994-A5
TRILOGY PKWY	Npmo	93444	755-C3
	SLOC	93420	755-C3
TRIMERA AV	SMRA	93458	796-E4
TRINIDAD DR	SLOC	93445	734-G1
TRINIDAD ST	MOBY	93442	611-D1
TRINITY AV	ARGD	93420	715-B6
	SLOC	93405	633-E5
TRINITY CT	PSRS	93446	514-B7
	PSRS	93446	534-B1
TRINITY DR	SMRA	93458	796-E4
TRISHA CT	SMRA	93455	796-J7
TRIUNFO AV	SMRA	93458	796-E4
TROCHA WY	StBC	93111	984-H7
TROPEA AV	SMRA	93458	796-E4
TROPIC DR	GOL	93117	984-E7
TROUP RD	SBAR	93117	994-B2
TROUVILLE AV	GBCH	93433	714-D5
TRUCKEE RD	SLOC	93405	653-J1
	SLOC	93405	654-A1
TRUDI CT	GOL	93117	984-E7
TRUDI DR	GOL	93117	984-D7
TRUDY CT	StBC	93455	816-H5
TRUMAN DR	SLOC	93445	714-D7
TUCKER AV	PSRS	93446	513-H5
TUCKERNUCK LN	StBC	93455	817-B7
TULARE AV	MOBY	93442	611-G7
	SLOC	93405	633-A5
TULARE ST	PBCH	93449	714-C1
TULEY CT	PSRS	93446	514-A3
TULIP CT	SLO	93401	674-C2
TULIP LN	SMRA	93455	796-J5
TULIP ST	SLOC	93445	734-H1
S TULIP ST	LMPC	93436	916-C2
TULIPWOOD DR	PSRS	93446	514-A7
	PSRS	93446	534-A1
TULLY PL	Cmbr	93428	548-G2
TULPEN DR	SLOC	93420	715-C1
TUMBLEWEED WY	SLOC	93446	471-D6
TUNITAS AV	ATAS	93422	573-J2
TUNNEL RD	StBC	93105	985-J6
TUNNELL ST	SMRA	93454	776-H7
	SMRA	93458	776-F7
TUOLUMNE DR	GOL	93117	993-G2
TUPELO CT	SMRA	93454	796-H2
TURKEY COVE LN	SLOC	93426	469-J2
TURKEY RANCH RD	SLOC	93465	553-C2
TURNER AV	SLO	93401	654-A3
	SLO	93405	654-A3
TURNPIKE RD	StBC	93111	984-J7
	StBC	93111	994-J2
TURNSTONE CIR	GDLP	93434	774-H6
TURNSTONE ST	SLOC	93420	734-J6
TURQUOISE CT	StBC	93455	817-B5
TURQUOISE DR	ARGD	93420	714-J7
TURRI RD	SLOC	93402	631-J3
	SLOC	93402	632-A3
	SLOC	93402	652-E1
	SLOC	93405	631-J3
	SLOC	93405	632-A3
	SLOC	93405	652-E1
TURRI RANCH RD	SLOC	93402	632-F7
	SLOC	93405	632-F7
TURTLE CREEK DR	StBC	93455	816-J1
TURTLE CREEK RD	PSRS	93446	514-B7
	PSRS	93446	534-B1
TUSCAN AV	MOBY	-	591-E7
	MOBY	93442	591-E7
	MOBY	93442	611-E1
	SLOC	-	591-E7
TV TOWER RD	SLOC	-	593-A7
	SLOC	-	614-A7
TWEED AV	Cmbr	93428	548-G2
TWELVE OAKS DR	SLOC	93446	533-D4
TWILIGHT CT	SMRA	93455	796-J7
	StBC	93437	855-F7
TWILIGHT LN	Npmo	93444	756-C5
TWINBERRY CIR	SLOC	93424	693-B2
TWIN CREEKS WY	SLOC	93401	674-G7
	SLOC	93401	694-F1
TWIN OAK DR	BLTN	93427	919-G5
TWIN OAKS RD	SLOC	93453	614-C4
TWIN RIDGE CT	SLO	93405	633-G7
	SLO	93405	653-G1
TWIN RIDGE DR	SLO	93405	653-G1
TWINRIDGE RD	StBC	93111	984-H4
TWITCHELL ST	StBC	93455	816-G5
TWITCHELL DAM RD	StBC	93454	777-H2
TYE RD	StBC	93105	985-H7
TYKES LN	SLOC	93401	693-F1
TYLER DR	SMRA	93454	777-B6
TYNDALL ST	StBC	93460	921-B5
TYRUS CT	Npmo	93444	756-A6
U			
N U ST	LMPC	93436	896-C7
	LMPC	93436	916-C1
S U ST	LMPC	93436	916-C2
UCEN RD	StBC	93106	994-C5
UHLAN CT	SBAR	93103	996-E3
UKIAH ST	StBC	93111	994-J2
UMBRA RD	StBC	93429	855-A2
UNION AV	StBC	93455	816-G6
UNION RD	PSRS	93446	513-G5
	PSRS	93446	514-B3
	SLOC	93446	514-G5
UNION ST	SBAR	93103	996-C4
UNION SUGAR AV	StBC	93436	895-E6
UNION VALLEY PKWY	SMRA	93455	816-F4
	StBC	93455	816-F4
	StBC	93455	817-A4
UNIVERSITY DR	LMPC	93436	916-E3
	SLOC	93405	653-J1
	StBC	93111	984-G7
UPHAM ST	SLO	93401	653-J5
	SLO	93401	654-A5
UPPER HYDE	StBC	93108	986-E6
UPPER LOS BERROS RD	Npmo	93444	735-H3
	Npmo	93444	736-A2
	SLOC	93420	735-H3
	SLOC	93420	736-A2
UPSON RD	StBC	93013	998-C5
URANUS AV	StBC	93436	896-D1
URANUS CT	Npmo	93444	756-A5
US GOVERNMENT RD	StBC	-	998-G6
	StBC	93013	998-G6
UTAH AV	SLOC	93445	734-D1
	StBC	93437	855-E6
	StBC	93437	875-E1
UTAH ST	StBC	93437	855-F6
V			
N V ST	LMPC	93436	896-C5
	LMPC	93436	916-C1
	StBC	93436	896-C7
S V ST	LMPC	93436	916-C2
	StBC	93436	916-C2
VACHELL LN	SLO	93401	673-H3
	SLOC	93401	673-H3
VALA DR	StBC	93111	984-J7
VALDEZ AV	ATAS	93422	573-G2
	GOL	93117	984-C7
	GOL	93117	994-C1
VALDIVIA DR	StBC	93110	995-A1
VALENCIA AV	StBC	93105	985-J5
VALENCIA DR	SBAR	93105	995-H1
VALENCIA RD	Summ	93067	997-D3
VALENTINA AV	ATAS	93422	573-J1
VALENTINE CT	SMRA	93454	796-H4
VALERIE ST	SMRA	93454	777-A6
VALERIO PL	SBAR	93103	996-A2
VALERIO ST	SBAR	93101	995-H4
	SBAR	93101	996-A2
	SBAR	93103	996-A2
VALES ST	SBAR	93109	995-H6
VALHALLA DR	SLVG	93463	940-E1
VALLE AV	ATAS	93422	574-A3
VALLECITO CT	CARP	93013	998-E6
	SLO	93405	653-E6
VALLECITO PL	CARP	93013	998-E6
VALLECITO RD	CARP	93013	998-E6
VALLEJO RD	SLOC	93402	651-E1
VALLE VISTA PL	SLOC	93405	653-C6
VALLEY DR	StBC	93455	817-A4
VALLEY LN	SLOC	93446	471-C5
VALLEY RD	ARGD	93420	714-J7
	SLOC	93420	714-J7
	SLOC	93420	734-J1
E VALLEY RD Rt#-192	StBC	93108	996-H2
	StBC	93108	997-B1
VALLEY CLUB RD	StBC	93108	997-B2
VALLEY DAIRY RD	BLTN	93427	919-G5
VALLEY OAK PL	SMRA	93454	777-A6
VALLEY QUAIL PL	SLOC	93446	493-C6
VALLEY STATION CIR	BLTN	93427	919-G5
VALLEY STATION DR	BLTN	93427	919-G5
VALLEY VIEW DR	LMPC	93436	916-G2
	PBCH	93449	714-D2
	StBC	93455	816-H6
VALLEY VIEW LN	SLOC	93402	651-J1
	SLOC	93402	652-A1
	SLOC	93424	693-B1
VALLEY VIEW PL	SLOC	93420	715-D2
VALLEY VISTA	SMRA	93458	796-G4
VALONIA LN	SMRA	93458	796-E4
VAL VERDE	SLVG	93463	940-D1
VAL VERDE LN	SLOC	93420	735-G5
VANDERLIP CT	PSRS	93446	514-A3
VANESSA WY	StBC	93455	817-C7
VAN GORDON CREEK RD	SLOC	93452	528-C1
VANGUARD DR	StBC	93436	876-D5
VAQUERITO PL	StBC	93111	984-J7
VAQUERO DR	SLOC	93465	533-G7
	SLOC	93465	553-G1
VAQUERO LN	ATAS	93422	574-B5
	StBC	93111	984-J7
VARD LOOMIS CT	ARGD	93420	715-C4
VARD LOOMIS LN	ARGD	93420	715-C4
VARDON CT	Npmo	93444	735-D7
VARIAN CIR	SLOC	93453	695-C3
VARLEY ST	Summ	93067	997-D3
VARNER CT	SMRA	93458	776-H3
VASHON ST	MOBY	93442	611-D1
VEGA AV	ATAS	93422	573-G3
	StBC	93436	876-C6
VEGA DR	GOL	93117	984-D7
	GOL	93117	994-D1
VEGA WY	SLO	93405	653-E6
VELA WY	StBC	93436	896-C1
VELOZ DR	StBC	93108	997-C1
VENABLE ST	SLO	93405	633-J3
VENADO AV	ATAS	93422	573-G3
VENADO DR	StBC	93111	984-J7
VENADO TR	SLOC	93401	673-F5
VENDELS CIR	PSRS	93446	533-F3
VENETTE LN	SMRA	93454	777-B5
VENICE LN	CARP	93013	998-B5
	StBC	93013	998-B5
VENITIA LN	SBAR	93105	995-E2
VENTANA CT	StBC	93437	855-E7
	StBC	93455	816-J2
VENTANA DR	PBCH	93449	714-E3
VENTANA DEL ROBLES LN	SLOC	93465	553-C2
VENTURA AV	SLOC	93405	633-A5
VENTURA DR	SBAR	93105	995-H1
VENTURA FRWY U.S.-101	StBC	-	1018-J3
	VeCo	-	1018-J3
VENTURA RD	SLOC	93422	572-J5
	SMRA	93455	796-H6
VENTURE DR	SLOC	93401	673-H3
VENUS AV	StBC	93436	896-D1
VENUS CT	Npmo	93444	756-A5
VERANO DR	CARP	93013	998-C6
	SBAR	93110	985-C7
VERANO WY	Npmo	93444	756-A6
VERBENA ST	Npmo	93444	755-J4
VERDE DR	SLO	93405	653-H2
VERDE PL	ARGD	93420	714-G7
	SLOC	93451	473-F2
VERDE CANYON RD	SLOC	93420	695-A5
VERDE MAR DR	SBAR	93103	996-E4
VERDE VISTA DR	SBAR	93105	995-G1
VERDON ST	MOBY	93442	611-E2
VERDUGO PL	StBC	93110	995-A2
VERDUGO RANCH WY	SLOC	93405	693-C1
VERDURA AV	GOL	93117	994-D1
VEREDA CORDILLERA	StBC	93117	993-D2
VEREDA DEL CIERVO	StBC	93117	983-D5
	StBC	93117	993-D1
VEREDA DEL PADRE	StBC	93117	993-C1
VEREDA ESCOLAR	StBC	93117	993-C1
VEREDA GALERIA	StBC	93117	993-C1
VEREDA LEYENDA	StBC	93117	983-C7
	StBC	93117	993-C1
VEREDA NUEVA	StBC	93117	983-D7
VEREDA PARQUE	StBC	93117	983-C7
VEREDA PRADERA	StBC	93117	993-D1
VEREDA VERDE LN	ATAS	93422	594-C2
VERHELLE RD	SBAR	93117	994-D2
VERNAL AV	SBAR	93105	995-H1
VERNALIS RD	ATAS	93422	574-B3
VERNON RD	SBAR	93105	995-G2
VERNON ST	ARGD	93420	714-J5
VERONA AV	GOL	93117	993-H1
VERONICA DR	PSRS	93446	513-J7
VERONICA LN	SMRA	93454	776-J5
	SMRA	93454	777-A4
VERONICA PL	SBAR	93105	995-F4
VERONICA SPRINGS RD	SBAR	93105	995-E3
	StBC	93105	995-E3
	StBC	93109	995-E5
VESTER HOF	SLVG	93463	940-D1
VESTER STED	SLVG	93463	940-D1
VETTER LN	SLOC	93449	694-G7
VIA AV	ATAS	93422	573-J2
VIA ABAJO	StBC	93110	994-J3
VIA ABRIGADA	StBC	93110	995-B3
VIA AIROSA	StBC	93110	995-B2
VIA ALBA	StBC	93111	984-H6
VIA ALEGRE	StBC	93110	995-B2
VIA ALICIA	SBAR	93108	996-E2
VIA ALTA	StBC	93455	817-A7
VIA ALTA CT	StBC	93437	855-E7
VIA ALTA MESA	Npmo	93444	755-G5
VIA ALTA ZORRO	SLOC	93446	513-D3
VIA ANDORRA	StBC	93110	985-C6
VIA ANZUELO	ATAS	93422	553-J7
VIA ARBOLITOS	SMRA	93458	796-E5
VIA ARLETA	StBC	93455	817-A7
VIA ARNEZ	StBC	93436	896-G2
VIA ARROYO	PSRS	93446	513-H4
VIA ARTURO	SLOC	93445	734-H1
VIA ASUETO	SMRA	93454	777-B6
S VIA AVANTE	ARGD	93420	715-A6
VIA BANDOLERO	ARGD	93420	714-H4
VIA BARBA	StBC	93436	896-G2
VIA BELIZ	SMRA	93454	777-B5
N VIA BELMONTE CT	ARGD	93420	715-A6
S VIA BELMONTE CT	ARGD	93420	715-A6
VIA BENDITA	StBC	93110	995-A4
VIA BERROS	ARGD	93420	714-J7
VIA BOLZANO	GOL	93111	984-F6
	GOL	93117	984-F6
	StBC	93111	984-F6
VIA BRIGITTE	StBC	93111	985-A5
VIA BRIZA CT	PSRS	93446	513-H4
VIA BROCHA	StBC	93110	994-J3
VIA CAMELIA	PSRS	93446	513-H4
VIA CAMPOBELLO	StBC	93111	984-H6
VIA CARISMA	SBAR	93109	995-H7
VIA CARRETAS	StBC	93110	995-A3
VIA CARRO	SMRA	93458	776-F4
VIA CARTA	SLO	93405	
	SLO	93405	
	SLOC	93405	
	SLOC	93405	
VIA CASA VISTA	SLOC	93420	
VIA CASTILLO	SMRA	93458	
VIA CAYENTE	StBC	93110	
VIA CHAPARRAL RD	StBC	93105	
	StBC	93110	
VIA CHORRO	StBC	93455	
VIA CHULA ROBLES	SLOC	93420	
VIA CIELO	ATAS	93422	
VIA CLARICE	StBC	93111	
VIA COLONIA CT	ATAS	93422	
VIA CONCHA RD	Npmo	93444	
	Npmo	93444	
VIA CONCHA WY	Npmo	93444	
	SLOC	93420	
VIA CONTENTO	SMRA	93454	
VIA CORONA	BLTN	93427	
	StBC	93110	
VIA CORTEZ	StBC	93436	
VIA COVELLO	StBC	93110	
VIA DE LA CRUZ	SMRA	93455	
VIA DE LA LUNA	StBC	93455	
VIA DEL CARMEL	StBC	93455	
VIA DEL CENTRO	SLOC	93445	
VIA DEL CIELO	SBAR	93109	
	SBAR	93109	
VIA DEL FLORISTA	StBC	93455	
VIA DELICIA	SMRA	93454	
VIA DEL MAR	StBC	93108	
VIA DEL NORTE	SLOC	93445	
VIA DE LOS RANCHOS	StBC	93441	
	StBC	93463	
	StBC	93463	
VIA DEL PALMA	StBC	93455	
VIA DEL REY	StBC	93117	
VIA DEL RIO	SLOC	93445	
VIA DEL SALINAS	SLOC	93446	
VIA DEL SOL	SLVG	93463	
VIA DEL SUENO	ATAS	93422	
VIA DI CAMPO	StBC	93455	
VIA DICHOSA	StBC	93110	
VIA DIEGO	SBAR	93110	
VIA DINERO	StBC	93463	
VIA DOCENA	StBC	93110	
VIA DONA	StBC	93436	
VIA ELBA	StBC	93436	
VIA EL CIELO	SLOC	93420	
VIA EL CUADRO	StBC	93111	
VIA EL ENCANTADOR	StBC	93111	
VIA EL RINCON	CARP	93013	
VIA ELSIE	CARP	93013	
VIA ENCANTO	SBAR	93108	
VIA ENSENADA	SLO	93401	
VIA ENTRADA	Npmo	93444	
	SLOC	93420	
VIA ESMERALDA	StBC	93455	
	StBC	93455	
VIA ESPARTO	StBC	93110	
VIA ESPERANZA	Npmo	93444	
	StBC	93110	
VIA ESTABLO	SMRA	93458	
VIA ESTEBAN	SLO	93401	
VIA ESTIO	SMRA	93454	
VIA ESTRELLA	ATAS	93422	
VIA FARGO	StBC	93455	
VIA FEDORA	StBC	93455	
VIA FELICE	SMRA	93454	
VIA FELIZ	StBC	93436	
VIA FIORI LN	GOL	93117	
N VIA FIRENZE CT	ARGD	93420	
S VIA FIRENZE CT	ARGD	93420	
VIA FLORA	PSRS	93446	
VIA FRUTERIA	StBC	93110	

STREET Name	City	ZIP	Pg-Grid
…CHSIA	PSRS	93446	513-H4
…AITERO	StBC	93105	985-C6
…ALA	StBC	93436	896-H1
…ENNITA	StBC	93111	985-A5
…ORIETA	StBC	93110	995-B3
…RANADA	SBAR	93103	995-J1
	SBAR	93103	996-A1
…STO	SMRA	93454	777-B6
…ELO	SMRA	93454	777-B6
…ERBA	StBC	93110	995-C2
…ERTO	StBC	93110	994-J3
	StBC	93110	995-A3
…ERTO CT	ATAS	93422	553-E7
…LA	StBC	93436	876-H7
…CINTO	StBC	93111	994-H2
…O DR	GOL	93117	993-F2
…ANA RD	StBC	93460	921-A6
… BARRANCA	ARGD	93420	715-A4
…GUNA DR	StBC	93110	995-D2
…GUNA VISTA	SLOC	93405	653-C6
…NTANA	PSRS	93446	513-G4
… PAZ	SLO	93401	653-J7
…RA LN	StBC	93111	994-H2
…S AGUILAS	ARGD	93420	714-H4
…S BRISAS	StBC	93110	985-E7
… SELVA	StBC	93463	921-A3
…TINA	StBC	93013	998-C5
…TO	StBC	93436	876-H7
	StBC	93436	896-H1
…E	StBC	93111	994-J1
…MORA	StBC	93117	984-E5
…NDA	CARP	93013	998-F7
	CARP	93013	1018-F1
…S PADRES	StBC	93111	984-J5
…S SANTOS	StBC	93111	984-H6
	StBC	93111	985-A6
…CERO	SBAR	93110	995-E1
…ADRONA	PSRS	93446	513-H4
…AGNOLIA	PSRS	93446	513-H4
…ANANA	StBC	93108	987-A7
…ANZANITA CT	PSRS	93446	513-H4
…ARCINA	StBC	93013	998-C5
…ARGARITA	StBC	93455	817-A7
…ARIA	CARP	93013	998-E7
	StBC	93111	985-B5
…AR SOL	SLOC	93449	714-F1
…AVIS	StBC	93455	817-A6
…AXWELL	Npmo	93444	755-H5
…ERANO	StBC	93111	984-F6
…ESSINA	GOL	93117	984-E5
…GUEL AV	StBC	93111	994-H3
…RA VALLE	Npmo	93444	755-G6
…TAD	StBC	93436	876-H7
…ONDO	StBC	93436	876-H7
…ETO	StBC	93110	994-J3
…NA	StBC	93455	817-A5
…STRE	Npmo	93444	735-H5
	SLOC	93420	735-H5
…JEVO	SMRA	93458	776-F4
…RILLA	StBC	93436	896-G1
…RQUIDIA	StBC	93111	985-A6
…ALO	Npmo	93444	755-D2
…ALOMA	SLOC	93446	533-G2
…APAGALLO	SLOC	93420	734-H5
…ARTE	StBC	93436	876-H7
…ARVA	StBC	93111	984-J6
…AVION	StBC	93455	817-A7
…CCOLI	StBC	93111	984-H6
…NTA	StBC	93455	817-A5
…OCA	ARGD	93420	714-H3
…RESADA	StBC	93110	995-C2
…RIVADO	SLOC	93449	714-F1
…ROMESA	Npmo	93444	755-J5
VIA PROMESA	PSRS	93446	513-H5
VIA PROMESA DR	PSRS	93446	513-G5
VIA QUANTICO	SMRA	93454	777-B6
VIA RAMONA	PSRS	93446	514-A7
	PSRS	93446	534-A1
VIA RANCHITOS	ATAS	93422	553-E6
VIA RAVENNA	GOL	93111	984-E6
	GOL	93117	984-E6
VIA REAL	CARP	93013	998-B6
	StBC	93013	997-H4
	StBC	93013	998-B6
	Summ	93067	997-E4
N VIA REAL	CARP	93013	1018-G1
	StBC	93013	1018-G1
VIA REGINA	StBC	93111	984-J6
VIA REPOSA	SLVG	93463	940-D1
VIA REPOSO	StBC	93111	984-G6
VIA RICARDO	CARP	93013	998-F7
VIA RICO	SMRA	93454	777-B6
VIA RIVIERA	StBC	93455	817-B7
VIA ROBLADA	StBC	93110	995-A3
VIA ROBLES	SLOC	93401	694-J2
	SLOC	93446	533-E5
VIA ROJAS	SLOC	93465	553-A3
VIA ROJO	SBAR	93110	985-E7
VIA ROMA	StBC	93110	995-A2
VIA ROSA	PSRS	93446	513-H4
	SBAR	93110	985-D7
	SMRA	93458	796-E4
VIA ROSITA	StBC	93110	995-C3
VIA RUBI	StBC	93111	985-A6
VIA RUBIO	CARP	93013	998-F7
VIA RUBIO DR	SMRA	93454	776-H5
VIA RUEDA	StBC	93110	995-A2
VIA SABROSA	SMRA	93454	777-B6
VIA SALADITA	StBC	93111	985-A5
VIA SALERNO	GOL	93111	984-E6
	GOL	93117	984-E6
VIA SAN BLAS	SLO	93401	653-J7
VIA SAN CARLOS	SLOC	93446	533-E5
	StBC	93463	920-F4
VIA SAN MIGUEL	SLOC	93446	533-E5
VIA SANTA BARBARA	SLOC	93446	533-E5
VIA SANTA MARIA	StBC	93455	817-A4
VIA SECO	Npmo	93444	755-G2
VIA SEMI	StBC	93436	896-H1
VIA SENDA	StBC	93110	995-D2
VIA SEVILLA	SBAR	93109	995-G7
VIA SINUOSA	StBC	93110	995-C2
VIA SOLANA	SLOC	93420	734-H5
VIA SPANISH OAKS	SLOC	93453	614-B4
VIA STEVARINO	CARP	93013	998-F7
VIA TARREGA	StBC	93111	994-H3
VIA TORTUGA	ATAS	93422	574-A6
VIA TRANQUILA	StBC	93110	995-C3
VIA TRENTO	GOL	93117	984-E6
VIA TREPADORA	StBC	93110	995-B2
VIA TROPICO	SMRA	93454	777-B6
VIA TUSA	SBAR	93105	985-G6
VIA UNDOSA	SMRA	93454	777-B5
VIA VALVERDE	StBC	93111	994-H3
VIA VAQUERO	ARGD	93420	714-H4
VIA VENADO	SLOC	93401	693-F1
VIA VENETO	StBC	93111	985-A5
VIA VENTANA	SMRA	93458	776-G3
VIA VERDE RD	Npmo	93444	755-D3
VIA VICENTE	Npmo	93444	755-H5
VIA VIENTO	ATAS	93422	553-E6
VIA VISALIA	SMRA	93458	776-F4
VIA VISTA	SMRA	93454	777-B5
VIA VISTA WY	SLOC	93432	574-E1
	SLOC	93465	574-E1
VIA VISTA VERDE	StBC	93455	816-J6
VIA VISTOSA	SLOC	93402	631-J7
	SLOC	93402	651-H1
	StBC	93110	995-B2
VIA YNEZ	SMRA	93454	777-B5
VIA ZACATA	SLOC	93420	755-B1
VIA ZORRO	StBC	93110	995-D1
VIBORG RD	SLOC	93446	493-E3
	SLVG	93463	920-F6
VICENTE DR	SLO	93405	653-F7
	SLO	93405	673-G1
VICENTI PL	StBC	93108	996-J4
VICKIE AV	SMRA	93454	776-H5
VICTORIA AV	SLO	93401	654-A6
VICTORIA CT	PSRS	93446	513-H3
VICTORIA PL	SMRA	93458	796-G2
VICTORIA ST	SBAR	93101	995-J4
	SBAR	93101	996-A3
	SBAR	93103	996-A3
VICTORIA WY	ARGD	93420	714-H7
	Cmbr	93428	548-F1
VICTORIAN CT	ARGD	93420	714-H6
VICTORY DR	BLTN	93427	919-H5
VICTORY WY	SLOC	93420	734-J7
VIDA AV	ATAS	93422	573-H2
VIEJA DR	StBC	93110	994-J3
	StBC	93110	995-B2
VIEJO RD	SLOC	93420	735-C5
VIEJO CAMINO	ATAS	93422	594-C1
	SLOC	93422	594-D2
VIENDRA DR	StBC	93441	920-B4
VIEW DR	StBC	93460	921-J2
VIEWMONT ST	SLO	93401	654-B5
VIEW PARK DR	StBC	93455	816-G6
VIGARD DR	SLVG	93463	920-F7
VIKING WY	SLVG	93463	920-E6
VILLA AV	SBAR	93101	995-H4
VILLA CT	PBCH	93449	714-D2
	SLO	93401	673-G2
VILLA DR	PSRS	93446	513-F4
VILLAGE CT	ARGD	93420	715-A6
	SMRA	93454	777-B6
	StBC	93455	817-A4
VILLAGE DR	StBC	93455	817-A4
VILLAGE GRN	SMRA	93455	796-G5
VILLAGE LN	Cmbr	93428	528-H7
	SLVG	93463	920-F7
	StBC	93110	994-J3
VILLAGE RD	SLOC	93446	471-A5
VILLAGE CIRCLE DR	LMPC	93436	916-C1
VILLAGE CREST	SLOC	93424	693-B2
VILLAGE GLEN DR	ARGD	93420	714-J3
	ARGD	93420	715-A3
VILLAGE KNOLL CT	StBC	93455	817-A4
VILLAGE KNOLL DR	StBC	93455	817-A4
VILLAGE MEADOWS DR	LMPC	93436	896-C6
VILLAGE TERRACE DR	GOL	93117	984-E7
VILLA LOTS RD	PSRS	93446	513-F1
	SLOC	93446	513-D1
VILLA NONA	Npmo	93444	755-G2
VILLA PARK WY	Npmo	93444	755-F5
VINA WY	SLOC	93451	473-D3
VINCENTE WY	SBAR	93105	995-E3
VINE AV	SBAR	93101	996-B3
VINE ST	PSRS	93446	513-F2
	SLOC	93402	631-G5
	SLOC	93446	513-F2
	SMRA	93454	776-H5
S VINE ST	PSRS	93446	513-F7
	PSRS	93446	533-F3
	SLOC	93446	513-F7
	SLOC	93446	533-F1
VINE HILL LN	SLOC	93446	513-A2
VINELAND DR	StBC	93455	816-H1
VINEYARD CIR	PSRS	93446	513-H2
VINEYARD DR	SLOC	93465	553-A3
VINEYARD RD	StBC	93111	984-G5
VINEYARD CANYON RD	MonC	-	453-H3
	SLOC	93451	453-F6
VINEYARD VIEW LN	SLOC	93420	694-J5
E VINTAGE ST	Npmo	93444	756-D2
VINTAGE WY	StBC	93440	878-H2
VINTAGE RANCH LN	StBC	93110	995-A2
VINTON LN	SLOC	93420	715-C2
VIOLA CT	Npmo	93444	756-A3
VIOLA LN	StBC	93108	987-H7
VIOLA WY	LMPC	93436	896-D6
VIOLET AV	Npmo	93444	756-B4
VIOLET LN	GOL	93117	993-H2
VIOLETA AV	ATAS	93422	573-H4
VIRGINIA DR	ARGD	93420	714-H7
VIRGINIA LN	StBC	93108	996-H4
VIRGINIA RD	StBC	93108	996-H4
VISALIA ST	PBCH	93449	714-C1
VISCAINO RD	SBAR	93103	996-B1
VISCANO AV	ATAS	93422	573-J1
VISTA CIR	ARGD	93420	714-H2
	SMRA	93458	796-G4
VISTA CT	PSRS	93446	513-F3
	SLOC	93402	631-F7
	SLOC	93446	533-E5
VISTA DR	ARGD	93420	714-H2
VISTA LN	SLO	93401	673-G2
VISTA RD	ATAS	93422	573-E7
	ATAS	93422	593-F1
VISTA ST	MOBY	93442	611-G7
	SLOC	93445	714-F7
VISTA ARROYO	SBAR	93109	995-E6
VISTA BAHIA	StBC	93111	984-G7
VISTA BUENA RD	StBC	93110	995-A1
VISTA CERRO DR	PSRS	93446	514-A5
VISTA CLARA RD	StBC	93110	995-C1
VISTA COLINA	PSRS	93446	514-A5
VISTA DE AVILA	SLOC	93424	693-B3
VISTA DE LA CUMBRE	SBAR	93105	985-G7
	SBAR	93105	995-G1
VISTA DE LA MESA DR	StBC	93110	994-J3
VISTA DE LA MONTANA	SLO	93405	653-E6
VISTA DE LA PLAYA LN	SBAR	93109	995-J6
VISTA DEL ARROYO	SLO	93405	653-E6
VISTA DEL ASTA	SLOC	93420	714-J2
VISTA DE LA VINA	SLOC	93446	534-A4
VISTA DEL BRISA	SLO	93405	653-E6
VISTA DEL CAMPO	SBAR	93101	995-G3
VISTA DEL COLLADOS	SLO	93405	653-E6
VISTA DE LEJOS DR	StBC	93110	994-J3
VISTA DEL LAGO	SLO	93405	653-F6
VISTA DEL MAR	PBCH	93449	693-G7
VISTA DEL MAR DR	SBAR	93109	995-F5
VISTA DEL MUNDO	SMRA	93458	776-F4
VISTA DEL ORO	SMRA	93458	796-G4
VISTA DEL OSOS	SLOC	93402	651-J1
VISTA DEL PUEBLO	Npmo	93444	776-G1
	SBAR	93101	995-J5
VISTA DEL RIO	Npmo	93444	756-G7
	Npmo	93444	776-G1
	SMRA	93458	776-F3
VISTA DEL RIO CT	PSRS	93446	513-H6
VISTA DEL ROBLES	SLOC	93420	694-G6
	SLOC	93449	694-G6
VISTA DEL SOL	Npmo	93444	776-G1
	SMRA	93458	776-F3
VISTA DE ROBLES PL	SLOC	93446	514-J7
VISTA ELEGANTE	SMRA	93455	796-J5
VISTA ELEVADA	StBC	93105	985-H6
VISTA GRANDE LN	SLOC	93449	694-G7
VISTA GRANDE ST	PSRS	93446	513-J4
	PSRS	93446	514-A5
VISTA LINDA LN	StBC	93108	997-G1
VISTA MADERA	SBAR	93101	995-G3
	SBAR	93105	995-G3
VISTA MONTANA	SMRA	93458	776-F4
VISTA OAKS WY	PSRS	93446	513-H3
VISTA OCEANO LN	Summ	93067	997-F4
VISTA PACIFICA	SBAR	93109	995-J6
VISTA PACIFICA CIR	PBCH	93449	714-E3
VISTA PROMESA	SMRA	93458	776-F3
VISTA SERRANO WY	SLOC	93446	493-A4
VISTA VALLEJO	SBAR	93105	995-F2
	StBC	93105	995-F2
VISTA VERDE LN	Npmo	93444	756-A4
VIVA WY	Npmo	93444	755-E5
VOLANS AV	StBC	93436	876-C6
VOLANTE PL	GOL	93117	984-D6
VOLPI YSABEL RD	SLOC	93446	533-F5
VOLUNTARIO ST	SBAR	93103	996-C2
VOYAGER RD	StBC	93436	896-D2
VULCAN DR	StBC	93436	876-D7
W			
W ST	LMPC	93436	916-C2
N W ST	LMPC	93436	896-C6
	LMPC	93436	916-C1
WADE CT	PSRS	93446	513-J7
	SBAR	93109	995-F6
	SMRA	93454	776-H4
WADE DR	PSRS	93446	513-H7
	PSRS	93446	533-H1
WADSWORTH AV	PBCH	93449	714-B1
WAGONEER RD	SLOC	93446	513-C6
WAGON WHEEL DR	GOL	93117	993-E1
WAGON WHEEL PL	SLOC	93446	534-J4
WAGON WHEEL RD	StBC	93437	875-F2
WAGON WHEEL WY	SLOC	93420	735-F5
WAH KON TAH LN	ATAS	93422	594-C2
	SLOC	93422	594-C2
WAILEA CT	SMRA	93455	796-G5
WAILEA WY	Npmo	93444	755-F1
WAITE ST	StBC	93440	878-G1
WAKE RD	StBC	93437	875-E2
WAKEFIELD RD	GOL	93117	984-E7
WALDRON AV	SBAR	93103	996-C2
WALES RD	Cmbr	93428	548-G2
WALKER ST	SLO	93401	653-H5
WALL ST	Cmbr	93428	528-G6
WALLACE AV	Cmbr	93428	548-H1
	Summ	93067	997-D4
WALLACE DR	PSRS	93446	514-A3
WALLACE PL	ARGD	93420	714-H6
WALLBRIDGE DR	Cmbr	93428	528-E7
WALLER LN	SMRA	93455	796-G7
	StBC	93455	796-G7
WALLIS AV	SMRA	93458	796-G3
WALNUT AV	CARP	93013	998-D7
	SBAR	93101	995-J4
	SLOC	93422	594-G5
	SLOC	93422	614-F1
E WALNUT AV	LMPC	93436	916-F1
W WALNUT AV	LMPC	93436	916-B1
WALNUT DR	PSRS	93446	513-J4
	SMRA	93458	776-G6
	SMRA	93458	796-G3
	StBC	93110	985-E6
WALNUT LN	BLTN	93427	919-G5
	StBC	93111	994-H1
WALNUT PL	StBC	93111	994-H2
WALNUT RD	StBC	93437	875-H1
WALNUT ST	ARGD	93420	714-H6
	MOBY	93442	611-F7
	SLO	93401	653-J3
WALNUT PARK DR	StBC	93111	984-H7
WALNUT PARK LN	StBC	93111	984-H7
WALTER WY	StBC	93455	816-H6
WALTER CREEK RD	SLOC	93405	632-H4
WARBLER CT	PSRS	93446	534-A2
WARD CT	SLOC	93465	553-D2
WARD DR	GOL	93111	994-F2
	StBC	93111	994-F3
WARD ST	SLO	93401	653-J5
WARM SPRINGS LN	SLOC	93446	533-J4
WARNER ST	SLOC	93445	714-F7
WARREN RD	Cmbr	93428	548-F1
	SLOC	93446	473-E6
WARREN WY	SLO	93405	653-G2
WARWICK PL	GOL	93117	993-F2
WARWICK ST	Cmbr	93428	528-D5
WASHINGTON AV	StBC	93437	855-B7
	StBC	93437	875-B1
WASHINGTON BLVD	SLOC	93451	453-A4
WASHINGTON CIR	SMRA	93458	776-G3
WASHINGTON ST	StBC	93254	806-C4
WASOIJA ST	StBC	93254	806-C2
WATER ST	PBCH	93449	693-H7
WATERCRESS WY	SLOC	93453	695-D3
WATERFALL LN	PSRS	93446	533-G1
WATERFALL RD	SLOC	93465	533-E7
	SLOC	93465	553-E1
WATERFORD CT	PSRS	93446	513-H2
WATER MILL LN	StBC	93460	921-A6
WATER VIEW DR	SLOC	93446	471-B5
WATERVIEW PL	Npmo	93444	755-C2
	SLOC	93420	755-C2
WATSON DR	SLOC	93405	632-J4
WAVE AV	PBCH	93449	714-D2
WAVERTREE ST	SLO	93401	674-D2
	SLOC	93401	674-D2
WAWONA AV	PBCH	93449	693-H7
WAYLAND DR	StBC	93437	855-D6
WAYLAND PL	StBC	93455	816-J4
WAYNE WY	SLOC	93420	715-C1
WAYPOINT DR	Npmo	93444	755-G3
WEATHERFORD DR	StBC	93436	896-G2
WEAVER LN	SLOC	93446	514-J4
WEDGEWOOD DR	SMRA	93455	796-F6
WEDGEWOOD LN	PSRS	93446	513-H2
WEDGEWOOD ST	Cmbr	93428	548-F2
WEEPING WILLOW WY	SLOC	93446	494-G7
WELDON PL	SBAR	93109	996-A5
WELDON RD	SBAR	93109	996-A6
WELL RD	SLOC	93446	469-D2
	SLOC	93465	553-B2
WELLINGTON AV	SBAR	93105	995-H2
WELLINGTON DR	StBC	93455	816-G4
WELLINGTON LN	Cmbr	93428	528-D6
WELLSONA RD	SLOC	93446	493-D2
	SLOC	93446	494-A3
WELSH CT	SLO	93405	653-F7
	SLO	93405	673-F1
WELSH LN	SLOC	93420	735-A2
WELSH WY	SLOC	93446	471-C4
WENDY CT	SMRA	93454	797-A1
WENDY WY	StBC	93455	816-J2
WENTWORTH AV	SBAR	93101	996-A5
WESLEY ST	ARGD	93420	714-J4
WESSELS WY	SLOC	93465	553-D1
WESSEX CT	GOL	93117	984-C7
WEST AV	MOBY	93442	611-F6
WEST MALL	ATAS	93422	573-J3
WEST ST	Cmbr	93428	528-G7
	SLO	93405	653-H3
	SMRA	93458	796-G4
WESTBROOK RD	LMPC	93436	896-D6
WESTBURY WY	SMRA	93455	796-G5
WESTCLIFF DR	CARP	93013	998-A5
WESTERLY RD	StBC	93441	922-A4
WESTERN AV	SBAR	93101	995-H4
	SMRA	93458	776-F4
	SMRA	93458	796-F1
WESTERN GULL DR	SLOC	93424	693-B3
WESTFIELD RD	PSRS	93446	534-B1
WESTGATE	BLTN	93427	919-G5
WESTGATE RD	SMRA	93455	796-E5
	SMRA	93458	796-E4
WESTHAMPTON DR	SLOC	93420	735-B6
WESTMINSTER LN	StBC	93455	816-G4
WESTMONT AV	SLO	93405	653-G1
WESTMONT RD	SBAR	93108	986-E7
	SBAR	93108	996-E1
WESTMORLAND PL	GOL	93117	984-C7
WESTON CT	SMRA	93458	776-F4
	StBC	93437	875-E1
WESTON DR	StBC	93437	875-E1
WESTWIND WY	Npmo	93444	755-F1
WESTWOOD DR	SBAR	93109	995-G6
WEYMOUTH CT	StBC	93455	816-F4
WEYMOUTH ST	Cmbr	93428	528-D5
WHIDBEY ST	MOBY	93442	611-D1
WHIDBEY WY	MOBY	93442	611-E1
WHIMBREL CT	Npmo	93444	755-H2
WHIPPOORWILL DR	SLOC	93455	816-J1
WHIPPOORWILL LN	SLOC	93465	553-B1
WHIPTAIL CT	SLOC	93426	470-A2
WHISPER LN	Npmo	93444	755-F2
WHISPERING MEADOW LN	Npmo	93444	735-J3
WHISPERING OAK WY	SLOC	93446	494-G7
	SLOC	93446	514-G1
WHISPERING PINE DR	StBC	93455	817-A3
WHITBY ST	Cmbr	93428	548-G1
WHITE AV	SBAR	93109	995-G6
WHITE CT	ARGD	93420	715-A3
	SMRA	93458	796-E1
WHITE BASS WY	SLOC	93446	469-G4
WHITECAP ST	PBCH	93449	714-D2
WHITE CHAPEL CT	StBC	93455	816-G4
WHITECLIFF PL	StBC	93455	816-F4
WHITE CLOVER LN	PSRS	93446	514-A6
WHITE DOVE CT	Npmo	93444	735-H4
N WHITE DOVE DR	StBC	93455	816-G2
S WHITE DOVE DR	StBC	93455	816-J1
WHITEFIELD CT	StBC	93455	816-F4
WHITEHALL AV	Cmbr	93428	528-E7
WHITELEY ST	ARGD	93420	715-A5
WHITE OAK AV	PBCH	93449	714-E3
WHITE OAK LN	SLOC	93401	674-D7
	SLOC	93465	553-A5
WHITE OAK RD	SLOC	93465	553-B6
	StBC	93460	941-D1
WHITEWATER RD	SLOC	93465	533-E7
WHITMAN ST	GOL	93117	993-J3
WHITNEY AV	Summ	93067	997-D3
WHITNEY CT	StBC	93111	994-H2
WHITTIER DR	GOL	93117	993-J3
	StBC	93117	993-J3
WICKENDEN ST	StBC	93440	878-H2
WICKSON WY	ATAS	93422	594-C2
WIDGEON WY	SLOC	93420	735-A6
WIDOW LN	Npmo	93444	756-C5
WILCOMBE DR	Cmbr	93428	548-G1
WILD DEER CT	PSRS	93446	513-F4
WILDERNESS LN	PSRS	93446	494-E4
	SLOC	93446	494-E4
WILD FLOWER RD	Npmo	93444	737-C6
WILD FOX	SLOC	93446	470-C4
WILDHAVEN CIR	StBC	93454	797-C7
WILD HORSE PL	SLOC	93446	534-J4
WILD HORSE WINERY CT	SLOC	93465	553-H5
WILDING LN	SLO	93401	654-B4
WILD MUSTARD LN	PSRS	93446	514-A6
WILD OATS WY	SLOC	93465	533-C6
WILD PIGEON WY	SLOC	93446	469-H5
WILD RICE LN	SLOC	93446	471-D6
WILD ROSE LN	SLOC	93446	493-E7
	SLOC	93446	513-E1
WILD RYE WY	SLOC	93453	695-D3
WILDWOOD DR	ARGD	93420	715-B4
	SLOC	93465	553-A2
WILDWOOD RD	SMRA	93454	776-J5
	SMRA	93454	777-A5
WILHELMINA AV	SLOC	93453	614-E4
WILL ST	SMRA	93454	777-A5
WILLETT WY	SLOC	93420	734-J5
	SLOC	93420	735-A5
WILLHOIT LN	SLOC	93465	553-D2
WILLIAM ST	SLOC	93465	553-D1
WILLIAMS ST	SMRA	93454	776-H5
	SMRA	93458	776-F5
WILLIAMS WY	StBC	93105	985-H6
WILLINA LN	StBC	93108	996-J3

STREET Name | City | ZIP | Pg-Grid

WILLITS LN
- PSRS 93446 513-G2

E WILLOW AV
- LMPC 93436 916-F3

W WILLOW AV
- LMPC 93436 916-C3
- StBC 93436 916-D3

WILLOW CIR
- SLO 93401 654-C7
- StBC 93460 921-B6

WILLOW CT
- ATAS 93422 574-B7

WILLOW DR
- SLOC 93402 631-J7
- SLOC 93402 632-A6
- SLVG 93463 940-E1

WILLOW LN
- ARGD 93420 714-H7
- BLTN 93427 919-G4

WILLOW PL
- CARP 93013 998-D7

WILLOW RD
- Npmo 93444 735-J7
- Npmo 93444 755-H1
- SLOC 93420 755-C1

WILLOW RD Rt#-1
- SLOC 93420 754-H1
- SLOC 93420 755-A1

WILLOW ST
- SLOC 93445 734-F2
- StBC 93437 875-H1
- StBC 93460 921-B4

WILLOW WK
- StBC 93117 994-A4

WILLOWBANK LN
- PSRS 93446 533-G1

WILLOWBROOK CT
- StBC 93437 855-F7

WILLOW BROOK LN
- SLOC 93446 471-D6

WILLOWGLEN DR
- StBC 93455 796-H7
- StBC 93455 816-H1

WILLOWGLEN PL
- SBAR 93105 985-E6

WILLOWGLEN RD
- SBAR 93105 985-E7

WILLOWGROVE DR
- GOL 93117 993-J4

WILLOW HILL DR
- StBC 93455 816-J2

WILLOWOOD RD
- StBC 93455 796-B7
- StBC 93455 816-B1

WILLOW SPRINGS LN
- GOL 93117 994-B2

WILLOW WALK WY
- SMRA 93454 776-J6

WILMA WY
- SMRA 93458 796-F4

WILMAR AV
- PBCH 93449 714-B2
- SLOC 93445 714-F7

WILSHIRE LN
- StBC 93455 796-H7

WILSHIRE ST
- SLOC 93420 714-H7

WILSON AV
- SBAR 93103 996-D3

WILSON CT
- ARGD 93420 714-G6
- StBC 93455 816-G5

WILSON DR
- StBC 93455 816-G5

WILSON ST
- SBAR 93101 996-B5
- SLO 93401 654-A3

N WILSON ST
- Npmo 93444 756-C2

S WILSON ST
- Npmo 93444 756-C2

WILTON DR
- Cmbr 93428 528-F7
- Cmbr 93428 548-G1

WILTON PL
- ARGD 93420 714-J5

WINCHESTER CIR
- GOL 93117 993-E2

WINCHESTER DR
- GOL 93117 993-E1

WINCHESTER PL
- GOL 93117 993-E2

WINCHESTER WY
- SMRA 93454 777-B6

WINCHESTER CANYON RD
- GOL 93117 993-E1
- StBC 93117 993-E1

WINDERMERE LN
- SLOC 93420 714-J2

WINDING WY
- StBC 93111 984-J7

WINDING BROOK RD
- PSRS 93446 534-C2

WINDING CREEK LN
- StBC 93108 987-D7
- StBC 93108 997-D1

WINDMILL CT
- SLVG 93463 920-F7

WINDMILL LN
- SLVG 93463 920-F7

WINDMILL PL
- SLOC 93446 534-J4

WINDMILL RD
- SLOC 93446 471-E5

WINDMILL WY
- SLOC 93401 674-D4

WINDRIDGE PL
- SLOC 93420 715-C3

WINDSONG LN
- Npmo 93444 756-B4

WINDSONG WY
- PSRS 93446 513-H4

WINDSOR AV
- GOL 93117 984-C7

WINDSOR BLVD
- Cmbr 93428 528-D6
- Cmbr 93428 548-F2

WINDSOR CT
- StBC 93111 984-F6

WINDSOR ST
- SMRA 93458 796-G3

WINDSOR WY
- StBC 93105 985-H7

WINDWARD AV
- PBCH 93449 693-H7

WINDWARD WY
- SLOC 93446 471-B5

WINDWOOD RD
- SLOC 93446 534-J2

WINDY COVE LN
- SLOC 93422 594-D2

WINE COUNTRY PL
- SLOC 93465 553-B2

WINEGRAPE CT
- SLOC 93465 533-C7

WINEMAN RD
- Npmo 93444 756-J7
- Npmo 93444 776-H1
- SLOC 93454 756-J7
- SLOC 93454 776-H1

WINFIELD PL
- StBC 93436 896-G2

WING WY
- PSRS 93446 494-C7

WINNELL AV
- SLOC 93402 631-H7

WINSTON DR
- SMRA 93458 776-F5

WINTER RD
- StBC 93455 816-H1

WINTERHAVEN WY
- SLOC 93420 734-J7
- SLOC 93420 754-J1

WINTER WHEAT PL
- PSRS 93446 534-C1

WINTHER WY
- StBC 93110 985-D6

WINTHROP CT
- StBC 93111 994-H3

WISTERIA CT
- StBC 93455 817-A3

WISTERIA DR
- SMRA 93455 796-G6

WISTERIA LN
- PSRS 93446 514-A2
- SLO 93401 674-C2
- SLOC 93446 514-A2
- StBC 93437 875-J3

WONG ST
- GDLP 93434 774-J6

WOOD DR
- Cmbr 93428 528-H7
- Cmbr 93428 548-H1

WOOD PL
- ARGD 93420 714-H6

WOODBINE LN
- Npmo 93444 756-C3

WOODBRIDGE CT
- StBC 93455 816-G4

WOODBRIDGE ST
- SLO 93401 653-J6
- SLO 93401 654-A6

WOODDALE LN
- SBAR 93103 986-B7

WOOD DUCK LN
- SLOC 93446 471-C6

WOODGREEN WY
- Npmo 93444 735-D7
- Npmo 93444 755-D1

WOODHAVEN CT
- PSRS 93446 533-J1
- StBC 93437 855-E7
- StBC 93455 816-J2

WOODHAVEN WY
- Npmo 93444 755-E5

WOODLAND CT
- ARGD 93420 714-J7
- SLO 93401 654-B4

WOODLAND DR
- ARGD 93420 714-H6
- SBAR 93108 996-E2
- SLO 93401 654-B4
- SLOC 93402 631-F6

WOODLAND RD
- SLOC 93446 493-E4

WOODLAND ST
- StBC 93455 816-J3

WOODLAND HILLS RD
- SLOC 93420 734-H5

WOODLAWN DR
- SMRA 93458 776-F5

WOODLEAF RD
- GOL 93117 993-J3

WOODLEY CT
- SBAR 93105 985-F7

WOODLEY RD
- StBC 93108 996-G2

WOODMANSEE WY
- SLOC 93451 473-D2

WOODMERE RD
- StBC 93455 816-J4
- StBC 93455 817-A4

WOOD MILL LN
- SMRA 93458 796-G4

WOODSIDE CT
- SMRA 93458 776-F5

WOODSIDE DR
- SLO 93401 654-C6

WOODSIDE LN
- StBC 93455 816-H3

WOODSTOCK RD
- StBC 93441 901-D2
- StBC 93460 901-C5

WOODVIEW AV
- Cmbr 93428 548-G1

WOODY POINT LN
- SLOC 93426 469-J2

WORCESTER DR
- Cmbr 93428 528-E7

WORCHESTER CT
- StBC 93455 817-B4

WRANGLER PL
- SLOC 93446 534-J4

WULLBRANDT WY
- CARP 93013 998-D7

WYANT RD
- StBC 93108 996-J3

WYE RD
- SBAR 93110 995-D1

WYOLA RD
- SBAR 93105 995-G2

WYOMING AV
- SLOC 93451 453-A4
- StBC 93437 855-D7

X

X ST
- LMPC 93436 916-C2

N X ST
- LMPC 93436 896-C6
- LMPC 93436 916-C1

XANDRIAS LN
- SLOC 93420 695-B5

Y

Y PL
- LMPC 93436 916-C2

Y ST
- LMPC 93436 916-C2

N Y ST
- LMPC 93436 896-C6
- LMPC 93436 916-C1

YALE PL
- SMRA 93458 796-G2

YAMA LN
- SLOC 93402 631-J5

YANKEE FARM RD
- SBAR 93109 995-E5

YANONALI ST
- SBAR 93101 996-C4
- SBAR 93103 996-D3

YAPLE AV
- StBC 93111 984-H7

YARROW CT
- SLO 93401 674-C2

YBARRA AV
- SMRA 93458 796-E4

YEDID HILLWAY
- GOL 93117 984-E7

YELLOW FEATHER CIR
- SLOC 93446 471-D6

YELLOW GOLD CIR
- SLOC 93446 471-D7

YERBA AV
- ATAS 93422 573-H1

YERBA BUENA AV
- SLOC 93422 614-F2
- SLOC 93453 614-F2

YERBA BUENA ST
- MOBY 93442 591-E7
- MOBY 93442 611-D1

YESAL AV
- ATAS 93422 574-B4

YOLO AV
- SLOC 93405 633-A5

YOLO LN
- GOL 93117 993-G2

YORK
- Cmbr 93428 528-D6

YORK AV
- SLOC 93445 714-D7

YORK LN
- SMRA 93455 796-H6

YORK PL
- GOL 93117 984-F7

YORKSHIRE CT
- StBC 93455 816-F4

YORKSHIRE ST
- Cmbr 93428 528-G7
- Cmbr 93428 548-G1

YOSHIDA DR
- SMRA 93454 776-J4

YSABEL AV
- PSRS 93446 513-G3

YUBA AV
- SLOC 93405 633-A5

YUBA LN
- GOL 93117 993-G2

YUCCA LN
- CARP 93013 998-D7

YUCCA ST
- StBC 93437 875-H1

Z

Z ST
- LMPC 93436 916-B2

N Z ST
- LMPC 93436 896-B7
- LMPC 93436 916-B1

ZACA LN
- SLO 93401 673-H1

ZACA PL
- SMRA 93458 776-G3

ZACA ST
- BLTN 93427 919-H5

ZACA STATION RD
- StBC 93440 900-C2
- StBC 93441 900-C2

ZACKERY CT
- StBC 93455 816-J4

ZANZIBAR ST
- MOBY 93442 591-E7
- MOBY 93442 611-D1
- SLOC - 591-E7
- SLOC - 611-D1
- SLOC 93442 591-E7

ZANZIBAR TER
- MOBY 93442 611-D1

ZENON WY
- SLOC 93420 735-C5

ZIA LUCIA LN
- Cmbr 93428 528-F7

ZINFANDEL CT
- SLOC 93465 553-A3

ZINK AV
- StBC 93111 994-J2

ZINK PL
- StBC 93111 994-J2

ZINNIA CT
- Npmo 93444 755-J4

ZION PL
- StBC 93455 816-H2

ZIRCON CT
- StBC 93455 817-B5

ZOGATA WY
- ARGD 93420 715-B3

#

1ST CT
- SLVG 93463 940-E2

1ST PL
- SLVG 93463 920-E7
- SLVG 93463 940-E1

N 1ST PL
- LMPC 93436 896-F6
- LMPC 93436 916-F2

1ST ST
- BLTN 93427 919-H5
- LMPC 93436 896-F7
- LMPC 93436 916-F1
- PSRS 93446 513-F7
- SLOC 93402 631-G4
- SLOC 93424 693-A4
- SLOC 93430 590-J2
- SLOC 93430 591-A2
- SLOC 93446 513-F7
- SLOC 93465 553-E1
- SLVG 93463 940-E1
- SMRA 93458 796-C4
- StBC 93455 816-G6

N 1ST ST
- GBCH 93433 714-D4

2ND PL
- SLVG 93463 920-E7

2ND ST
- BLTN 93427 919-F4
- GDLP 93434 774-J6
- GDLP 93434 775-A6
- LMPC 93436 896-F6
- LMPC 93436 916-F1
- PSRS 93446 513-F7
- SLOC 93402 631-G4
- SLOC 93420 734-H7
- SLOC 93424 693-A4
- SLOC 93430 591-A2
- SLOC 93465 553-E2
- SLVG 93463 940-E1

N 2ND ST
- GBCH 93433 714-D4

3RD ST
- CARP 93013 998-C7
- GDLP 93434 774-J6
- GDLP 93434 775-A6
- LMPC 93436 896-F6
- LMPC 93436 916-F1
- PSRS 93446 513-F7
- SLOC 93402 631-G5
- SLOC 93420 754-H1
- SLOC 93465 553-E2
- SLVG 93463 940-D1

N 3RD ST
- GBCH 93433 714-D4
- SLOC 93430 591-A2

S 3RD ST
- GBCH 93433 714-D5
- SLOC 93430 591-A2

4TH PL
- SLVG 93463 920-E7
- SLVG 93463 940-E1

4TH ST
- CARP 93013 998-C7
- GDLP 93434 775-A6
- LMPC 93436 896-F7
- LMPC 93436 916-F1
- PSRS 93446 513-F6
- SLOC 93402 631-G5
- SLOC 93430 591-A2
- SLOC 93446 513-E6
- SLOC 93465 553-E2
- StBC 93437 875-E3

N 4TH ST
- GBCH 93433 714-D4
- PBCH 93449 714-E4

S 4TH ST
- GBCH 93433 714-D5
- GBCH 93445 714-E7
- SLOC 93433 714-D5
- SLOC 93445 714-E7

W 4TH ST
- SLOC 93446 513-E6

5TH ST
- CARP 93013 998-C7
- GDLP 93434 774-J5
- GDLP 93434 775-A5
- LMPC 93436 896-G7
- LMPC 93436 916-G1
- PSRS 93446 513-F6
- SLOC 93402 631-G5
- SLOC 93430 591-A2
- SLOC 93465 553-D2
- SLVG 93463 920-D7
- SLVG 93463 940-D1
- StBC 93434 774-J5
- StBC 93437 875-E3

N 5TH ST
- GBCH 93433 714-D4

S 5TH ST
- GBCH 93433 714-D5

6TH ST
- CARP 93013 998-D7
- CARP 93013 1018-D1
- GDLP 93434 775-A5
- LMPC 93436 896-G6
- LMPC 93436 916-G1
- PSRS 93446 513-F6
- SLOC 93402 631-H5
- SLOC 93430 591-A2
- SLOC 93465 553-D2
- StBC 93437 875-E3

N 6TH ST
- GBCH 93433 714-E4

S 6TH ST
- GBCH 93433 714-E5

7TH ST
- CARP 93013 998-D7
- GDLP 93434 775-A5
- LMPC 93436 896-G6
- LMPC 93436 916-G2
- PSRS 93446 513-F6
- SLOC 93402 631-H5
- SLOC 93430 591-A2
- SLOC 93465 553-D2
- StBC 93437 875-D3

N 7TH ST
- GBCH 93433 714-E4

S 7TH ST
- GBCH 93433 714-E5

8TH ST
- CARP 93013 998-D6
- GDLP 93434 775-A5
- LMPC 93436 896-G7
- LMPC 93436 916-G1
- PSRS 93446 513-F6
- SLOC 93402 631-H5
- SLOC 93430 591-A2
- SLOC 93465 553-D2
- StBC 93437 875-D3

N 8TH ST
- GBCH 93433 714-E5

S 8TH ST
- GBCH 93433 714-E5

9TH ST
- CARP 93013 998-C6
- GDLP 93434 775-A5
- LMPC 93436 896-G7
- LMPC 93436 916-G1
- PSRS 93446 513-F6
- SLOC 93402 631-H6
- SLOC 93430 591-A2
- SLOC 93451 473-F3
- StBC 93434 774-J4
- StBC 93434 775-A5
- StBC 93437 875-D3

N 9TH ST
- GBCH 93433 714-E4

S 9TH ST
- GBCH 93433 714-E5

10TH ST
- GDLP 93434 775-A5
- LMPC 93436 896-G7
- PSRS 93446 513-F6
- SLOC 93402 631-H5
- SLOC 93430 591-A2
- SLOC 93451 473-D2
- StBC 93437 875-D4

N 10TH ST
- GBCH 93433 714-E4

S 10TH ST
- GBCH 93433 714-E5

11TH ST
- GDLP 93434 775-A4
- PSRS 93446 513-F5
- SLOC 93402 631-H6
- SLOC 93430 591-A3
- SLOC 93451 473-F2
- SMRA 93455 816-C1
- StBC 93434 775-B5
- StBC 93437 875-D4
- StBC 93455 816-C1

N 11TH ST
- GBCH 93433 714-E4

S 11TH ST
- GBCH 93433 714-E6

12TH ST
- GDLP 93434 775-A4
- LMPC 93436 916-G1
- PSRS 93446 513-E5
- SLOC 93402 631-H5
- SLOC 93430 591-A3
- SLOC 93451 473-F2
- StBC 93437 875-D4

N 12TH ST
- GBCH 93433 714-F4

S 12TH ST
- GBCH 93433 714-E5

12TH STEX
- PSRS 93446 513-D5
- SLOC 93446 513-D5

13TH ST
- PSRS 93446 513-F5
- SLOC 93402 631-H5
- SLOC 93430 591-B2
- SLOC 93445 714-E7
- SLOC 93451 473-F2
- StBC 93436 895-C3
- StBC 93437 855-A6
- StBC 93437 875-B1
- StBC 93437 895-C3

N 13TH ST
- GBCH 93433 714-F4

S 13TH ST
- GBCH 93433 714-E6

14TH ST
- PSRS 93446 513-F5
- SLOC 93402 631-J5
- SLOC 93430 591-A3
- SLOC 93445 714-E7
- SLOC 93451 473-F2
- StBC 93437 875-D4

N 14TH ST
- GBCH 93433 714-F5

S 14TH ST
- GBCH 93433 714-F6

15TH ST
- PSRS 93446 513-E5
- SLOC 93402 631-J5
- SLOC 93430 591-A3
- SLOC 93445 714-F7
- SLOC 93445 734-F1
- SLOC 93451 473-F2
- StBC 93437 875-D4

16TH ST
- PSRS 93446 513-F5
- SLOC 93402 631-J5
- SLOC 93430 591-A3
- SLOC 93445 714-F7
- SLOC 93451 473-F1
- StBC 93437 875-C4

N 16TH ST
- GBCH 93433 714-F5

S 16TH ST
- GBCH 93433 714-F5

NW 17TH PL
- StBC 93455 816-H3

17TH ST
- PSRS 93446 513-E5
- SLOC 93402 631-J5
- SLOC 93430 591-B3
- SLOC 93445 714-F7
- SLOC 93445 734-F1
- SLOC 93451 473-F1
- StBC 93437 875-C4

18TH ST
- PSRS 93446 513-F4
- SLOC 93402 631-J5
- SLOC 93430 591-B3
- SLOC 93445 714-F7
- SLOC 93451 473-F1
- StBC 93437 875-C4

19TH ST
- PSRS 93446 513-F4
- SLOC 93430 591-B3
- SLOC 93445 714-F7
- SLOC 93445 734-F1
- SLOC 93451 473-F1
- StBC 93437 875-C4

20TH CT
- SLOC 93445 714-F7

20TH ST
- PSRS 93446 513-F4
- SLOC 93430 591-B3
- SLOC 93445 714-F7
- SLOC 93451 473-F1
- StBC 93437 875-C4

21ST CT
- SLOC 93445 714-F7

21ST ST
- PSRS 93446 513-E4
- SLOC 93430 591-B3
- SLOC 93445 714-F7
- SLOC 93445 734-F1
- SLOC 93446 513-E4
- StBC 93437 875-C4

22ND ST
- PSRS 93446 513-F4
- SLOC 93430 591-B3
- SLOC 93445 714-F7
- SLOC 93445 734-F1
- StBC 93437 875-B5

23RD ST
- PSRS 93446 513-F4
- SLOC 93430 591-B3
- SLOC 93445 714-G7
- SLOC 93445 734-G1
- StBC 93437 875-C5

24TH ST
- PSRS 93446 513-F4
- SLOC 93430 591-B3
- SLOC 93445 714-G7
- SLOC 93445 734-G1
- StBC 93437 875-B5

25TH ST
- SLOC 93445 714-G7
- SLOC 93445 734-G1
- StBC 93437 875-B5

26TH ST
- PSRS 93446 513-F3

28TH ST
- PSRS 93446 513-F3
- StBC 93437 875-B5

29TH ST
- StBC 93437 875-B5

30TH ST
- PSRS 93446 513-F3
- StBC 93437 875-B6

31ST ST
- StBC 93437 875-B6

32ND ST
- PSRS 93446 513-F2
- StBC 93437 875-B6

33RD ST
- StBC 93437 875-A6

34TH ST
- PSRS 93446 513-F2
- StBC 93437 875-A6

35TH ST
- StBC 93437 875-A6

36TH ST
- PSRS 93446 513-F2

38TH ST
- PSRS 93446 513-F2

Rt#-G14 NACIMIENTO LAKE DR
- PSRS 93446 513-E3
- SLOC 93446 471-C1
- SLOC 93446 493-A5
- SLOC 93446 513-B1

Rt#-1 CABRILLO HWY
- Cmbr 93428 528-B2
- Cmbr 93428 548-J1
- GBCH 93433 714-C4
- GBCH 93449 714-C4
- GDLP 93434 775-A3
- LMPC 93436 916-H1
- MOBY - 591-C6
- MOBY 93430 591-C6
- MOBY 93442 591-C6
- MOBY 93442 611-E4
- MOBY 93442 612-A6
- Npmo 93444 755-B2
- Npmo 93444 775-A3
- PBCH 93449 714-C4
- SLO 93405 633-F6
- SLO 93405 653-H1
- SLOC - 591-C6
- SLOC - 612-A6
- SLOC 93405 612-A6
- SLOC 93405 632-F1
- SLOC 93405 633-B4
- SLOC 93405 653-H1
- SLOC 93420 734-H1
- SLOC 93420 754-H1
- SLOC 93420 755-A1
- SLOC 93430 590-E1
- SLOC 93430 591-C6
- SLOC 93433 714-C4
- SLOC 93442 591-C6
- SLOC 93442 611-G6
- SLOC 93442 612-A6
- SLOC 93445 714-C4
- SLOC 93445 734-H1
- SLOC 93445 755-B6
- SLOC 93445 775-A3
- SLOC 93452 528-B2
- StBC 93429 816-B4
- StBC 93429 855-G6
- StBC 93434 775-A7
- StBC 93434 795-A2
- StBC 93436 916-H1
- StBC 93437 855-G6
- StBC 93455 795-C5
- StBC 93455 816-B4

Rt#-1 CIENAGA ST
- SLOC 93420 734-H1
- SLOC 93445 734-H1

Rt#-1 DOLLIVER ST
- GBCH 93433 714-C3
- GBCH 93449 714-C3
- PBCH 93449 714-C3

Rt#-1 FRONT ST
- SLOC 93445 714-E7
- SLOC 93445 734-E1

Rt#-1 GUADALUPE RD
- SLOC 93420 755-B2

Rt#-1 GUADALUPE ST
- GDLP 93434 775-A6

Rt#-1 N H ST
- LMPC 93436 896-E5
- LMPC 93436 916-E1
- StBC 93436 896-E5

Rt#-1 LOMPOC CASMALIA RD
- LMPC 93436 896-D1
- StBC 93436 876-A4
- StBC 93436 896-D1
- StBC 93437 855-G7
- StBC 93437 875-G1
- StBC 93437 876-A4

Rt#-1 MESA VIEW DR
- SLOC 93420 734-H5

Rt#-1 E OCEAN AV
- LMPC 93436 916-F1

Rt#-1 PACIFIC BLVD
- GBCH 93433 714-D5
- SLOC 93433 714-D5
- SLOC 93445 714-D5

Rt#-1 SANTA ROSA ST
- SLO 93401 653-H2
- SLO 93405 653-H2
- SLOC 93405 653-H2

Rt#-1 WILLOW RD
- SLOC 93420 754-H1
- SLOC 93420 755-A1

Rt#-41 ATASCADERO RD
- MOBY 93442 611-G3
- SLOC 93442 611-G3
- SLOC 93442 612-A1

Rt#-41 CRESTON EUREKA RD
- ATAS 93422 574-E1
- SLOC 93422 574-E1
- SLOC 93432 574-E1
- SLOC 93465 574-E1

Rt#-41 MERCEDES AV
- ATAS 93422
- ATAS 93422

Rt#-41 MORRO RD
- ATAS 93422
- ATAS 93422
- SLOC -
- SLOC 93422
- SLOC 93422
- SLOC 93422

Rt#-41 SANTA YSABEL AV
- ATAS 93422

Rt#-46 HIGHWAY
- PSRS 93446
- PSRS 93446
- PSRS 93446
- SLOC 93446
- SLOC 93446
- SLOC 93465

Rt#-58 CALF CANYON HWY
- SLOC 93422
- SLOC 93453

Rt#-58 EL CAMINO REAL
- SLOC 93453

Rt#-58 ESTRADA AV
- SLOC 93453

Rt#-58 G ST
- SLOC 93453

Rt#-135 BELL ST
- StBC 93440

Rt#-135 N BROADWAY
- SMRA 93454

Rt#-135 S BROADWAY
- SMRA 93454
- SMRA 93454
- SMRA 93455

Rt#-135 HIGHWAY
- StBC 93440

Rt#-135 ORCUTT EXWY
- SMRA 93455
- SMRA 93455
- StBC 93455
- StBC 93455

Rt#-144 E MASON ST
- SBAR 93103

Rt#-144 N MILPAS ST
- SBAR 93103

Rt#-144 S MILPAS ST
- SBAR 93103

Rt#-144 N SALINAS ST
- SBAR 93103

Rt#-144 SYCAMORE CANYON RD
- SBAR 93108

Rt#-150 CASITAS PASS RD
- StBC 93013
- VeCo -
- VeCo 93001

Rt#-150 HIGHWAY
- CARP 93013
- StBC 93013

Rt#-150 RINCON RD
- StBC 93013

Rt#-154 CALLE REAL
- SBAR 93110
- StBC 93110

Rt#-154 HIGHWAY
- StBC 93440
- StBC 93441
- StBC 93460
- StBC 93460
- StBC 93460
- StBC 93460

Rt#-154 SAN MARCOS PASS RD
- SBAR 93110
- SBAR 93110
- StBC 93105
- StBC 93105
- StBC 93105
- StBC 93110
- StBC 93111

Rt#-166 CUYAMA HWY
- Npmo 93444
- SLOC 93454
- SLOC 93454

Rt#-166 HIGHWAY
- StBC 93254

Rt#-166 IRVINE STOVALL MEM HY
- Npmo 93444
- SLOC 93454
- SLOC 93454

Rt#-166 E MAIN ST
- SMRA 93454
- SMRA 93454

Rt#-166 W MAIN ST
- GDLP 93434
- SMRA 93454
- SMRA 93458
- StBC 93434
- StBC 93458
- StBC 93458

Rt#-192 CASITAS PASS RD
- StBC 93013
- StBC 93013

Rt#-192 CATHEDRAL OAKS RD
- StBC 93110

Rt#-192 FOOTHILL RD
- CARP 93013
- SBAR 93105
- SBAR 93105
- SBAR 93110
- StBC 93013
- StBC 93013
- StBC 93105
- StBC 93105
- StBC 93110

Rt#-192 MISSION RIDGE RD
- SBAR 93103
- SBAR 93103

Rt#-192 MOUNTAIN DR
- SBAR 93103
- SBAR 93105

Rt#-192 STANWOOD DR
- SBAR 93103
- SBAR 93103
- SBAR 93108

Rt#-192 SYCAMORE CANYON RD
- SBAR 93108

STREET Name	City	ZIP	Pg-Grid
2 SYCAMORE ON RD			
	SBAR	93108	**996-F1**
	StBC	93108	**986-D7**
	StBC	93108	**996-F1**
2 TORO ON RD			
	StBC	93013	**997-G3**
	StBC	93108	**997-G3**
2 E VALLEY RD			
	StBC	93108	**996-H2**
	StBC	93108	**997-B1**
7 CLARENCE MEM BL			
	GOL	93111	**994-E3**
	GOL	93117	**994-E3**
	SBAR	93117	**994-E3**
	StBC	93106	**994-E3**
	StBC	93111	**994-E3**
	StBC	93117	**994-E3**
5 CASTILLO ST			
	SBAR	93101	**996-B5**
5 CLIFF DR			
	SBAR	93101	**996-A6**
	SBAR	93109	**995-F6**
	SBAR	93109	**996-A6**
	StBC	93105	**995-F6**
	StBC	93109	**995-F6**
5 LAS AS RD			
	SBAR	93105	**995-F4**
	StBC	93105	**995-F4**
5 W ECITO ST			
	SBAR	93101	**996-B5**
	SBAR	93109	**996-A5**
7 ARROYO DE SLO RD			
	ARGD	93420	**715-A3**
	SLOC	93420	**715-A3**
7 E BRANCH ST			
	ARGD	93420	**715-A5**
7 W BRANCH ST			
	ARGD	93420	**714-J5**
	ARGD	93420	**715-A5**
7 BROAD ST			
	SLO	93401	**654-A6**
	SLO	93401	**674-B1**
	SLOC	93401	**654-A6**
	SLOC	93401	**674-B1**
7 CARPENTER ON RD			
	SLOC	93401	**694-G1**
	SLOC	93420	**694-G3**
	SLOC	93420	**695-A6**
	SLOC	93420	**715-A1**
7 CORBETT ON RD			
	ARGD	93420	**715-A4**
7 EDNA RD			
	SLOC	93401	**674-D4**
	SLOC	93401	**694-F1**
7 E GRAND AV			
	ARGD	93420	**714-J5**
7 HIGUERA ST			
	SLO	93401	**653-H6**
27 MADONNA RD			
	SLO	93401	**653-G6**
	SLO	93405	**653-G6**
27 SOUTH ST			
	SLO	93401	**653-J5**
	SLO	93401	**654-A5**
46 BUELLTON OC RD			
	StBC	93436	**896-H7**
	StBC	93436	**916-H1**
46 HIGHWAY			
	BLTN	-	**919-H5**
	BLTN	-	**920-A6**
	BLTN	93427	**919-F4**
	BLTN	93427	**920-A6**
	StBC	93427	**919-E4**
	StBC	93436	**919-B4**
	StBC	93463	**920-A6**
46 MISSION DR			
	SLVG	93463	**920-F7**
	SLVG	93463	**940-C1**
	StBC	93460	**921-A6**
	StBC	93463	**920-F7**
	StBC	93463	**921-A6**
46 E OCEAN AV			
	LMPC	93436	**916-H1**
	StBC	93436	**916-H1**
01 EL CAMINO			
	ARGD	-	**714-J5**
	ARGD	-	**715-B6**
	ATAS	-	**553-D3**
	BLTN	-	**919-J3**
	CARP	-	**998-A6**
	CARP	-	**1018-F1**
	GBCH	-	**714-F3**
	GOL	-	**993-A1**
	GOL	-	**994-E1**
	MonC	-	**453-B3**
	Npmo	-	**735-H6**
	Npmo	-	**736-A7**
	Npmo	-	**756-D4**
	Npmo	-	**776-H4**
	PBCH	-	**693-E3**
	PBCH	-	**714-F3**
	PSRS	-	**513-F2**
	PSRS	-	**533-F3**
	SBAR	-	**995-D1**
	SBAR	-	**996-E3**
	SLO	-	**653-H5**
	SLO	-	**654-B2**
	SLO	-	**673-F4**
	SLOC	-	**453-B3**
	SLOC	-	**473-E5**
	SLOC	-	**493-F3**
	SLOC	-	**513-F2**
	SLOC	-	**533-F3**
	SLOC	-	**553-D3**
	SLOC	-	**594-C3**
	SLOC	-	**614-C6**
	SLOC	-	**653-H5**
	SLOC	-	**654-B2**
	SLOC	-	**673-F4**
	SLOC	-	**693-E3**
	SLOC	-	**714-A1**
	SLOC	-	**715-B6**
	SLOC	-	**735-E2**
	SLOC	-	**776-H4**
	SMRA	-	**776-H4**
	SMRA	-	**777-A6**
	SMRA	-	**797-A7**
	StBC	-	**797-A7**
	StBC	-	**817-B4**
U.S.-101 EL CAMINO REAL			
	StBC	-	**878-H1**
	StBC	-	**900-C1**
	StBC	-	**919-H7**
	StBC	-	**939-H3**
	StBC	-	**981-A5**
	StBC	-	**982-E6**
	StBC	-	**992-J1**
	StBC	-	**993-A1**
	StBC	-	**994-E1**
	StBC	-	**995-D1**
	StBC	-	**996-E3**
	StBC	-	**997-C3**
	StBC	-	**998-A6**
	StBC	-	**1018-F1**
	Summ	-	**997-C3**
	VeCo	-	**1018-F1**
U.S.-101 FRWY			
	ATAS	-	**553-E5**
	ATAS	-	**573-F1**
	ATAS	-	**574-A4**
	ATAS	-	**594-B1**
	SLOC	-	**553-E5**
	SLOC	-	**594-C3**
U.S.-101 VENTURA FRWY			
	StBC	-	**1018-J3**
	VeCo	-	**1018-J3**

AIRPORTS

FEATURE NAME Address City, ZIP Code	PAGE-GRID
LOMPOC, LMPC	896 - C5
NEW CUYAMA, StBC	806 - B2
OCEANO COUNTY, SLOC	714 - D7
PASO ROBLES MUNICIPAL, PSRS	494 - D6
SAN LUIS OBISPO, SLOC	674 - B2
SANTA BARBARA MUNICIPAL, SBAR	994 - B3
SANTA MARIA, SMRA	796 - E7
SANTA YNEZ VALLEY, StBC	921 - C6

BEACHES, HARBORS & WATER REC

FEATURE NAME Address City, ZIP Code	PAGE-GRID
ARROYO BURRO BEACH COUNTY PK, SBAR	995 - E6
AVILA BEACH, SLOC	693 - A4
BUTTERFLY BEACH, StBC	996 - G4
CARPINTERIA CITY BEACH, CARP	998 - C7
CARPINTERIA ST BCH, CARP	1018 - C1
CAYUCOS ST BCH, SLOC	590 - J2
EAST BEACH, SBAR	996 - E4
EL CAPITAN ST BCH, StBC	981 - H5
GOLETA BEACH COUNTY PK, StBC	994 - E4
ISLA VISTA BEACH, StBC	993 - J5
LAKE NACIMIENTO, SLOC	470 - H3
LEADBETTER BEACH, SBAR	996 - A6
LEFFINGWELL LANDING BEACH, Cmbr	528 - C5
LOOKOUT PK, Summ	997 - D4
MOONSTONE BEACH, Cmbr	528 - D5
MORRO BAY YACHT CLUB, MOBY	611 - F7
MORRO ROCK BEACH, MOBY	611 - D5
MORRO STRAND ST BCH, MOBY	611 - D3
MORRO STRAND ST BCH, SLOC	591 - B4
OCEAN BEACH PK, StBC	894 - G1
PISMO STATE BCH, SLOC	714 - D6
RANCHO GUADALUPE DUNES COUNTY PK, StBC	774 - A5
REFUGIO ST BCH, StBC	981 - D5
RINCON BEACH, StBC	1018 - H3
SAN SIMEON ST BCH, Cmbr	528 - B2
SANTA BARBARA SHORES PK, GOL	993 - F3
SANTA BARBARA YACHT CLUB, SBAR	996 - B6
WEST BEACH, SBAR	996 - B5

BUILDINGS - GOVERNMENTAL

FEATURE NAME Address City, ZIP Code	PAGE-GRID
FOR DOWNTOWN BLDGS SEE PAGE F	-
ARROYO GRANDE CITY HALL 214 E BRANCH ST, ARGD, 93420	715 - A5
ATASCADERO CITY HALL 6907 EL CAMINO REAL, ATAS, 93422	573 - J3
BUELLTON CITY HALL 107 W HWY 246, BLTN, 93427	919 - H5
CALIFORNIA MENS COLONY COLONY DR, SLOC, 93405	633 - F5
CARPINTERIA CITY HALL 5775 CARPINTERIA AV, CARP, 93013	1018 - E1
EL PASO DE ROBLES YOUTH CORR FACILITY 4545 AIRPORT RD, PSRS, 93446	494 - B7
FIRE TRAINING FACILITY 30 S OLIVE ST, SBAR, 93103	996 - C4
GOLETA CITY HALL 130 CREMONA DR, GOL, 93117	994 - A2
GROVER BEACH BRANCH 214 S 16TH ST, GBCH, 93433	714 - F5
GROVER BEACH CITY HALL 154 S 8TH ST, GBCH, 93433	714 - E5
GUADALUPE CITY HALL 918 OBISPO ST, GDLP, 93434	775 - A5
JUVENILE HALL 4500 HOLLISTER AV, StBC, 93110	995 - B1
JUVENILE HALL 812 W FOSTER RD, SMRA, 93455	816 - F3
LOMPOC CITY HALL 100 CIVIC CENTER PZ, LMPC, 93436	916 - F2
LOMPOC COURTHOUSE 115 CIVIC CENTER PZ, LMPC, 93436	916 - F2
LOMPOC FEDERAL CORRECTIONAL COMPLEX 3901 KLEIN BLVD, LMPC, 93436	895 - H2
MORRO BAY CITY HALL 595 HARBOR ST, MOBY, 93442	611 - F6
PASO ROBLES CITY HALL 1000 SPRING ST, PSRS, 93446	513 - F6
PISMO BEACH CITY HALL 760 MATTIE RD, PBCH, 93449	693 - H7
SAN LUIS OBISPO CITY HALL 990 PALM ST, SLO, 93401	653 - J4
SAN LUIS OBISPO COUNTY COURTHOUSE 1050 MONTEREY ST, SLO, 93401	653 - J4
SANTA BARBARA CITY HALL 735 ANACAPA ST, SBAR, 93101	996 - B4
SANTA BARBARA COUNTY ADMIN 105 ANAPAMU ST, SBAR, 93101	996 - A3
SANTA BARBARA COUNTY COURTHOUSE 1110 ANACAPA ST, SBAR, 93101	996 - A3
SANTA BARBARA COUNTY FIRE-HEADQUARTERS 4410 CATHEDRAL OAKS RD, StBC, 93110	985 - C6
SANTA BARBARA COUNTY GOVERNMENT CTR 2125 S CENTERPOINTE PKWY, SMRA, 93455	796 - H4
SANTA BARBARA COUNTY GOVERNMENT-OFFICES 511 LAKESIDE PKWY, SMRA, 93454	796 - J4
SANTA BARBARA COUNTY HONOR FARM 4436 CL REAL, StBC, 93110	985 - B7
SANTA BARBARA COUNTY JAIL 4436 CL REAL, StBC, 93110	985 - B7
SANTA MARIA CITY HALL 110 E COOK ST, SMRA, 93454	796 - H1
SANTA MARIA COURTHOUSE 312 E COOK ST, SMRA, 93454	796 - H1
SOLVANG CITY HALL 1644 OAK ST, SLVG, 93463	940 - E1
SOLVANG COURTHOUSE 1745 MISSION DR, SLVG, 93463	940 - F1
SOUTH ADMINISTRATIVE AREA ARGUELLO BLVD, StBC, 93437	895 - A4
WATERFRONT DEPARTMENT 132 HARBOR WY, SBAR, 93109	996 - B6

CASINOS

FEATURE NAME Address City, ZIP Code	PAGE-GRID
CHUMASH CASINO 3400 MISSION DR, StBC, 93460	921 - B6

CEMETERIES

FEATURE NAME Address City, ZIP Code	PAGE-GRID
ARROYO GRANDE DIST CEM, ARGD	714 - H5
CALVARY CEM, SBAR	985 - E7
CAMBRIA CEM, Cmbr	528 - F5
CARPINTERIA CEM, StBC	998 - A5
CAYUCOS MORRO BAY CEM, SLOC	591 - B3
GOLETA CEM, StBC	995 - A1
GUADALUPE DISTRICT CEM, GDLP	775 - A6
LADY FAMILY SUTCLIFFE CEM, SLO	653 - H6
LOMPOC EVERGREEN CEM, StBC	916 - F3
LOS OSOS VALLEY MEM PK, SLOC	632 - B7
OAK HILL CEM, StBC	920 - H3
OLD MISSION CATHOLIC CEM, SLO	653 - H6
PASO ROBLES DISTRICT CEM, SLOC	513 - E3
PINE MOUNTAIN PARK CEM, ATAS	574 - A2
SANTA BARBARA CEM, StBC	996 - F4
SANTA MARIA CEM, SMRA	796 - J2

COLLEGES & UNIVERSITIES

FEATURE NAME Address City, ZIP Code	PAGE-GRID
ANTIOCH UNIV 801 GARDEN ST, SBAR, 93101	996 - B3
BROOKS INSTITUTE OF PHOTOGRAPHY 801 ALSTON RD, SBAR, 93108	996 - F2
CALIFORNIA POLYTECHNIC STATE UNIV 1 GRAND AV, SLOC, 93405	633 - J7
CUESTA COLLEGE EDUCATION DR, SLOC, 93405	632 - J4
CUESTA COLLEGE - NORTH COUNTY CAMPUS 2800 BUENA VISTA DR, PSRS, 93446	513 - J2
HANCOCK, ALLAN COLLEGE - LMPC CAMPUS 1 HANCOCK DR, LMPC, 93436	896 - D3
HANCOCK, ALLAN COLLEGE - SMRA CAMPUS 800 COLLEGE DR, SMRA, 93454	796 - J3
MUSIC ACADEMY OF THE WEST 1070 FAIRWAY RD, StBC, 93108	996 - G4
SAINT MARYS SEMINARY 1964 LAS CANOAS RD, SBAR, 93105	986 - B5
SANTA BARBARA CITY COLLEGE 721 CLIFF DR, SBAR, 93109	996 - A6
UNIV OF CALIF SANTA BARBARA END OF WARD MEMORIAL BLVD, StBC, 93106	994 - C5
UC SANTA BARBARA WEST CAMPUS EL COLEGIO RD & STORKE RD, StBC, 93117	993 - H5
WESTMONT COLLEGE 955 LA PAZ RD, StBC, 93108	986 - F7

ENTERTAINMENT & SPORTS

FEATURE NAME Address City, ZIP Code	PAGE-GRID
ARLINGTON THEATRE 1317 STATE ST, SBAR, 93101	996 - A3
BEATIE, GEORGE C SKATEPARK 5493 TRAFFIC WY, ATAS, 93422	573 - J2
CLARK CTR FOR THE PERF ARTS 487 FAIR OAKS AV, ARGD, 93420	714 - J6
COHAN, CHRISTOPHER CTR TAHOE RD & GRAND AV, SLOC, 93405	654 - A2
GRANADA THEATER 1216 STATE ST, SBAR, 93101	996 - A3
LA PLAYA STADIUM 721 CLIFF DR, SBAR, 93109	996 - B6
LOBERO THEATER 33 CANON PERDIDO ST, SBAR, 93101	996 - A4
LOS OSOS SKATEPARK 2180 PALISADES AV, SLOC, 93402	631 - H6
MORRO BAY SKATEPARK COLEMAN DR, MOBY, 93442	611 - E5
PASO ROBLES EVENTS CTR 2198 RIVERSIDE AV, PSRS, 93446	513 - G4
PASO ROBLES SKATEPARK 19TH ST & RIVERSIDE AV, PSRS, 93446	513 - G4
PEABODY STADIUM ANAPAMU ST, SBAR, 93103	996 - B2
SAN LUIS OBISPO SKATEPARK SANTA ROSA ST & OAK ST, SLO, 93405	653 - J3
SANTA BARBARA COUNTY BOWL 1122 MILPAS ST, SBAR, 93103	996 - B2
SANTA BARBARA - SKATERS POINT CABRILLO BLVD & GARDEN ST, SBAR, 93101	996 - C5
SANTA MARIA FAIRPARK 937 THORNBURG ST, SMRA, 93458	796 - G2
SANTA MARIA YMCA SKATEPARK 3400 SKYWAY DR, StBC, 93455	816 - G1
SOUTH COUNTY SKATEPARK 1750 RAMONA AV, GBCH, 93433	714 - F5
TEMPLETON SKATEPARK 599 S MAIN ST, SLOC, 93465	553 - E2
WARREN, EARL SHOWGROUNDS 3400 CL REAL, StBC, 93105	995 - F2

GOLF COURSES

FEATURE NAME Address City, ZIP Code	PAGE-GRID
ALISAL GUEST RANCH & GC, SLVG	940 - D4
AVILA BEACH RESORT GC, SLOC	693 - B3
BIRNAM WOOD GC, StBC	997 - C2
BLACKLAKE GOLF RESORT, Npmo	735 - D7
CHALK MOUNTAIN GC, ATAS	574 - B6
CYPRESS RIDGE GC, SLOC	734 - J6
DAIRY CREEK GC, SLOC	632 - J3
GLEN, ANNIE GC, StBC	993 - G7
HIDDEN OAKS CC, StBC	994 - J2
HUNTER RANCH GC, PSRS	514 - E2
LA CUMBRE GOLF & CC, StBC	995 - D2
LAGUNA LAKE GC, SLO	653 - E7
LINKS AT VISTA DEL HOMBRE, THE, PSRS	494 - G5
MONARCH DUNES GC, Npmo	755 - D3
MONTECITO CC, SBAR	996 - F3
MORRO BAY GC, MOBY	611 - G7
OCEAN MEADOWS GC, StBC	993 - H4
PASO ROBLES GC, PSRS	513 - J7
PISMO BEACH GC, GBCH	714 - C4
RANCHO MARIA GC, StBC	816 - B5
RIVER COURSE AT THE ALISAL, StBC	940 - F2
SANDPIPER GC, GOL	993 - E3
SAN LUIS OBISPO CC, SLOC	674 - D6
SANTA BARBARA GC, SBAR	995 - F2
SANTA MARIA CC, SMRA	796 - G6
SEA PINES GC, SLOC	631 - E6
SUNSET RIDGE GC, SMRA	796 - D6
TWIN LAKES GC, SBAR	994 - D1
VALLEY CLUB GC, StBC	997 - D2
VILLAGE CC, THE, StBC	876 - E5
ZACA CREEK GC, BLTN	919 - G6

HISTORIC SITES

FEATURE NAME Address City, ZIP Code	PAGE-GRID
CARILLO ADOBE 11 E CARILLO ST, SBAR, 93101	996 - A3
CASA DE LA GUERRA 15 E DE LA GUERRA ST, SBAR, 93101	996 - A4
CHUMASH PAINTED CAVE ST HIST PARK PAINTED CAVE RD, StBC, 93105	964 - J6
COLD SPRINGS TAVERN 5995 STAGECOACH RD, StBC, 93105	964 - C4
DE LA GUERRA PLAZA DE LA GUERRA ST, SBAR, 93101	996 - A4
EL PRESIDIO DE STB ST HIST PK 123 CANON PERDIDO ST, SBAR, 93101	996 - A3
FERNALD MNSN & TRUSSELL-WINCHESTER-ADBE 414 W MONTECITO ST, SBAR, 93101	996 - A5
HASTINGS ADOBE 412 W MONTECITO ST, SBAR, 93101	996 - B5
LA PURISIMA MISSION STATE HIST PK 2295 PURISIMA RD, StBC, 93436	876 - J7
MISSION LA PURISIMA 2295 PURISIMA RD, StBC, 93436	896 - J4
MISSION SAN LUIS OBISPO DE TOLOSA 751 PALM ST, SLO, 93401	653 - J4
MISSION SAN MIGUEL ARCANGEL 775 MISSION ST, SLOC, 93451	473 - F3
MISSION SANTA BARBARA 2201 LAGUNA ST, SBAR, 93105	99
MISSION SANTA INES 1760 MISSION DR, SLVG, 93463	94
RIOS CALEDONIA ADOBE 700 MISSION ST, SLOC, 93451	47

HOSPITALS

FEATURE NAME Address City, ZIP Code	PAGE
ARROYO GRANDE COMM HOSP 345 S HALCYON RD, ARGD, 93420	71
ATASCADERO STATE HOSP 10333 EL CAMINO REAL, ATAS, 93422	57
FRENCH HOSP MED CTR 1911 JOHNSON AV, SLO, 93401	65
GOLETA VALLEY COTTAGE HOSP 351 S PATTERSON AV, GOL, 93111	99
LOMPOC HEALTHCARE DIST 508 E HICKORY AV, LMPC, 93436	91
MARIAN MED CTR 1400 E CHURCH ST, SMRA, 93454	77
SAN LUIS OBISBO GENERAL HOSP 2180 JOHNSON AV, SLO, 93401	65
SANTA BARBARA COTTAGE HOSP PUEBLO ST & BATH ST, SBAR, 93105	99
SANTA YNEZ VALLEY COTTAGE HOSP 700 ALAMO PINTADO RD, SLVG, 93463	92
SIERRA VISTA REGL MED CTR 1010 MURRAY ST, SLO, 93405	65
TWIN CITIES COMM HOSP 1100 LAS TABLAS RD, SLOC, 93465	55

HOTELS

FEATURE NAME Address City, ZIP Code	PAGE
APPLE FARM INN 2015 MONTEREY ST, SLO, 93401	65
BACARA RESORT 8301 HOLLISTER AV, GOL, 93117	99
BEST WESTERN BIG AMERICA 1725 N BROADWAY, SMRA, 93454	77
BEST WESTERN BLACK OAK MOTOR LODGE 1135 24TH ST, PSRS, 93446	51
BEST WESTERN CARPINTERIA INN 4558 CARPINTERIA AV, CARP, 93013	99
BEST WESTERN COLONY INN 3600 EL CAMINO REAL, ATAS, 93422	57
BEST WESTERN ENCINA LODGE 2220 BATH ST, SBAR, 93105	99
BEST WESTERN FIRESIDE INN 6700 MOONSTONE BEACH DR, Cmbr, 93428	52
BEST WESTERN KING FREDERIK MOTEL 1617 COPENHAGEN DR, SLVG, 93463	94
BEST WESTERN KRONBERG INN 1440 MISSION DR, SLVG, 93463	94
BEST WESTERN OCARINS INN 940 E OCEAN AV, LMPC, 93436	91
BEST WESTERN PEA SOUP ANDERSENS INN 51 E HWY 246, BLTN, 93427	91
BEST WESTERN PEPPER TREE INN 3850 STATE ST, SBAR, 93110	99
BEST WESTERN ROYAL OAK 214 MADONNA RD, SLO, 93405	653
BEST WESTERN SAN MARCOS 250 PACIFIC ST, MOBY, 93442	611
BEST WESTERN SHELTER COVE LODGE 2651 PRICE ST, PBCH, 93449	693
BEST WESTERN SHORE CLIFF LODGE 2555 PRICE ST, PBCH, 93449	714
BEST WESTERN SOMERSET INN 1895 MONTEREY ST, SLO, 93401	654
BEST WESTERN SOUTH COAST INN 5620 CL REAL, GOL, 93117	994
CAMBRIA PINES LODGE 2905 BURTON DR, Cmbr, 93428	52
CLIFFS RESORT 2757 SHELL BEACH RD, PBCH, 93449	693
DAYS INN 114 E HWY 246, BLTN, 93427	919
EMBASSY SUITES HOTEL 1117 N H ST, LMPC, 93436	896
EMBASSY SUITES HOTEL 333 MADONNA RD, SLO, 93405	653
FESS PARKERS DOUBLETREE RESORT STB 633 E CABRILLO BLVD, SBAR, 93103	996
FOUR SEASONS BILTMORE HOTEL 1260 CHANNEL DR, StBC, 93108	996
HOLIDAY INN 2100 N BROADWAY, SMRA, 93454	776
HOLIDAY INN EXPRESS 1800 MONTEREY ST, SLO, 93401	654
HOLIDAY INN SANTA BARBARA/GOLETA 5650 CL REAL, GOL, 93117	994
HOTEL MARMONTE 1111 E CABRILLO BLVD, SBAR, 93103	996
INN AT MORRO BAY 60 STATE PARK RD, MOBY, 93442	631
KON TIKI INN 1621 PRICE ST, PBCH, 93449	714
MADONNA INN 100 MADONNA RD, SLO, 93405	653
MONTECITO INN 1295 COAST VILLAGE RD, SBAR, 93108	996
MOONSTONE INN MOTEL 5860 MOONSTONE BEACH DR, Cmbr, 93428	528
OLIVE TREE RAMADA INN 1000 OLIVE ST, SLO, 93405	653
OXFORD SUITES RESORT 651 FIVE CITIES DR, PBCH, 93449	714
PACIFICA SUITES 5490 HOLLISTER AV, GOL, 93111	994
PETERSEN VILLAGE INN 1576 MISSION DR, SLVG, 93463	940
QUALITY INN & EXECUTIVE SUITES 1621 N H ST, LMPC, 93436	896
QUALITY SUITES 1631 MONTEREY ST, SLO, 93401	654
RADISSON HOTEL AT SANTA MARIA 3455 SKYWAY DR, SMRA, 93455	816
RAMADA LIMITED 4770 CALLE REAL, StBC, 93110	984
ROYAL SCANDINAVIAN INN 400 ALISAL RD, SLVG, 93463	940
SANTA INEZ MARRIOTT 555 MCMURRAY RD, BLTN, 93427	919
SANTA MARIA INN 801 S BROADWAY, SMRA, 93458	796
SEA CREST RESORT 2241 PRICE ST, PBCH, 93449	714
SEA PINES GOLF RESORT 1945 SOLANO ST, SLOC, 93402	631
SYCAMORE MINERAL SPRINGS RESORT 1215 AVILA BEACH DR, SLOC, 93424	693
UPHAM HOTEL 1404 DE LA VINA ST, SBAR, 93101	995

LAW ENFORCEMENT

FEATURE NAME Address City, ZIP Code	PAGE
ARROYO GRANDE POLICE DEPT 200 N HALCYON RD, ARGD, 93420	714

RE NAME ss City, ZIP Code	PAGE-GRID
ADERO POLICE STA EL CAMINO REAL, ATAS, 93422	573 - H3
TON POLICE DEPT / HWY 246 HWY, BLTN, 93427	919 - H5
RNIA HIGHWAY PATROL OTTI DR & NOBLE WY, SMRA, 93454	776 - J5
RNIA HIGHWAY PATROL AL, GOL, 93117	994 - B1
RNIA HIGHWAY PATROL AN RD, SLOC, 93465	553 - D1
RNIA HIGHWAY PATROL STRIAL WY, BLTN, 93427	919 - G5
RNIA HIGHWAY PATROL ORNIA BLVD, SLO, 93401	654 - A3
R CITY POLICE STA OCKAWAY AV, GBCH, 93433	714 - E5
ALUPE POLICE DEPT 10TH ST, GDLP, 93434	775 - A5
OC POLICE STA IVIC CENTER PZ, LMPC, 93436	916 - E2
O BAY POLICE STA IORRO BAY BLVD, MOBY, 93442	611 - G6
ROBLES POLICE STA ARK ST, PSRS, 93446	513 - G6
BEACH POLICE STA BELLO ST, PBCH, 93449	714 - C2
IS OBISPO COUNTY SHRIFF DEPT FRONT ST, SLOC, 93445	714 - E7
IS OBISPO POLICE DEPT WALNUT ST, SLO, 93401	653 - J3
BARBARA POLICE STA FIGUEROA ST, SBAR, 93101	996 - A3
MARIA POLICE STA COOK ST, SMRA, 93454	796 - H1
HERIFF DEPT MAIN STA KANSAS AV, SLOC, 93405	633 - B5
HERIFF DEPT NORTH STA MAIN ST, SLOC, 93465	533 - E7
HERIFF DEPT CARPINTERIA STA CARPINTERIA AV, CARP, 93013	1018 - E1
HERIFF DEPT COAST STA 0TH ST, SLOC, 93402	631 - H6
HERIFF DEPT ISLA VISTA STA PARDALL RD, StBC, 93117	994 - B5
HERIFF DEPT LOMPOC STA URTON MESA BLVD, StBC, 93436	896 - F1
HERIFF DEPT NEW CUYAMA STA IEWSOME ST, StBC, 93254	806 - C1
HERIFF DEPT SANTA MARIA STA / FOSTER RD, SMRA, 93455	816 - F3
HERIFF DEPT SOLVANG STA MISSION DR, SLVG, 93463	940 - F1
HERIFF MAIN STATION CL REAL, StBC, 93110	995 - B1

LIBRARIES

YO GRANDE / BRANCH ST, ARGD, 93420	714 - H5
ADERO MORRO RD, ATAS, 93422	573 - J4
TON / HWY 246, BLTN, 93427	919 - H5
RIA MAIN ST, Cmbr, 93428	528 - F6
NTERIA CARPINTERIA AV, CARP, 93013	998 - D7
OS OCEAN AV, SLOC, 93430	591 - A2
MA 166 & NEWSOME ST, StBC, 93254	806 - C1
DE MONTECITO ST, SBAR, 93103	996 - D3
A VALLEY FAIRVIEW AV, GOL, 93117	984 - D7
ER BEACH ST & RAMONA AV, GBCH, 93433	714 - E5
ALUPE BRANCH W MAIN ST, GDLP, 93434	774 - J6
OC NORTH AV, LMPC, 93436	896 - F6
LIVOS BRANCH ALAMO PINTADO AV, StBC, 93441	900 - H5
SOS PALISADES AV, SLOC, 93402	631 - G6
 LIFF DR, SBAR, 93109	996 - A6
ECITO E VALLEY RD, StBC, 93108	996 - J1
O BAY HARBOR ST, MOBY, 93442	611 - G6
MO / TEFFT ST, Npmo, 93444	756 - A4
NO 17TH ST, SLOC, 93445	714 - F7
TT E CLARK AV, StBC, 93455	817 - A5
ROBLES SPRING ST, PSRS, 93446	513 - F5
UIS OBISPO PALM ST, SLO, 93401	653 - J4
IIGUEL 3TH ST, SLOC, 93451	473 - F2
BARBARA CENTRAL NAPAMU ST, SBAR, 93101	996 - A3
MARGARITA MURPHY AV, SLOC, 93453	614 - F3
MARIA GUADALUPE ST, GDLP, 93434	775 - A5
MARIA BROADWAY, SMRA, 93454	796 - H1
YNEZ BRANCH SAGUNTO ST, StBC, 93460	921 - C5
BEACH EEWARD AV, PBCH, 93449	693 - H7
ANG MISSION DR, SLVG, 93463	940 - F1
ENBERG VILLAGE CONSTELLATION RD, StBC, 93436	876 - D7

MILITARY INSTALLATIONS

ROBERTS MILITARY RESV C, 93451	453 - B1
SAN LUIS OBISPO MILITARY RESV RILLO HWY, SLOC, 93405	612 - J7
ENBERG AIR FORCE BASE 1, StBC, 93429	855 - D3
ENBERG AIR FORCE BASE AIRFIELD IELD RD, StBC, 93437	875 - B3

MUSEUMS

RSEN, HANS CHRISTIAN MUS MISSION DR, SLVG, 93463	940 - E1
RAL COAST VETERANS MEM MUS GRAND AV, SLO, 93401	654 - A3
EMPORARY ARTS FORUM PASEO NUEVO, SBAR, 93101	996 - A4

FEATURE NAME Address City, ZIP Code	PAGE-GRID
EXPLORATION STA 867 RAMONA AV, GBCH, 93433	714 - E5
KARPELES MANUSCRIPT MUS 21 W ANAPAMU ST, SBAR, 93101	996 - A3
LOMPOC MUS 200 S H ST, LMPC, 93436	916 - E2
MUS OF NATURAL HIST 20 STATE PARK RD, MOBY, 93442	631 - G2
PRICE HOUSE MUS FRADY LN & BELLO ST, PBCH, 93449	714 - D2
SAN LUIS OBISPO ART CTR 1010 BROAD ST, SLO, 93401	653 - J4
SAN LUIS OBISPO CHILDRENS MUS 1010 NIPOMO ST, SLO, 93401	653 - J4
SAN LUIS OBISPO CO HIST MUS 696 MONTEREY ST, SLO, 93401	653 - J4
SANTA BARBARA HIST SOCIETY MUS 136 E DE LA GUERRA ST, SBAR, 93101	996 - B4
SANTA BARBARA MARITIME MUS 113 HARBOR WY, SBAR, 93109	996 - B6
SANTA BARBARA MUS OF ART 1130 STATE ST, SBAR, 93101	996 - A3
SANTA BARBARA MUS OF NATURAL HIST 2559 PUESTA DEL SOL RD, SBAR, 93105	995 - J1
SANTA MARIA MUS OF FLIGHT 3015 AIR PARK DR, SMRA, 93455	796 - E7
SANTA MARIA NATURAL HIST MUS 412 S MCCLELLAND ST, SMRA, 93454	796 - H1
SEA CTR MARINE MUS 211 STEARNS WHARF, SBAR, 93101	996 - C5
SOUTH COAST RAILROAD MUS 300 LOS CARNEROS RD, GOL, 93117	994 - B1
STOW HOUSE 304 LOS CARNEROS RD, GOL, 93117	994 - B1

OPEN SPACE

ANDRE CLARK BIRD REFUGE, SBAR	996 - F4
BELLA VISTA OPEN SPACE, GOL	993 - G1
BISHOP PEAK NATURAL RESERVE, SLO	633 - F7
CAMINO CORTO OPEN SPACE, StBC	993 - J4
CARPINTERIA BLUFFS PUB OPEN SPACE, CARP	1018 - F1
CARPINTERIA SALT MARSH RESERVE, StBC	998 - B6
CERRO SAN LUIS NATURAL RESERVE, SLO	653 - H4
CLOISTERS OPEN SPACE, THE, MOBY	611 - E3
DOUGLAS FAMILY PRESERVE, SBAR	995 - E6
DUNE RESTORATION AREA, MOBY	611 - E3
ELFIN FOREST ECOLOGICAL PRESERVE, SLOC	631 - H3
EMERALD TERRACE OPEN SPACE, GOL	984 - E7
EVERGREEN OPEN SPACE, GOL	993 - F1
IRISH HILLS NATURAL RESERVE, SLO	653 - C7
ISLAY HILL OPEN SPACE, SLO	674 - E2
KELLOGG OPEN SPACE, StBC	984 - F6
LET IT BE NATURE PRESERVE, SLO	653 - E5
LOS OSOS OAKS STATE RESERVE, SLOC	631 - J7
MONARCH GROVE NATURAL AREA, SLOC	631 - E7
MORRO ROCK NATURAL PRESERVE, MOBY	611 - D5
NORTH POINT NATURAL AREA, MOBY	591 - D7
RESERVOIR CANYON NATURAL RESERVE, SLOC	654 - C3
SAN LUIS CREEK OPEN SPACE, SLO	653 - H5
SAN MIGUEL OPEN SPACE, GOL	993 - E1
SOUTH HILLS OPEN SPACE, SLO	653 - J6
STONEBROOK OPEN SPACE, StBC	816 - G4
STOW CANYON OPEN SPACE, GOL	984 - C7
SUMMERLAND GREENWELL PRESERVE, Summ	997 - E3
SWEET SPRINGS NATURE RESERVE, SLOC	631 - G5
TERRACE HILL OPEN SPACE, SLO	654 - A5
UNIV CIRCLE OPEN SPACE, StBC	984 - F7
WINCHESTER OPEN SPACE, GOL	993 - F2

OTHER

BOY SCOUT COUNTY HEADQUARTERS 4000 MODOC RD, StBC, 93110	995 - D2
BRAILLE INSTITUTE 2031 DE LA VINA ST, SBAR, 93105	995 - H2
LA CASA DE MARIA CTR 801 LADERA LN, StBC, 93108	997 - F1
MORETON BAY FIG TREE CHAPALA ST & MONTECITO ST, SBAR, 93101	996 - B5
MOUNT CALVARY MONASTERY 2501 MT GIBRALTER RD, StBC, 93105	986 - C5
PADDOCK, CHARLES ZOO 9305 PISMO AV, ATAS, 93422	573 - H6
SANTA BARBARA BOTANIC GARDENS 1212 MISSION CANYON RD, StBC, 93105	985 - J6
SANTA BARBARA POLO FIELD 3375 FOOTHILL RD, StBC, 93013	997 - H4
SANTA BARBARA ZOOLOGICAL GARDENS 500 NINOS DR, SBAR, 93103	996 - E4

PARK & RIDE

ARROYO GRANDE 101, ARGD	714 - H5
ATASCADERO 101, ATAS	574 - A5
ATASCADERO 101, ATAS	594 - C3
ATASCADERO 101, ATAS	573 - J4
BOB JONES TRAIL, SLOC	693 - E3
BUELLTON, BLTN	919 - H6
HWY 58/101 LOT, SLOC	614 - D4
OCEANO LOT, SLOC	714 - E7
ORCUTT 101, StBC	817 - C6
ORCUTT 135, StBC	816 - H5
ORCUTT 135, StBC	816 - H6
PARK & RIDE, LMPC	916 - G2
PARK & RIDE, SLOC	553 - C1
PARK & RIDE, SLOC	553 - D1
PARK & RIDE, PSRS	513 - G7
PARK & RIDE, SLOC	631 - J4
PASO ROBLES, PSRS	513 - G6
PISMO BEACH, PBCH	714 - D3
SAINT WILLIAMS CHURCH, ATAS	573 - J3
SANTA ROSA LOT, ATAS	574 - B7
SANTA YNEZ 154, StBC	921 - E6
WALMART, ARGD	714 - H4

PARKS & RECREATION

16TH STREET PK, GBCH	714 - F6
ADAM, KEN PK, LMPC	896 - E3
ADAM PK, SMRA	796 - G3
ADAMS, SPENCER PK, SBAR	995 - J3
ALAMEDA PK, SBAR	996 - A3
ALISAL COMMONS PK, SLVG	940 - E1
AMBASSADOR PK, SBAR	996 - B5
ANDERSEN, HANS CHRISTIAN PK, SLVG	920 - D7
ANDREW, PAUL PK, SLOC	591 - A2
ANHOLM PK, SLO	653 - J3
APPLE VALLEY PK, ATAS	553 - E7
ARMSTRONG PK, SMRA	776 - J7
ATASCADERO LAKE PK, ATAS	573 - J6
ATKINSON PK, SMRA	776 - G6
AVILA BEACH COMM PK, SLOC	693 - A4
BARTON PK, LMPC	896 - D6
BAYSHORE BLUFFS PK, MOBY	611 - F7
BEATTIE PK, LMPC	916 - G3
BERRY GARDENS PK, ARGD	714 - G5
BIDDLE REGL PK, SLOC	695 - H4
BOHNETT PK, SBAR	995 - J4

FEATURE NAME Address City, ZIP Code	PAGE-GRID
BOOSINGER PK, PBCH	714 - C1
BUELLTON PK, BLTN	919 - H4
BUENA VISTA PK, SMRA	796 - G1
BUENA VISTA PK, SLO	654 - B2
CABRILLO BALL PK, SBAR	996 - D4
CAMINO PASCADERO PK, StBC	994 - A5
CENTENNIAL PK, PSRS	513 - J6
CHASE PALM PK, SBAR	996 - C5
CHENG PK, SLO	654 - A4
CHILDRENS PK, StBC	994 - A5
CHUMASH PK, PBCH	714 - E3
CITY PK, PSRS	513 - F5
CLOISTERS COMM PK, MOBY	611 - E3
COASTAL DUNES RV PK, SLOC	714 - D6
COLEMAN PK, MOBY	611 - E5
COLLEGE PK REC AREA, LMPC	896 - E7
COLONY PK, ATAS	573 - J2
COSTA BELLA PK, GBCH	714 - F6
CREEKSIDE PLACE PK, SLVG	920 - G7
CUESTA COUNTY PK, SLOC	654 - B2
DAMON GARCIA SPORTS FIELDS, SLO	674 - B1
DE ANZA PK, ATAS	553 - F5
DEL MAR PK, MOBY	611 - E2
DINOSAUR CAVES PK, PBCH	693 - J7
DON ROBERTS FIELD, ARGD	714 - F6
DOWER WAYSIDE PK, ARGD	715 - A5
DUNES STREET PK, MOBY	611 - F6
EAST SIDE NEIGHBORHOOD PK, SBAR	996 - D3
EL CARRO PK, CARP	998 - E6
EL CHORRO REGL PK, SLOC	633 - B3
ELDWAYEN OCEAN PK, PBCH	693 - G7
ELINGS PK, StBC	995 - F5
ELLSFORD PK, SLO	654 - A3
ELM STREET PK, ARGD	714 - G6
EMERSON PK, SLO	653 - J5
ESCONDIDO PK, SBAR	995 - G5
ESTERO PK, StBC	993 - J5
EVERS SPORTS PK, SLOC	553 - E1
FERINI PK, StBC	878 - G1
FLETCHER PK, SMRA	796 - J5
FRANCESCHI PK, SBAR	996 - B1
FRANKLIN PK, CARP	998 - D6
FRENCH PK, SLO	674 - C2
GAFFNEY PK, StBC	993 - J5
GIRSH PK, GOL	993 - H3
GOLDEN WEST PK, GBCH	714 - F7
GOULD PK (UNDEVELOPED), StBC	986 - G4
GREEK PK, StBC	994 - B5
GROGAN PK, SMRA	776 - F4
GROVER HEIGHTS PK, GBCH	714 - E4
HAGERMAN COMPLEX, SMRA	796 - G7
HALE PK (UNDEVELOPED), SBAR	996 - F2
HARDIE PK, SLOC	590 - J1
HARRINGTON, MARY PK, PBCH	714 - C3
HART-COLLETT VFM PK, ARGD	715 - A5
HEATH RANCH PARK & ADOBE, CARP	998 - D5
HEILMAN GROVE, ATAS	574 - C4
HEILMANN REGL PK, ATAS	574 - B5
HERO COMM PK, GBCH	714 - F6
HIDDEN VALLEY PK, SBAR	995 - E3
HIGHLAND PK, PBCH	714 - D3
HONDA VALLEY PK (UNDEVELOPED), SBAR	995 - H5
HOOSGOW PK, ARGD	715 - A4
JERMIN,TOM JR COMM PK, SLOC	553 - B1
ISLAY HILL PK, SLO	674 - D1
JOHNS-MANVILLE PK, LMPC	916 - F1
JOHNSON PK, SLO	654 - B6
KECK, ALICE PK MEM GARDEN, SBAR	995 - J2
KEISER PK, MOBY	611 - E4
KIWANIS PK, ARGD	715 - A5
LA CORONILLA PK (UNDEVELOPED), SBAR	995 - H6
LAGUNA HILLS PK, SLO	653 - E6
LAGUNA LAKE PARK & NATURAL RESERVE, SLO	653 - F5
LAKE CACHUMA REC AREA, StBC	922 - H7
LA MESA PK, SBAR	995 - H7
LAMPTON CLIFFS COUNTY PK, Cmbr	548 - F3
LAS PRADERAS PK, SLO	673 - G2
LAUREL CANYON PK (UNDEVELOPED), SBAR	985 - G6
LEASE, IRA PK, PBCH	714 - C3
LENCO PK, PSRS	513 - H7
LEROY PK, GDLP	775 - A4
LIONS PK, StBC	998 - G6
LITTLE ACORN PK, StBC	994 - A5
LOPEZ LAKE REC AREA, SLOC	695 - H1
LOS ALAMOS PK, StBC	878 - G2
LOS CARNEROS PK, GOL	984 - B7
LOS OSOS COMM PK, SLOC	631 - H6
LOS PADRES NATL FOREST, SLOC	572 - C6
LOS ROBLES PK, SBAR	985 - D7
MACKENZIE PK, SBAR	995 - F1
MANNING PK, StBC	996 - J2
MARAMONTE PK (NORTH), SMRA	796 - H6
MARAMONTE PK (SOUTH), SMRA	796 - H7
MARTIN, PRIOLO PK, SLO	653 - E6
MEADOW PK, SLO	653 - J6
MELODY PK, PSRS	513 - J7
MEM PK, SMRA	776 - G7
MEM PK, CARP	998 - C6
MEMORY PK, PBCH	693 - F7
MENTONE BASIN PK, GBCH	714 - F6
MIGUELITO COUNTY PK, StBC	916 - D7
MINAMI PK, SMRA	796 - G3
MISSION PK, SBAR	995 - J1
MITCHELL PK, SLO	654 - A4
MONTANA DE ORO STATE PK, SLOC	631 - D4
MONTE VISTA PK, CARP	1018 - G1
MONTE VISTA PK, StBC	998 - G7
MOORE, LAWRENCE PK, PSRS	513 - G7
MORRO BAY PK, MOBY	611 - G6
MORRO BAY STATE PK, MOBY	611 - H7
MORRO BAY STATE PK, SLOC	631 - H2
MURPHY, DWIGHT FIELD, SBAR	996 - E4
NIPOMO COMM PK, Npmo	755 - J3
NORTH PREISKER RANCH PK, SMRA	776 - F3
OAK CREEK PK, PSRS	534 - A1
OAKLEY PK, SMRA	776 - F6
OAK PK, SBAR	995 - G2
OCEANO COUNTY PK, SLOC	714 - D7
OCEANO DUNES STATE VEHICLE REC AREA, - SLOC	734 - D4
OCEANO MEM PK, SLOC	714 - D7
OCEAN VIEW PK, Summ	997 - E4
OCONNELL, JACK PK, GDLP	774 - H6
ORPET PK, SBAR	996 - A1
ORTEGA PK, SBAR	996 - B3
PALISADES BLUFF WALKWAY, PBCH	693 - E5
PALISADES PK, PBCH	693 - E5
PALOMA CREEK PK, ATAS	594 - D1
PARADISE PK, StBC	964 - F1
PARMA PK (UNDEVELOPED), SBAR	986 - D7
PARQUE DE LOS NINOS, SBAR	996 - A5
PELICAN PK, StBC	994 - B5
PERLMAN PK, SMRA	776 - H7
PERSHING PK, SBAR	996 - B5
PILGRIM TERRACE PK, SBAR	995 - G3
PIONEER PK, LMPC	896 - G7
PIONEER PK, SMRA	816 - F3
PIONEER PK, PSRS	513 - G4
PISMO BEACH SPORTS COMPLEX, PBCH	714 - C2

FEATURE NAME Address City, ZIP Code	PAGE-GRID
PLAZA DEL MAR PK, SBAR	996 - B5
PLAZA VERA CRUZ, SBAR	996 - B4
PREISKER PK, SMRA	776 - G3
PRICE REGL PK, PBCH	714 - D2
RAMONA GARDEN PK, GBCH	714 - E5
RANCHO GRANDE PK, ARGD	714 - J3
RATTLESNAKE CANYON PK, StBC	986 - C4
RAY, HILDA PK, SBAR	995 - H5
RICE PK, SMRA	776 - J6
RICHARDSON COUNTY PK, StBC	806 - C2
RINCON BEACH PK, StBC	1018 - H2
RIVERBEND PK, StBC	896 - F5
RIVER OAKS PK, SMRA	776 - J4
RIVER PK, StBC	896 - G7
RIVER VIEW PK, BLTN	919 - F5
ROBINS FIELD, PSRS	513 - F6
ROCKY NOOK PK, StBC	985 - J7
RODENBERGER PK, SMRA	796 - H6
ROTARY CENTENNIAL PK, SMRA	796 - J6
ROYAL OAK MEADOWS PK, PSRS	534 - C1
RUSSELL PK, SMRA	776 - F7
RYON PK, LMPC	916 - D2
SALT MARSH NATURE PK, CARP	998 - C7
SAN MIGUEL PK, SLOC	473 - F2
SAN ROQUE PK, SBAR	985 - F7
SAN SIMEON STATE BCH, Cmbr	528 - C2
SANTA MARGARITA COMM PK, SLOC	614 - G2
SANTA ROSA PK, SLO	653 - J3
SANTA YNEZ PK, StBC	921 - B5
SCHWARTZ, BARNEY SPORTS PK, PSRS	514 - B4
SEA LOCKOUT PK, StBC	993 - J5
SHAMEL PK, Cmbr	528 - D6
SHERWOOD PK, PSRS	534 - A1
SHORELINE PK, SBAR	995 - J7
SIERRA VISTA PK, SMRA	777 - B6
SIMAS BASIN PK, SMRA	796 - H1
SINSHEIMER PK, SLO	654 - B6
SKATERS POINT, SBAR	996 - C5
SKOFIELD PK, SBAR	986 - B6
SMITH PK, SLO	653 - F7
SOLVANG PK, SLVG	940 - E1
SOTO SPORTS COMPLEX, ARGD	714 - G6
SPYGLASS PK, PBCH	693 - F7
STADIUM PK, ATAS	574 - A3
STANLEY, MARILYN PK, SMRA	796 - G6
STEVENS PK, SBAR	985 - F6
STONE RIDGE PK, SLO	654 - A7
STOW GROVE PK, GOL	984 - C7
STROTHER PK, ARGD	715 - C4
SUENO PK, StBC	994 - A5
SUNFLOWER PK, SBAR	996 - D3
SUNKEN GARDENS, ATAS	573 - J3
SUNNY FIELDS PK, SLVG	920 - G6
TAR PITS PK, CARP	1018 - E1
TEMPLETON COUNTY PK, SLOC	553 - D2
TERRA DE ORO PK, ARGD	715 - B3
THOMPSON PK, LMPC	896 - C7
THORNBURY PK (UNDEVELOPED), SBAR	995 - J5
THROOP PK, SLO	653 - H2
TIDELANDS PK, MOBY	611 - F7
TIGER TAIL PK, ARGD	714 - J7
TORO CANYON PK, StBC	997 - J2
TREFTS, ALICE PK, SMRA	796 - J2
TRIANGLE PK, SLO	654 - A4
TRIGO PASADO PK, StBC	994 - A5
TUCKERS GROVE PK, StBC	984 - J6
TUNNELL PK, SMRA	777 - A6
TURTLE CREEK PK, PSRS	514 - B7
VILLAGE GREEN PK, ARGD	715 - A5
VISTA DEL LAGO PK, SLO	653 - F6
WALLER PK, StBC	796 - G7
WESTGATE PK, SMRA	796 - E4
WESTVALE PK, LMPC	916 - C2
WHITE, JOE PK, SMRA	797 - A1
WILLOWGLEN PK, SBAR	985 - E7
WINDOW TO THE SEA PK, StBC	994 - A5
WOODLAND PK, ARGD	714 - H7
YOUNG, MONTE PK, MOBY	611 - F7

POST OFFICES

FEATURE NAME Address City, ZIP Code	PAGE-GRID
ARROYO GRANDE 250 TRAFFIC WY, ARGD, 93420	715 - A5
ATASCADERO 9800 EL CAMINO REAL, ATAS, 93422	573 - J3
ATASCADERO EL CAMINO REAL, ATAS, 93422	574 - B7
AVILA BEACH 191 SAN MIGUEL ST, SLOC, 93424	693 - A4
BUELLTON 140 W HWY 246, BLTN, 93427	919 - H5
CAMBRIA 4100 BRIDGE ST, Cmbr, 93428	528 - G7
CARPINTERIA 5425 CARPINTERIA AV, CARP, 93013	998 - D7
CAYUCOS 97 ASH AV, SLOC, 93430	590 - J1
ELLWOOD 7127 HOLLISTER AV, GOL, 93117	993 - H3
GOLETA 130 PATTERSON AV, GOL, 93111	994 - G2
GROVER BEACH 917 W GRAND AV, GBCH, 93433	714 - E5
GUADALUPE 1030 GUADALUPE ST, GDLP, 93434	775 - A4
HALCYON 936 S HALCYON RD, SLOC, 93420	714 - H7
LOMPOC 801 W OCEAN AV, LMPC, 93436	916 - D1
LOS ALAMOS 497 BELL ST, StBC, 93440	878 - G1
LOS OLIVOS 2880 GRAND AV, StBC, 93441	900 - H5
LOS OSOS 1189 LOS OSOS VALLEY RD, SLOC, 93402	631 - H7
MILPAS 18 S MILPAS ST, SBAR, 93103	996 - D4
MISSION SAN LUIS OBISPO 893 MARSH ST, SLO, 93401	653 - J4
MONTECITO 1470 E VALLEY RD, StBC, 93108	996 - J1
MORRO BAY 898 NAPA AV, MOBY, 93442	611 - F6
NEW CUYAMA 4855 PRIMERO ST, StBC, 93254	806 - C1
NIPOMO 630 W TEFFT ST, Npmo, 93444	756 - B3
OCEANO 1800 BEACH ST, SLOC, 93445	734 - F1
ORCUTT 155 S 1ST ST, StBC, 93455	816 - G6
PASO ROBLES 800 6TH ST, PSRS, 93446	513 - G6
PISMO BEACH 100 CREST DR, PBCH, 93449	714 - G3
SAN MIGUEL 1185 MISSION ST, SLOC, 93451	473 - F2
SAN LUIS OBISPO 1655 DALIDIO DR, SLO, 93405	653 - G7
SAN ROQUE 3345 STATE ST, SBAR, 93105	995 - F1
SANTA BARBARA 836 ANACAPA ST, SBAR, 93101	996 - A4
SANTA MARGARITA 22360 EL CAMINO REAL, SLOC, 93453	614 - F3
SANTA MARIA 201 E BATTLES RD, SMRA, 93454	796 - H3
SANTA YNEZ 3564 SAGUNTO ST, StBC, 93460	921 - C5
SHELL BEACH 1301 SHELL BEACH RD, PBCH, 93449	693 - H7
SOLVANG 430 ALISAL RD, SLVG, 93463	940 - E1
SUMMERLAND 2245 LILLIE AV, Summ, 93067	997 - D3
TEMPLETON 101 N MAIN ST, SLOC, 93465	553 - E1
VANDENBERG AFB 100 COMMUNITY LP, StBC, 93437	875 - E2

SCHOOLS

FEATURE NAME Address City, ZIP Code	PAGE-GRID
ADAM ELEM 500 WINDSOR ST, SMRA, 93458	796 - G3
ADAMS ELEM 2701 LAS POSITAS RD, SBAR, 93105	995 - F2
ADVANCED CHRISTIAN TRAINING HIGH 3025 ADELAIDA RD, SLOC, 93446	513 - A2
ADVANCED CHRISTIAN TRAINING ELEM 3025 ADELAIDA RD, SLOC, 93446	513 - A2
ALISO ELEM 4545 CARPINTERIA AV, CARP, 93013	998 - C6
ALVIN ELEM 301 E ALVIN AV, SMRA, 93454	776 - H6
ARELLANES ELEM 1890 SANDALWOOD DR, StBC, 93455	816 - B1
ARELLANES JR HIGH 1890 SANDALWOOD DR, StBC, 93455	816 - B1
ARROYO GRANDE HIGH 495 VALLEY RD, ARGD, 93420	714 - J6
ATASCADERO FINE ARTS ACADEMY 6100 OLMEDA AV, ATAS, 93422	573 - J3
ATASCADERO HIGH 1 HIGH SCHOOL HILL RD, ATAS, 93422	573 - H4
ATASCADERO JR HIGH 6501 LEWIS AV, ATAS, 93422	573 - J3
BALLARD ELEM 2425 SCHOOL ST, StBC, 93463	920 - H2
BATTLES, GEORGE W ELEM 605 E BATTLES RD, SMRA, 93454	796 - H3
BAUER-SPECK ELEM 401 17TH ST, PSRS, 93446	513 - F4
BAYWOOD ELEM 1330 9TH ST, SLOC, 93402	631 - H4
BELLEVUE-SANTA FE ELEM 1401 SAN LUIS BAY DR, SLOC, 93405	693 - C2
BISHOP GARCIA DIEGO HIGH 4000 LA COLINA RD, SBAR, 93110	985 - D7
BISHOPS PEAK ELEM 451 JAYCEE DR, SLO, 93405	653 - G2
BLAIR, RITA 1250 E GRAND AV, ARGD, 93420	714 - G5
BONITA ELEM 2715 W MAIN ST, StBC, 93458	775 - H6
BRANCH ELEM 970 SCHOOL RD, SLOC, 93420	715 - F2
BRANDON 195 BRANDON DR, GOL, 93117	993 - F2
BROWN, GEORGIA ELEM 525 36TH ST, PSRS, 93446	513 - F2
BRUCE, ROBERT ELEM 601 W ALVIN AV, SMRA, 93458	776 - G6
BUENA VISTA ELEM 100 ALDEBARAN AV, StBC, 93436	876 - D6
BUREN, MARY ELEM 1050 PERALTA ST, GDLP, 93434	775 - A5
BUTLER, PAT ELEM 700 NICKLAUS ST, PSRS, 93446	513 - H7
CABRILLO HIGH 4350 CONSTELLATION RD, StBC, 93436	876 - C6
CAMBRIA ELEM 1350 MAIN ST, Cmbr, 93428	528 - F7
CANALINO ELEM 1480 LINDEN AV, CARP, 93013	998 - D6
CARPINTERIA HIGH 4810 FOOTHILL RD, CARP, 93013	998 - D5
CARPINTERIA MID 5351 CARPINTERIA AV, CARP, 93013	998 - D7
CATE HIGH 1960 CATE MESA RD, StBC, 93013	998 - J6
CAYUCOS ELEM 301 CAYUCOS DR, SLOC, 93430	590 - J1
CHAVEZ ESTRADA CHARTER ELEM 1102 YANONALI ST, SBAR, 93103	996 - D3
CHRISTIAN LIFE ELEM 709 CURRYER ST, SMRA, 93458	776 - G6
CLEVELAND ELEM 123 ALAMEDA PADRE SERRA, SBAR, 93103	996 - D2
COASTAL CHRISTIAN ELEM 1220 FARROLL AV, ARGD, 93420	714 - G6
COASTAL CHRISTIAN HIGH 1220 FARROLL AV, ARGD, 93420	714 - G6
COASTLINE CHRISTIAN ACADEMY 5950 CATHEDRAL OAKS RD, GOL, 93117	984 - E6
COAST UNION HIGH 2950 SANTA ROSA CREEK RD, Cmbr, 93428	528 - J6
COLD SPRING ELEM 2243 SYCAMORE CANYON RD, StBC, 93108	996 - F1
COLLEGE ELEM 3525 PINE ST, StBC, 93460	921 - C5
CRANE ELEM 1795 SAN LEANDRO LN, StBC, 93108	997 - A3
CRESTVIEW ELEM UTAH AV, StBC, 93437	855 - F6
CULVER, CAPPY ELEM 11011 HERITAGE RANCH RD, SLOC, 93446	471 - D3
CUYAMA ELEM 2300 HWY 166, StBC, 93254	806 - C1
CUYAMA VALLEY HIGH 4500 HWY 166, StBC, 93254	806 - D1
DANA ELEM 920 W TEFFT ST, Npmo, 93444	756 - A4
DEL MAR ELEM 501 SEQUOIA ST, MOBY, 93442	611 - E2
DEL RIO HIGH 4507 DEL RIO RD, ATAS, 93422	553 - G7
DELTA HIGH 251 E CLARK AV, StBC, 93455	816 - G6
DEVEREUX CALIFORNIA 6875 EL COLEGIO RD, StBC, 93117	993 - H5
DOS PUEBLOS HIGH 7266 ALAMEDA AV, GOL, 93117	993 - H1
DUNLAP, RALPH ELEM 1220 OAK KNOLL RD, StBC, 93455	817 - A5
DUNN COLLEGE PREP HIGH 2555 HWY 154, StBC, 93460	900 - J6
EL CAMINO ELEM 5020 SAN SIMEON DR, StBC, 93111	994 - H1
EL CAMINO JR HIGH 219 EL CAMINO ST, SMRA, 93458	77
EL CAMINO MID 320 N J ST, LMPC, 93436	91
ELLWOOD ELEM 7686 HOLLISTER AV, GOL, 93117	99
EL MONTECITO EARLY 1455 E VALLEY RD, StBC, 93108	99
FAIRLAWN ELEM 120 MARY DR, SMRA, 93458	77
FESLER, ISAAC JR HIGH 1100 E FESLER ST, SMRA, 93454	77
FILLMORE, LEONORA ELEM 1211 E PINE AV, LMPC, 93436	89
FITZGERALD COMM 402 FARNEL RD, SMRA, 93458	79
FLAMSON, GEORGE MID 655 24TH ST, PSRS, 93446	51
FOOTHILL ELEM 711 RIBERA RD, StBC, 93111	98
FRANKLIN ELEM 1111 MASON ST, SBAR, 93103	99
GOLETA VALLEY JR HIGH 6100 STOW CANYON RD, GOL, 93117	98
GRISHAM, MAY ELEM 610 PINAL AV, StBC, 93455	81
GROVER BEACH ELEM 365 S 10TH ST, GBCH, 93433	71
GROVER HEIGHTS ELEM 770 N 8TH ST, GBCH, 93433	71
HAPGOOD, ARTHUR ELEM 324 S A ST, LMPC, 93436	91
HARDING ELEM 1625 ROBBINS ST, SBAR, 93101	99
HARLOE ELEM 901 FAIR OAKS AV, ARGD, 93420	71
HAWTHORNE ELEM 2125 STORY ST, SLO, 93401	65
HOLLISTER ELEM 4950 ANITA LN, StBC, 93111	99
HOPE ELEM 3970 LA COLINA RD, SBAR, 93110	98
ISLA VISTA ELEM 6875 EL COLEGIO RD, StBC, 93117	99
JONATA ELEM 301 2ND ST, BLTN, 93427	91
JUDKINS MID 680 WADSWORTH AV, PBCH, 93449	71
KELLOGG ELEM 475 CAMBRIDGE DR, GOL, 93117	98
KING, KERMIT ELEM 700 SCHOOLHOUSE CIR, PSRS, 93446	51
KUNST, TOMMIE JR HIGH 930 HIDDEN PINES WY, SMRA, 93458	77
LA CANADA ELEM 621 W NORTH AV, LMPC, 93436	89
LA COLINA JR HIGH 4025 FOOTHILL RD, SBAR, 93110	98
LA CUESTA HIGH 905 NOPAL ST, SBAR, 93103	99
LA CUMBRE JR HIGH 2255 MODOC RD, SBAR, 93101	99
LAGUNA BLANCA ELEM 4125 PALOMA DR, StBC, 93110	99
LAGUNA BLANCA HIGH 4125 PALOMA DR, StBC, 93110	99
LAGUNA MID 11050 LOS OSOS VALLEY RD, SLO, 93405	65
LA HONDA ELEM 1213 N A ST, LMPC, 93436	89
LAKEVIEW JR HIGH 3700 ORCUTT RD, StBC, 93455	81
LANG, DORTHEA ELEM 1661 VIA ALTA MESA, Npmo, 93444	75
LA PATERA ELEM 555 LA PATERA LN, GOL, 93117	98
LA PURISIMA CONCEPCION ELEM 219 W OLIVE AV, LMPC, 93436	91
LARSEN, LILLIAN ELEM 1601 L ST, SLOC, 93451	47
LAUREATE 880 LAUREATE LN, SLOC, 93405	65
LEWIS, DANIEL MID 900 CRESTON RD, PSRS, 93446	51
LIBERTY HIGH 810 NIBLICK RD, PSRS, 93446	51
LIBERTY ELEM 1300 W SONYA LN, SMRA, 93458	79
LOMPOC HIGH 515 W COLLEGE AV, LMPC, 93436	89
LOMPOC VALLEY MID 234 S N ST, LMPC, 93436	91
LOPEZ HIGH 1055 MESA VIEW DR, SLOC, 93420	73
LOS BERROS ELEM 3745 VIA LATO, StBC, 93436	89
LOS OLIVOS ELEM 2540 ALAMO PINTADO AV, StBC, 93441	90
LOS OSOS MID 1555 EL MORRO AV, SLOC, 93402	63
LOS PADRES ELEM 990 MOUNTAIN VIEW BLVD, StBC, 93437	85
LOS RANCHOS ELEM 5785 LOS RANCHOS RD, SLOC, 93401	67
MAIN ELEM 5241 8TH ST, CARP, 93013	99
MAPLE HIGH 1 CAROB ST, StBC, 93437	87
MARYMOUNT ELEM 2130 MISSION RIDGE RD, SBAR, 93103	99
MARYMOUNT JR HIGH 2130 MISSION RIDGE RD, SBAR, 93103	99
MCKENZIE, KERMIT JR HIGH 4710 W MAIN ST, StBC, 93434	77
MCKINLEY ELEM 350 LOMA ALTA DR, SBAR, 93101	99
MESA MID 2555 HALCYON RD, SLOC, 93420	73
MIGUELITO ELEM 1600 W OLIVE AV, LMPC, 93436	91
MILLER ELEM 410 E CM COLEGIO, SMRA, 93454	79
MISSION COLLEGE PREP HIGH 682 PALM ST, SLO, 93401	65
MONARCH GROVE ELEM 348 LOS OSOS VALLEY RD, SLOC, 93402	63
MONROE ELEM 431 FLORA VISTA DR, SBAR, 93109	99
MONTECITO ELEM 385 SAN YSIDRO RD, StBC, 93108	99
MONTEREY ROAD ELEM 3355 MONTEREY RD, ATAS, 93422	57
MONTESSORI CTR 401 N FAIRVIEW AV, GOL, 93117	98
MONTE VISTA ELEM 730 N HOPE AV, SBAR, 93105	98
MORRO BAY HIGH 235 ATASCADERO RD, MOBY, 93442	61

SANTA BARBARA & SAN LUIS OBISPO COUNTIES POINTS OF INTEREST

RE NAME ss City, ZIP Code	PAGE-GRID
AIN VIEW ELEM QUEEN ANN LN, StBC, 93111	**984 - F6**
NGALE, JOE ELEM INTER RD, StBC, 93455	**816 - H1**
O ELEM PRICE ST, Npmo, 93444	**756 - D2**
O HIGH THOMPSON AV, Npmo, 93444	**756 - B1**
COUNTY CHRISTIAN ELEM ATASCADERO MALL, ATAS, 93422	**573 - J4**
COUNTY CHRISTIAN HIGH ATASCADERO MALL, ATAS, 93422	**573 - J4**
OCEANO ELEM THE PIKE, GBCH, 93433	**714 - G7**
DAME MICHELTORENA ST, SBAR, 93101	**995 - J3**
Y ELEM W HARDING AV, SMRA, 93458	**776 - F6**
O ELEM 17TH ST, SLOC, 93445	**714 - F7**
VIEW ELEM LINDA DR, ARGD, 93420	**714 - G5**
SSION ROAD ST, SLO, 93401	**653 - J4**
SSION ELEM ROAD ST, SLO, 93401	**653 - J4**
EROS ELEM ANCHO VERDE, SMRA, 93458	**776 - F4**
LTERNATIVE FOOTHILL RD, SBAR, 93110	**985 - D7**
T JR HIGH INAL AV, StBC, 93455	**816 - G6**
ADY OF MT CARMEL ELEM OT SPRINGS RD, StBC, 93108	**996 - H1**
CO ELEM UESTA DR, SLO, 93405	**653 - H2**
C CHRISTIAN ELEM SANTA MARIA WY, StBC, 93455	**816 - J1**
OBLES HIGH IBLICK RD, PSRS, 93446	**513 - J6**
RSON RD ELEM ATTERSON RD, StBC, 93455	**816 - H5**
NG MID ROWN HILL ST, ARGD, 93420	**715 - A4**
DY ELEM CL NOGUERA, SBAR, 93105	**995 - G1**
SON, VIRGINIA ELEM BEECHWOOD DR, PSRS, 93446	**534 - A2**
WINIFRED ELEM CRESTON RD, PSRS, 93446	**514 - A6**
ROVE ELEM RICE RANCH RD, StBC, 93455	**817 - A7**
ER VALLEY HIGH REMONT ST, SMRA, 93454	**777 - B6**
ANT VALLEY ELEM RANCHITA CANYON RD, SLOC, 93451	**494 - F1**
OLGA ELEM ENTENNIAL ST, StBC, 93440	**878 - G2**
LEM ICKIE AV, SMRA, 93454	**776 - J5**
TI, ERNEST HIGH FOSTER RD, StBC, 93455	**816 - J3**
VELT ELEM LAGUNA ST, SBAR, 93103	**995 - J1**
OAKS CHRISTIAN ELEM AK PARK BLVD, ARGD, 93420	**714 - G3**
CLARENCE ELEM W ST, LMPC, 93436	**916 - C1**
JOSEPH HIGH BRADLEY RD, StBC, 93455	**817 - A3**
LOUIS DE MONTFORT ELEM HARP RD, StBC, 93455	**817 - A6**
MARY OF THE ASSUMPTION CYPRESS ST, SMRA, 93454	**796 - H1**
PATRICK ELEM / BRANCH ST, ARGD, 93420	**714 - H4**
RAPHAEL ELEM AINT JOSEPHS ST, GOL, 93111	**994 - F1**
ROSE OF LIMA UCKER AV, PSRS, 93446	**513 - H6**
ENITO ELEM SAN BENITO RD, ATAS, 93422	**553 - G7**
EZ, DAVID J ELEM / LIBERTY ST, SMRA, 93458	**796 - F2**
ABRIEL ELEM SAN GABRIEL RD, ATAS, 93422	**593 - J1**
JIS OBISPO COMM CONT HS VICENTE DR, SLO, 93405	**673 - F1**
JIS OBISPO HIGH SAN LUIS DR, SLO, 93401	**654 - B3**
ARCOS HIGH HOLLISTER AV, StBC, 93110	**994 - J1**
OQUE ELEM CL CEDRO, SBAR, 93105	**985 - G7**
BARBARA CHARTER ELEM STOW CANYON RD, GOL, 93117	**984 - D7**
BARBARA CHARTER MID STOW CANYON RD, GOL, 93117	**984 - D7**
BARBARA CHRISTIAN MODOC RD, SBAR, 93105	**995 - E2**
BARBARA COMM ACADEMY ORTEGA ST, SBAR, 93101	**996 - B4**
BARBARA HIGH NAPAMU ST, SBAR, 93103	**996 - B2**
BARBARA JR HIGH OTA ST, SBAR, 93103	**996 - C3**
BARBARA MID A GARDEN ST, SBAR, 93105	**995 - J1**
BARBARA MONTESSORI MIRANO DR, GOL, 93117	**993 - G1**
LUCIA MID SCHOOLHOUSE LN, Cmbr, 93428	**528 - H7**
MARGARITA ELEM H ST, SLOC, 93453	**614 - G2**
MARIA HIGH BROADWAY, SMRA, 93458	**796 - G2**
ROSA ACADEMIC ACADEMY SANTA ROSA RD, ATAS, 93422	**574 - A7**
YNEZ ELEM PINE ST, StBC, 93460	**921 - B5**
YNEZ VALLEY CHARTER PINE ST, StBC, 93460	**921 - C5**
YNEZ VALLEY CHRISTIAN ACADEMY EFUGIO RD, StBC, 93463	**921 - A6**
YNEZ VALLEY HIGH E HWY 246, StBC, 93463	**921 - A6**
ALICE ELEM AHLIA PL, StBC, 93455	**816 - J2**
BEACH ELEM SHELL BEACH RD, PBCH, 93449	**693 - G7**
EIMER ELEM AUGUSTA ST, SLO, 93401	**654 - B6**
, C L ELEM BALBOA ST, SLO, 93405	**653 - F6**
NG ELEM TTERDAG RD, SLVG, 93463	**920 - E7**
NG MID TTERDAG RD, SLVG, 93463	**920 - E7**

FEATURE NAME Address City, ZIP Code	PAGE-GRID
SUMMERLAND 135 VALENCIA RD, Summ, 93067	**997 - D4**
TAYLOR, IDA REDMOND ELEM 1921 N CARLOTTI DR, SMRA, 93454	**776 - J4**
TEACH, CHARLES ELEM 375 FERRINI RD, SLO, 93405	**653 - H2**
TEMPLETON ELEM 215 8TH ST, SLOC, 93465	**553 - D2**
TEMPLETON HIGH 1200 S MAIN ST, SLOC, 93465	**553 - D3**
TEMPLETON MID 925 OLD COUNTY RD, SLOC, 93465	**553 - D2**
TRINITY LUTHERAN 940 CRESTON RD, PSRS, 93446	**513 - J6**
TUNNELL ELEM 1248 E DENA WY, SMRA, 93454	**777 - A6**
VALLEY CHRISTIAN ACADEMY ELEM 2970 SANTA MARIA WY, SMRA, 93455	**796 - H7**
VALLEY CHRISTIAN ACADEMY HIGH 2970 SANTA MARIA WY, SMRA, 93455	**796 - H7**
VALLEY VIEW ACADEMY ELEM 230 VERNON ST, ARGD, 93420	**714 - J5**
VANDENBERG MID 1145 MOUNTAIN VIEW BLVD, StBC, 93437	**855 - G7**
VIEJA VALLEY ELEM 434 NOGAL DR, StBC, 93110	**995 - B2**
WALDORF OF SANTA BARBARA 2300-B GARDEN ST, SBAR, 93105	**995 - J1**
WASHINGTON ELEM 290 LIGHTHOUSE RD, SBAR, 93109	**995 - H7**

SHOPPING CENTERS

FEATURE NAME Address City, ZIP Code	PAGE-GRID
BROADWAY PLAZA 1450 S BROADWAY, SMRA, 93454	**796 - H3**
CAMINO REAL MARKETPLACE STORKE RD & HOLLISTER AV, GOL, 93117	**993 - H3**
LA CUMBRE PLAZA 140 S HOPE AV, SBAR, 93105	**995 - E1**
MADONNA PLAZA 221 MADONNA RD, SLO, 93405	**653 - H6**
PASEO NUEVO 651 PASEO NUEVO, SBAR, 93101	**996 - A4**
SANTA MARIA CTR 1425 S BROADWAY, SMRA, 93458	**796 - G3**
SANTA MARIA TOWN CTR EAST S BROADWAY & COOK ST, SMRA, 93454	**776 - H7**
SANTA MARIA TOWN CTR WEST S BROADWAY & COOK ST, SMRA, 93458	**776 - G7**
SLO PROMENADE 321 MADONNA RD, SLO, 93405	**653 - G7**

TRANSPORTATION

FEATURE NAME Address City, ZIP Code	PAGE-GRID
AMTRAK CARPINTERIA STA, CARP	**998 - D7**
AMTRAK GOLETA STA, GOL	**994 - C1**
AMTRAK GROVER BEACH STA, GBCH	**714 - D5**
AMTRAK RAIL STA, GDLP	**775 - A6**
AMTRAK SAN LUIS OBISPO STA, SLO	**654 - A4**
AMTRAK SANTA BARBARA STA, SBAR	**996 - B5**
AMTRAK STA, StBC	**894 - F2**
GREYHOUND TERMINAL, SLO	**653 - H5**
GREYHOUND TERMINAL, SMRA	**776 - H7**
GREYHOUND TERMINAL, SBAR	**996 - A4**
GREYHOUND TERMINAL, PSRS	**513 - G6**
GREYHOUND TERMINAL, ATAS	**573 - J3**

VISITOR INFORMATION

FEATURE NAME Address City, ZIP Code	PAGE-GRID
SAN LUIS OBISPO CO VISITORS CTR 1037 MILL ST, SLO, 93401	**653 - J4**
SOLVANG VISITORS BUREAU 1511 MISSION DR, SLVG, 93463	**940 - E1**
VISITOR BUREAU 1639 COPENHAGEN DR, SLVG, 93463	**940 - E1**
VISITORS CTR 1 GARDEN ST, SBAR, 93101	**996 - C5**

WINERIES

FEATURE NAME Address City, ZIP Code	PAGE-GRID
ARTHUR EARL 90 EASY ST, BLTN, 93427	**919 - J4**
BAILEYANA 4915 ORCUTT RD, SLOC, 93401	**674 - F3**
BECKMEN VINEYARDS 2670 ONTIVEROS RD, StBC, 93460	**900 - H7**
BRANDER VINEYARD, THE 2401 REFUGIO RD, StBC, 93460	**901 - A6**
BRIDLEWOOD ESTATE 3555 ROBLAR AV, StBC, 93460	**901 - B7**
BUTTONWOOD FARM 1500 ALAMO PINTADO RD, StBC, 93463	**920 - H3**
CLAUTIERE VINEYARD PENMAN SPRINGS RD, SLOC, 93446	**514 - F6**
COTTONWOOD CANYON 4330 SANTA FE RD, SLOC, 93401	**674 - A2**
DOMAINE ALFRED 7525 ORCUTT RD, SLOC, 93401	**695 - A1**
EBERLE HIGHWAY 46, PSRS, 93446	**514 - D2**
EDNA VALLEY 2585 BIDDLE RANCH RD, SLOC, 93401	**674 - F6**
EOS ESTATE HWY 46 E, SLOC, 93446	**514 - E2**
FETZER FIVE RIVERS RANCH N RIVER RD, SLOC, 93451	**473 - H6**
FOLEY ESTATES VINEYARD 1711 ALAMO PINTADO RD, StBC, 93463	**920 - G2**
FRATELLI PERATA ARBOR RD, SLOC, 93446	**533 - C1**
GAINEY VINEYARD, THE 3950 E HWY 246, StBC, 93460	**921 - D6**
HALL, ROBERT 3443 MILL RD, SLOC, 93446	**514 - D3**
KELSEY SEE CANYON VINEYARDS 1947 SEE CANYON RD, SLOC, 93405	**693 - D1**
LAETITIA VINEYARD 453 LAETITIA VINEYARD DR, SLOC, 93420	**735 - E2**
LINCOURT VINEYARDS 343 N REFUGIO RD, StBC, 93463	**941 - A1**
LOHR, J VINEYARD 6169 AIRPORT RD, SLOC, 93446	**494 - C3**
LOS OLIVOS VINTNERS 2923 GRAND AV, StBC, 93441	**900 - H5**
MARTIN & WEYRICH 2610 BUENA VISTA DR, SLOC, 93446	**513 - J1**
MIDNIGHT CELLARS 2925 ANDERSON RD, SLOC, 93446	**533 - A5**
MOSBY 9496 SANTA ROSA RD, StBC	**919 - H7**
PEACHY CANYON 1480 N BETHEL RD, SLOC, 93446	**533 - C5**
PENMAN SPRINGS VINEYARD 1985 PENMAN SPRINGS RD, SLOC, 93446	**514 - F5**
PRETTY-SMITH 13350 N RIVER RD, SLOC, 93451	**473 - H2**
RIO SECO VINEYARD UNION RD, SLOC, 93446	**514 - D4**

FEATURE NAME Address City, ZIP Code	PAGE-GRID
ROSS-KELLER 985 ORCHARD AV, Npmo, 93444	**756 - C6**
RUSACK VINEYARDS 1819 BALLARD CANYON RD, StBC, 93441	**920 - D2**
SANFORD 7250 SANTA ROSA RD, StBC, 93427	**919 - B7**
SANTA BARBARA 202 ANACAPA ST, SBAR, 93101	**996 - B4**
STEARNS WHARF VINTNERS 217 STEARNS WHARF, SBAR, 93101	**996 - C5**
SUMMERWOOD 2175 ARBOR RD, SLOC, 93446	**533 - C4**
SUNSTONE VINEYARDS 125 REFUGIO RD, StBC, 93463	**940 - J2**
SYLVESTER 5115 BUENA VISTA DR, SLOC, 93446	**493 - J6**
TALLEY VINEYARDS 3031 LOPEZ DR, SLOC, 93453	**695 - F5**
WILD HORSE 1437 WILD HORSE WINERY CT, SLOC, 93465	**553 - J4**
WINDWARD VINEYARD 1380 LIVE OAK RD, SLOC, 93446	**533 - C3**
ZENAIDA CELLARS 1550 HIGHWAY 46 W, SLOC, 93446	**533 - B5**

Note Page

Note Page

The Thomas Guide®

Thank you for purchasing this Rand McNally Thomas Guide! We value your comments and suggestions.

Please help us serve you better by completing this postage-paid reply card.
This information is for internal use ONLY and will not be distributed or sold to any external third party.

Missing pages? Maybe not... Please refer to the "Using Your Street Guide" page for further explanation.

Thomas Guide Title: Easy-to-Read Santa Barbara & San Luis Obispo Counties ISBN-13# 978-0-5288-6852-8 MKT: LA

Today's Date: ____________ Gender: ☐M ☐F Age Group: ☐18-24 ☐25-31 ☐32-40 ☐41-50 ☐51-64 ☐65

1. What type of industry do you work in?
   ☐Real Estate ☐Trucking ☐Delivery ☐Construction ☐Utilities ☐Governme
   ☐Retail ☐Sales ☐Transportation ☐Landscape ☐Service & Repair
   ☐Courier ☐Automotive ☐Insurance ☐Medical ☐Police/Fire/First Response
   ☐Other, please specify: ____________
2. What type of job do you have in this industry? ____________
3. Where did you purchase this Thomas Guide? (store name & city) ____________
4. Why did you purchase this Thomas Guide? ____________
5. How often do you purchase an updated Thomas Guide? ☐Annually ☐2 yrs. ☐3-5 yrs. ☐Other: ____________
6. Where do you use it? ☐Primarily in the car ☐Primarily in the office ☐Primarily at home ☐Other: ____________
7. How do you use it? ☐Exclusively for business ☐Primarily for business but also for personal or leisure use
   ☐Both work and personal evenly ☐Primarily for personal use ☐Exclusively for personal use
8. What do you use your Thomas Guide for?
   ☐Find Addresses ☐In-route navigation ☐Planning routes ☐Other: ____________
   Find points of interest: ☐Schools ☐Parks ☐Buildings ☐Shopping Centers ☐Other: ____________
9. How often do you use it? ☐Daily ☐Weekly ☐Monthly ☐Other: ____________
10. Do you use the internet for maps and/or directions? ☐Yes ☐No
11. How often do you use the internet for directions? ☐Daily ☐Weekly ☐Monthly ☐Other: ____________
12. Do you use any of the following mapping products in addition to your Thomas Guide?
    ☐Folded paper maps ☐Folded laminated maps ☐Wall maps ☐GPS ☐PDA ☐In-car navigation ☐Phone maps
13. What features, if any, would you like to see added to your Thomas Guide? ____________
14. What features or information do you find most useful in your Rand McNally Thomas Guide? (please specify) ____________
15. Please provide any additional comments or suggestions you have. ____________

We strive to provide you with the most current updated information available if you know a map correction, please notify us here.

Where is the correction? Map Page #: ________ Grid #: ________ Index Page #: ________

Nature of the correction: ☐Street name missing ☐Street name misspelled ☐Street information incorrect
☐Incorrect location for point of interest ☐Index error ☐Other: ____________

Detail: ____________

I would like to receive information about updated editions and special offers from Rand McNally
☐via e-mail E-mail address: ____________
☐via postal mail
Your Name: ____________ Company (if used for work): ____________
Address: ____________ City/State/ZIP: ____________

Thank you for your time and help. We are working to serve you better.
This information is for internal use ONLY and will not be distributed or sold to any external third party.

CUT ALONG DOTTED LINE

CUT ALONG DOTTED LINE

TAPE SHUT

get directions at
randmcnally.com

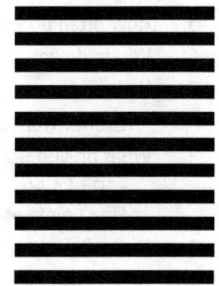

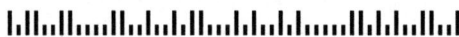

CUT ALONG DOTTED LINE

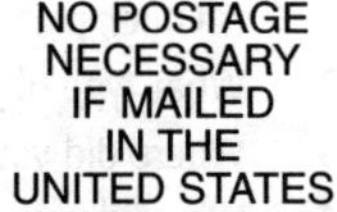
NO POSTAGE
NECESSARY
IF MAILED
IN THE
UNITED STATES

BUSINESS REPLY MAIL

FIRST-CLASS MAIL PERMIT NO. 388 CHICAGO IL

POSTAGE WILL BE PAID BY ADDRESSEE

RAND MCNALLY
CONSUMER AFFAIRS
PO BOX 7600
CHICAGO IL 60680-9915

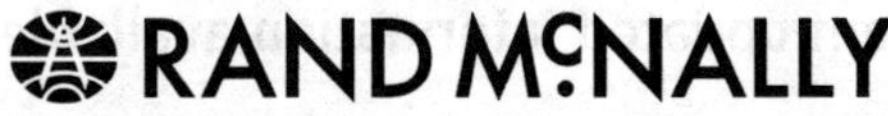
RAND McNALLY

The most trusted name on the map.

You'll never need to ask for directions again with these Rand McNally products!

- EasyFinder® Laminated Maps
- Folded Maps
- Street Guides
- Wall Maps
- CustomView Wall Maps
- Road Atlases
- Motor Carriers' Road Atlases

CUT ALONG DOTTED LINE

SGTG_07

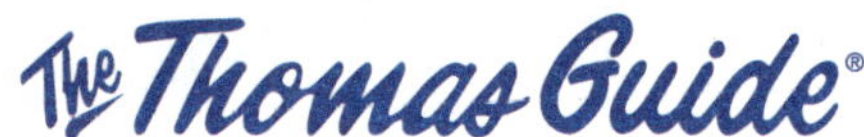
The Thomas Guide®

Easy-to-Read Ventura County street guide

TELL US WHAT YOU THINK
comment card on last page

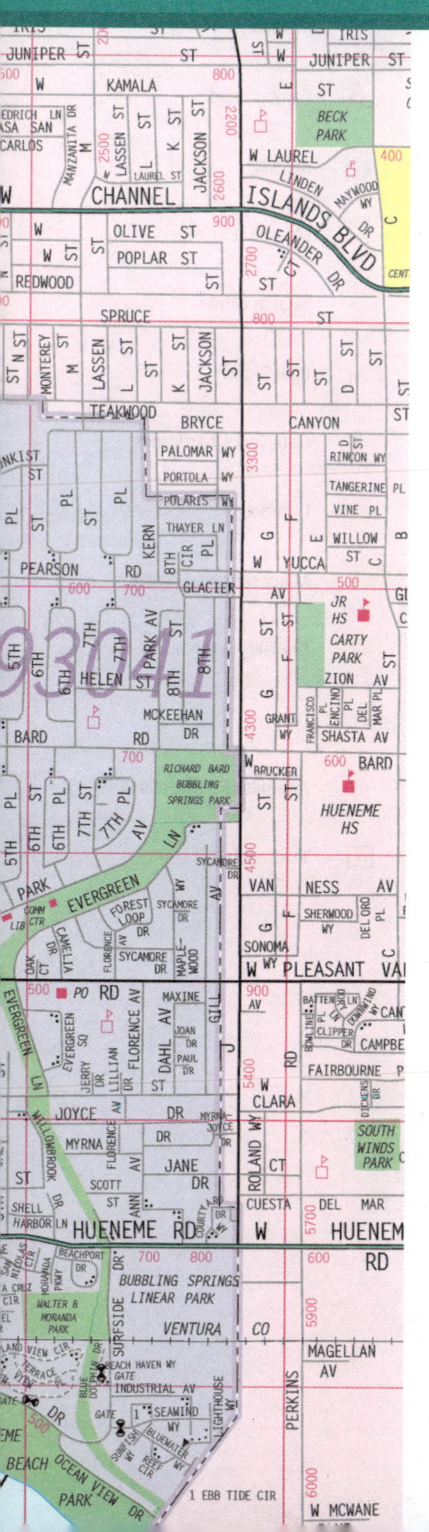
JUNIPER ST
KAMALA
CHANNEL
OLIVE ST
POPLAR ST
REDWOOD
SPRUCE
TEAKWOOD
BRYCE
CANYON
BECK PARK
W LAUREL
ISLANDS BLVD
OLEANDER
PALOMAR WY
PORTOLA WY
POLARIS WY
THAYER LN
PEARSON
GLACIER
93041
HELEN
MCKEEHAN
BARD
RICHARD BARD BUBBLING SPRINGS PARK
JR HS
CARTY PARK
ZION AV
SHASTA AV
HUENEME HS
EVERGREEN
VAN NESS AV
W PLEASANT VALLEY
SOUTH WINDS PARK
HUENEME RD
BUBBLING SPRINGS LINEAR PARK
VENTURA
MAGELLAN AV
PERKINS
OCEAN VIEW DR
BEACH PARK
1 EBB TIDE CIR
W MCWANE

Contents

Introduction

Using Your Street Guide	A
PageFinder™ Map	B
Legend	D
We've Got You Covered	E

Maps

Downtown Map	F
Street Guide Detail Maps	441-625
Vicinity Map	Inside back cover

Lists and Indexes

Cities & Communities Index	626
List of Abbreviations	627
Street Index and Points of Interest Index	628
Comment Card	Last page

PageFinder™ Map U.S. Patent No. 5,419,586
Canadian Patent No. 2,116,425
Patente Mexicana No. 188186

Published in U.S.A. Printed in U.S.A.

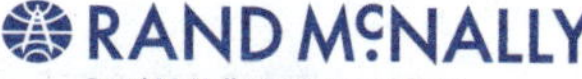
RAND McNALLY

Rand McNally Consumer Affairs
P.O. Box 7600
Chicago, IL 60680-9915
randmcnally.com
For comments or suggestions, please call (800) 777-MAPS (-6277)
or email us at:
consumeraffairs@randmcnally.com

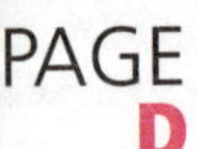
PAGE
D

Legend

- Freeway
- Interchange/ramp
- Highway
- Primary road
- Secondary road
- Minor road
- Restricted road
- Alley
- Unpaved road
- Tunnel
- Toll road
- High occupancy vehicle lane
- Stacked multiple roadways
- Proposed road
- Proposed freeway
- Freeway under construction
- One-way road
- Two-way road
- Trail, walkway
- Stairs
- Railroad
- Rapid transit
- Rapid transit, underground
- Ferry
- City boundary
- County boundary
- State boundary
- International boundary
- Military base, Indian reservation
- Township, range, rancho
- River, creek, shoreline
- 98607 ZIP code boundary, ZIP code
- 5 Interstate
- 5 Interstate (Business)
- 3 U.S. highway
- 1 4 8 9 State highways
- Carpool lane
- A Street list marker
- Street name continuation
- Street name change
- Station (train, bus)
- Building (see List of Abbreviations page)
- Building footprint
- Public elementary school
- Public high school
- Private elementary school
- Private high school
- Fire station
- Library
- Mission
- Campground
- H Hospital
- Mountain
- Section corner
- Boat launch
- Gate, locks, barricades
- Lighthouse
- Major shopping center
- Dry lake, beach
- Dam
- Intermittent lake, marsh
- 29 Exit number

we've got you COVERED

Rand McNally's broad selection of products is perfect for your every need. Whether you're looking for the convenience of write-on wipe-off laminated maps, extra maps for every car, or a Road Atlas to plan your next vacation or to use as a reference, Rand McNally has you covered.

Street Guides

Los Angeles & Orange Counties
Los Angeles & Orange Counties - Pro Series Laminated Edition
Los Angeles & San Bernardino Counties
Los Angeles & Ventura Counties
Los Angeles County
Los Angeles County - Easy to Read
Orange County
Orange County - Easy to Read
Riverside & Orange Counties
Riverside & San Diego Counties
Riverside County
Riverside County - Easy to Read
San Bernardino & Riverside Counties
San Bernardino & Riverside Counties - Pro Series Laminated Edition
San Bernardino County
San Bernardino County - Easy to Read
San Diego & Orange Counties
San Diego County
Santa Barbara & San Luis Obispo Counties - Easy to Read
Santa Barbara, San Luis Obispo & Ventura Counties - Easy to Read
Ventura County
Ventura County - Easy to Read

Folded Maps

EasyFinder Laminated Maps:
Los Angeles & Vicinity
Los Angeles to San Diego Regional
Los Angeles/ Hollywood
Palm Springs
Pomona/Ontario
Riverside
San Diego
San Diego & Vicinity
Southern California
West LA/ Santa Monica

Paper Maps:
Anaheim/ Fullerton
Hemet/ Perris
Lancaster/ Palmdale
Long Beach/ Carson/ Torrance
Los Angeles
Los Angeles & Vicinity
Moreno Valley/ Banning
North San Diego/ Encinitas
Oceanside/ Escondido
Ontario/ Pomona
Orange County, Central
Orange County, Northern
Orange County, Southern
Palm Springs/ Desert Cities
River Cities
Riverside
San Bernardino/ Fontana
San Diego
San Fernando Valley
San Gabriel Valley/ Pasadena
Santa Clarita Valley
Southern California Freeways
Temecula/ Murrieta
Thousand Oaks/ Simi Valley
Ventura/ Oxnard
Victorville/ Barstow

Wall Maps

California State
Southern California Arterial

Road Atlases

California Road Atlas
Road Atlas
Road Atlas & Travel Guide
Large Scale Road Atlas
Midsize Road Atlas
Deluxe Midsize Road Atlas
Pocket Road Atlas

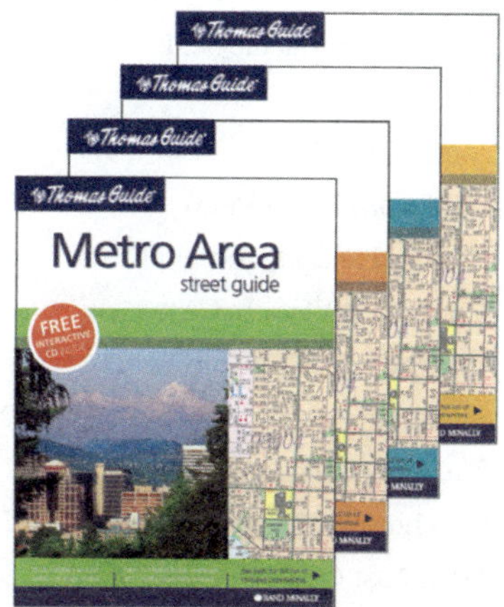
Thomas Guide
Metro Area
street guide
FREE

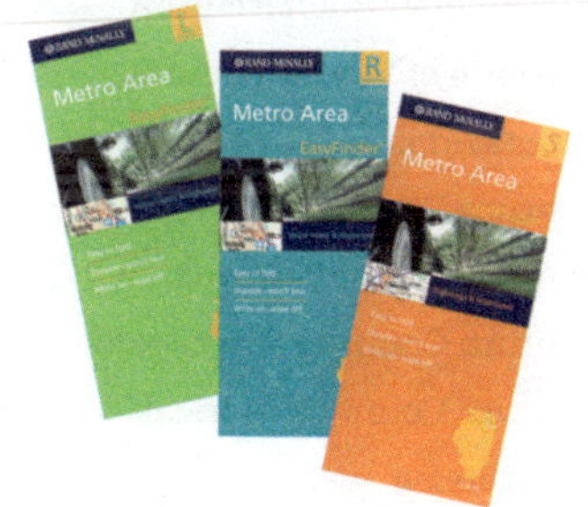
Metro Area
Metro Area
Metro Area

Wherever Rand McNally products are sold or at
www.randmcnally.com

PAGE
F

Downtown Ventura

Points of Interest

1	A J Comstock Fire Museum	C2
2	Albinger Archaeological Museum	C2
3	Amtrak Station	C2
4	California Street Plaza	D2
5	Channel Islands National Park HQ & Visitors Center	G7
6	Crowne Plaza Ventura Beach	C2
7	E P Foster Library	D2
8	Father Serra Cross	C1
9	Greyhound Bus Station	C2
10	Main Post Office	D2
11	Marriott Hotel	F4
12	Mission San Buenaventura	C2
13	Museum of Ventura County	C2
14	Ortega Adobe	B1
15	Ventura City Hall	D1
16	Ventura Concert Theater	D2
17	Ventura County Fairgrounds	B3
18	Ventura County Historical Courthouse	D1
19	Ventura Historical Pier	D3
20	Visitors Bureau	C2

Map Scale

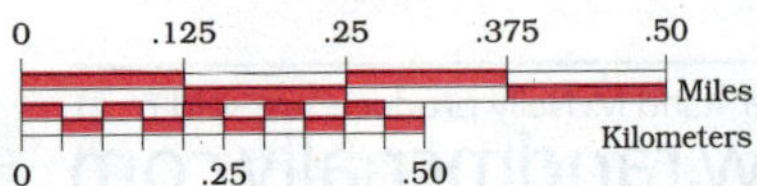
0
.125
.25
.375
.50
Miles
Kilometers
0
.25
.50

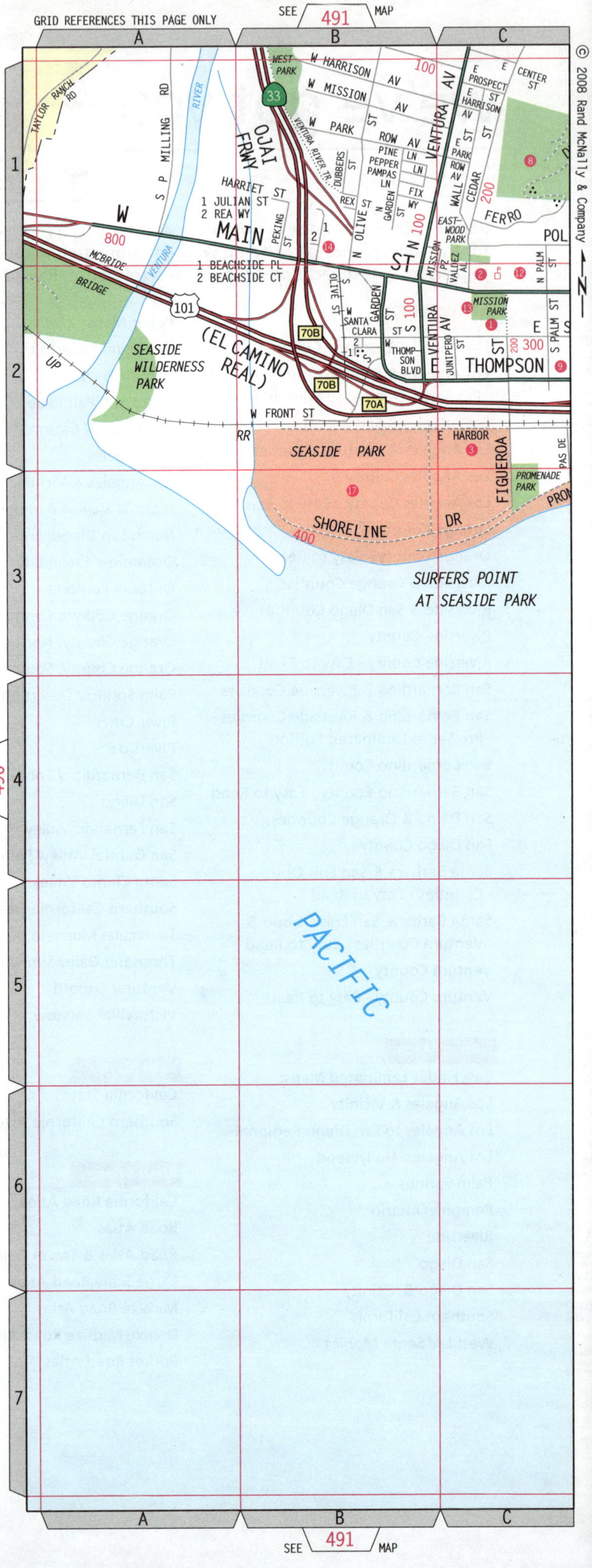

GRID REFERENCES THIS PAGE ONLY

SEE 491 MAP

A B C
1 2 3 4 5 6 7

TAYLOR RANCH RD
S P MILLING RD
VENTURA RIVER
W HARRISON AV
W MISSION AV
W PARK ROW AV
OJAI FRWY
HARRIET ST
1 JULIAN ST
2 REA WY
W MAIN ST
PEKING ST
MCBRIDE BRIDGE
1 BEACHSIDE PL
2 BEACHSIDE CT
SEASIDE WILDERNESS PARK
(EL CAMINO REAL)
W FRONT ST
SEASIDE PARK
SHORELINE DR
SURFERS POINT AT SEASIDE PARK
E HARBOR
FIGUEROA ST
PROMENADE PARK
E THOMPSON BLVD
N VENTURA AV
MISSION PARK
EASTWOOD PARK
FERRO
PACIFIC

SEE 490 MAP

SEE 491 MAP

SEE 491 MAP

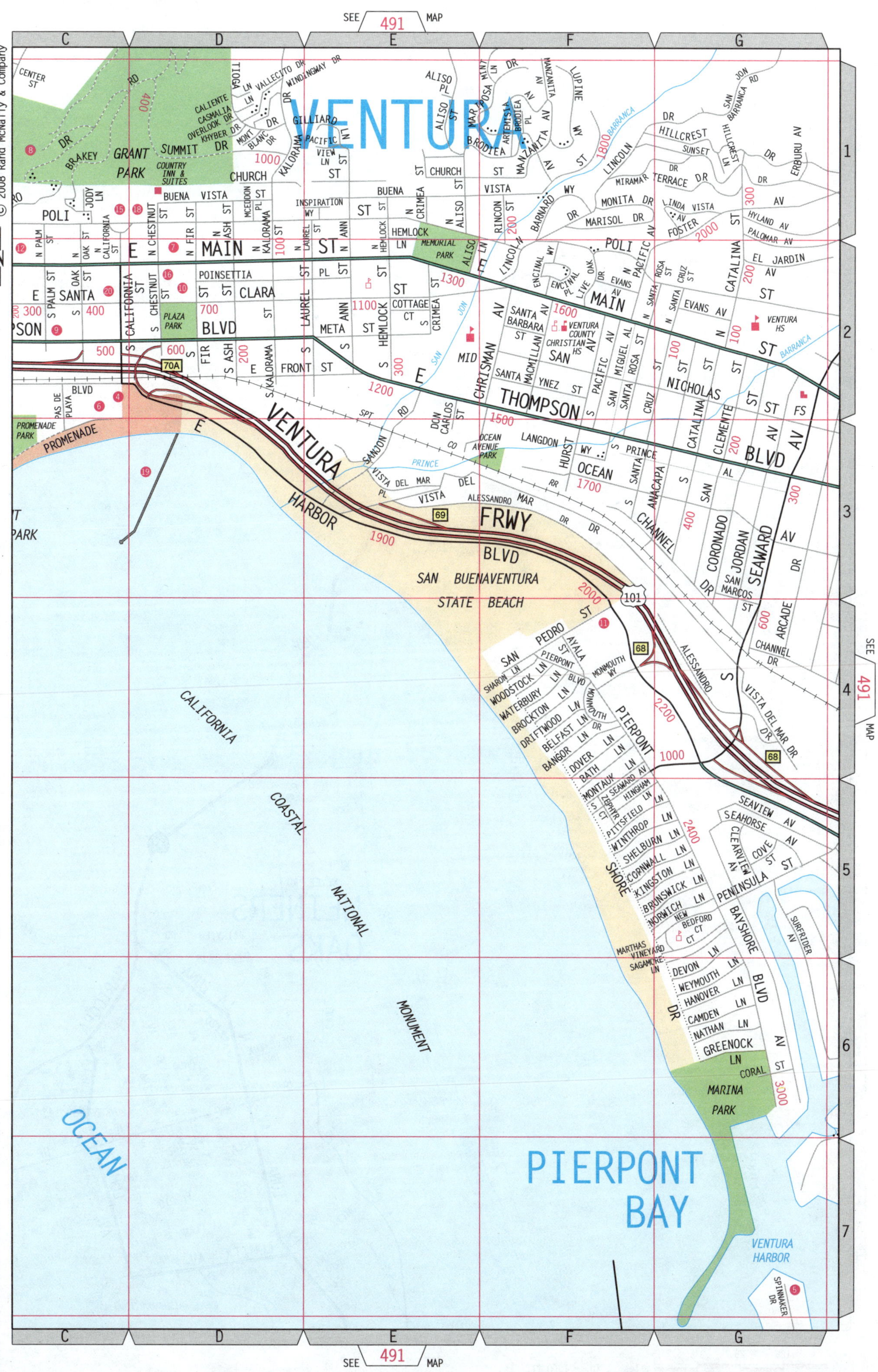
VENTURA
C
D
E
F
G
1
2
3
4
5
6
7
GRANT PARK
SUMMIT DR
BRAKEY DR
COUNTRY INN & SUITES
CHURCH ST
BUENA VISTA ST
POLI ST
E MAIN ST
E SANTA CLARA ST
E THOMPSON BLVD
POINSETTIA PL
PLAZA PARK
FRONT ST
MEMORIAL PARK
HEMLOCK
MID
VENTURA COUNTY CHRISTIAN HS
VENTURA HS
FS
VENTURA FRWY
HARBOR BLVD
PROMENADE PARK
PROMENADE
PAS DE PLAYA
OCEAN AVENUE PARK
PRINCE BARRANCA
SAN JON
SAN BUENAVENTURA STATE BEACH
SAN PEDRO ST
PIERPONT BLVD
SEAWARD AV
ALESSANDRO DR
VISTA DEL MAR DR
CHANNEL DR
PENINSULA ST
BAYSHORE
SHORE DR
GREENOCK LN
CORAL ST
MARINA PARK
VENTURA HARBOR
SPINNAKER DR
SURFRIDER AV
CALIFORNIA COASTAL NATIONAL MONUMENT
OCEAN
PIERPONT BAY
101
70A
69
68
1000
1100
1200
1300
1500
1600
1700
1800
1900
2000
2200
2400
3000

SEE 491 MAP
SEE 491 MAP

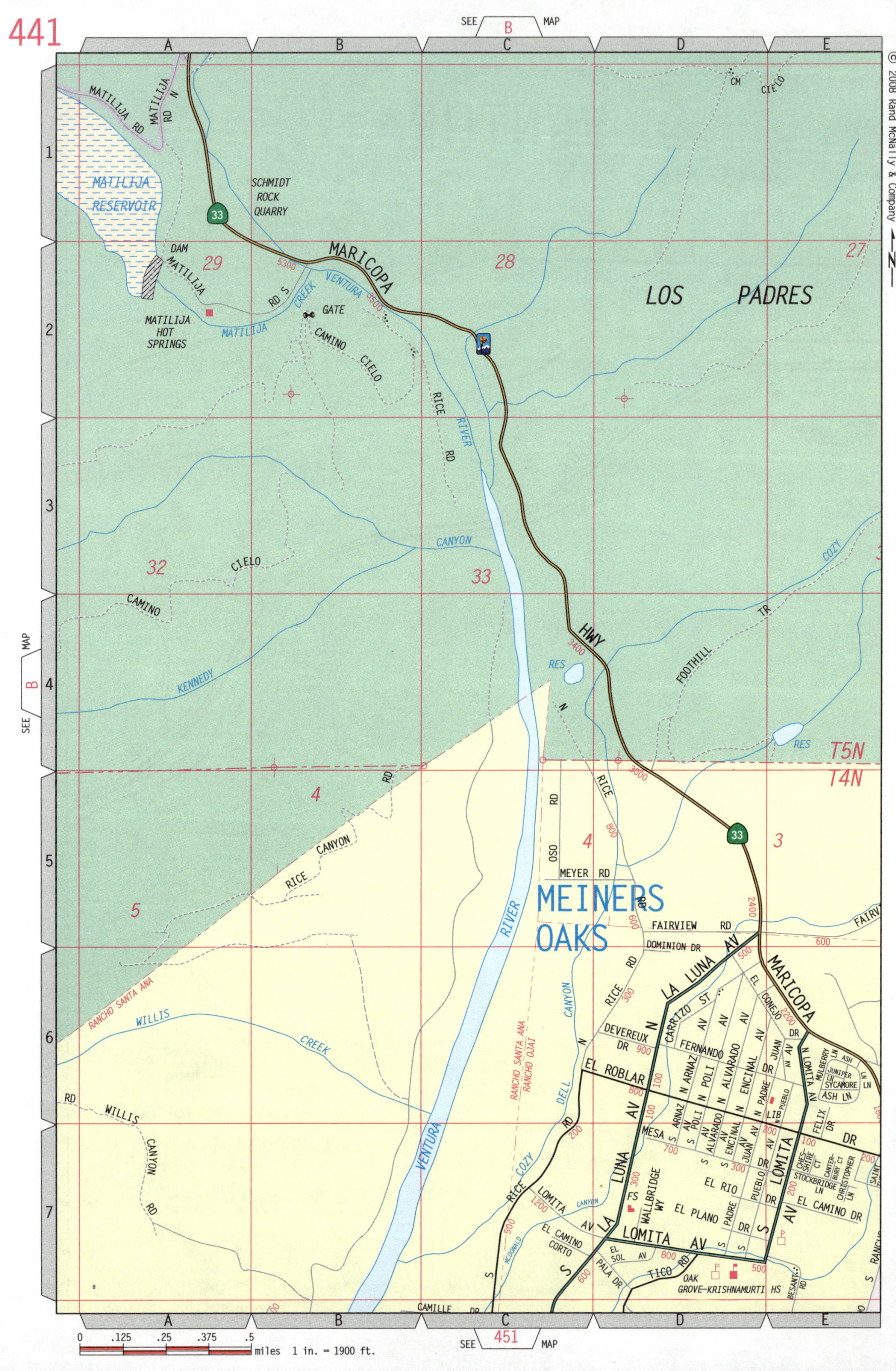
SEE B MAP
MATILIJA RD
MATILIJA RD N
MATILIJA RESERVOIR
SCHMIDT ROCK QUARRY
33
DAM
MATILIJA RD S
29
MARICOPA
VENTURA
28
27
LOS PADRES
MATILIJA HOT SPRINGS
MATILIJA CREEK
GATE
CAMINO CIELO
RICE RD
RIVER
CM
CIELO
CANYON
32
CIELO
CAMINO
33
HWY
KENNEDY
RES
FOOTHILL TR
COZY
T5N
T4N
4
RICE CANYON RD
5
OSO RD
MEYER RD
MEINERS OAKS
FAIRVIEW RD
DOMINION DR
3
RANCHO SANTA ANA
WILLIS CREEK
WILLIS CANYON RD
VENTURA RIVER
RANCHO SANTA ANA
RANCHO OJAI
DELL
N LA LUNA AV
CARRIZO ST
DEVEREUX DR
FERNANDO
EL ROBLAR DR
N ARNAZ AV
N POLI AV
N ALVARADO AV
N ENCINAL AV
N PADRE
N JUAN DR
EL CONEJO DR
MARICOPA
N LOMITA AV
MULBERRY LN
ASH LN
JUNIPER LN
SYCAMORE LN
FELIX DR
LIB
MESA
S ARNAZ AV
S POLI AV
S ALVARADO AV
S ENCINAL AV
S JUAN AV
S PADRE DR
S LOMITA AV
CHESHIRE CT
STOCKBRIDGE LN
CHRISTOPHER LN
EL RIO
EL CAMINO DR
FS
WALLBRIDGE WY
EL PLANO DR
S LA LUNA
LOMITA AV
RICE RD
COZY CANYON
EL CAMINO CORTO
EL SOL AV
PALA DR
TICO RD
OAK GROVE-KRISHNAMURTI HS
BESANT RD
CAMILLE DR
SEE 451 MAP
0 .125 .25 .375 .5 miles 1 in. = 1900 ft.

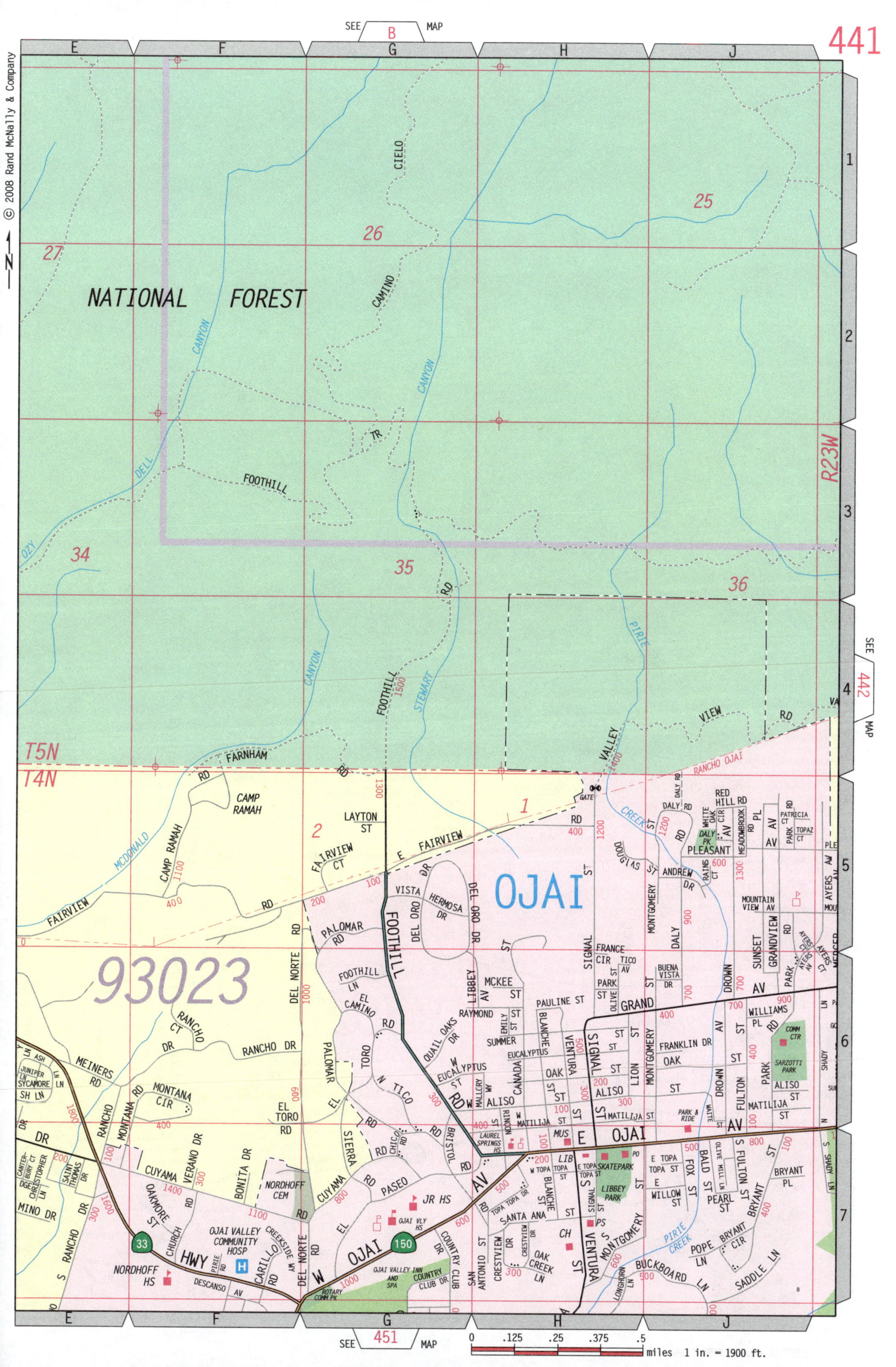

SEE B MAP
SEE 442 MAP
SEE 451 MAP
E
F
G
H
J
1
2
3
4
5
6
7
NATIONAL FOREST
OJAI
93023
T5N
T4N
R23W
27
26
25
34
35
36
1
2
CIELO
CAMINO
TR
FOOTHILL
RD
CANYON
DELL
OZY
STEWART
PIRIE CREEK
MCDONALD
FARNHAM RD
CAMP RAMAH
CAMP RAMAH RD
FAIRVIEW RD
FAIRVIEW CT
E FAIRVIEW
LAYTON ST
VALLEY VIEW RD
RANCHO OJAI
GATE
DALY RD
RED HILL RD
WHITE OAK CIR
MEADOWBROOK RD
DALY PK
PLEASANT
ANDREW DR
RAINS CT
DOUGLAS ST
MOUNTAIN VIEW AV
GRANDVIEW AV
SUNSET AV
AYERS AV
PATRICIA CT
TOPAZ CT
FOOTHILL
VISTA
HERMOSA DR
DEL ORO DR
PALOMAR RD
DEL NORTE RD
FOOTHILL LN
EL CAMINO RD
MCKEE ST
LIBBEY AV
SIGNAL ST
FRANCE CIR
TICO AV
PARK ST
OLIVE ST
BUENA VISTA DR
MONTGOMERY
DALY
DROWN
GRAND AV
WILLIAMS PL
COMM CTR
SARZOTTI PARK
ALISO ST
MATILIJA ST
FULTON ST
PAULINE ST
RAYMOND ST
EMILY ST
SUMMER
EUCALYPTUS
QUAIL OAKS DR
BLANCHE ST
VENTURA ST
CANADA ST
OAK ST
FRANKLIN DR
LION ST
RANCHO CT
RANCHO DR
MEINERS RD
MONTANA RD
MONTANA CIR
EL TORO RD
TORO
N TICO RD
SIERRA
CHICO RD
BRISTOL RD
MALLORY WY
RINCON ST
W MATILIJA
LAUREL SPRINGS HS
MUS
LIB
E OJAI AV
PARK & RIDE
SKATEPARK
PO
E TOPA TOPA ST
FOX ST
BALD ST
PEARL ST
OLIVE MILL LN
S FULTON ST
BRYANT PL
BRYANT ST
LIBBEY PARK
WILLOW ST
S SIGNAL ST
PS
MONTGOMERY
PIRIE CREEK
POPE LN
BRYANT CIR
SADDLE LN
BUCKBOARD LN
LONGHORN LN
S VENTURA ST
OAK CREEK LN
CH
SANTA ANA
CRESTVIEW DR
SAN ANTONIO ST
COUNTRY CLUB DR
OJAI VALLEY INN AND SPA
COUNTRY CLUB DR
ROTARY COMM PK
W OJAI AV
OJAI VLY HS
JR HS
PASEO
CUYAMA RD
NORDHOFF CEM
BONITA DR
VERANO DR
CUYAMA
OAKMORE ST
CHURCH RD
OJAI VALLEY COMMUNITY HOSP
H
CARILLO RD
CREEKSIDE WY
HWY
PIRIE RD
DESCANSO AV
NORDHOFF HS
33
150
S RANCHO DR
MINO DR
SAINT THOMAS DR
CHRISTOPHER LN
CANTERBURY CT
SYCAMORE LN
JUNIPER LN
ASH LN
SHADY LN
0 .125 .25 .375 .5 miles 1 in. = 1900 ft.

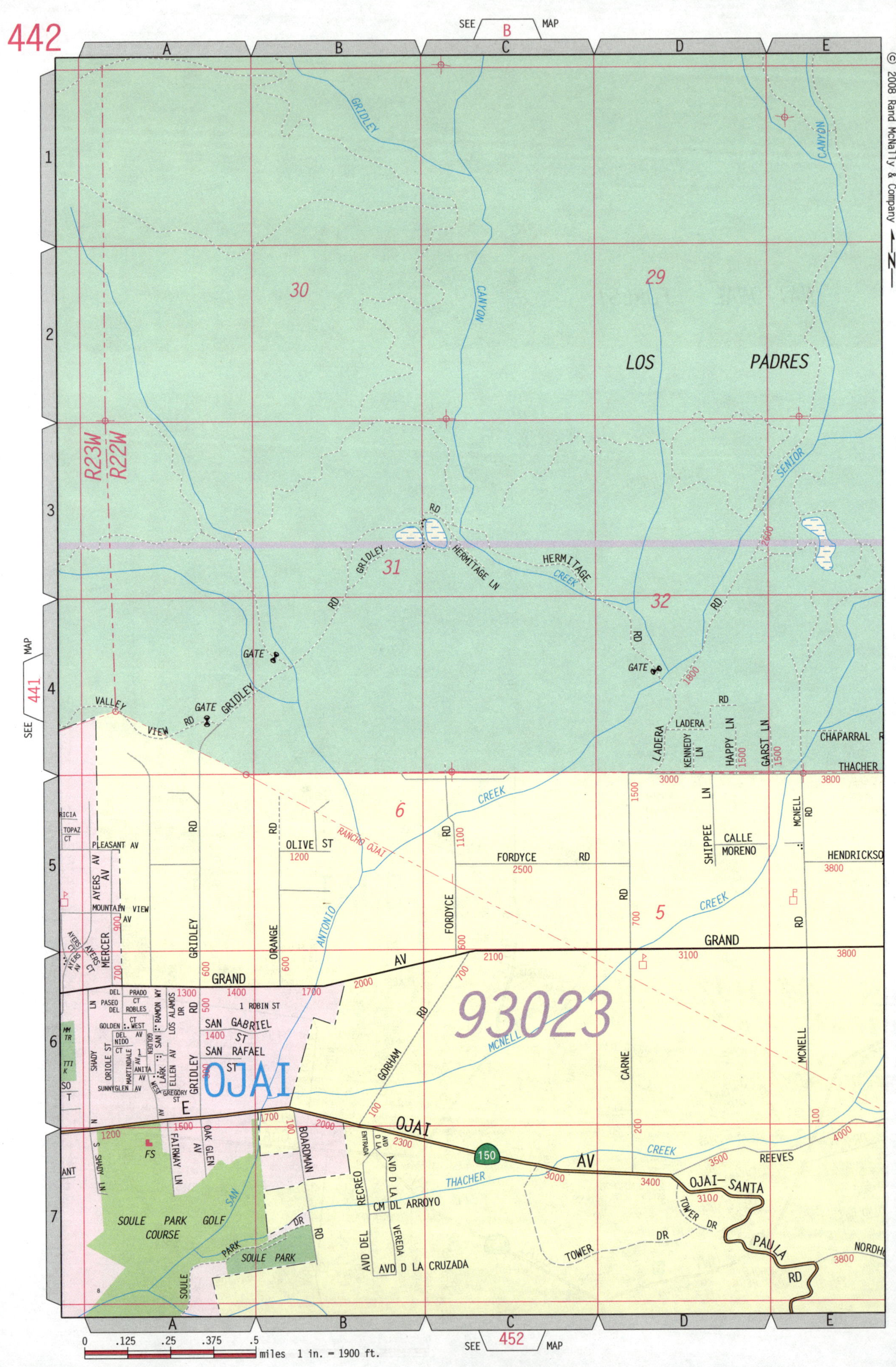

SEE B MAP
SEE 441 MAP
SEE 452 MAP
LOS PADRES
OJAI
93023
GRIDLEY CANYON
SENIOR CANYON
HERMITAGE CREEK
HERMITAGE LN
GRIDLEY RD
VALLEY VIEW RD
GATE
R23W
R22W
LADERA RD
KENNEDY LN
HAPPY LN
GARST LN
CHAPARRAL RD
THACHER RD
MCNELL RD
FORDYCE RD
GRAND AV
OJAI AV
OJAI-SANTA PAULA RD
REEVES CREEK
THACHER CREEK
SAN ANTONIO CREEK
MCNELL CREEK
SHIPPEE LN
CALLE MORENO
HENDRICKSON
CARNE RD
GORHAM RD
ORANGE RD
OLIVE ST
PLEASANT AV
AYERS AV
MOUNTAIN VIEW AV
MERCER AV
SAN GABRIEL ST
SAN RAFAEL ST
ROBIN ST
LOS ALAMOS DR
BOARDMAN RD
TOWER DR
NORDHOFF
SOULE PARK GOLF COURSE
SOULE PARK
FAIRWAY LN
OAK GLEN AV
AVD DEL RECREO
CM DL ARROYO
AVD D LA VEREDA
AVD D LA CRUZADA
FS
150

0 .125 .25 .375 .5 miles 1 in. = 1900 ft.

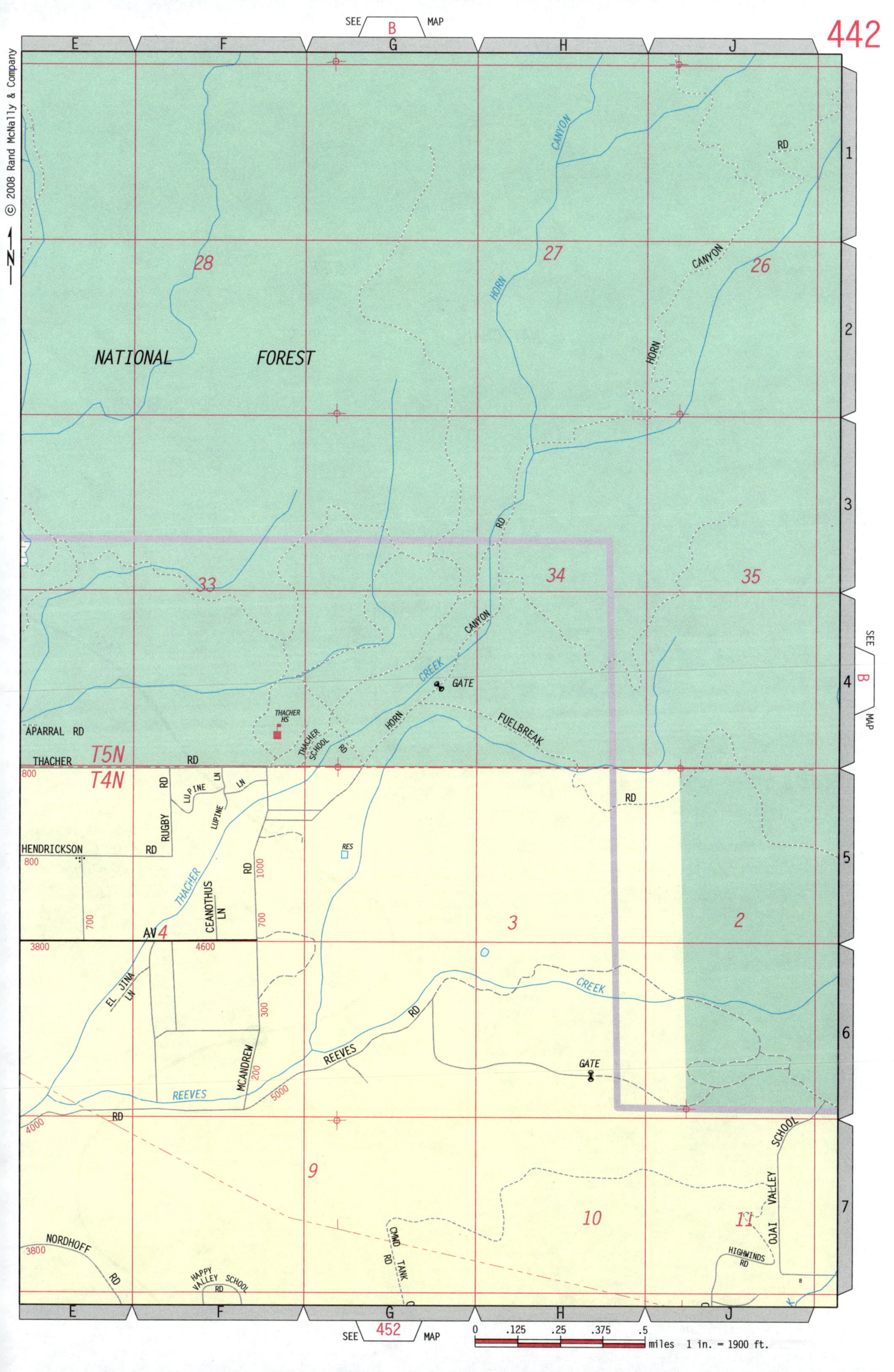

SEE B MAP
E
F
G
H
J
1
2
3
4
5
6
7
CANYON
RD
28
27
26
HORN
CANYON
NATIONAL
FOREST
HORN
33
34
35
RD
CANYON
CREEK
GATE
HORN
FUELBREAK
THACHER HS
THACHER SCHOOL RD
APARRAL RD
THACHER
RD
T5N
T4N
800
RUGBY RD
LUPINE LN
LN
LUPINE
HENDRICKSON
RD
800
RES
THACHER
CEANOTHUS LN
RD
1000
700
700
AV
4
3
2
3800
4600
EL JINA LN
CREEK
300
RD
REEVES
MCANDREW
200
GATE
REEVES
5000
RD
4000
SCHOOL
9
VALLEY
OJAI
10
11
NORDHOFF RD
3800
CMWD TANK RD
HIGHWINDS RD
HAPPY VALLEY SCHOOL RD
SEE B MAP
SEE 452 MAP
0 .125 .25 .375 .5
miles 1 in. = 1900 ft.

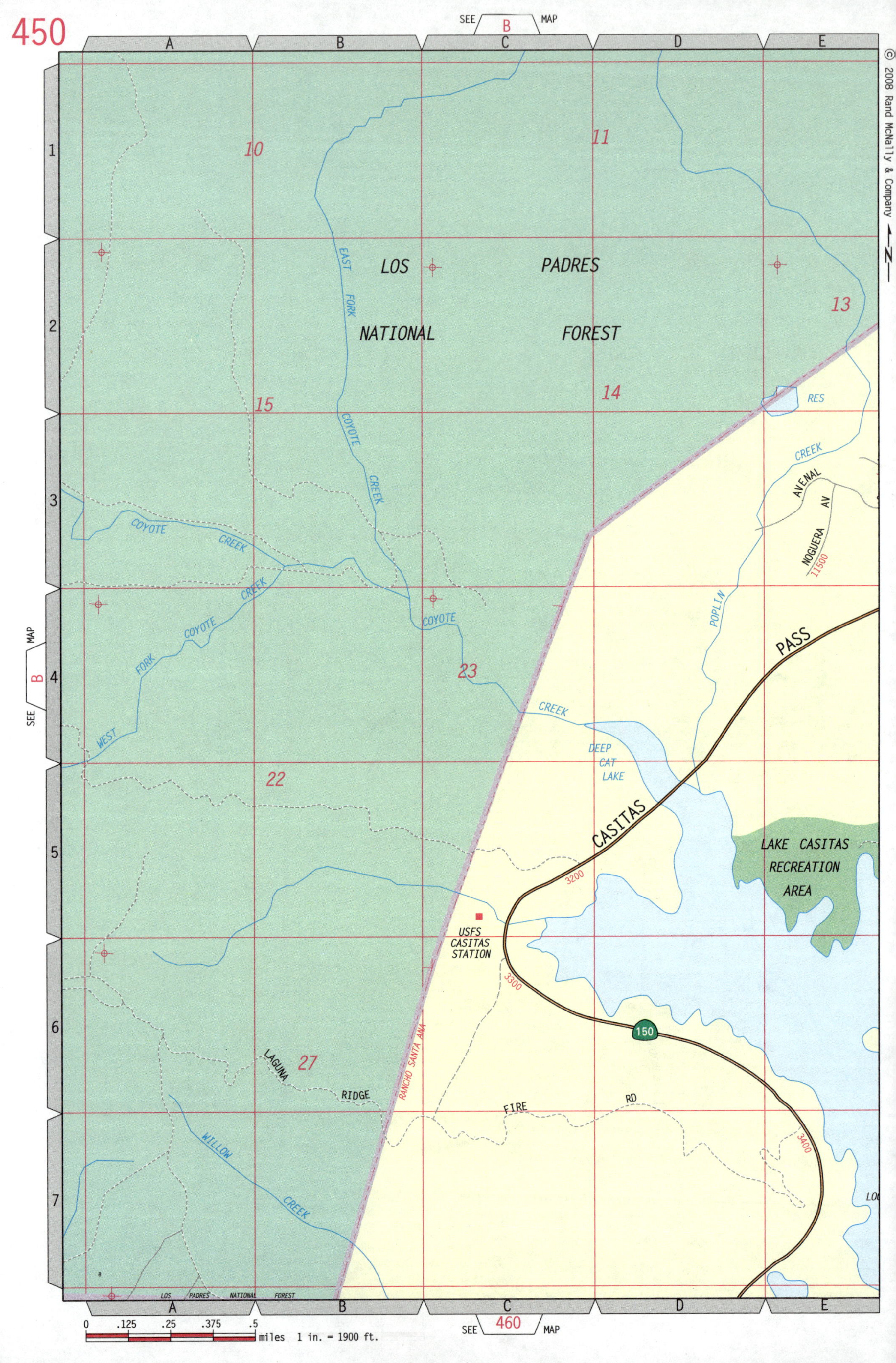
SEE B MAP
A
B
C
D
E
1
2
3
4
5
6
7
10
11
13
14
15
22
23
27
LOS
PADRES
NATIONAL
FOREST
EAST FORK
COYOTE CREEK
COYOTE CREEK
WEST FORK COYOTE CREEK
COYOTE CREEK
RES
CREEK
AVENAL
NOGUERA AV
11500
POPLIN
PASS
CASITAS
DEEP CAT LAKE
LAKE CASITAS RECREATION AREA
3200
USFS CASITAS STATION
3300
150
3400
RANCHO SANTA ANA
LAGUNA RIDGE
FIRE RD
WILLOW CREEK
LOS PADRES NATIONAL FOREST
SEE B MAP
SEE 460 MAP
0 .125 .25 .375 .5
miles 1 in. = 1900 ft.

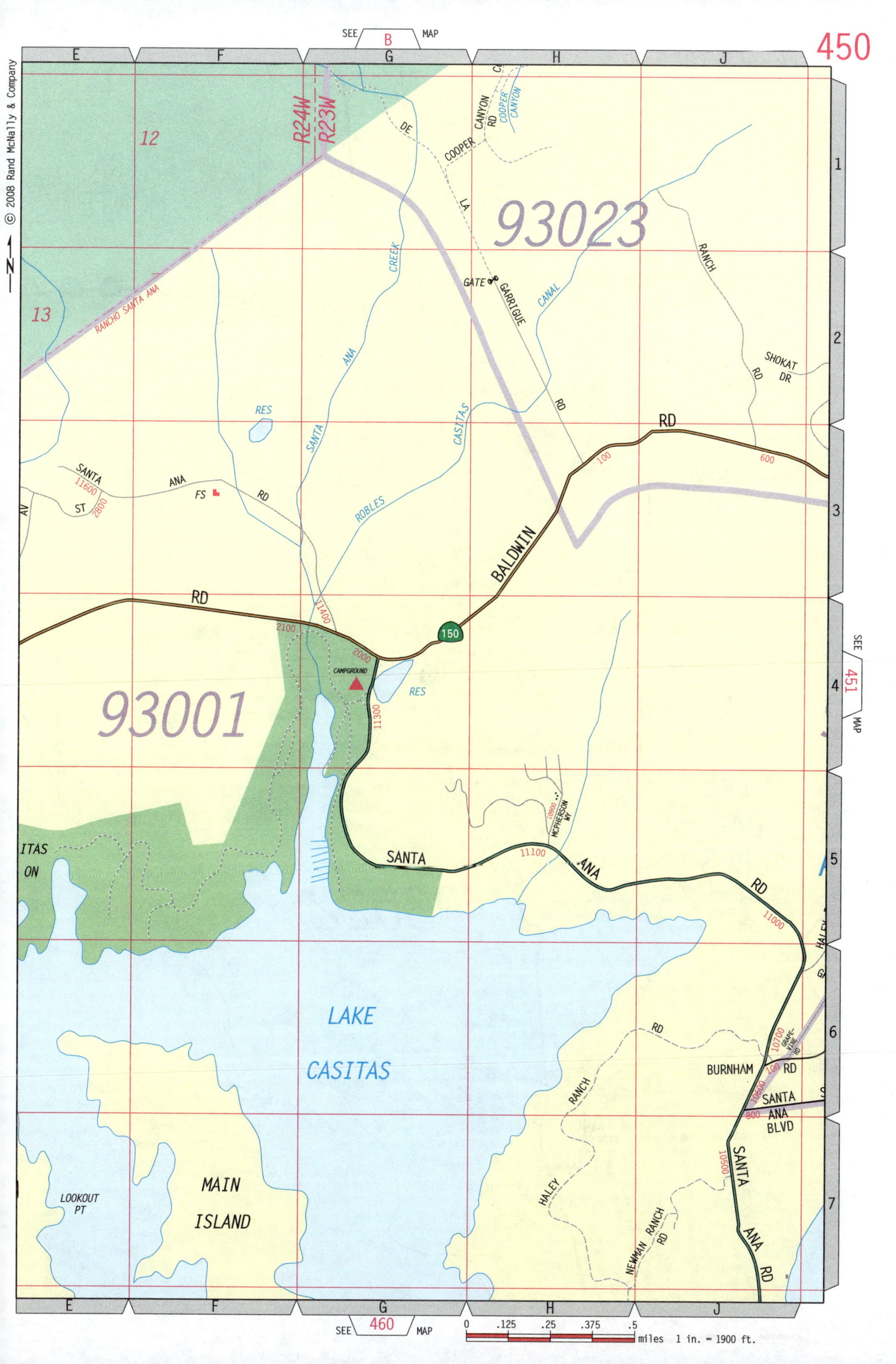
SEE B MAP
E
F
G
H
J
12
13
R24W
R23W
93023
93001
DE
COOPER
LA
COOPER CANYON RD
COOPER CANYON
GATE
GARRIGUE
RD
CANAL
RANCH
SHOKAT DR
RD
RANCHO SANTA ANA
SANTA ANA CREEK
RES
CASITAS
ROBLES
SANTA
11600
ST
2800
ANA
FS
RD
AV
RD
100
600
BALDWIN
RD
2100
11400
150
2000
CAMPGROUND
RES
11300
MCPHERSON WY
10900
SANTA
11100
ANA
RD
11000
ITAS
ON
LAKE
CASITAS
MAIN
ISLAND
LOOKOUT
PT
RD
RANCH
HALEY
NEWMAN RANCH RD
BURNHAM
100
RD
10700
GRAPE-VINE RD
10600
SANTA
800
ANA
BLVD
10500
SANTA
ANA
RD
1
2
3
4
5
6
7
SEE 451 MAP
SEE 460 MAP
0 .125 .25 .375 .5 miles 1 in. = 1900 ft.

SEE 441 MAP

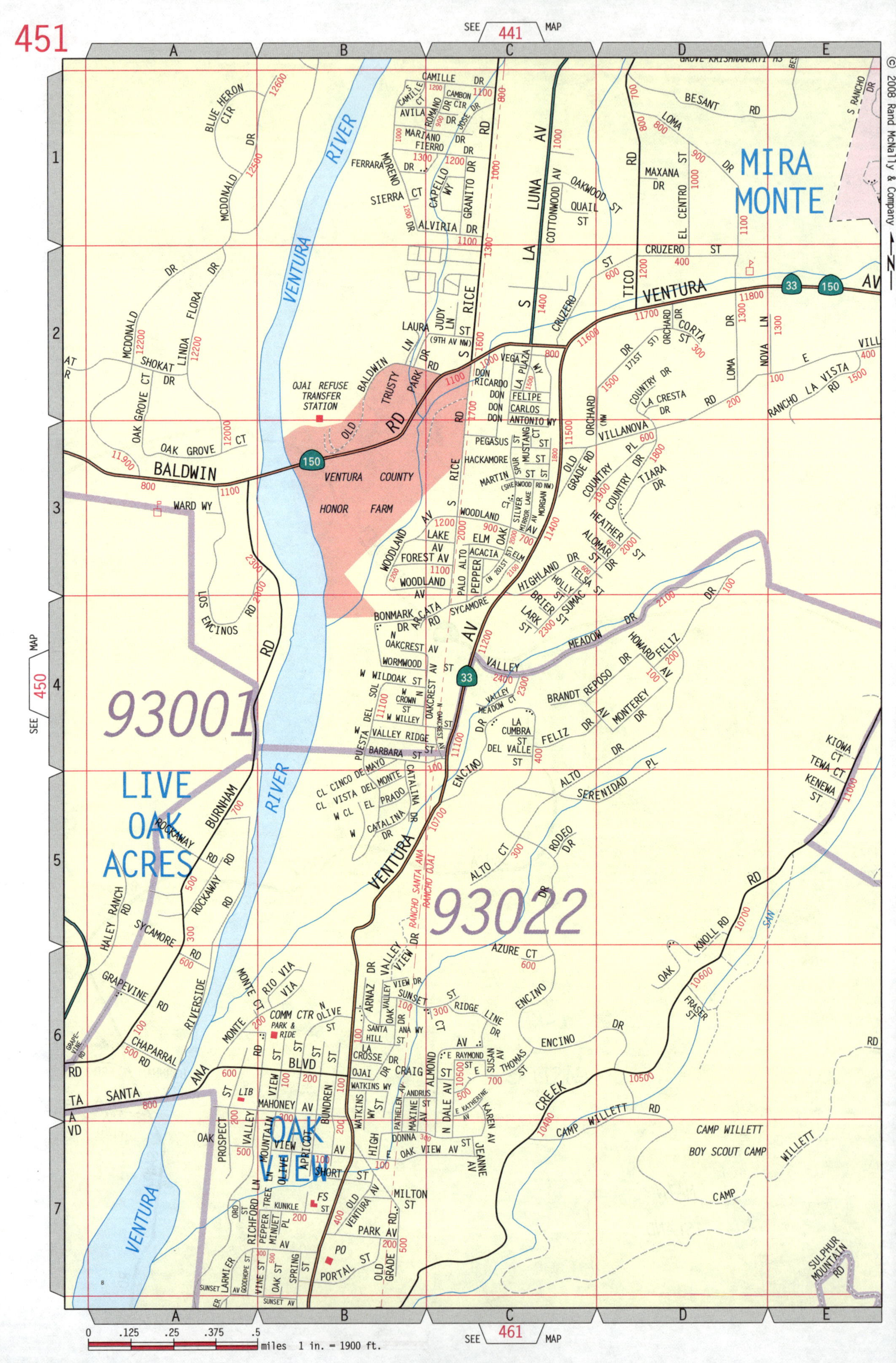

MIRA MONTE
LIVE OAK ACRES
OAK VIEW
93001
93022
VENTURA RIVER
VENTURA COUNTY HONOR FARM
OJAI REFUSE TRANSFER STATION
CAMP WILLETT BOY SCOUT CAMP
BALDWIN RD
VENTURA AV
S RICE RD
S LA LUNA AV
BLUE HERON CIR
MCDONALD DR
LINDA FLORA DR
SHOKAT DR
OAK GROVE CT
WARD WY
LOS ENCINOS RD
BURNHAM RD
ROCKAWAY RD
HALEY RANCH RD
SYCAMORE RD
GRAPEVINE RD
CHAPARRAL RD
RIVERSIDE RD
SANTA ANA BLVD
CREEK RD
CAMP WILLETT RD
VALLEY MEADOW DR
ENCINO DR
SERENIDAD PL
ALTO DR
AZURE CT
OAK KNOLL RD
SULPHUR MOUNTAIN RD
CRUZERO ST
BESANT RD
LOMA DR
MAXANA DR
EL CENTRO ST
TICO RD
VILLANOVA RD
COUNTRY DR
RANCHO LA VISTA RD
OLD GRADE RD
HIGHLAND DR
MEADOW DR
REPOSO DR
FELIZ DR
MONTEREY DR
KIOWA CT
TEWA CT
KENEWA ST
LIB
FS
PO
PARK & RIDE
COMM CTR

SEE 450 MAP

SEE 461 MAP

0 .125 .25 .375 .5 miles 1 in. = 1900 ft.

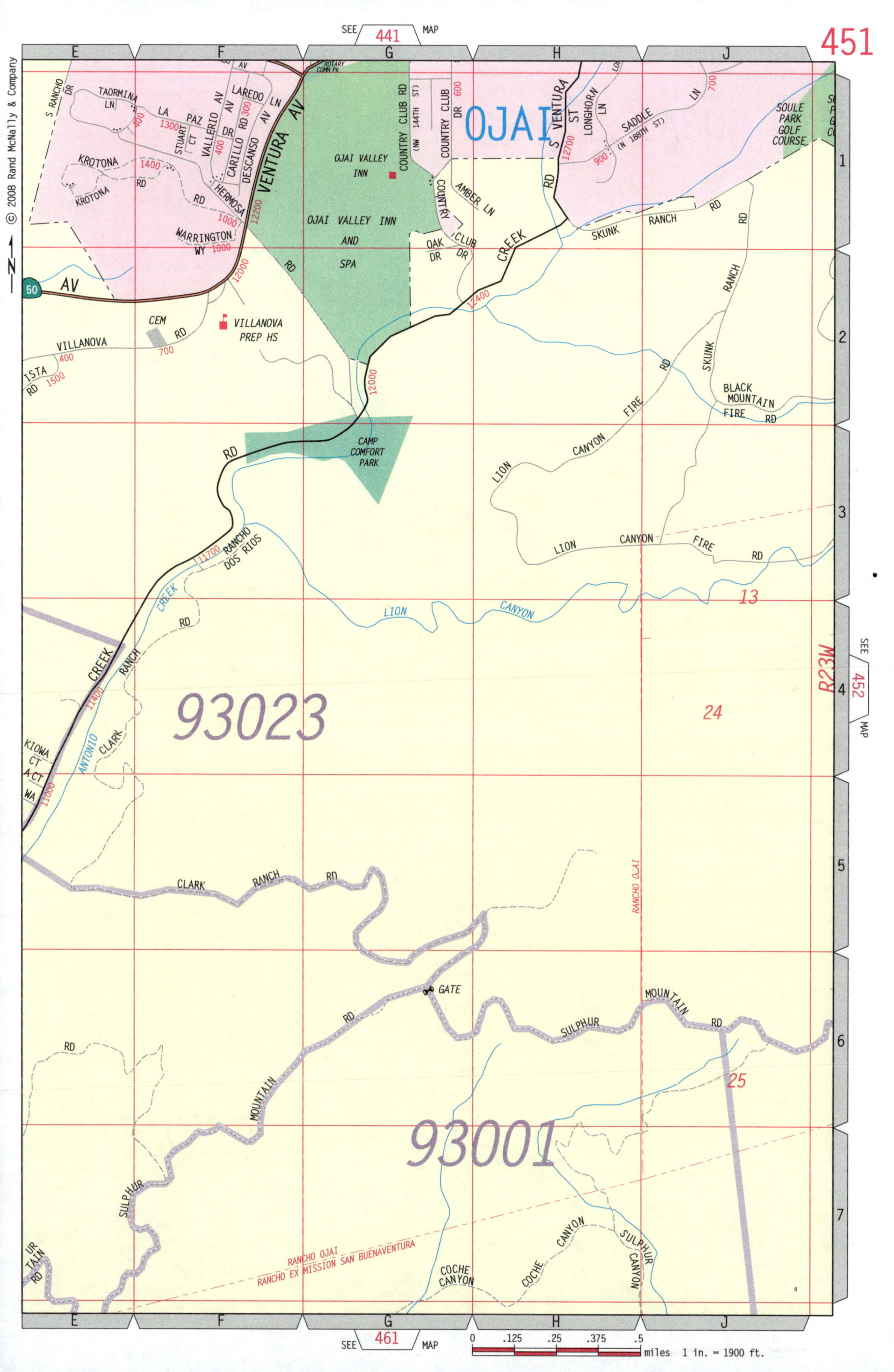

SEE 441 MAP
E
F
G
H
J
OJAI
VENTURA AV
S VENTURA ST
S RANCHO DR
TAORMINA LN
LA PAZ
LAREDO LN
VALLERIO AV
STUART CT
CARILLO RD
DESCANSO AV
HERMOSA RD
KROTONA
KROTONA RD
WARRINGTON WY
COUNTRY CLUB RD
(NW 144TH ST)
COUNTRY CLUB DR
OJAI VALLEY INN
OJAI VALLEY INN AND SPA
ROTARY COMM PK
AMBER LN
OAK DR
COUNTRY CLUB DR
LONGHORN LN
SADDLE LN
(N 188TH ST)
SOULE PARK GOLF COURSE
SKUNK RANCH RD
CREEK RD
50
AV
CEM RD
VILLANOVA PREP HS
VILLANOVA
ISTA RD
BLACK MOUNTAIN FIRE RD
LION CANYON FIRE RD
CAMP COMFORT PARK
RANCHO DOS RIOS
CREEK
LION CANYON
13
24
R23W
SEE 452 MAP
93023
CREEK RANCH RD
ANTONIO
CLARK
KIOWA CT
ACT
WA
RANCHO OJAI
CLARK RANCH RD
GATE
MOUNTAIN
SULPHUR MOUNTAIN RD
25
93001
SULPHUR
COCHE CANYON
SULPHUR CANYON
RANCHO OJAI
RANCHO EX MISSION SAN BUENAVENTURA
1
2
3
4
5
6
7

0 .125 .25 .375 .5 miles 1 in. = 1900 ft.

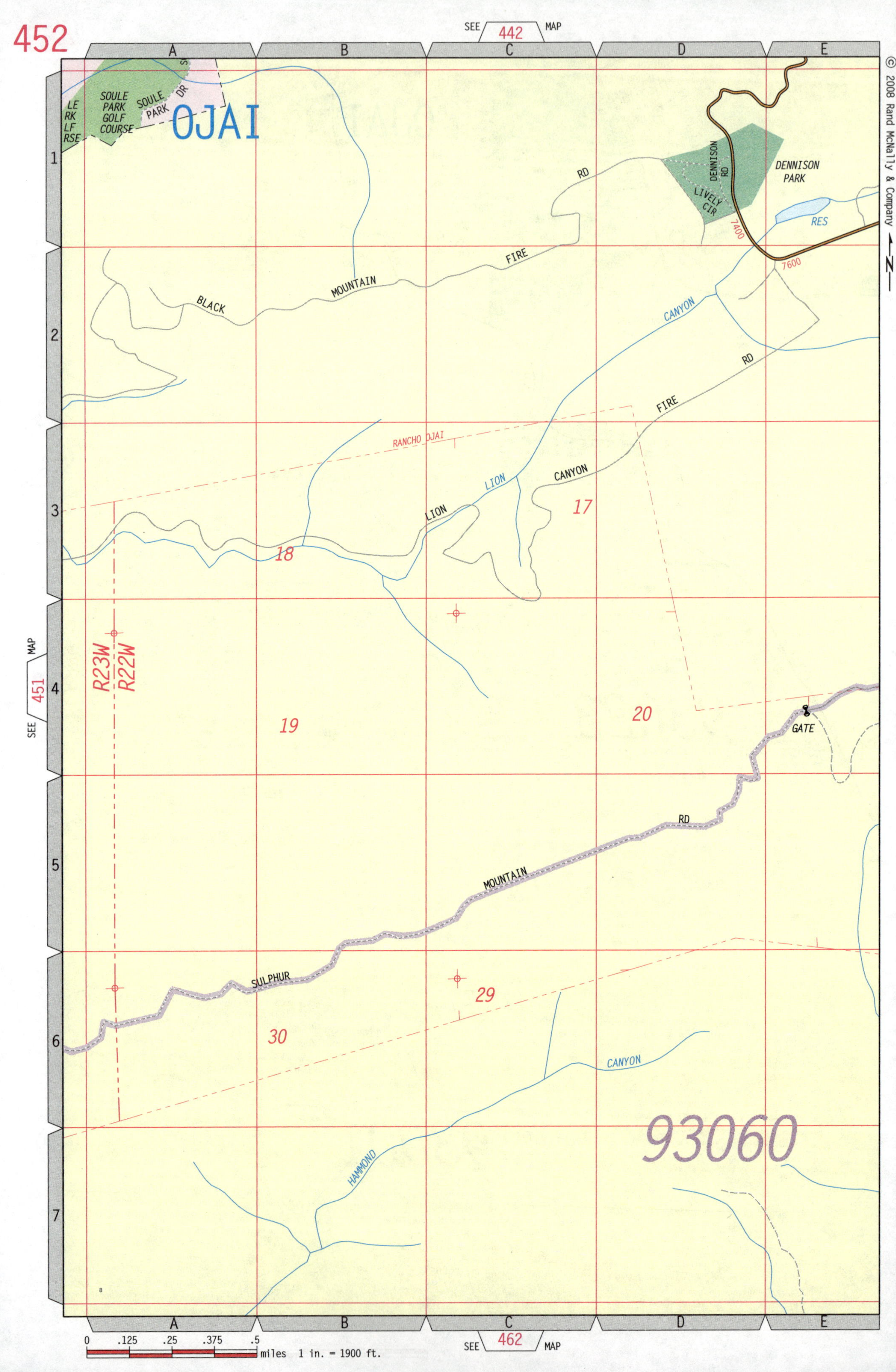
SEE 442 MAP
SOULE PARK GOLF COURSE
SOULE PARK DR
OJAI
DENNISON PARK
DENNISON RD
LIVELY CIR
RES
7400
7600
RD
BLACK MOUNTAIN FIRE
CANYON
RD
FIRE
RANCHO OJAI
CANYON
LION
LION
17
18
R23W
R22W
SEE 451 MAP
19
20
GATE
RD
MOUNTAIN
SULPHUR
29
30
CANYON
HAMMOND
93060
SEE 462 MAP
0 .125 .25 .375 .5
miles 1 in. = 1900 ft.

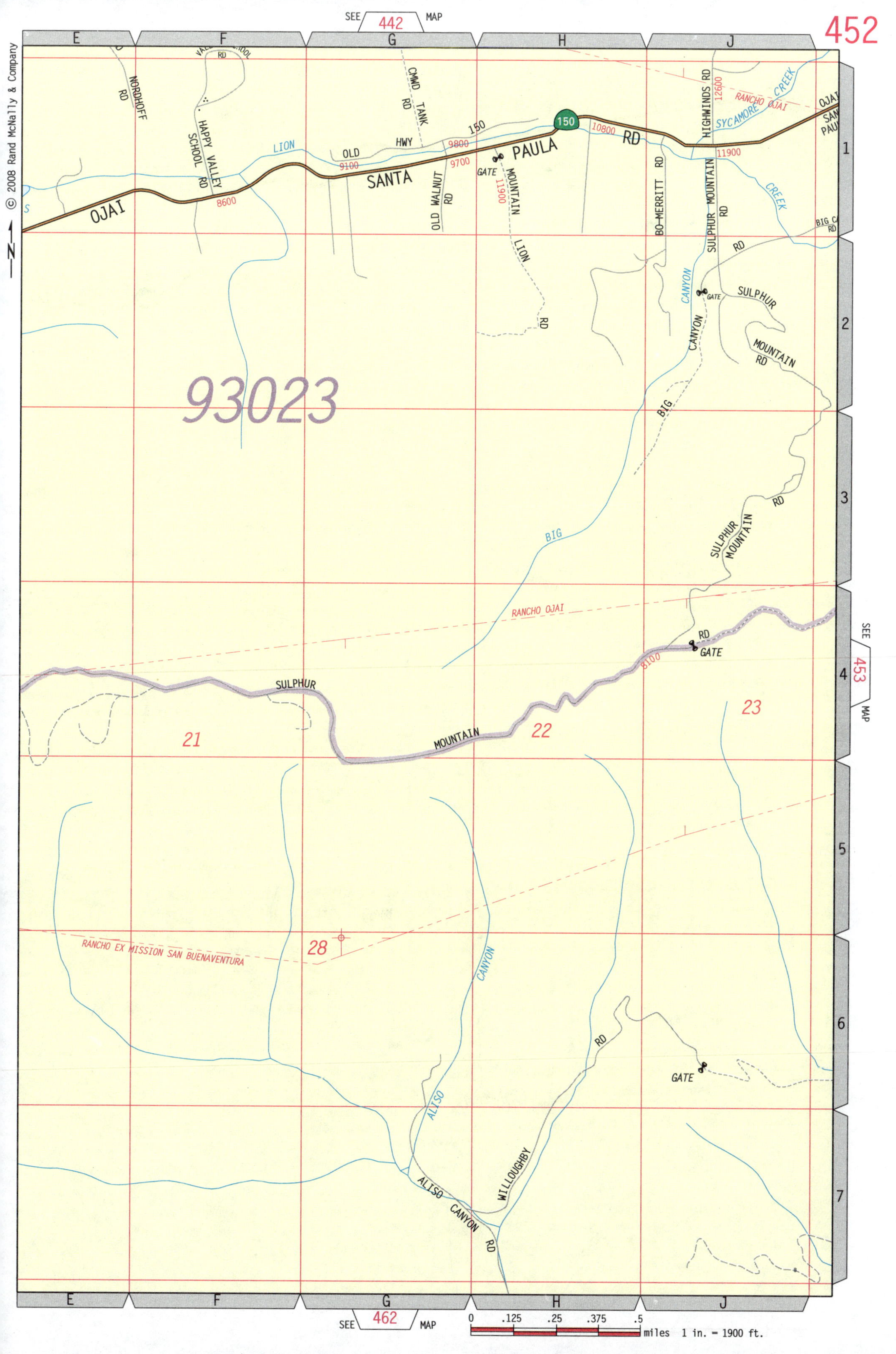
SEE 442 MAP
E
F
G
H
J
NORDHOFF RD
HAPPY VALLEY SCHOOL RD
CMWD TANK RD
OLD HWY 150
LION
9100
9800
9700
SANTA PAULA RD
OJAI
8600
150
10800
GATE
MOUNTAIN
11900
LION RD
OLD WALNUT RD
BO-MERRITT RD
HIGHWINDS RD
12600
RANCHO OJAI
SYCAMORE CREEK
SULPHUR MOUNTAIN RD
11900
CREEK
BIG CANYON RD
CANYON
GATE
SULPHUR MOUNTAIN RD
93023
BIG
SULPHUR MOUNTAIN RD
RANCHO OJAI
RD
GATE
8100
SULPHUR
MOUNTAIN
21
22
23
SEE 453 MAP
RANCHO EX MISSION SAN BUENAVENTURA
28
CANYON
RD
GATE
ALISO
WILLOUGHBY
ALISO CANYON RD
1
2
3
4
5
6
7
SEE 462 MAP
0 .125 .25 .375 .5 miles 1 in. = 1900 ft.

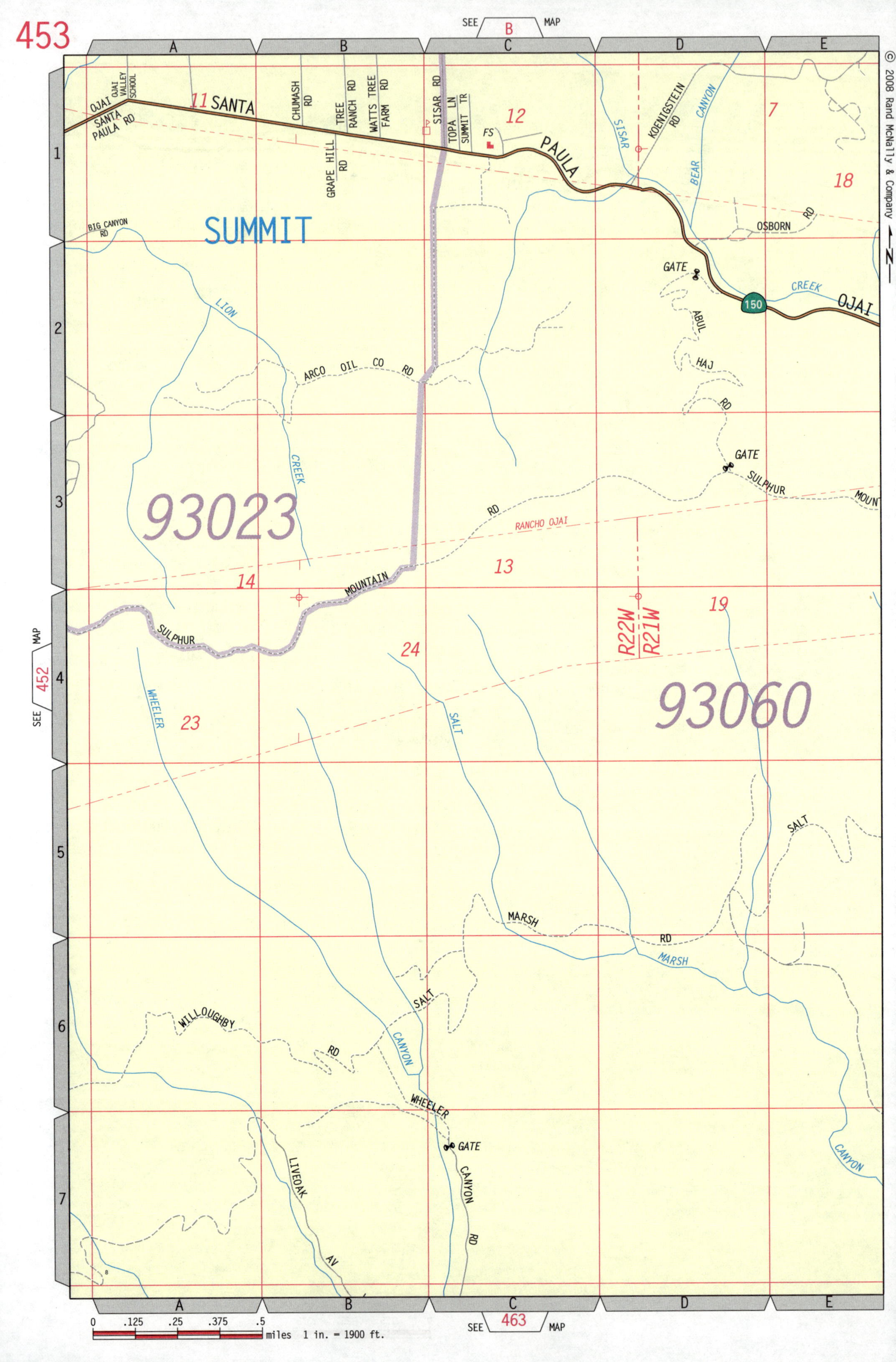

SEE B MAP
A
B
C
D
E
1
2
3
4
5
6
7
OJAI
OJAI VALLEY SCHOOL
SANTA PAULA RD
11
SANTA
CHUMASH RD
TREE RANCH RD
WATTS TREE FARM RD
GRAPE HILL RD
SISAR RD
TOPA LN
SUMMIT TR
12
FS
PAULA
SISAR
KOENIGSTEIN RD
BEAR
CANYON
7
18
OSBORN
RD
BIG CANYON RD
SUMMIT
GATE
CREEK
OJAI
150
LION
ABUL
HAJ
RD
ARCO OIL CO RD
CREEK
GATE
SULPHUR
MOUNT
93023
RD
RANCHO OJAI
13
14
MOUNTAIN
SULPHUR
19
R22W
R21W
24
SEE 452 MAP
WHEELER
SALT
93060
23
SALT
MARSH
RD
MARSH
SALT
WILLOUGHBY
RD
CANYON
WHEELER
GATE
LIVEOAK AV
CANYON RD
CANYON

SEE 463 MAP

0 .125 .25 .375 .5 miles 1 in. = 1900 ft.

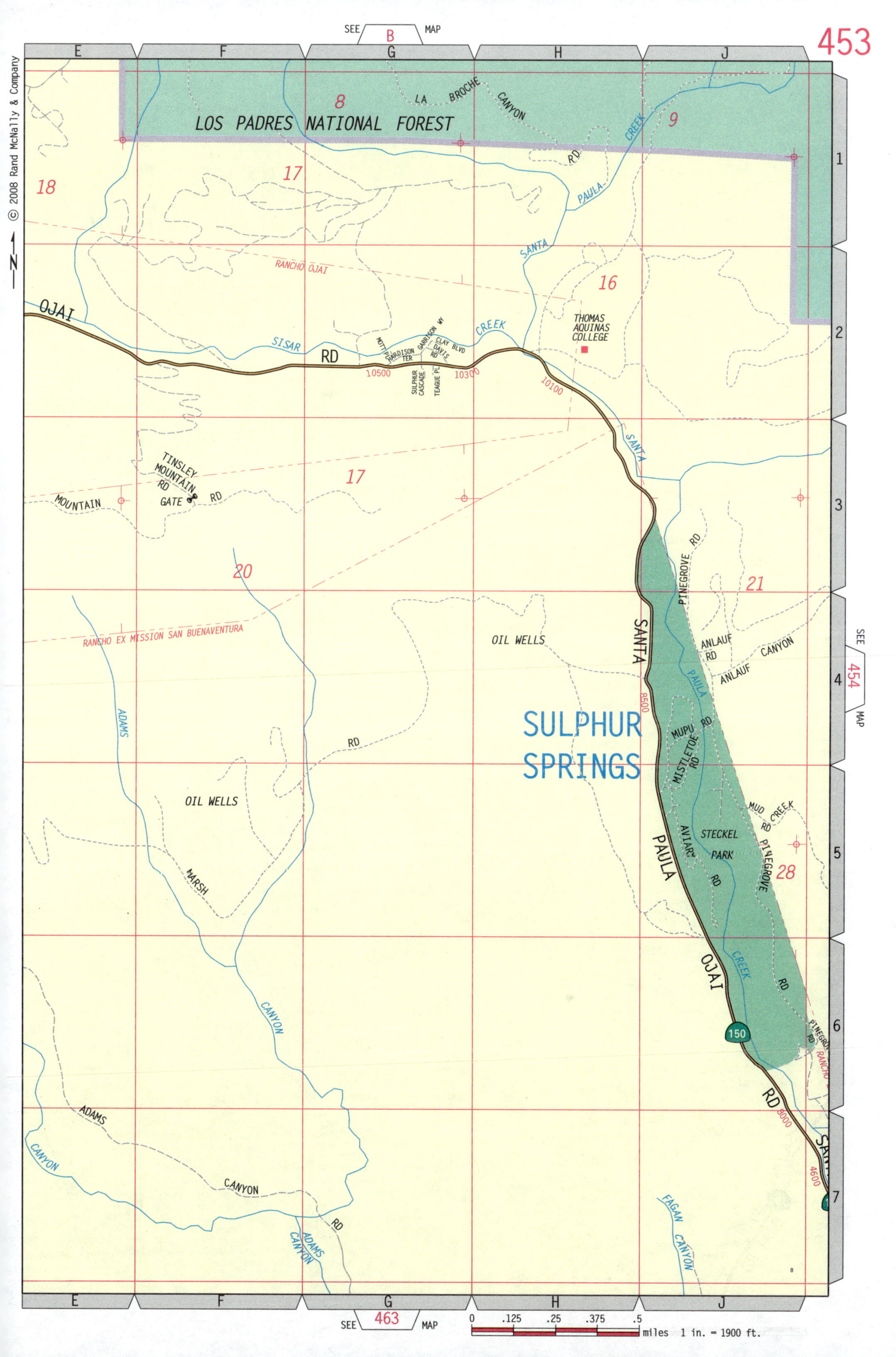

SEE B MAP
E
F
G
H
J
LOS PADRES NATIONAL FOREST
8
9
LA BROCHE CANYON RD
PAULA CREEK
SANTA
18
17
RANCHO OJAI
16
THOMAS AQUINAS COLLEGE
OJAI
SISAR CREEK
RD
MOTT PL
HARDISON TER
GARRISON WY
CLAY BLVD
DAVIS RD
SULPHUR CASCADE
TEAGUE PL
10500
10300
10100
SANTA
TINSLEY MOUNTAIN RD
MOUNTAIN
GATE
RD
17
20
PINEGROVE RD
21
RANCHO EX MISSION SAN BUENAVENTURA
OIL WELLS
SANTA
ANLAUF RD
ANLAUF CANYON
PAULA
8500
ADAMS
SULPHUR SPRINGS
MUPU RD
MISTLETOE RD
RD
OIL WELLS
MUD CREEK RD
AVIARY RD
STECKEL PARK
PINEGROVE
28
PAULA
MARSH
OJAI
CREEK
RD
CANYON
150
PINEGROVE RD
RANCHO
RD
8000
SANTA
4600
ADAMS
CANYON
CANYON
RD
ADAMS CANYON
CANYON
FAGAN CANYON
1
2
3
4
5
6
7
SEE 454 MAP
SEE 463 MAP
0 .125 .25 .375 .5 miles 1 in. = 1900 ft.

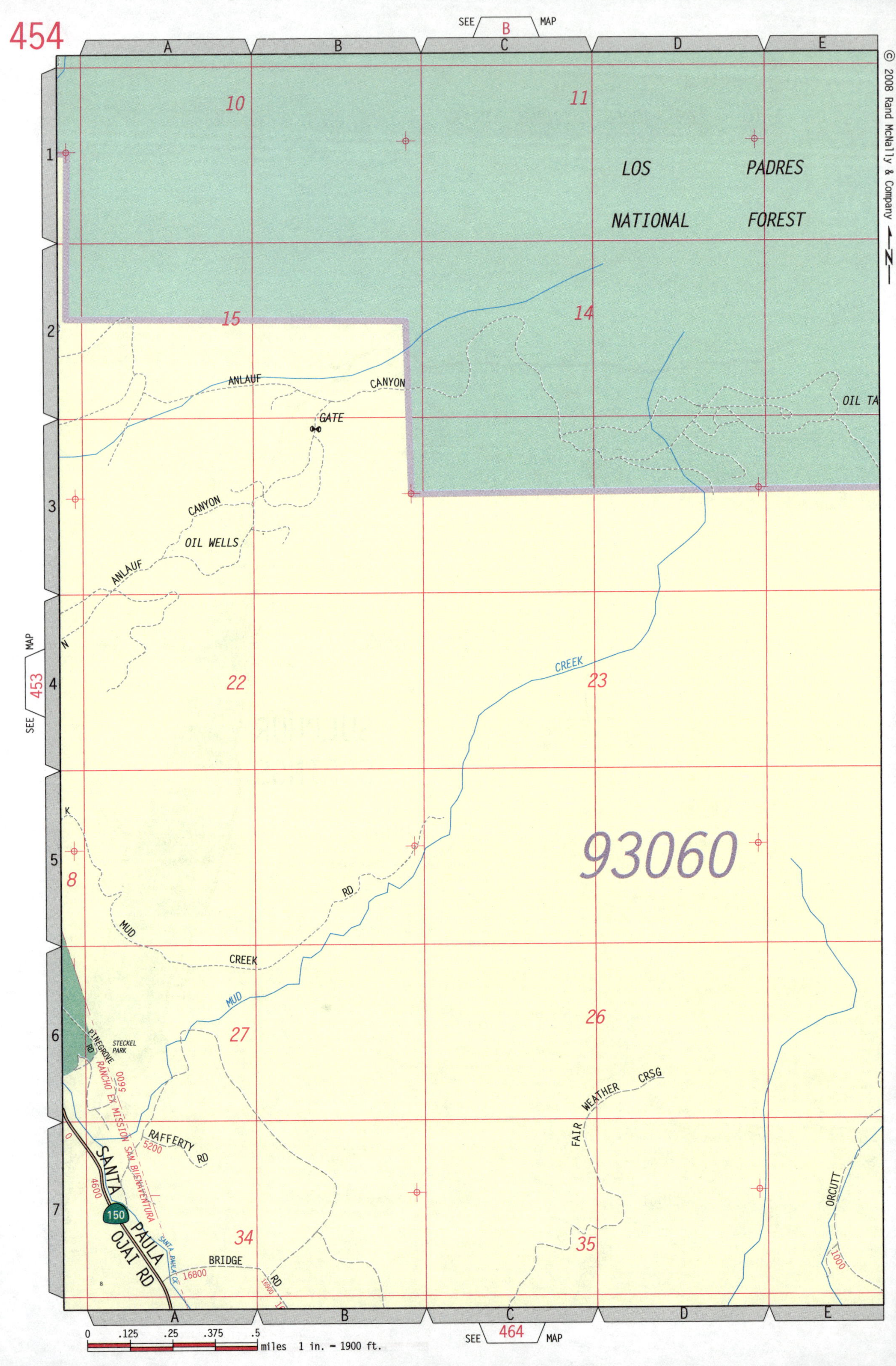

SEE B MAP
A
B
C
D
E
© 2008 Rand McNally & Company
10
11
LOS PADRES
NATIONAL FOREST
15
14
ANLAUF
CANYON
GATE
OIL TA
CANYON
OIL WELLS
ANLAUF
N
SEE 453 MAP
22
23
CREEK
K
8
93060
RD
MUD
CREEK
MUD
27
26
PINEGROVE RD
STECKEL PARK
RANCHO EX MISSION SAN BUENAVENTURA
5900
RAFFERTY RD
5200
FAIR WEATHER CRSG
SANTA PAULA OJAI RD
4600
150
SANTA PAULA CK
BRIDGE
16800
RD
16800
34
35
ORCUTT
1000
0 .125 .25 .375 .5
miles 1 in. = 1900 ft.
SEE 464 MAP

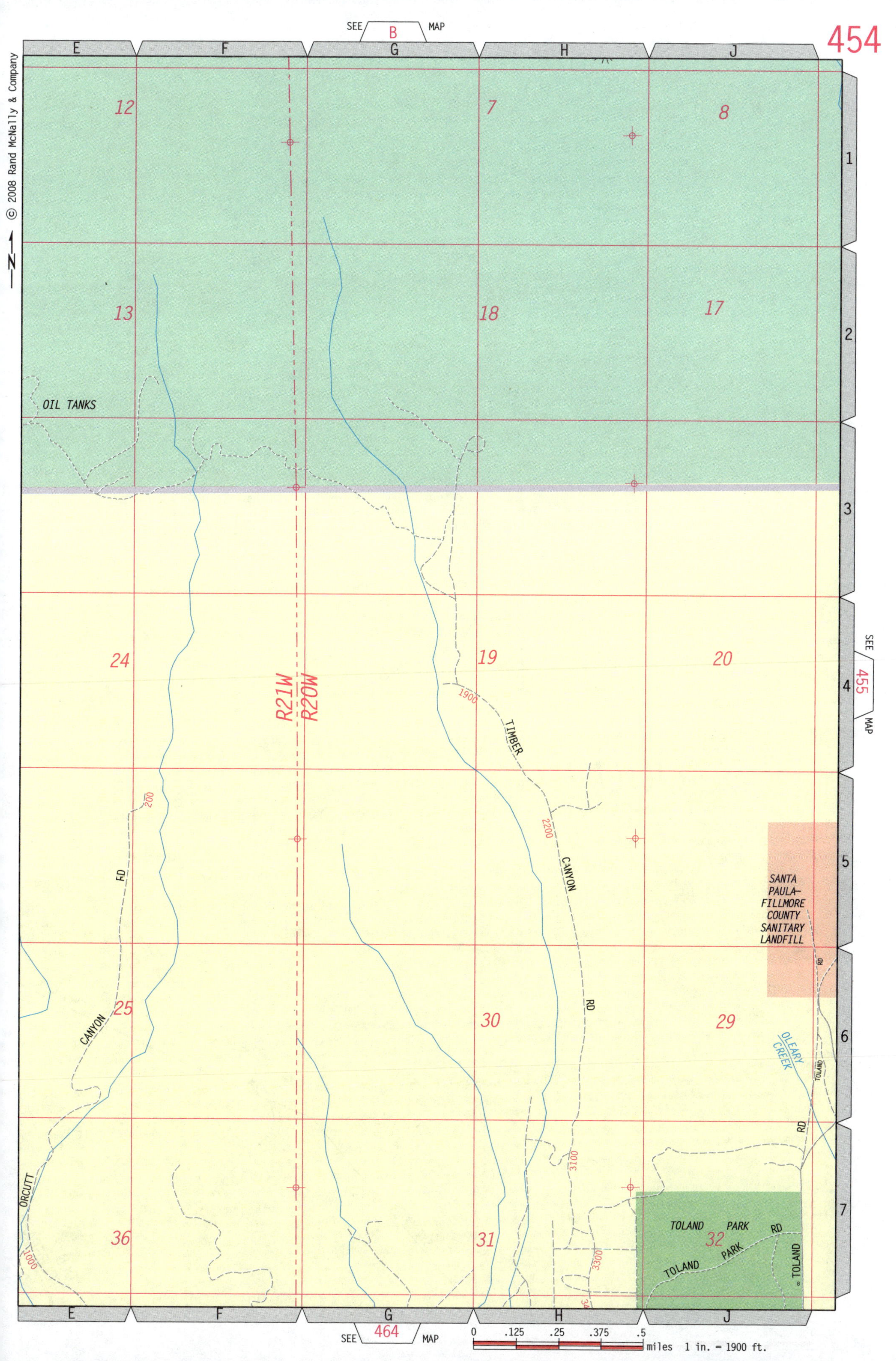

SEE B MAP
E
F
G
H
J
12
7
8
13
18
17
OIL TANKS
1
2
3
4
5
6
7
24
19
20
R21W
R20W
1900
TIMBER
CANYON
RD
2200
200
RD
SEE 455 MAP
SANTA PAULA-FILLMORE COUNTY SANITARY LANDFILL
CANYON
25
30
29
OLEARY CREEK
TOLAND
RD
ORCUTT
3100
TOLAND PARK RD
32
TOLAND PARK
TOLAND
36
31
1000
3300
SEE 464 MAP
0 .125 .25 .375 .5
miles 1 in. = 1900 ft.

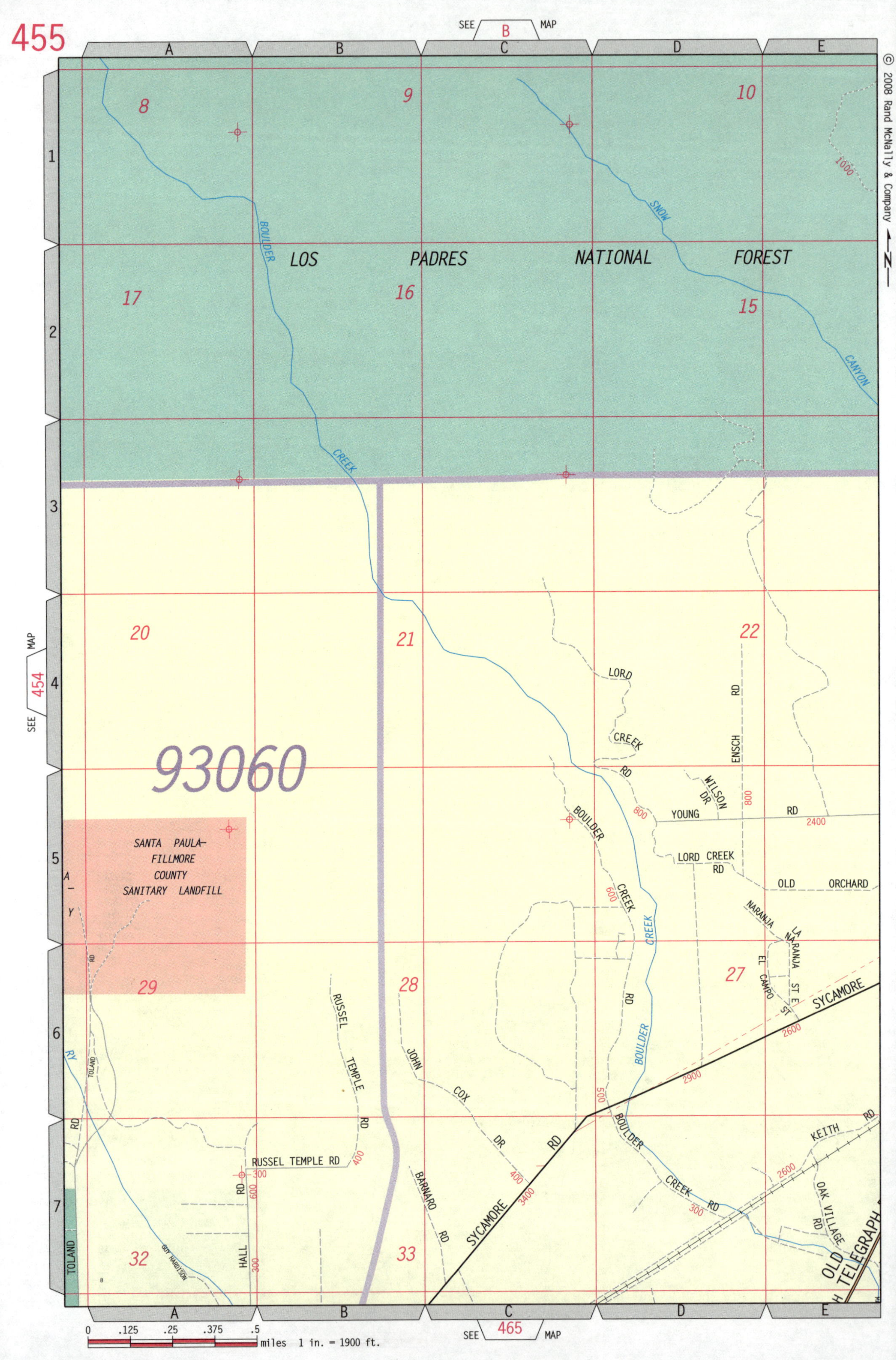

SEE B MAP
A
B
C
D
E
1
2
3
4
5
6
7
8
9
10
17
16
15
20
21
22
28
27
29
32
33
LOS PADRES NATIONAL FOREST
BOULDER
CREEK
SNOW
CANYON
1000
93060
SANTA PAULA-FILLMORE COUNTY SANITARY LANDFILL
LORD CREEK RD
ENSCH RD
WILSON DR
YOUNG RD
800
2400
BOULDER CREEK RD
LORD CREEK RD
OLD ORCHARD
600
NARANJA
LA NARANJA ST E
EL CAMPO ST
SYCAMORE
2600
2900
BOULDER
RUSSEL TEMPLE RD
JOHN COX DR
RUSSEL TEMPLE RD
400
300
600
500
HALL RD
300
BARNARO RD
SYCAMORE RD
3400
KEITH RD
OAK VILLAGE RD
OLD TELEGRAPH
TOLAND RD
TOLAND
GUY HARDISON
SEE 454 MAP
SEE 465 MAP
0 .125 .25 .375 .5 miles 1 in. = 1900 ft.

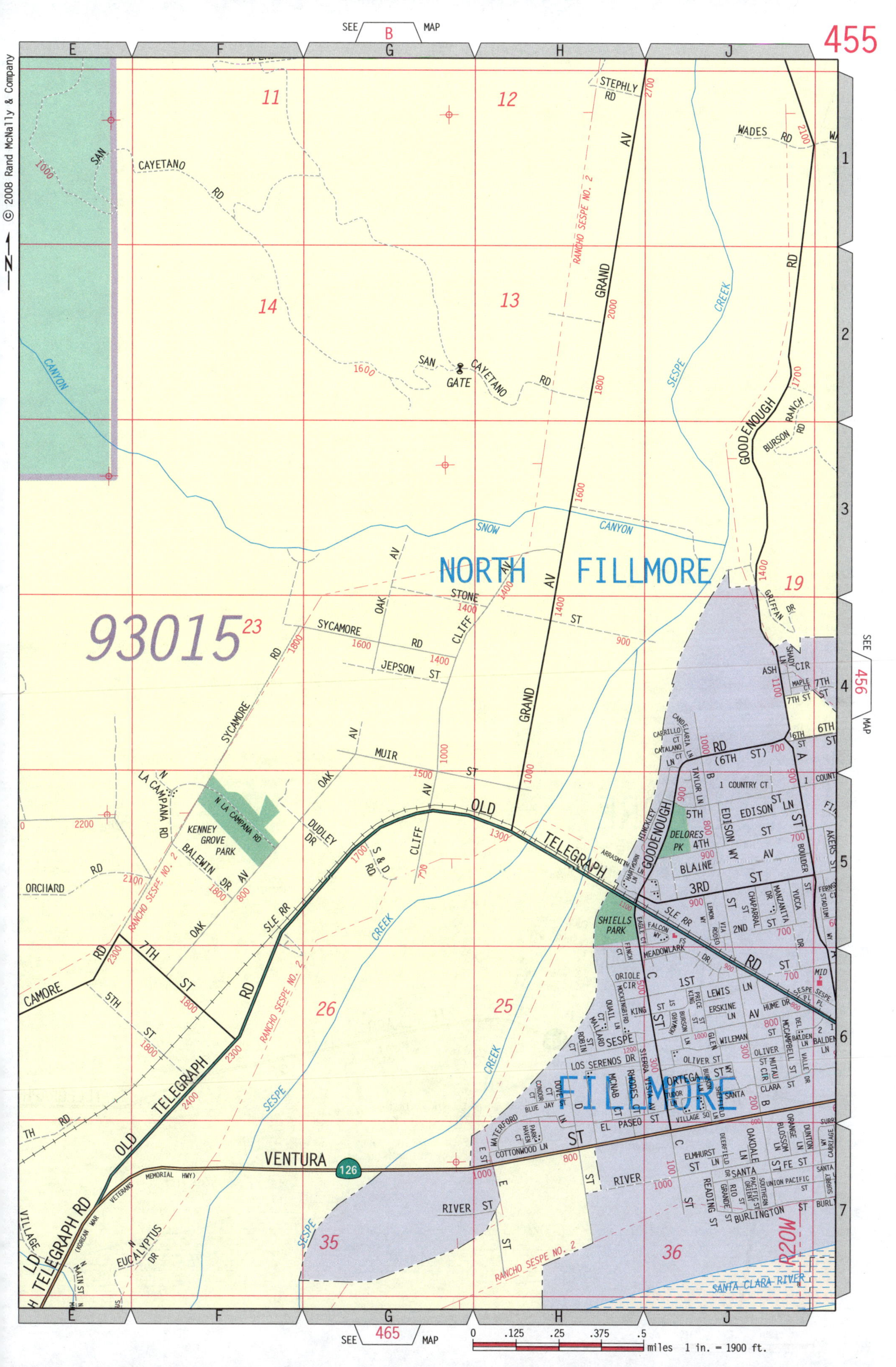

SEE B MAP
SEE 456 MAP
SEE 465 MAP
NORTH FILLMORE
FILLMORE
93015
GRAND AV
GOODENOUGH RD
SESPE CREEK
SNOW CANYON
CANYON
SAN CAYETANO RD
SAN CAYETANO GATE
STEPHLY RD
WADES RD
BURSON RANCH RD
GRIFFAN DR
STONE ST
SYCAMORE RD
JEPSON ST
OAK AV
CLIFF AV
MUIR ST
OLD TELEGRAPH RD
SLE RR
KENNEY GROVE PARK
N LA CAMPANA RD
BALEWIN DR
ORCHARD RD
DUDLEY DR
S & D RD
7TH ST
5TH ST
RANCHO SESPE NO. 2
VENTURA 126
VETERANS MEMORIAL HWY
(KOREAN WAR
TELEGRAPH RD
N EUCALYPTUS DR
VILLAGE
N MAIN ST
RIVER ST
E ST
SANTA CLARA RIVER
R20W
SHIELLS PARK
DELORES PK
EDISON ST
EDISON WY
BLAINE AV
3RD ST
2ND ST
1ST ST
4TH ST
5TH ST
6TH ST
SESPE AV
OLIVER ST
ORTEGA ST
SANTA CLARA ST
EL PASEO ST
LOS SERENOS DR
RIVER ST
SANTA FE ST
BURLINGTON ST
ELMHURST ST
OAKDALE LN
MEADOWLARK DR
WILEMAN ST
LEWIS LN
ERSKINE LN
HUME DR
BOULDER ST
MANZANITA DR
YUCCA DR
AKERS ST
ASH
SHADY LN
MAPLE CT
7TH ST
CIR
1 COUNTRY CT
TAYLOR LN
HINCKLEY
ARRASMITH
FALCON WY
EAGLE CT
FINCH CT
ORIOLE CIR
QUAIL LN
MOCKINGBIRD LN
KING ST
MALLARD CT
ROBIN CT
MCNAB CT
RHODES CT
SIERRA VISTA AV
CONDOR CT
BLUE JAY CT
DOVE LN
WATERFORD
PARK HAVEN CT
COTTONWOOD LN
1 in. = 1900 ft.
© 2008 Rand McNally & Company

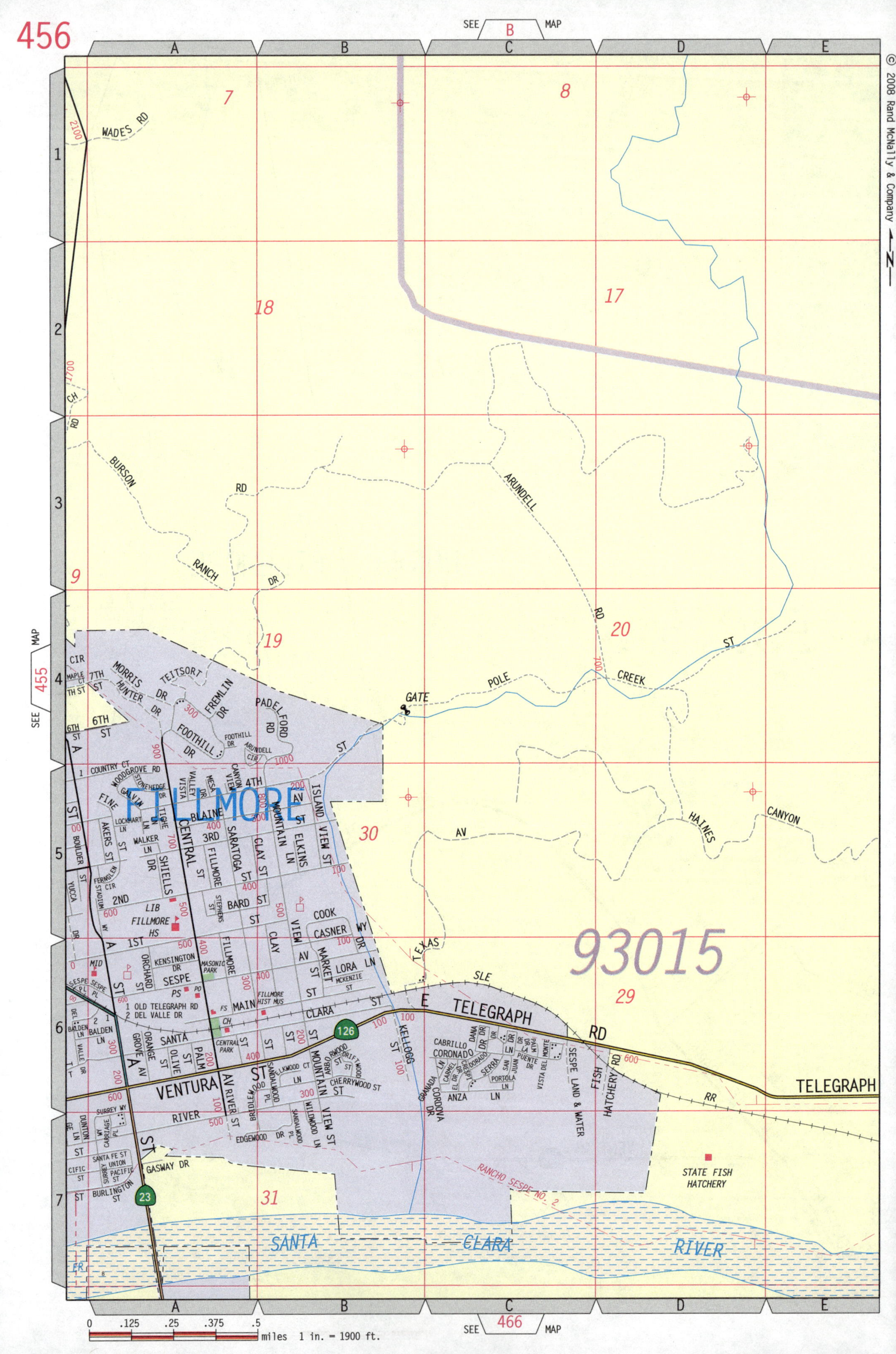
SEE B MAP
SEE 455 MAP
SEE 466 MAP
FILLMORE
93015
WADES RD
BURSON RANCH RD
DR
ARUNDELL RD
POLE CREEK ST
GATE
HAINES CANYON AV
TEXAS
SLE
E TELEGRAPH RD
TELEGRAPH
RR
STATE FISH HATCHERY
RANCHO SESPE NO. 2
SANTA CLARA RIVER
VENTURA ST
CENTRAL AV
A ST
RIVER ST
KELLOGG ST
MOUNTAIN VIEW ST
SESPE AV
SANTA CLARA ST
MAIN ST
FILLMORE HS
LIB
FILLMORE HIST MUS
MASONIC PARK
CENTRAL PARK
GASWAY DR
EDGEWOOD DR
FISH HATCHERY RD
SESPE LAND & WATER
CABRILLO
CORONADO
ANZA LN
SERRA
PORTOLA
CORDOVA DR
GRANADA
126
23
FR
© 2008 Rand McNally & Company
0 .125 .25 .375 .5 miles 1 in. = 1900 ft.

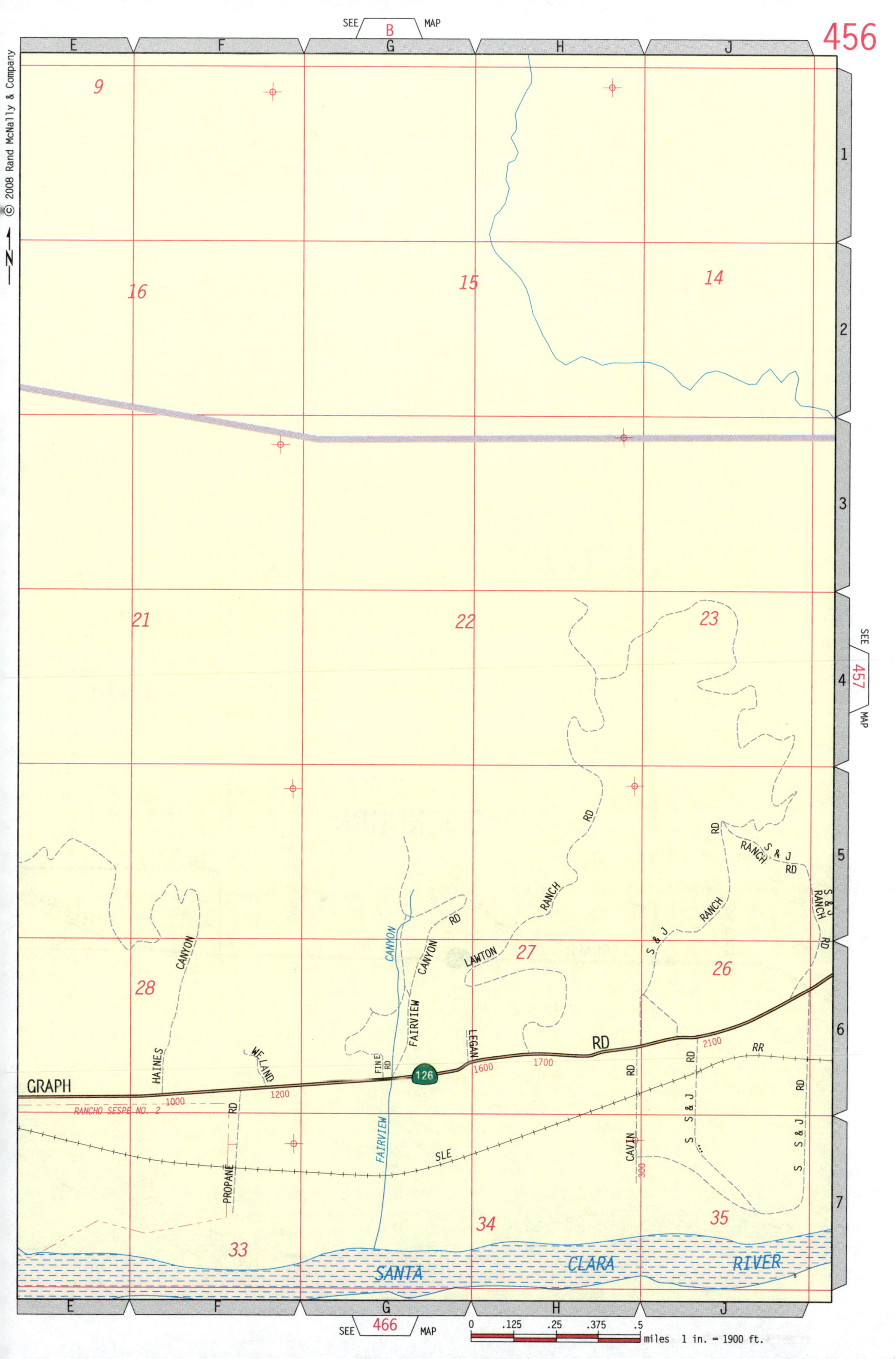
SEE B MAP
E
F
G
H
J
9
16
15
14
21
22
23
28
27
26
33
34
35
1
2
3
4
5
6
7
SEE 457 MAP
HAINES
CANYON
WELAND
PROPANE
RD
FAIRVIEW
CANYON
FINE RD
FAIRVIEW
CANYON
RD
LAWTON
RANCH
RD
LEGAN
RD
S & J
RANCH
RD
RANCH
S & J
RD
S & J
RANCH
RD
CAVIN
S S & J
S S & J
RD
RD
RR
SLE
GRAPH
126
1000
1200
1600
1700
2100
300
RANCHO SESPE NO. 2
SANTA
CLARA
RIVER
SEE 466 MAP
0 .125 .25 .375 .5 miles 1 in. = 1900 ft.

SEE B MAP

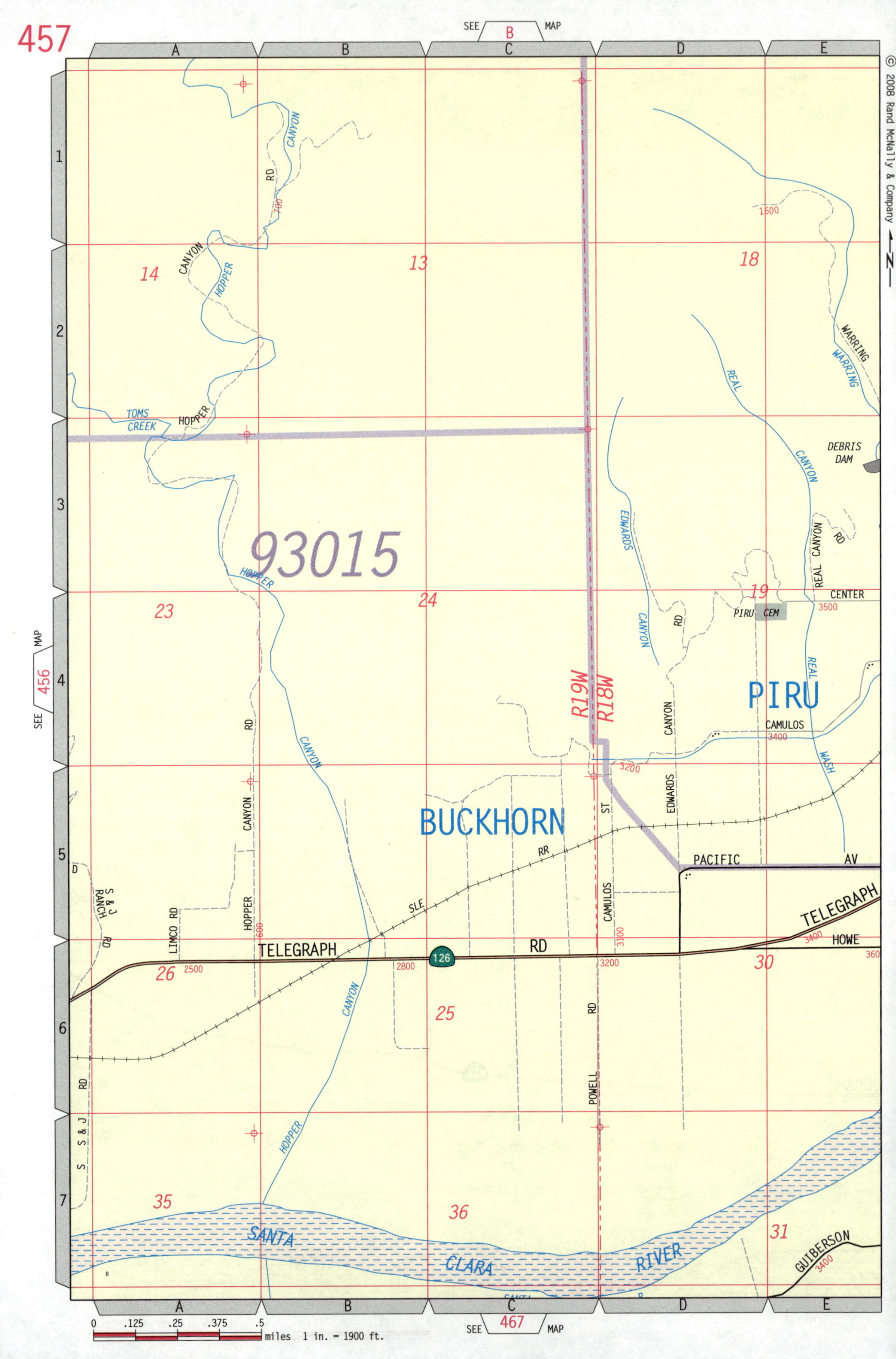

A
B
C
D
E
1
2
3
4
5
6
7
CANYON
RD
700
CANYON
HOPPER
14
13
18
1600
TOMS
CREEK
HOPPER
WARRING
WARRING
REAL
CANYON
DEBRIS
DAM
93015
HOPPER
EDWARDS
CANYON
REAL
CANYON
RD
23
24
19
CENTER
3500
PIRU
CEM
CANYON
RD
RD
REAL
R19W
R18W
PIRU
CANYON
CAMULOS
3400
WASH
3200
CANYON
BUCKHORN
ST
EDWARDS
RR
PACIFIC
AV
D
S & J
RANCH
RD
LIMCO RD
HOPPER
1600
SLE
CAMULOS
3100
TELEGRAPH
TELEGRAPH
RD
126
HOWE
3400
360
26
2500
2800
3200
30
CANYON
25
RD
RD
POWELL
S
S & J
HOPPER
35
36
31
SANTA
CLARA
RIVER
GUIBERSON
3400

SEE 456 MAP

0 .125 .25 .375 .5 miles 1 in. = 1900 ft.

SEE 467 MAP

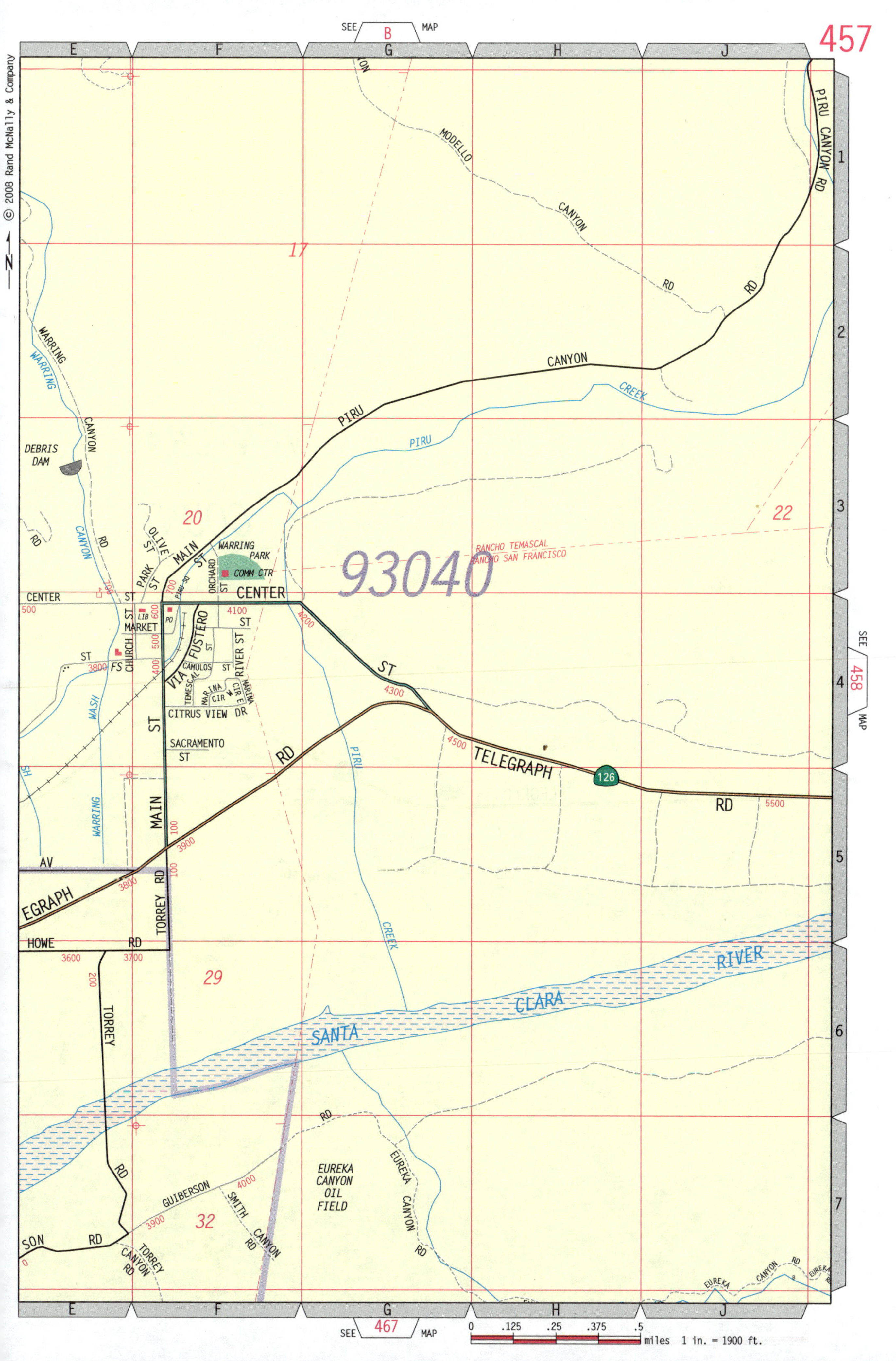
SEE B MAP
E
F
G
H
J
1
2
3
4
5
6
7
PIRU CANYON RD
MODELLO CANYON RD
RD
17
WARRING CANYON RD
WARRING
PIRU CANYON RD
CREEK
PIRU
DEBRIS DAM
20
22
93040
RANCHO TEMASCAL
RANCHO SAN FRANCISCO
OLIVE ST
MAIN ST
WARRING PARK
COMM CTR
PARK ST
ORCHARD ST
PIRU SQ
CENTER ST
CENTER
500
700
600
500
400
4100
4200
LIB
PO
MARKET
ST
CHURCH
FS
3800
WASH
VIA FUSTERO
RIVER ST
CAMULOS
TEMESCAL
MARINA
CIR W
CIR E
MARINA
CITRUS VIEW DR
SACRAMENTO ST
4300
4500
TELEGRAPH RD
126
5500
PIRU CREEK
WARRING
MAIN ST
100
3900
100
AV
TELEGRAPH
3800
TORREY RD
HOWE RD
3600
3700
200
TORREY RD
29
SANTA CLARA RIVER
EUREKA CANYON OIL FIELD
EUREKA CANYON RD
GUIBERSON RD
4000
3900
SMITH CANYON RD
32
TORREY CANYON RD
0
EUREKA CANYON RD
EUREKA RD
SEE 458 MAP
SEE 467 MAP
0 .125 .25 .375 .5 miles 1 in. = 1900 ft.

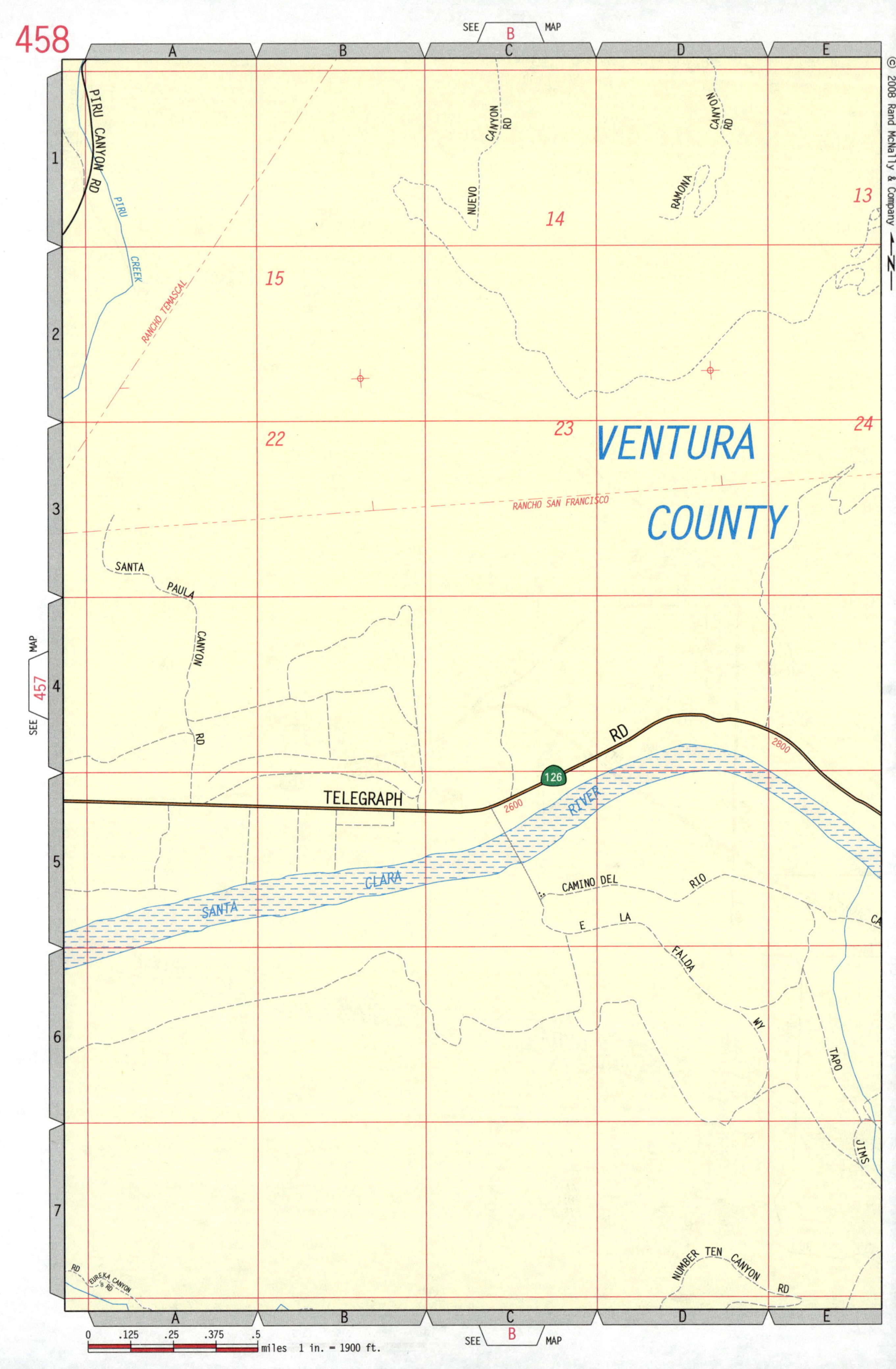
SEE B MAP
A
B
C
D
E
1
2
3
4
5
6
7
PIRU CANYON RD
PIRU CREEK
NUEVO CANYON RD
CANYON RD
RAMONA
14
13
15
RANCHO TEMASCAL
22
23
24
VENTURA
COUNTY
RANCHO SAN FRANCISCO
SANTA PAULA CANYON RD
SEE 457 MAP
TELEGRAPH RD
126
2600
2800
SANTA CLARA RIVER
CAMINO DEL RIO
E LA FALDA WY
TAPO
JIMS
NUMBER TEN CANYON RD
EUREKA CANYON RD
RD
0 .125 .25 .375 .5 miles 1 in. = 1900 ft.
SEE B MAP

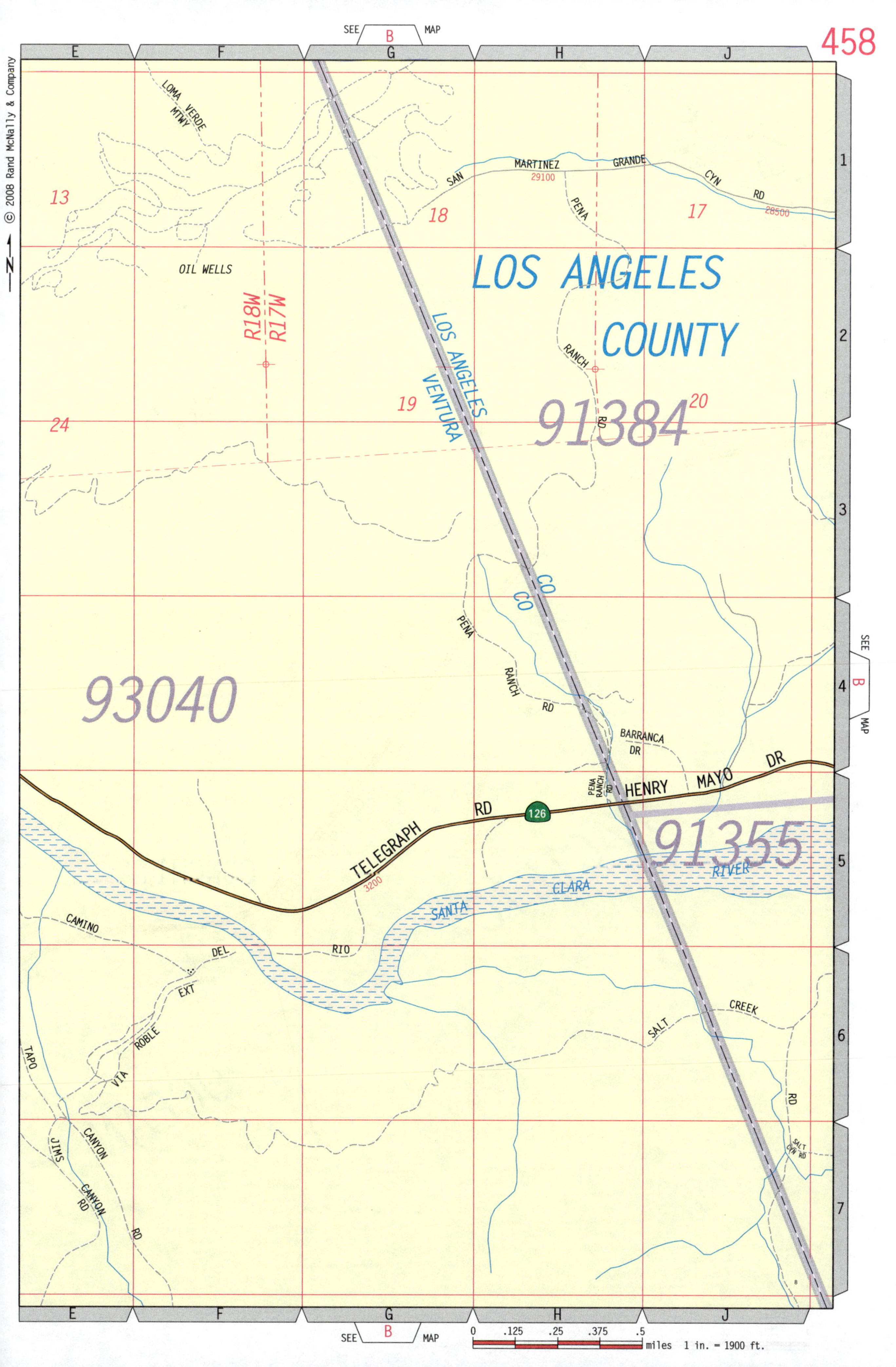
SEE B MAP
E
F
G
H
J
1
2
3
4
5
6
7
LOMA VERDE MTWY
OIL WELLS
R18W
R17W
SAN MARTINEZ GRANDE CYN RD
29100
28500
PENA RANCH RD
13
18
17
24
19
20
LOS ANGELES COUNTY
LOS ANGELES
VENTURA
CO
CO
91384
93040
91355
BARRANCA DR
HENRY MAYO DR
TELEGRAPH RD
3200
126
SANTA CLARA RIVER
CAMINO DEL RIO EXT
VIA ROBLE
TAPO CANYON RD
JIMS CANYON RD
SALT CREEK RD
SALT CYN RD
0 .125 .25 .375 .5 miles 1 in. = 1900 ft.

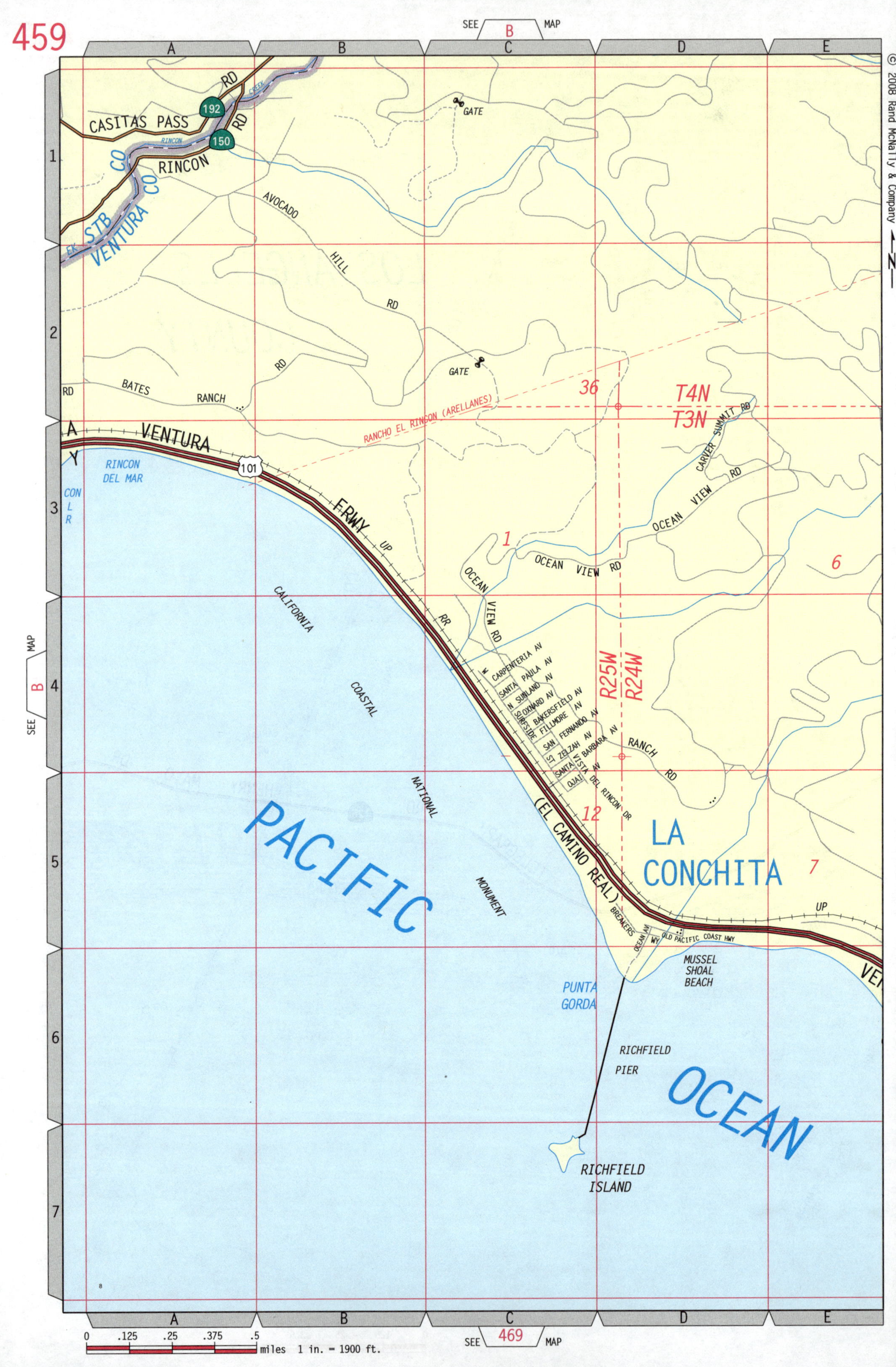
SEE B MAP
SEE B MAP
SEE 469 MAP
CASITAS PASS RD
RINCON RD
192
150
101
STB CO
VENTURA CO
AVOCADO HILL RD
BATES RANCH RD
GATE
GATE
RANCHO EL RINCON (ARELLANES)
36
T4N
T3N
CARVER SUMMIT RD
OCEAN VIEW RD
OCEAN VIEW RD
OCEAN VIEW RD
1
6
VENTURA FRWY
UP
RR
RINCON DEL MAR
CON L R
CALIFORNIA COASTAL NATIONAL MONUMENT
W CARPENTERIA AV
SANTA PAULA AV
N SUNLAND AV
OXNARD AV
SURFSIDE
BAKERSFIELD AV
FILLMORE AV
SAN FERNANDO AV
ST ZELZAH AV
SANTA BARBARA AV
VISTA DEL RINCON DR
OJAI AV
R25W
R24W
RANCH RD
12
7
(EL CAMINO REAL)
LA CONCHITA
BREAKERS WY
OCEAN AV
OLD PACIFIC COAST HWY
MUSSEL SHOAL BEACH
PUNTA GORDA
RICHFIELD PIER
RICHFIELD ISLAND
PACIFIC OCEAN
0 .125 .25 .375 .5 miles 1 in. = 1900 ft.

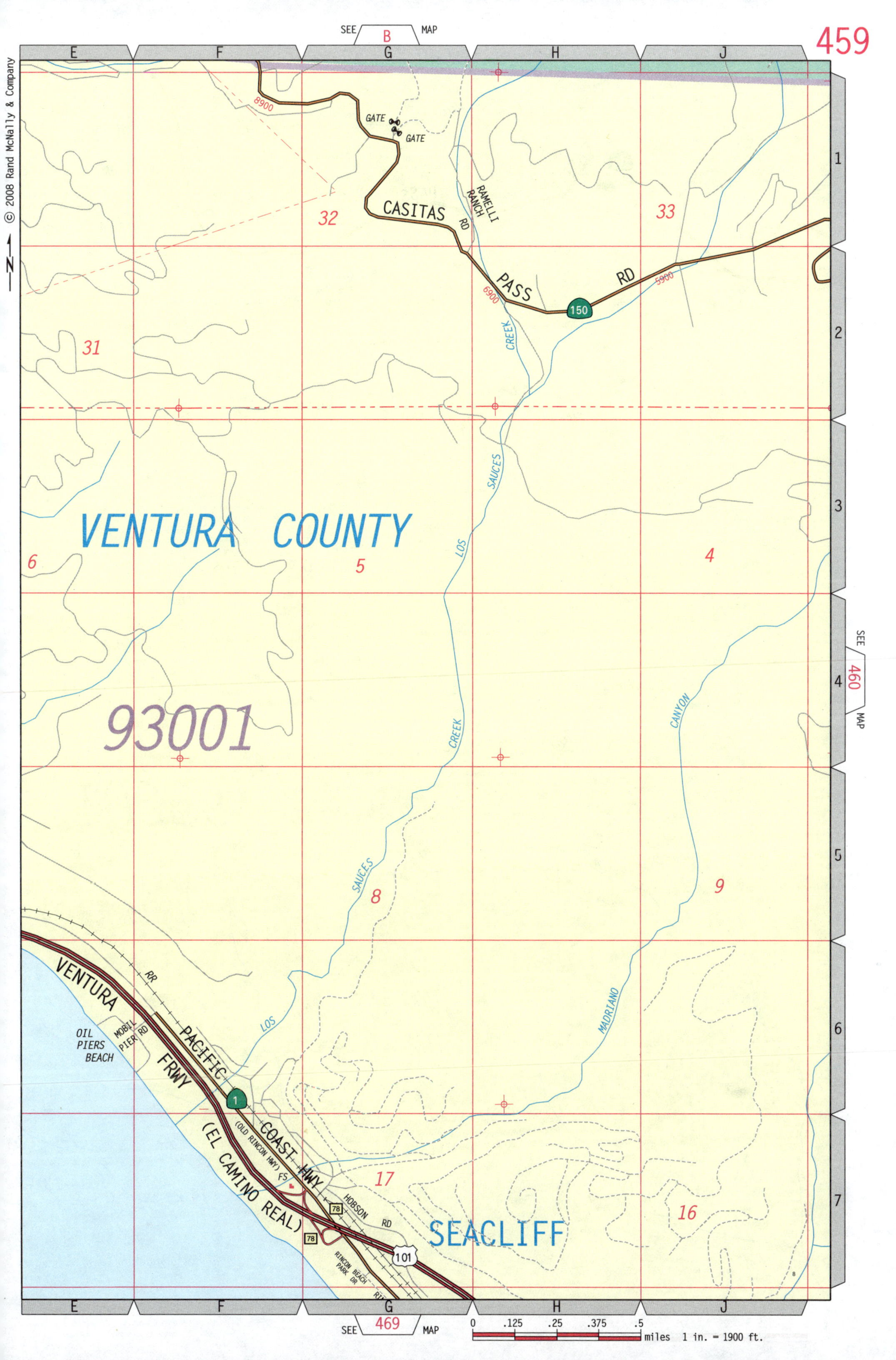
SEE B MAP
E
F
G
H
J
1
2
3
4
5
6
7
GATE
GATE
8900
CASITAS
RD
RAMELLI RANCH
32
33
PASS
RD
6900
5900
150
CREEK
31
SAUCES
VENTURA COUNTY
LOS
6
5
4
SEE 460 MAP
CANYON
93001
CREEK
SAUCES
8
9
RR
VENTURA
LOS
MADRIANO
OIL PIERS BEACH
MOBIL PIER RD
PACIFIC
FRWY
1
COAST
(EL CAMINO REAL)
(OLD RINCON HWY)
FS
HWY
17
HOBSON
RD
78
78
SEACLIFF
16
101
RINCON BEACH PARK DR
SEE 469 MAP
0 .125 .25 .375 .5
miles 1 in. = 1900 ft.

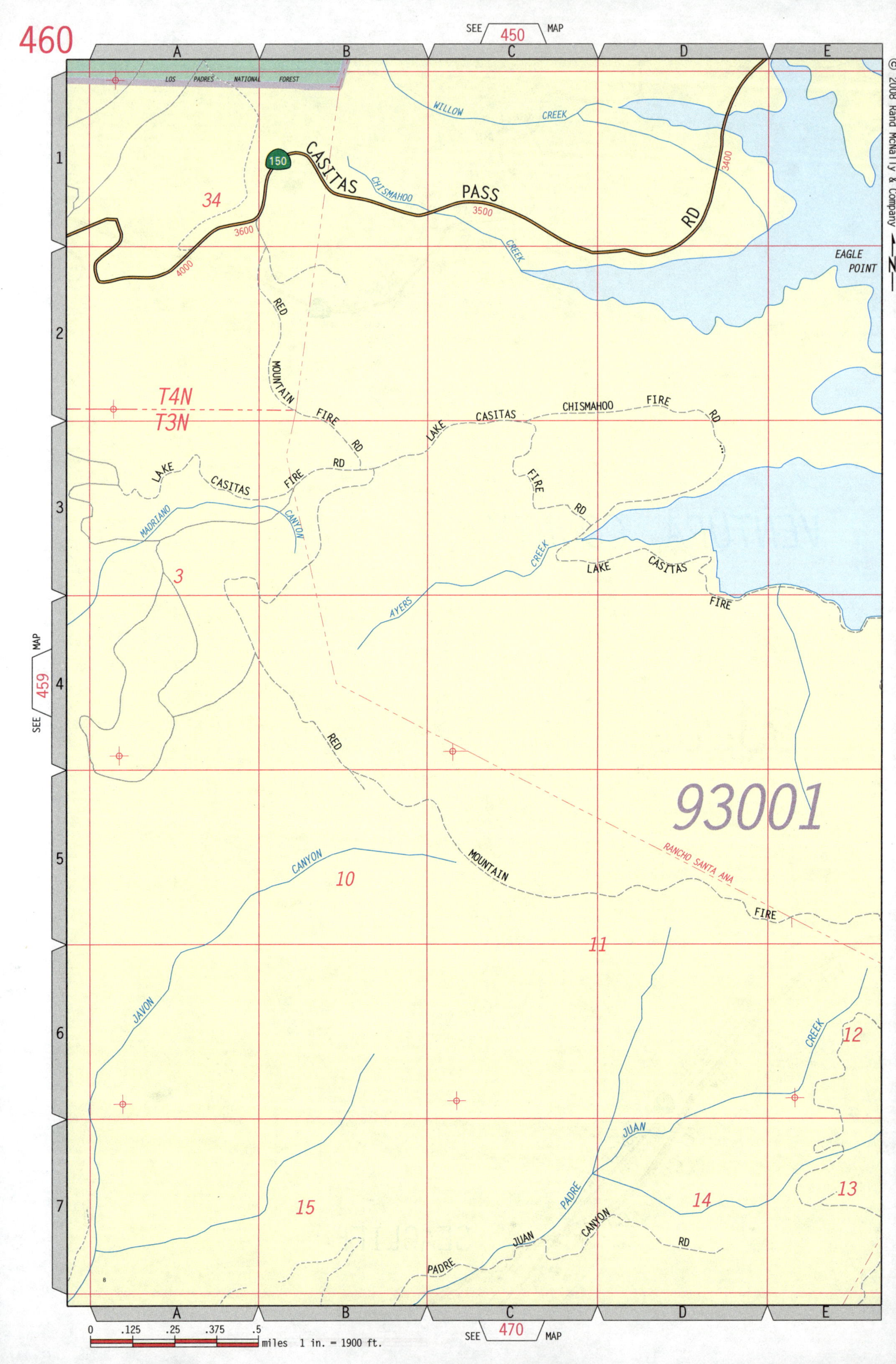
SEE 450 MAP
A
B
C
D
E
1
2
3
4
5
6
7
LOS PADRES NATIONAL FOREST
WILLOW CREEK
150
CASITAS PASS RD
CHISMAHOO CREEK
3400
3500
3600
4000
34
EAGLE POINT
RED MOUNTAIN FIRE RD
T4N
T3N
CHISMAHOO FIRE RD
LAKE CASITAS FIRE RD
MADRIANO CANYON
3
AYERS CREEK
SEE 459 MAP
93001
RANCHO SANTA ANA
RED MOUNTAIN FIRE
CANYON
10
11
JAVON
CREEK
12
JUAN
PADRE
14
13
15
PADRE JUAN CANYON RD
SEE 470 MAP
0 .125 .25 .375 .5 miles 1 in. = 1900 ft.

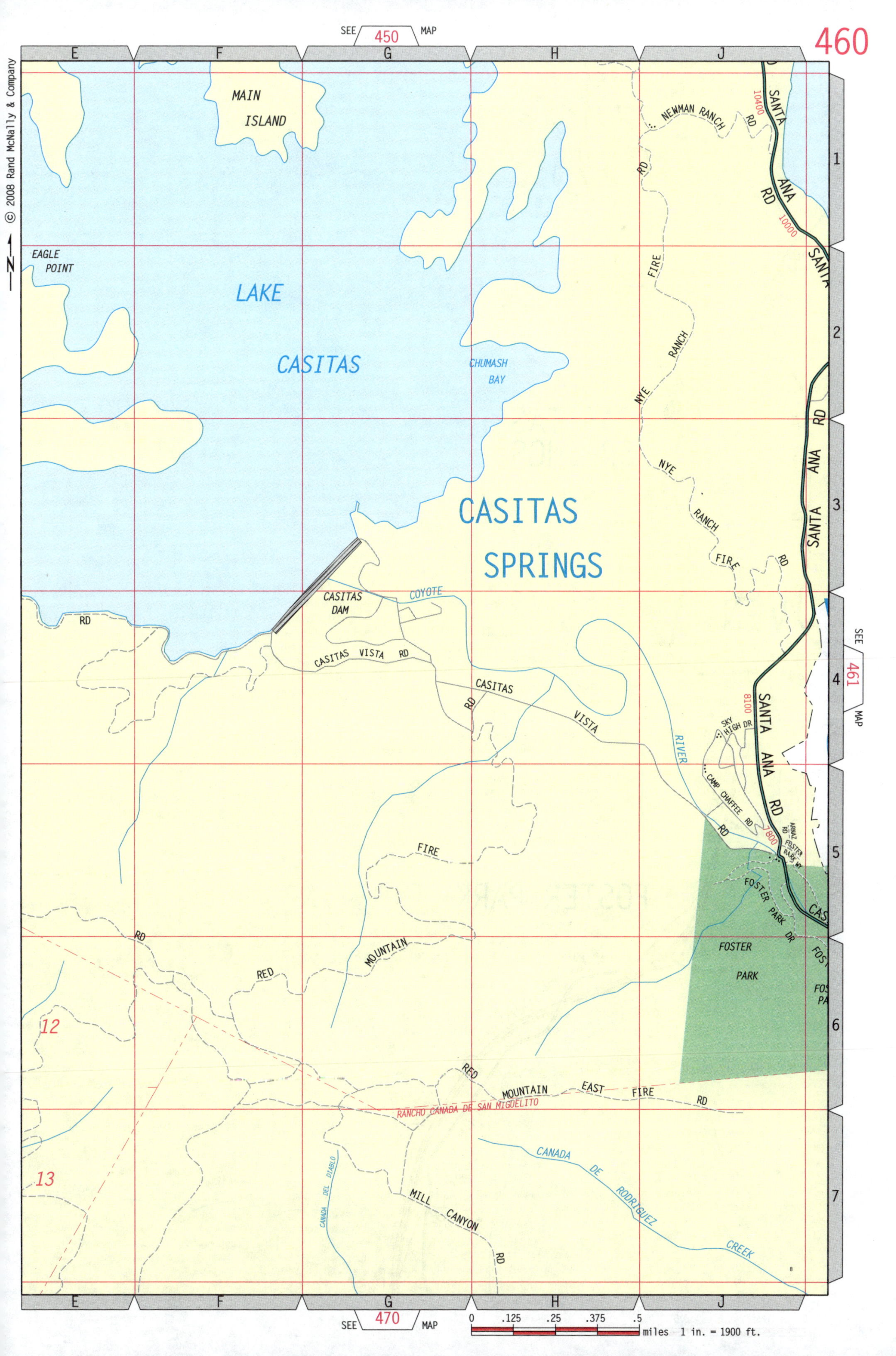
SEE 450 MAP
E
F
G
H
J
MAIN
ISLAND
EAGLE
POINT
LAKE
CASITAS
CHUMASH
BAY
CASITAS
SPRINGS
CASITAS
DAM
COYOTE
CASITAS VISTA RD
CASITAS
RD
VISTA
RIVER
NEWMAN RANCH
RD
FIRE
RANCH
NYE
NYE
RANCH
FIRE
RD
SANTA
ANA
RD
10400
10000
SANTA
ANA
RD
SANTA
ANA
RD
8100
7800
SKY HIGH DR
CAMP CHAFFEE RD
RD
FOSTER PARK DR
FOSTER
PARK
FIRE
RD
MOUNTAIN
RED
RED
MOUNTAIN
EAST
FIRE
RD
RANCHO CANADA DE SAN MIGUELITO
CANADA DEL DIABLO
MILL
CANYON
RD
CANADA
DE
RODRIGUEZ
CREEK
12
13
1
2
3
4
5
6
7
SEE 461 MAP
SEE 470 MAP
0
.125
.25
.375
.5
miles 1 in. = 1900 ft.

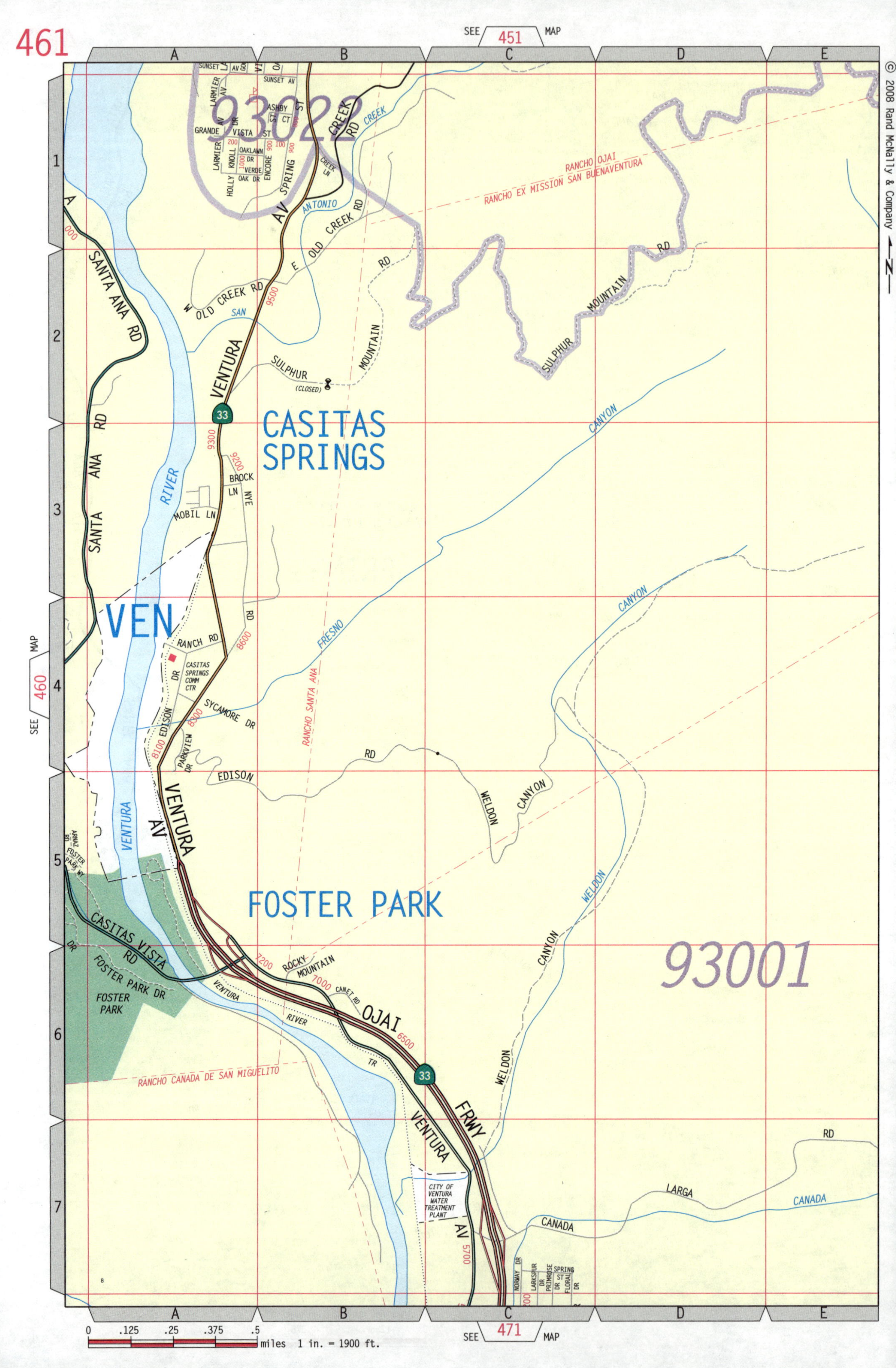

SEE 451 MAP
93022
CASITAS SPRINGS
VEN
FOSTER PARK
93001
VENTURA AV
33
SANTA ANA RD
OLD CREEK RD
SAN ANTONIO CREEK
SULPHUR MOUNTAIN RD
RANCHO OJAI
RANCHO EX MISSION SAN BUENAVENTURA
FRESNO CANYON
RANCHO SANTA ANA
CASITAS SPRINGS COMM CTR
SYCAMORE DR
EDISON RD
WELDON CANYON
CASITAS VISTA RD
FOSTER PARK DR
FOSTER PARK
VENTURA RIVER
OJAI FRWY
ROCKY MOUNTAIN
RANCHO CANADA DE SAN MIGUELITO
CITY OF VENTURA WATER TREATMENT PLANT
CANADA LARGA RD
SEE 460 MAP
SEE 471 MAP
miles 1 in. = 1900 ft.

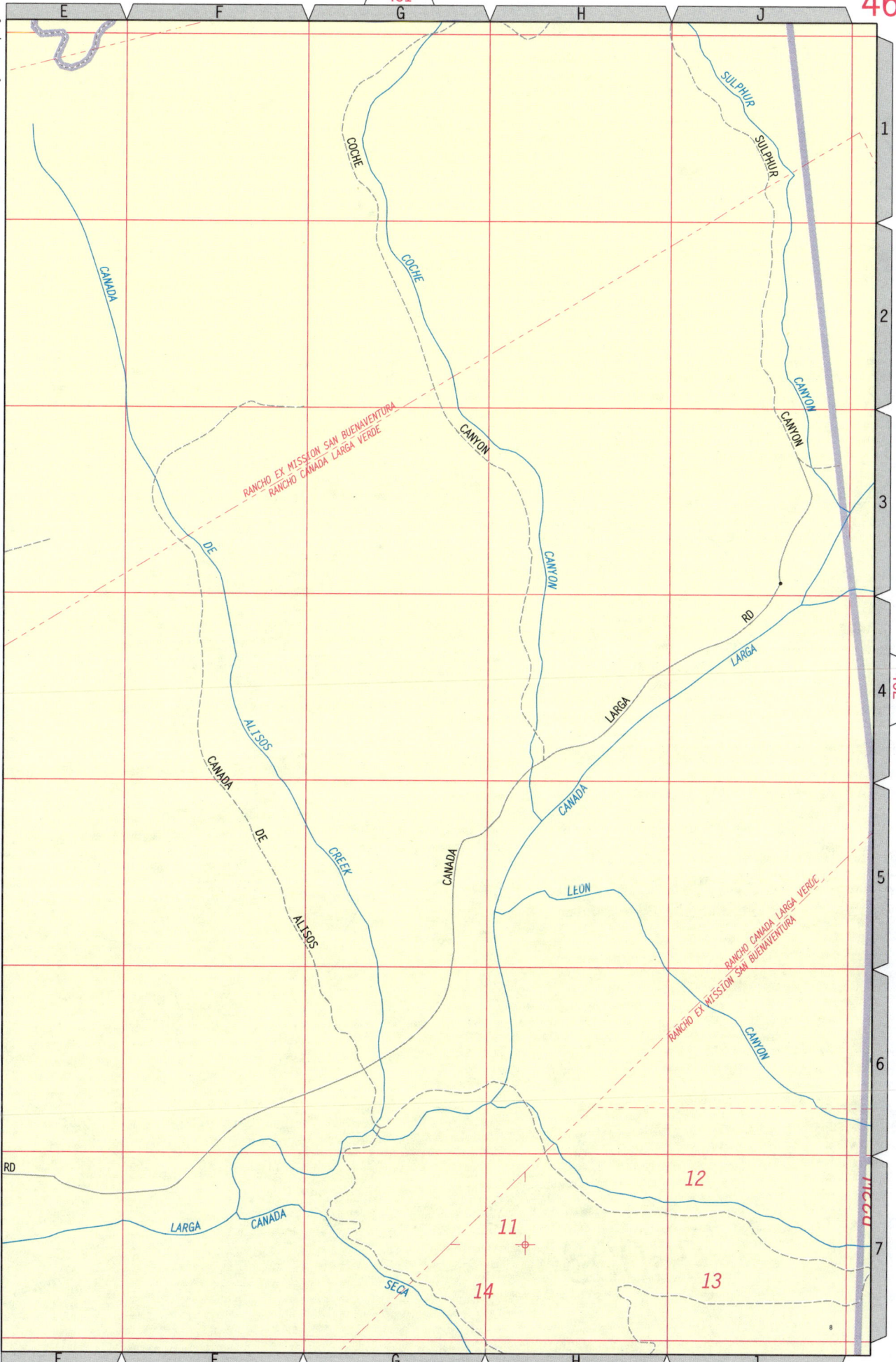

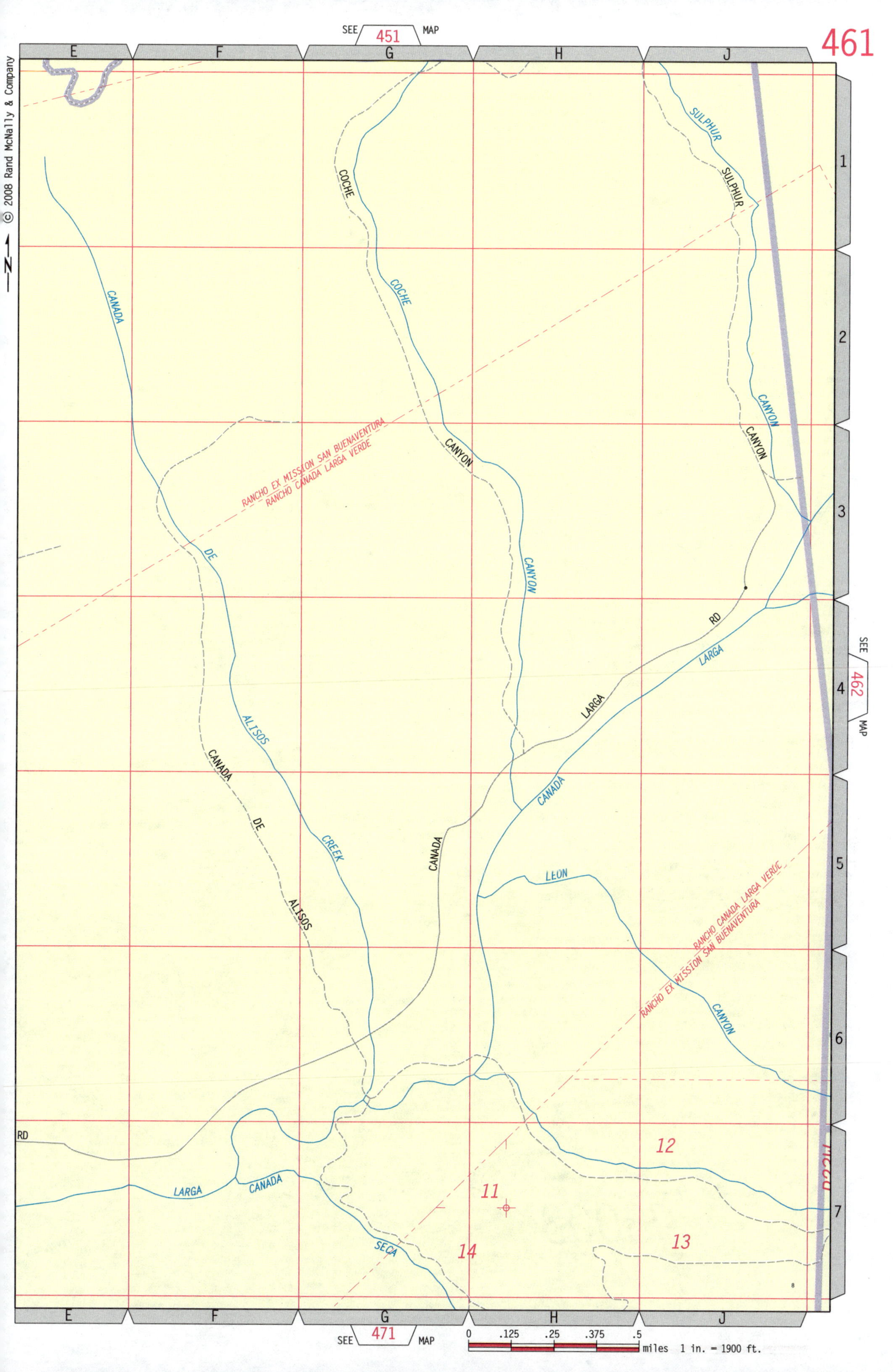
SEE 451 MAP
E
F
G
H
J
1
2
3
4
5
6
7
SEE 462 MAP
CANADA
COCHE
COCHE
SULPHUR
SULPHUR
CANYON
CANYON
CANYON
CANYON
RANCHO EX MISSION SAN BUENAVENTURA
RANCHO CANADA LARGA VERDE
DE
ALISOS
CREEK
CANADA
DE
ALISOS
RD
LARGA
LARGA
CANADA
CANADA
LEON
CANYON
RANCHO CANADA LARGA VERDE
RANCHO EX MISSION SAN BUENAVENTURA
RD
LARGA
CANADA
SECA
12
11
14
13
SEE 471 MAP
0 .125 .25 .375 .5 miles 1 in. = 1900 ft.

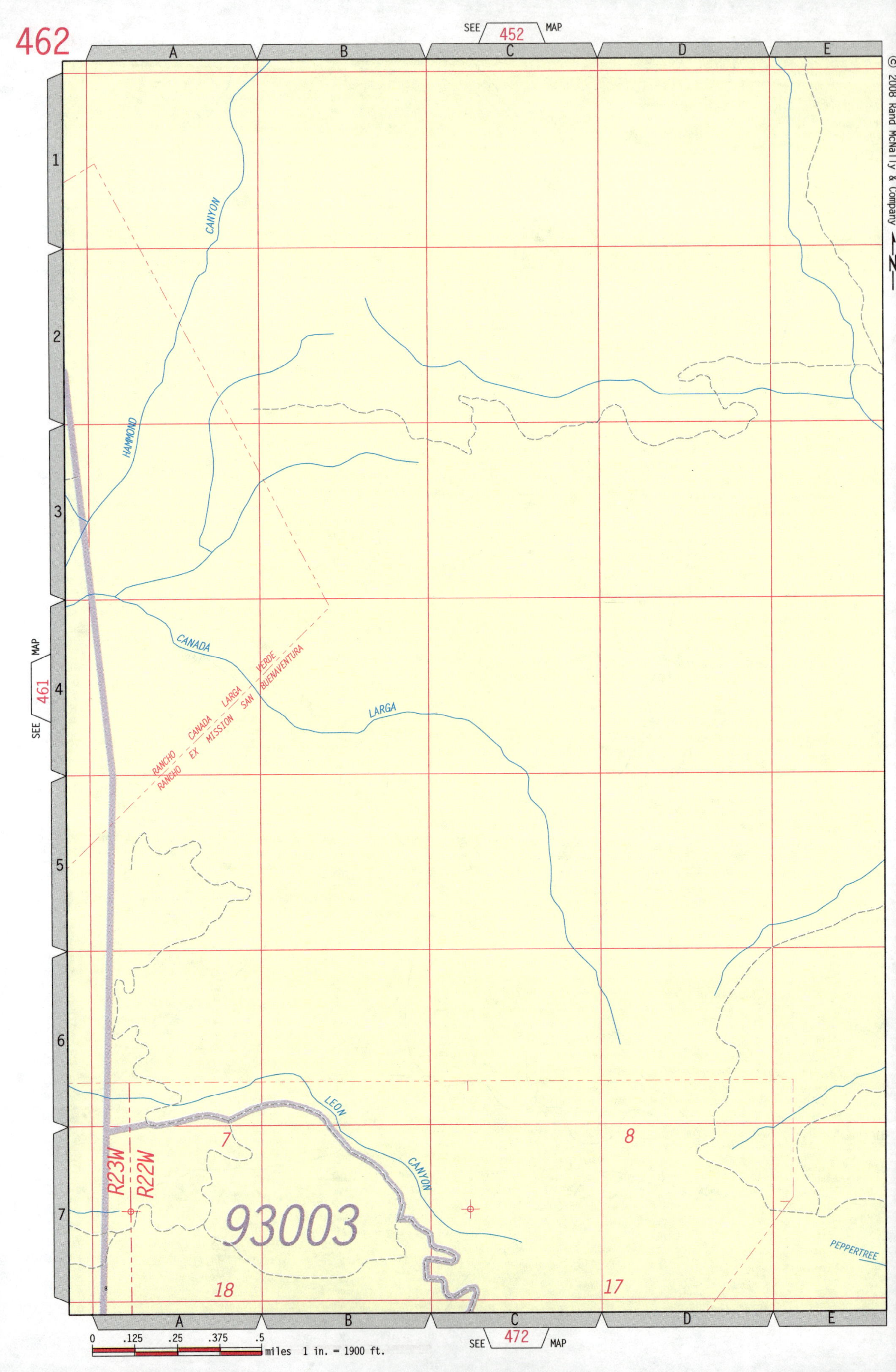
SEE 452 MAP
A
B
C
D
E
1
2
3
4
5
6
7
CANYON
HAMMOND
CANADA
LARGA
RANCHO CANADA LARGA VERDE
RANCHO EX MISSION SAN BUENAVENTURA
SEE 461 MAP
LEON
CANYON
7
8
R23W
R22W
93003
18
17
PEPPERTREE
SEE 472 MAP
0 .125 .25 .375 .5
miles 1 in. = 1900 ft.

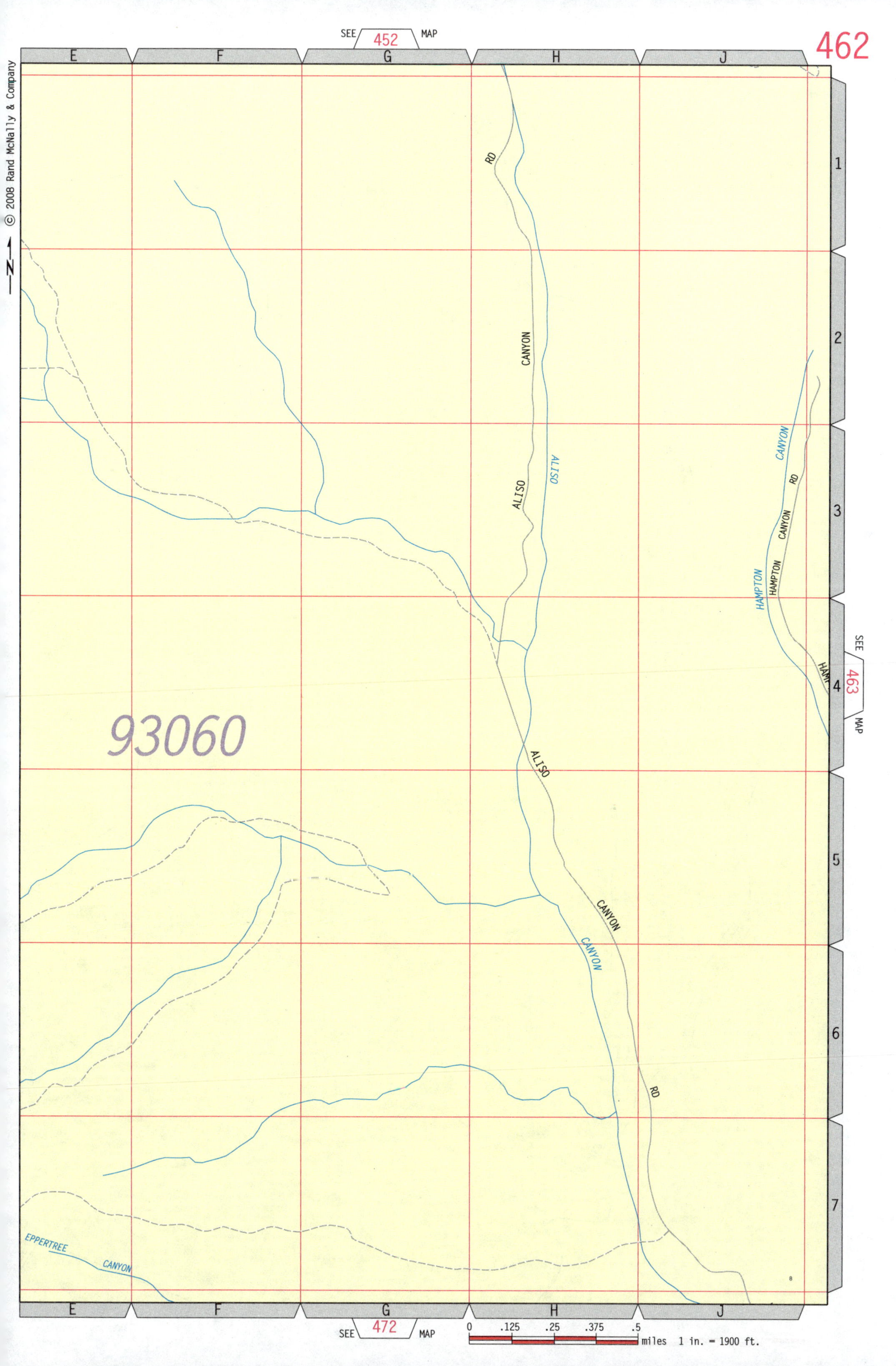
SEE 452 MAP
E
F
G
H
J
1
2
3
4
5
6
7
RD
CANYON
ALISO
ALISO
CANYON
HAMPTON
CANYON
RD
CANYON
HAMPTON
HAMPTON
SEE 463 MAP
ALISO
93060
CANYON
CANYON
RD
EPPERTREE
CANYON
SEE 472 MAP
0 .125 .25 .375 .5
miles 1 in. = 1900 ft.

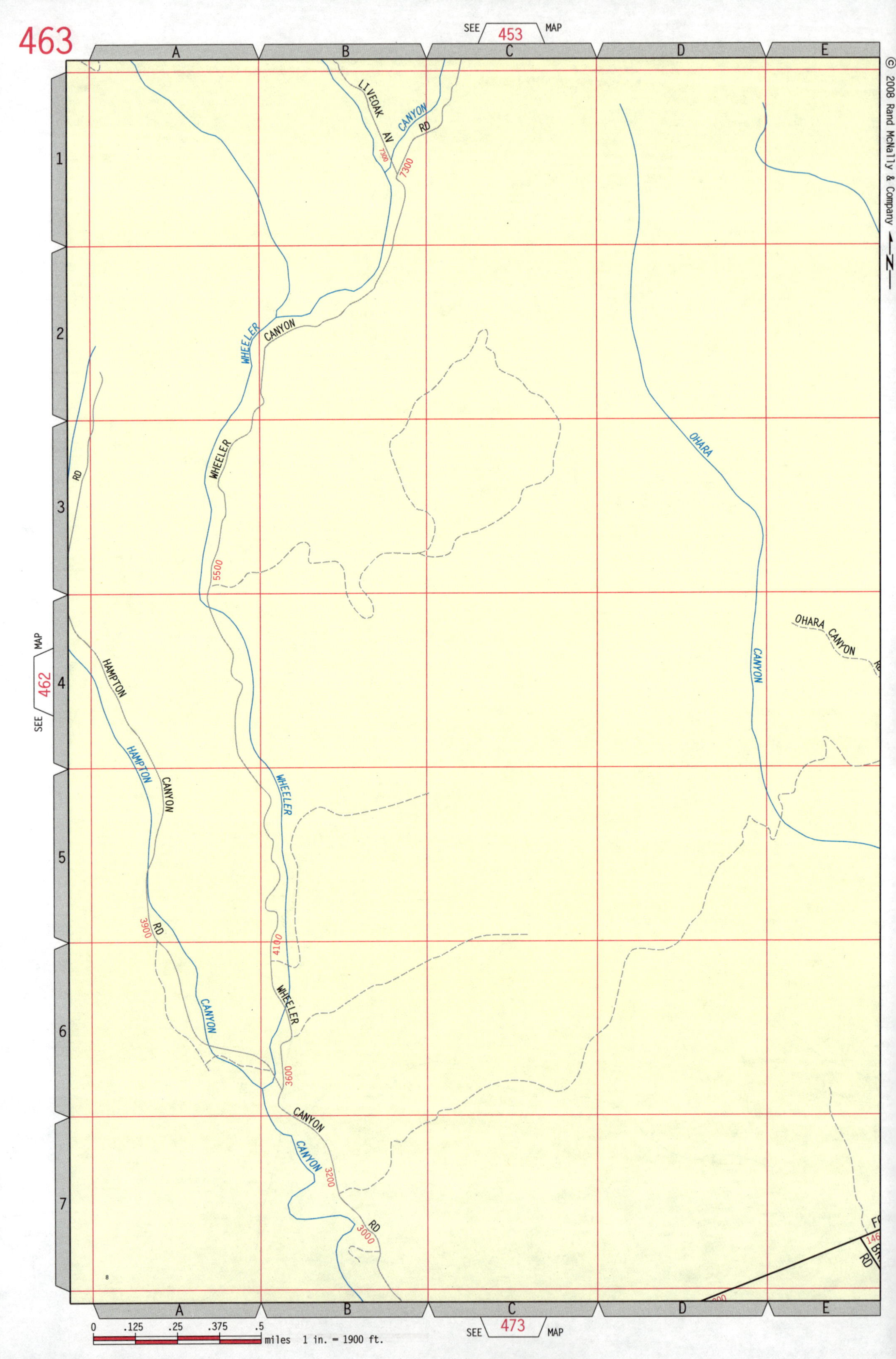

SEE 453 MAP
A
B
C
D
E
1
2
3
4
5
6
7
LIVEOAK
AV
CANYON
RD
7300
7300
WHEELER
CANYON
WHEELER
5500
RD
OHARA
CANYON
OHARA CANYON
HAMPTON
HAMPTON
CANYON
WHEELER
3900
RD
4100
CANYON
WHEELER
3600
CANYON
CANYON
3200
RD
3000
SEE 462 MAP
SEE 473 MAP
0 .125 .25 .375 .5
miles 1 in. = 1900 ft.

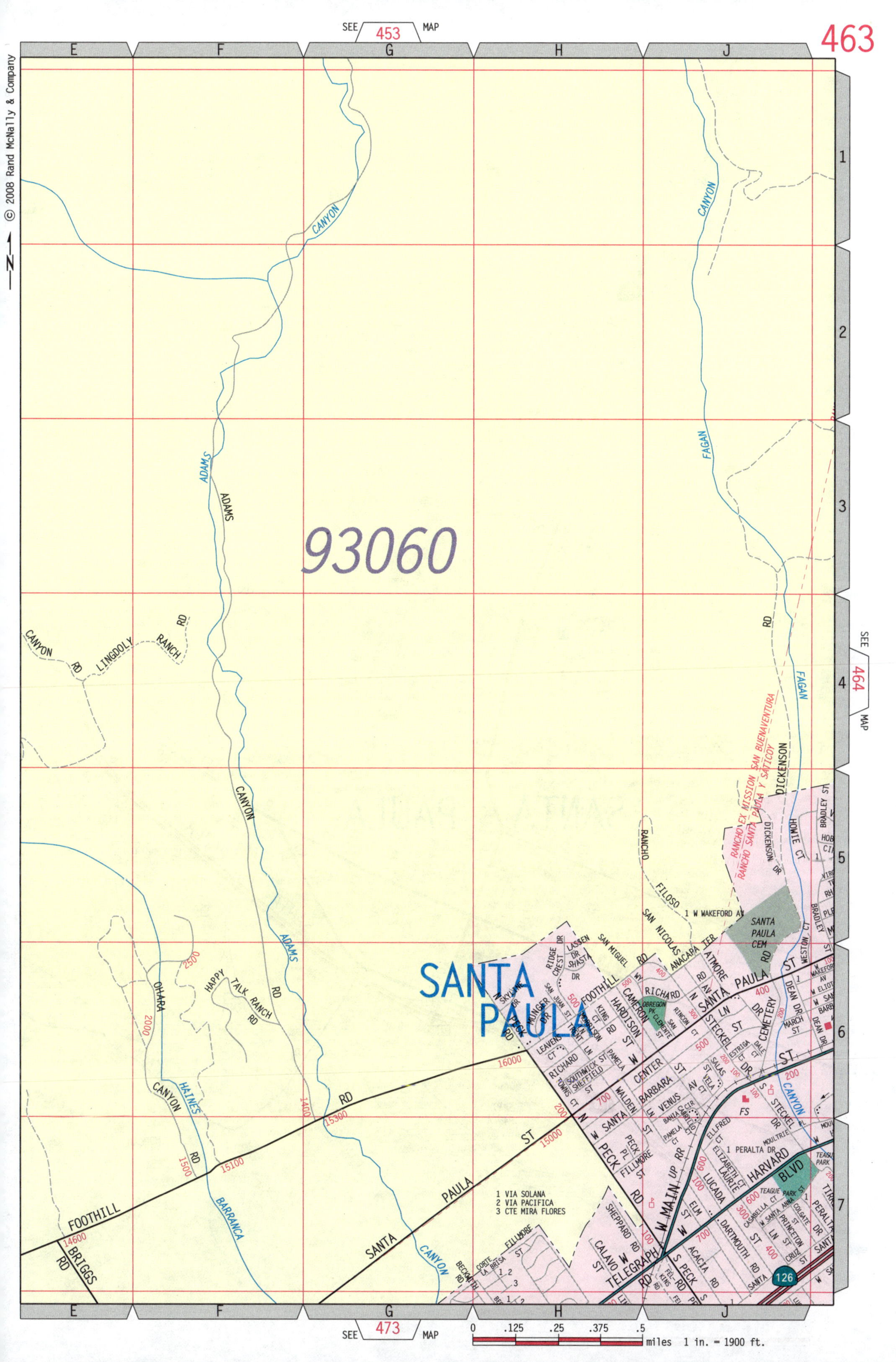
SEE 453 MAP
93060
SANTA PAULA
CANYON
ADAMS
FAGAN
LINGDOLY RANCH RD
CANYON RD
OHARA
HAPPY TALK RANCH RD
HAINES
BARRANCA
FOOTHILL RD
BRIGGS RD
SANTA PAULA ST
RANCHO EX MISSION SAN BUENAVENTURA
RANCHO SANTA PAULA Y SATICOY
DICKENSON
SANTA PAULA CEM
OBREGON PK
1 W WAKEFORD AV
1 PERALTA DR
TEAGUE PARK
1 VIA SOLANA
2 VIA PACIFICA
3 CTE MIRA FLORES
SEE 464 MAP
SEE 473 MAP
miles 1 in. = 1900 ft.

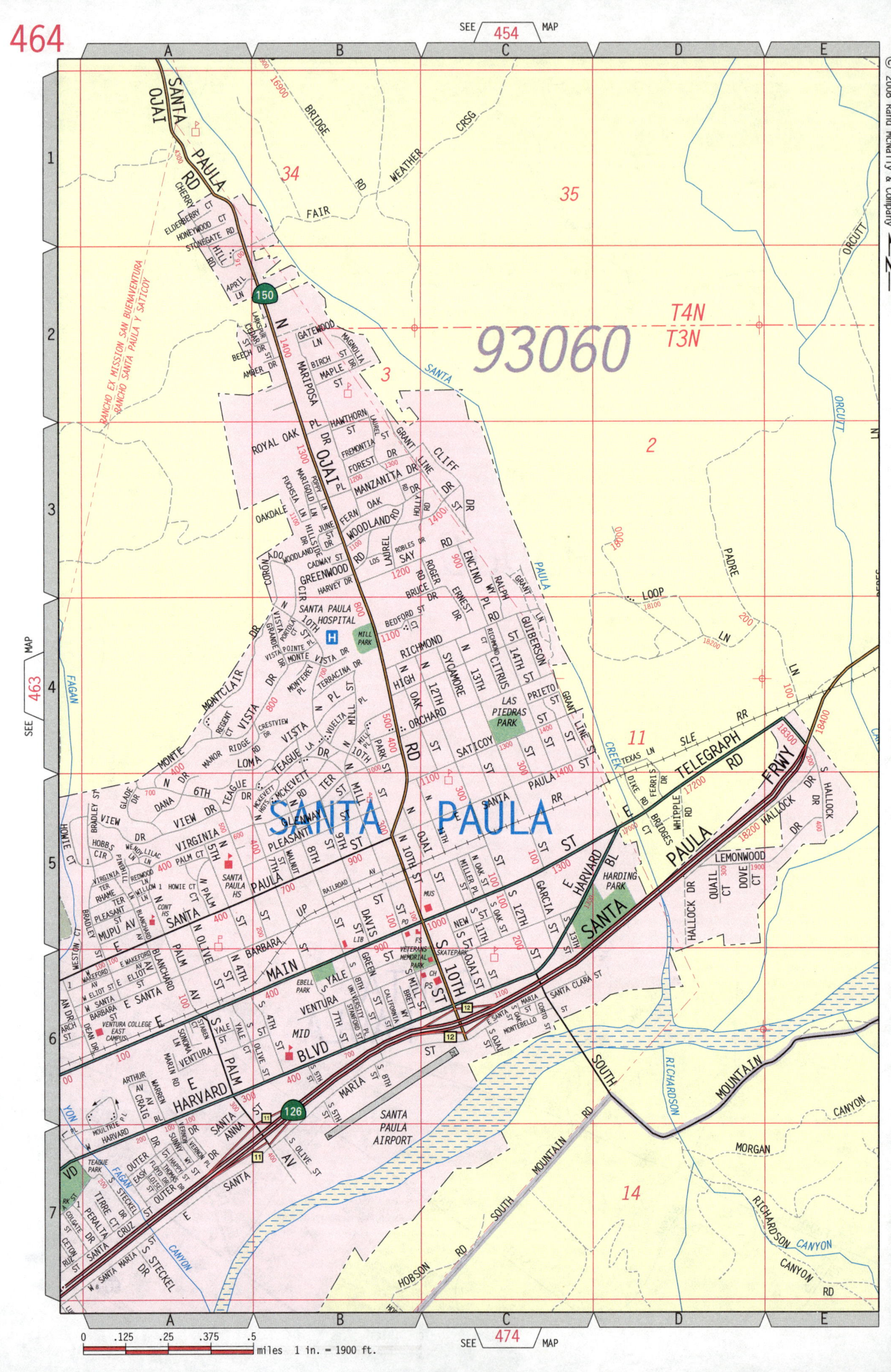

SEE 454 MAP
SEE 463 MAP
SEE 474 MAP
A
B
C
D
E
1
2
3
4
5
6
7
SANTA PAULA
93060
T4N
T3N
34
35
3
2
11
14
SANTA PAULA HOSPITAL
MILL PARK
LAS PIEDRAS PARK
SANTA PAULA HS
CONT HS
VENTURA COLLEGE EAST CAMPUS
EBELL PARK
VETERANS MEMORIAL PARK
SKATEPARK
HARDING PARK
TEAGUE PARK
SANTA PAULA AIRPORT
MUS
LIB
PO
FS
CH
PS
OJAI SANTA PAULA RD
N OJAI RD
S 10TH ST
SANTA PAULA FRWY
TELEGRAPH RD
E HARVARD BL
E MAIN ST
E SANTA BARBARA ST
E SANTA PAULA ST
VENTURA ST
MID BLVD
SANTA CLARA ST
SOUTH MOUNTAIN RD
HOBSON RD
MORGAN CANYON
RICHARDSON CANYON RD
ORCUTT
PADRE LN
LOOP
BRIDGE
WEATHER CRSG
FAIR
CHERRY
ELDERBERRY CT
HONEYWOOD CT
STONEGATE RD
HILL RD
APRIL LN
LARKSPUR
CEDAR ST
BEECH DR
AMBER DR
GATEWOOD LN
MAGNOLIA
BIRCH ST
MAPLE ST
MARIPOSA DR
ROYAL OAK PL
HAWTHORN ST
FREMONTIA
FOREST DR
MANZANITA DR
LAUREL
GRANT LINE
CLIFF DR
FUCHSIA LN
MARIGOLD LN
POPPY
OAKDALE
HILLSIDE DR
JUNE ST
FERN
OAK
WOODLAND RD
CADWAY ST
GREENWOOD CIR
HARVEY DR
SAY RD
ROBLES DR
ROGER ST
BRUCE DR
ENCINO DR
ERNEST PL
RALPH WY
GUIBERSON
BEDFORD ST
RICHMOND
SYCAMORE
CITRUS
13TH
14TH
12TH
HIGH
ORCHARD
SATICOY ST
PRIETO
MONTECITO
VISTA GRANDE DR
VISTA POINTE PL
MONTE VISTA DR
MONTEREY DR
TERRACINA DR
MONTCLAIR DR
REGENT CT
CRESTVIEW DR
MANOR RIDGE
LOMA
TEAGUE DR
MCKEVETT
GLENWAY
PLEASANT
MILL
PARK ST
10TH
9TH
8TH
7TH
6TH
5TH
4TH
DANA DR
GLADE
VIEW DR
BRADLEY ST
HOBBS CIR
VIRGINIA TER
RHAME TER
MUPU AV
PALM
OLIVE
BLANCHARD
WALNUT
RAILROAD AV
DAVIS
GREEN
UNIVERSITY
STANFORD
CALIFORNIA
BRETT
NEW ST
MILLER PL
GARCIA ST
TEXAS LN
DIKE RD
FERRIS DR
WHIPPLE RD
BRIDGES CT
HALLOCK DR
LEMONWOOD
QUAIL CT
DOVE CT
YALE
SONOMA LN
STABEN CT
ARTHUR AV
WARREN
CRAIG
HARVARD
MOULTRIE PL
OUTER
EASY
FLOYD
LOISE
THOMAS
HAPPY
SUNNY
VERNON DR
SANTA ANNA
TIRRE CT
PERALTA DR
COLGATE
CETON
STECKEL DR
SANTA CRUZ
SANTA MARIA
MONTEBELLO
CORTO
MARIA
FAGAN CANYON
SANTA PAULA CREEK
RANCHO EX MISSION SAN BUENAVENTURA
RANCHO SANTA PAULA Y SATICOY
150
126
12
11
0 .125 .25 .375 .5
miles 1 in. = 1900 ft.

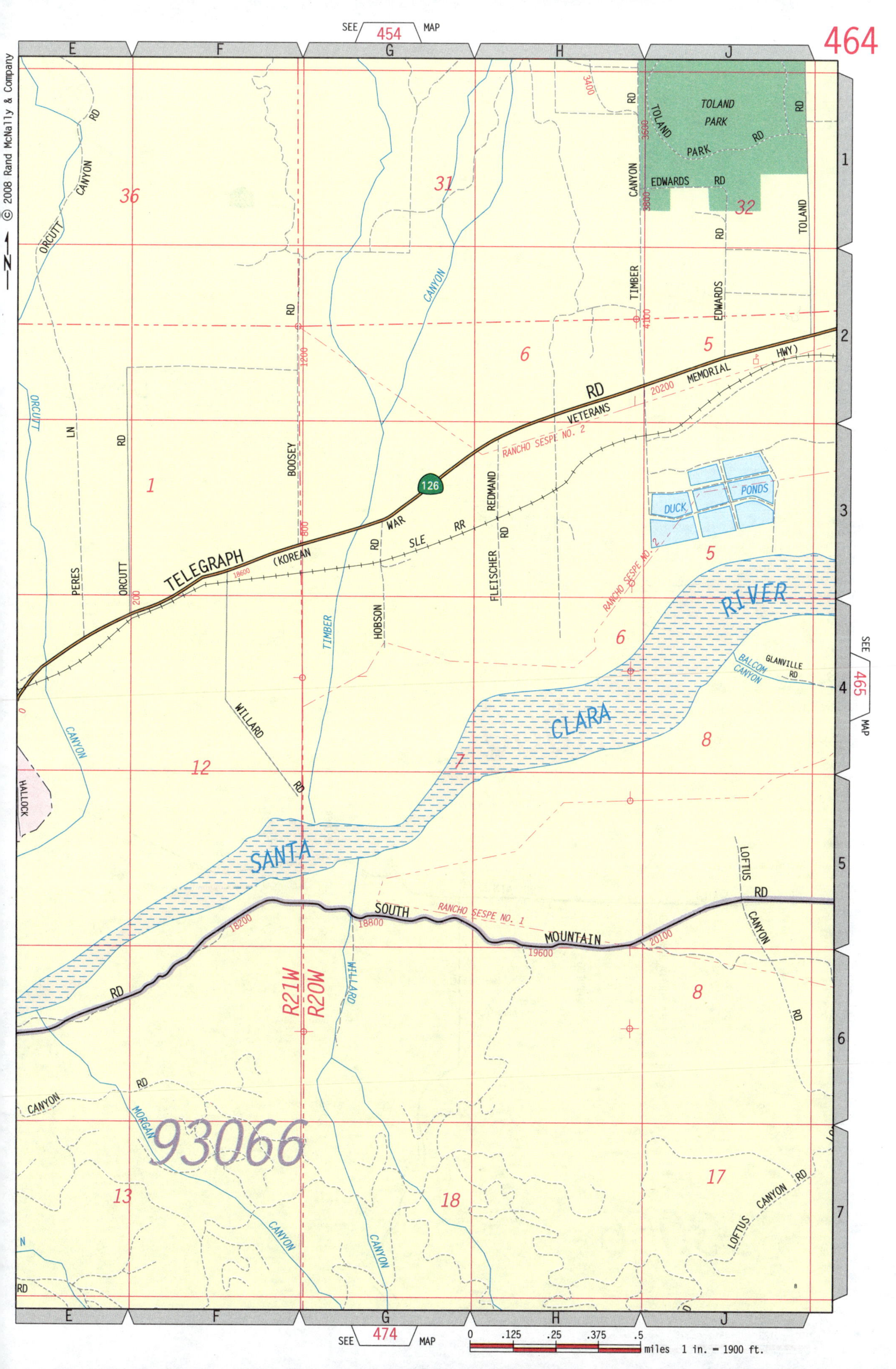

SEE 454 MAP
TOLAND PARK
TOLAND PARK RD
EDWARDS RD
TIMBER CANYON RD
TELEGRAPH RD
VETERANS MEMORIAL HWY
(KOREAN WAR
126
SLE RR
RANCHO SESPE NO. 2
DUCK PONDS
SANTA CLARA RIVER
SOUTH MOUNTAIN RD
RANCHO SESPE NO. 1
ORCUTT CANYON RD
PERES LN
ORCUTT RD
BOOSEY RD
HOBSON RD
REDMAND RD
FLEISCHER RD
WILLARD RD
GLANVILLE RD
BALCOM CANYON
SEE 465 MAP
HALLOCK
LOFTUS CANYON RD
MORGAN CANYON RD
WILLARD CANYON
R21W
R20W
93066
SEE 474 MAP
0 .125 .25 .375 .5 miles 1 in. = 1900 ft.

SEE 455 MAP

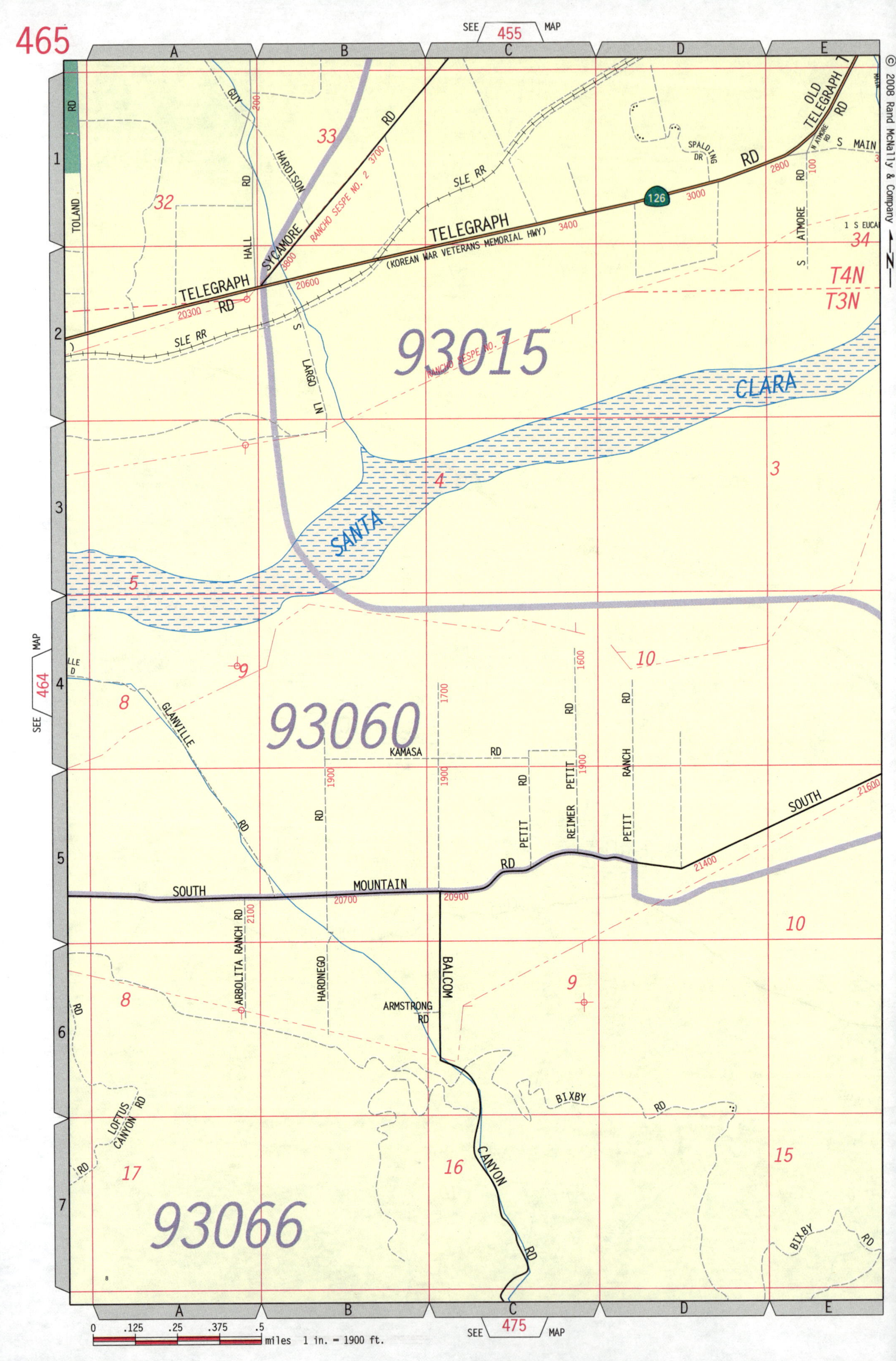
TELEGRAPH RD
(KOREAN WAR VETERANS MEMORIAL HWY)
OLD TELEGRAPH RD
SLE RR
RANCHO SESPE NO. 2
SYCAMORE RD
HARDISON
GUY
HALL RD
TOLAND RD
S LARGO LN
SPALDING DR
S ATMORE RD
S MAIN
126
SANTA CLARA
93015
93060
93066
T4N
T3N
GLANVILLE RD
KAMASA RD
PETIT RD
REIMER PETIT
RANCH RD
SOUTH MOUNTAIN RD
ARBOLITA RANCH RD
HARDNEGO RD
BALCOM
ARMSTRONG RD
CANYON RD
BIXBY RD
LOFTUS CANYON RD

SEE 464 MAP

SEE 475 MAP

0 .125 .25 .375 .5 miles 1 in. = 1900 ft.

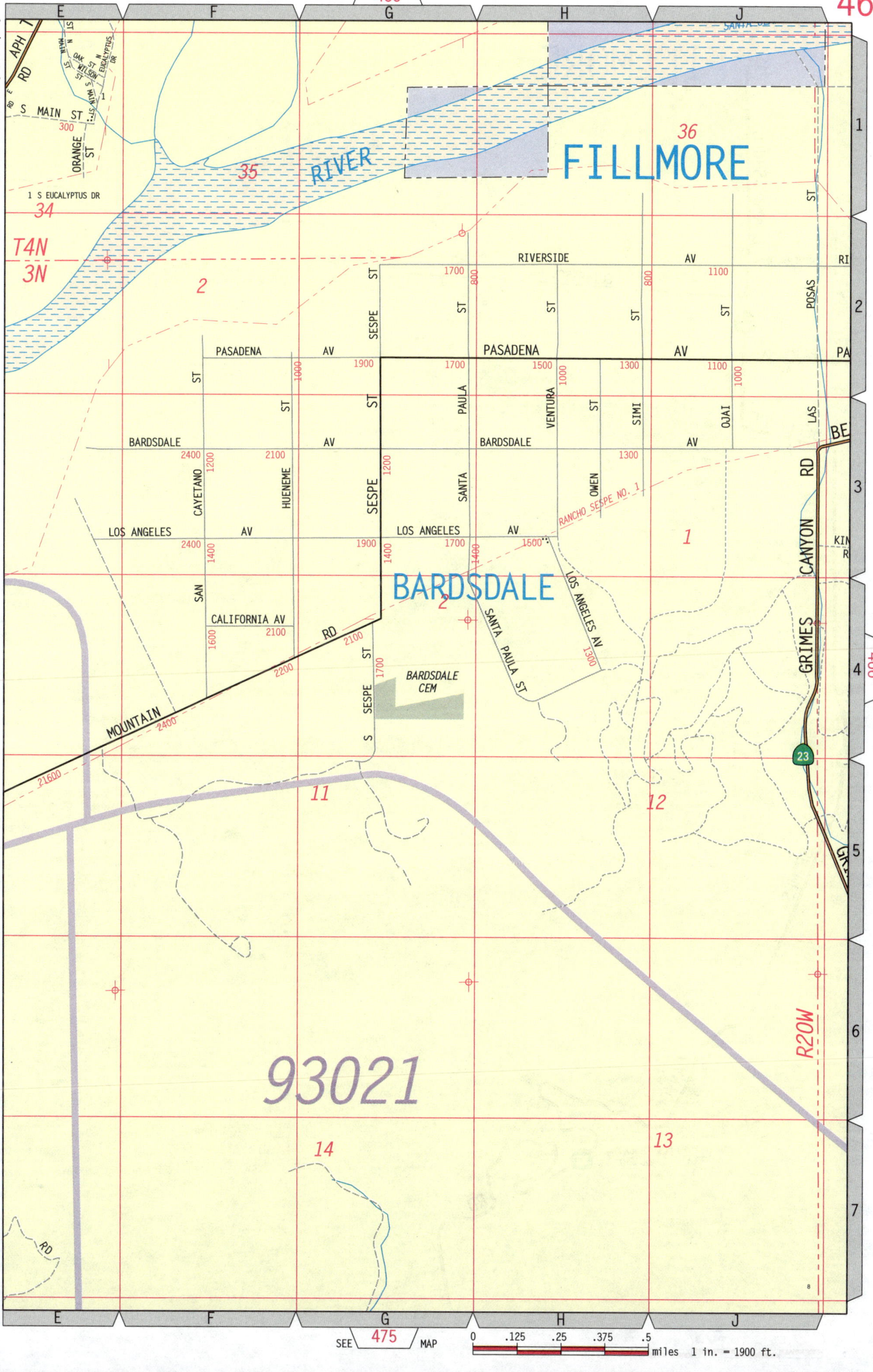

SEE 455 MAP

FILLMORE
BARDSDALE
RIVER
SANTA CLARA
RIVERSIDE AV
PASADENA AV
BARDSDALE AV
LOS ANGELES AV
CALIFORNIA AV
MOUNTAIN RD
SESPE ST
S SESPE ST
SANTA PAULA ST
VENTURA ST
OWEN ST
SIMI ST
OJAI ST
CAYETANO ST
SAN ST
HUENEME ST
LAS POSAS ST
GRIMES CANYON RD
S MAIN ST
ORANGE ST
OAK ST
WILSON ST
N MAIN ST
S MAIN ST
N EUCALYPTUS DR
1 S EUCALYPTUS DR
RANCHO SESPE NO. 1
BARDSDALE CEM
LOS ANGELES AV
T4N
3N
R20W
93021
23
34
35
36
2
1
11
12
13
14

SEE 466 MAP

SEE 475 MAP

0 .125 .25 .375 .5 miles 1 in. = 1900 ft.

SEE 456 MAP

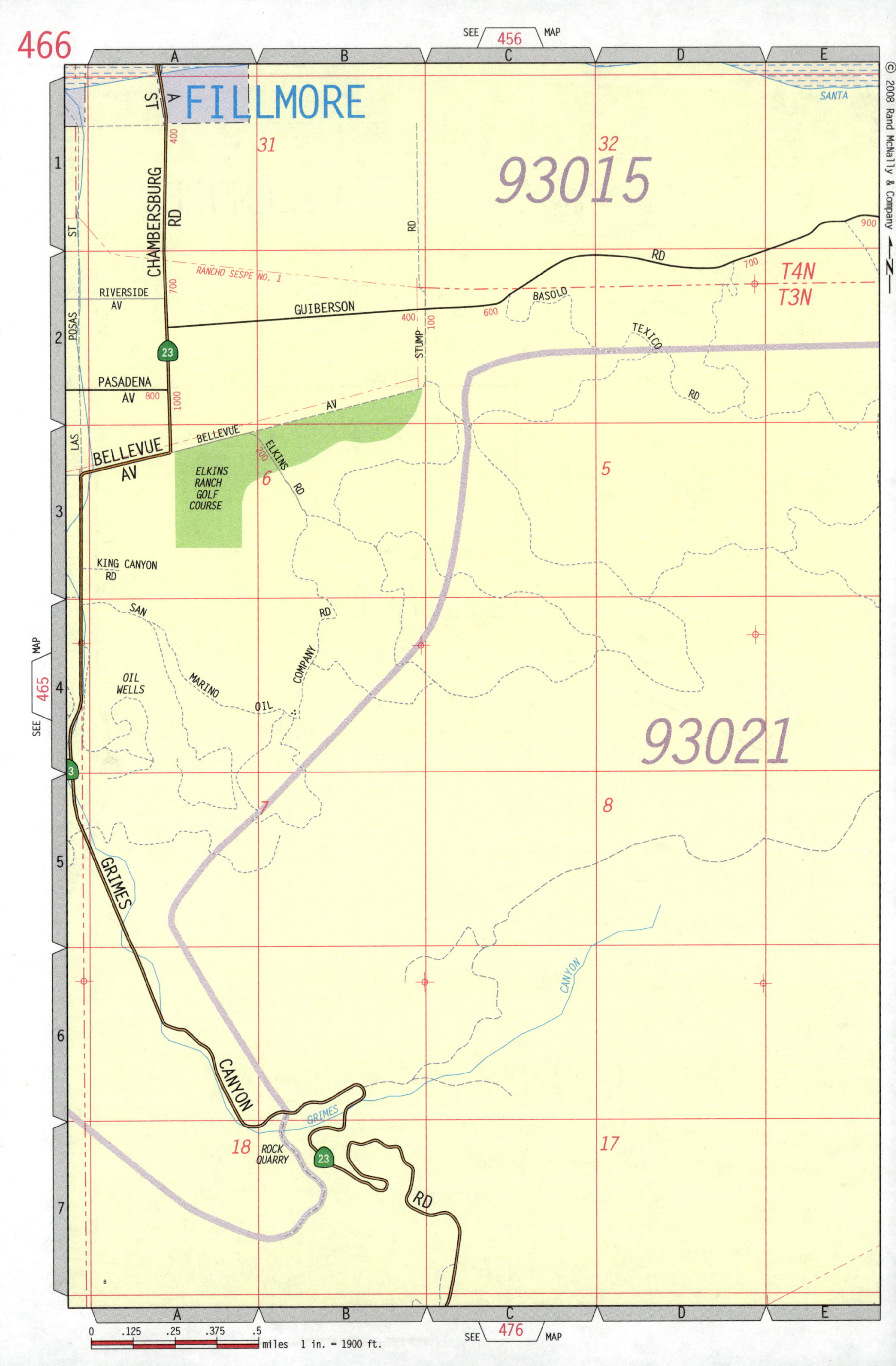

FILLMORE
A ST
CHAMBERSBURG RD
31
32
93015
RD
RD
RANCHO SESPE NO. 1
T4N
T3N
RIVERSIDE AV
GUIBERSON
BASOLO
TEXICO
RD
STUMP
POSAS
PASADENA AV
LAS
BELLEVUE AV
BELLEVUE AV
ELKINS RD
ELKINS RANCH GOLF COURSE
6
5
KING CANYON RD
SAN MARINO OIL COMPANY RD
OIL WELLS
93021
7
8
GRIMES CANYON RD
CANYON
GRIMES
18
ROCK QUARRY
17
SANTA
23
3
A B C D E
1 2 3 4 5 6 7

SEE 465 MAP

SEE 476 MAP

0 .125 .25 .375 .5 miles 1 in. = 1900 ft.

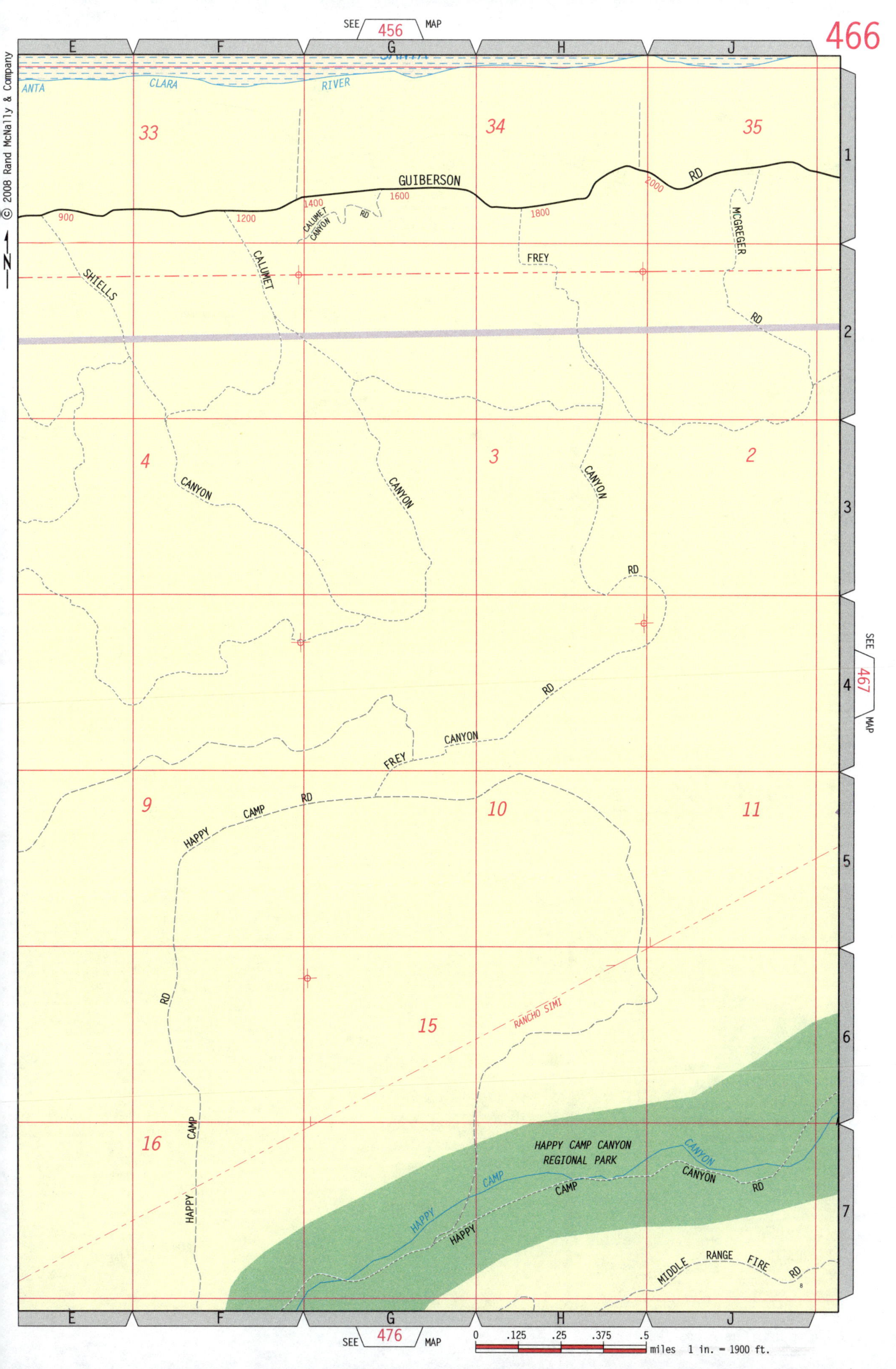
SEE 456 MAP
E
F
G
H
J
CLARA
RIVER
ANTA
33
34
35
GUIBERSON
RD
900
1200
1400
1600
1800
2000
CALUMET CANYON
RD
MCGREGER
FREY
SHIELLS
CALUMET
RD
4
3
2
CANYON
CANYON
CANYON
RD
RD
CANYON
FREY
9
10
11
HAPPY
CAMP
RD
RD
RANCHO SIMI
15
16
CAMP
HAPPY
HAPPY CAMP CANYON
REGIONAL PARK
CANYON
CANYON
RD
CAMP
CAMP
HAPPY
HAPPY
MIDDLE
RANGE
FIRE
RD
1
2
3
4
5
6
7
SEE 467 MAP
SEE 476 MAP
0
.125
.25
.375
.5
miles 1 in. = 1900 ft.

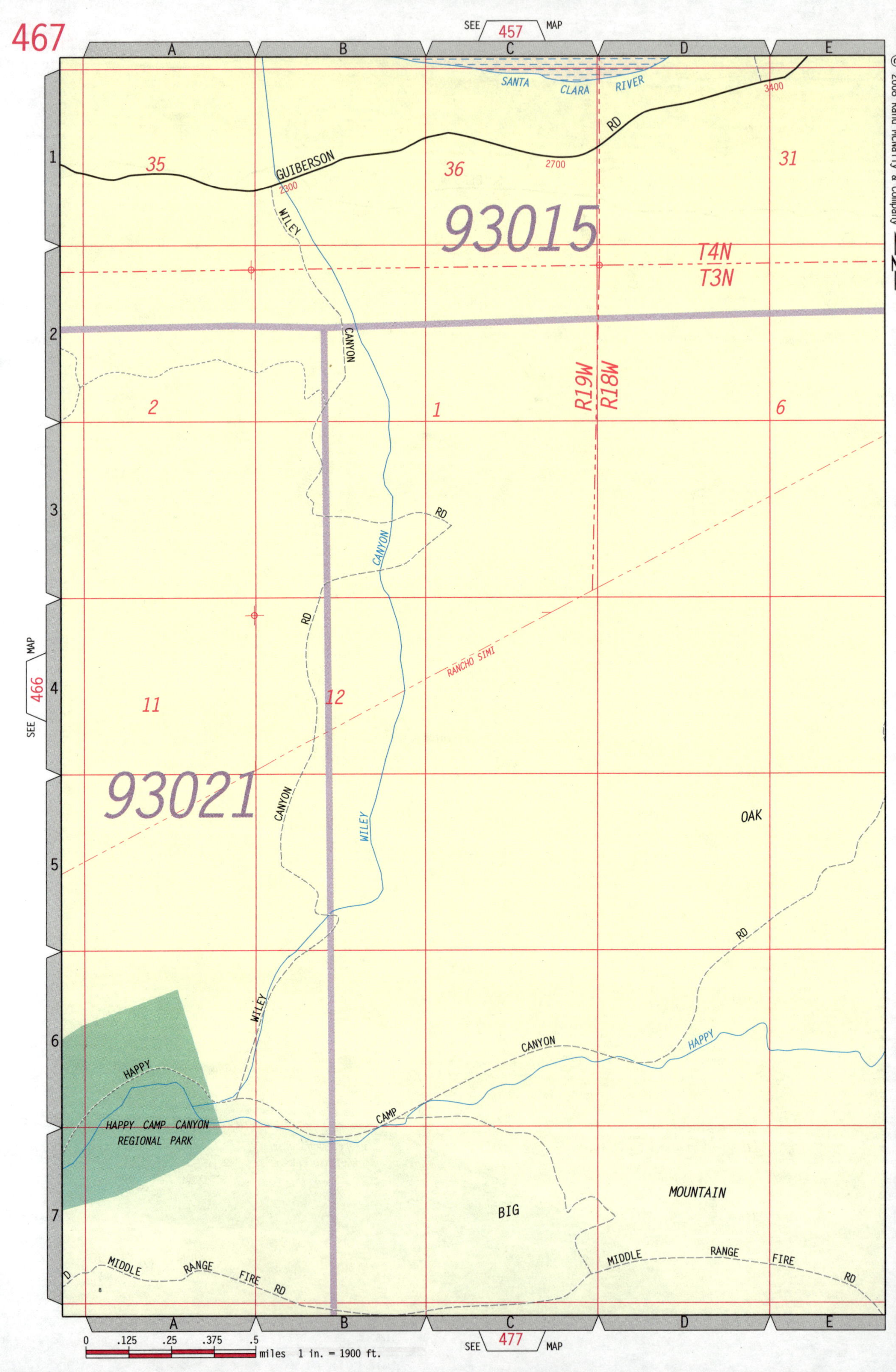
SEE 457 MAP
SANTA CLARA RIVER
GUIBERSON RD
2300
2700
3400
35
36
31
93015
WILEY CANYON RD
T4N
T3N
R19W
R18W
2
1
6
RANCHO SIMI
11
12
93021
CANYON
WILEY
OAK
RD
HAPPY
CANYON
CAMP
HAPPY CAMP CANYON REGIONAL PARK
BIG
MOUNTAIN
MIDDLE RANGE FIRE RD
SEE 466 MAP
SEE 477 MAP
0 .125 .25 .375 .5 miles 1 in. = 1900 ft.

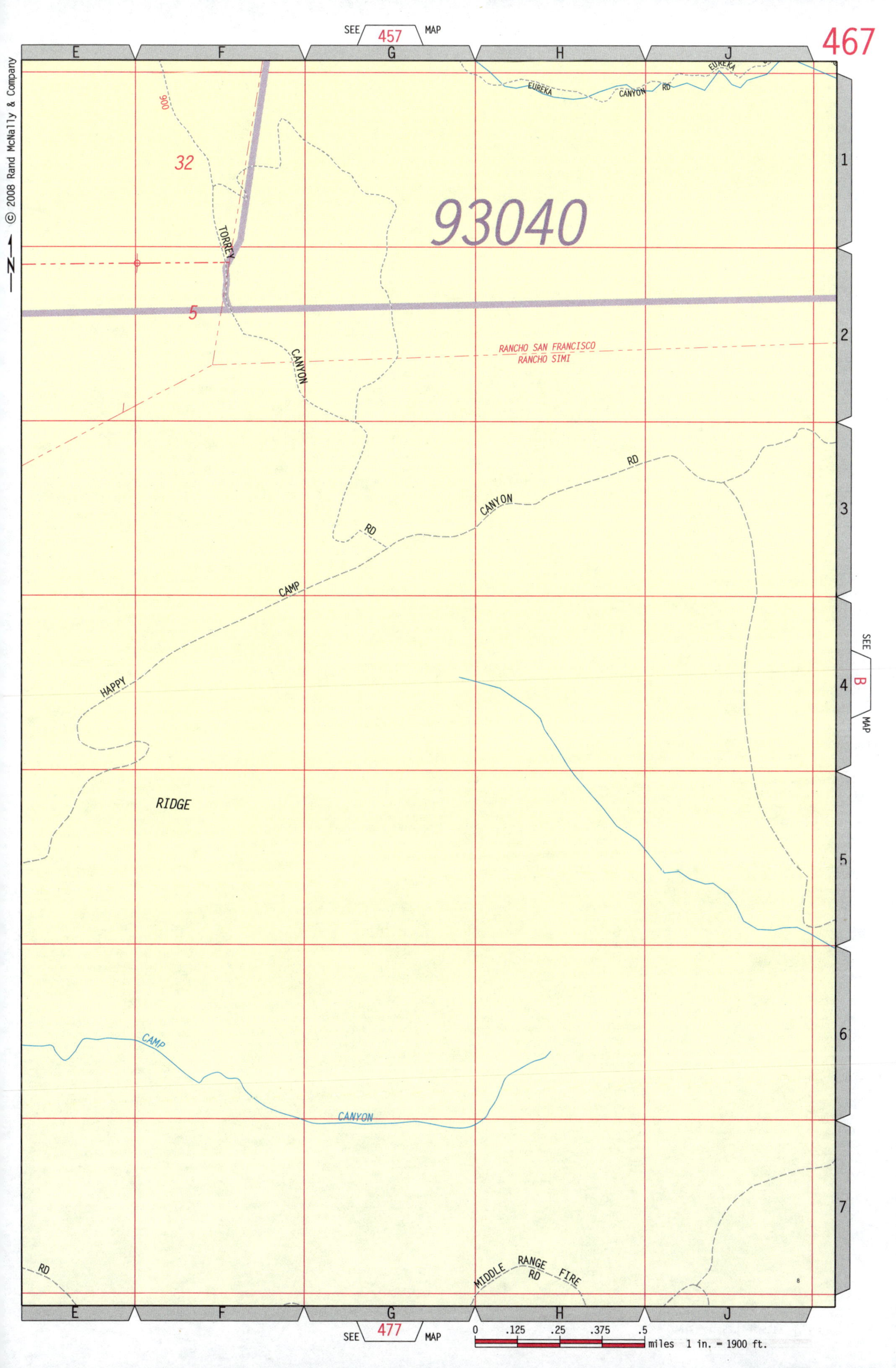
SEE 457 MAP
E
F
G
H
J
1
2
3
4
5
6
7
93040
32
5
900
TORREY
CANYON
EUREKA
CANYON RD
EUREKA
RANCHO SAN FRANCISCO
RANCHO SIMI
RD
CANYON
RD
CAMP
HAPPY
RIDGE
SEE B MAP
CAMP
CANYON
RD
MIDDLE
RANGE
RD
FIRE
SEE 477 MAP
0 .125 .25 .375 .5
miles 1 in. = 1900 ft.

SEE 459 MAP

A B C D E

1
2
3
4
5
6
7

SEE B MAP

A B C D E

8

SEE B MAP

0 .125 .25 .375 .5 miles 1 in. = 1900 ft.

N

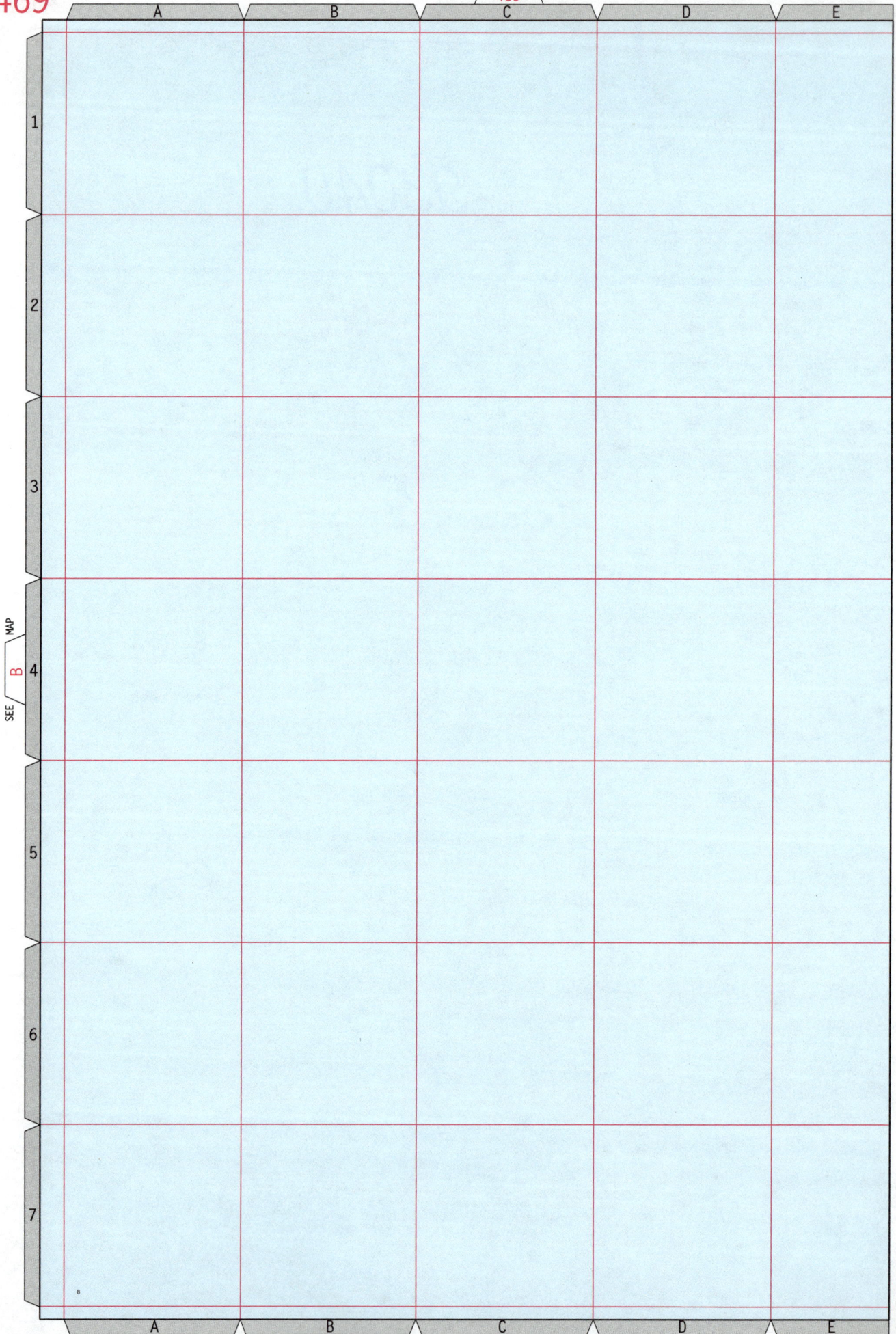

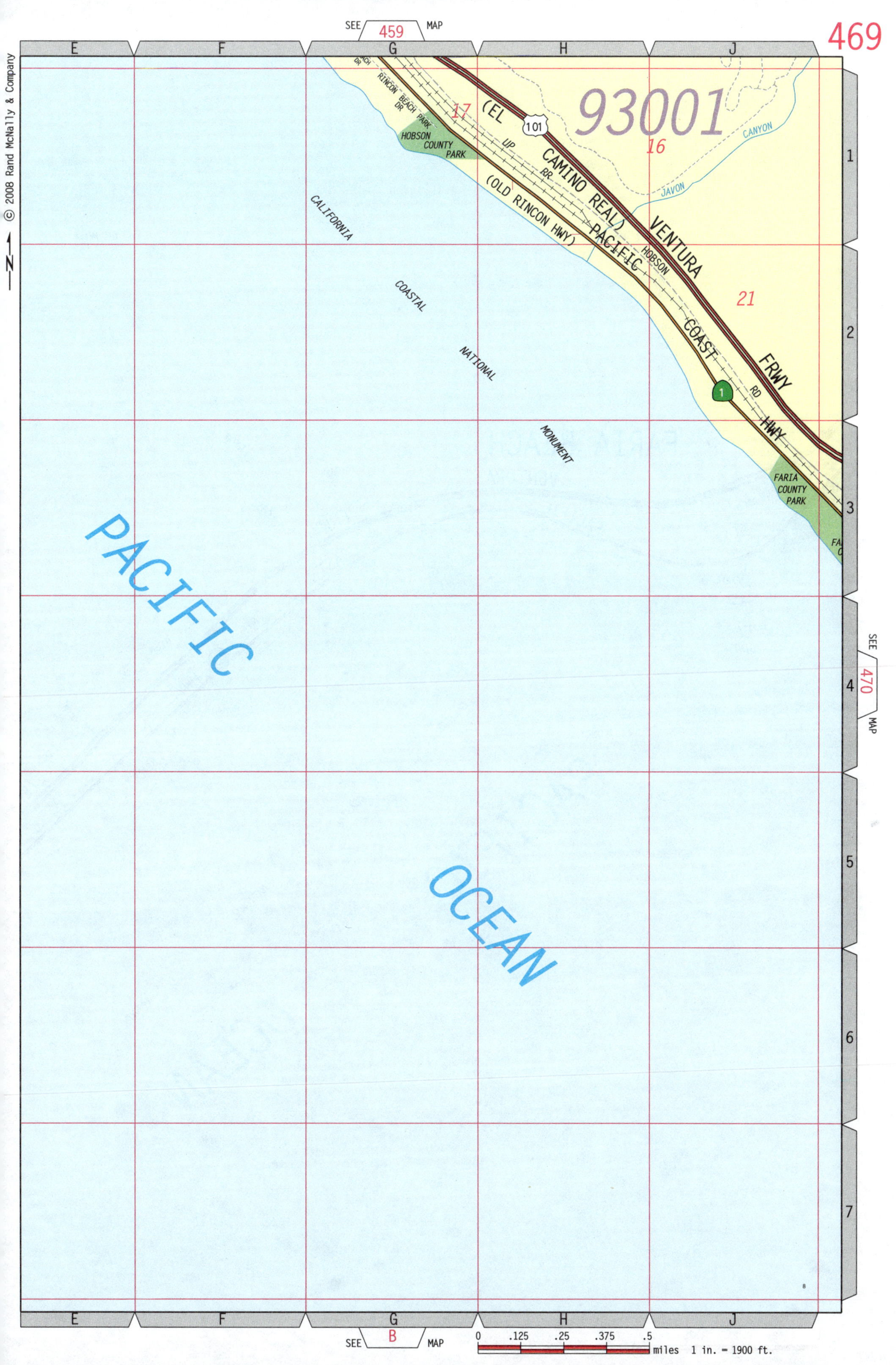

SEE 459 MAP
E
F
G
H
J
1
2
3
4
5
6
7
93001
17
16
21
(EL
101
CAMINO REAL)
VENTURA
FRWY
CANYON
JAVON
UP
RR
HOBSON
RD
RINCON BEACH PARK DR
HOBSON COUNTY PARK
(OLD RINCON HWY)
PACIFIC
COAST
HWY
1
FARIA COUNTY PARK
CALIFORNIA
COASTAL
NATIONAL
MONUMENT
PACIFIC
OCEAN
SEE 470 MAP
SEE B MAP
0
.125
.25
.375
.5
miles 1 in. = 1900 ft.

SEE 460 MAP

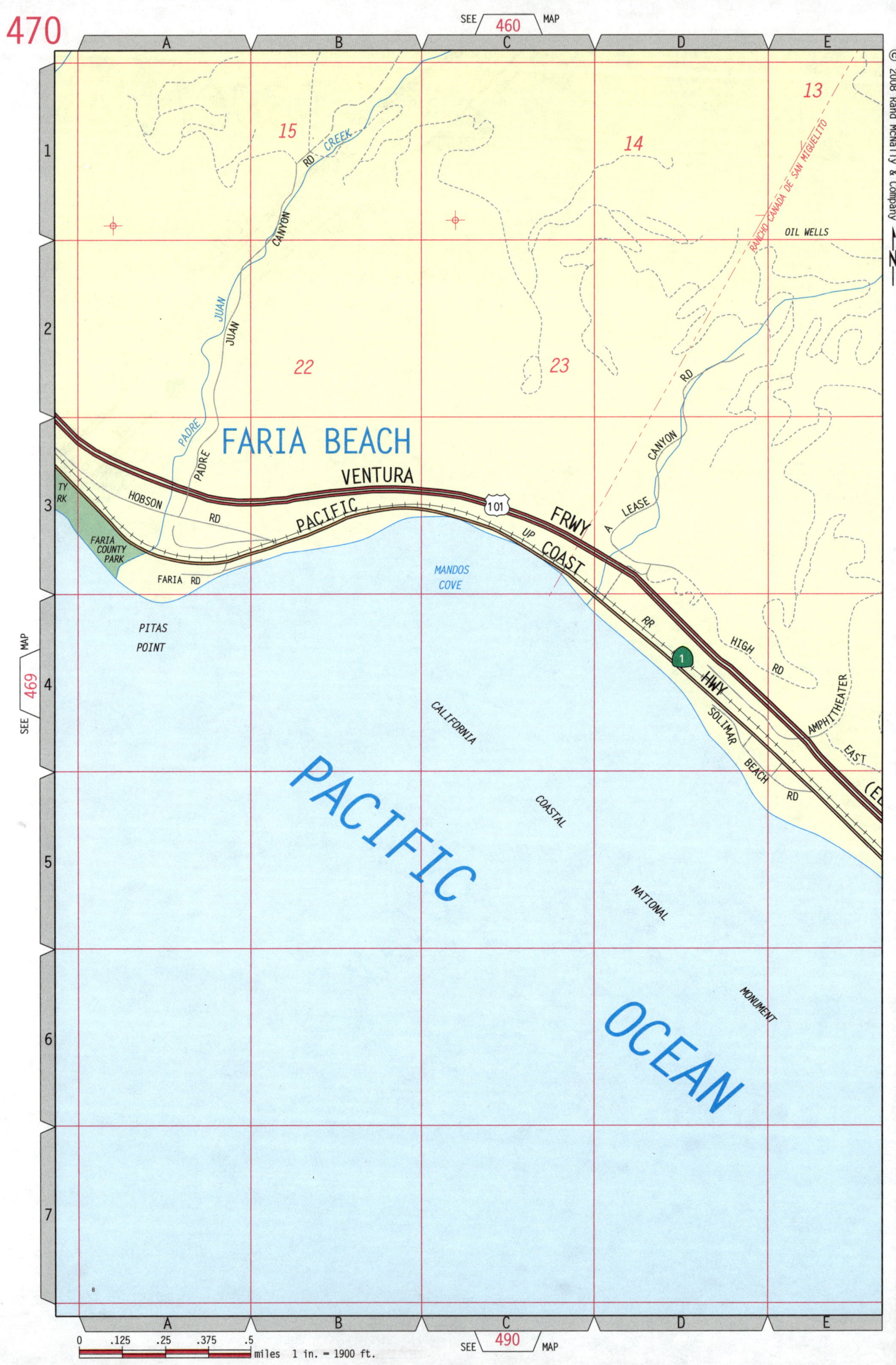

A
B
C
D
E
1
2
3
4
5
6
7
15
14
13
22
23
CREEK
RD
CANYON
JUAN
JUAN
PADRE
PADRE
RANCHO CANADA DE SAN MIGUELITO
OIL WELLS
RD
CANYON
FARIA BEACH
VENTURA
HOBSON
RD
PACIFIC
101
FRWY
UP
COAST
LEASE
A
FARIA COUNTY PARK
FARIA RD
MANDOS COVE
PITAS POINT
RR
1
HIGH
RD
HWY
SOLIMAR
BEACH
RD
AMPHITHEATER
EAST
CALIFORNIA
COASTAL
NATIONAL
MONUMENT
PACIFIC
OCEAN
0 .125 .25 .375 .5 miles 1 in. = 1900 ft.

SEE 469 MAP

SEE 490 MAP

SEE 460 MAP

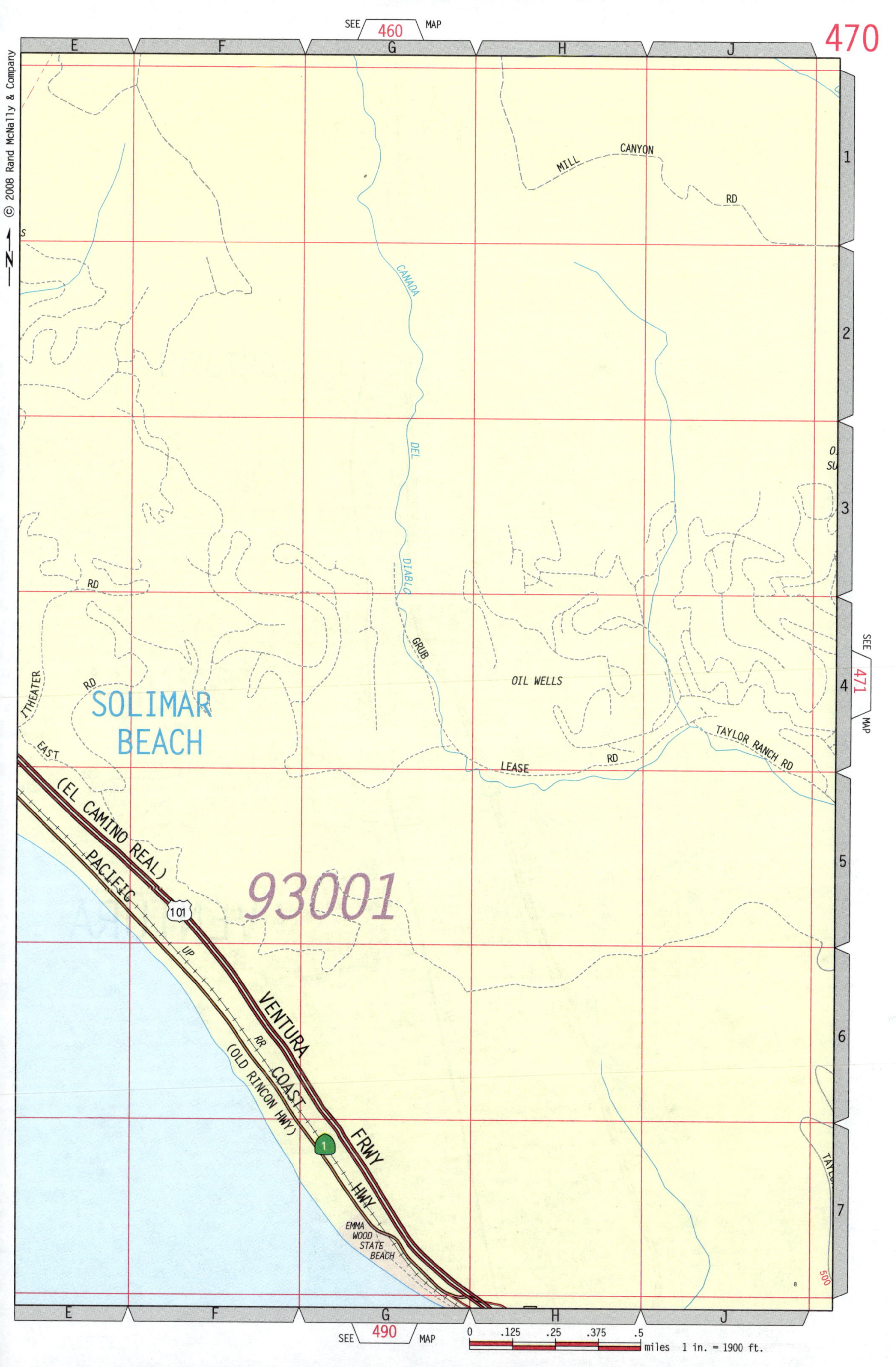
E
F
G
H
J
1
2
3
4
5
6
7
MILL CANYON RD
CANADA DEL DIABLO
GRUB
OIL WELLS
LEASE RD
TAYLOR RANCH RD
RD
THEATER
RD
EAST
SOLIMAR BEACH
93001
(EL CAMINO REAL)
PACIFIC
101
UP
VENTURA
RR
COAST
(OLD RINCON HWY)
FRWY
1
HWY
EMMA WOOD STATE BEACH
500
0 .125 .25 .375 .5 miles 1 in. = 1900 ft.

SEE 471 MAP
SEE 490 MAP

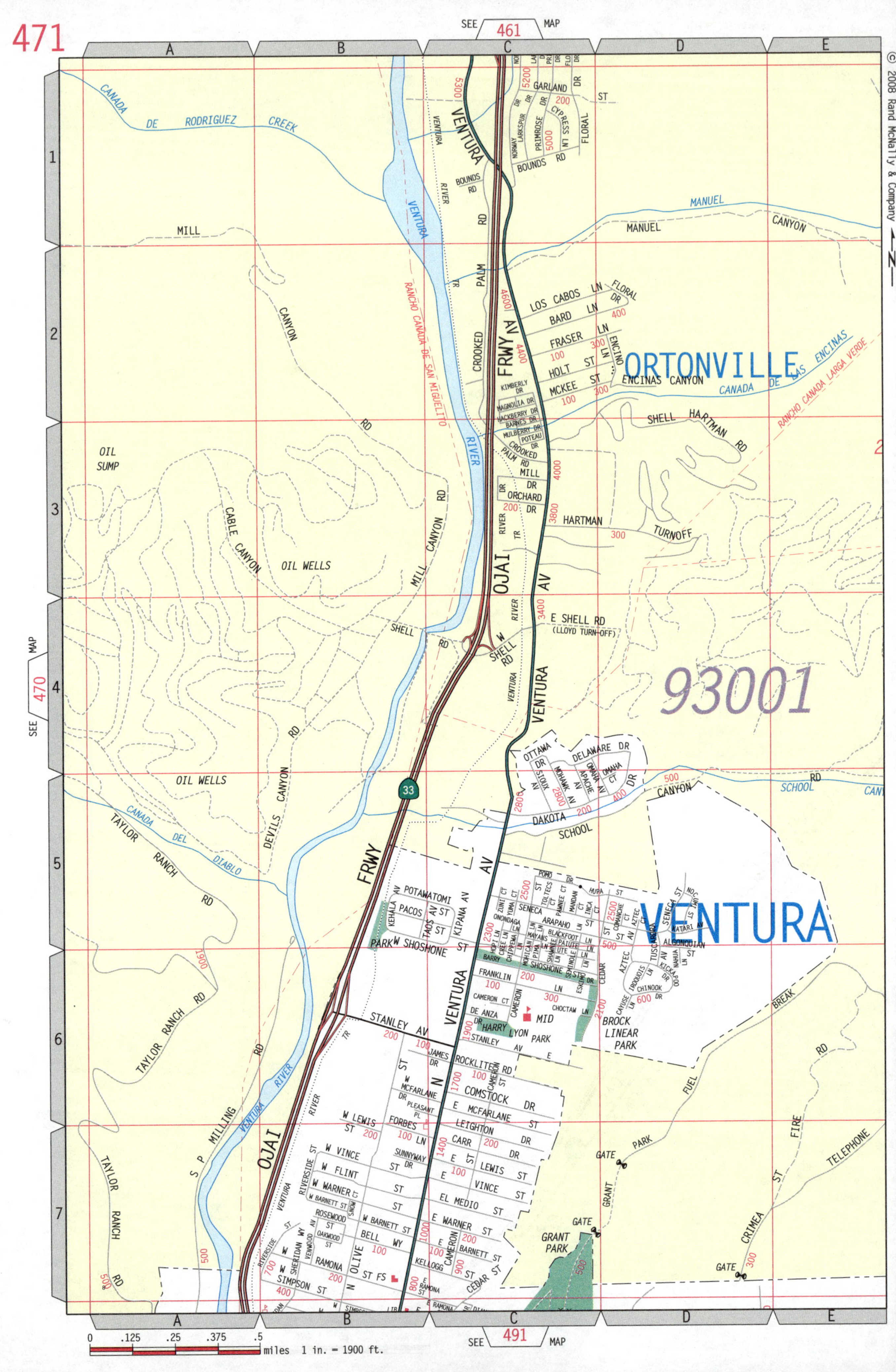
SEE 461 MAP
SEE 470 MAP
SEE 491 MAP
A
B
C
D
E
1
2
3
4
5
6
7
CANADA DE RODRIGUEZ CREEK
VENTURA RIVER
MANUEL CANYON
MILL CANYON RD
RANCHO CANADA DE SAN MIGUELITO
RANCHO CANADA LARGA VERDE
ORTONVILLE
CANADA DE LAS ENCINAS
ENCINAS CANYON
SHELL HARTMAN RD
HARTMAN TURNOFF
E SHELL RD
(LLOYD TURN-OFF)
W SHELL RD
OIL SUMP
OIL WELLS
CABLE CANYON
DEVILS CANYON RD
CANADA DEL DIABLO
TAYLOR RANCH RD
S P MILLING RD
93001
VENTURA
VENTURA AV
OJAI FRWY
33
GARLAND ST
BOUNDS RD
LOS CABOS LN
BARD LN
FRASER LN
HOLT ST
MCKEE ST
CROOKED PALM RD
ORCHARD DR
MILL DR
DAKOTA
SCHOOL CANYON RD
OTTAWA DR
DELAWARE DR
POTAWATOMI
W SHOSHONE ST
STANLEY AV
HARRY LYON PARK
MID
BROCK LINEAR PARK
JAMES DR
ROCKLITE RD
COMSTOCK DR
E MCFARLANE ST
LEIGHTON DR
CARR DR
LEWIS ST
VINCE ST
EL MEDIO ST
E WARNER ST
BARNETT ST
KELLOGG ST
CEDAR ST
W LEWIS ST
W VINCE ST
W FLINT ST
W WARNER ST
W BARNETT ST
BELL WY
RAMONA ST
SIMPSON ST
OLIVE ST
GRANT PARK
GATE
FUEL BREAK RD
FIRE RD
TELEPHONE
CRIMEA ST
0 .125 .25 .375 .5 miles 1 in. = 1900 ft.

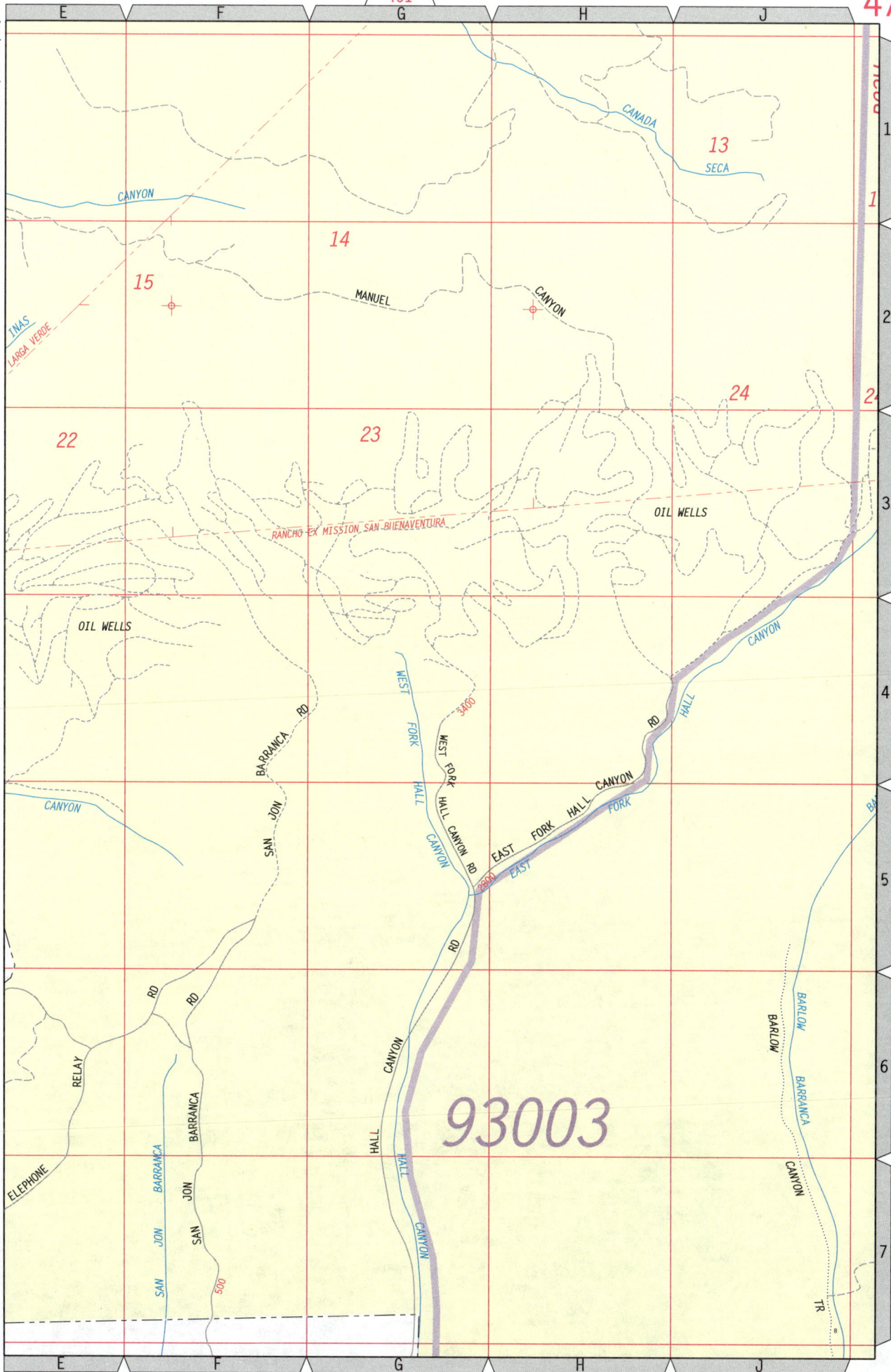

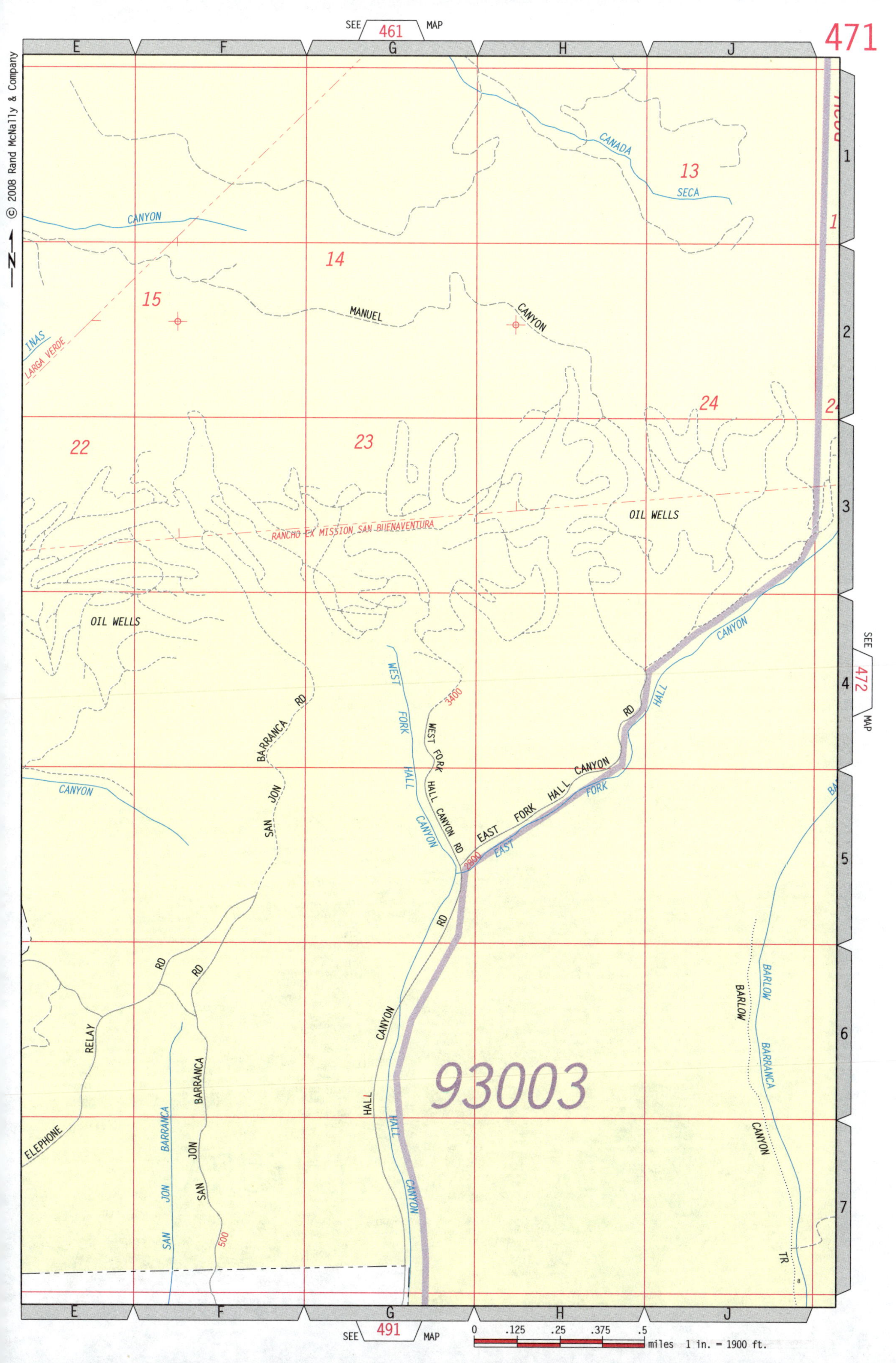
SEE 461 MAP
E
F
G
H
J
1
2
3
4
5
6
7
13
14
15
22
23
24
CANYON
CANADA
SECA
MANUEL
CANYON
INAS
LARGA VERDE
RANCHO EX MISSION SAN BUENAVENTURA
OIL WELLS
OIL WELLS
BARRANCA
RD
SAN JON
WEST FORK HALL CANYON
WEST FORK HALL CANYON RD
3400
EAST FORK HALL CANYON RD
EAST FORK
2800
HALL CANYON
CANYON
RD
RD
RD
RELAY
ELEPHONE
SAN JON BARRANCA
SAN JON BARRANCA
500
HALL CANYON RD
HALL CANYON
93003
BARLOW
BARLOW BARRANCA
CANYON
TR
SEE 472 MAP
SEE 491 MAP
0 .125 .25 .375 .5
miles 1 in. = 1900 ft.

SEE 462 MAP

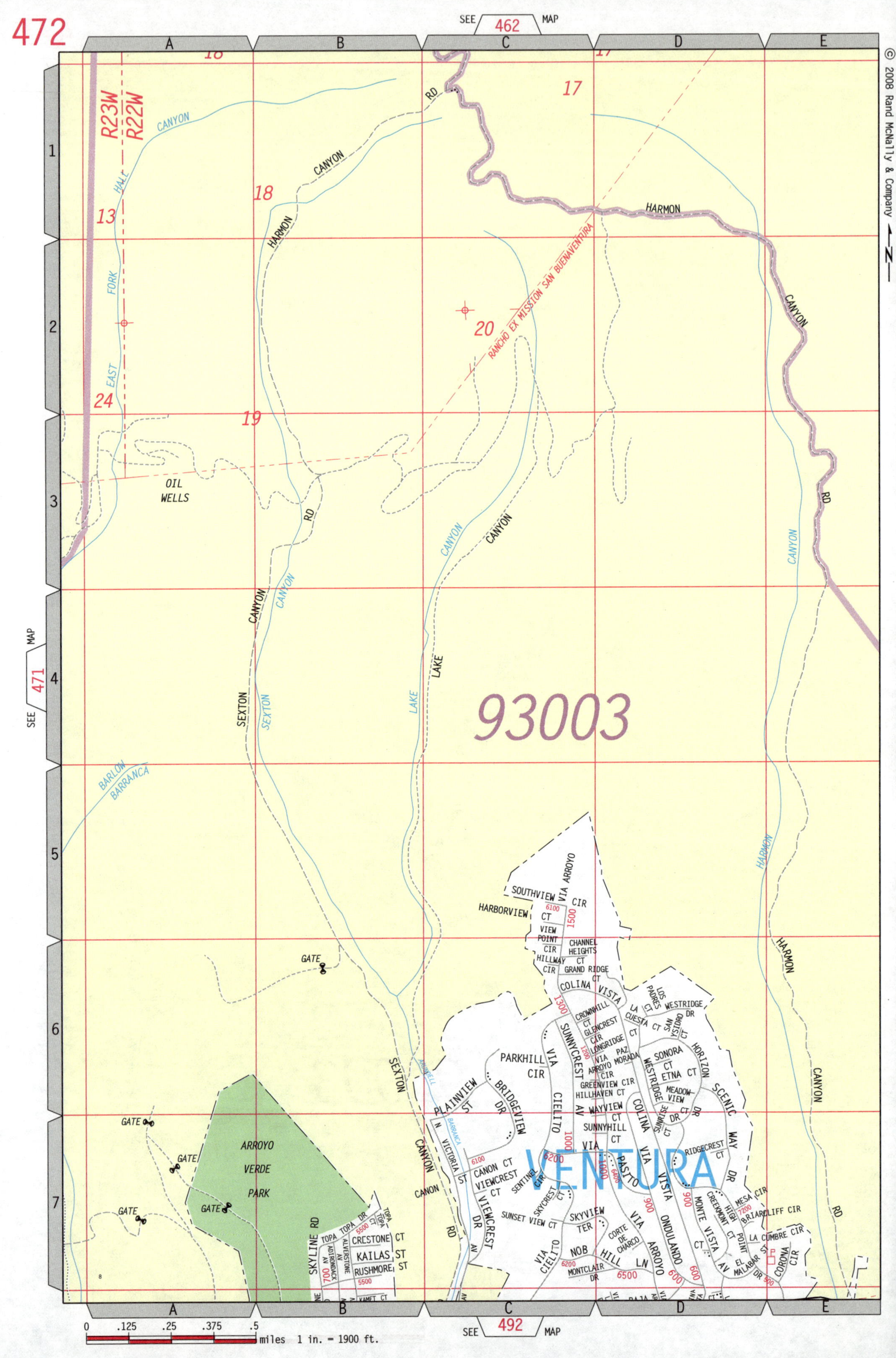
A
B
C
D
E
1
2
3
4
5
6
7
R23W
R22W
HALL
CANYON
EAST
FORK
13
24
18
19
20
17
HARMON
CANYON
RD
RANCHO EX MISSION SAN BUENAVENTURA
OIL
WELLS
SEXTON
CANYON
LAKE
93003
BARLOW
BARRANCA
GATE
ARROYO
VERDE
PARK
SOUTHVIEW
VIA ARROYO
CIR
HARBORVIEW
CT
VIEW
POINT
CIR
CHANNEL
HEIGHTS
HILLWAY
GRAND RIDGE
COLINA
VISTA
LOS
PADRES
WESTRIDGE
DR
CROWNHILL
GLENCREST
LONGRIDGE
LA
CUESTA
SAN
YSIDRO
HORIZON
SONORA
ETNA
PARKHILL
VIA
CIELITO
SUNNYCREST
AV
PAZ
MORADA
ARROYO
GREENVIEW CIR
HILLHAVEN CT
MEADOW-
VIEW
SCENIC
WAY
PLAINVIEW
ST
BRIDGEVIEW
WAYVIEW
SUNNYHILL
SUNRISE
RIDGECREST
VENTURA
VICTORIA
N
BARRANCA
CANON CT
VIEWCREST
SENTINEL
PASITO
ONDULANDO
CREEKMONT
MONTE VISTA
HIGH
POINT
MESA CIR
BRIARCLIFF CIR
SKYCREST
SUNSET VIEW CT
SKYVIEW
TER
CORTE
DE
CHARCO
NOB
HILL
LN
MONTCLAIR
EL
MALABAR
LA CUMBRE CIR
CORONA
SKYLINE RD
TOPA TOPA DR
CRESTONE CT
KAILAS ST
RUSHMORE ST
ADIRONDACK AV
ALVERSTONE AV
KAMET CT
1500
6100
1300
1200
1000
6200
900
600
7200
6500
5500
700
© 2008 Rand McNally & Company
N
0 .125 .25 .375 .5
miles 1 in. = 1900 ft.

SEE 471 MAP

SEE 492 MAP

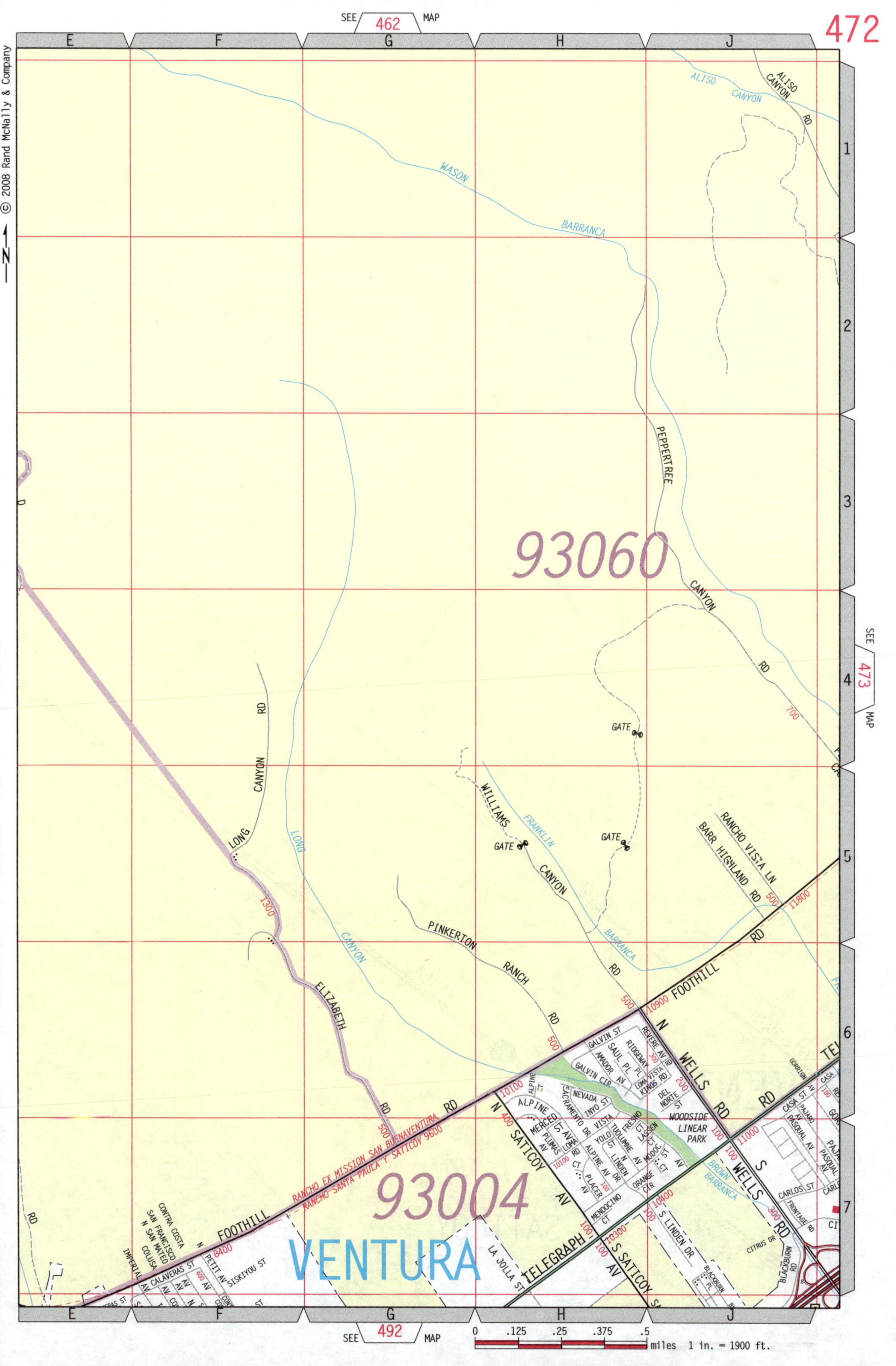

SEE 462 MAP
SEE 473 MAP
SEE 492 MAP
© 2008 Rand McNally & Company
93060
93004
VENTURA
ALISO CANYON RD
WASON BARRANCA
PEPPERTREE CANYON RD
LONG CANYON RD
WILLIAMS CANYON RD
FRANKLIN BARRANCA
PINKERTON RANCH RD
ELIZABETH RD
RANCHO VISTA LN
BARR HIGHLAND RD
FOOTHILL RD
N WELLS RD
S WELLS RD
N SATICOY AV
S SATICOY AV
TELEGRAPH RD
WOODSIDE LINEAR PARK
BROWN BARRANCA
RANCHO EX MISSION SAN BUENAVENTURA
RANCHO SANTA PAULA Y SATICOY 9600
GATE
miles 1 in. = 1900 ft.
0 .125 .25 .375 .5

SEE 463 MAP

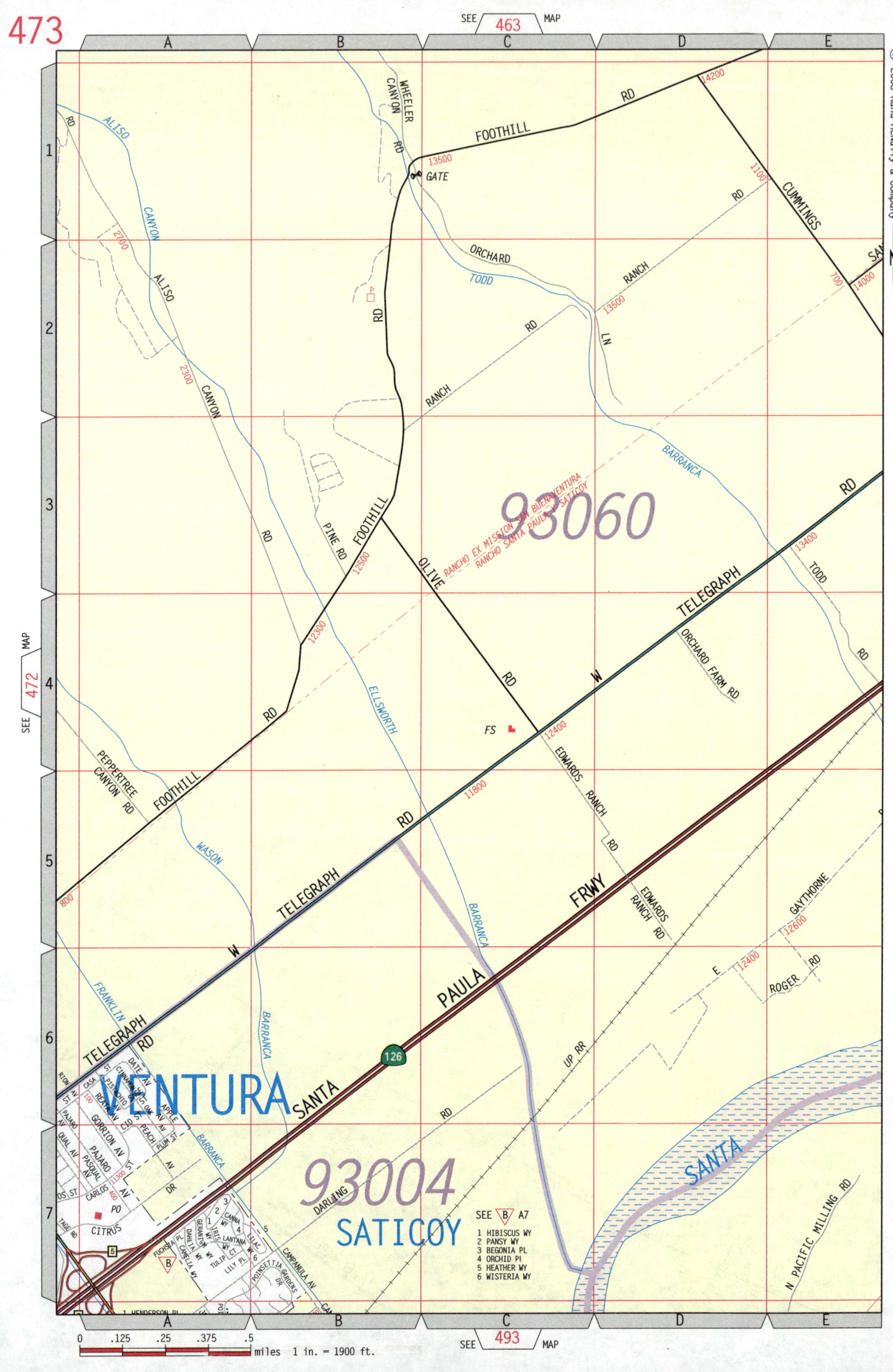

93060
93004
VENTURA
SATICOY
FOOTHILL RD
W TELEGRAPH RD
SANTA PAULA FRWY
126
OLIVE RD
ALISO CANYON RD
WHEELER CANYON RD
CUMMINGS RD
RANCH RD
ORCHARD
TODD LN
TODD RD
PINE RD
EDWARDS RANCH RD
ORCHARD FARM RD
PEPPERTREE CANYON RD
GAYTHORNE
E ROGER RD
DARLING RD
N PACIFIC MILLING RD
UP RR
GATE
FS
PO
CITRUS
ALISO CANYON
BARRANCA
ELLSWORTH
WASON
FRANKLIN
SANTA
RANCHO EX MISSION SAN BUENAVENTURA
RANCHO SANTA PAULA Y SATICOY
SEE B A7
1 HIBISCUS WY
2 PANSY WY
3 BEGONIA PL
4 ORCHID PL
5 HEATHER WY
6 WISTERIA WY
1 HENDERSON PL
0 .125 .25 .375 .5 miles 1 in. = 1900 ft.

SEE 472 MAP

SEE 493 MAP

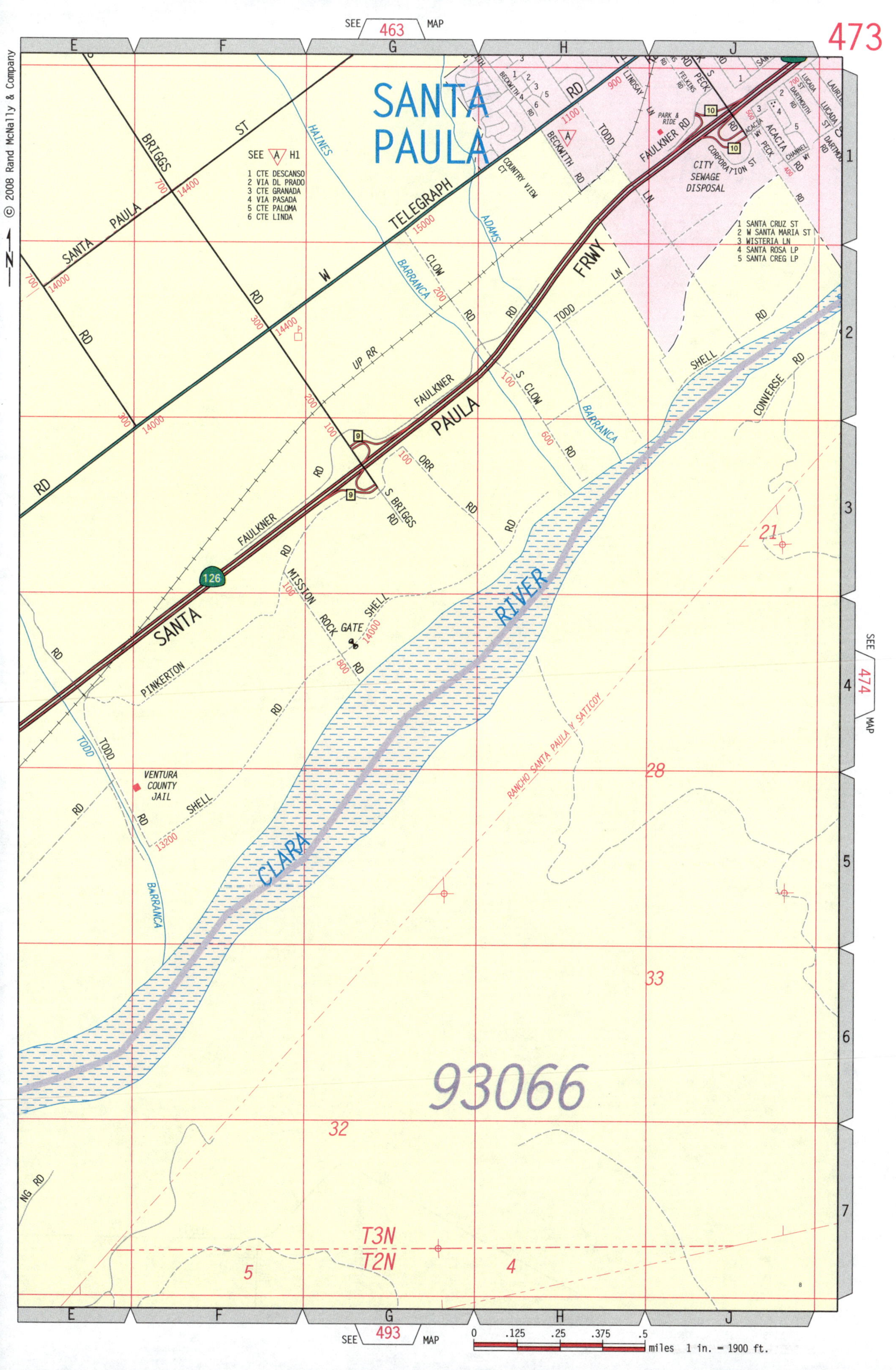
SEE 463 MAP
SANTA PAULA
SEE A H1
1 CTE DESCANSO
2 VIA DL PRADO
3 CTE GRANADA
4 VIA PASADA
5 CTE PALOMA
6 CTE LINDA
1 SANTA CRUZ ST
2 W SANTA MARIA ST
3 WISTERIA LN
4 SANTA ROSA LP
5 SANTA CREG LP
CITY SEWAGE DISPOSAL
PARK & RIDE
W TELEGRAPH RD
SANTA PAULA ST
BRIGGS RD
HAINES BARRANCA
ADAMS BARRANCA
SANTA PAULA FRWY
FAULKNER RD
UP RR
S CLOW RD
ORR RD
S BRIGGS RD
MISSION ROCK RD
SHELL RD
GATE
PINKERTON RD
TODD RD
TODD BARRANCA
VENTURA COUNTY JAIL
CONVERSE RD
SANTA CLARA RIVER
RANCHO SANTA PAULA Y SATICOY
93066
T3N
T2N
SEE 474 MAP
SEE 493 MAP
0 .125 .25 .375 .5 miles 1 in. = 1900 ft.

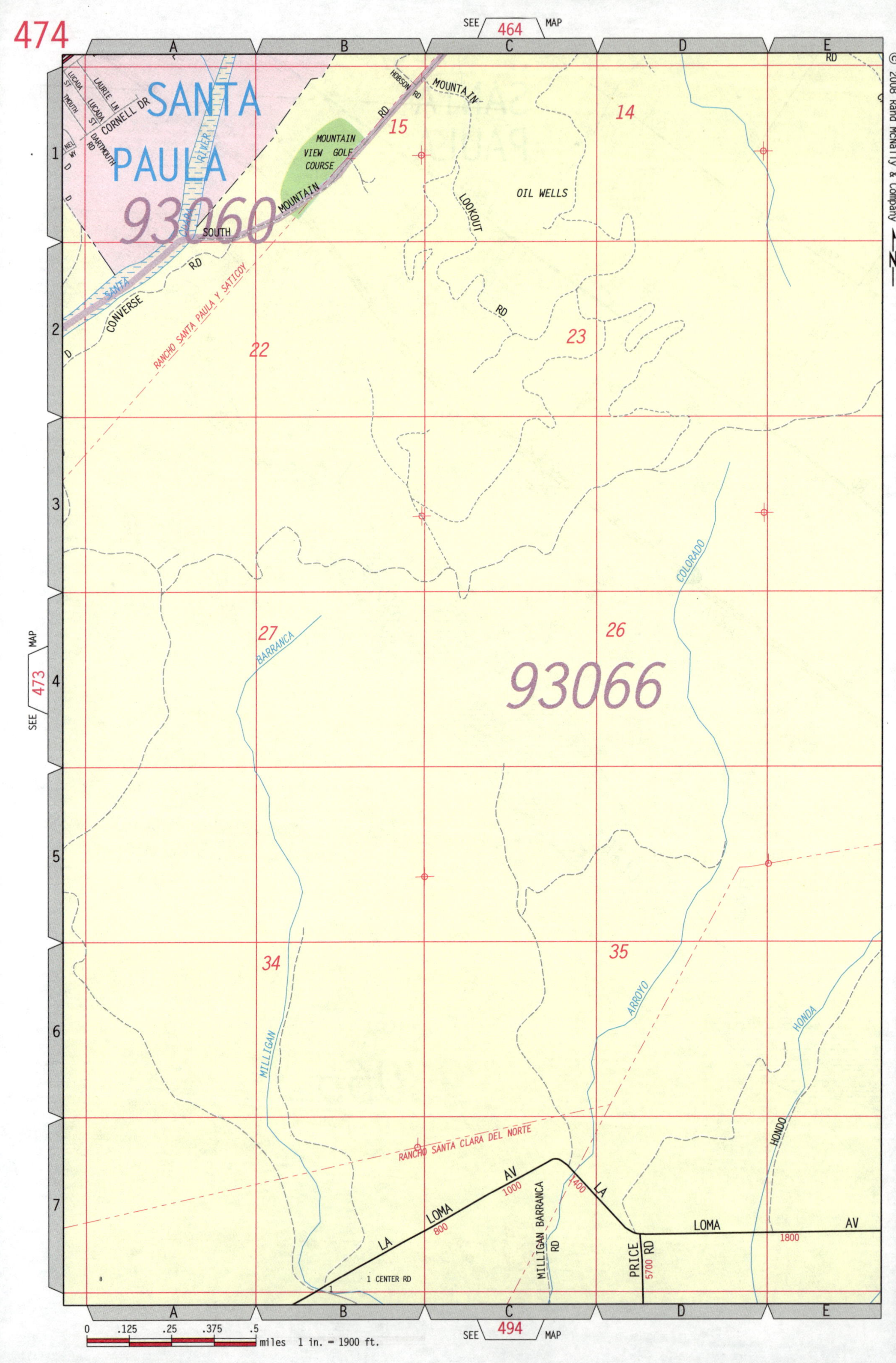

SEE 464 MAP
SANTA PAULA
93060
LUCADA ST
LAURIE LN
CORNELL DR
DARTMOUTH RD
RIVER
MOUNTAIN VIEW GOLF COURSE
HOBSON RD
MOUNTAIN RD
15
14
OIL WELLS
LOOKOUT RD
SOUTH MOUNTAIN
SANTA
CONVERSE RD
RANCHO SANTA PAULA Y SATICOY
22
23
27
26
BARRANCA
COLORADO
93066
SEE 473 MAP
34
35
MILLIGAN
ARROYO
HONDA
HONDO
RANCHO SANTA CLARA DEL NORTE
LA LOMA AV
800
1000
1400
MILLIGAN BARRANCA RD
PRICE RD
5700
LOMA AV
1800
1 CENTER RD
SEE 494 MAP
0 .125 .25 .375 .5
miles 1 in. = 1900 ft.

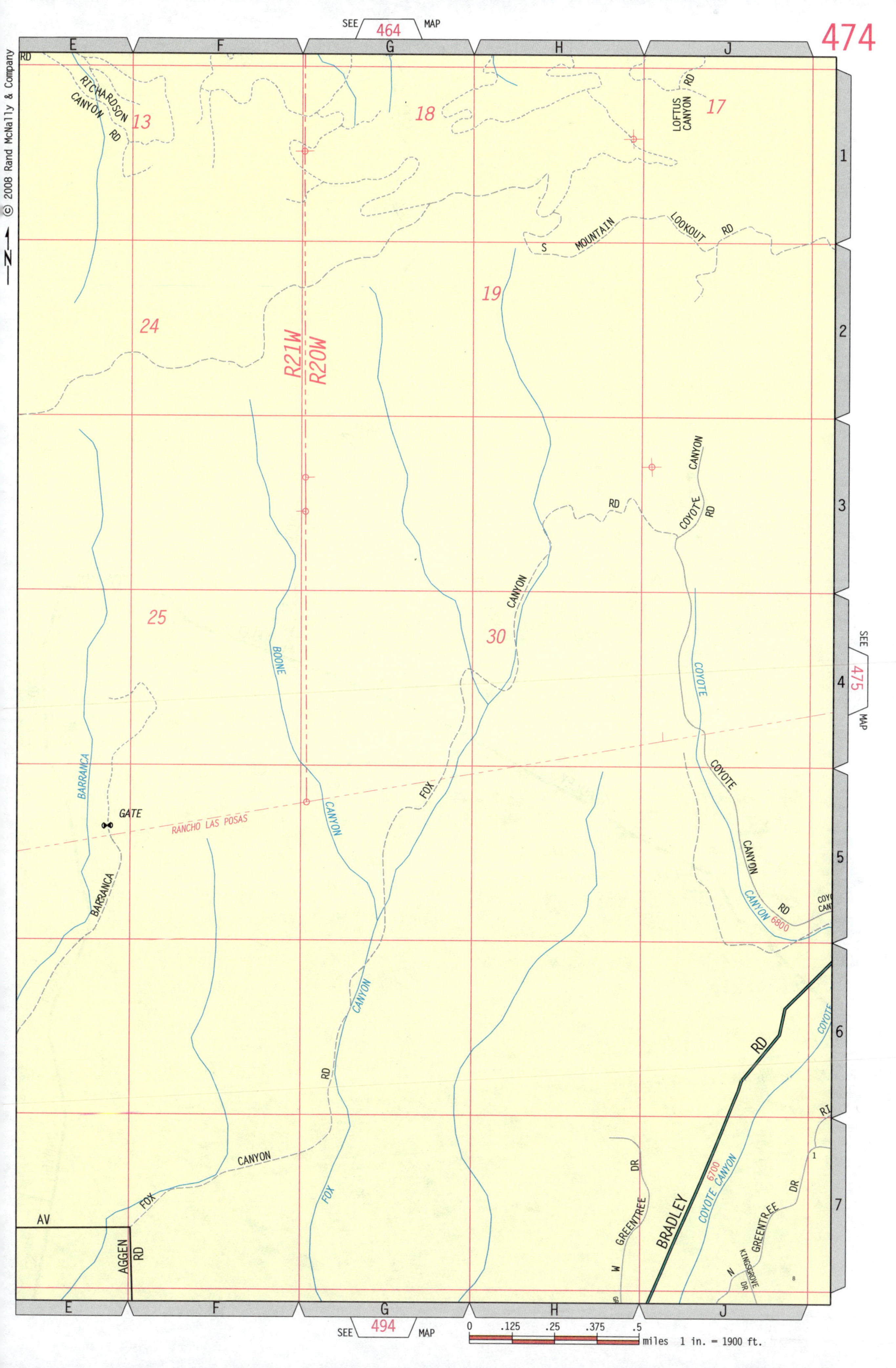
SEE 464 MAP
RD
RICHARDSON CANYON RD
13
18
17
LOFTUS CANYON RD
S MOUNTAIN LOOKOUT RD
24
19
R21W
R20W
CANYON
COYOTE RD
RD
25
30
CANYON
BOONE
COYOTE
SEE 475 MAP
BARRANCA
GATE
RANCHO LAS POSAS
FOX
CANYON
COYOTE
CANYON
BARRANCA
CANYON
RD
COYOTE CANYON
6800
CANYON
FOX
RD
COYOTE
RD
CANYON
FOX
DR
GREENTREE
W
6700
COYOTE CANYON
BRADLEY
GREENTREE DR
N KINGSGROVE DR
AV
AGGEN RD
FOX
SEE 494 MAP
0 .125 .25 .375 .5 miles 1 in. = 1900 ft.

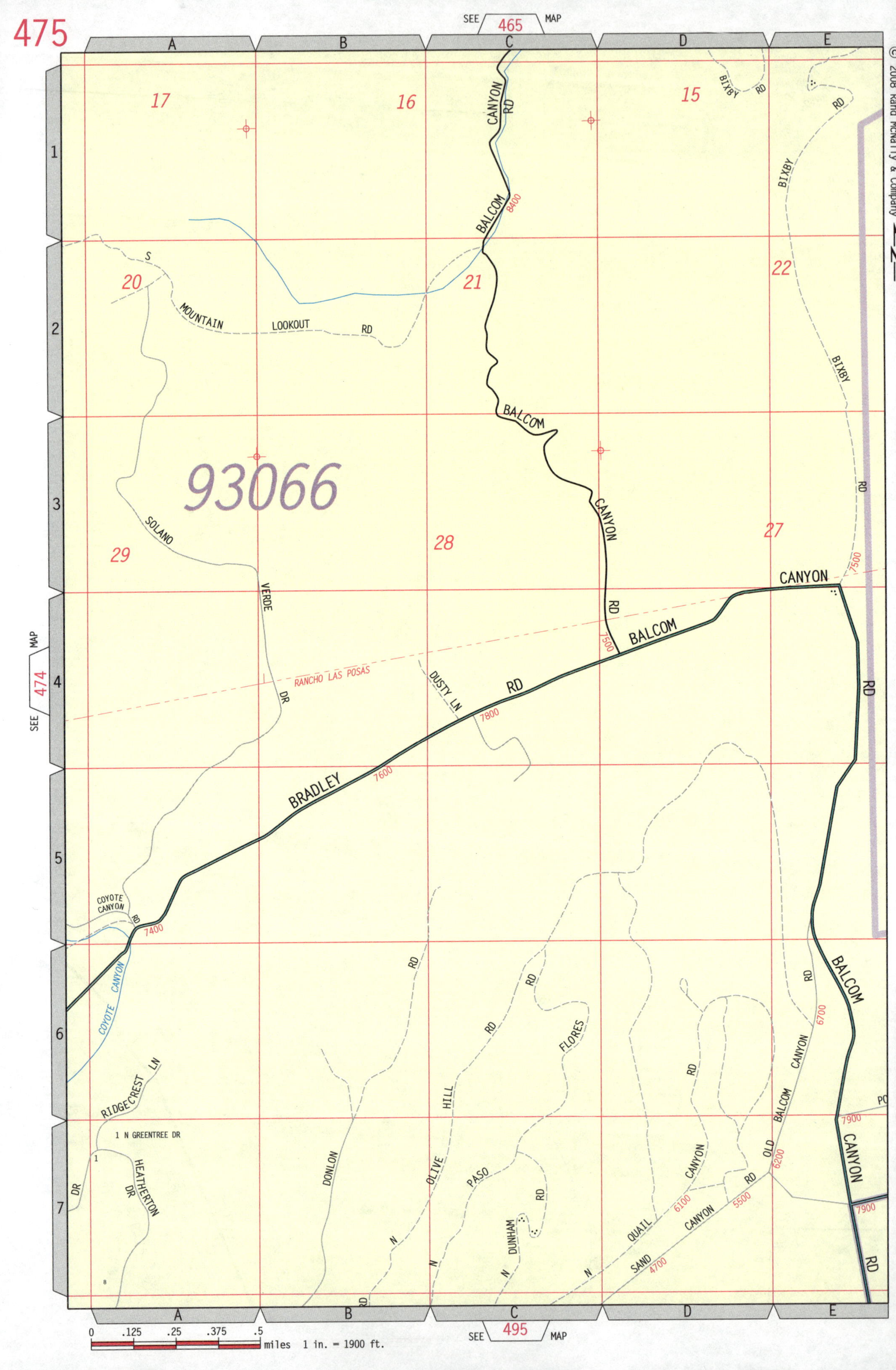
SEE 465 MAP
A
B
C
D
E
1
2
3
4
5
6
7
17
16
15
22
20
21
28
29
27
93066
CANYON RD
BALCOM
8400
BIXBY RD
RD
BIXBY
S MOUNTAIN LOOKOUT RD
BALCOM
CANYON
RD
SOLANO
VERDE DR
BIXBY RD
7500
CANYON
BALCOM
7500
RANCHO LAS POSAS
DUSTY LN
RD
7800
BRADLEY
7600
RD
COYOTE CANYON RD
7400
COYOTE CANYON
BALCOM
CANYON
RD
6700
RD
RD
RD
FLORES
RD
HILL
OLIVE
N
RIDGECREST LN
1 N GREENTREE DR
1
HEATHERTON DR
DR
DONLON
PASO
N
DUNHAM
N
RD
RD
QUAIL
N
CANYON
6100
BALCOM
OLD
6200
RD
5500
CANYON
SAND
4700
7900
CANYON
7900
RD
PO
SEE 474 MAP
SEE 495 MAP
0 .125 .25 .375 .5
miles 1 in. = 1900 ft.

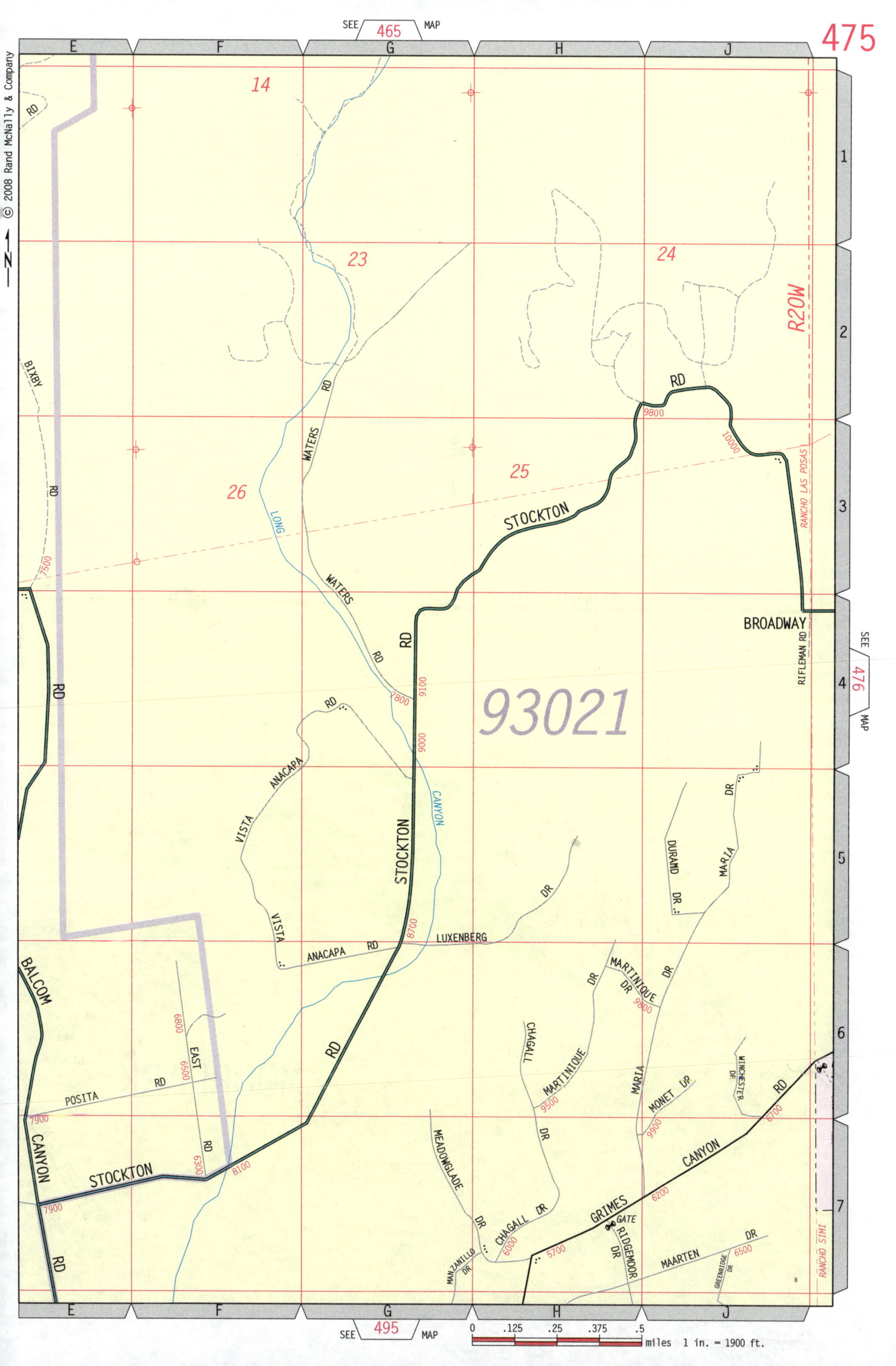
SEE 465 MAP
E
F
G
H
J
1
2
3
4
5
6
7
14
23
24
25
26
R20W
RD
BIXBY
RD
7500
RD
WATERS
RD
WATERS
RD
LONG
CANYON
STOCKTON
RD
9800
10000
RANCHO LAS POSAS
BROADWAY
RIFLEMAN RD
SEE 476 MAP
93021
STOCKTON
RD
7800
9100
9000
8700
VISTA
ANACAPA
RD
VISTA
ANACAPA
RD
LUXENBERG
DR
DURAND
DR
MARIA
DR
MARTINIQUE
DR
9800
DR
DR
CHAGALL
MARTINIQUE
9500
DR
MARIA
MONET DR
9900
WINCHESTER DR
RD
6700
CANYON
6200
GRIMES
GATE
RIDGEMOOR
DR
MAARTEN
DR
6500
GREENRIDGE DR
MEADOWGLADE
DR
CHAGALL DR
6000
5700
MANZANILLO DR
RANCHO SIMI
BALCOM
CANYON
RD
7900
7900
POSITA
RD
EAST
6800
6500
6300
RD
STOCKTON
8100
RD
SEE 495 MAP
0 .125 .25 .375 .5
miles 1 in. = 1900 ft.

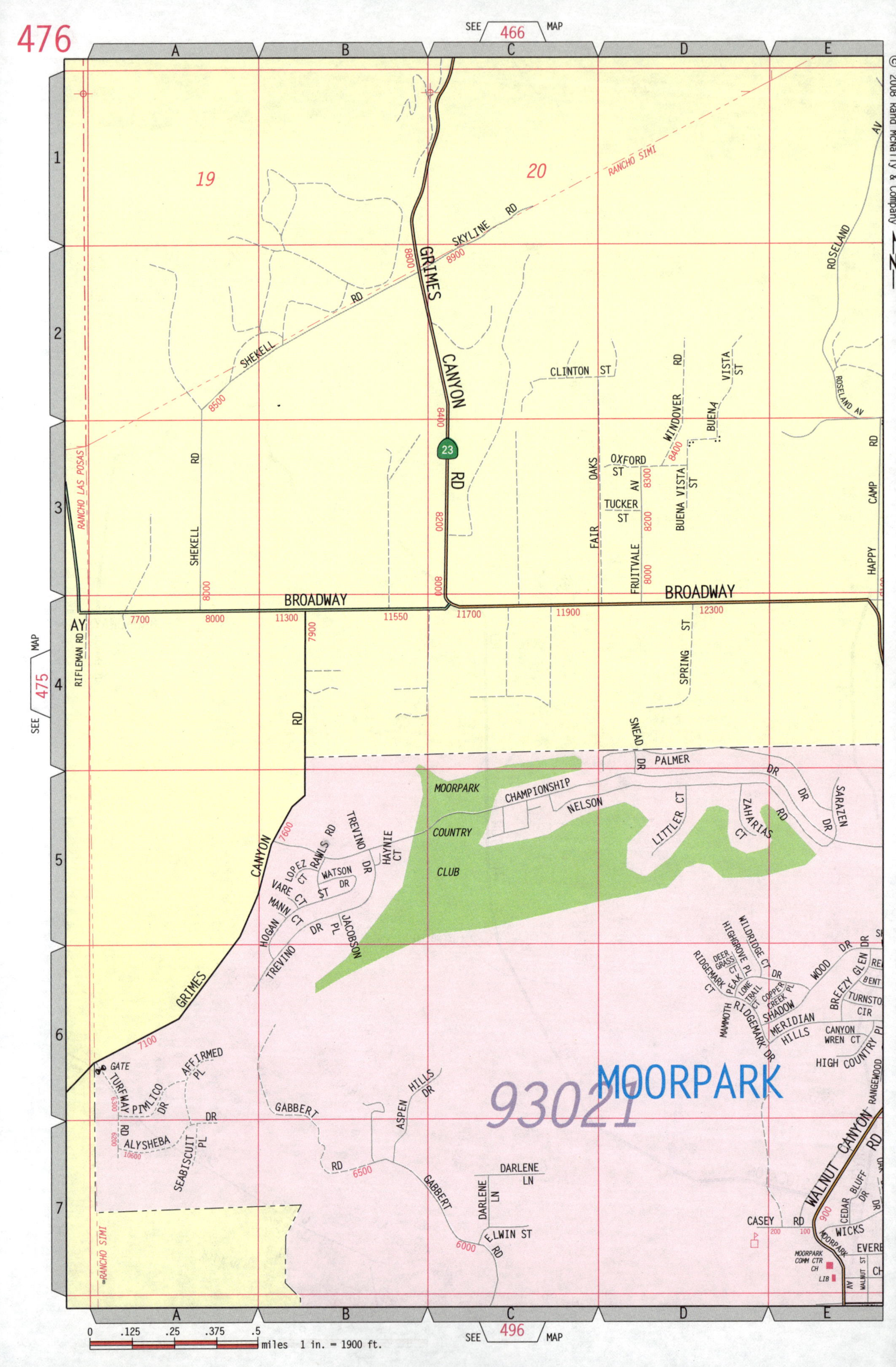
SEE 466 MAP
A
B
C
D
E
1
2
3
4
5
6
7
19
20
RANCHO SIMI
SKYLINE RD
8900
8800
GRIMES CANYON RD
SHEKELL
RD
8500
SHEKELL RD
8000
RANCHO LAS POSAS
8400
23
8200
8000
CLINTON ST
WINDOVER RD
VISTA ST
BUENA
OXFORD ST
TUCKER ST
FAIR OAKS AV
8300
8200
8000
FRUITVALE
BUENA VISTA ST
8400
ROSELAND AV
ROSELAND AV
HAPPY CAMP RD
BROADWAY
7700
8000
11300
11550
11700
11900
12300
BROADWAY
7900
RIFLEMAN RD
AY
SEE 475 MAP
SPRING ST
SNEAD DR
PALMER DR
SARAZEN DR
DR
CHAMPIONSHIP
NELSON
LITTLER CT
ZAHARIAS CT
RD
MOORPARK COUNTRY CLUB
GRIMES CANYON RD
7600
RAWLS RD
TREVINO DR
HAYNIE CT
LOPEZ CT
WATSON DR
ST
VARE CT
MANN CT
HOGAN CT
DR
JACOBSON PL
TREVINO
GRIMES
7100
GATE
TURFWAY RD
6300
6200
PIMLICO DR
AFFIRMED PL
DR
ALYSHEBA
10600
SEABISCUIT PL
GABBERT RD
6500
ASPEN HILLS DR
GABBERT RD
6000
DARLENE LN
DARLENE LN
ELWIN ST
MOORPARK
93021
WILDRIDGE CT
HIGHGROVE PL
DEER GRASS CT
RIDGEMARK CT
PEAK
LONE TRAIL CT
COPPER CREEK PL
SHADOW
WOOD DR
DR
BREEZY GLEN DR
BENT
TURNSTONE CIR
MAMMOTH
RIDGEMARK DR
MERIDIAN HILLS
CANYON WREN CT
HIGH COUNTRY PL
RANGEWOOD
WALNUT CANYON RD
900
CEDAR BLUFF DR
CASEY RD
200
100
WICKS
MOORPARK
EVERE
MOORPARK COMM CTR
CH
LIB
WALNUT ST
AV
RANCHO SIMI
SEE 496 MAP
0 .125 .25 .375 .5 miles 1 in. = 1900 ft.

SEE 466 MAP

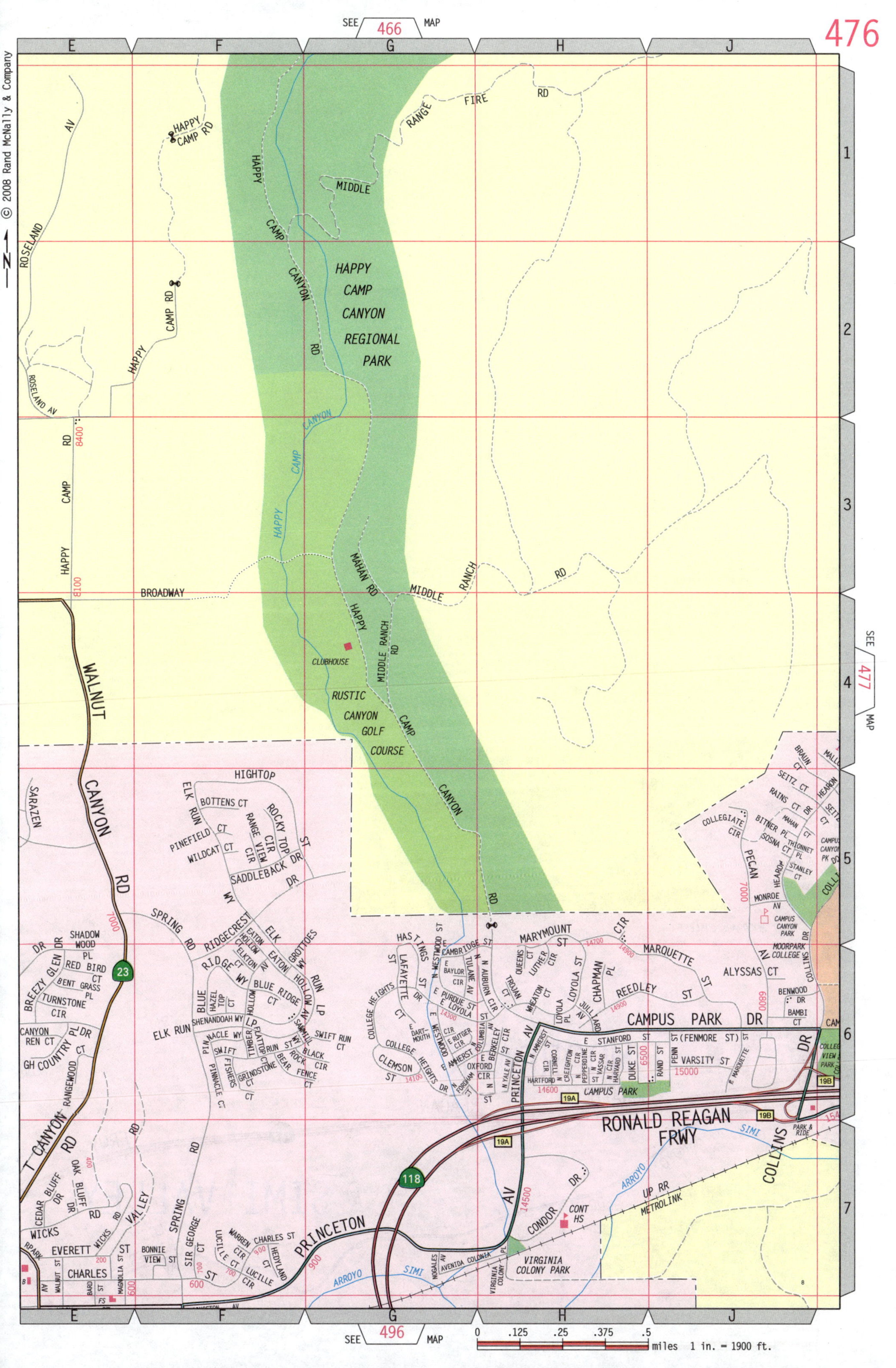
HAPPY CAMP CANYON REGIONAL PARK
CLUBHOUSE
RUSTIC CANYON GOLF COURSE
HAPPY CAMP CANYON RD
MIDDLE RANGE FIRE RD
MIDDLE RANCH RD
MAHAN RD
BROADWAY
WALNUT CANYON RD
ROSELAND AV
HAPPY CAMP RD
SPRING RD
ELK RUN
HIGHTOP
PRINCETON AV
CAMPUS PARK DR
CAMPUS PARK
MARYMOUNT ST
MARQUETTE ST
REEDLEY ST
COLLEGE HEIGHTS DR
RONALD REAGAN FRWY
COLLINS
ARROYO SIMI
UP RR METROLINK
CONDOR DR
CONT HS
VIRGINIA COLONY PARK
PRINCETON
CHARLES ST
EVERETT ST
WICKS RD
VALLEY RD
SIR GEORGE ST
CAMPUS CANYON PARK
MOORPARK COLLEGE
PARK & RIDE
23
118
19A
19B
© 2008 Rand McNally & Company

SEE 477 MAP

SEE 496 MAP

0 .125 .25 .375 .5 miles 1 in. = 1900 ft.

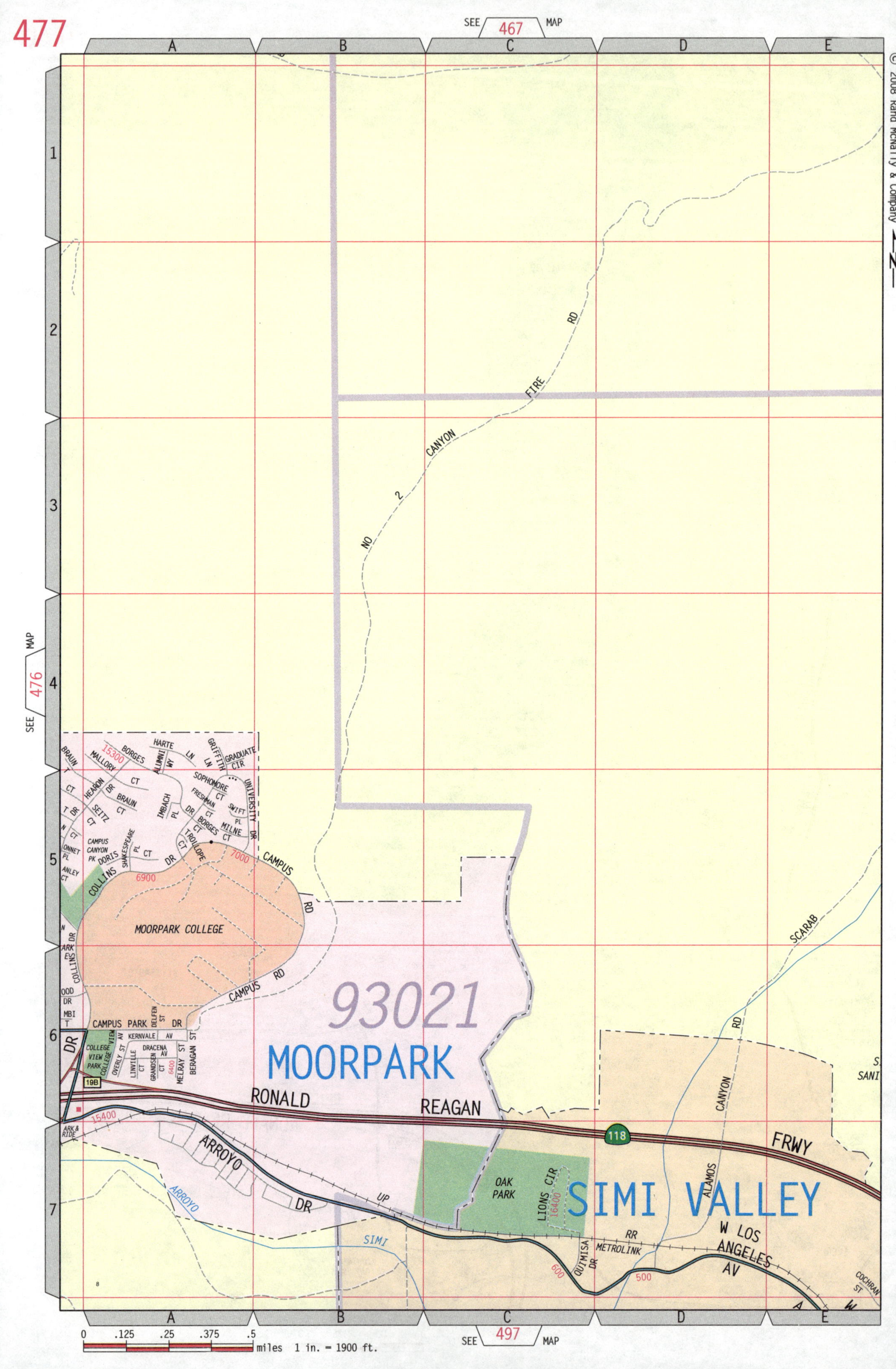

SEE 467 MAP
SEE 476 MAP
SEE 497 MAP
93021
MOORPARK
SIMI VALLEY
MOORPARK COLLEGE
CAMPUS RD
RONALD REAGAN FRWY
118
NO 2 CANYON FIRE RD
SCARAB
ALAMOS CANYON RD
ARROYO DR
ARROYO
SIMI
OAK PARK
LIONS CIR
W LOS ANGELES AV
METROLINK RR
UP
QUIMISA DR
COCHRAN ST
CAMPUS PARK DR
KERNVALE AV
COLLEGE VIEW PARK
COLLINS DR
BORGES
MALLORY
HARTE LN
GRIFFITH LN
GRADUATE CIR
ALUMNI WY
UNIVERSITY DR
SOPHOMORE CT
FRESHMAN CT
SWIFT PL
MILNE CT
TROLLOPE CT
IMBACH PL
HEARON DR
BRAUN CT
SEITZ CT
SHAKESPEARE PL
DORIS CT
CAMPUS CANYON PK
DELFEN ST
BERAGAN ST
MELRAY ST
DRACENA AV
GRANDSEN CT
LINVILLE CT
OVERLY ST
COLLEGE VIEW AV
15300
7000
6900
6400
16400
15400
600
500
19B
0 .125 .25 .375 .5 miles 1 in. = 1900 ft.

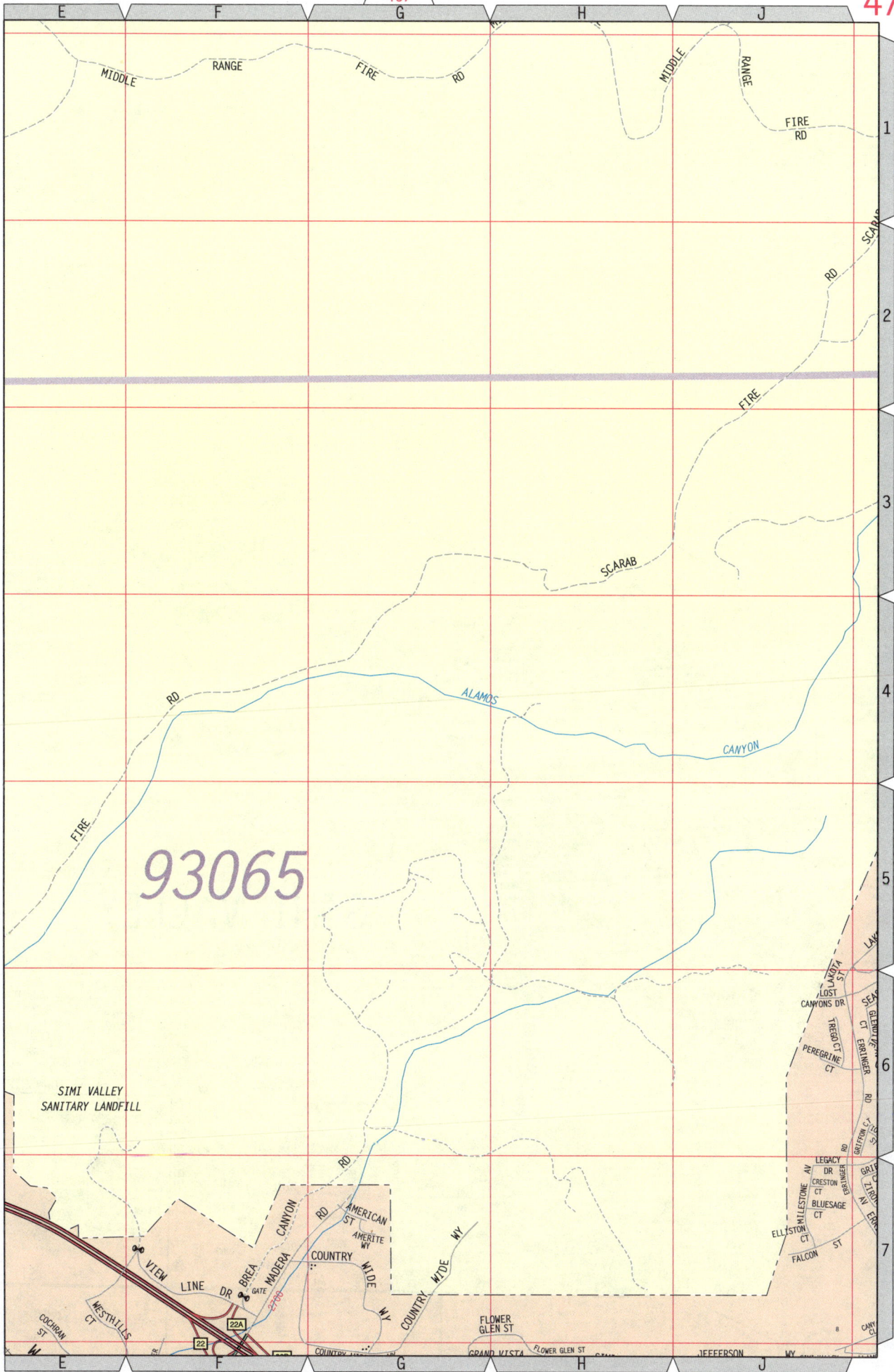

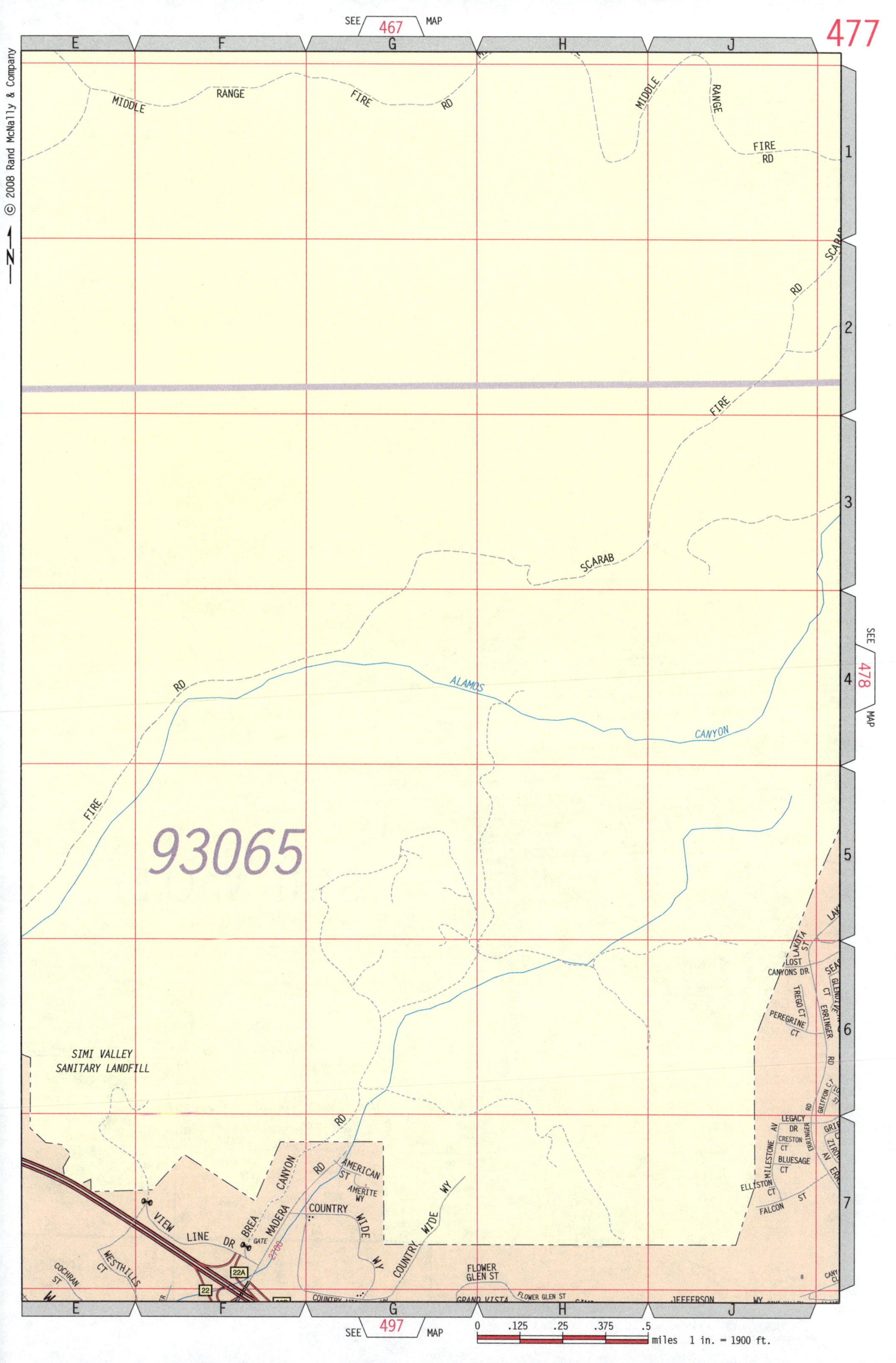

SEE 467 MAP
E
F
G
H
J
MIDDLE
RANGE
FIRE
RD
MIDDLE
RANGE
FIRE
RD
1
SCARAB
RD
2
FIRE
3
SCARAB
RD
ALAMOS
CANYON
4
SEE 478 MAP
FIRE
93065
5
SIMI VALLEY
SANITARY LANDFILL
LAKOTA ST
LOST CANYONS DR
TREGO CT
PEREGRINE CT
ERRINGER
RD
6
LEGACY DR
CRESTON CT
BLUESAGE CT
MILESTONE AV
ELLISTON CT
FALCON ST
7
RD
CANYON
AMERICAN ST
AMERITE WY
COUNTRY
WIDE
WY
COUNTRY WIDE WY
MADERA
BREA
GATE
VIEW
LINE DR
WESTHILLS CT
COCHRAN ST
22A
22
FLOWER GLEN ST
GRAND VISTA
JEFFERSON
WY
SEE 497 MAP
0 .125 .25 .375 .5
miles 1 in. = 1900 ft.

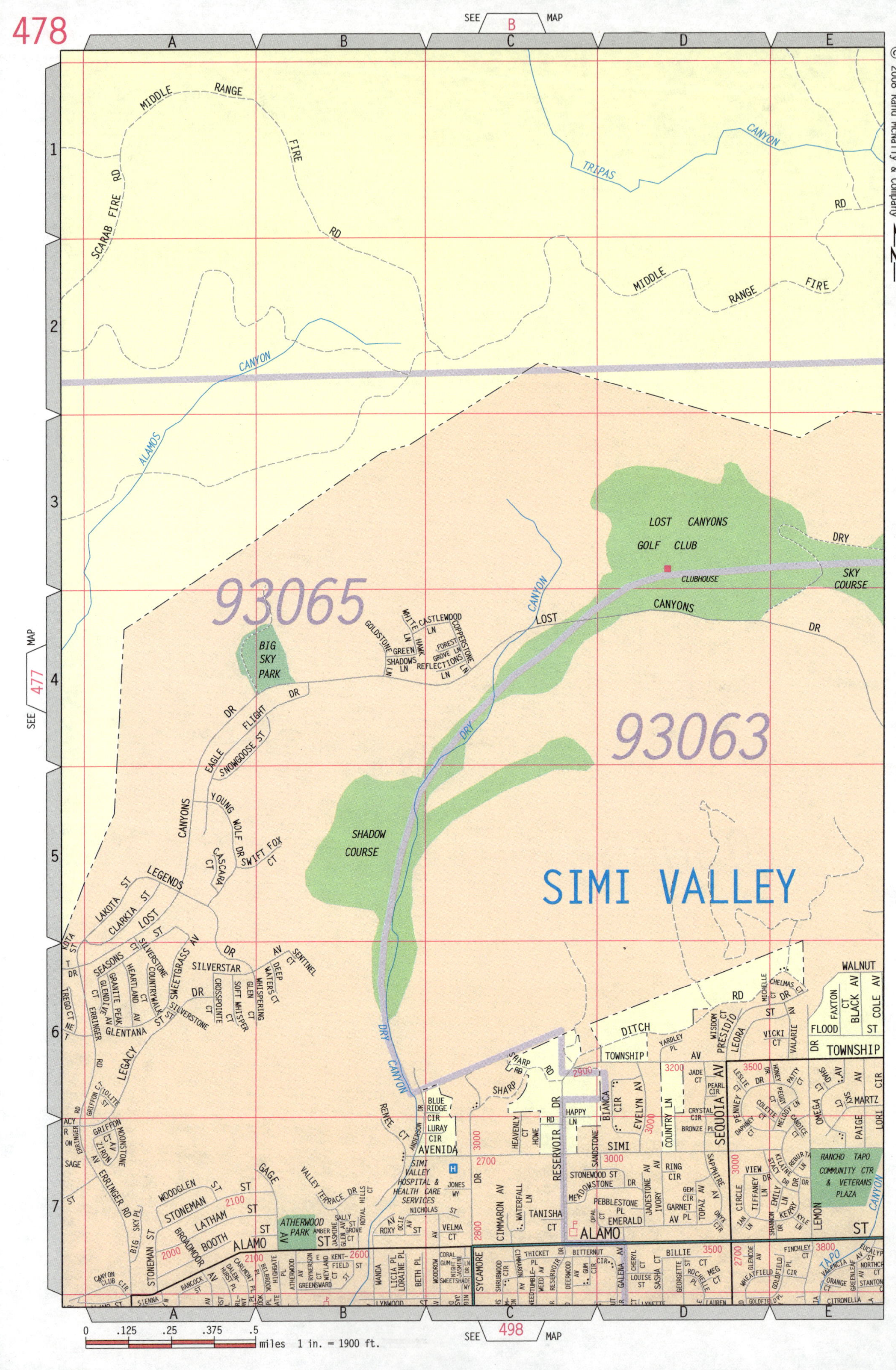
SEE B MAP
SEE 477 MAP
SEE 498 MAP
© 2008 Rand McNally & Company
MIDDLE RANGE FIRE RD
SCARAB FIRE RD
TRIPAS CANYON
ALAMOS CANYON
93065
93063
LOST CANYONS GOLF CLUB
CLUBHOUSE
SKY COURSE
LOST CANYONS DR
BIG SKY PARK
SHADOW COURSE
DRY CANYON
SIMI VALLEY
EAGLE FLIGHT DR
SNOWGOOSE ST
YOUNG WOLF DR
SWIFT FOX CT
CASCARA CT
LEGENDS
LAKOTA ST
CLARKIA ST
SILVERSTAR
SWEETGRASS AV
LEGACY
ERRINGER RD
GLENTANA ST
TOWNSHIP AV
DITCH RD
SEQUOIA AV
RESERVOIR DR
ALAMO ST
AVENIDA
SIMI VALLEY HOSPITAL & HEALTH CARE SERVICES
ATHERWOOD PARK
RANCHO TAPO COMMUNITY CTR & VETERANS PLAZA
TAPO CANYON
WALNUT
FLOOD ST
LEMON ST
STONEMAN ST
LATHAM ST
BOOTH ST
GAGE ST
VALLEY TERRACE DR
SYCAMORE DR
CIMMARON AV
BIANCA CIR
EVELYN AV
COUNTRY LN
0 .125 .25 .375 .5 miles 1 in. = 1900 ft.

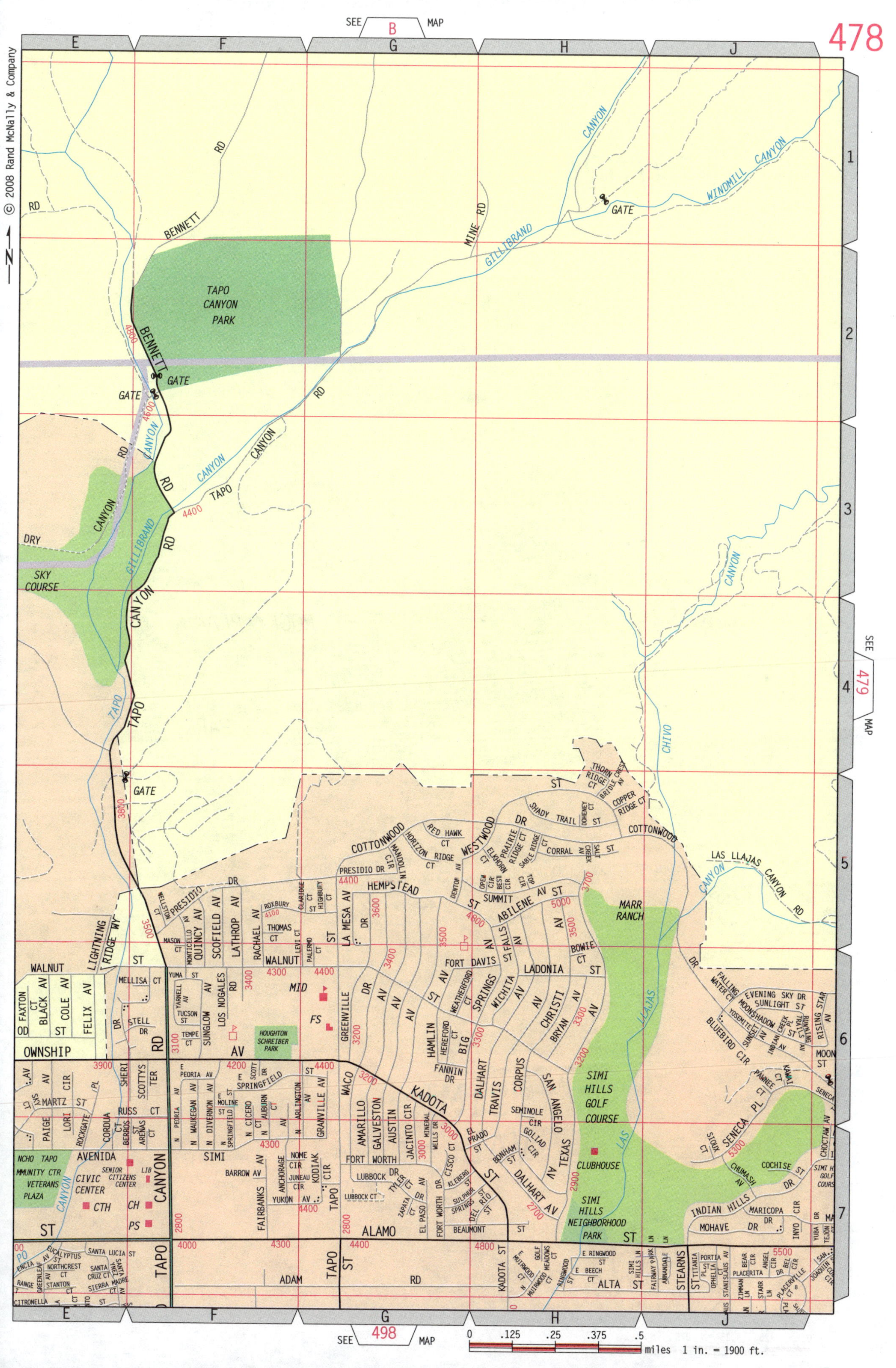

SEE B MAP
TAPO CANYON PARK
BENNETT RD
GATE
MINE RD
GILLIBRAND CANYON
WINDMILL CANYON
TAPO CANYON RD
DRY CANYON
SKY COURSE
MARR RANCH
SIMI HILLS GOLF COURSE
CLUBHOUSE
SIMI HILLS NEIGHBORHOOD PARK
HOUGHTON SCHREIBER PARK
CIVIC CENTER
SENIOR CITIZENS CENTER
VETERANS PLAZA
LAS LLAJAS CANYON RD
CHIVO CANYON
COTTONWOOD DR
KADOTA ST
ALAMO ST
WALNUT ST
ADAM RD
ALTA ST
STEARNS ST
SEE 479 MAP
SEE 498 MAP
miles 1 in. = 1900 ft.

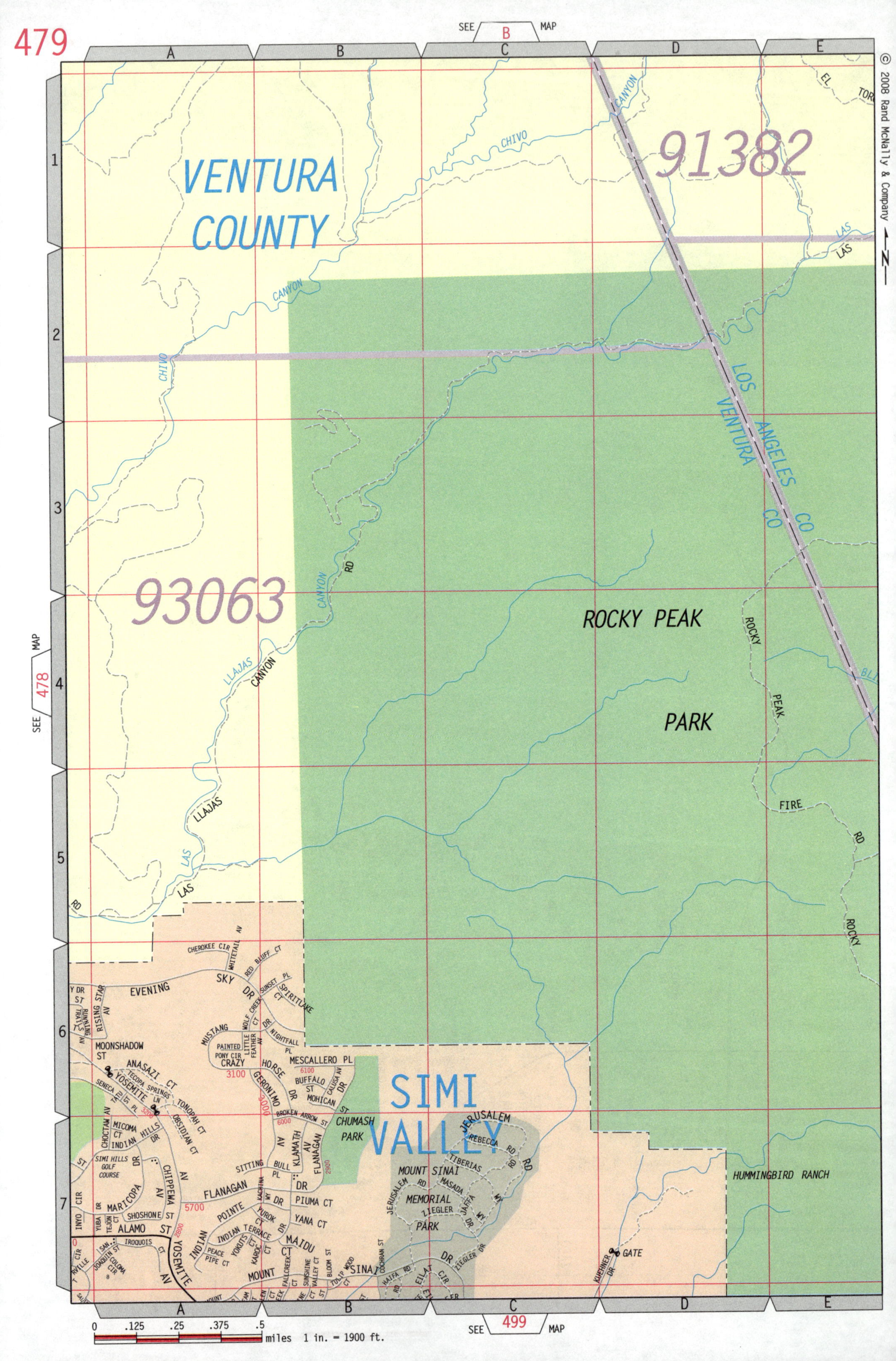

SEE B MAP
A
B
C
D
E
1
2
3
4
5
6
7
VENTURA COUNTY
91382
93063
CHIVO
CANYON
LAS
LOS ANGELES CO
VENTURA CO
ROCKY PEAK
PARK
ROCKY
PEAK
FIRE
RD
LLAJAS
CANYON
SEE 478 MAP
SIMI VALLEY
CHUMASH PARK
MOUNT SINAI
MEMORIAL PARK
HUMMINGBIRD RANCH
GATE
EVENING SKY DR
MOONSHADOW ST
ANASAZI CT
YOSEMITE AV
TONOPAH CT
OBSIDIAN CT
MICOMA CT
INDIAN HILLS DR
SIMI HILLS GOLF COURSE
CHIPPEWA AV
MARICOPA DR
SHOSHONE CT
ALAMO ST
IROQUOIS
FLANAGAN DR
POINTE DR
INDIAN TERRACE
MAIDU CT
MOUNT SINAI DR
KLAMATH AV
SITTING BULL PL
BROKEN ARROW ST
GERONIMO DR
CRAZY HORSE DR
MESCALLERO PL
BUFFALO ST
MOHICAN ST
PIUMA CT
YANA CT
JERUSALEM RD
REBECCA RD
TIBERIAS
MASADA
JAFFA WY
LIEGLER DR
EILAT CIR
HAIFA RD
KUEHNER DR
COCHRAN ST
3100
6000
5700
2800

0 .125 .25 .375 .5 miles 1 in. = 1900 ft.

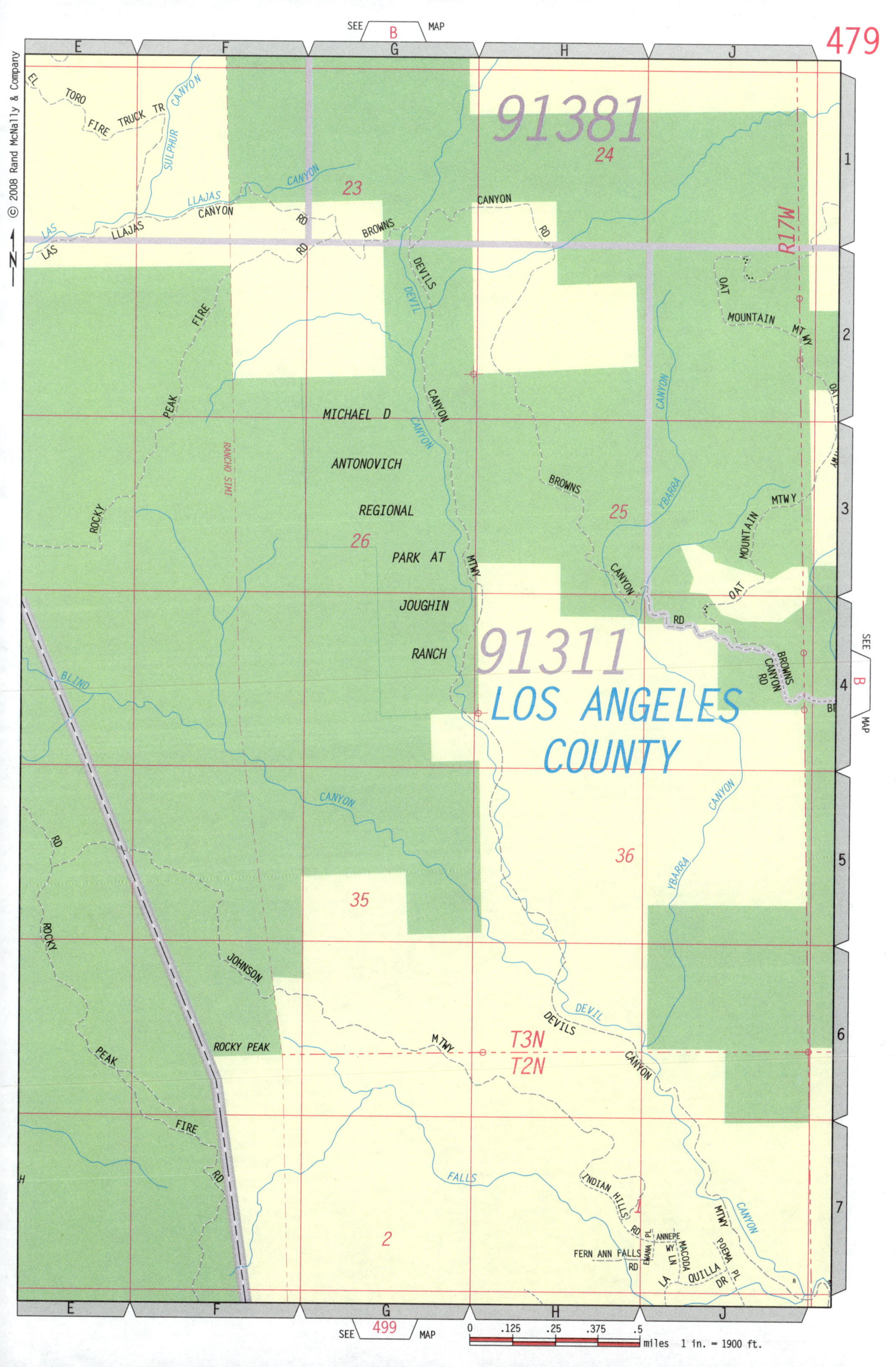
SEE B MAP
E
F
G
H
J
1
2
3
4
5
6
7
91381
91311
LOS ANGELES COUNTY
MICHAEL D ANTONOVICH REGIONAL PARK AT JOUGHIN RANCH
EL TORO FIRE TRUCK TR
SULPHUR CANYON
LLAJAS CANYON
LAS LLAJAS CANYON RD
BROWNS CANYON RD
DEVILS CANYON MTWY
DEVIL CANYON
ROCKY PEAK FIRE RD
RANCHO SIMI
BLIND CANYON
YBARRA CANYON
OAT MOUNTAIN MTWY
JOHNSON
ROCKY PEAK
FALLS
INDIAN HILLS RD
FERN ANN FALLS RD
EMANA PL
ANNEPE WY
MACODA LN
LA QUILLA DR
POEMA PL
R17W
T3N
T2N
23
24
25
26
35
36
2
SEE B MAP
SEE 499 MAP
0 .125 .25 .375 .5 miles 1 in. = 1900 ft.

SEE 470 MAP
A
B
C
D
E
1
2
3
4
5
6
7
SEE B MAP
0 .125 .25 .375 .5 miles 1 in. = 1900 ft.
SEE B MAP
© 2008 Rand McNally & Company
N

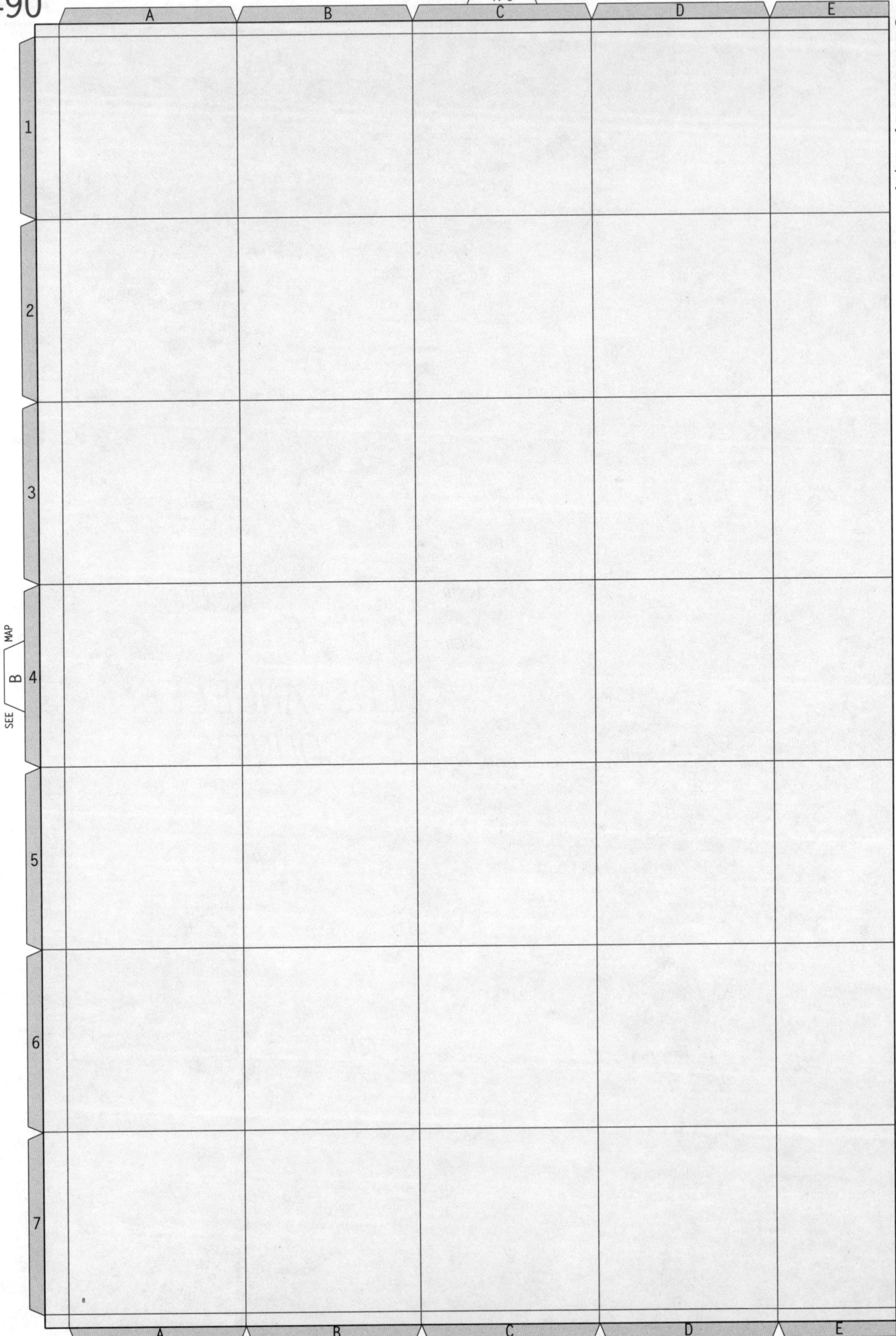

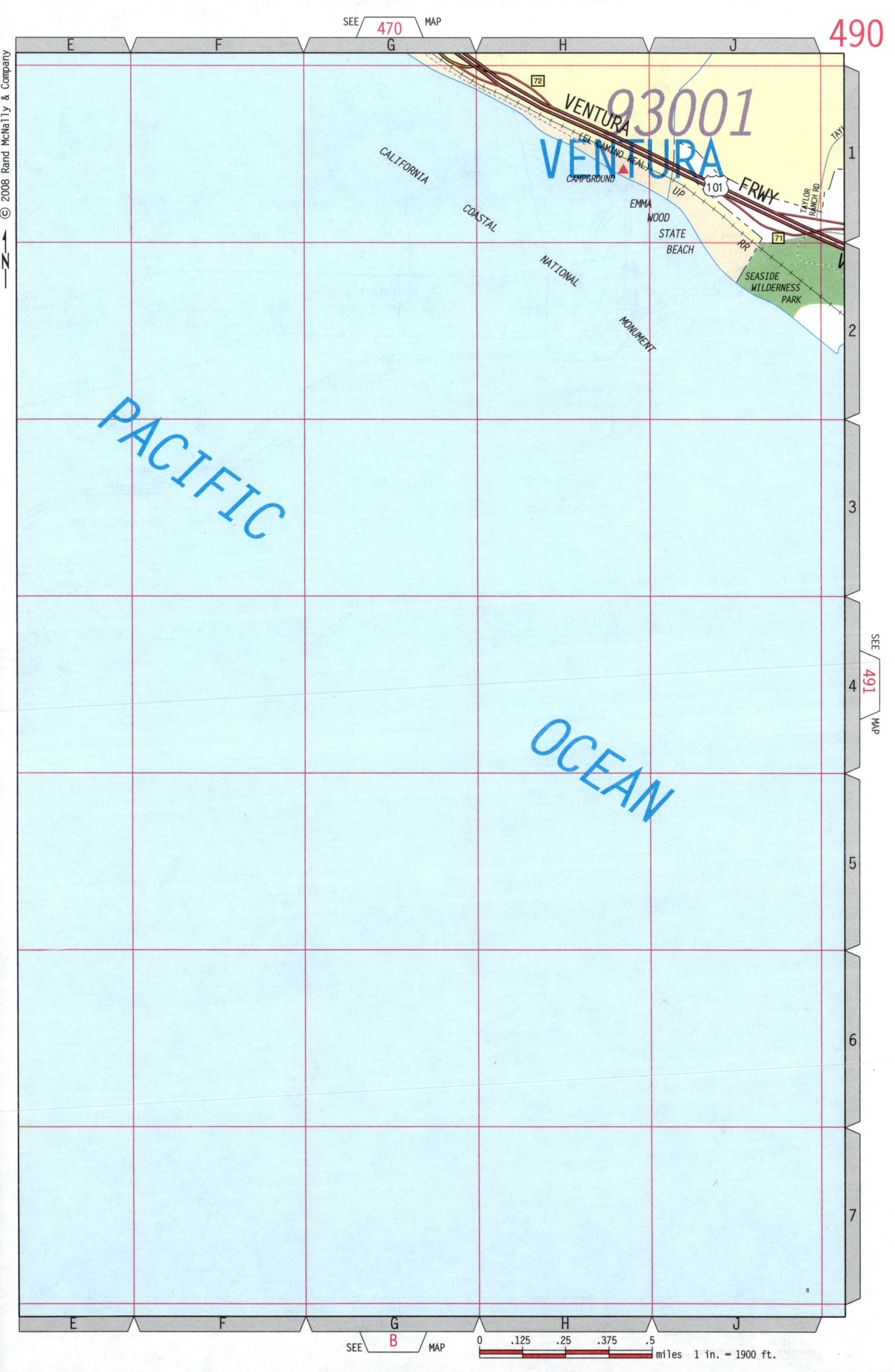

SEE 470 MAP
E
F
G
H
J
93001
VENTURA
VENTURA
FRWY
(EL CAMINO REAL)
72
101
71
CAMPGROUND
EMMA
WOOD
STATE
BEACH
UP
RR
SEASIDE
WILDERNESS
PARK
TAYLOR
RANCH RD
CALIFORNIA
COASTAL
NATIONAL
MONUMENT
PACIFIC
OCEAN
1
2
3
4
5
6
7
SEE 491 MAP
SEE B MAP
0
.125
.25
.375
.5
miles 1 in. = 1900 ft.

SEE 471 MAP

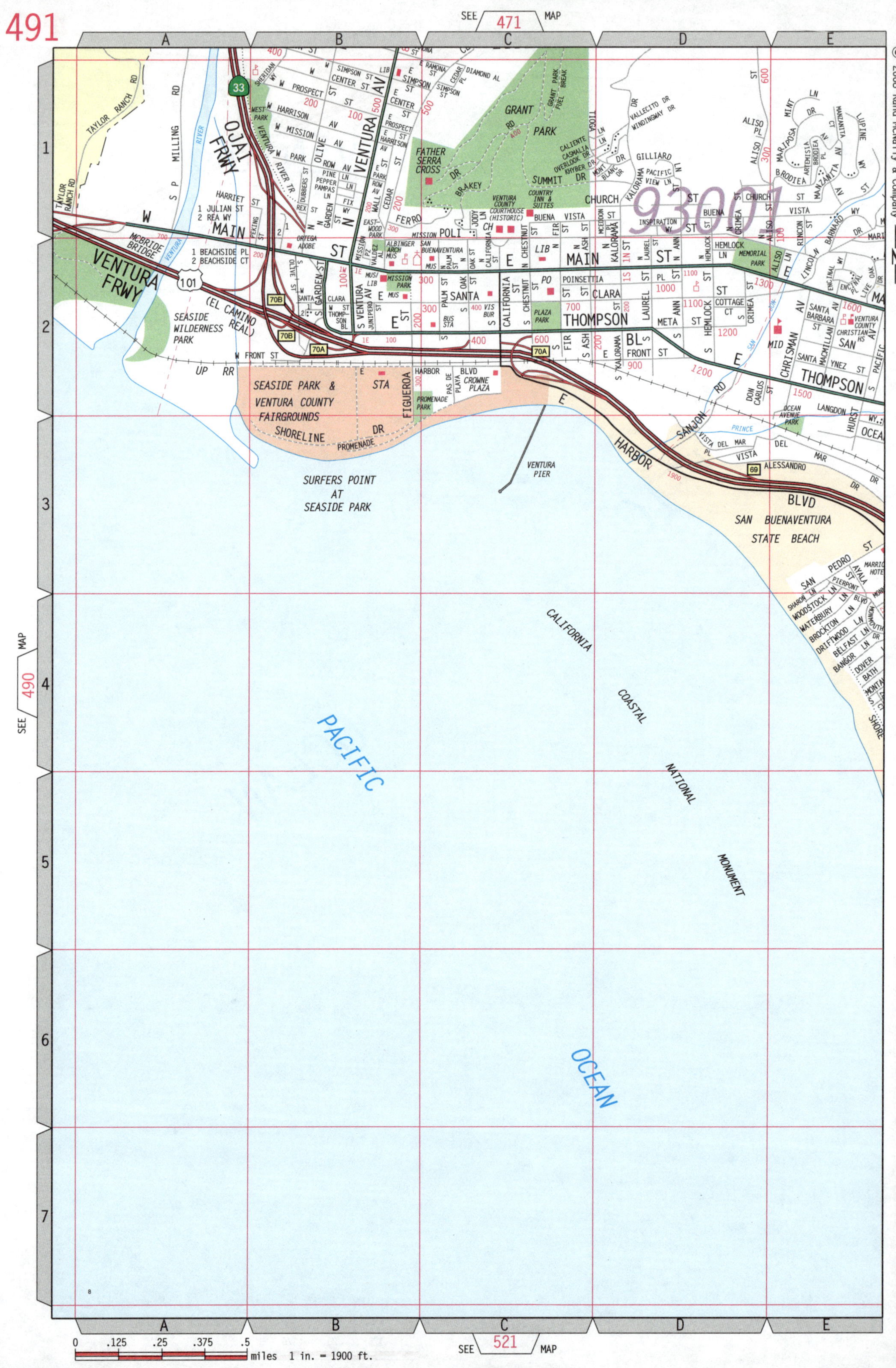
A
B
C
D
E
1
2
3
4
5
6
7
93001
TAYLOR RANCH RD
MILLING RD
S P
VENTURA RIVER
OJAI FRWY
33
W MAIN ST
MCBRIDE BRIDGE
VENTURA FRWY
101
(EL CAMINO REAL)
SEASIDE WILDERNESS PARK
1 JULIAN ST
2 REA WY
1 BEACHSIDE PL
2 BEACHSIDE CT
ORTEGA ADOBE
70B
70A
W FRONT ST
UP RR
SEASIDE PARK & VENTURA COUNTY FAIRGROUNDS
SHORELINE DR
PROMENADE
FIGUEROA
HARBOR BLVD
PAS DE PLAYA
CROWNE PLAZA
PROMENADE PARK
STA
SURFERS POINT AT SEASIDE PARK
VENTURA PIER
E HARBOR BLVD
W PROSPECT ST
W HARRISON AV
W MISSION AV
W PARK ROW AV
PEPPER LN
PAMPAS LN
FIX WY
OLIVE ST
GARDEN ST
REX ST
DUBBERS ST
VENTURA RIVER TR
N VENTURA AV
W SIMPSON ST
CENTER ST
E SIMPSON ST
E CENTER ST
E PROSPECT ST
E HARRISON ST
E PARK ROW AV
WALL ST
CEDAR ST
FERRO DR
MISSION AV
MISSION PZ
VALDEZ AL
ALBINGER ARCH MUS
SAN BUENAVENTURA MUS
MISSION PARK
E SANTA CLARA ST
E THOMPSON BL
S VENTURA AV
JUNIPERO ST
W SANTA CLARA ST
PALM ST
OAK ST
BUS STA
VIS BUR
CALIFORNIA ST
CHESTNUT ST
PLAZA PARK
PO
LIB
E MAIN ST
POLI ST
JODY LN
FATHER SERRA CROSS
BRAKEY RD
GRANT PARK
GRANT PARK FUEL BREAK
SUMMIT DR
VENTURA COUNTY COURTHOUSE (HISTORIC)
COUNTRY INN & SUITES
BUENA VISTA ST
CHURCH ST
CALIENTE
CASMALIA
OVERLOOK DR
KHYBER DR
MONT BLANC DR
GILLIARD DR
PACIFIC VIEW LN
VALLECITO DR
WINDINGWAY DR
INSPIRATION WY
KALORAMA ST
LAUREL ST
ANN ST
HEMLOCK ST
CRIMEA ST
ALISO ST
ALISO PL
MARIPOSA DR
MINT LN
BRODIEA AV
MANZANITA AV
LUPINE WY
ARTEMISIA
RINCON ST
BARNARD
LINCOLN DR
ENCINAL WY
LIVE OAK DR
MEMORIAL PARK
FIR ST
ASH ST
POINSETTIA PL
FRONT ST
META ST
COTTAGE CT
SANJON RD
DON CARLOS DR
CHRISMAN AV
SANTA BARBARA ST
MACMILLAN AV
SANTA YNEZ ST
CHRISTIAN HS
VENTURA COUNTY
PACIFIC AV
E THOMPSON BL
MID
OCEAN AVENUE PARK
LANGDON
HURST AV
PRINCE BARRANCA
SAN JON BARRANCA
VISTA DEL MAR
ALESSANDRO DR
69
SAN BUENAVENTURA STATE BEACH
SAN PEDRO ST
AYALA
PIERPONT BLVD
SHARON LN
WOODSTOCK LN
WATERBURY LN
BROCKTON LN
DRIFTWOOD LN
BELFAST LN
BANGOR LN
DOVER
BATH
SHORE
MARRIOTT HOTEL
PACIFIC OCEAN
CALIFORNIA COASTAL NATIONAL MONUMENT
0 .125 .25 .375 .5 miles 1 in. = 1900 ft.

SEE 490 MAP

SEE 521 MAP

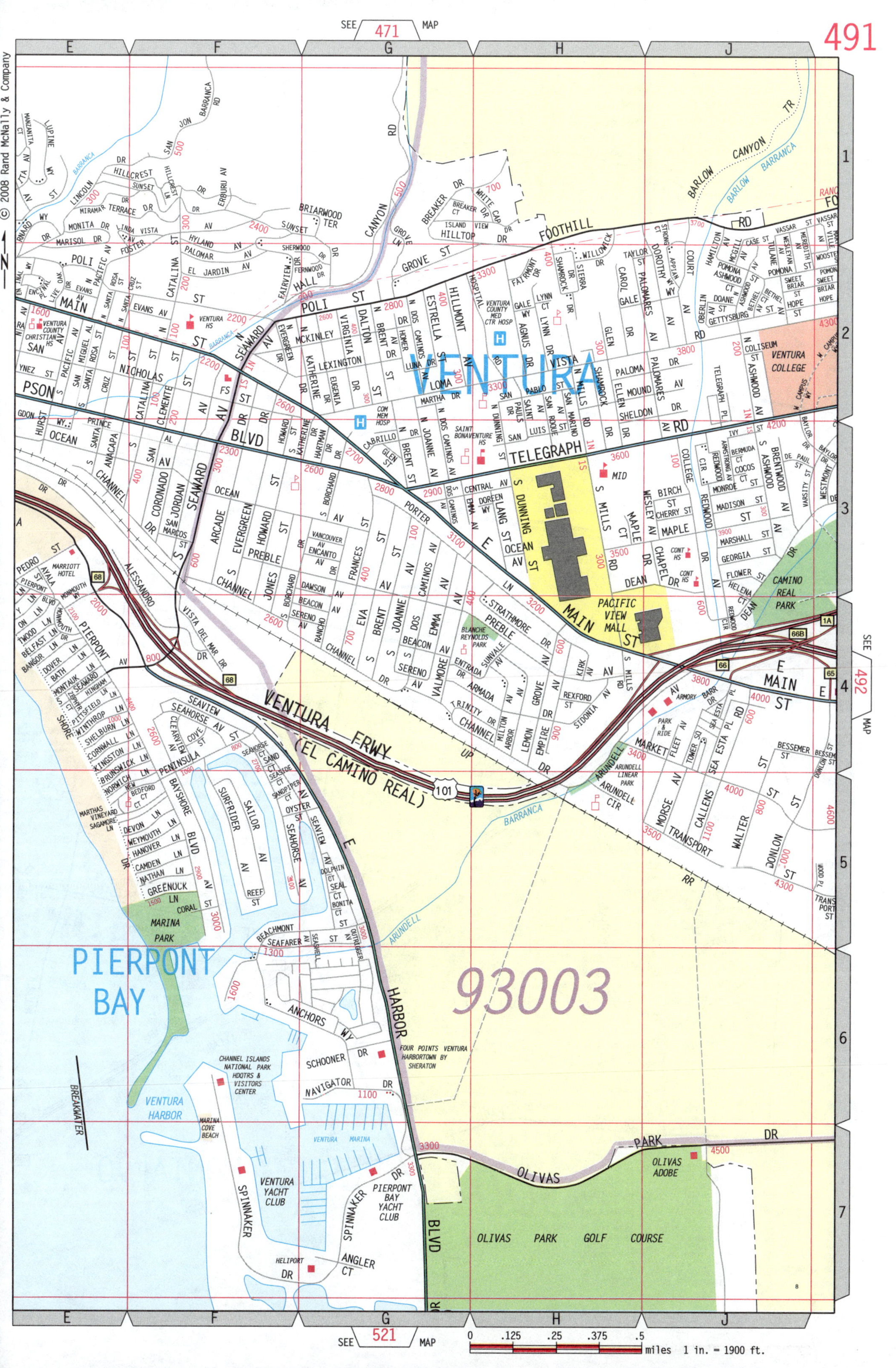
SEE 471 MAP
SEE 492 MAP
SEE 521 MAP
VENTURA
93003
PIERPONT BAY
VENTURA HARBOR
BREAKWATER
MARINA PARK
VENTURA COLLEGE
PACIFIC VIEW MALL
CAMINO REAL PARK
OLIVAS PARK GOLF COURSE
OLIVAS ADOBE
VENTURA YACHT CLUB
PIERPONT BAY YACHT CLUB
CHANNEL ISLANDS NATIONAL PARK HDQTRS & VISITORS CENTER
FOUR POINTS VENTURA HARBORTOWN BY SHERATON
MARRIOTT HOTEL
VENTURA FRWY (EL CAMINO REAL)
101
HARBOR BLVD
OLIVAS PARK DR
TELEGRAPH RD
FOOTHILL RD
MAIN ST
E MAIN ST
THOMPSON BLVD
POLI ST
SEAWARD AV
TELEPHONE RD
BARLOW CANYON TR
CANYON RD
VENTURA COUNTY MED CTR HOSP
COM MEM HOSP
VENTURA HS
VENTURA COUNTY CHRISTIAN HS
SAINT BONAVENTURE HS
0 .125 .25 .375 .5 miles 1 in. = 1900 ft.

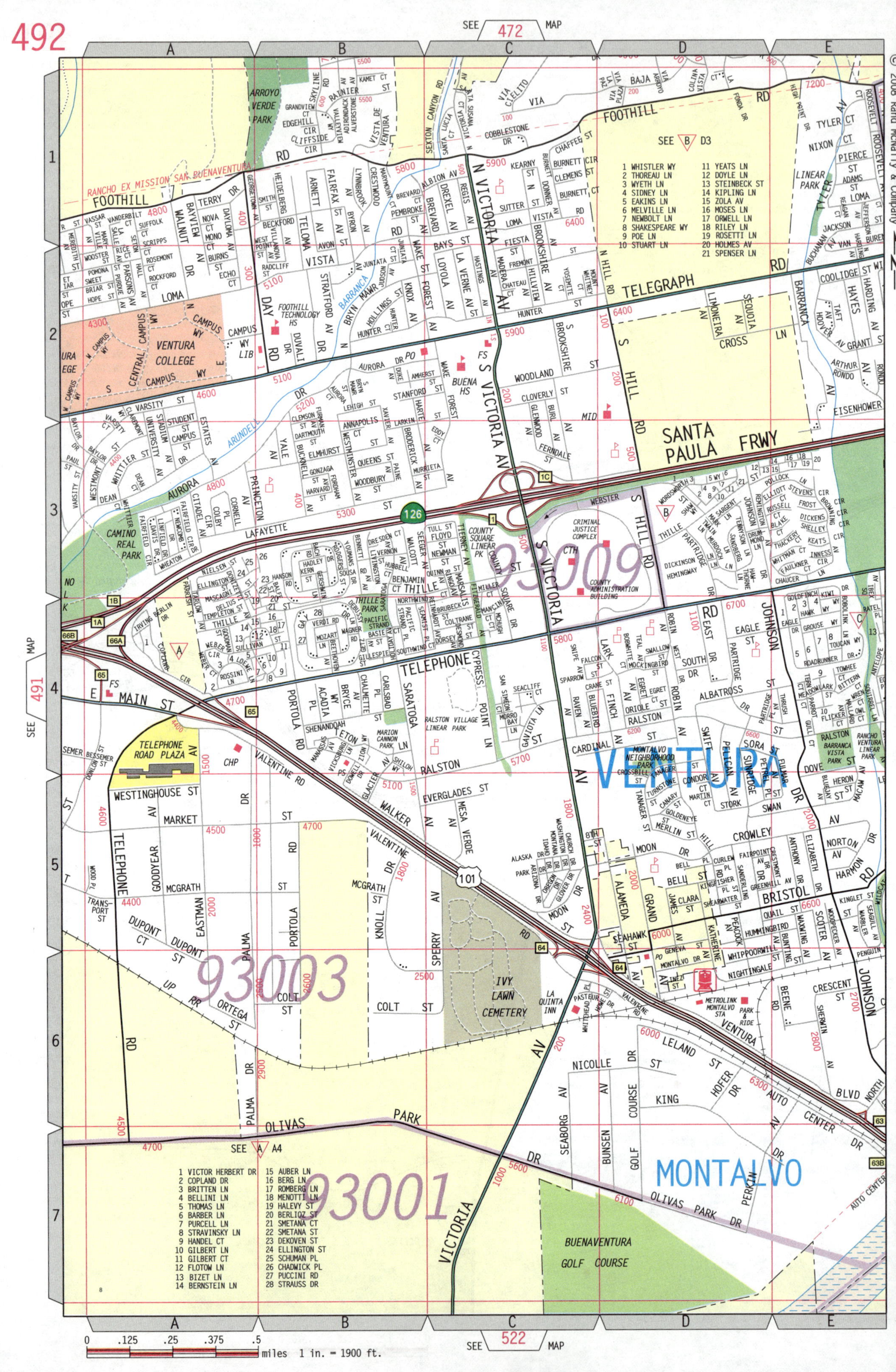
SEE 472 MAP
SEE 491 MAP
SEE 522 MAP
SEE B D3
1 WHISTLER WY
2 THOREAU LN
3 WYETH LN
4 SIDNEY LN
5 EAKINS LN
6 MELVILLE LN
7 NEWBOLT LN
8 SHAKESPEARE WY
9 POE LN
10 STUART LN
11 YEATS LN
12 DOYLE LN
13 STEINBECK ST
14 KIPLING LN
15 ZOLA AV
16 MOSES LN
17 ORWELL LN
18 RILEY LN
19 ROSETTI LN
20 HOLMES AV
21 SPENSER LN
SEE A A4
1 VICTOR HERBERT DR
2 COPLAND DR
3 BRITTEN LN
4 BELLINI LN
5 THOMAS LN
6 BARBER LN
7 PURCELL LN
8 STRAVINSKY LN
9 HANDEL CT
10 GILBERT LN
11 GILBERT CT
12 FLOTOW LN
13 BIZET LN
14 BERNSTEIN LN
15 AUBER LN
16 BERG LN
17 ROMBERG LN
18 MENOTTI LN
19 HALEVY ST
20 BERLIOZ ST
21 SMETANA CT
22 SMETANA ST
23 DEKOVEN ST
24 ELLINGTON ST
25 SCHUMAN PL
26 CHADWICK PL
27 PUCCINI RD
28 STRAUSS DR
VENTURA
MONTALVO
93003
93009
93001
VENTURA COLLEGE
ARROYO VERDE PARK
FOOTHILL TECHNOLOGY HS
BUENA HS
CAMINO REAL PARK
TELEPHONE ROAD PLAZA
IVY LAWN CEMETERY
BUENAVENTURA GOLF COURSE
CRIMINAL JUSTICE COMPLEX
COUNTY ADMINISTRATION BUILDING
COUNTY SQUARE LINEAR PK
RALSTON VILLAGE LINEAR PARK
MONTALVO NEIGHBORHOOD PARK
METROLINK MONTALVO STA
LINEAR PARK
SANTA PAULA FRWY
FOOTHILL RD
TELEGRAPH RD
TELEPHONE RD
VICTORIA AV
OLIVAS PARK DR
RANCHO EX MISSION SAN BUENAVENTURA
0 .125 .25 .375 .5 miles 1 in. = 1900 ft.

SEE 472 MAP

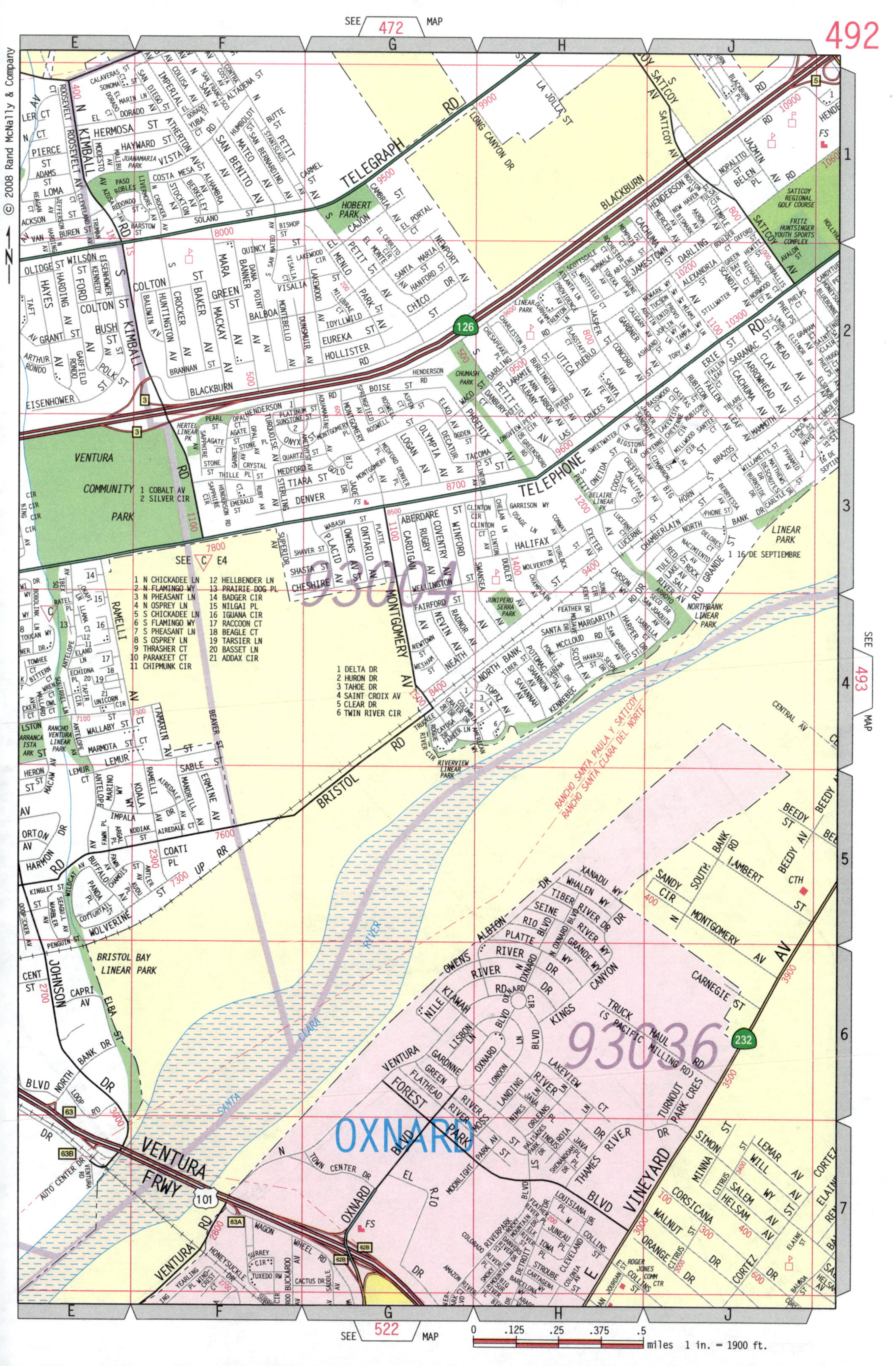

E
F
G
H
J
1
2
3
4
5
6
7
TELEGRAPH RD
BLACKBURN RD
TELEPHONE RD
KIMBALL RD
SATICOY AV
HOBERT PARK
CHUMASH PARK
VENTURA COMMUNITY PARK
1 COBALT AV
2 SILVER CIR
LINEAR PARK
SATICOY REGIONAL GOLF COURSE
FRITZ HUNTSINGER YOUTH SPORTS COMPLEX
93004
MONTGOMERY AV
BRISTOL RD
NORTHBANK LINEAR PARK
JUNIPERO SERRA PARK
1 N CHICKADEE LN
2 N FLAMINGO WY
3 N PHEASANT LN
4 N OSPREY LN
5 S CHICKADEE LN
6 S FLAMINGO WY
7 S PHEASANT LN
8 S OSPREY LN
9 THRASHER CT
10 PARAKEET CT
11 CHIPMUNK CIR
12 HELLBENDER LN
13 PRAIRIE DOG PL
14 BADGER CIR
15 NILGAI PL
16 IGUANA CIR
17 RACCOON CT
18 BEAGLE CT
19 TARSIER LN
20 BASSET LN
21 ADDAX CIR
1 DELTA DR
2 HURON DR
3 TAHOE DR
4 SAINT CROIX AV
5 CLEAR DR
6 TWIN RIVER CIR
1 16 DE SEPTIEMBRE
RIVERVIEW LINEAR PARK
RANCHO SANTA PAULA Y SATICOY
RANCHO SANTA CLARA DEL NORTE
SANTA CLARA RIVER
BRISTOL BAY LINEAR PARK
JOHNSON DR
VENTURA FRWY
101
126
232
OXNARD
93036
N OXNARD BLVD
VINEYARD AV
CENTRAL AV
BEEDY ST
SOUTH BANK RD
MONTGOMERY AV
CARNEGIE ST
TRUCK HAUL RD (S PACIFIC MILLING RD)
TURNOUT PARK CRES
RIVER PARK BLVD
N VENTURA RD
TOWN CENTER DR
EL RIO DR
ROGER JONES COMM CTR

SEE 493 MAP

SEE 522 MAP

0 .125 .25 .375 .5 miles 1 in. = 1900 ft.

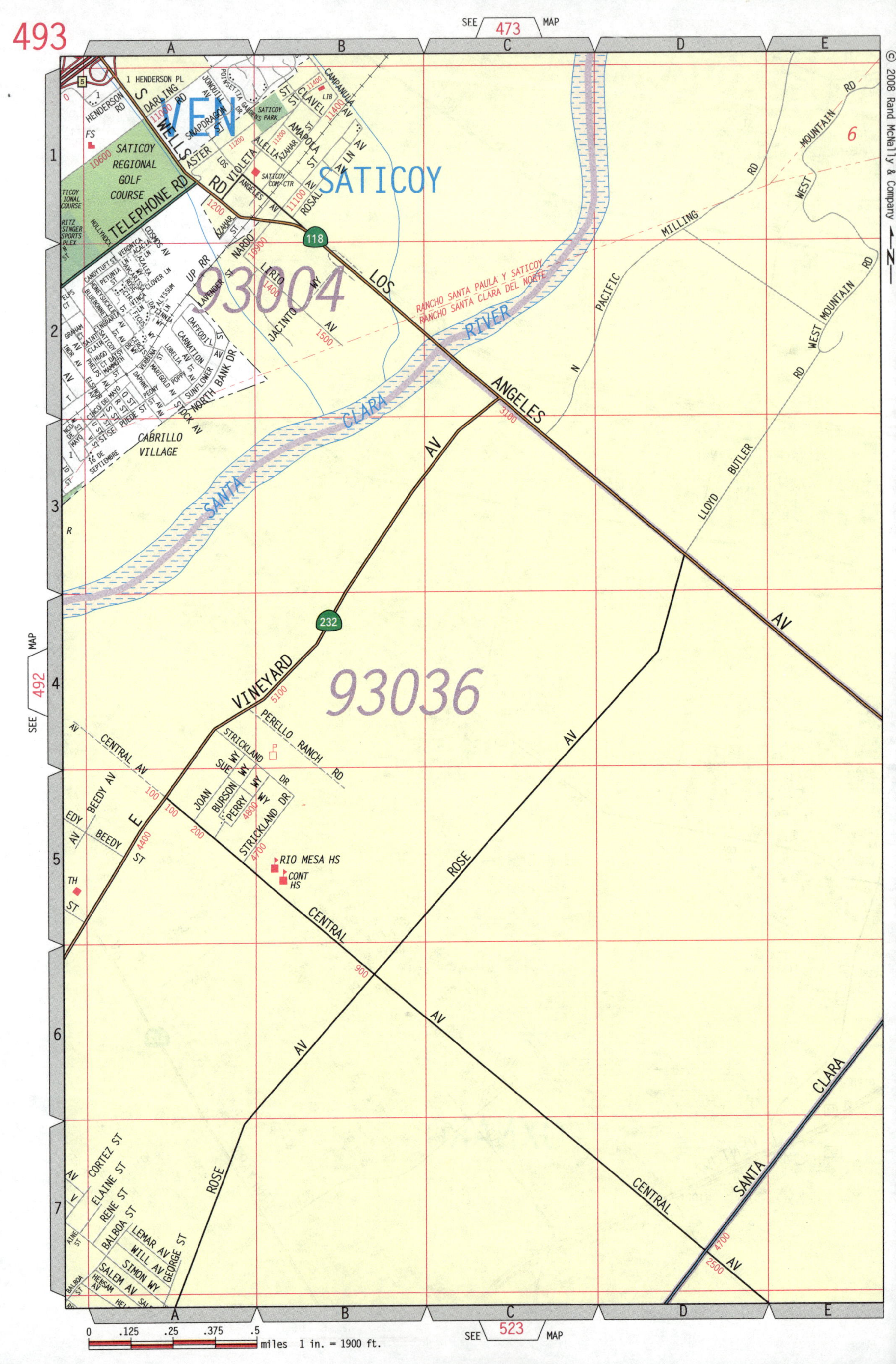
SEE 473 MAP
SATICOY
VEN
93004
93036
SATICOY REGIONAL GOLF COURSE
TELEPHONE RD
WELLS RD
LOS ANGELES AV
SANTA CLARA RIVER
RANCHO SANTA PAULA Y SATICOY
RANCHO SANTA CLARA DEL NORTE
VINEYARD AV
CENTRAL AV
ROSE AV
LLOYD BUTLER RD
WEST MOUNTAIN RD
MILLING RD
N PACIFIC
PERELLO RANCH RD
STRICKLAND DR
RIO MESA HS
CONT HS
CABRILLO VILLAGE
E ST
BEEDY AV
SANTA CLARA
SEE 492 MAP
SEE 523 MAP
© 2008 Rand McNally & Company

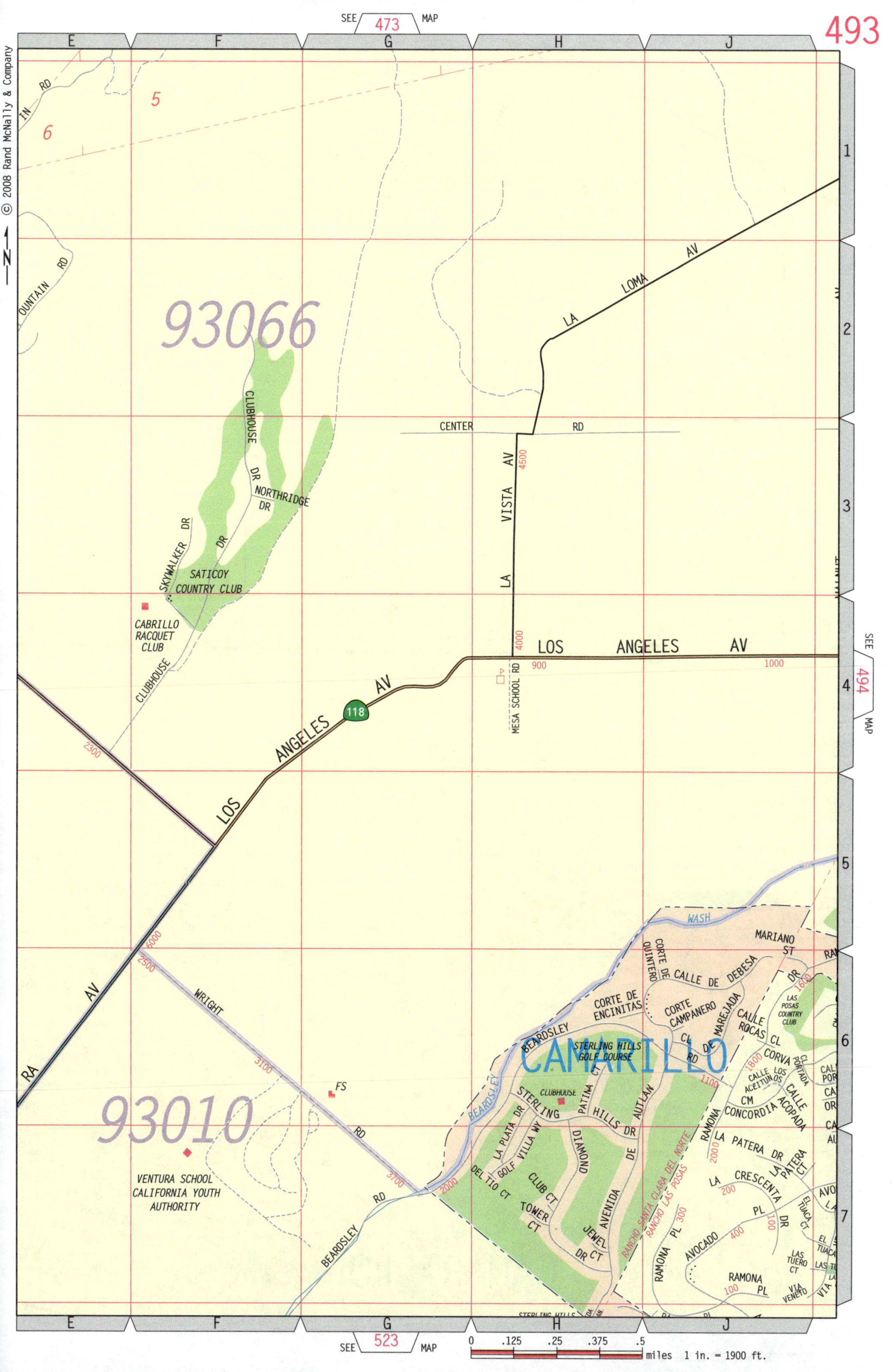

SEE 473 MAP
E
F
G
H
J
1
2
3
4
5
6
7
93066
93010
LA LOMA AV
CENTER RD
LA VISTA AV
4500
4000
CLUBHOUSE DR
NORTHRIDGE DR
SKYWALKER DR
SATICOY COUNTRY CLUB
CABRILLO RACQUET CLUB
CLUBHOUSE
LOS ANGELES AV
118
900
1000
MESA SCHOOL RD
2300
6000
2500
WRIGHT RD
3100
3700
FS
VENTURA SCHOOL CALIFORNIA YOUTH AUTHORITY
BEARDSLEY RD
2000
CAMARILLO
WASH
MARIANO ST
CORTE DE QUINTERO
CALLE DE DEBESA
CORTE DE ENCINITAS
CORTE CAMPANERO
MAREJADA
CALLE ROCAS
CL DE RD
BEARDSLEY
STERLING HILLS GOLF COURSE
CLUBHOUSE
STERLING HILLS DR
PATIMA CT
AUTLAN
LA PLATA DR
GOLF VILLA WY
DIAMOND
DE
DEL TIO CT
CLUB CT
TOWER CT
AVENIDA
JEWEL CT DR
RANCHO SANTA CLARA DEL NORTE
RANCHO LAS POSAS
RAMONA
RAMONA PL
300
AVOCADO
400
LA PATERA DR
LA PATERA CT
LA CRESCENTA DR
200
100
PL
RAMONA PL
LAS POSAS COUNTRY CLUB
CORVA
CALLE ACOPADA
CM CONCORDIA
CALLE LOS ACEITUNOS
1600
1800
1100
2000
EL TUACA CT
LAS TUERO CT
VIA VENETO
SEE 494 MAP
SEE 523 MAP
0 .125 .25 .375 .5 miles 1 in. = 1900 ft.

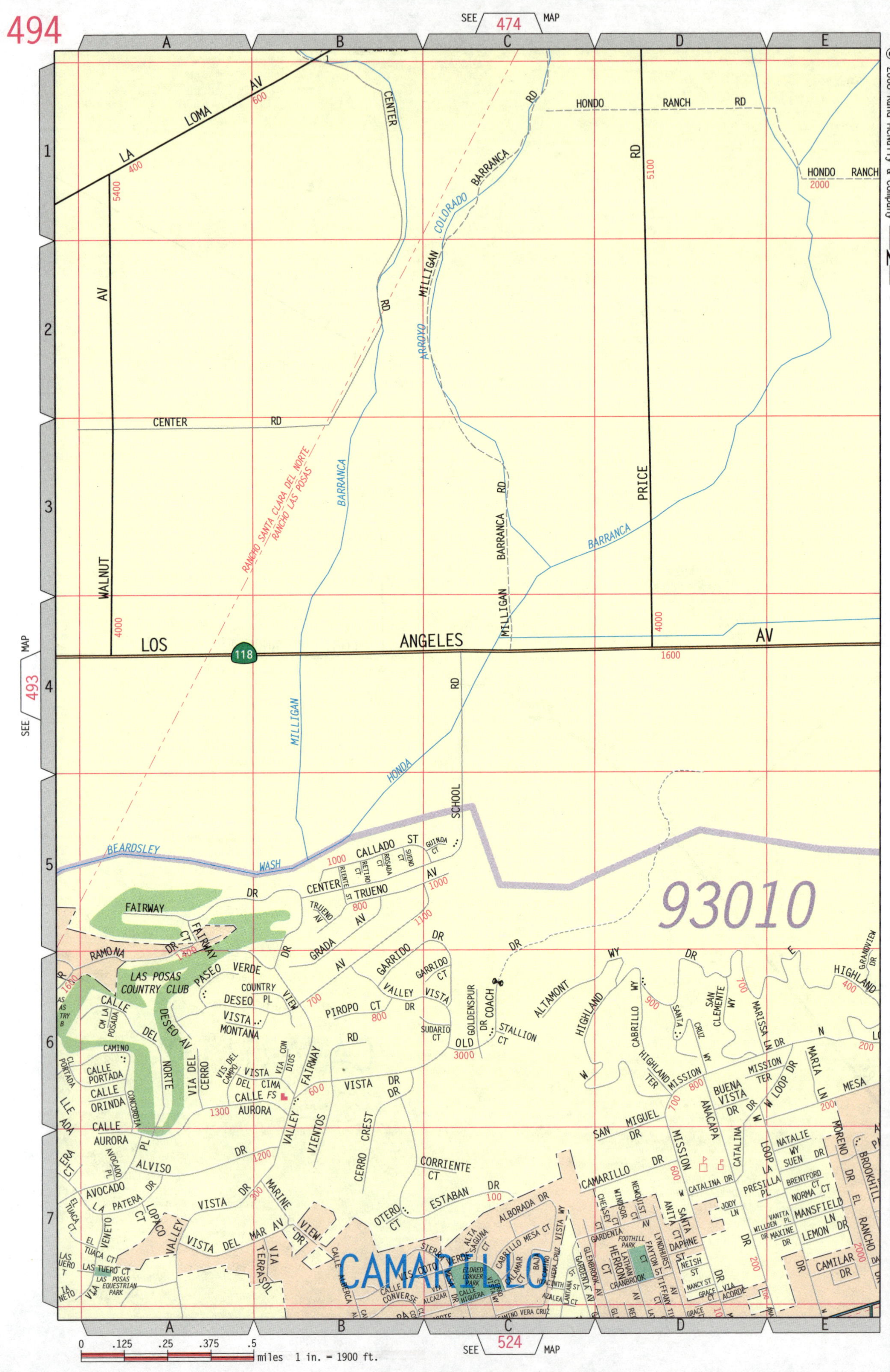

SEE 474 MAP
SEE 493 MAP
SEE 524 MAP
© 2008 Rand McNally & Company
LA LOMA AV
WALNUT AV
CENTER RD
HONDO RANCH RD
PRICE RD
BARRANCA RD
MILLIGAN BARRANCA
ARROYO COLORADO
BARRANCA
RANCHO SANTA CLARA DEL NORTE
RANCHO LAS POSAS
LOS ANGELES AV
118
HONDA
SCHOOL RD
BEARDSLEY WASH
93010
CALLADO ST
CENTER DR
TRUENO AV
FAIRWAY DR
RAMONA DR
LAS POSAS COUNTRY CLUB
PASEO VERDE
GRADA AV
GARRIDO DR
VALLEY VISTA DR
PIROPO CT
GOLDENSPUR DR
COACH
STALLION CT
ALTAMONT DR
HIGHLAND WY
CABRILLO WY
SANTA CRUZ WY
SAN CLEMENTE WY
MARISSA LN
HIGHLAND DR
MISSION DR
BUENA VISTA DR
ANACAPA DR
SAN MIGUEL DR
CATALINA DR
LOOP DR
MESA DR
CAMARILLO DR
VIENTOS
CERRO CREST DR
CORRIENTE CT
ESTABAN DR
ALBORADA DR
VISTA DEL MAR AV
MARINE VIEW DR
ALVISO DR
AVOCADO CT
LA PATERA DR
LAS POSAS EQUESTRIAN PARK
ELDRED LOKKER PARK
FOOTHILL PARK
CAMARILLO
miles 1 in. = 1900 ft.

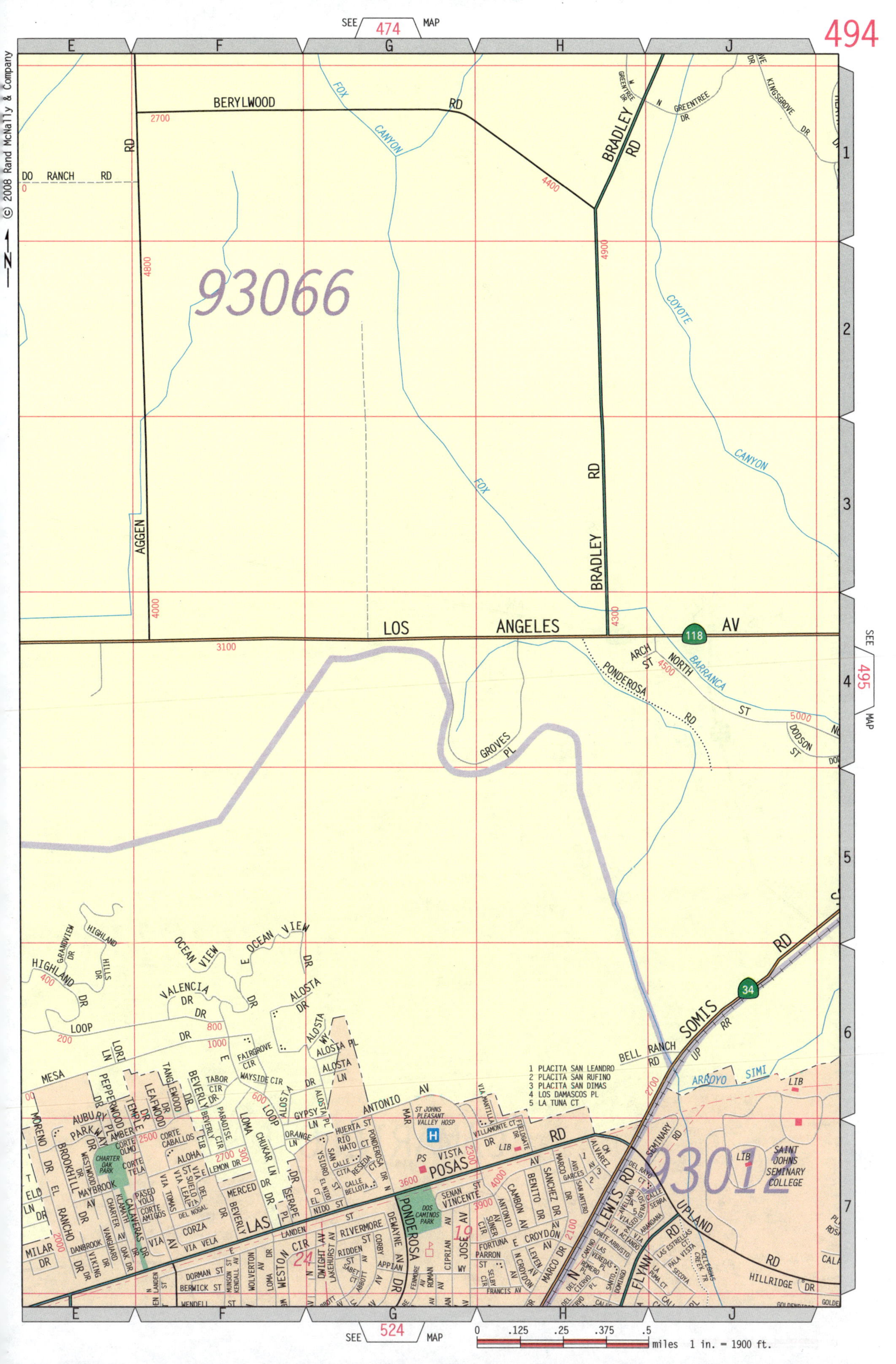
SEE 474 MAP
SEE 495 MAP
SEE 524 MAP
93066
93012
BERYLWOOD RD
BRADLEY RD
AGGEN RD
FOX CANYON
COYOTE CANYON
LOS ANGELES AV
118
BARRANCA
NORTH ST
ARCH ST
PONDEROSA RD
GROVES PL
DODSON ST
SOMIS RD
34
UP RR
BELL RANCH RD
ARROYO SIMI
LAS POSAS RD
LEWIS RD
UPLAND RD
HILLRIDGE DR
SEMINARY RD
SAINT JOHNS SEMINARY COLLEGE
ST JOHNS PLEASANT VALLEY HOSP
DOS CAMINOS PARK
CHARTER OAK PARK
ANTONIO AV
VISTA
1 PLACITA SAN LEANDRO
2 PLACITA SAN RUFINO
3 PLACITA SAN DIMAS
4 LOS DAMASCOS PL
5 LA TUNA CT
OCEAN VIEW DR
HIGHLAND DR
VALENCIA DR
LOOP DR
MESA
ALOSTA DR
FAIRGROVE CIR
WAYSIDE CIR
0 .125 .25 .375 .5 miles 1 in. = 1900 ft.

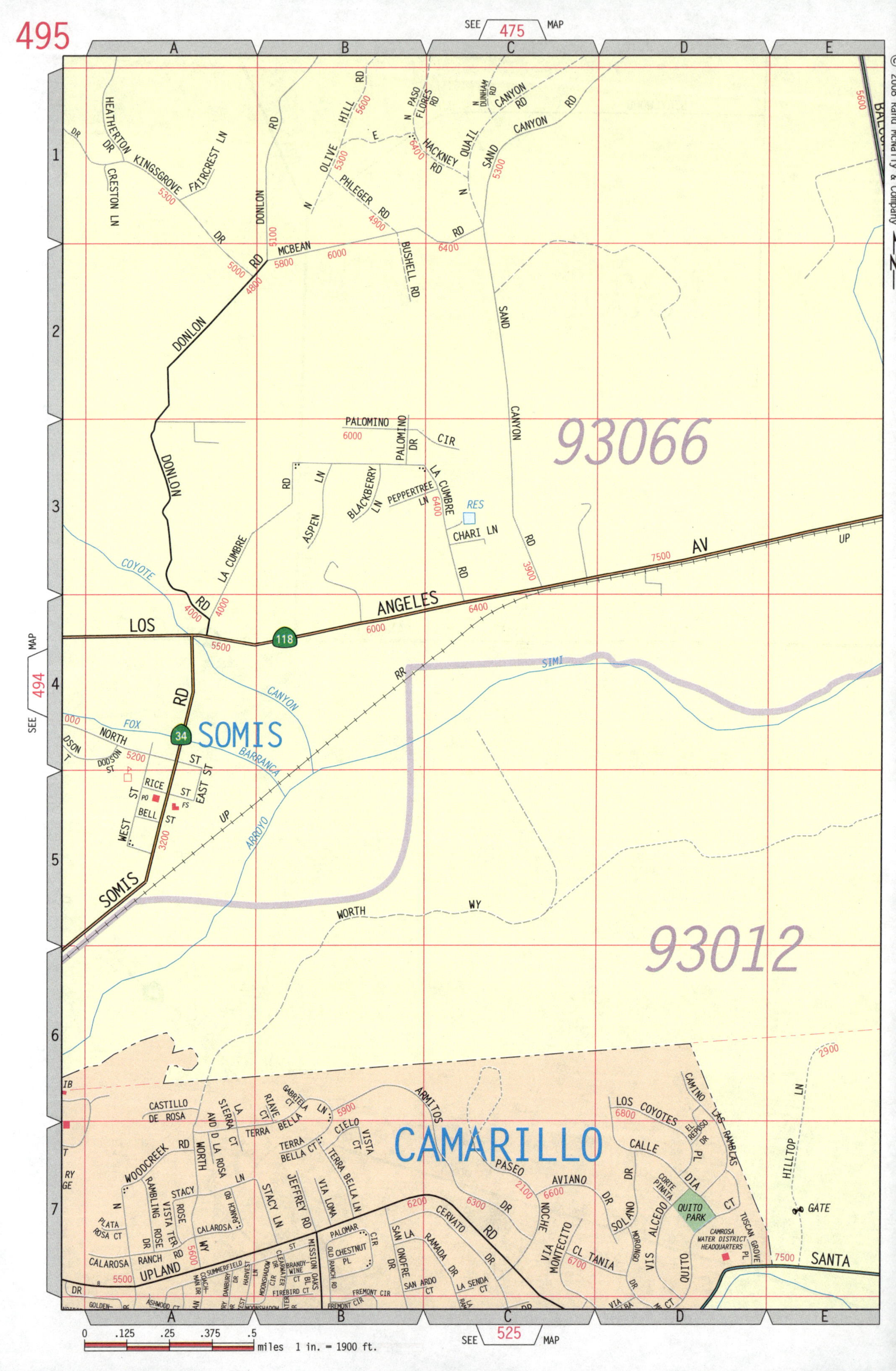
SEE 475 MAP
SEE 494 MAP
SEE 525 MAP
93066
93012
SOMIS
CAMARILLO
LOS ANGELES AV
DONLON RD
SOMIS RD
SAND CANYON RD
LA CUMBRE RD
MCBEAN
PALOMINO CIR
QUITO PARK
CAMROSA WATER DISTRICT HEADQUARTERS
SANTA
UPLAND RD
WORTH WY
GATE
0 .125 .25 .375 .5 miles 1 in. = 1900 ft.

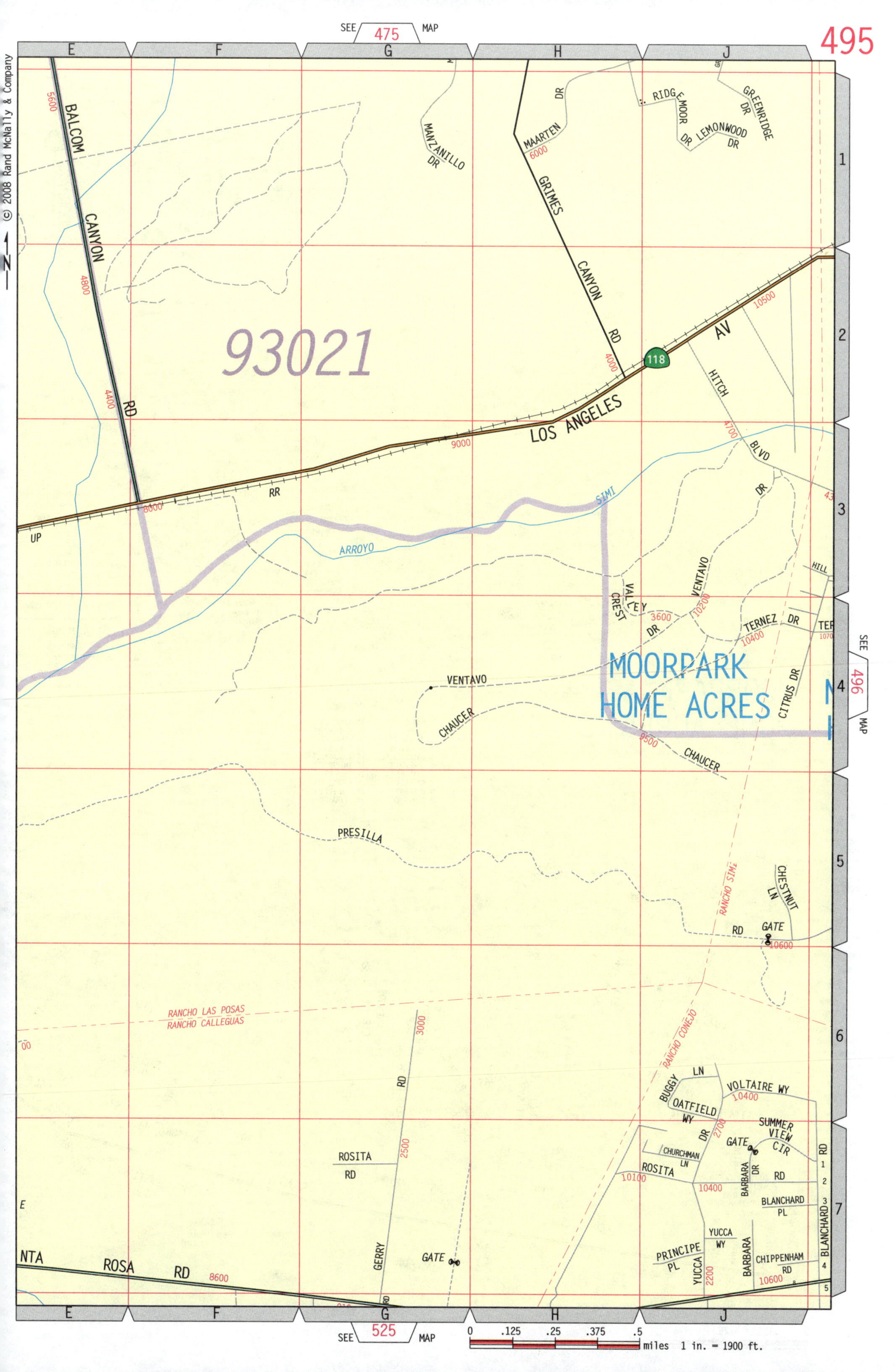
SEE 475 MAP
E
F
G
H
J
1
2
3
4
5
6
7
93021
BALCOM
CANYON
RD
5600
4800
4400
MANZANILLO
DR
MAARTEN
DR
6000
GRIMES
CANYON
RD
4000
RIDGEMOOR
DR
LEMONWOOD
DR
GREENRIDGE
DR
118
LOS ANGELES
AV
10500
9000
8000
HITCH
BLVD
4700
RR
UP
SIMI
ARROYO
VALLEY
CREST
DR
3600
VENTAVO
10200
DR
HILL
TERNEZ
DR
10400
MOORPARK
HOME ACRES
CITRUS DR
SEE 496 MAP
VENTAVO
CHAUCER
9500
CHAUCER
PRESILLA
RANCHO SIMI
CHESTNUT
LN
RD
GATE
10600
RANCHO LAS POSAS
RANCHO CALLEGUAS
RANCHO CONEJO
3000
RD
BUGGY
LN
VOLTAIRE WY
10400
OATFIELD
WY
DR
2700
SUMMER
VIEW
CIR
GATE
CHURCHMAN
LN
ROSITA
RD
10100
10400
BARBARA
DR
RD
BLANCHARD
PL
ROSITA
RD
2500
YUCCA
WY
PRINCIPE
PL
YUCCA
2200
BARBARA
CHIPPENHAM
RD
10600
BLANCHARD
RD
GERRY
RD
GATE
NTA
ROSA
RD
8600
SEE 525 MAP
0
.125
.25
.375
.5
miles 1 in. = 1900 ft.

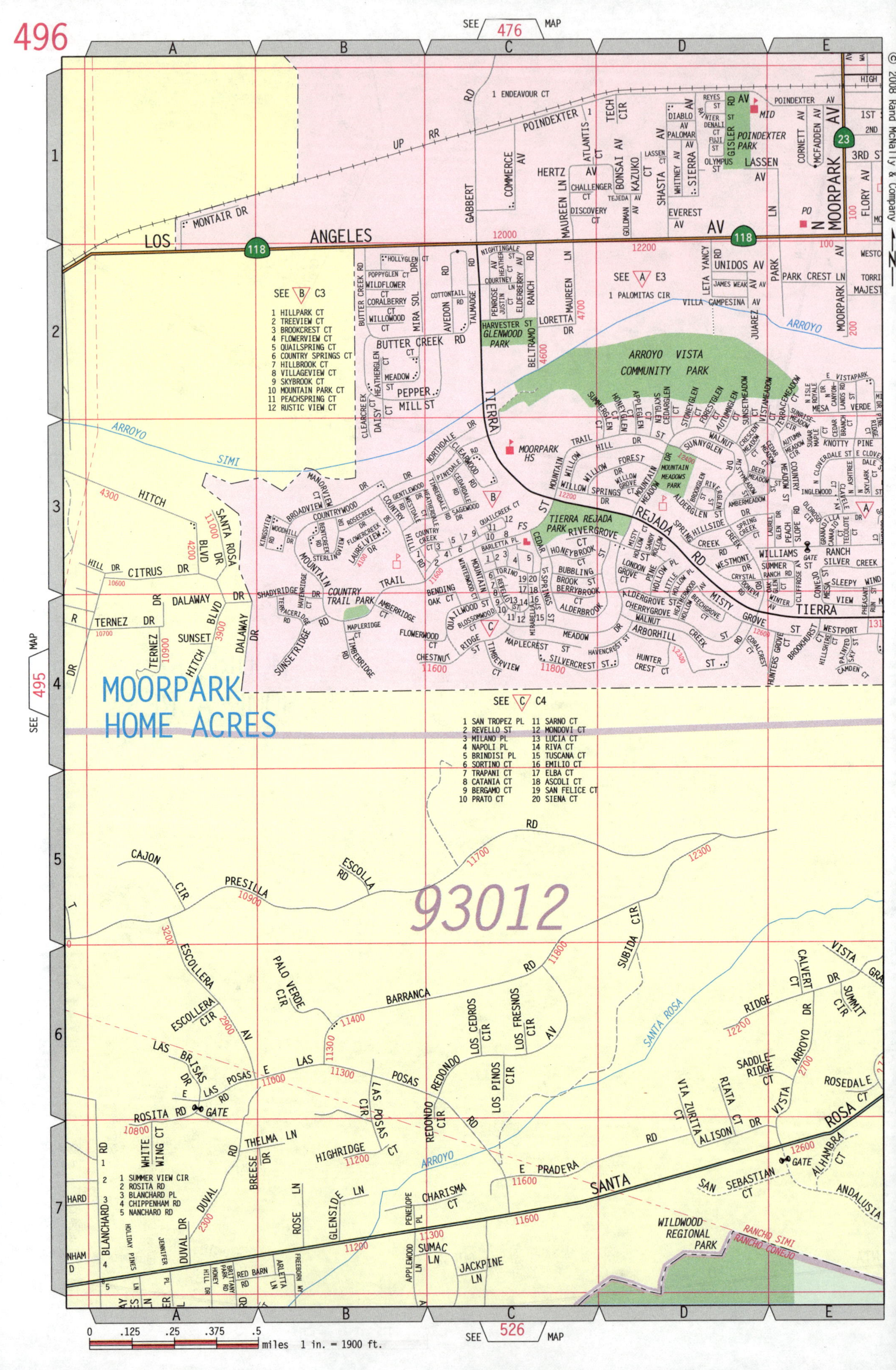
SEE 476 MAP
SEE 526 MAP
SEE 495 MAP
MOORPARK HOME ACRES
93012
LOS ANGELES AV
118
23
N MOORPARK AV
POINDEXTER AV
UP RR
1 ENDEAVOUR CT
GABBERT RD
COMMERCE AV
HERTZ AV
MAUREEN LN
ATLANTIS AV
TECH CIR
CHALLENGER CT
DISCOVERY CT
BONSAI AV
KAZUKO CT
TEJEDA AV
GOLDMAN AV
SHASTA AV
EVEREST AV
SIERRA AV
WHITNEY AV
OLYMPUS ST
LASSEN AV
GISLER RD
POINDEXTER PARK
REYES ST
DIABLO AV
PALOMAR AV
CORNETT AV
MCFADDEN AV
MONTAIR DR
SEE B C3
1 HILLPARK CT
2 TREEVIEW CT
3 BROOKCREST CT
4 FLOWERVIEW CT
5 QUAILSPRING CT
6 COUNTRY SPRINGS CT
7 HILLBROOK CT
8 VILLAGEVIEW CT
9 SKYBROOK CT
10 MOUNTAIN PARK CT
11 PEACHSPRING CT
12 RUSTIC VIEW CT
BUTTER CREEK RD
MIRA SOL
AVEDON RD
TALMADGE
GLENWOOD PARK
HARVESTER ST
BELTRAMO RANCH RD
LORETTA DR
SEE A E3
1 PALOMITAS CIR
UNIDOS AV
VILLA CAMPESINA AV
PARK CREST LN
JUAREZ PARK LN
ARROYO VISTA COMMUNITY PARK
ARROYO SIMI
TIERRA REJADA RD
MOORPARK HS
TIERRA REJADA PARK
MOUNTAIN MEADOWS PARK
COUNTRY TRAIL PARK
MOUNTAIN TRAIL
WILLIAMS RANCH RD
SILVER CREEK
MISTY GROVE ST
WESTPORT
HITCH
SANTA ROSA DR
CITRUS DR
DALAWAY DR
TERNEZ DR
SUNSET HITCH BLVD
SEE C C4
1 SAN TROPEZ PL
2 REVELLO ST
3 MILANO PL
4 NAPOLI PL
5 BRINDISI PL
6 SORTINO CT
7 TRAPANI CT
8 CATANIA CT
9 BERGAMO CT
10 PRATO CT
11 SARNO CT
12 MONDOVI CT
13 LUCIA CT
14 RIVA CT
15 TUSCANA CT
16 EMILIO CT
17 ELBA CT
18 ASCOLI CT
19 SAN FELICE CT
20 SIENA CT
CAJON CIR
PRESILLA RD
ESCOLLA RD
ESCOLLERA AV
ESCOLLERA CIR
PALO VERDE CIR
BARRANCA RD
SUBIDA CIR
LOS CEDROS CIR
LOS FRESNOS CIR
LAS BRISAS DR
E LAS POSAS RD
LAS POSAS CIR
REDONDO CIR
LOS PINOS CIR
ROSITA RD
GATE
THELMA LN
HIGHRIDGE CT
BREESE DR
WHITE WING CT
SANTA ROSA
VIA ZURITA CT
RIATA CT
ALISON DR
SADDLE RIDGE CT
ARROYO DR
VISTA
CALVERT CT
SUMMIT CIR
ROSEDALE CT
ALHAMBRA CT
SAN SEBASTIAN CT
ANDALUSIA
E PRADERA
SANTA ROSA RD
ARROYO
CHARISMA CT
GLENSIDE LN
ROSE LN
DUVAL DR
BLANCHARD RD
WILDWOOD REGIONAL PARK
RANCHO SIMI
RANCHO CONEJO
SUMAC LN
JACKPINE LN
APPLEWOOD LN
1 SUMMER VIEW CIR
2 ROSITA RD
3 BLANCHARD PL
4 CHIPPENHAM RD
5 NANCHARO RD
© 2008 Rand McNally & Company
0 .125 .25 .375 .5 miles 1 in. = 1900 ft.

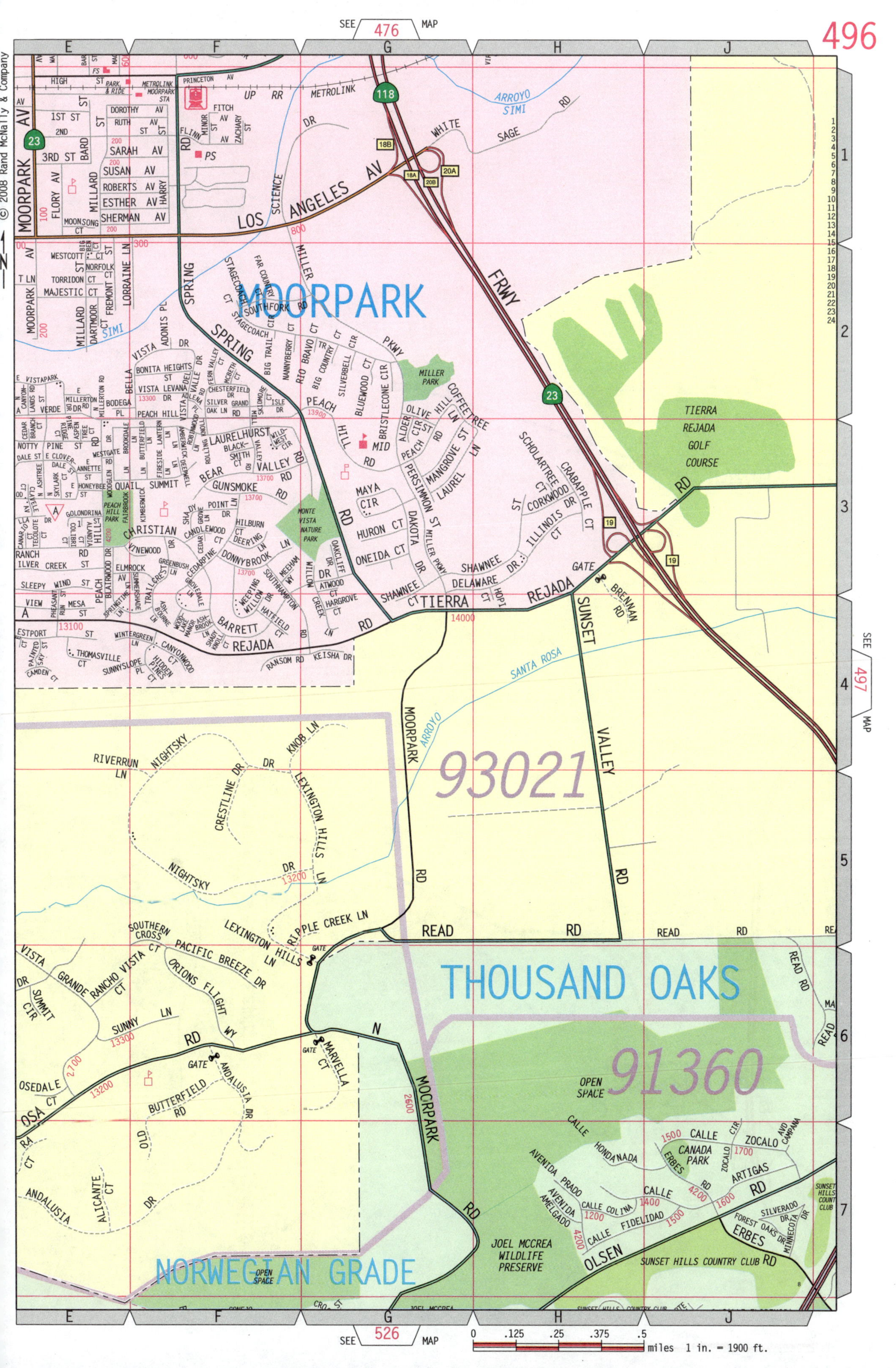

496
SEE 476 MAP
SEE 526 MAP
SEE 497 MAP
© 2008 Rand McNally & Company
MOORPARK
THOUSAND OAKS
NORWEGIAN GRADE
93021
91360
TIERRA REJADA GOLF COURSE
MILLER PARK
MONTE VISTA NATURE PARK
PEACH HILL PARK
CANADA PARK
JOEL MCCREA WILDLIFE PRESERVE
OPEN SPACE
SUNSET HILLS COUNTRY CLUB
ARROYO SIMI
SANTA ROSA
ARROYO
METROLINK
LOS ANGELES AV
SPRING RD
TIERRA REJADA RD
MOORPARK RD
SUNSET VALLEY RD
READ RD
OLSEN RD
FRWY
PEACH HILL RD
PRINCETON AV
WHITE SAGE RD
LEXINGTON HILLS LN
NIGHTSKY DR
CRESTLINE DR
KNOB LN
RIVERRUN LN
SOUTHERN CROSS CT
PACIFIC BREEZE DR
ORIONS FLIGHT WY
RANCHO VISTA CT
VISTA GRANDE DR
SUNNY LN
MARVELLA CT
ANDALUSIA DR
BUTTERFIELD RD
ALICANTE CT
CALLE ZOCALO
AVENIDA PRADO
CALLE FIDELIDAD
SUNSET HILLS COUNTRY CLUB RD
0 .125 .25 .375 .5 miles 1 in. = 1900 ft.

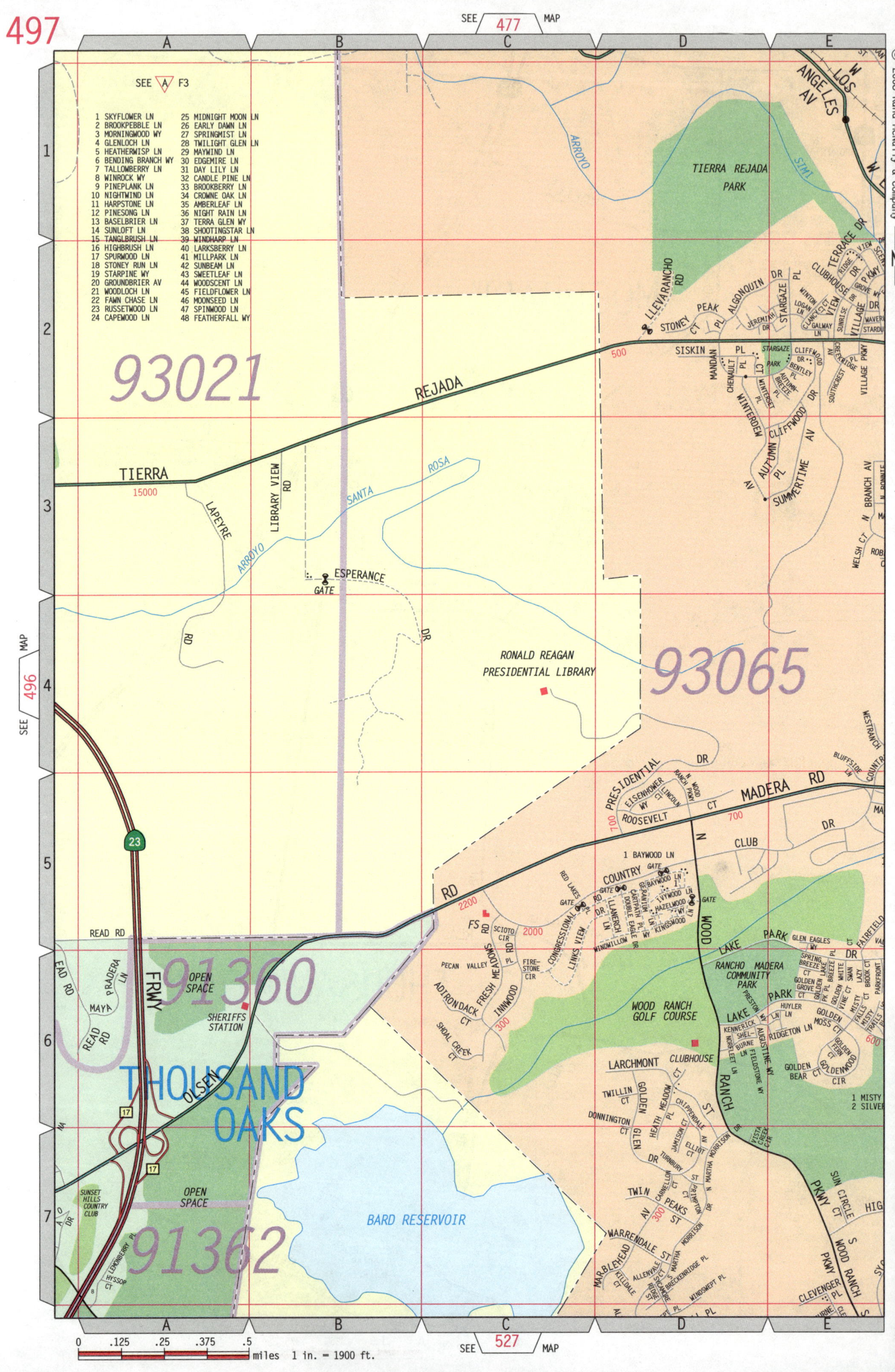
SEE 477 MAP
SEE A F3
1 SKYFLOWER LN
2 BROOKPEBBLE LN
3 MORNINGWOOD WY
4 GLENLOCH LN
5 HEATHERWISP LN
6 BENDING BRANCH WY
7 TALLOWBERRY LN
8 WINROCK WY
9 PINEPLANK LN
10 NIGHTWIND LN
11 HARPSTONE LN
12 PINESONG LN
13 BASELBRIER LN
14 SUNLOFT LN
15 TANGLBRUSH LN
16 HIGHBRUSH LN
17 SPURWOOD LN
18 STONEY RUN LN
19 STARPINE WY
20 GROUNDBRIER AV
21 WOODLOCH LN
22 FAWN CHASE LN
23 RUSSETWOOD LN
24 CAPEWOOD LN
25 MIDNIGHT MOON LN
26 EARLY DAWN LN
27 SPRINGMIST LN
28 TWILIGHT GLEN LN
29 MAYWIND LN
30 EDGEMIRE LN
31 DAY LILY LN
32 CANDLE PINE LN
33 BROOKBERRY LN
34 CROWNE OAK LN
35 AMBERLEAF LN
36 NIGHT RAIN LN
37 TERRA GLEN WY
38 SHOOTINGSTAR LN
39 WINDHARP LN
40 LARKSBERRY LN
41 MILLPARK LN
42 SUNBEAM LN
43 SWEETLEAF LN
44 WOODSCENT LN
45 FIELDFLOWER LN
46 MOONSEED LN
47 SPINWOOD LN
48 FEATHERFALL WY
93021
93065
91360
91362
TIERRA REJADA PARK
TIERRA REJADA
W LOS ANGELES AV
ARROYO SIMI
LLEVARANCHO RD
ARROYO SANTA ROSA
LIBRARY VIEW RD
LAPEYRE RD
ESPERANCE DR
GATE
RONALD REAGAN PRESIDENTIAL LIBRARY
PRESIDENTIAL DR
MADERA RD
COUNTRY CLUB DR
WOOD RANCH PKWY
RANCHO MADERA COMMUNITY PARK
LAKE PARK DR
WOOD RANCH GOLF COURSE
CLUBHOUSE
OPEN SPACE
SHERIFFS STATION
THOUSAND OAKS
OLSEN RD
FRWY
READ RD
BARD RESERVOIR
SUNSET HILLS COUNTRY CLUB
23
17
SEE 496 MAP
SEE 527 MAP
0 .125 .25 .375 .5 miles 1 in. = 1900 ft.
© 2008 Rand McNally & Company

SEE 477 MAP

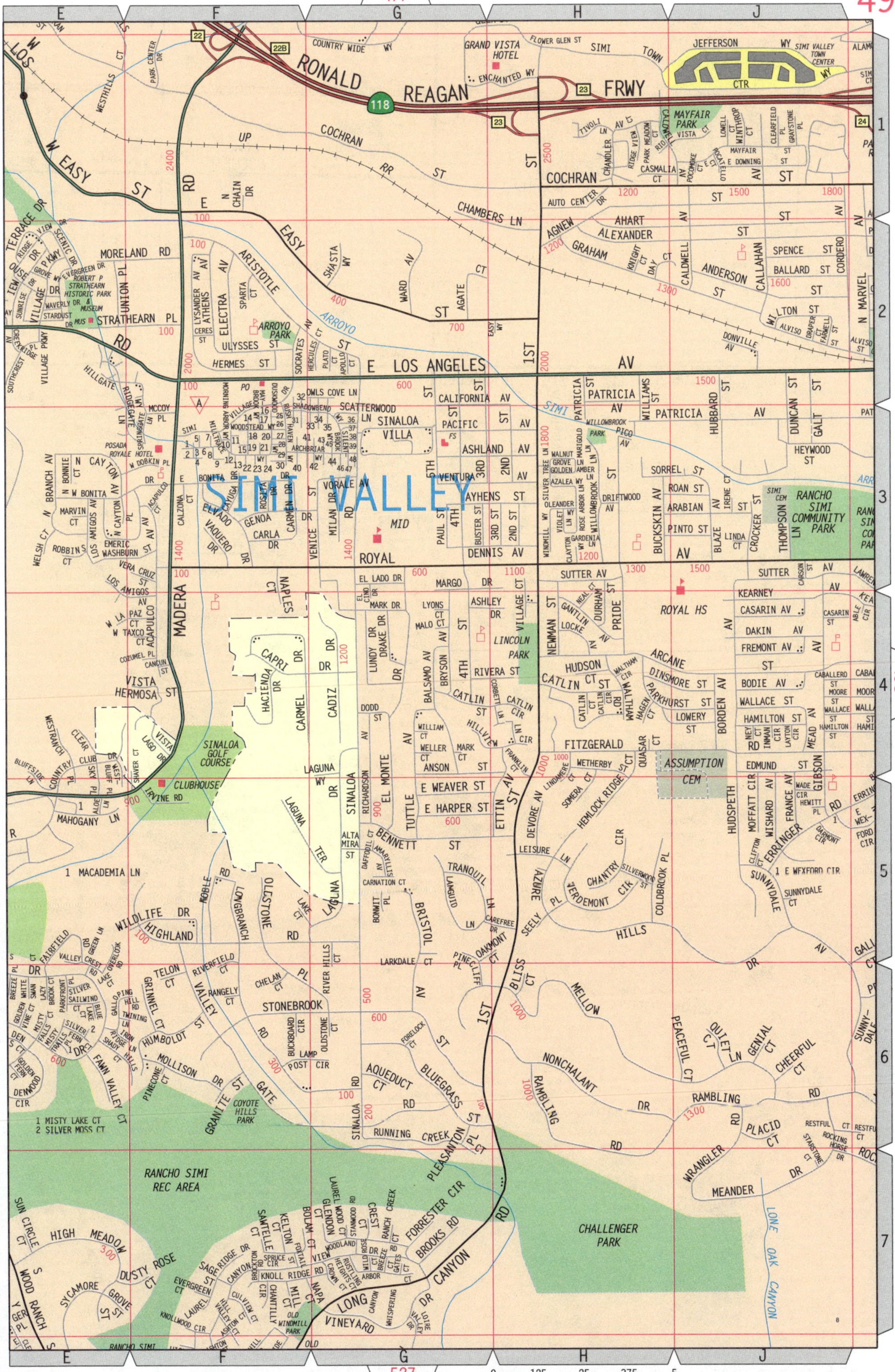

SEE 498 MAP

E F G H J

1 2 3 4 5 6 7

SIMI VALLEY

RONALD REAGAN FRWY
118
22 22B 23 24
COUNTRY WIDE WY
GRAND VISTA HOTEL
ENCHANTED WY
FLOWER GLEN ST
SIMI TOWN
JEFFERSON WY
SIMI VALLEY TOWN CENTER
CTR WY
MAYFAIR PARK
VISTA CT
COCHRAN ST
CHAMBERS LN
AUTO CENTER DR
AHART ST
ALEXANDER ST
GRAHAM
ANDERSON ST
SPENCE ST
BALLARD ST
CORDERO
N MARVEL
WILTON ST
DONVILLE AV
W LOS ANGELES AV
W EASY ST
E EASY ST
UP
RR
MORELAND RD
ROBERT P STRATHEARN HISTORIC PARK & MUSEUM
STRATHEARN PL
UNION PL
ARISTOTLE
ARROYO PARK
ARROYO SIMI
SHASTA WY
WARD AV
AGATE CT
ULYSSES ST
HERMES ST
E LOS ANGELES AV
1ST ST
EASY WY
PATRICIA AV
WILLIAMS ST
HUBBARD ST
DUNCAN ST
GALT ST
HEYWOOD ST
WILLOWBROOK PARK
PICO AV
OWLS COVE LN
SCATTERWOOD LN
SINALOA VILLA
CALIFORNIA AV
PACIFIC AV
ASHLAND AV
VENTURA
AYHENS ST
MCCOY PL
POSADA ROYALE HOTEL
N CAYTON AV
N BRANCH AV
W BONITA
MARVIN CT
EMERIC
WASHBURN ST
ROBBINS CT
WELSH CT
MID
ROYAL AV
DENNIS AV
PAUL ST
4TH ST
BUSTER ST
3RD ST
2ND ST
DRIFTWOOD AV
SORREL ST
ROAN ST
ARABIAN
PINTO ST
BUCKSKIN AV
IRENE CT
LINDA CT
BLAZE
CROCKER ST
THOMPSON LN
SIMI CEM
RANCHO SIMI COMMUNITY PARK
GENOA
CARLA DR
CARMEN DR
VENICE ST
MILAN DR
VAQUERO DR
ELVADO
CALZONA ST
MADERA RD
SUTTER AV
ROYAL HS
KEARNEY
CASARIN AV
DAKIN AV
FREMONT AV
BODIE AV
WALLACE ST
HAMILTON ST
EL LADO DR
MARGO DR
ASHLEY DR
LYONS
MARK DR
LUNDY DR
DRAKE DR
LINCOLN PARK
NEWMAN ST
DURHAM
PRIDE ST
GANTLIN
LOCKE
HUDSON
CATLIN CT
ARCANE
DINSMORE ST
PARKHURST ST
LOWERY ST
BORDEN AV
FITZGERALD
ASSUMPTION CEM
WETHERBY
QUASAR CT
EDMUND ST
GIBSON
MEAD AV
CAPRI DR
HACIENDA DR
CARMEL
CADIZ
LAGUNA WY
SINALOA DR
NAPLES CT
VISTA HERMOSA ST
ACAPULCO
LOS AMIGOS
VERA CRUZ
W LA PAZ
W TAXCO
SINALOA GOLF COURSE
CLUBHOUSE
IRVINE RD
MAHOGANY LN
MACADEMIA LN
COUNTRY CLUB
WESTRANCH
BALSAMO AV
BRYSON AV
RIVERA ST
WILLIAM CT
WELLER CT
ANSON
MARK CT
HILLVIEW
E WEAVER ST
E HARPER ST
TUTTLE
EL MONTE
RICHARDSON
BENNETT ST
ETTIN AV
DEVORE AV
LINDMERE
SOMERA CT
HEMLOCK RIDGE
LEISURE LN
CHANTRY CIR
SILVERWOOD
VERDEMONT CIR
COLDBROOK PL
HUDSPETH
MOFFATT CIR
WISHARD AV
FRANCE AV
ERRINGER RD
E WEXFORD CIR
SUNNYDALE CT
TRANQUIL
LANGUID
CAREFREE
OAKMONT
BRISTOL
LARKDALE CT
PINECLIFF
BLISS CT
SEELY PL
AZURE
HILLS AV
WILDLIFE DR
HIGHLAND
NOBLE
LONGBRANCH
OLSTONE RD
TELON CT
RIVERFIELD CT
RANGELY CT
CHELAN CT
STONEBROOK
RIVER HILLS CT
HUMBOLDT ST
MOLLISON DR
GRINNELL CT
BUCKBOARD CIR
LAMP POST CIR
AQUEDUCT CT
BLUEGRASS ST
FORELOCK CT
MELLOW
PEACEFUL CT
QUIET CT
GENTIAL CT
CHEERFUL CT
NONCHALANT DR
RAMBLING RD
PLACID CT
WRANGLER RD
MEANDER DR
RESTFUL CT
ROCKING HORSE RD
COYOTE HILLS PARK
GRANITE ST
GATE
RUNNING CREEK
PLEASANTON PL
SINALOA RD
1 MISTY LAKE CT
2 SILVER MOSS CT
FAWN VALLEY CT
PINECONE CT
RANCHO SIMI REC AREA
FORRESTER CIR
BROOKS RD
CHALLENGER PARK
LONE OAK CANYON
LONG CANYON RD
VINEYARD
HIGH MEADOW
DUSTY ROSE CT
SYCAMORE
GROVE ST
WOOD RANCH
SUN CIRCLE
EVERGREEN CT
KNOLL RIDGE RD
SAGE RIDGE DR
OLD WINDMILL PARK
RANCHO SIMI

SEE 527 MAP

0 .125 .25 .375 .5 miles 1 in. = 1900 ft.

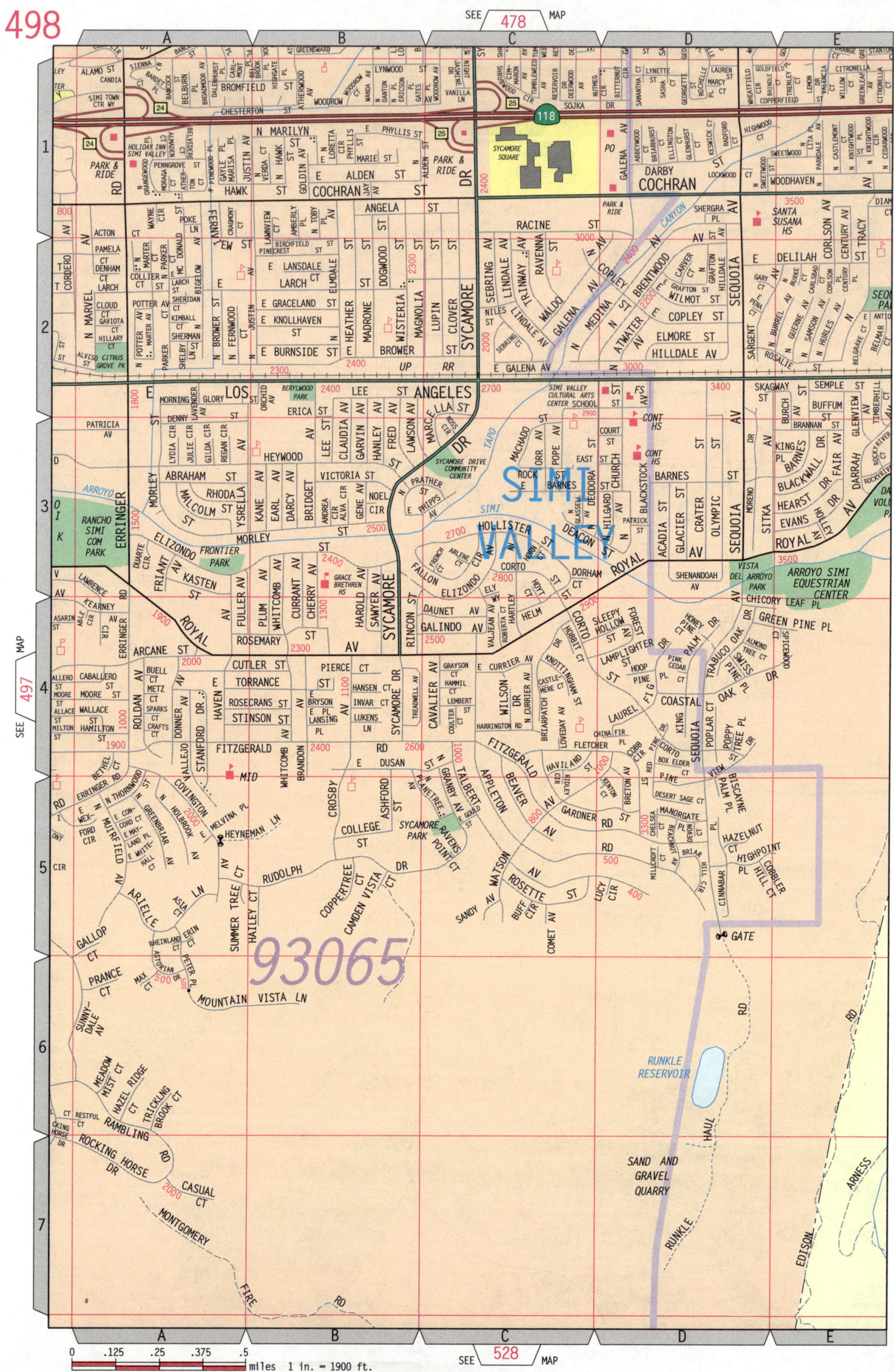

SEE 478 MAP
SEE 497 MAP
SEE 528 MAP
SIMI VALLEY
93065
118
SYCAMORE SQUARE
SANTA SUSANA HS
RANCHO SIMI COM PARK
FRONTIER PARK
SYCAMORE DRIVE COMMUNITY CENTER
SIMI VALLEY CULTURAL ARTS CENTER
GRACE BRETHREN HS
CONT HS
ARROYO SIMI EQUESTRIAN CENTER
VISTA DEL ARROYO PARK
SYCAMORE PARK
RUNKLE RESERVOIR
SAND AND GRAVEL QUARRY
GATE
MID
PARK & RIDE
COCHRAN
LOS ANGELES AV
ROYAL AV
SYCAMORE DR
SEQUOIA AV
ERRINGER RD
FITZGERALD RD
MORLEY ST
ELIZONDO
MOUNTAIN VISTA LN
ROCKING HORSE DR
RAMBLING RD
MONTGOMERY FIRE RD
RUNKLE HAUL RD
EDISON RD
ARROYO SIMI
TAPO CANYON
0 .125 .25 .375 .5 miles 1 in. = 1900 ft.

SEE 478 MAP

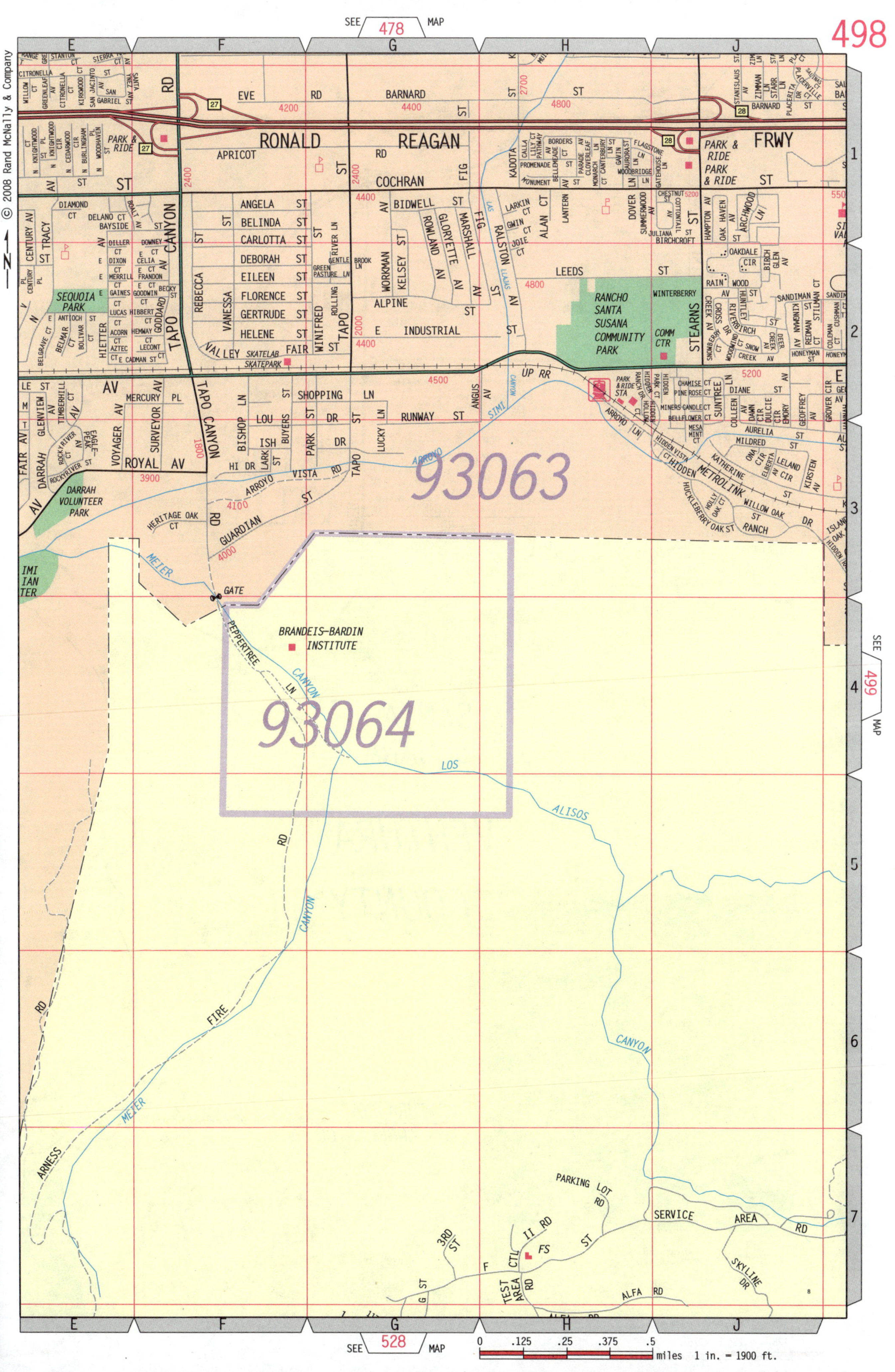

RONALD REAGAN FRWY
RONALD
REAGAN
FRWY
BARNARD
EVE RD
APRICOT
COCHRAN ST
TAPO CANYON RD
PARK & RIDE
ANGELA ST
BELINDA ST
CARLOTTA ST
DEBORAH ST
EILEEN ST
FLORENCE ST
GERTRUDE ST
HELENE ST
VALLEY FAIR ST
REBECCA ST
VANESSA
WINIFRED
ROLLING
TAPO
SKATELAB SKATEPARK
BIDWELL ST
ROWLAND AV
GLORYETTE AV
MARSHALL ST
WORKMAN AV
KELSEY ST
ALPINE ST
E INDUSTRIAL ST
RALSTON AV
KADOTA
FIG
LEEDS ST
ALAN CT
LANTERN
DOVER
SUMMERWOOD
STEARNS ST
RANCHO SANTA SUSANA COMMUNITY PARK
COMM CTR
WINTERBERRY
SEQUOIA PARK
DIAMOND CT
DELANO CT
BAYSIDE
CENTURY AV
TRACY ST
DARRAH VOLUNTEER PARK
DARRAH AV
FAIR AV
GLENVIEW AV
VOYAGER AV
SURVEYOR AV
MERCURY PL
ROYAL AV
BISHOP LN
LOU
ISH
BUYERS
SHOPPING LN
PARK DR
RUNWAY ST
ANGUS AV
LUCKY LN
UP RR
SIMI ARROYO
ARROYO VISTA RD
HERITAGE OAK CT
GUARDIAN ST
HI DR
METROLINK
PARK & RIDE STA
RANCH DR
HIDDEN RANCH
WILLOW OAK DR
KATHERINE
MILDRED ST
AURELIA ST
DIANE ST
COLLEEN AV
SUNTREE LN
GEOFFREY AV
ARCHWOOD LN
OAKDALE CIR
SANDIMAN ST
HONEYMAN ST
93063
93064
GATE
BRANDEIS-BARDIN INSTITUTE
PEPPERTREE LN
CANYON
LOS ALISOS CANYON
METER
FIRE RD
ARNESS
PARKING LOT RD
SERVICE AREA RD
SKYLINE DR
FS
TEST AREA
CTL II RD
F ST
G ST
3RD ST
ALFA RD
4200
4400
4800
2400
2700
4500
5200
2000
1800
3900
4100
4000
E F G H J
1 2 3 4 5 6 7
0 .125 .25 .375 .5 miles 1 in. = 1900 ft.

SEE 499 MAP

SEE 528 MAP

SEE 479 MAP

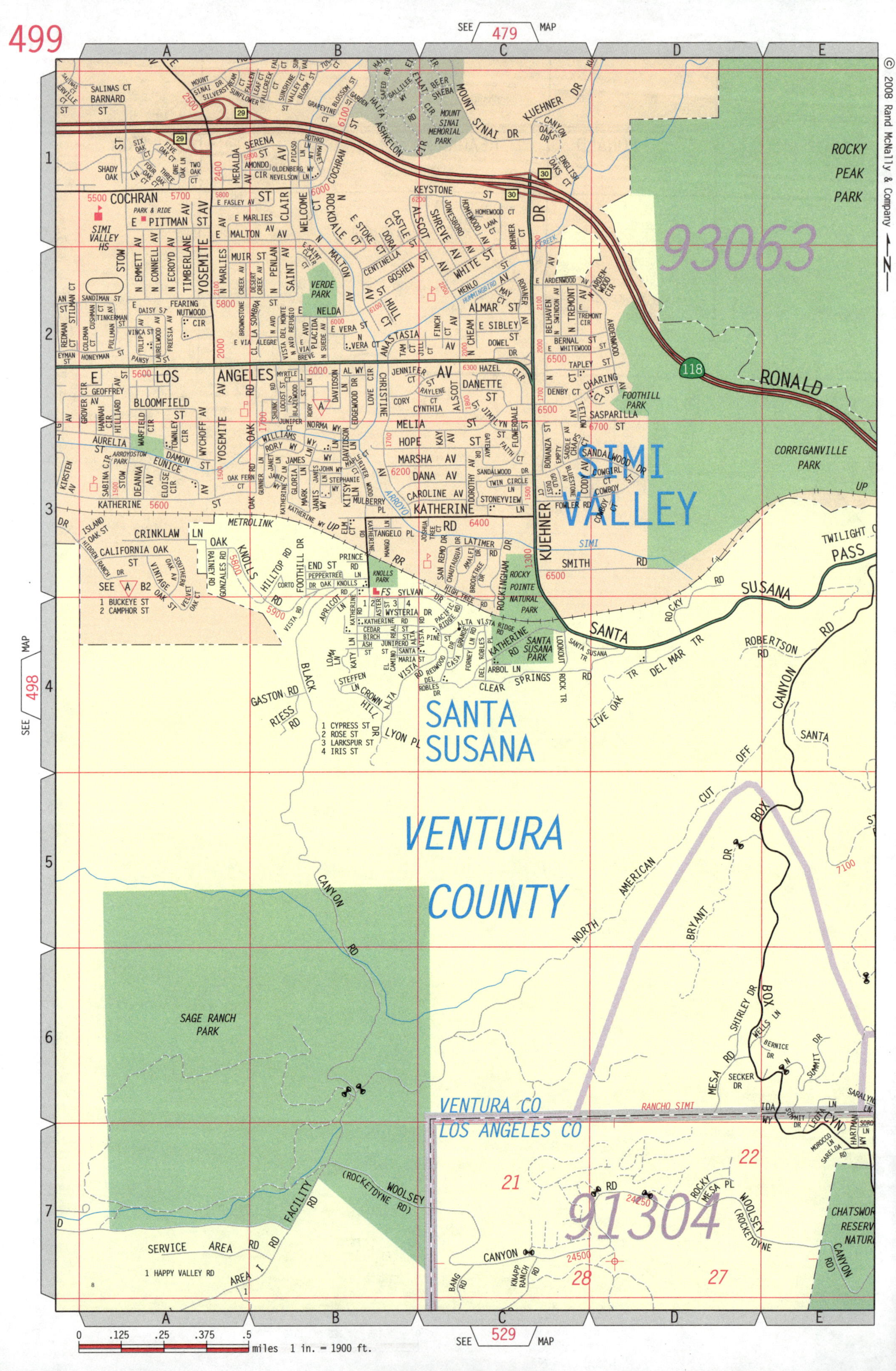

A
B
C
D
E
1
2
3
4
5
6
7
ROCKY PEAK PARK
93063
SIMI VALLEY
COCHRAN ST
LOS ANGELES AV
KATHERINE RD
KUEHNER DR
RONALD
118
29
30
SIMI VALLEY HS
VERDE PARK
FOOTHILL PARK
CORRIGANVILLE PARK
METROLINK
KNOLLS PARK
ROCKY POINTE NATURAL PARK
SANTA SUSANA PARK
SANTA SUSANA PASS RD
TWILIGHT PASS
ROCKY RD
ROBERTSON RD
SANTA SUSANA
VENTURA COUNTY
BLACK CANYON RD
GASTON RD
RIESS RD
LYON PL
CLEAR SPRINGS RD
LIVE OAK TR
DEL MAR TR
CUT OFF
BOX CANYON RD
NORTH AMERICAN
BRYANT DR
SHIRLEY DR
MESA RD
SAGE RANCH PARK
VENTURA CO
LOS ANGELES CO
RANCHO SIMI
91304
WOOLSEY CANYON RD
(ROCKETDYNE RD)
ROCKY MESA PL
FACILITY RD
SERVICE AREA RD
1 HAPPY VALLEY RD
CHATSWORTH RESERVOIR NATURE
SEE A B2
1 BUCKEYE ST
2 CAMPHOR ST
1 CYPRESS ST
2 ROSE ST
3 LARKSPUR ST
4 IRIS ST
21
22
27
28
0 .125 .25 .375 .5 miles 1 in. = 1900 ft.

SEE 498 MAP

SEE 529 MAP

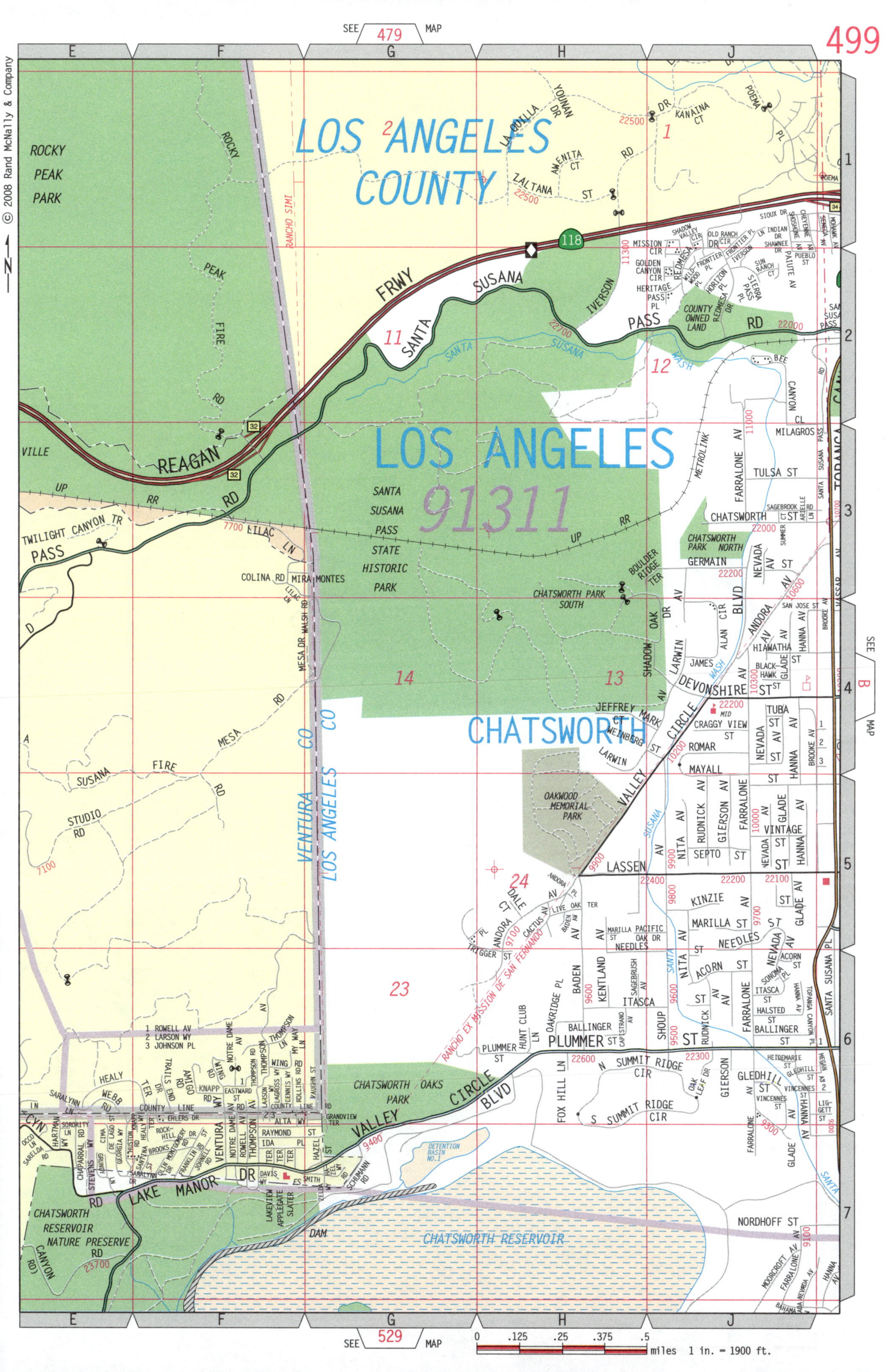
SEE 479 MAP
LOS ANGELES COUNTY
ROCKY PEAK PARK
LOS ANGELES
91311
SANTA SUSANA PASS STATE HISTORIC PARK
CHATSWORTH
CHATSWORTH PARK SOUTH
CHATSWORTH PARK NORTH
OAKWOOD MEMORIAL PARK
COUNTY OWNED LAND
CHATSWORTH OAKS PARK
CHATSWORTH RESERVOIR NATURE PRESERVE
CHATSWORTH RESERVOIR
DETENTION BASIN NO.1
RONALD REAGAN FRWY
SANTA SUSANA PASS RD
DEVONSHIRE ST
CHATSWORTH ST
LASSEN ST
PLUMMER ST
NORDHOFF ST
VALLEY CIRCLE BLVD
TOPANGA CANYON BLVD
VENTURA CO
LOS ANGELES CO
RANCHO SIMI
RANCHO EX MISSION DE SAN FERNANDO
METROLINK
UP RR
SEE B MAP
SEE 529 MAP
0 .125 .25 .375 .5 miles 1 in. = 1900 ft.

SEE 491 MAP
A
B
C
D
E
1
2
3
4
5
6
7
SEE B MAP
PACIFIC
OCEAN
0 .125 .25 .375 .5
miles 1 in. = 1900 ft.
SEE 551 MAP

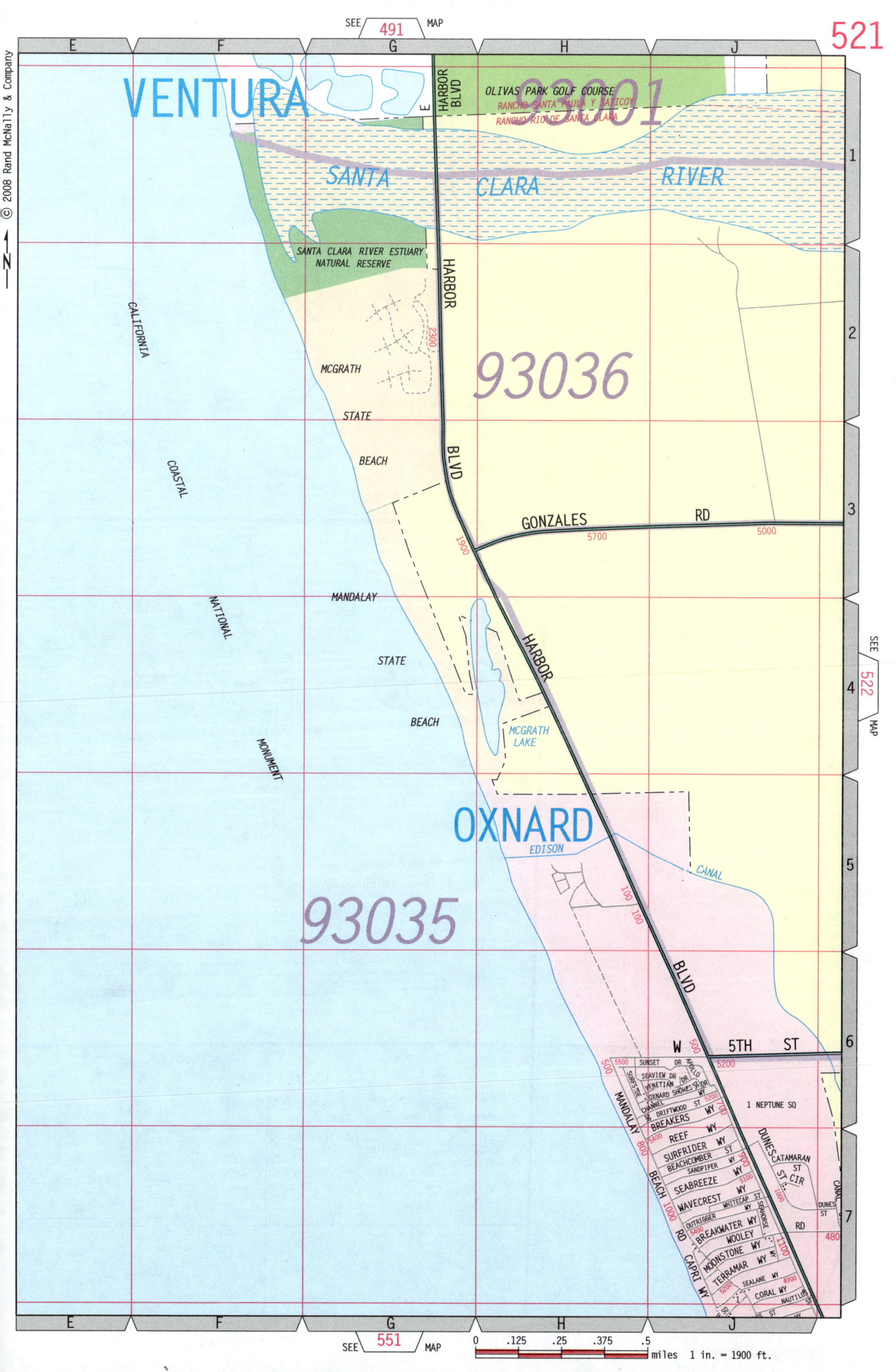
SEE 491 MAP
E
F
G
H
J
VENTURA
93001
HARBOR BLVD
OLIVAS PARK GOLF COURSE
RANCHO SANTA PAULA Y SATICOY
RANCHO RIO DE SANTA CLARA
SANTA CLARA RIVER
SANTA CLARA RIVER ESTUARY NATURAL RESERVE
HARBOR
CALIFORNIA
2300
MCGRATH
93036
STATE
BEACH
COASTAL
BLVD
GONZALES RD
5700
5000
1900
MANDALAY
NATIONAL
HARBOR
STATE
BEACH
MCGRATH LAKE
MONUMENT
OXNARD
EDISON
CANAL
93035
100
BLVD
W 5TH ST
500
5200
SUNSET DR
SEAVIEW DR
VENETIAN DR
OXNARD SHORES DR
CHANNEL
DRIFTWOOD ST
BREAKERS WY
REEF WY
SURFRIDER WY
BEACHCOMBER ST
SANDPIPER WY
SEABREEZE WY
WAVECREST WY
WHITECAP ST
OUTRIGGER WY
BREAKWATER WY
WOOLEY
MOONSTONE WY
TERRAMAR WY
SEALANE WY
CORAL WY
NAUTILUS
1 NEPTUNE SQ
DUNES ST
CATAMARAN ST CIR
MANDALAY BEACH RD
800
1000
CAPRI WY
RD
480
1
2
3
4
5
6
7
SEE 522 MAP
SEE 551 MAP
0 .125 .25 .375 .5 miles 1 in. = 1900 ft.

SEE 492 MAP

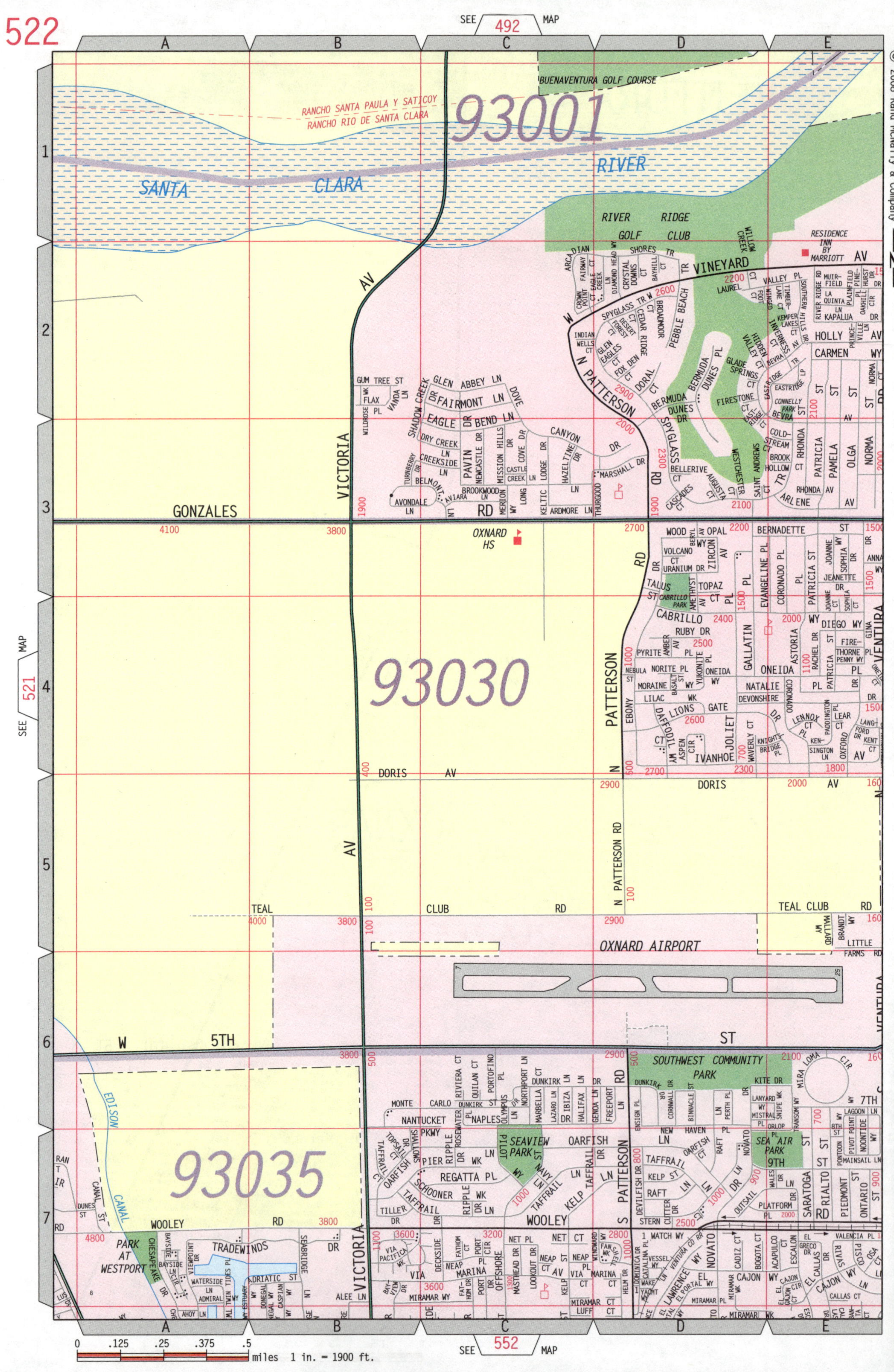
93001
93030
93035
SANTA CLARA RIVER
RANCHO SANTA PAULA Y SATICOY
RANCHO RIO DE SANTA CLARA
BUENAVENTURA GOLF COURSE
RIVER RIDGE GOLF CLUB
RESIDENCE INN BY MARRIOTT
VINEYARD AV
VICTORIA AV
GONZALES RD
N PATTERSON RD
OXNARD HS
CABRILLO PARK
DORIS AV
TEAL CLUB RD
OXNARD AIRPORT
W 5TH ST
SOUTHWEST COMMUNITY PARK
SEAVIEW PARK
SEA AIR PARK
WOOLEY RD
EDISON CANAL
PARK AT WESTPORT
TRADEWINDS DR
S PATTERSON RD
MIRAMAR WY
VENTURA RD
CAJON WY

0 .125 .25 .375 .5 miles 1 in. = 1900 ft.

SEE 521 MAP

SEE 552 MAP

SEE 492 MAP

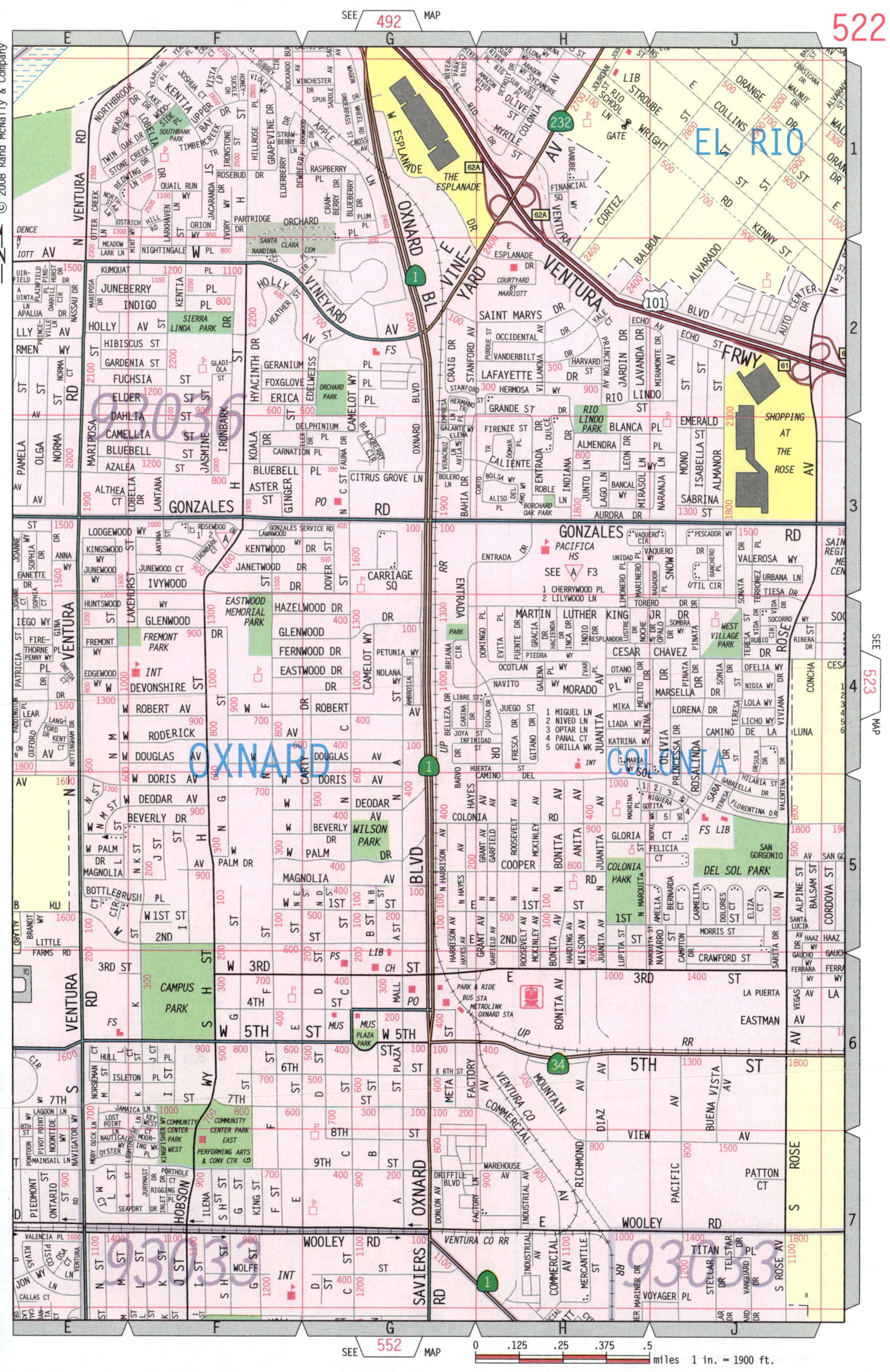
EL RIO
OXNARD
COLONIA
93036
93033
THE ESPLANADE
SHOPPING AT THE ROSE
SIERRA LINDA PARK
ORCHARD PARK
RIO LINDO PARK
EASTWOOD MEMORIAL PARK
FREMONT PARK
WEST VILLAGE PARK
WILSON PARK
COLONIA PARK
DEL SOL PARK
CAMPUS PARK
COMMUNITY CENTER PARK
PLAZA PARK
PACIFICA HS
COURTYARD BY MARRIOTT
CARRIAGE SQ
METROLINK OXNARD STA
PARK & RIDE
BUS STA
PERFORMING ARTS & CONV CTR
WAREHOUSE
OXNARD BL
VENTURA FRWY
GONZALES RD
SAVIERS RD
WOOLEY RD
5TH ST
3RD ST
VINEYARD AV
ROSE AV
VENTURA RD
OXNARD BLVD
ROSE AV
101
1
232
34
E F G H J
1 2 3 4 5 6 7

SEE 523 MAP

SEE 552 MAP

0 .125 .25 .375 .5 miles 1 in. = 1900 ft.

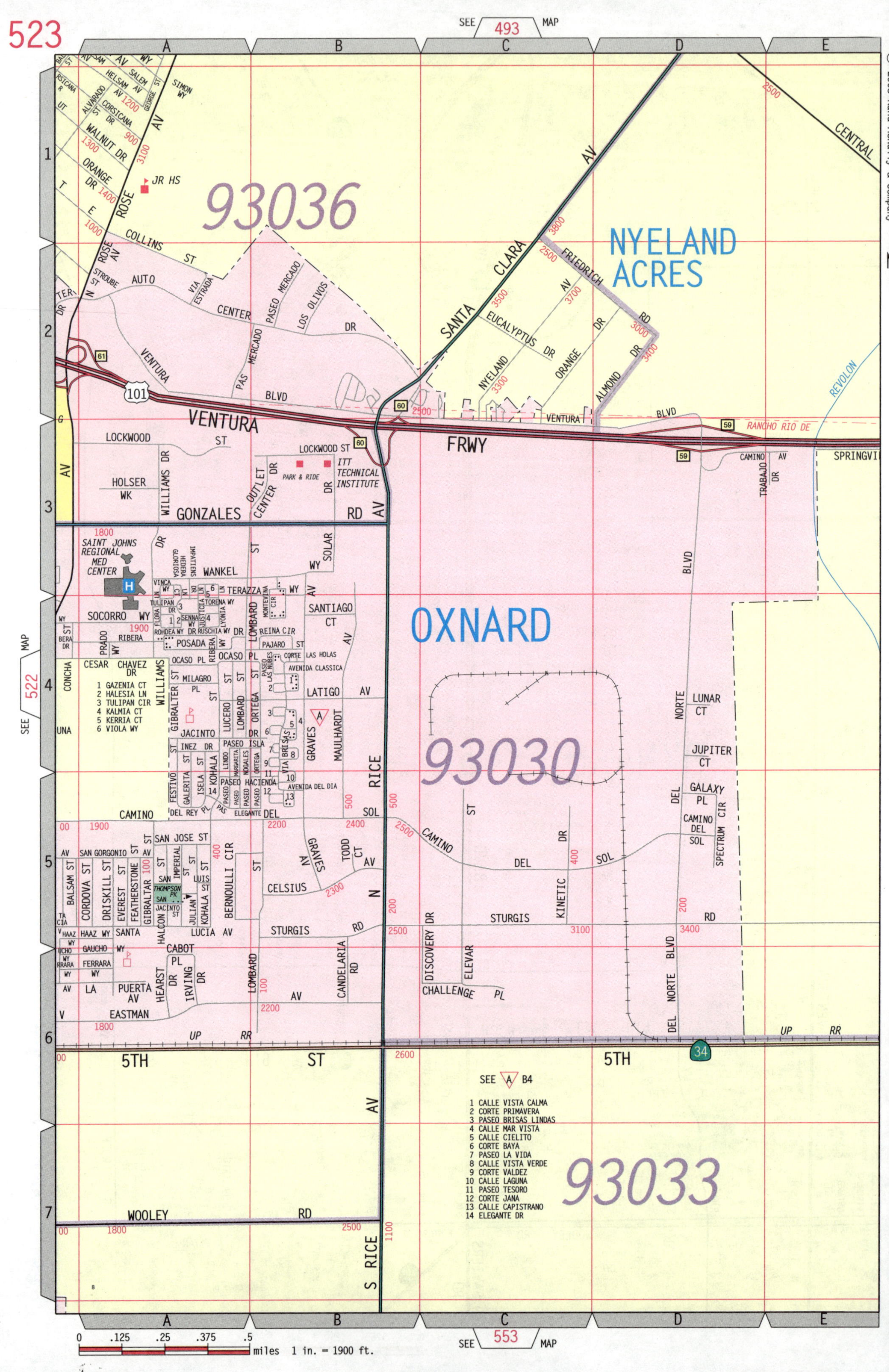

SEE 493 MAP
A
B
C
D
E
1
2
3
4
5
6
7
93036
NYELAND ACRES
OXNARD
93030
93033
SANTA CLARA AV
FRIEDRICH RD
EUCALYPTUS DR
NYELAND AV
ORANGE DR
ALMOND DR
CENTRAL
REVOLON
ROSE AV
N ROSE AV
JR HS
COLLINS ST
STROUBE ST
AUTO CENTER DR
VIA ESTRADA
PASEO MERCADO
LOS OLIVOS
PAS MERCADO
VENTURA BLVD
VENTURA FRWY
101
61
60
59
34
RANCHO RIO DE
SPRINGVI
CAMINO TRABAJO DR
LOCKWOOD ST
LOCKWOOD ST
PARK & RIDE
ITT TECHNICAL INSTITUTE
HOLSER WK
WILLIAMS DR
GONZALES RD
OUTLET CENTER DR
SAINT JOHNS REGIONAL MED CENTER
WANKEL WY
SOLAR
TERAZZA
SANTIAGO CT
SOCORRO WY
POSADA
RIBERA
PRADO
CESAR CHAVEZ DR
CONCHA
OCASO PL
MILAGRO PL
GIBRALTER ST
LATIGO AV
JACINTO DR
INEZ DR
PASEO ISLA
VIA BRISAS
GRAVES
MAULHARDT
LUCERO
LOMBARD
ORTEGA
KOHALA
AVENIDA DEL DIA
AVENIDA CLASSICA
CORTE LAS HOLAS
PAJARO
REINA CIR
FESTIVO
GALERITA
ISELA
PASEO HACIENDA
ELEGANTE
CAMINO DEL SOL
N RICE AV
SAN JOSE ST
SAN GORGONIO
BALSAM ST
CORDOVA ST
DRISKILL ST
EVEREST ST
FEATHERSTONE ST
GIBRALTAR ST
THOMPSON PK
IMPERIAL
SAN LUIS
JULIAN ST
KOHALA ST
BERNOULLI CIR
GRAVES AV
TODD CT
CELSIUS
STURGIS RD
SANTA LUCIA AV
HAAZ WY
GAUCHO WY
FERRARA WY
CABOT PL
HALCON
HEARST DR
IRVING DR
PUERTA AV
LA
EASTMAN AV
CANDELARIA RD
DISCOVERY DR
ELEVAR
CHALLENGE PL
KINETIC DR
NORTE BLVD
DEL NORTE BLVD
LUNAR CT
JUPITER CT
GALAXY PL
CAMINO DEL SOL
SPECTRUM CIR
UP RR
5TH ST
5TH
S RICE AV
WOOLEY RD
SEE A B4
1 CALLE VISTA CALMA
2 CORTE PRIMAVERA
3 PASEO BRISAS LINDAS
4 CALLE MAR VISTA
5 CALLE CIELITO
6 CORTE BAYA
7 PASEO LA VIDA
8 CALLE VISTA VERDE
9 CORTE VALDEZ
10 CALLE LAGUNA
11 PASEO TESORO
12 CORTE JANA
13 CALLE CAPISTRANO
14 ELEGANTE DR
1 GAZENIA CT
2 HALESIA LN
3 TULIPAN CIR
4 KALMIA CT
5 KERRIA CT
6 VIOLA WY
SEE 522 MAP
SEE 553 MAP
0 .125 .25 .375 .5 miles 1 in. = 1900 ft.

SEE 493 MAP

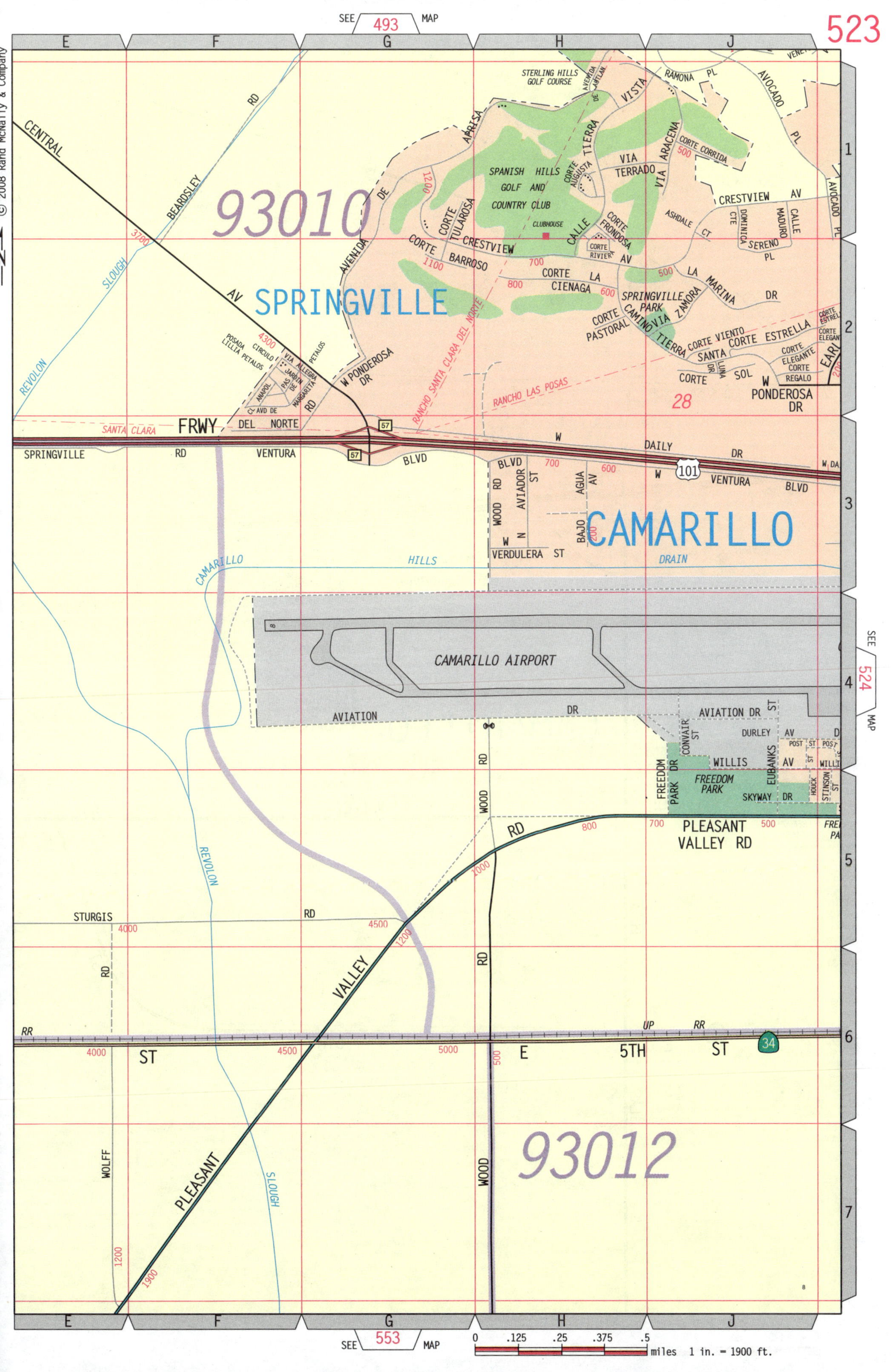

93010
SPRINGVILLE
CAMARILLO
93012
SPANISH HILLS GOLF AND COUNTRY CLUB
CLUBHOUSE
STERLING HILLS GOLF COURSE
CAMARILLO AIRPORT
FREEDOM PARK
SPRINGVILLE PARK
CENTRAL AV
BEARDSLEY RD
REVOLON SLOUGH
CAMARILLO HILLS DRAIN
SANTA CLARA FRWY
DEL NORTE
SPRINGVILLE RD
VENTURA BLVD
W VENTURA BLVD
W DAILY DR
W PONDEROSA DR
AVENIDA DE APRISA
RANCHO SANTA CLARA DEL NORTE
RANCHO LAS POSAS
CRESTVIEW AV
CORTE BARROSO
CORTE TULAROSA
CALLE CORTE RIVIERA
LA CIENAGA
LA MARINA DR
CAMINO TIERRA
VIA ZAMORA
CORTE PASTORAL
CORTE ESTRELLA
CORTE VIENTO
SANTA LUNA DR
CORTE SOL
CORTE REGALO
CORTE ELEGANTE
VIA TERRADO
VIA ARACENA
CORTE CORRIDA
VISTA TIERRA
RAMONA PL
AVOCADO PL
ASHDALE CT
DOMINICA
MADURO
CALLE SERENO PL
CORTE AUGUSTA
CORTE FRONDOSA
AVENIDA DE ANTLAN
POSADA CIRCULO
LILLIA PETALOS
VIA ALLEGRA
JARDIN DE MARGARITA
PAS DE
AMAPOL
CL AVD DE
PETALOS
WOOD RD
N AVIADOR ST
AGUA AV
BAJO
W VERDULERA ST
AVIATION DR
CONVAIR ST
DURLEY AV
WILLIS AV
EUBANKS ST
POST ST
STINSON ST
HOUCK
SKYWAY DR
FREEDOM PARK DR
PLEASANT VALLEY RD
STURGIS RD
WOLFF RD
E 5TH ST
UP RR
28
57
101
34

SEE 524 MAP

SEE 553 MAP

0 .125 .25 .375 .5 miles 1 in. = 1900 ft.

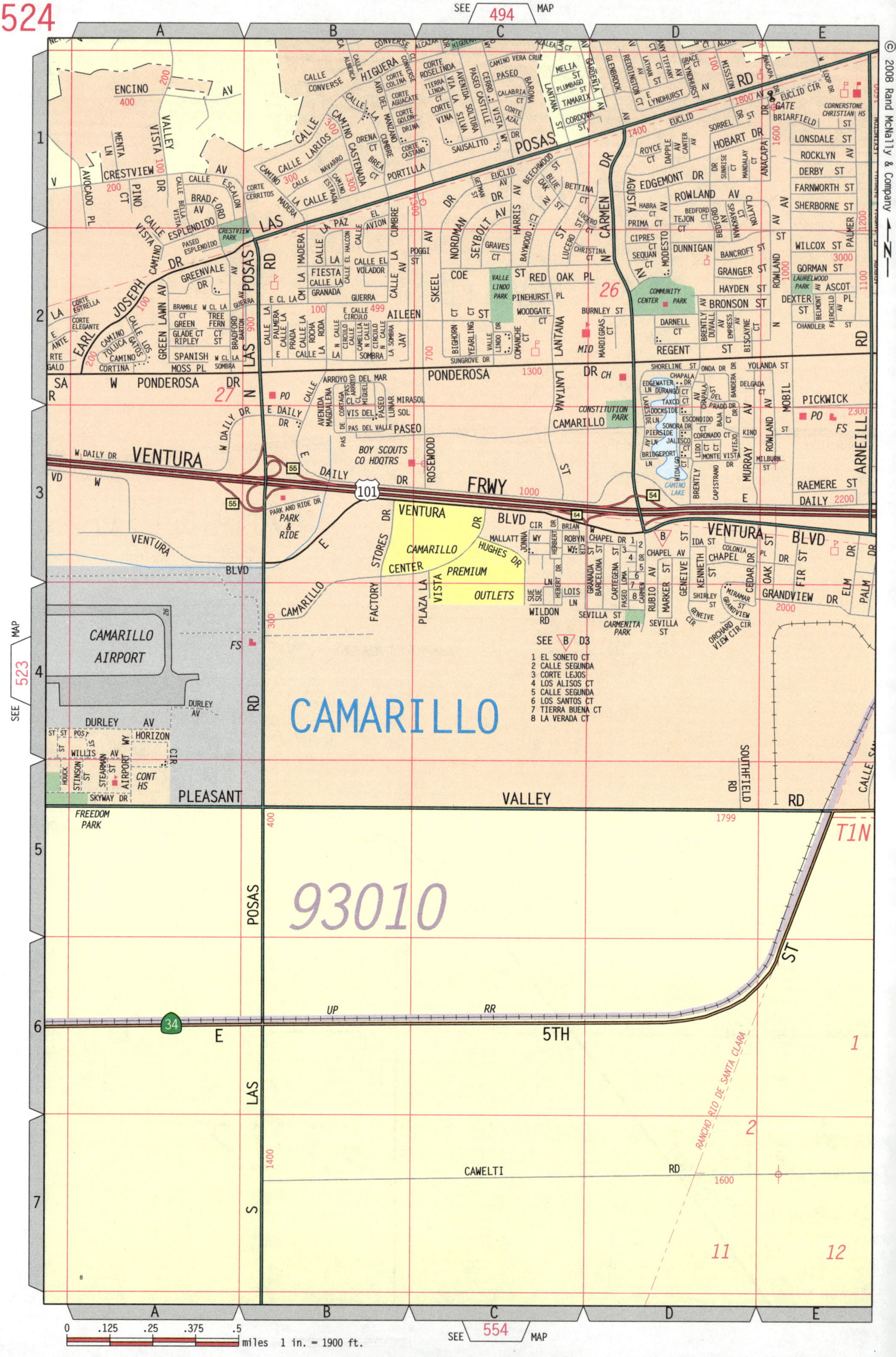

SEE 494 MAP

A B C D E

CAMARILLO

93010

ENCINO AV
VALLEY VISTA DR
MENTA LN
CRESTVIEW AV
AVOCADO PL
PINO CT
CALLE ESCALON
BRADFORD AV
CALLE BELLA VISTA
CALLE ESPLENDIDO
PASEO ESPLENDIDO
CAMINO VISTA
CRESTVIEW PARK
EARL JOSEPH DR
GREENVALE DR
GREEN LAWN AV
BRAMBLE CT
W CL LA GUERRA
TREE FERN CT
GLADE CT
RIPLEY ST
SPANISH W CL LA SOMBRA
MOSS PL
CAMINO TOLUCA
CALLE LOS GATOS
CAMINO CORTINA
CORTE ESTRELLA
CORTE ELEGANTE
BRADFORD BARTON
W PONDEROSA DR
W DAILY DR
E DAILY DR
VENTURA FRWY
VENTURA BLVD
CALLE CONVERSE
HIGUERA
CALLE ALBERCA
CALLE LA CUMBRE
AVD DEL MANZANO
CORTE COLINA
CORTE AGUACATE
CORTE GOLON
DRINA
CORTE CASTANO
CAMINO CASTENADA
CALLE LARIOS
ORENA CT
BREA CT
PORTILLA
CAMINO MADERA
CALLE NAVARRO
CAMINO ESTRADA
CORTE CERRITOS
CORTE ROSELINDA
TIERRA LINDA CT
CORTE VINA
VIA LA SILVA
AVENIDA SOLTURA
PASEO CASTILLE
CERRO VISTA WY
CAMINO VERA CRUZ
PASEO CALABRIA CT
CORTE AZAL
BARONA
SAUSALITO
LAS POSAS RD
MELIA CT
PLUMBAGO ST
TAMARIX ST
CORDOVA ST
LANTANA ST
GARDENIA AV
GLENBROOK
REDDINGTON CT
LATHAN CT
TIFFANY CT
WYNDHURST AV
GRACE CT
LYNDHURST CT
MISSION
EUCLID AV
EUCLID CIR
GATE
ANACAPA DR
CORNERSTONE CHRISTIAN HS
BRIARFIELD ST
LONSDALE ST
ROCKLYN AV
DERBY ST
FARNWORTH ST
SHERBORNE ST
WILCOX ST
GORMAN ST
LAURELWOOD PARK
ASCOT
DEXTER ST
BELMONT AV
FAIRCHILD AV
CHANDLER ST
PALMER
ARNEILL RD
ROYCE CT
DAPPLE AV
CANTER AV
SORREL CT
HOBART DR
EDGEMONT DR
ROWLAND AV
SUNRISE CT
MANDALAY CT
AGUSTA AV
HABRA CT
PRIMA CT
CIPRES CT
SEQUAN CT
MODESTO
BEDFORD CT
TEJON CT
SPARKMAN CT
CLAYTON CT
DUNNIGAN
BANCROFT ST
GRANGER ST
HAYDEN ST
BRONSON ST
COMMUNITY CENTER PARK
DARNELL CT
BRENTLY AV
DUVALL AV
EMPRESS AV
BISCAYNE CT
REGENT ST
ROWLAND
N CARMEN DR
BETTINA CT
LUCERO
CHRISTINA CT
BEECHWOOD
BLUE OAK ST
RED OAK PL
BURNLEY ST
MARDIGRAS CT
MID
PINEHURST PL
WOODGATE CT
VALLE LINDO PARK
HARRIS AV
BAYWOOD CT
GRAVES CT
SEYBOLT AV
NORDMAN DR
GETMAN ST
COE
SKEEL AV
POGGI ST
BIGHORN CT
YEARLING CT
VALLE LINDO DR
COMANCHE CT
SUNGROVE DR
CALLE LA PAZ
EL AVION
CALLE LA MADERA
CALLE EL HALCON
CALLE EL VOLADOR
FIESTA CALLE LA GRANADA
GUERRA
E CL LA
E CALLE CIRCULO
AILEEN
JAY AV
CALLE LA PALMERA
CALLE LA PRADA
CALLE LA ROCHA
LA RODA
N CALLE CIRCULO
CAMELLIA
LA SOMBRA
SOMBRA
PONDEROSA DR
CH
PO
ARROYO DEL MAR
AVENIDA MAGDALENA
PAS DE CORTAGA
CL MIGUEL
LUNAR PASEO
MIRASOL
SOL
VIS DEL
PAS DEL VALLE
PASEO
BOY SCOUTS CO HDQTRS
ROSEWOOD
CONSTITUTION PARK
CAMARILLO ST
SHORELINE ST
ONDA DR
YOLANDA ST
CHAPALA DR
DELGADA CT
EDGEWATER LN
DURANGO CT
DOCKSIDE LN
TAXCO CT
LAKESIDE LN
PRADO DR
ESCONDIDO
SONORA DR
PIERSIDE LN
BRIDGEPORT LN
CORONADO CT
JALISCO
LIDO CT
MONTE CT
BAJA
VIEJO
VISTA DR
KINO
MILBURN ST
MURRAY AV
MOBIL AV
PICKWICK
FS
HIDALGO
CAMINO LAKE
BRENTLY
CAPISTRANO
RAEMERE ST
DAILY
PARK AND RIDE DR
PARK & RIDE
E CAMARILLO
VENTURA STORES DR
CAMARILLO CENTER
FACTORY
PLAZA LA VISTA
PREMIUM OUTLETS
HUGHES DR
MALLATT
JONNA CIR
BRIAN WY
HERBERT DR
ROBYN CIR WY
W CHAPEL DR
CHAPEL AV
GRANADA
BARCELONA ST
CARTEGENA ST
PASEO LOMA
CARMEN
RUBIO AV
MARKER ST
GENEIVE ST
IDA ST
KENNETH ST
COLONIA
CHAPEL
CEDAR DR
OAK ST
FIR ST
ELM DR
PALM
GRANDVIEW DR
SHIRLEY ST
GENEIVE CIR
MIRAMAR ST
GRANDVIEW CIR
ORCHARD VIEW CIR
SUE LN
HEBERT
LOIS LN
WILDON RD
SEVILLA ST
CARMENITA PARK
CAMARILLO AIRPORT
DURLEY AV
HORIZON
POST ST
WILLIS AV
STEARMAN ST
AIRPORT WY
STINSON ST
HOUCK
CONT HS
SKYWAY DR
CIR
PLEASANT VALLEY RD
SOUTHFIELD RD
FREEDOM PARK
T1N
UP RR
E 5TH ST
CALLE
LAS POSAS S
CAWELTI RD
RANCHO RIO DE SANTA CLARA

SEE B D3
1 EL SONETO CT
2 CALLE SEGUNDA
3 CORTE LEJOS
4 LOS ALISOS CT
5 CALLE SEGUNDA
6 LOS SANTOS CT
7 TIERRA BUENA CT
8 LA VERADA CT

SEE 523 MAP

0 .125 .25 .375 .5 miles 1 in. = 1900 ft.

SEE 554 MAP

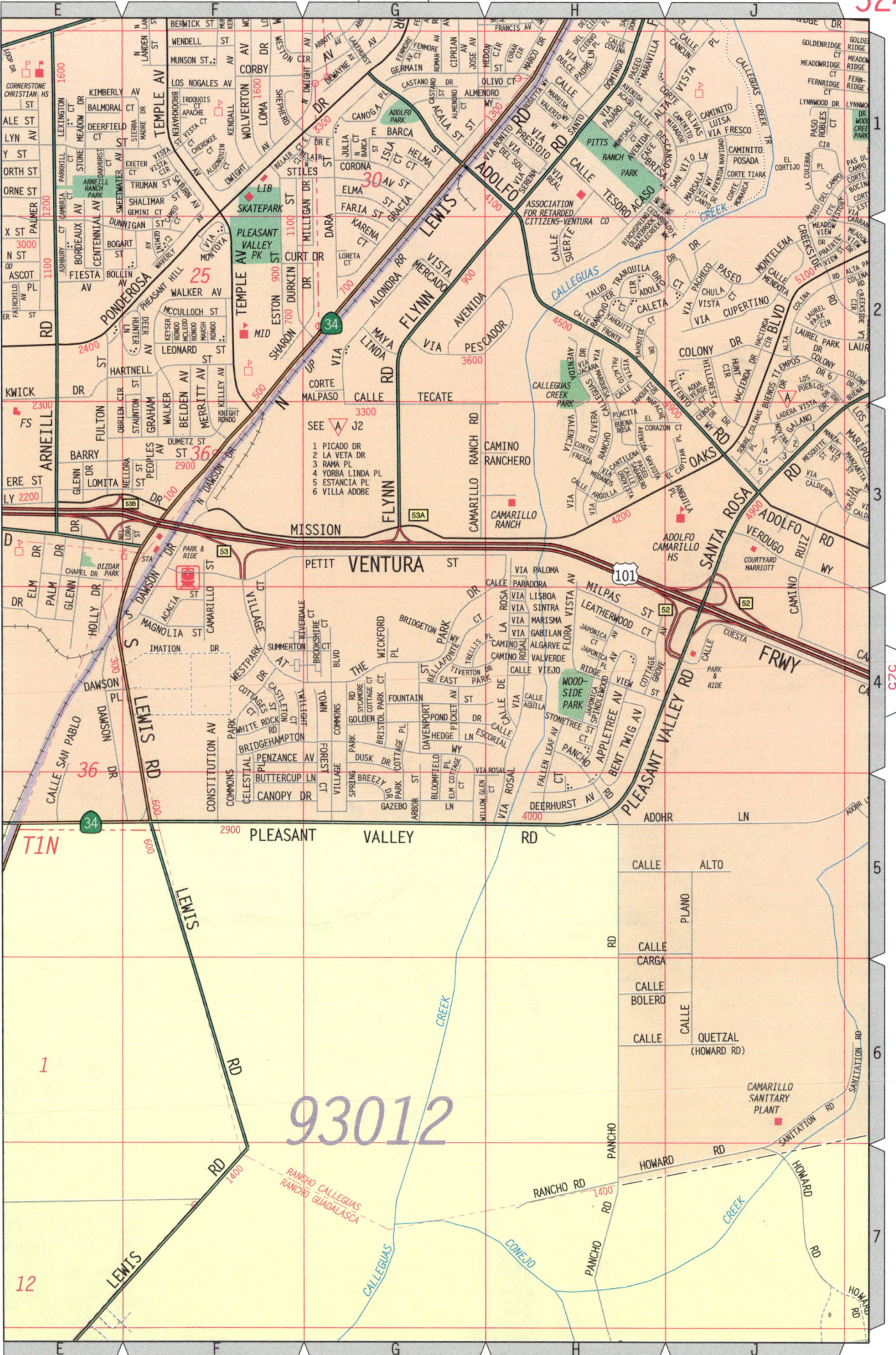

SEE 494 MAP

E F G H J

CORNERSTONE CHRISTIAN HS
KIMBERLY AV
BALMORAL CT
DEERFIELD CT
TEMPLE AV
BERWICK ST
WENDELL ST
MUNSON ST
CORBY
LOS NOGALES AV
IROQUOIS
APACHE
CHEROKEE
ALGONQUIN
DWIGHT
KENDALL
WOLVERTON AV
LOMA DR
SHEPHERD
WESTON CIR
N DWIGHT AV
ABBOTT
DEWAYNE AV
LAKEHURST
FENMORE CT
GERMAIN
ROMAN AV
CIPRIAN AV
JOSE AV
MEDON CIR
FORAD CT
MARCO DR
FRANCIS AV
CASTANO DR
ALMENDRO
OLIVO CT
CANOGA PL
ADOLFO PARK
E BARCA
ACALA ST
HELMA ST
JULIA CT
ISLA CT
CORONA
STILES
ELMA
FARIA ST
GRACIA
KARENA CT
DARA
LORETA CT
CURT DR
MILLIGAN DR
DURKIN DR
ESTON
SHARON
LIB
SKATEPARK
PLEASANT VALLEY PK
LEXINGTON CT
MEADOW DR
STONE CT
OAKHURST
ARNEILL RANCH PARK
EXETER CT
VISTA CIR
TRUMAN ST
SHALIMAR
GEMINI CT
DUNNIGAN
BOGART
SATURN AV
BORDEAUX AV
CENTENNIAL AV
FIESTA
BOLLIN
PONDEROSA
PLEASANT HILL
WAVERLY
VIA MONTOYA
WALKER AV
MCCULLOCH ST
LEONARD ST
HARTNELL
DEER HUNTER LN
KEYSER
MID
PALMER
ASCOT
ARNEILL RD
KWICK DR
FS
FULTON
OBRIEN CIR
STAUNTON ST
GRAHAM AV
WALKER AV
BELDEN AV
MERRITT AV
KELLEY AV
KNIGHT RONDO
DUMETZ ST
PEOPLES AV
BARRY
GLENN DR
LOMITA
NELLORA
N DAWSON DR
VIA ALONDRA
LEWIS RD
VISTA MERCADO
AVENIDA
FLYNN RD
MAYA LINDA
VIA PESCADOR
CORTE MALPASO
CALLE TECATE
SEE A J2
1 PICADO DR
2 LA VETA DR
3 RAMA PL
4 YORBA LINDA PL
5 ESTANCIA PL
6 VILLA ADOBE
CAMARILLO RANCH RD
CAMINO RANCHERO
CAMARILLO RANCH
ADOLFO RD
VIA PRESIDIO
VIA BONITO
VIA DEL SOL
SANTO RD
CALLE TESORO
ACASO
PITTS RANCH PARK
ASSOCIATION FOR RETARDED CITIZENS–VENTURA CO
CALLE SUERTE
CALLEGUAS CREEK
CALLEGUAS CREEK PARK
DOMINGO
PASEO
MARAVILLA
CORTE VISTA
CALLE CANCUN
CAMINITO LUISA
VIA FRESCO
CAMINITO POSADA
CORTE TIARA
EL CORTIJO
GOLDENRIDGE DR
MEADOWRIDGE CT
FERNRIDGE CT
LYNNWOOD DR
PASO ROBLES CT
PASEO
CHULA VISTA
CUPERTINO
MONTELENA
CALLE MENDOTA
CREEKSIDE
COLONY DR
HILLCREST CIR
HUNT CIR
HACIENDA DR
BUENOS TIEMPOS
BLVD
LAUREL PARK
LOS PUEBLOS
LADERA VISTA
GALANO
OAKS
AGUA VERDE
VIA VALENCIA
OLIVERA
RANCHO
PLACITA
BUENA ROSA
EL CORAZON
EL CAPITAN
ANGUILA
ADOLFO CAMARILLO HS
SANTA ROSA RD
ADOLFO RD
VERDUGO WY
RUIZ
CAMINO
COURTYARD MARRIOTT
MISSION
PETIT VENTURA ST
VIA PALOMA
CALLE PARADORA
VIA LISBOA
VIA SINTRA
VIA MARISMA
VIA GABILAN
VIA ALGARVE
VIA VALVERDE
CALLE VIEJO
LA ROSA
FLORA VISTA AV
MILPAS ST
LEATHERWOOD CT
CUESTA
FRWY
101
PARK & RIDE
CHAPEL DR
DIZDAR PARK
ELM DR
PALM DR
GLENN DR
HOLLY DR
S DAWSON DR
ACACIA
MAGNOLIA ST
CAMARILLO ST
VILLAGE CT
IMATION DR
DAWSON PL
S LEWIS RD
CALLE SAN PABLO
DAWSON DR
36
CONSTITUTION AV
COMMONS
WESTPARK DR
CASTLETON
COTTAGES
WHITE ROCK
BRIDGEHAMPTON
PENZANCE AV
BUTTERCUP LN
CANOPY DR
SUMMERTON
RIVERDALE
BROOKSHIRE CT
TWILIGHT
TOWN
FOREST CT
THE
WICKFORD PL
BRIDGETON PARK
FOUNTAIN
GOLDEN
BRISTOL PARK CT
SYCAMORE CT
COTTAGE PL
DUSK DR
BREEZY
SPRING
GAZEBO
ARBOR
DAVENPORT
POND
HEDGE
BLOOMFIELD
ELM COTTAGE
WILLOW GLEN CT
TIVERTON DR
EAST PARK
CAMINO ROSAL
CALLE DE
VIA ROSAL
ESCORIAL
WOODSIDE PARK
STONETREE
FALLEN LEAF AV
PANCHO
APPLETREE AV
BENT TWIG AV
DEERHURST AV
RIDGE
VIEW
COTTAGE GROVE
PLEASANT VALLEY RD
ADOHR LN
34
PLEASANT VALLEY RD
T1N
LEWIS RD
CALLE ALTO
PLANO
CALLE CARGA
CALLE BOLERO
CALLE QUETZAL (HOWARD RD)
CAMARILLO SANITARY PLANT
SANITATION RD
HOWARD RD
RANCHO RD
PANCHO RD
93012
RANCHO CALLEGUAS
RANCHO GUADALASCA
CALLEGUAS
CONEJO
CREEK
1
12
25
30

SEE 525 MAP

SEE 554 MAP

0 .125 .25 .375 .5 miles 1 in. = 1900 ft.

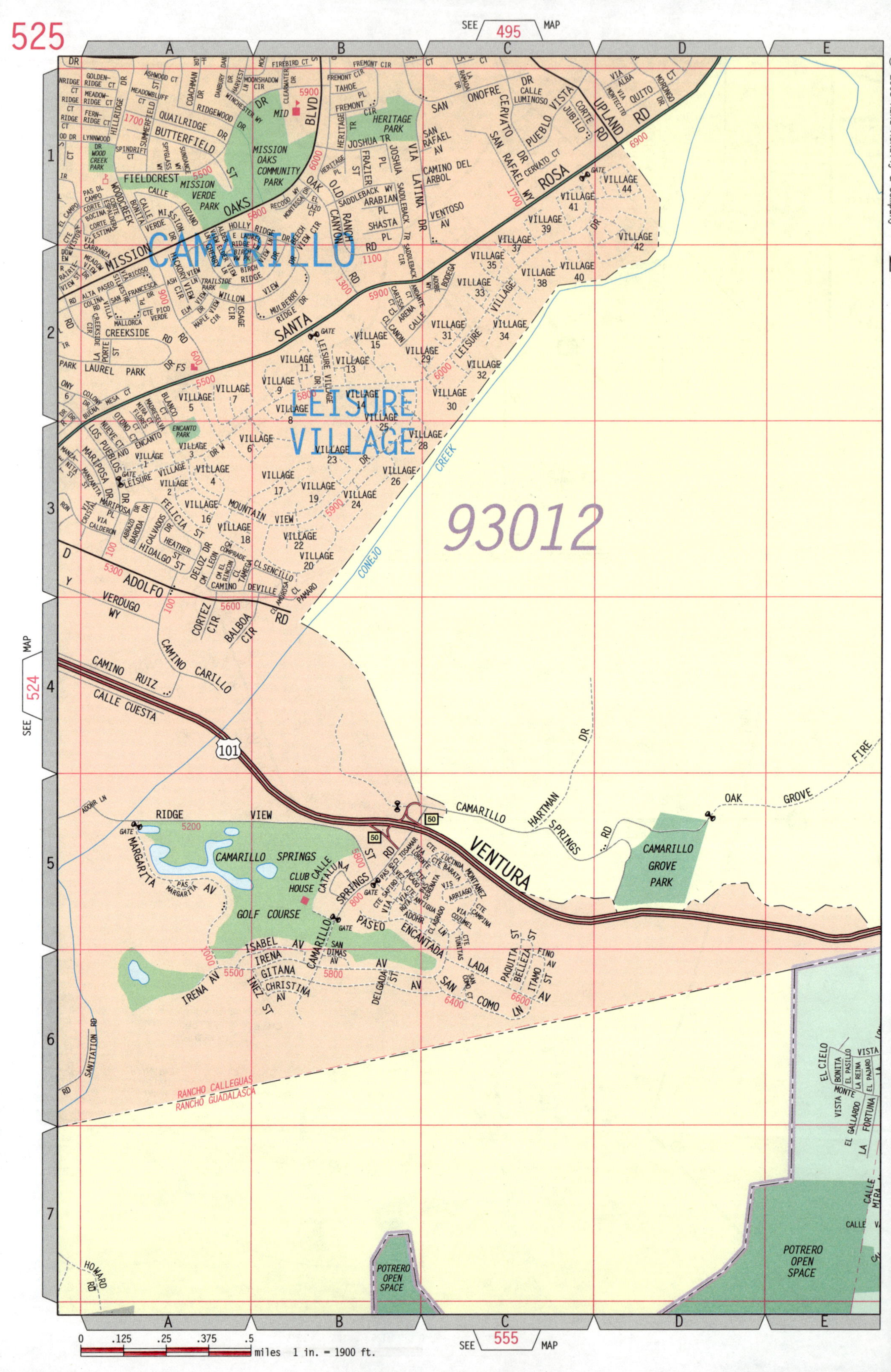
SEE 495 MAP
A
B
C
D
E
1
2
3
4
5
6
7
CAMARILLO
LEISURE VILLAGE
93012
MISSION OAKS
MISSION OAKS COMMUNITY PARK
MISSION VERDE PARK
HERITAGE PARK
WOOD CREEK PARK
ENCANTO PARK
SANTA ROSA RD
UPLAND RD
ADOLFO RD
VERDUGO WY
CAMINO RUIZ
CALLE CUESTA
CAMINO CARILLO
CONEJO CREEK
VENTURA
101
50
RIDGE VIEW
CAMARILLO SPRINGS RD
CAMARILLO SPRINGS GOLF COURSE
CLUB HOUSE
HARTMAN DR
OAK GROVE FIRE
CAMARILLO GROVE PARK
POTRERO OPEN SPACE
RANCHO CALLEGUAS
RANCHO GUADALASCA
SANITATION RD
HOWARD RD
SEE 524 MAP
SEE 555 MAP
0 .125 .25 .375 .5 miles 1 in. = 1900 ft.

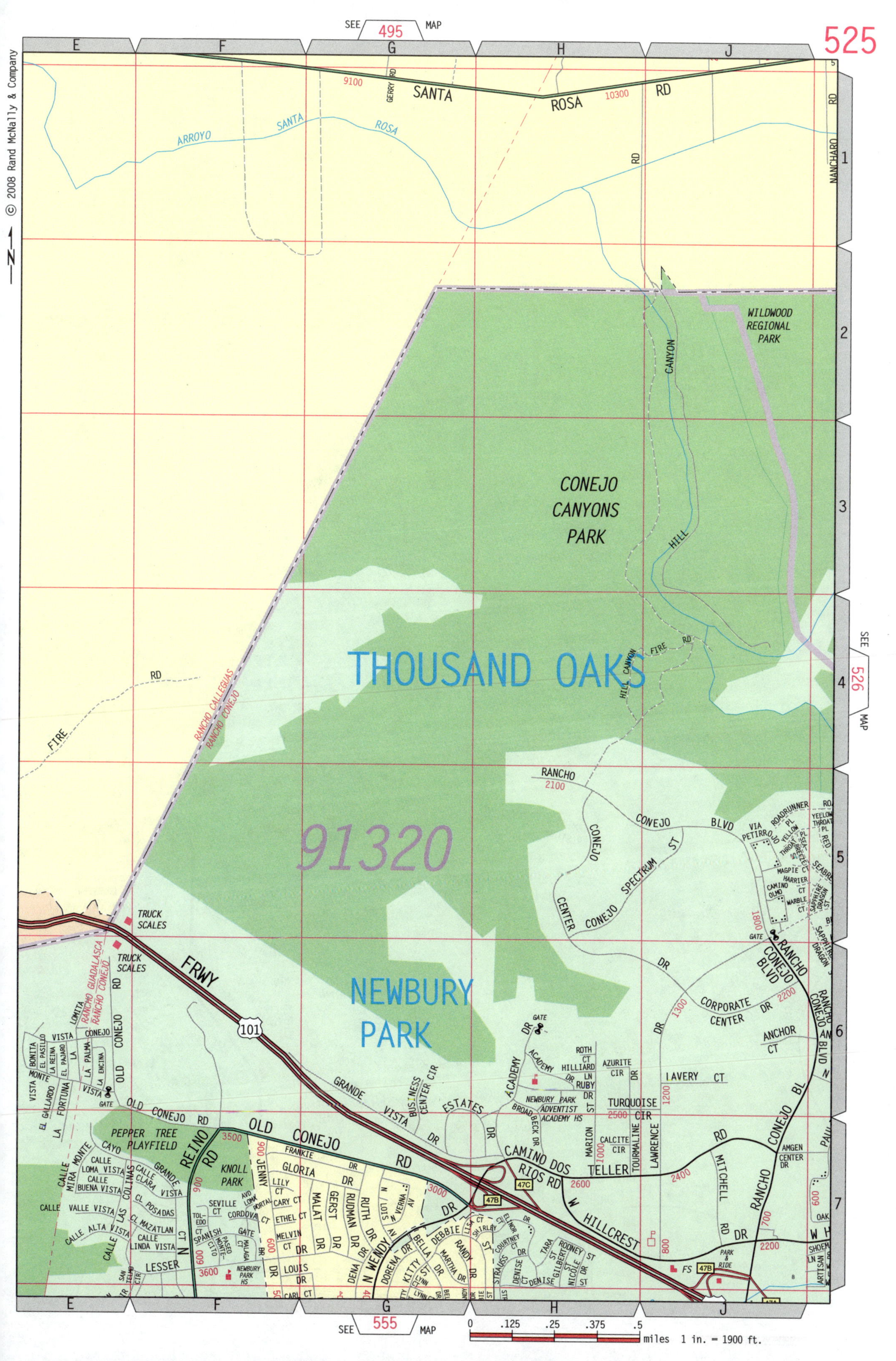
SEE 495 MAP
SANTA ROSA RD
ARROYO SANTA ROSA
WILDWOOD REGIONAL PARK
CONEJO CANYONS PARK
THOUSAND OAKS
91320
NEWBURY PARK
HILL CANYON FIRE RD
RANCHO CONEJO BLVD
CONEJO SPECTRUM ST
CONEJO CENTER DR
CORPORATE CENTER DR
TRUCK SCALES
FRWY
101
OLD CONEJO RD
PEPPER TREE PLAYFIELD
KNOLL PARK
REINO RD
CAMINO DOS RIOS
W HILLCREST DR
TELLER RD
GRANDE VISTA DR
NEWBURY PARK ADVENTIST ACADEMY HS
NEWBURY PARK HS
SEE 526 MAP
SEE 555 MAP
miles 1 in. = 1900 ft.

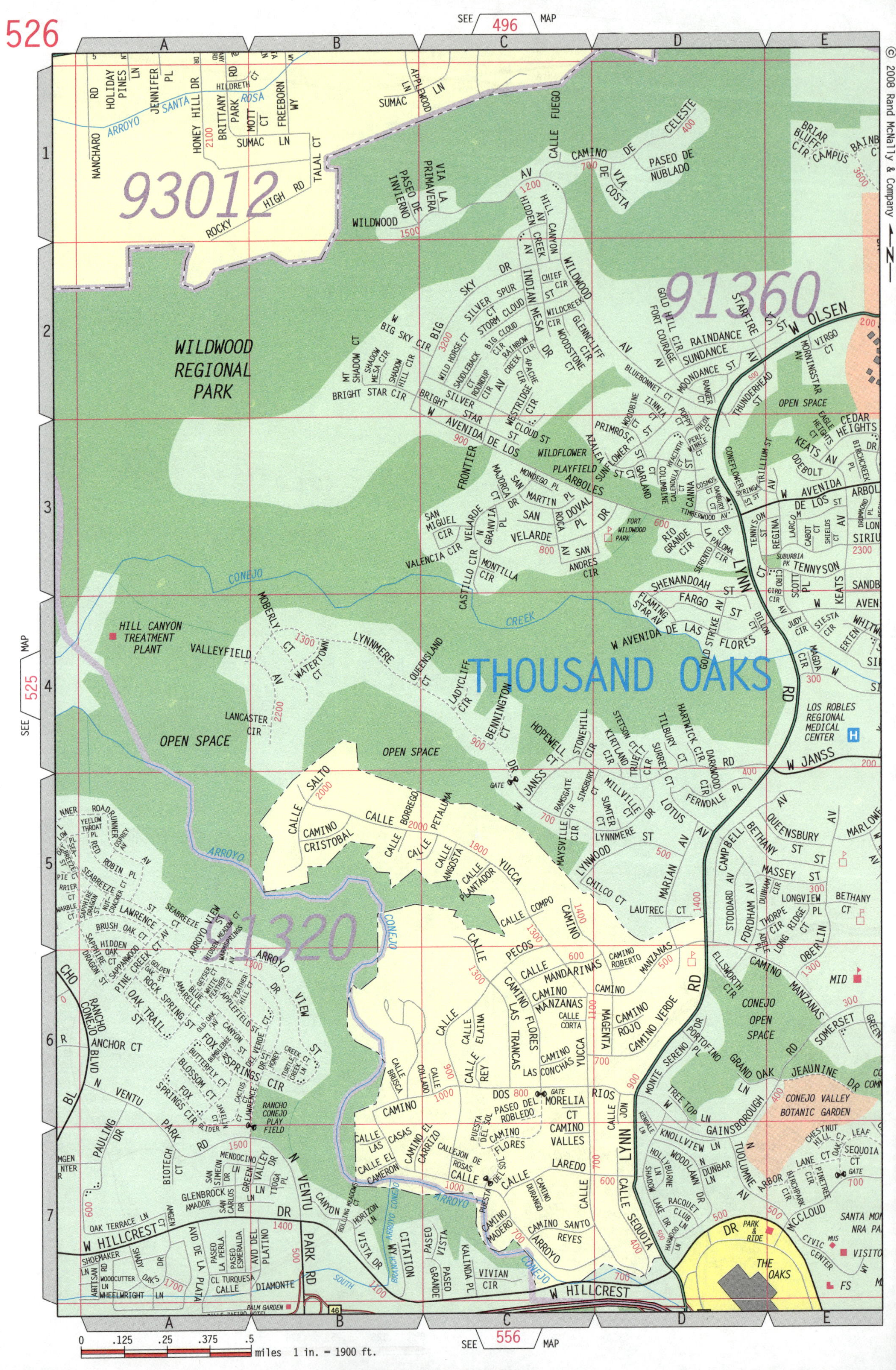

SEE 496 MAP
SEE 525 MAP
SEE 556 MAP
© 2008 Rand McNally & Company
A
B
C
D
E
1
2
3
4
5
6
7
93012
91360
91320
THOUSAND OAKS
WILDWOOD REGIONAL PARK
OPEN SPACE
HILL CANYON TREATMENT PLANT
LOS ROBLES REGIONAL MEDICAL CENTER
CONEJO OPEN SPACE
CONEJO VALLEY BOTANIC GARDEN
RANCHO CONEJO PLAY FIELD
FORT WILDWOOD PARK
THE OAKS
PARK & RIDE
SANTA MONICA NRA PA
ARROYO SANTA ROSA
CONEJO CREEK
ARROYO CONEJO
SOUTH BRANCH ARROYO CONEJO
W OLSEN RD
LYNN RD
W JANSS RD
W HILLCREST DR
W AVENIDA DE LOS ARBOLES
W AVENIDA DE LAS FLORES
N VENTU PARK RD
RANCHO CONEJO BLVD
CAMINO DOS RIOS
MOORPARK RD
VALLEYFIELD AV
LYNNMERE DR
CALLE YUCCA
MANZANAS
HOLIDAY PINES LN
JENNIFER PL
HONEY HILL DR
BRITTANY PARK RD
SUMAC LN
TALAL CT
ROCKY HIGH RD
NANCHARO RD
APPLEWOOD LN
SUMAC LN
WILDWOOD AV
CALLE FUEGO
PASEO DE NUBLADO
VIA DE COSTA
CELESTE
HILL CANYON AV
BIG SKY DR
SILVER SPUR CT
BRIGHT STAR CIR
MT SHADOW CT
FRONTIER
SAN MIGUEL CIR
VELARDE
VALENCIA CIR
MONTILLA CIR
CASTILLO CIR
SAN ANDRES CIR
RIO GRANDE CIR
SHENANDOAH ST
FARGO ST
GOLD STRIKE AV
MOBERLY CT
WATERTOWN CT
QUEENSLAND CT
LADYCLIFF CIR
BENNINGTON CT
LANCASTER CIR
HOPEWELL CT
STONEHILL CIR
KIRTLAND CIR
TILBURY CT
HARTWICK CIR
DARKWOOD CIR
FERNDALE PL
LOTUS AV
MARIAN AV
LAUTREC CT
CHILCO CT
LYNWOOD ST
CALLE SALTO
CAMINO CRISTOBAL
CALLE BORREGO
CALLE PETALUMA
CALLE ANGOSTA
CALLE PLANTADOR
CALLE COMPO
CALLE PECOS
CAMINO MANZANAS
CAMINO ROJO
CAMINO VERDE
CAMINO MORELIA
CAMINO VALLES
LAREDO
CALLE SEQUOIA
CAMINO SANTO REYES
CAMINO ARROYO
CAMINO MADERO
VIVIAN CIR
KALINDA PL
PASEO GRANDE
PASEO VISTA
CITATION
VISTA DR
HORIZON LN
OAK TERRACE LN
SHOEMAKER
WOODCUTTER LN
WHEELWRIGHT LN
AVD DE LA PLATA
PASEO LA PERLA
PASEO ESMERALDA
AVD DEL PLATINO
CL TURQUESA
CALLE DIAMONTE
PALM GARDEN HOTEL
PAULING DR
BIOTECH CT
GLENBROCK
MENDOCINO
TIOGA PL
FOX SPRINGS CIR
ANCHOR CT
OAK TRAIL ST
ARROYO VIEW DR
SEABREEZE CT
LAWRENCE ST
BRUSH OAK CT
ROBIN PL
MONTE SERENO
PORTOFINO PL
GRAND OAK LN
JEAUNINE DR
TREE TOP LN
GAINSBOROUGH
KNOLLVIEW LN
WOODLAWN DR
DUNBAR LN
TUOLUMNE AV
RACQUET CLUB LN
ARBOR LN
MCCLOUD
CHESTNUT HILL CT
SEQUOIA CT
CIVIC CENTER
QUEENSBURY ST
BETHANY ST
MASSEY ST
LONGVIEW PL
OBERLIN
STODDARD AV
FORDHAM AV
ELLSWORTH CIR
CAMPBELL
SOMERSET
TENNYSON ST
KEATS AV
MAGDA CIR
SIESTA CIR
JUDY CIR
CEDAR HEIGHTS
VIRGO CT
MORNINGSTAR AV
THUNDERHEAD ST
STARFIRE ST
RAINDANCE ST
SUNDANCE
MOONDANCE ST
GOLD HILL CIR
FORT COURAGE AV
BLUEBONNET CT
BRIAR BLUFF CIR
CAMPUS
MID
FS

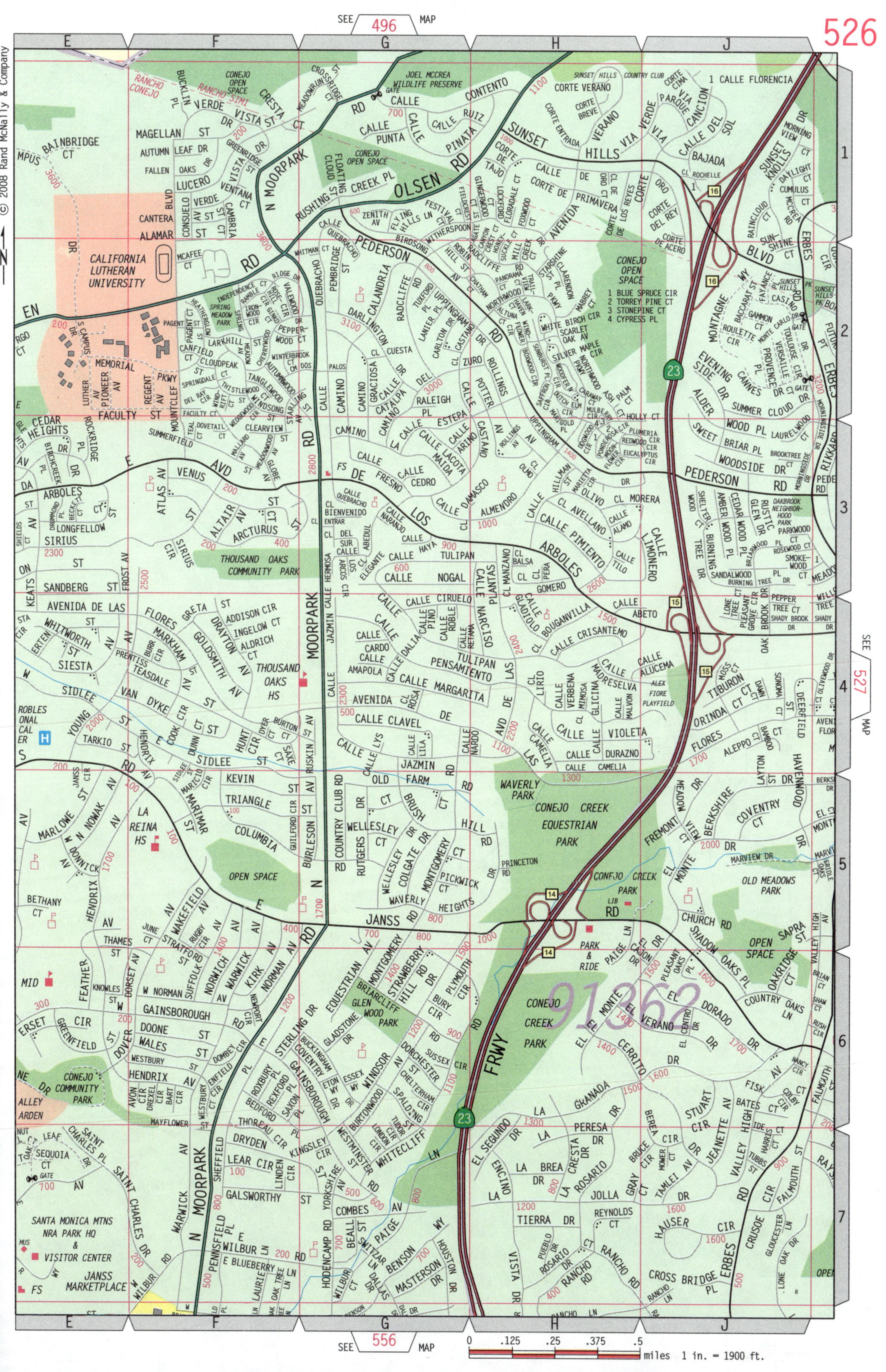
SEE 496 MAP
SEE 556 MAP
SEE 527 MAP
E
F
G
H
J
1
2
3
4
5
6
7
CALIFORNIA LUTHERAN UNIVERSITY
MEMORIAL PKWY
JOEL MCCREA WILDLIFE PRESERVE
CONEJO OPEN SPACE
SUNSET HILLS COUNTRY CLUB
OLSEN RD
N MOORPARK RD
PEDERSON RD
SUNSET HILLS BLVD
AVD DE LOS ARBOLES
THOUSAND OAKS COMMUNITY PARK
THOUSAND OAKS HS
ALEX FIORE PLAYFIELD
SIDLEE ST
JANSS RD
LA REINA HS
OPEN SPACE
WAVERLY PARK
CONEJO CREEK EQUESTRIAN PARK
CONEJO CREEK PARK
OLD MEADOWS PARK
GLEN WOOD PARK
CONEJO COMMUNITY PARK
PARK & RIDE
FRWY
91362
SANTA MONICA MTNS NRA PARK HQ & VISITOR CENTER
JANSS MARKETPLACE
HAUSER CIR
ERBES RD
RANCHO RD
CROSS BRIDGE PL
TIERRA DR
VISTA DR
LA BREA DR
EL SEGUNDO DR
1 BLUE SPRUCE CIR
2 TORREY PINE CT
3 STONEPINE CT
4 CYPRESS PL
1 CALLE FLORENCIA
0 .125 .25 .375 .5
miles 1 in. = 1900 ft.

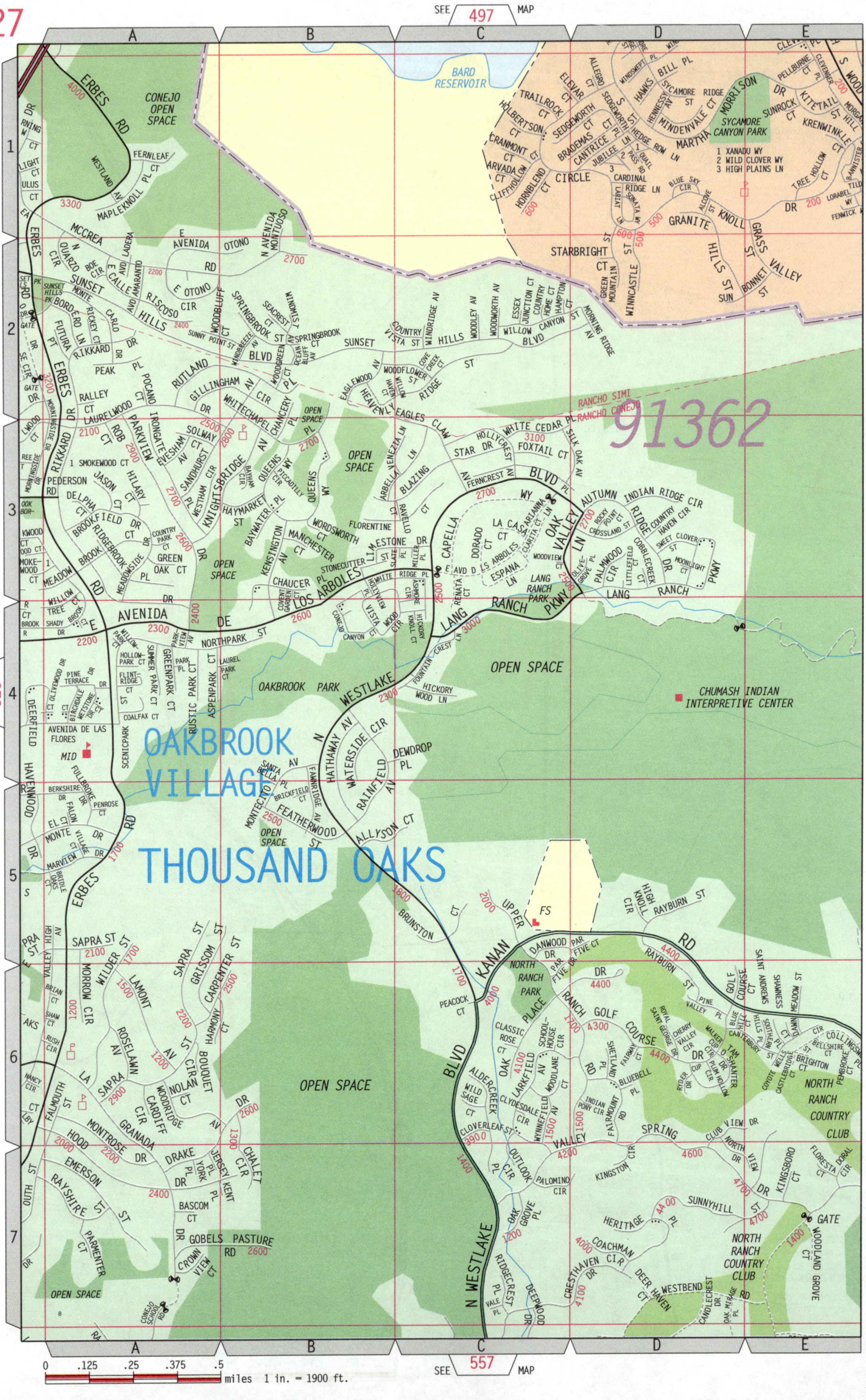

SEE 497 MAP

A B C D E

1 2 3 4 5 6 7

CONEJO OPEN SPACE

BARD RESERVOIR

SYCAMORE CANYON PARK

1 XANADU WY
2 WILD CLOVER WY
3 HIGH PLAINS LN

91362

RANCHO SIMI
RANCHO CONEJO

OPEN SPACE

OAKBROOK PARK

OAKBROOK VILLAGE

THOUSAND OAKS

CHUMASH INDIAN INTERPRETIVE CENTER

LANG RANCH PARK

NORTH RANCH PARK

NORTH RANCH COUNTRY CLUB

FS

MID

1 SMOKEWOOD CT

ERBES RD
MAPLEKNOLL PL
FERNLEAF CT
WESTLAND AV
MCCREA
AVENIDA OTONO
N AVENIDA MONTUOSO
SUNSET HILLS BLVD
E CALLE RISCOSO
RIKKARD DR
RALLEY CT
LAURELWOOD
ROB CT
PARKVIEW
HILARY
RUTLAND
GILLINGHAM AV
WHITECHAPEL CIR
CHANCERY PL
KNIGHTSBRIDGE AV
QUEENS WY
HAYMARKET ST
BAYWATER PL
KENSINGTON AV
MANCHESTER
WORDSWORTH
CHAUCER PL
LOS ARBOLES
FLORENTINE
LIMESTONE DR
CAPELLA
HEAVENLY
EAGLES CLAW
STAR DR
HOLLYCREST
FOXTAIL CT
WHITE CEDAR PL
SILK OAK AV
OAK VALLEY LN
AUTUMN RIDGE
INDIAN RIDGE CIR
COUNTRY HAVEN CIR
LANG RANCH PKWY
AVENIDA DE LAS FLORES
NORTHPARK ST
N WESTLAKE BLVD
HICKORY WOOD LN
HATHAWAY AV
WATERSIDE CIR
DEWDROP PL
RAINFIELD AV
ALLYSON CT
FEATHERWOOD ST
BRUNSTON CT
UPPER
KANAN RD
RAYBURN ST
HIGH KNOLL CIR
DANWOOD PAR
FIVE CT
RANCH PLACE
GOLF COURSE DR
SPRING VALLEY
CLUB VIEW DR
KINGSTON CIR
PALOMINO CIR
SUNNYHILL ST
HERITAGE PL
COACHMAN CIR
CRESTHAVEN DR
DEER HAVEN CT
WESTBEND RD
RIDGECREST
DEEPWOOD DR
OAK GROVE PL
WOODLAND GROVE CT
KINGSBORO CT
GATE
SAPRA ST
WILDER
LAMONT
ROSELAWN AV
MORROW CIR
GRISSOM ST
CARPENTER ST
HARMONY CT
BOUQUET CIR
NOLAN CT
CARDIFF CIR
WOODRIDGE AV
GRANADA DR
MONTROSE
HOOD
DRAKE
YORK PL
JERSEY KENT PL
CHALET CIR
EMERSON
RAYSHIRE ST
PARMENTER CT
BASCOM CT
GOBELS PASTURE RD
CROWN VIEW CT
TRAILROCK CT
ELEVAR
HOLBERTSON
CRANMONT CT
HORNBLEND CT
CIRCLE
SEDGEWORTH
BRADEMAS CT
HAWKS BILL PL
MINDENVALE CT
MARTHA MORRISON DR
SUNROCK CT
KITE TAIL
KRENWINKLE CT
TREE HOLLOW CT
GRANITE HILLS ST
KNOLL
GRASS VALLEY
STARBRIGHT CT
GREEN MOUNTAIN
WINNCASTLE ST
BONNET ST
SUN

SEE 557 MAP

SEE 526 MAP

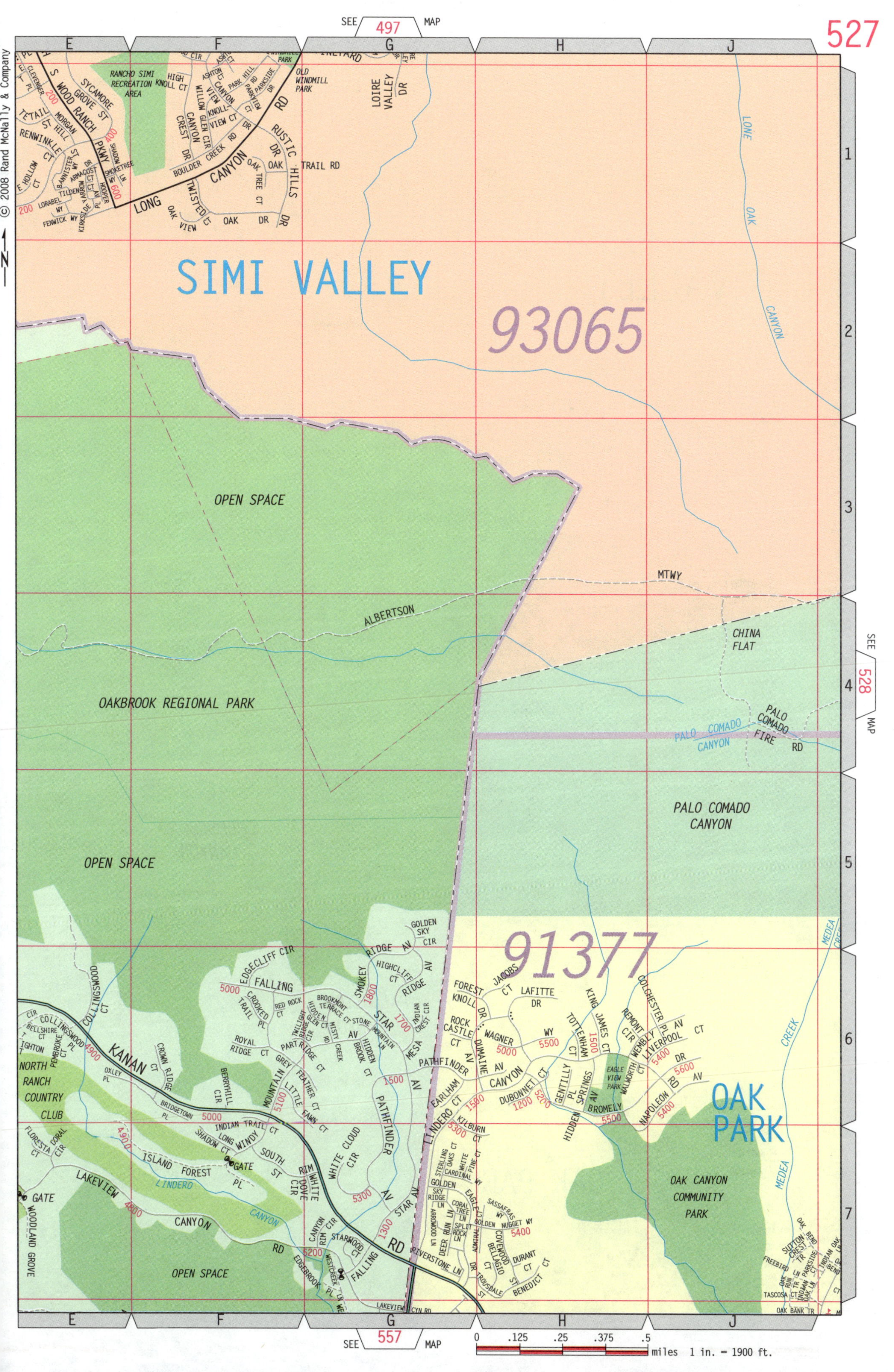
SEE 497 MAP
SEE 528 MAP
SEE 557 MAP
SIMI VALLEY
93065
91377
OAK PARK
OPEN SPACE
OAKBROOK REGIONAL PARK
PALO COMADO CANYON
CHINA FLAT
OAK CANYON COMMUNITY PARK
NORTH RANCH COUNTRY CLUB
RANCHO SIMI RECREATION AREA
OLD WINDMILL PARK
LONG CANYON RD
KANAN RD
LINDERO CANYON RD
ALBERTSON MTWY
PALO COMADO FIRE RD
LONE OAK CANYON
MEDEA CREEK
LINDERO CANYON
LAKEVIEW CANYON RD
PATHFINDER AV
RUSTIC HILLS DR
OAK TRAIL RD
LOIRE VALLEY DR
S WOOD RANCH PKWY
0 .125 .25 .375 .5 miles 1 in. = 1900 ft.

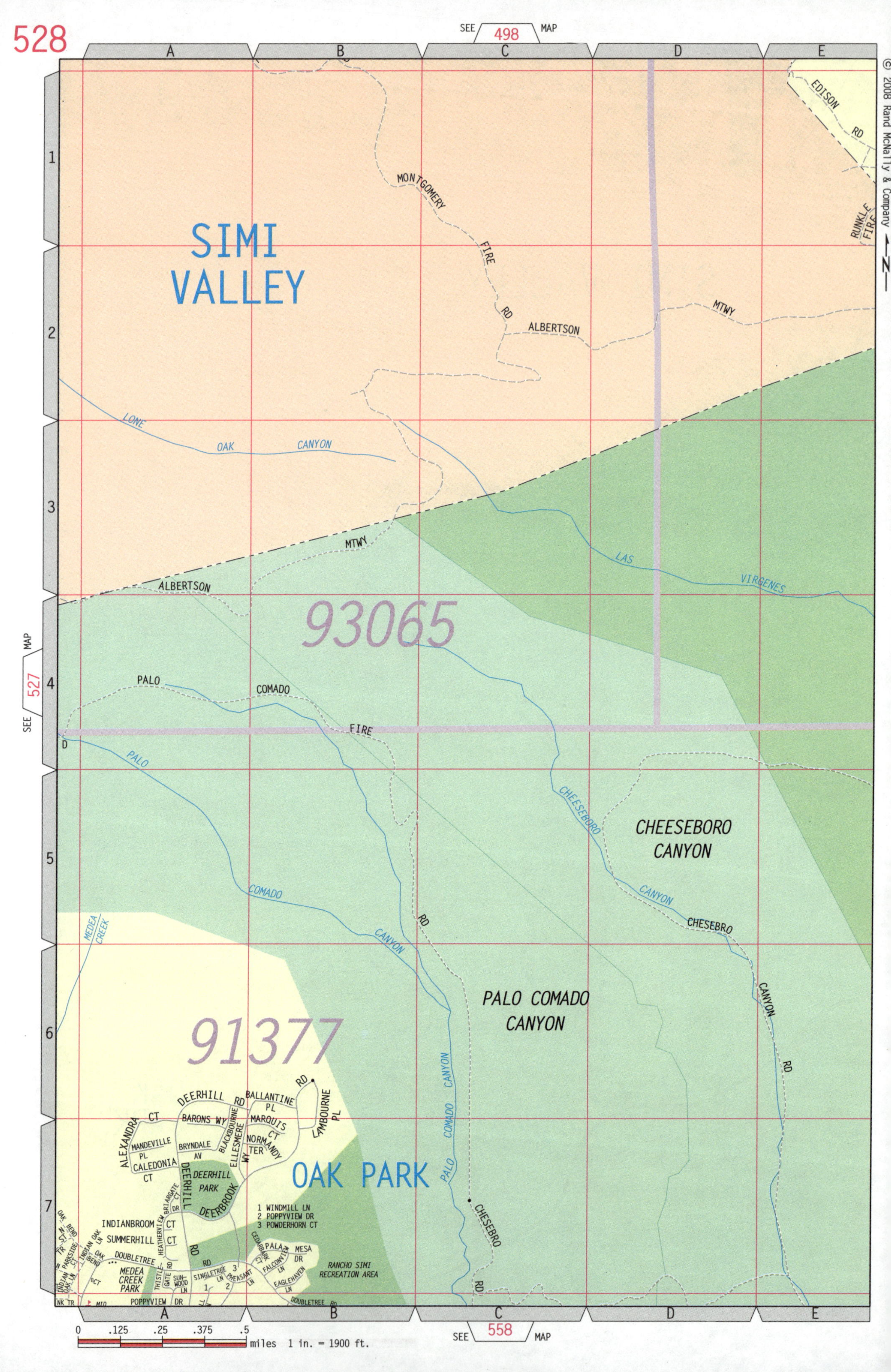
SEE 498 MAP
SEE 527 MAP
SEE 558 MAP
SIMI VALLEY
93065
91377
OAK PARK
CHEESEBORO CANYON
PALO COMADO CANYON
RANCHO SIMI RECREATION AREA
DEERHILL PARK
MEDEA CREEK PARK
MONTGOMERY FIRE RD
ALBERTSON MTWY
EDISON RD
RUNKLE FIRE
LONE OAK CANYON
LAS VIRGENES
PALO COMADO FIRE RD
PALO COMADO CANYON
CHEESEBORO CANYON
CHESEBRO CANYON RD
CHESEBRO RD
MEDEA CREEK
1 WINDMILL LN
2 POPPYVIEW DR
3 POWDERHORN CT
0 .125 .25 .375 .5 miles 1 in. = 1900 ft.

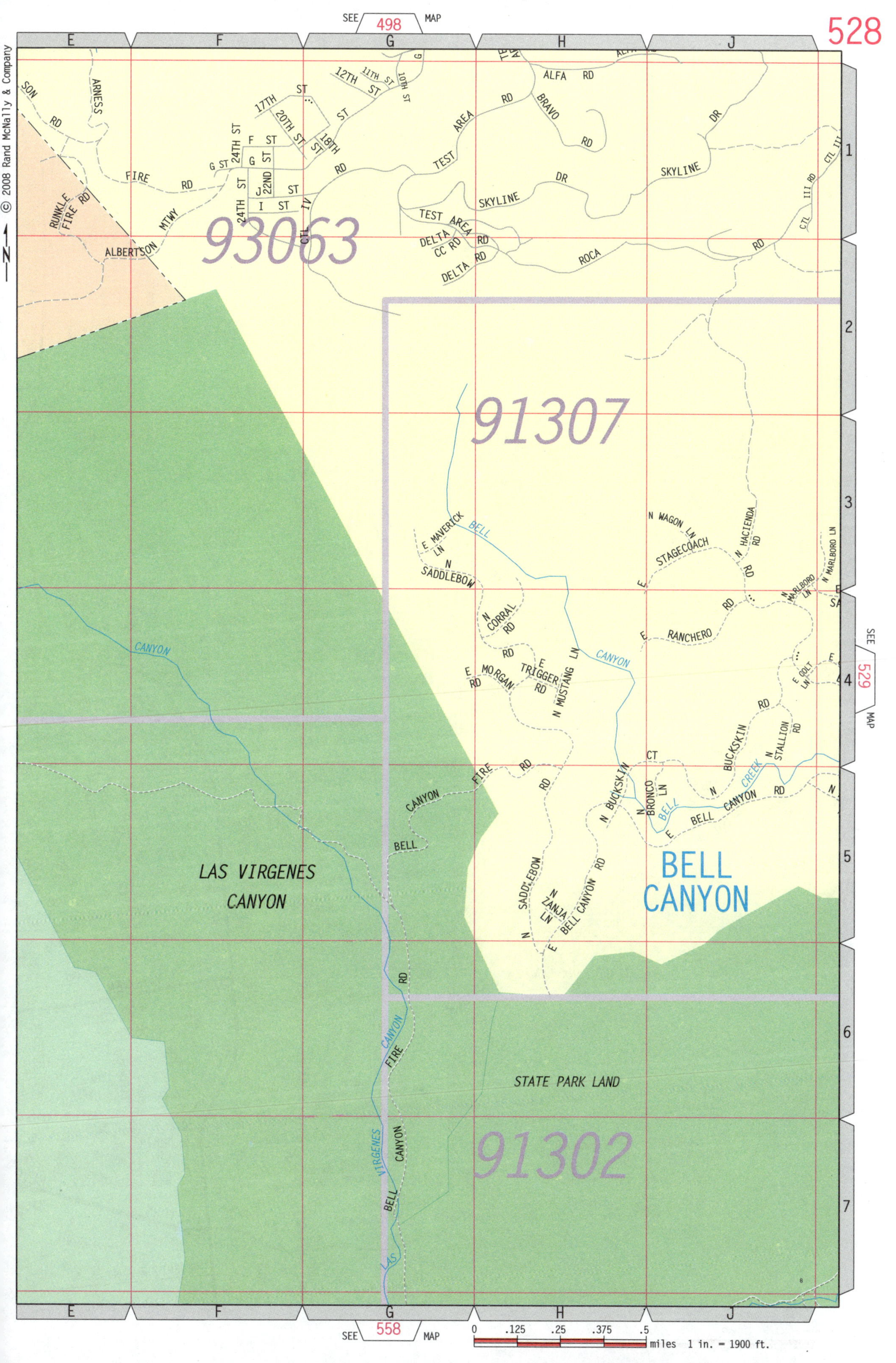

SEE 498 MAP
93063
91307
91302
BELL CANYON
LAS VIRGENES CANYON
STATE PARK LAND
SKYLINE DR
ALFA RD
BRAVO RD
TEST AREA RD
FIRE RD
ALBERTSON MTWY
RUNKLE FIRE RD
DELTA RD
CC RD
ROCA RD
CTL III RD
N WAGON LN
STAGECOACH
N HACIENDA RD
E MAVERICK LN
N SADDLEBOW
N CORRAL RD
E MORGAN RD
E TRIGGER RD
N MUSTANG LN
E RANCHERO RD
N MARLBORO LN
E COLT LN
N BUCKSKIN RD
N STALLION RD
N BUCKSKIN CT
N BRONCO LN
BELL CREEK
E BELL CANYON RD
N ZANJA LN
E BELL CANYON RD
BELL CANYON FIRE RD
LAS VIRGENES CANYON
SEE 529 MAP
SEE 558 MAP
0 .125 .25 .375 .5 miles 1 in. = 1900 ft.

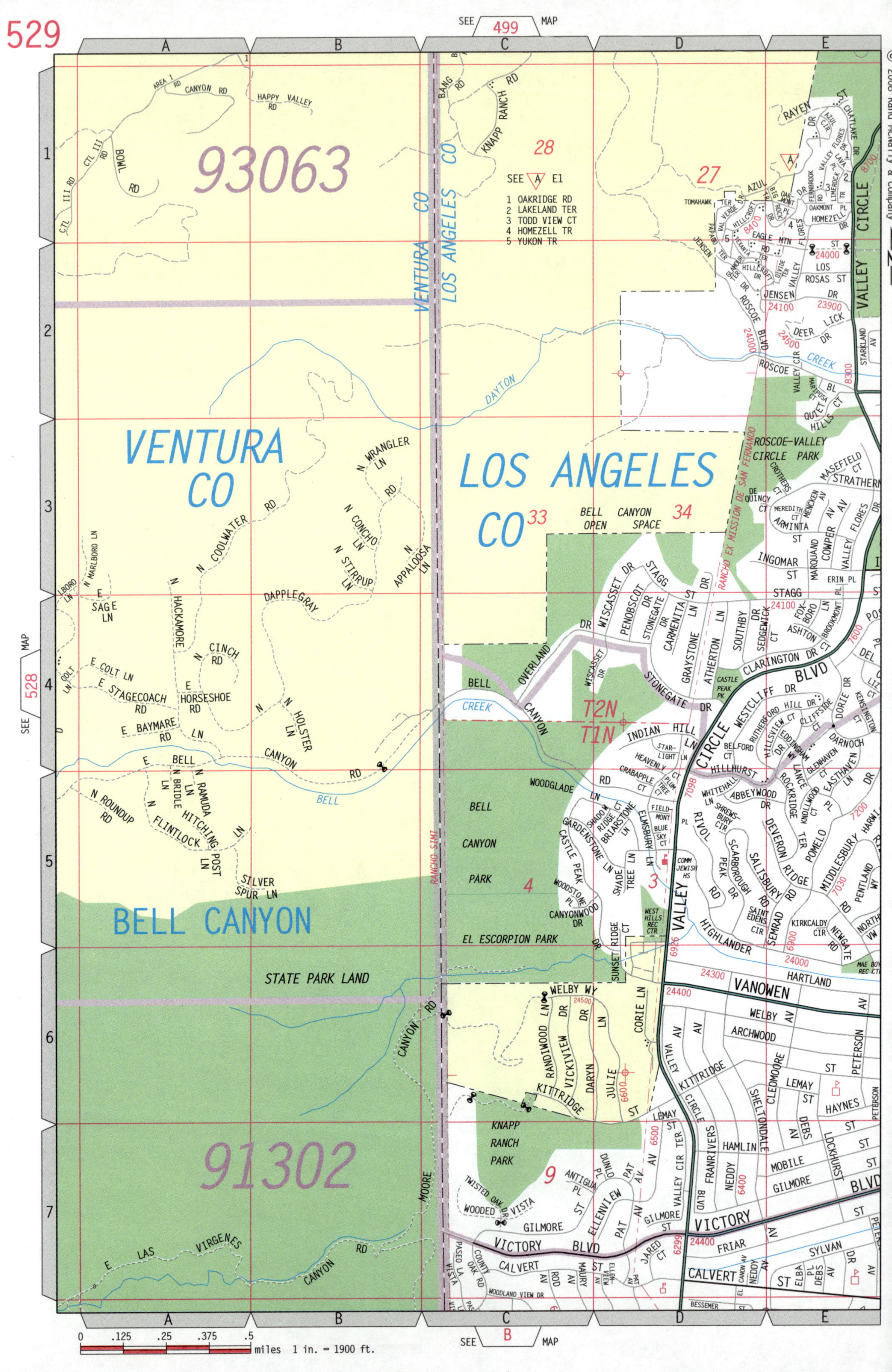
93063
VENTURA CO
LOS ANGELES CO
BELL CANYON
91302
SEE 499 MAP
SEE 528 MAP
SEE B MAP
SEE A E1
1 OAKRIDGE RD
2 LAKELAND TER
3 TODD VIEW CT
4 HOMEZELL TR
5 YUKON TR
ROSCOE-VALLEY CIRCLE PARK
BELL CANYON OPEN SPACE
BELL CANYON PARK
EL ESCORPION PARK
STATE PARK LAND
KNAPP RANCH PARK
VALLEY CIRCLE BLVD
VICTORY BLVD
VANOWEN
ROSCOE BLVD
T2N
T1N
0 .125 .25 .375 .5 miles 1 in. = 1900 ft.
© 2008 Rand McNally & Company

SEE 499 MAP

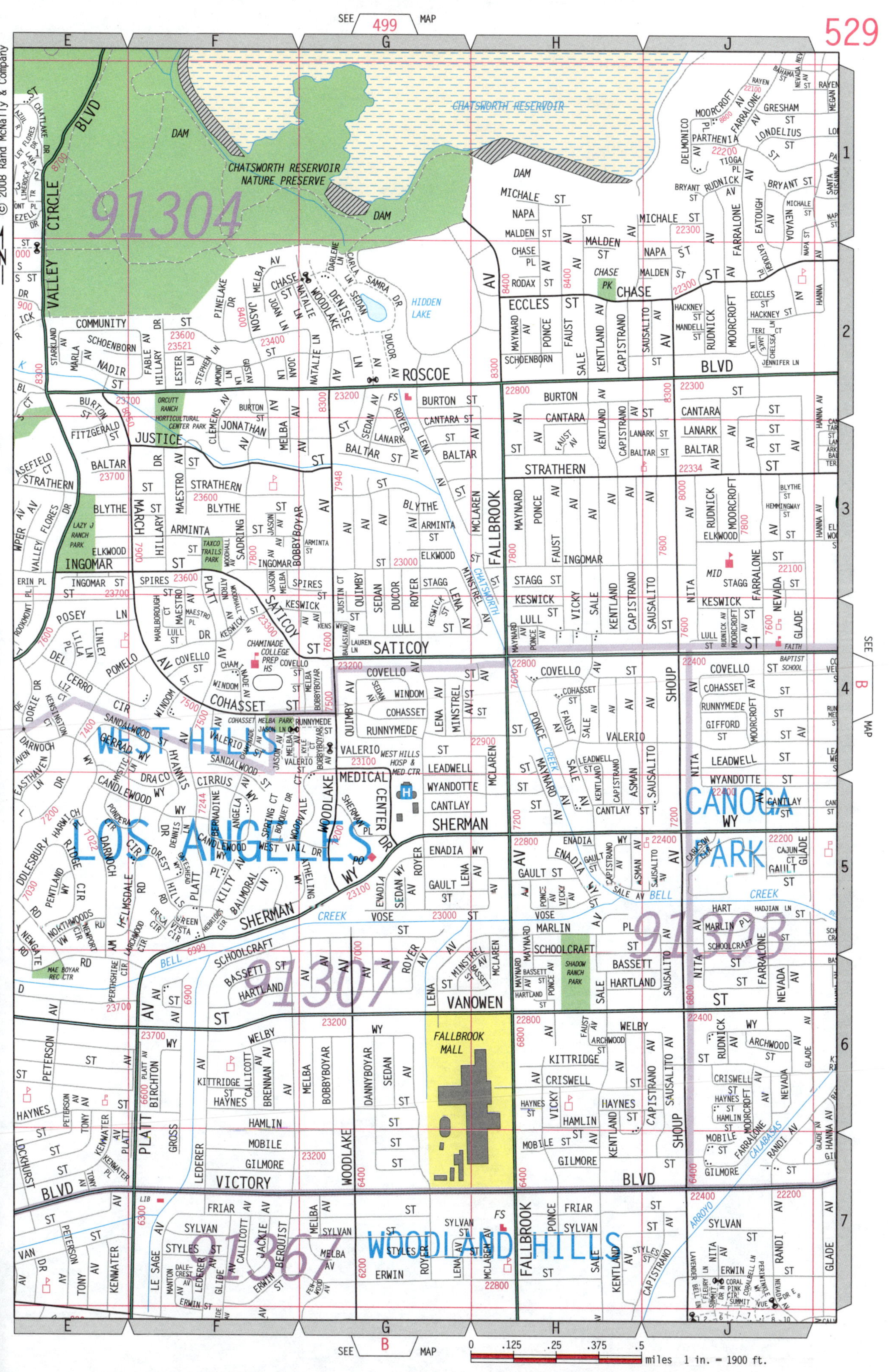
E
F
G
H
J
1
2
3
4
5
6
7
CHATSWORTH RESERVOIR
CHATSWORTH RESERVOIR NATURE PRESERVE
DAM
91304
VALLEY CIRCLE BLVD
HIDDEN LAKE
ROSCOE BLVD
ORCUTT RANCH HORTICULTURAL CENTER PARK
CHASE PK
LAZY J RANCH PARK
TAXCO TRAILS PARK
CHAMINADE COLLEGE PREP HS
SATICOY ST
FALLBROOK AV
SHERMAN WY
WEST HILLS
WEST HILLS HOSP & MED CTR
LOS ANGELES
CANOGA PARK
BELL CREEK
91303
91307
SHADOW RANCH PARK
MAE BOYAR REC CTR
VANOWEN ST
FALLBROOK MALL
VICTORY BLVD
91367
WOODLAND HILLS
ARROYO CALABASAS
SHOUP AV
TOPANGA CANYON
MID STAGG
FAITH BAPTIST SCHOOL

SEE B MAP

SEE B MAP

0 .125 .25 .375 .5 miles 1 in. = 1900 ft.

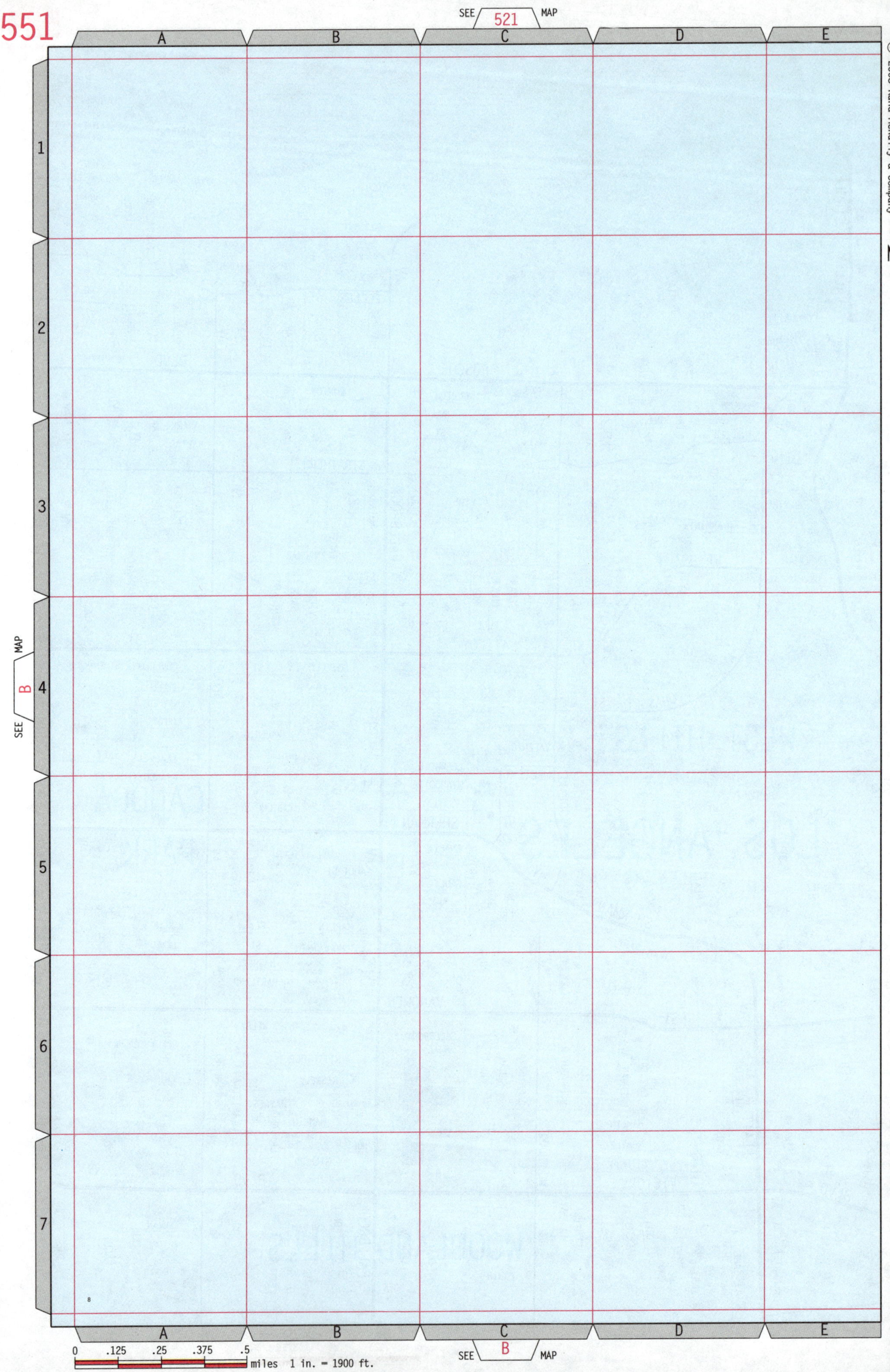
SEE 521 MAP
A
B
C
D
E
1
2
3
4
5
6
7
SEE B MAP
SEE B MAP
0 .125 .25 .375 .5
miles 1 in. = 1900 ft.

SEE 521 MAP

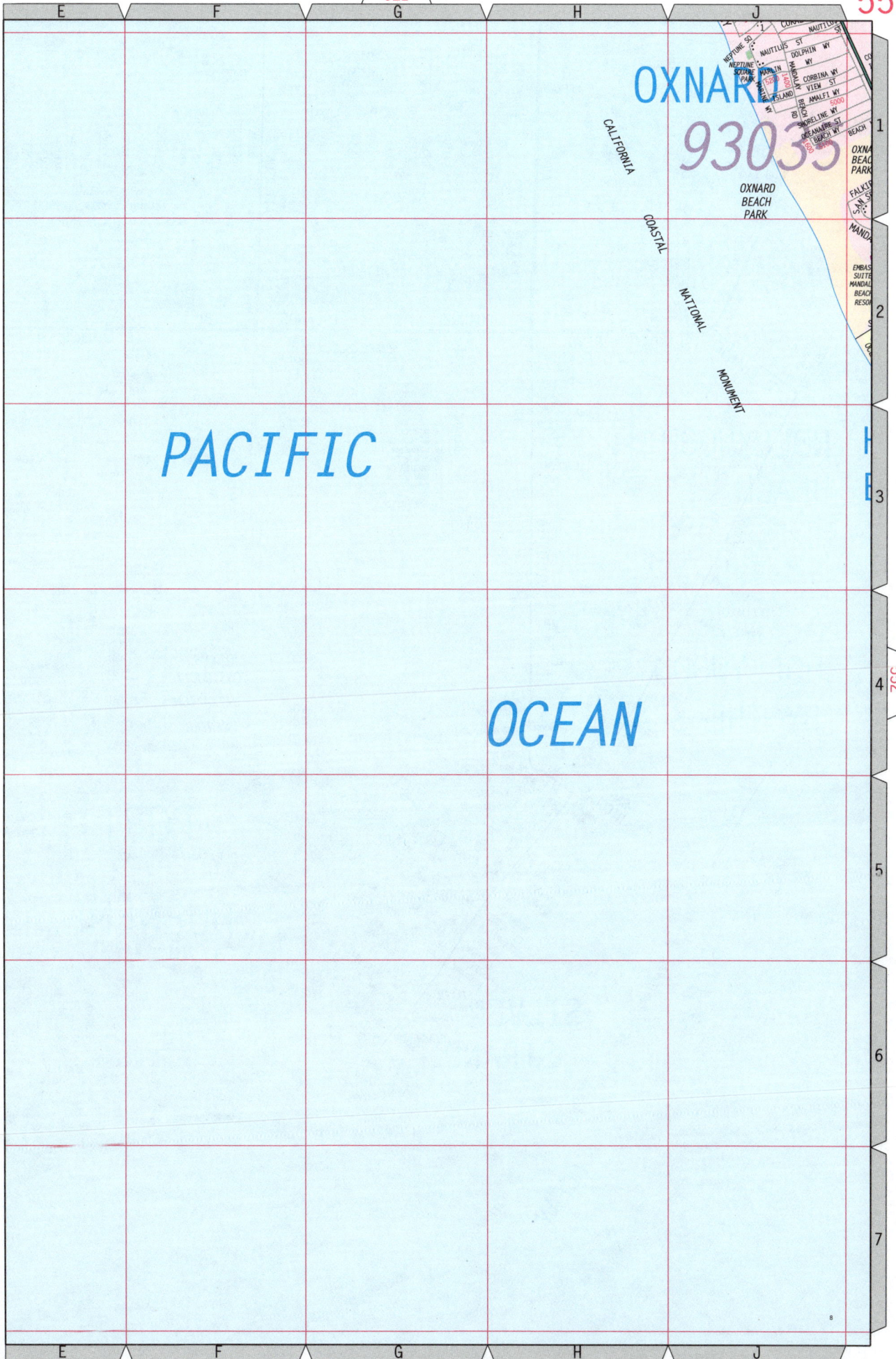

E F G H J

OXNARD

93035

CALIFORNIA COASTAL NATIONAL MONUMENT

OXNARD BEACH PARK

NEPTUNE SQUARE PARK

NAUTILUS ST

DOLPHIN WY

MARLIN WY

CORBINA WY

VIEW ST

AMALFI WY

ISLAND

MANDALAY BEACH RD

SHORELINE WY

OCEANAIRE ST

BEACH WY

PACIFIC OCEAN

1 2 3 4 5 6 7

SEE 552 MAP

SEE B MAP

0 .125 .25 .375 .5 miles 1 in. = 1900 ft.

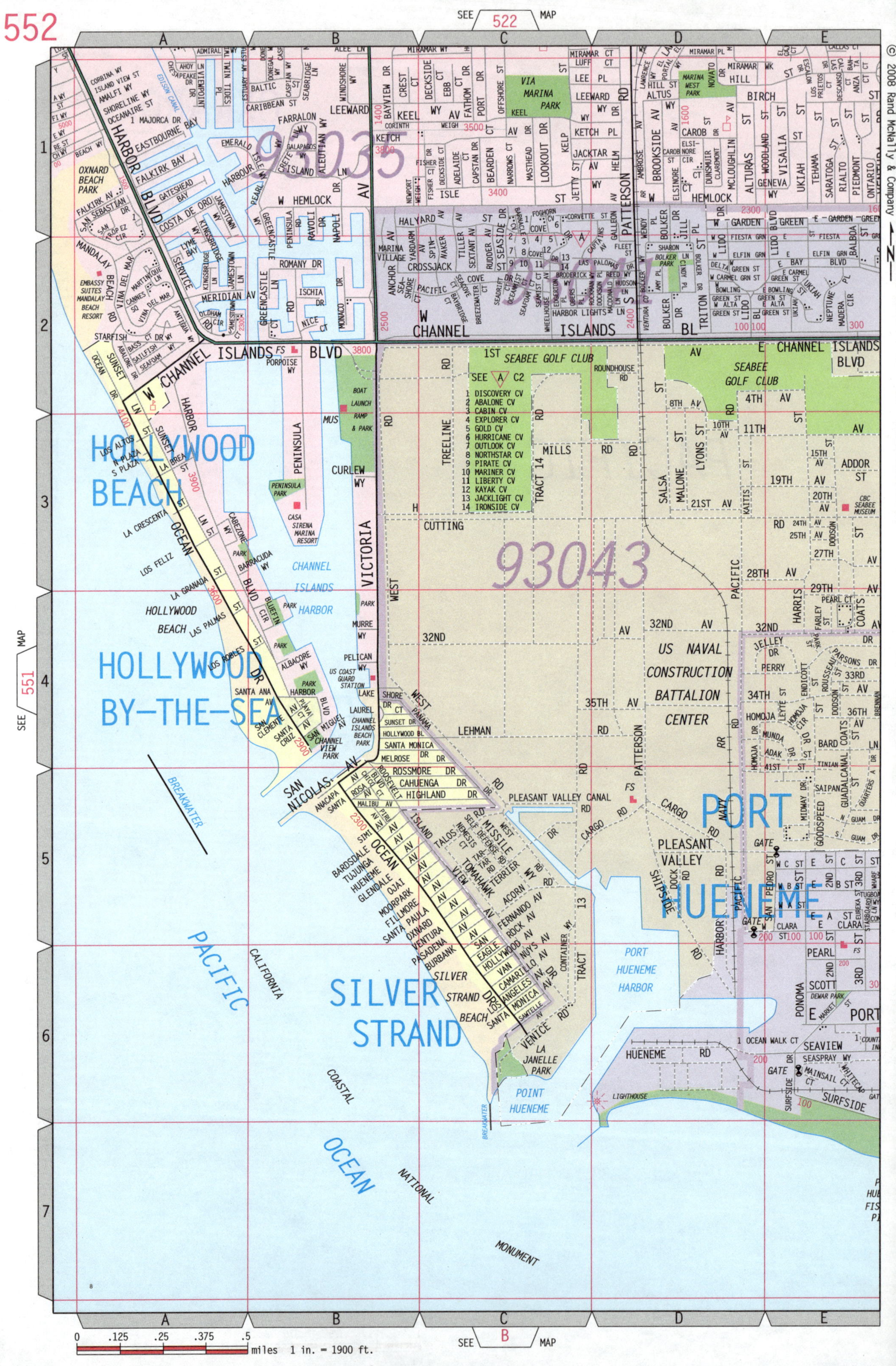

SEE 522 MAP
SEE 551 MAP
SEE B MAP
© 2008 Rand McNally & Company
93035
93041
93043
HOLLYWOOD BEACH
HOLLYWOOD BY-THE-SEA
SILVER STRAND
PORT HUENEME
OXNARD BEACH PARK
EMBASSY SUITES MANDALAY BEACH RESORT
CHANNEL ISLANDS HARBOR
PENINSULA PARK
CASA SIRENA MARINA RESORT
BOAT LAUNCH RAMP & PARK
US COAST GUARD STATION
CHANNEL ISLANDS BEACH PARK
CHANNEL VIEW PARK
VIA MARINA PARK
MARINA WEST PARK
BOLKER PARK
SEABEE GOLF CLUB
CBC SEABEE MUSEUM
US NAVAL CONSTRUCTION BATTALION CENTER
PLEASANT VALLEY CANAL
PORT HUENEME HARBOR
POINT HUENEME
LA JANELLE PARK
LIGHTHOUSE
BREAKWATER
PACIFIC OCEAN
CALIFORNIA COASTAL NATIONAL MONUMENT
HARBOR BLVD
W CHANNEL ISLANDS BLVD
E CHANNEL ISLANDS BLVD
VICTORIA AV
PATTERSON RD
OCEAN DR
HUENEME RD
SURFSIDE DR
PLEASANT VALLEY RD
SEE A C2
1 DISCOVERY CV
2 ABALONE CV
3 CABIN CV
4 EXPLORER CV
5 GOLD CV
6 HURRICANE CV
7 OUTLOOK CV
8 NORTHSTAR CV
9 PIRATE CV
10 MARINER CV
11 LIBERTY CV
12 KAYAK CV
13 JACKLIGHT CV
14 IRONSIDE CV
0 .125 .25 .375 .5 miles 1 in. = 1900 ft.

SEE 522 MAP

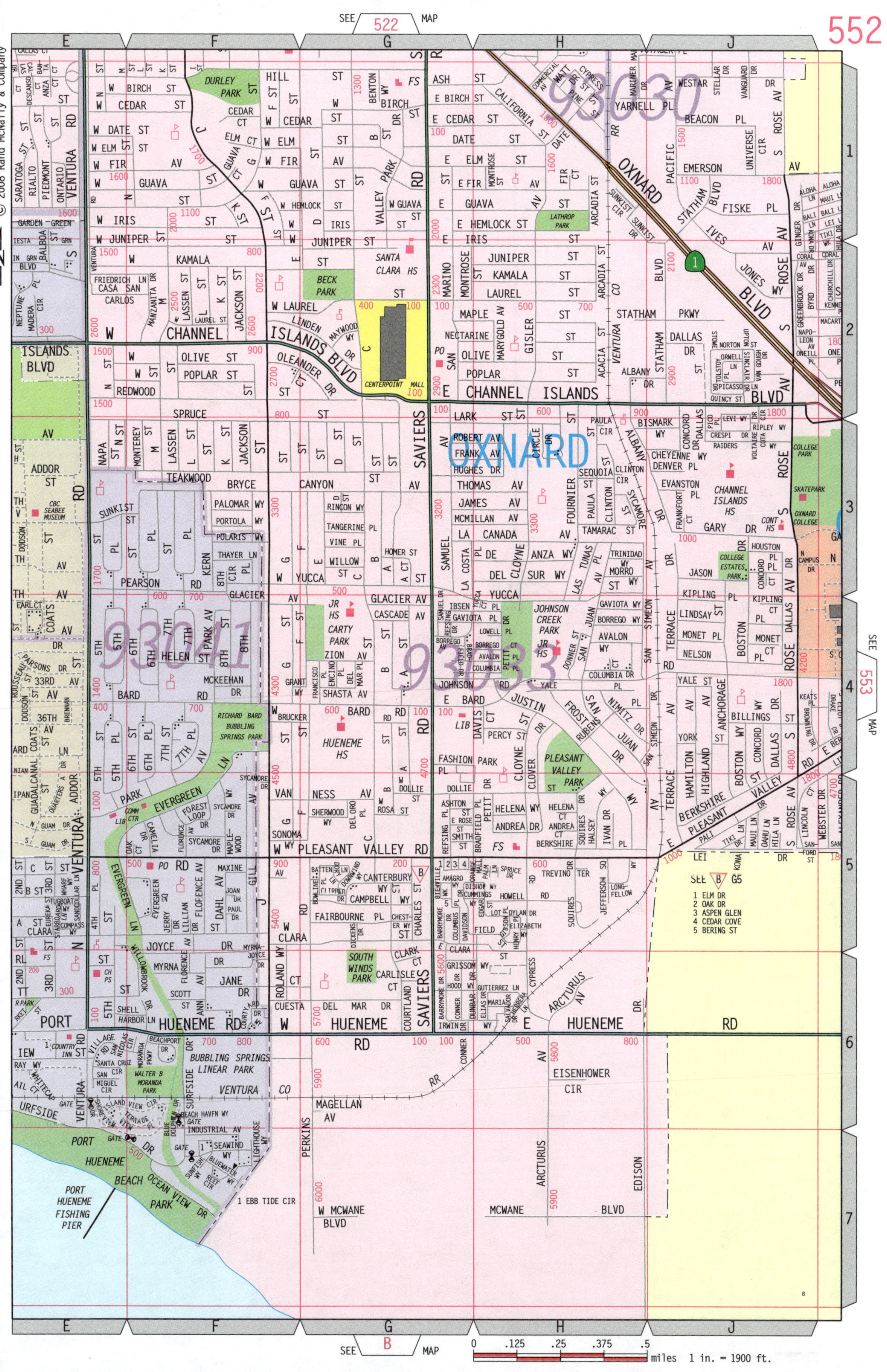

OXNARD
93030
93033
93041
CHANNEL ISLANDS BLVD
OXNARD BLVD
SAVIERS RD
VENTURA RD
ROSE AV
PLEASANT VALLEY RD
HUENEME RD
BARD RD
W HUENEME RD
E HUENEME RD
W MCWANE BLVD
MCWANE BLVD
MAGELLAN AV
EISENHOWER CIR
ARCTURUS AV
PERKINS
EDISON
CENTERPOINT MALL
DURLEY PARK
BECK PARK
LATHROP PARK
SANTA CLARA HS
CHANNEL ISLANDS HS
COLLEGE PARK
OXNARD COLLEGE
SKATEPARK
COLLEGE ESTATES PARK
JOHNSON CREEK PARK
CARTY PARK
HUENEME HS
PLEASANT VALLEY PARK
RICHARD BARD BUBBLING SPRINGS PARK
SOUTH WINDS PARK
BUBBLING SPRINGS LINEAR PARK
WALTER B MORANDA PARK
CBC SEABEE MUSEUM
PORT HUENEME BEACH OCEAN VIEW PARK
PORT HUENEME FISHING PIER
1 EBB TIDE CIR
SEE B G5
1 ELM DR
2 OAK DR
3 ASPEN GLEN
4 CEDAR COVE
5 BERING ST
0 .125 .25 .375 .5
miles 1 in. = 1900 ft.

SEE 553 MAP

SEE B MAP

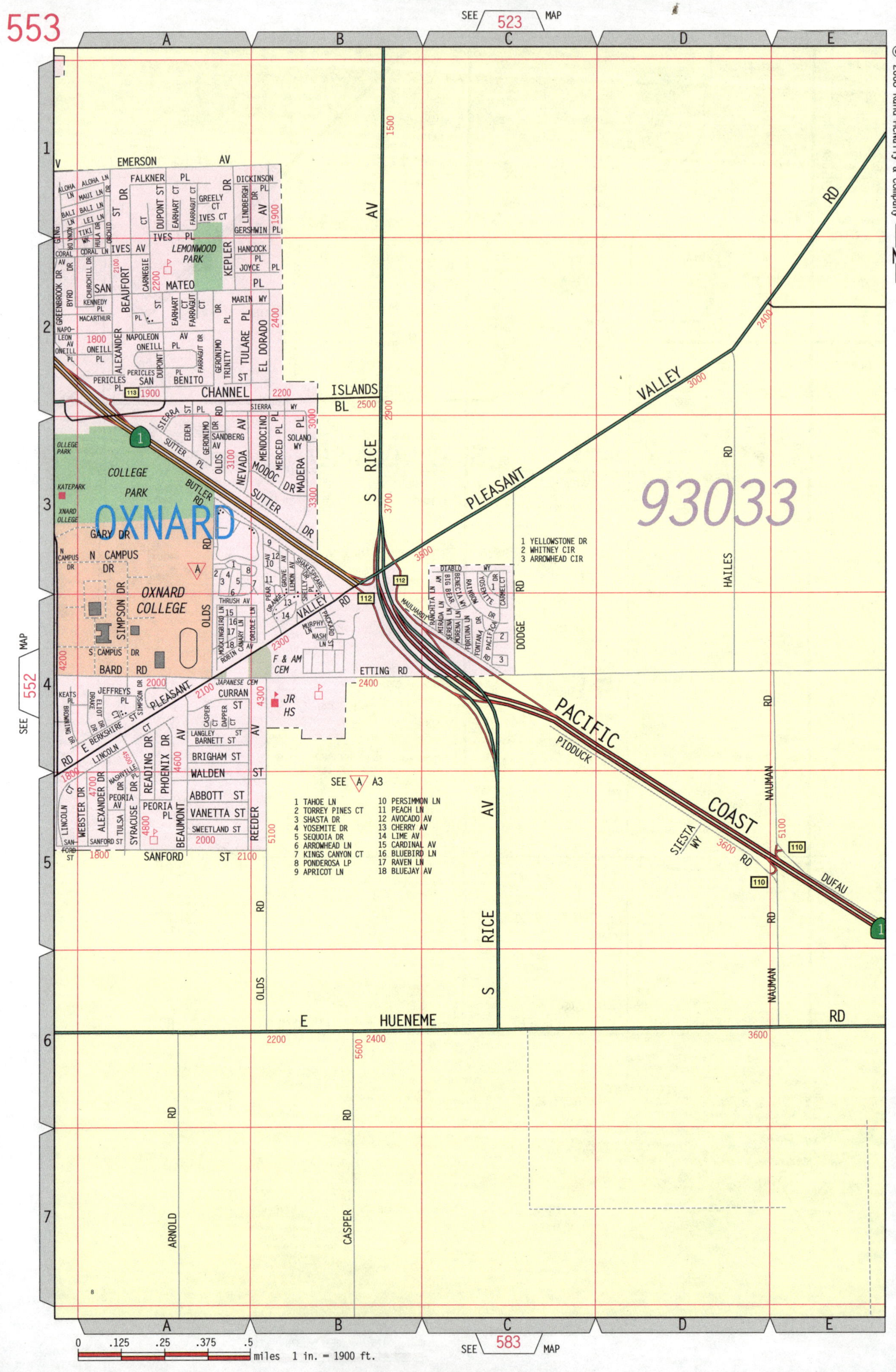
SEE 523 MAP
A
B
C
D
E
1
2
3
4
5
6
7
EMERSON AV
FALKNER PL
DICKINSON
ALOHA LN
MAUI LN
BALI LN
LEI LN
TIKI WK
HULA DR
ORCHID
CORAL LN
GREELY CT
IVES CT
DUPONT ST
EARHART CT
FARRAGUT CT
LINDBERGH DR
GERSHWIN PL
IVES PL
IVES AV
LEMONWOOD PARK
HANCOCK PL
JOYCE PL
KEPLER
CHURCHILL DR
BEAUFORT
CARNEGIE
SAN MATEO
GREENBROOK DR
BYRD
KENNEDY PL
MACARTHUR
MARIN WY
TULARE PL
EL DORADO
NAPOLEON AV
ONEILL PL
NAPOLEON
ALEXANDER DR
GERONIMO
TRINITY
PERICLES PL
SAN BENITO
CHANNEL ISLANDS BL
1800
1900
2200
2500
1500
1900
2400
2900
113
1
SIERRA PL
SIERRA WY
EDEN
GERONIMO DR
SANDBERG AV
OLDS
NEVADA AV
MENDOCINO PL
MERCED PL
MODOC DR
MADERA
SOLANO WY
SUTTER PL
SUTTER DR
BUTLER RD
3000
3100
3300
COLLEGE PARK
KATE PARK
XNARD COLLEGE
OXNARD
GARY DR
N CAMPUS DR
OXNARD COLLEGE
SIMPSON DR
S CAMPUS DR
BARD RD
4200
THRUSH AV
MOCKINGBIRD LN
CANARY LN
ORIOLE LN
ROBIN LN
PEAR AV
ORANGE
GROVE AV
LEMON AV
SHAKESPEARE DR
SHELLY PL
PLEASANT VALLEY RD
MURPHY LN
NASH LN
PACKARD ST
F & AM CEM
ETTING RD
2300
2400
112
S RICE AV
3700
3500
3000
2400
RD
1 YELLOWSTONE DR
2 WHITNEY CIR
3 ARROWHEAD CIR
DIABLO WY
RANCHITA LN
MIRADA LN
BIG BEAR
BENECIA WY
SERENA LN
MORENA LN
FORTUNA LN
RAINBOW
FONTANA DR
YOSEMITE DR
PACIFICA DR
CARMEL CT
MAULHARDT
DODGE RD
HAILES RD
93033
JEFFREYS PL
KEATS PL
DRAKE
ELIOT DR
BROWNING DR
E BERKSHIRE ST
SIMPSON DR
CURRAN ST
JAPANESE CEM
JR HS
CASPER CT
DAPPER CT
LANGLEY ST
BARNETT ST
BRIGHAM ST
WALDEN ST
ABBOTT ST
VANETTA ST
SWEETLAND ST
LINCOLN CT
LINCOLN
WEBSTER DR
ALEXANDER DR
NASHVILLE
PEORIA DR
TULSA
SYRACUSE DR
READING DR
PHOENIX DR
PEORIA PL
BEAUMONT
REEDER AV
SANFORD ST
2000
2100
4300
4500
4600
4700
4800
5100
SEE A A3
1 TAHOE LN
2 TORREY PINES CT
3 SHASTA DR
4 YOSEMITE DR
5 SEQUOIA DR
6 ARROWHEAD LN
7 KINGS CANYON CT
8 PONDEROSA LP
9 APRICOT LN
10 PERSIMMON LN
11 PEACH LN
12 AVOCADO AV
13 CHERRY AV
14 LIME AV
15 CARDINAL AV
16 BLUEBIRD LN
17 RAVEN LN
18 BLUEJAY AV
PACIFIC COAST
PIDDUCK
SIESTA WY
3600
DUFAU RD
NAUMAN RD
110
OLDS RD
E HUENEME RD
2200
2400
5600
3600
ARNOLD RD
CASPER RD
SEE 552 MAP
SEE 583 MAP
0 .125 .25 .375 .5 miles 1 in. = 1900 ft.

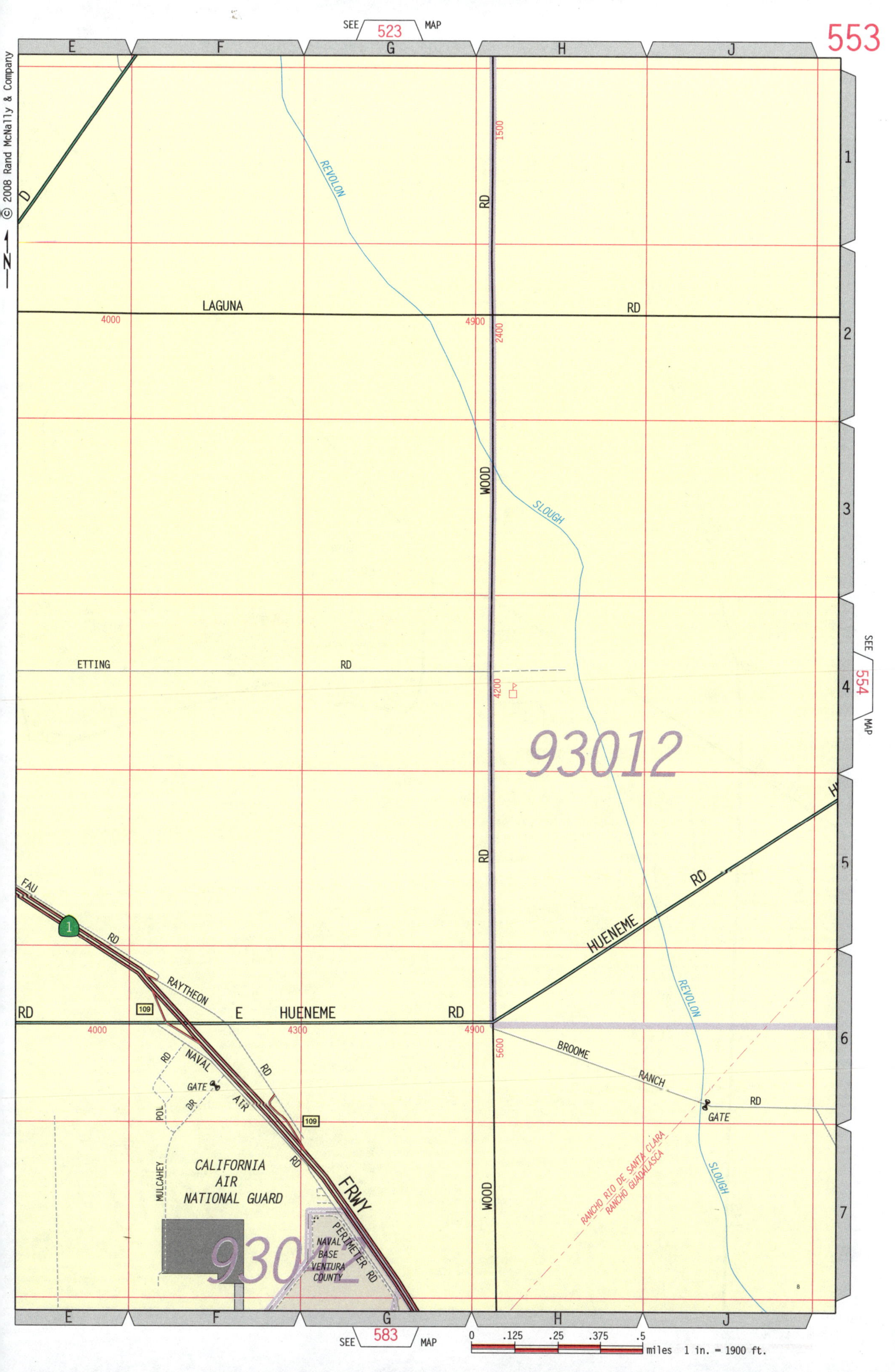

SEE 523 MAP
SEE 554 MAP
SEE 583 MAP
E
F
G
H
J
1
2
3
4
5
6
7
LAGUNA
RD
4000
4900
2400
1500
WOOD
RD
REVOLON
SLOUGH
ETTING
RD
4200
93012
HUENEME
RD
FAU
RD
RAYTHEON
RD
E
HUENEME
RD
4000
4300
4900
5600
109
BROOME
RANCH
RD
GATE
NAVAL
AIR
RD
POL
DR
MULCAHEY
CALIFORNIA
AIR
NATIONAL GUARD
FRWY
PERIMETER
RD
NAVAL
BASE
VENTURA
COUNTY
RANCHO RIO DE SANTA CLARA
RANCHO GUADALASCA
0
.125
.25
.375
.5
miles 1 in. = 1900 ft.

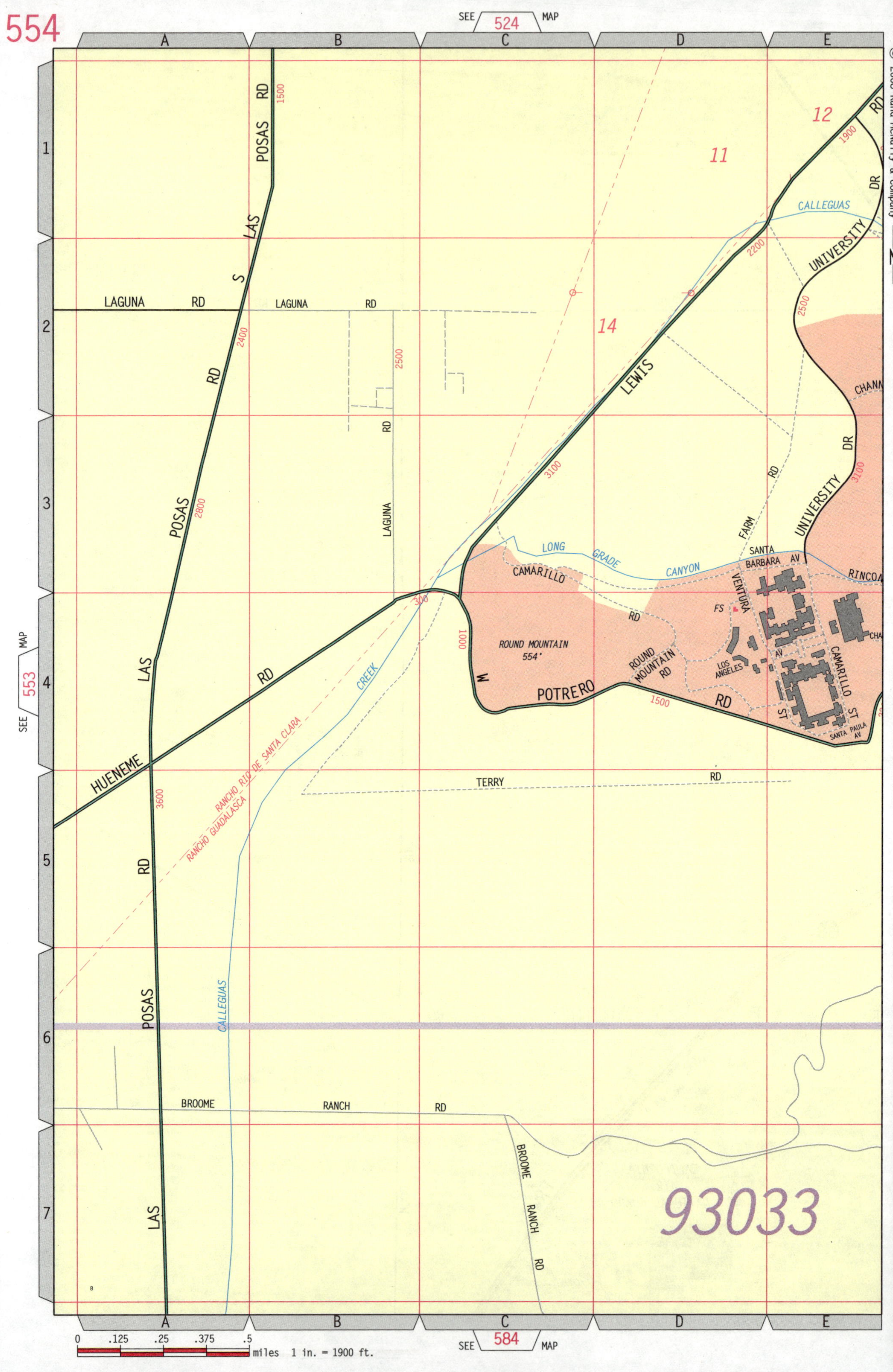
SEE 524 MAP
A
B
C
D
E
1
2
3
4
5
6
7
SEE 553 MAP
LAS POSAS RD
S LAS POSAS RD
1500
2400
2800
3600
LAGUNA RD
LAGUNA RD
LAGUNA RD
2500
LEWIS RD
2200
3100
1900
11
12
14
CALLEGUAS
UNIVERSITY DR
2500
3100
CHANNEL
FARM RD
SANTA BARBARA AV
VENTURA
LONG GRADE CANYON
CAMARILLO RD
RINCON
FS
LOS ANGELES AV
CAMARILLO ST
SANTA PAULA AV
ST
ROUND MOUNTAIN 554'
ROUND MOUNTAIN RD
W POTRERO RD
1500
1000
300
HUENEME RD
CREEK
RANCHO RIO DE SANTA CLARA
RANCHO GUADALASCA
TERRY RD
CALLEGUAS
BROOME RANCH RD
BROOME RANCH RD
93033
SEE 584 MAP
0 .125 .25 .375 .5 miles 1 in. = 1900 ft.

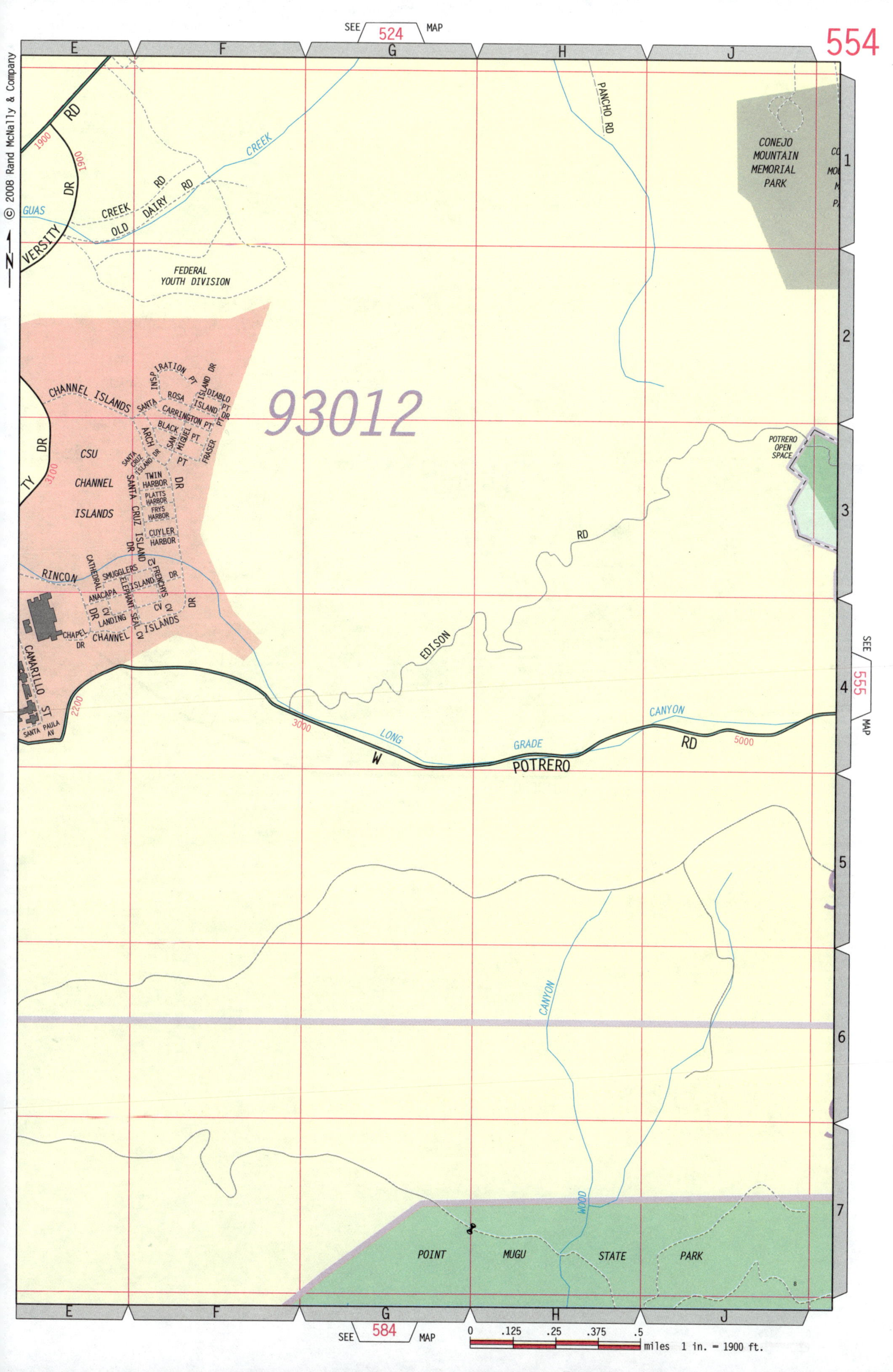
SEE 524 MAP
E
F
G
H
J
1
2
3
4
5
6
7
RD
1900
1900
DR
GUAS
CREEK
OLD
DAIRY
RD
RD
CREEK
VERSITY
FEDERAL
YOUTH DIVISION
PANCHO RD
CONEJO
MOUNTAIN
MEMORIAL
PARK
93012
CHANNEL ISLANDS
CSU
CHANNEL
ISLANDS
RINCON
CHAPEL DR
CHANNEL ISLANDS
CAMARILLO ST
SANTA PAULA AV
2200
3100
POTRERO
OPEN
SPACE
RD
EDISON
W
POTRERO
RD
LONG
GRADE
CANYON
3000
5000
CANYON
WOOD
POINT
MUGU
STATE
PARK
SEE 555 MAP
SEE 584 MAP
0 .125 .25 .375 .5
miles 1 in. = 1900 ft.

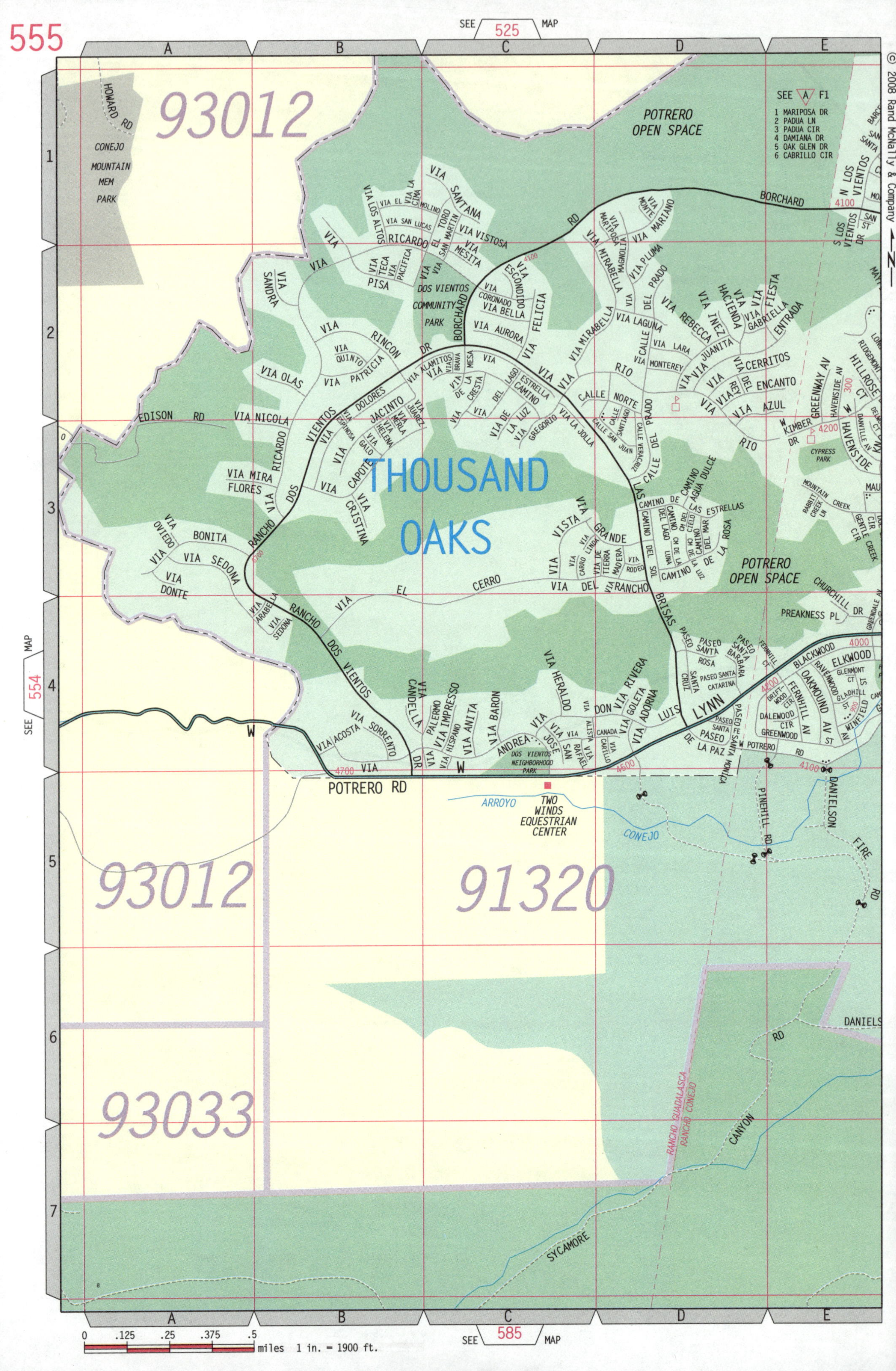
SEE 525 MAP
SEE 554 MAP
SEE 585 MAP
A
B
C
D
E
1
2
3
4
5
6
7
© 2008 Rand McNally & Company
93012
93012
93033
91320
THOUSAND OAKS
HOWARD RD
CONEJO MOUNTAIN MEM PARK
POTRERO OPEN SPACE
POTRERO OPEN SPACE
SEE A F1
1 MARIPOSA DR
2 PADUA LN
3 PADUA CIR
4 DAMIANA DR
5 OAK GLEN DR
6 CABRILLO CIR
BORCHARD RD
DOS VIENTOS COMMUNITY PARK
DOS VIENTOS NEIGHBORHOOD PARK
CYPRESS PARK
EDISON RD
RANCHO DOS VIENTOS
VIA EL CERRO
VIA DEL RANCHO
LAS BRISAS
LYNN RD
W POTRERO RD
POTRERO RD
TWO WINDS EQUESTRIAN CENTER
ARROYO CONEJO
PINEHILL RD
DANIELSON FIRE RD
DANIELS RD
CANYON
SYCAMORE
RANCHO GUADALASCA
RANCHO CONEJO
PREAKNESS PL
CHURCHILL DR
BLACKWOOD
ELKWOOD
OAKMOUND AV
FERNHILL AV
GREENWOOD
DALEWOOD CIR
HAVENSIDE
GREENWAY AV
KIMBER DR
RIO
MOUNTAIN CREEK
0 .125 .25 .375 .5 miles 1 in. = 1900 ft.

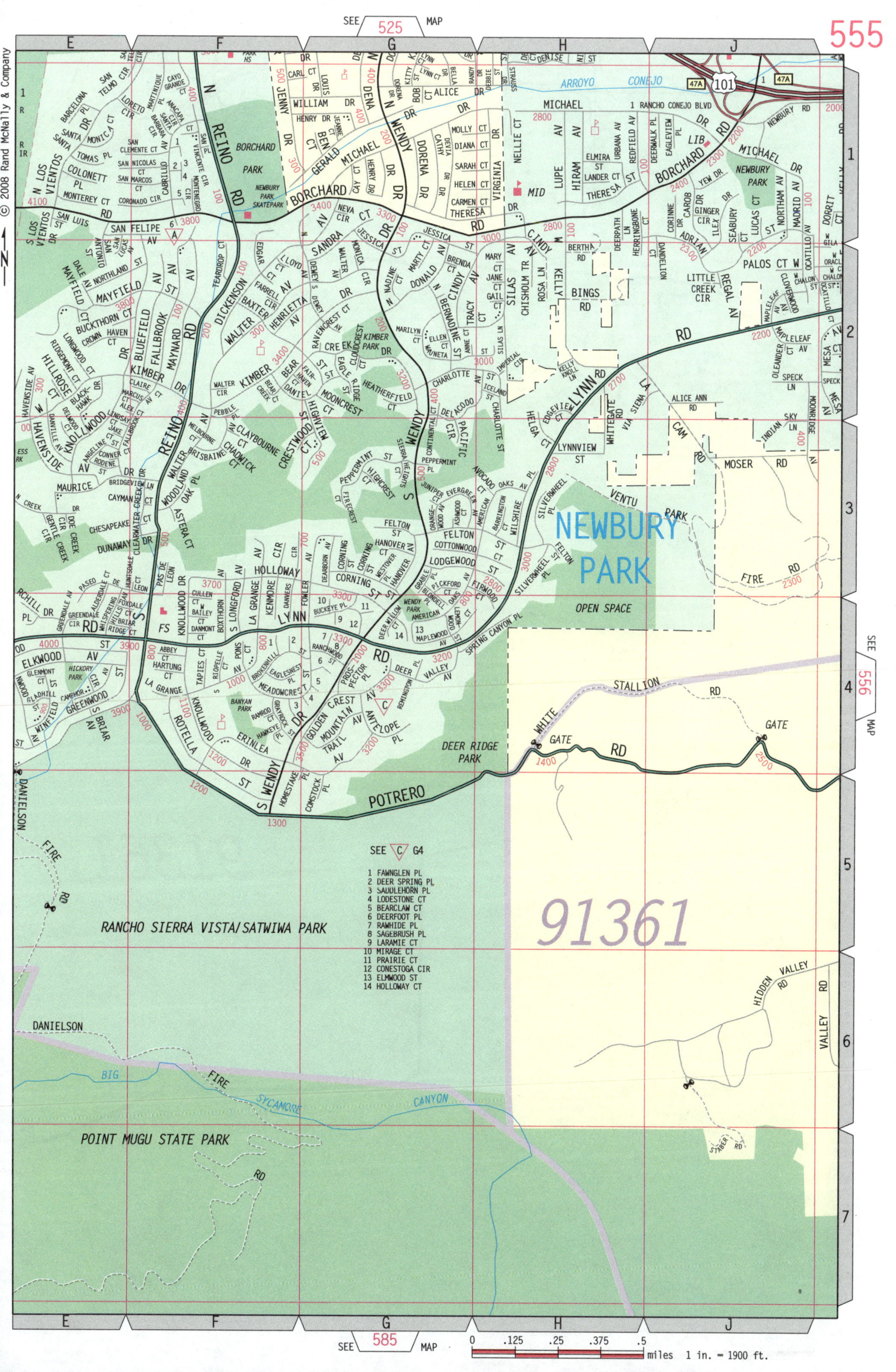

SEE 525 MAP
SEE 556 MAP
SEE 585 MAP
NEWBURY PARK
91361
NEWBURY PARK OPEN SPACE
BORCHARD PARK
NEWBURY PARK SKATEPARK
NEWBURY PARK
KIMBER PARK
WENDY PARK
DEER RIDGE PARK
BANYAN PARK
HICKORY PARK
RANCHO SIERRA VISTA/SATWIWA PARK
POINT MUGU STATE PARK
ARROYO CONEJO
BIG SYCAMORE CANYON
BORCHARD RD
LYNN RD
POTRERO RD
N REINO RD
N WENDY DR
S WENDY DR
MICHAEL DR
STALLION RD
WHITE GATE RD
HIDDEN VALLEY RD
VALLEY RD
DANIELSON FIRE RD
VENTU PARK RD
MOSER RD
SEE C G4
1 FAWNGLEN PL
2 DEER SPRING PL
3 SADDLEHORN PL
4 LODESTONE CT
5 BEARCLAW CT
6 DEERFOOT PL
7 RAWHIDE PL
8 SAGEBRUSH PL
9 LARAMIE CT
10 MIRAGE CT
11 PRAIRIE CT
12 CONESTOGA CIR
13 ELMWOOD ST
14 HOLLOWAY CT
0 .125 .25 .375 .5 miles 1 in. = 1900 ft.

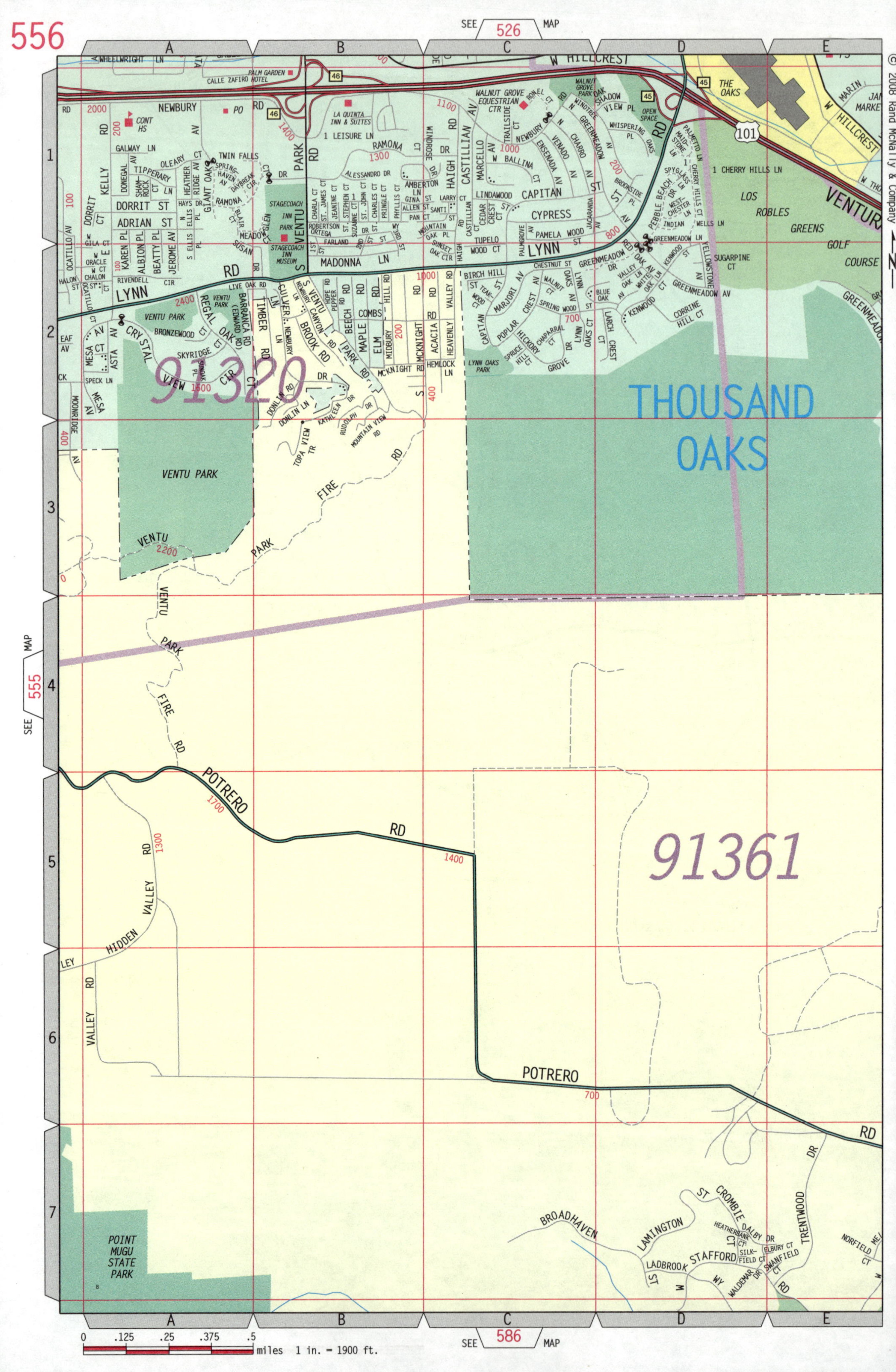
SEE 526 MAP
SEE 555 MAP
SEE 586 MAP
A
B
C
D
E
1
2
3
4
5
6
7
W HILLCREST
NEWBURY
PALM GARDEN
CALLE ZAFIRO HOTEL
CONT HS
PO
LA QUINTA INN & SUITES
WALNUT GROVE EQUESTRIAN CTR
WALNUT GROVE PARK
OPEN SPACE
THE OAKS
101
45
46
1 LEISURE LN
RAMONA
KELLY
DONEGAL
TIPPERARY
GALWAY LN
OLEARY CT
TWIN FALLS
GIANT OAK
DORRIT ST
ADRIAN ST
STAGECOACH INN PARK
STAGECOACH INN MUSEUM
VENTU PARK RD
MADONNA LN
LYNN RD
LIVE OAK RD
CAPITAN
CYPRESS
TUPELO
LINDAWOOD
PAMELA WOOD ST
CASTILLIAN AV
HAIGH RD
MARCELLO
BALLINA
GREENMEADOW
SHADOW VIEW PL
WHISPERING OAKS
1 CHERRY HILLS LN
LOS ROBLES GREENS GOLF COURSE
VENTURA
SUGARPINE CT
GREENMEADOW AV
CORRINE HILL CT
KENWOOD
PEBBLE BEACH
YELLOWSTONE
BIRCH HILL
MARJORI AV
POPLAR
HICKORY
SPRING WOOD
LARCH CREST
LYNN OAKS PARK
HEMLOCK LN
MCKNIGHT RD
ACACIA
HEAVENLY VALLEY RD
MIDBURY
ELM
MAPLE
BEECH
COMBS
BROOK RD
TIMBER RD
REGAL OAK
CRYSTAL VIEW CIR
BRONZEWOOD CT
SKYRIDGE CT
VENTU PARK
MESA AV
SPECK LN
MOONRIDGE AV
DONLIN LN
KATHLEEN DR
RUDOLPH DR
MOUNTAIN VIEW RD
TOPA VIEW TR
91320
THOUSAND OAKS
VENTU PARK FIRE RD
POTRERO RD
1700
1400
700
HIDDEN VALLEY RD
1300
91361
POINT MUGU STATE PARK
BROADHAVEN
LAMINGTON
CROMBIE ST
STAFFORD
LADBROOK
DALBY DR
TRENTWOOD DR
SWANFIELD
WALDEMAR DR
NORFIELD CT
0 .125 .25 .375 .5 miles 1 in. = 1900 ft.

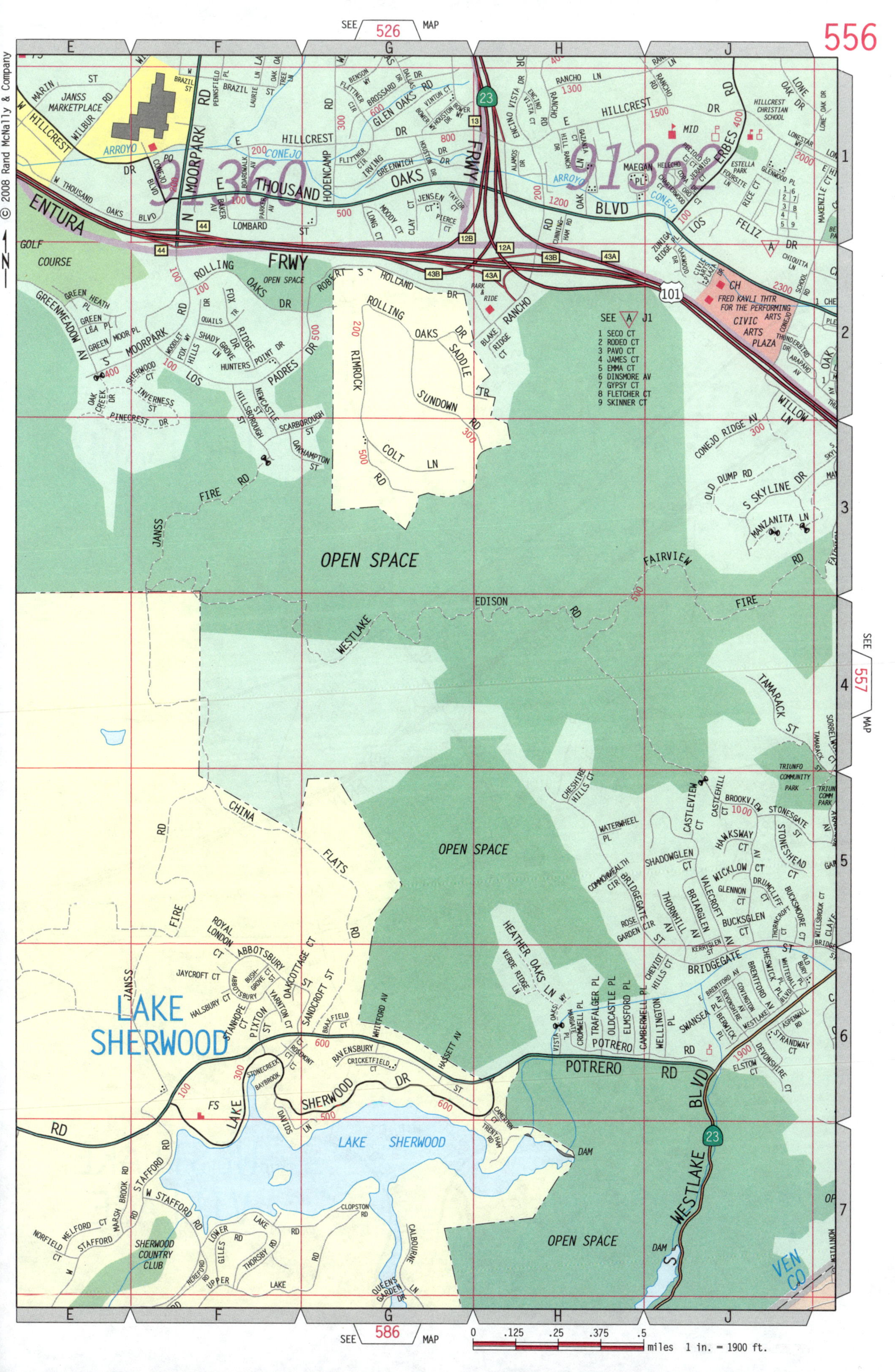
SEE 526 MAP
SEE 586 MAP
SEE 557 MAP
JANSS MARKETPLACE
HILLCREST
THOUSAND OAKS BLVD
VENTURA FRWY
MOORPARK RD
91360
91362
GOLF COURSE
OPEN SPACE
ROLLING OAKS DR
HODENCAMP RD
ERBES RD
HILLCREST CHRISTIAN SCHOOL
ESTELLA PARK
FRED KAVLI THTR FOR THE PERFORMING ARTS
CIVIC ARTS PLAZA
SEE A J1
1 SECO CT
2 RODEO CT
3 PAVO CT
4 JAMES CT
5 EMMA CT
6 DINSMORE AV
7 GYPSY CT
8 FLETCHER CT
9 SKINNER CT
PARK & RIDE
RANCHO RD
JANSS FIRE RD
FAIRVIEW FIRE RD
EDISON RD
WESTLAKE
TAMARACK ST
TRIUNFO COMMUNITY PARK
CHINA FLATS RD
LAKE SHERWOOD
LAKE SHERWOOD DR
POTRERO RD
WESTLAKE BLVD
SHERWOOD COUNTRY CLUB
DAM
VEN CO
0 .125 .25 .375 .5 miles 1 in. = 1900 ft.

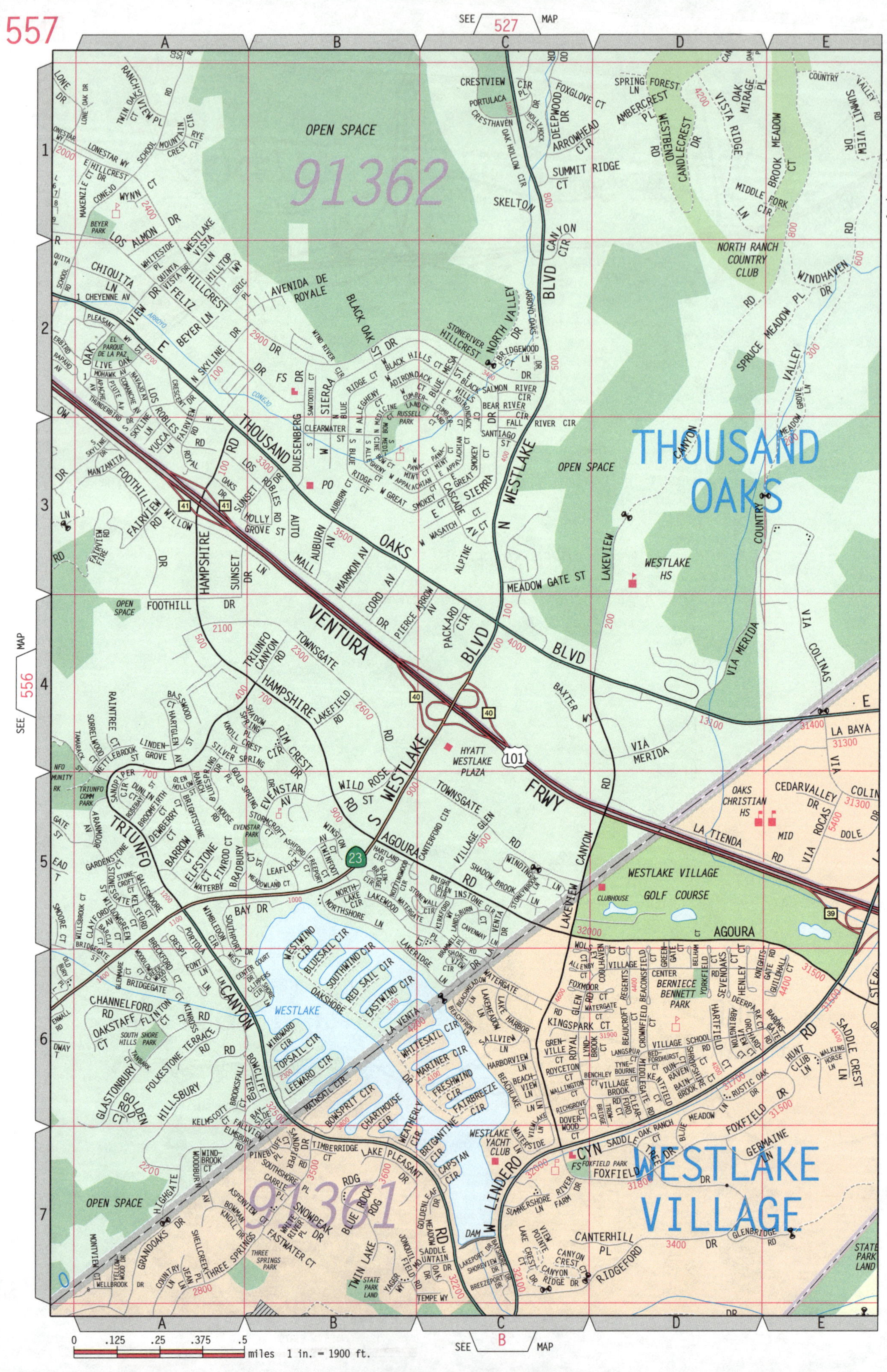

SEE 527 MAP
SEE 556 MAP
SEE B MAP
OPEN SPACE
91362
91361
THOUSAND OAKS
WESTLAKE VILLAGE
NORTH RANCH COUNTRY CLUB
WESTLAKE HS
HYATT WESTLAKE PLAZA
WESTLAKE VILLAGE GOLF COURSE
CLUBHOUSE
OAKS CHRISTIAN HS
BERNIECE BENNETT PARK
WESTLAKE
WESTLAKE YACHT CLUB
FOXFIELD PARK
SOUTH SHORE HILLS PARK
THREE SPRINGS PARK
STATE PARK LAND
BEYER PARK
RUSSELL PARK
EVENSTAR PARK
TRIUNFO COMM PARK
VENTURA FRWY
THOUSAND OAKS BLVD
N WESTLAKE BLVD
S WESTLAKE BLVD
AGOURA RD
LAKEVIEW CANYON RD
TRIUNFO CANYON RD
LINDERO CYN RD
HAMPSHIRE RD
FOOTHILL DR
TOWNSGATE RD
VIA MERIDA
VIA COLINAS
LA TIENDA RD
101
23
40
41
39
miles 1 in. = 1900 ft.
0 .125 .25 .375 .5

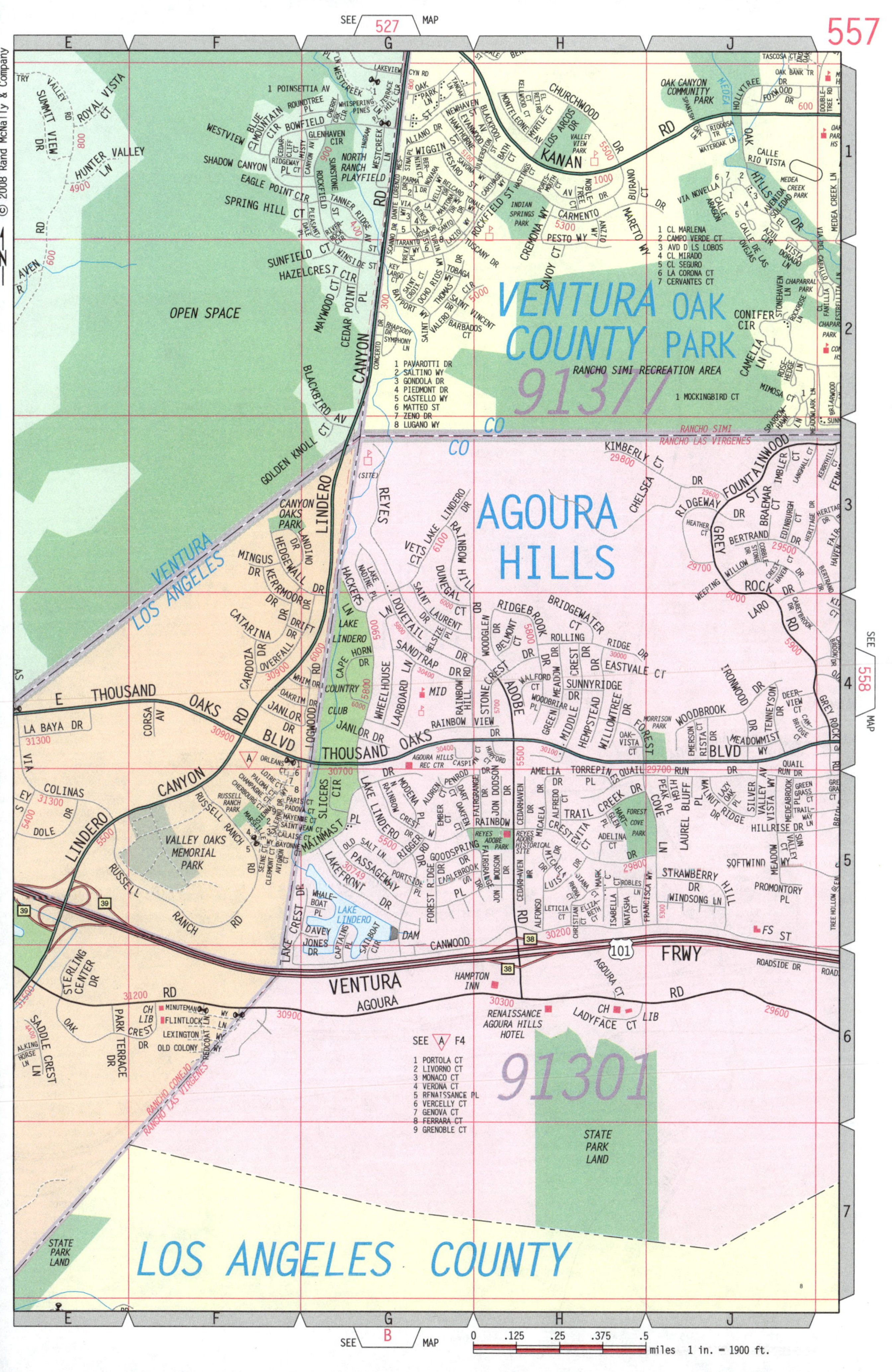
SEE 527 MAP
VENTURA COUNTY
OAK PARK
91377
RANCHO SIMI RECREATION AREA
OAK CANYON COMMUNITY PARK
AGOURA HILLS
OPEN SPACE
VENTURA
LOS ANGELES
THOUSAND OAKS BLVD
CANYON OAKS PARK
VALLEY OAKS MEMORIAL PARK
LAKE LINDERO
VENTURA FRWY
101
AGOURA RD
RENAISSANCE AGOURA HILLS HOTEL
HAMPTON INN
91301
STATE PARK LAND
LOS ANGELES COUNTY
1 PAVAROTTI DR
2 SALTINO WY
3 GONDOLA DR
4 PIEDMONT DR
5 CASTELLO WY
6 MATTEO ST
7 ZENO DR
8 LUGANO WY
1 CL MARLENA
2 CAMPO VERDE CT
3 AVD D LS LOBOS
4 CL MIRADO
5 CL SEGURO
6 LA CORONA CT
7 CERVANTES CT
SEE A F4
1 PORTOLA CT
2 LIVORNO CT
3 MONACO CT
4 VERONA CT
5 RENAISSANCE PL
6 VERCELLY CT
7 GENOVA CT
8 FERRARA CT
9 GRENOBLE CT
SEE 558 MAP
SEE B MAP
0 .125 .25 .375 .5 miles 1 in. = 1900 ft.

SEE 528 MAP

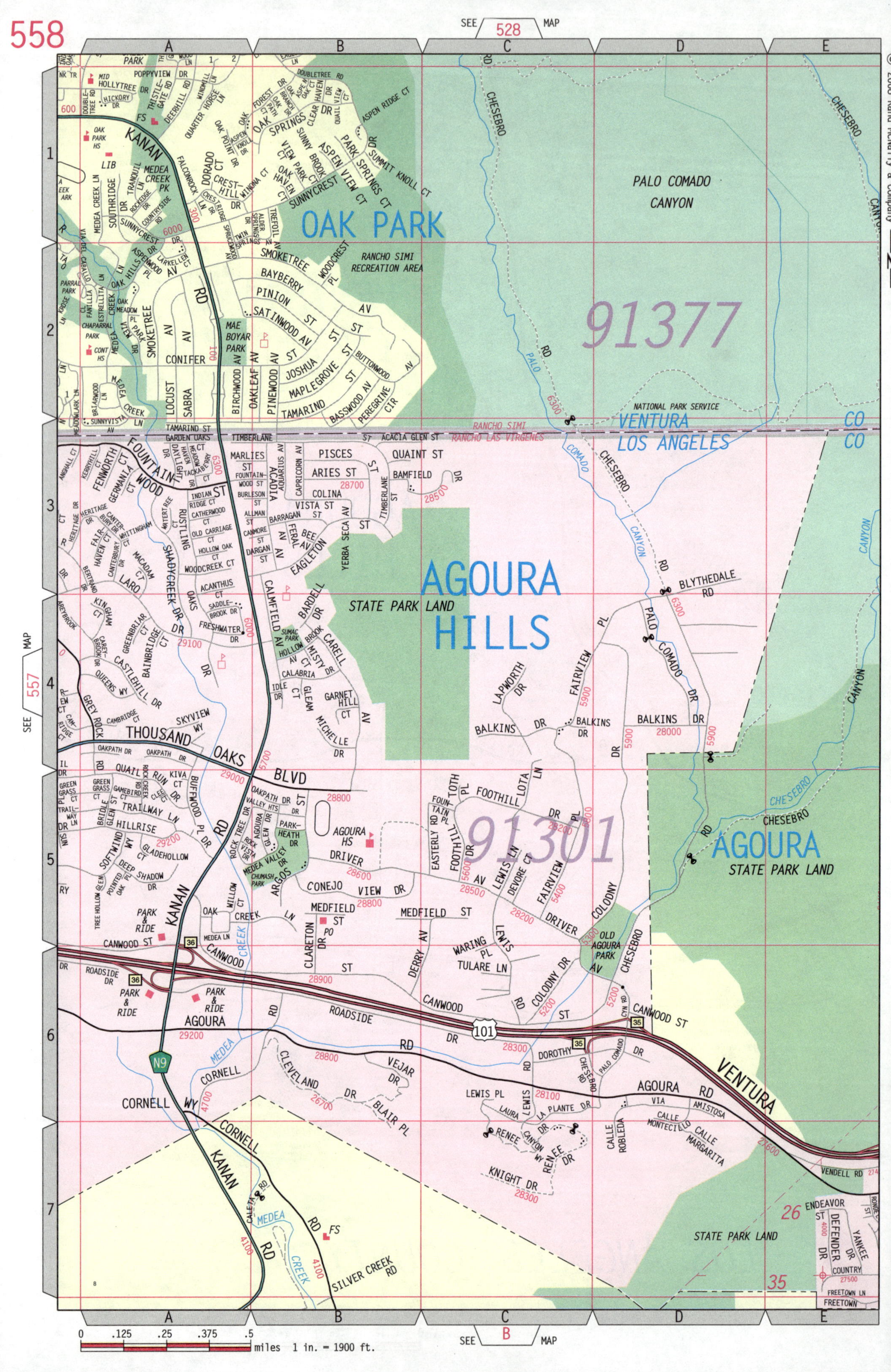
OAK PARK
AGOURA HILLS
AGOURA
91377
91301
PALO COMADO CANYON
RANCHO SIMI RECREATION AREA
STATE PARK LAND
VENTURA
LOS ANGELES
NATIONAL PARK SERVICE
THOUSAND OAKS BLVD
KANAN RD
AGOURA RD
CANWOOD ST
CORNELL WY
CHESEBRO RD
VENTURA
miles 1 in. = 1900 ft.

SEE 557 MAP

SEE B MAP

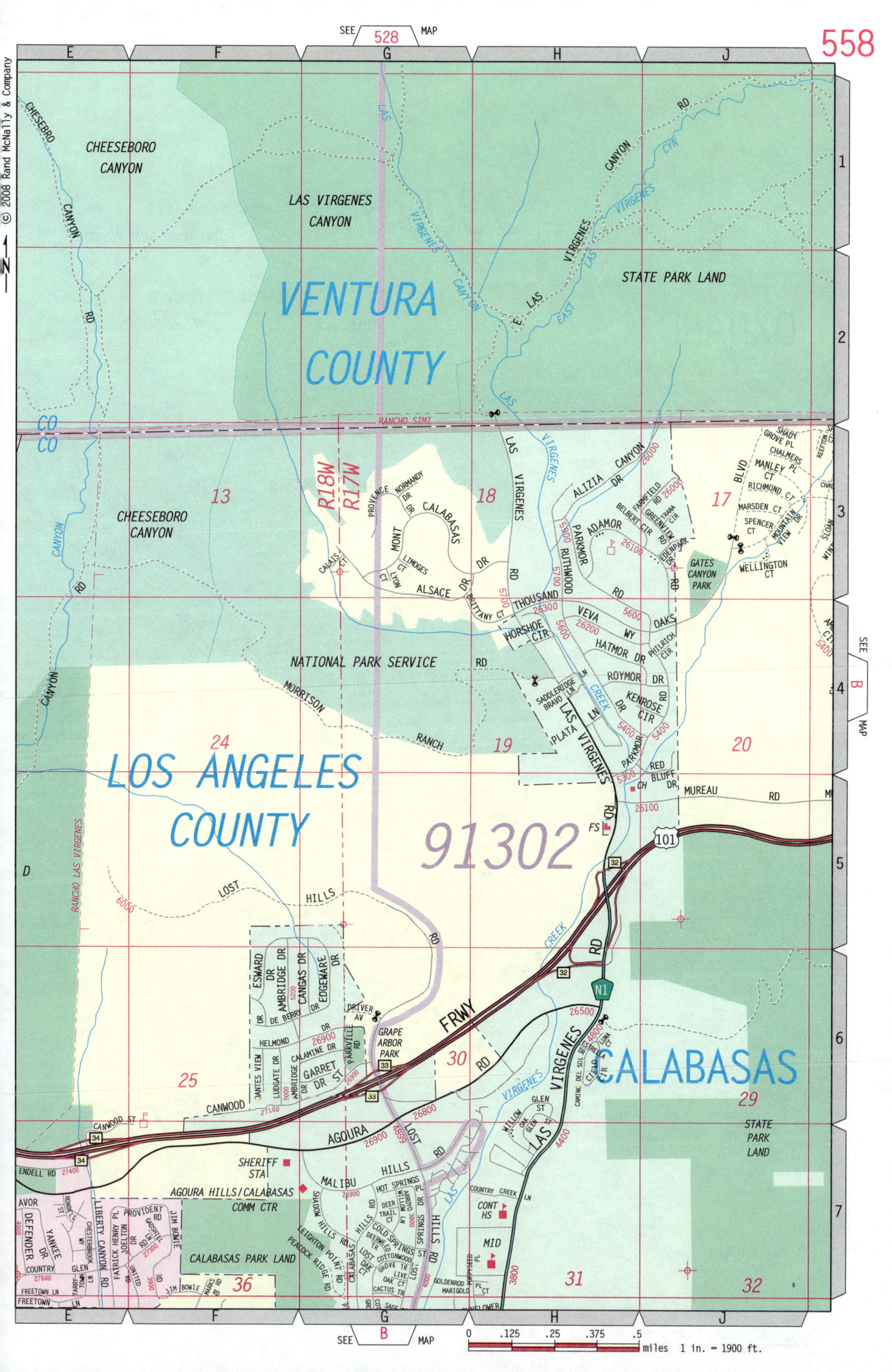
SEE 528 MAP
VENTURA COUNTY
LOS ANGELES COUNTY
CALABASAS
91302
CHEESEBORO CANYON
LAS VIRGENES CANYON
STATE PARK LAND
NATIONAL PARK SERVICE
GATES CANYON PARK
GRAPE ARBOR PARK
SHERIFF STA
AGOURA HILLS/CALABASAS COMM CTR
CALABASAS PARK LAND
CONT HS
MID
RANCHO SIMI
R18W
R17W
LAS VIRGENES RD
THOUSAND OAKS BLVD
MUREAU RD
LOST HILLS RD
AGOURA RD
MALIBU HILLS RD
VENTURA FRWY
CANWOOD ST
MORRISON RANCH RD
CHESEBRO CANYON RD
SEE B MAP
miles 1 in. = 1900 ft.

SEE B MAP

SEE 553 MAP

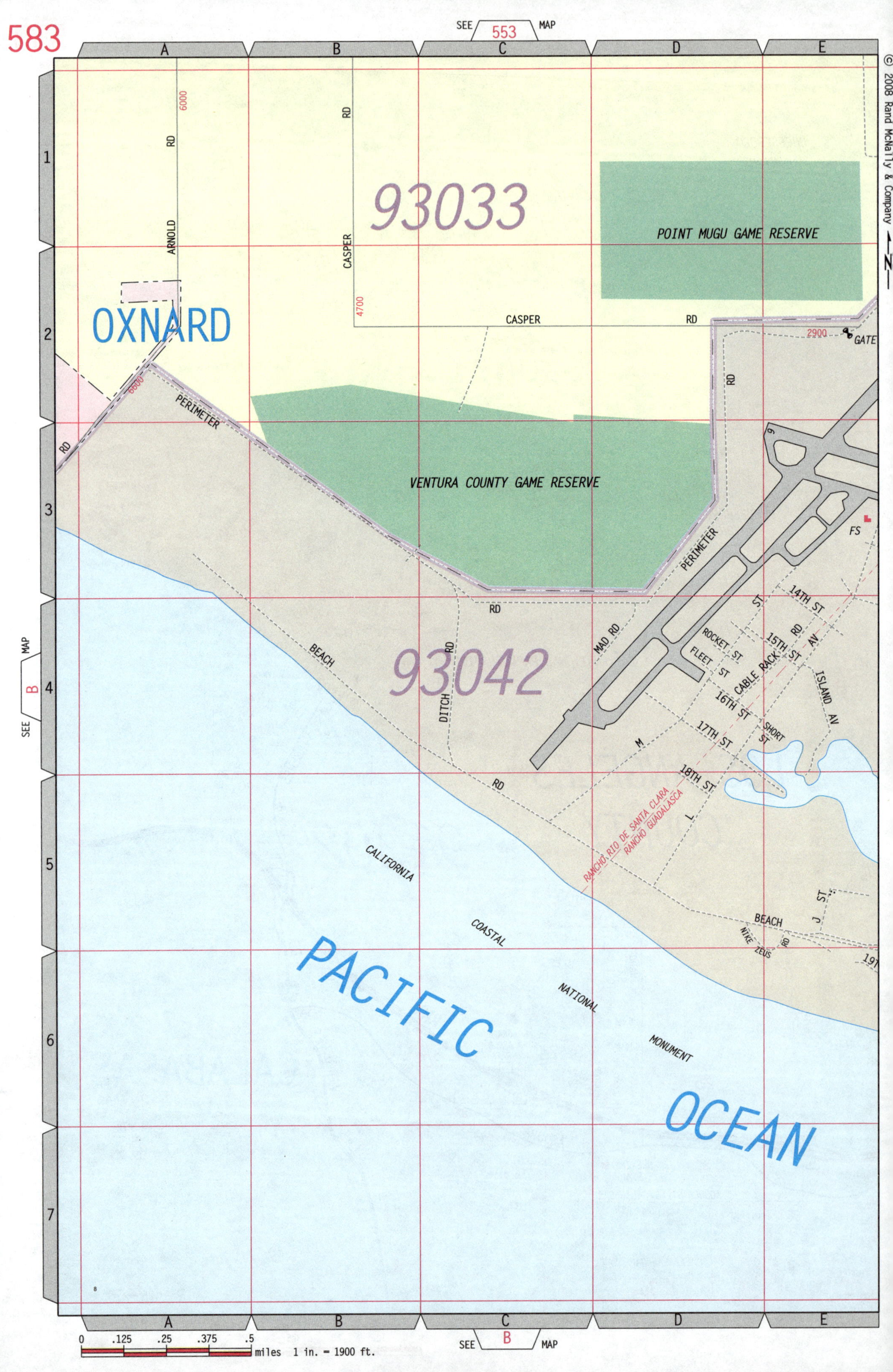
93033
POINT MUGU GAME RESERVE
ARNOLD RD
6000
CASPER RD
4700
CASPER RD
2900
GATE
OXNARD
6600
PERIMETER RD
VENTURA COUNTY GAME RESERVE
PERIMETER RD
FS
14TH ST
15TH ST
16TH ST
17TH ST
18TH ST
ROCKET ST
FLEET ST
CABLE RACK RD
ISLAND AV
SHORT ST
MAD RD
93042
DITCH RD
BEACH RD
M
L
RANCHO RIO DE SANTA CLARA
RANCHO GUADALASCA
CALIFORNIA COASTAL NATIONAL MONUMENT
PACIFIC OCEAN
BEACH RD
NIKE ZEUS RD
J ST
© 2008 Rand McNally & Company

SEE B MAP

0 .125 .25 .375 .5 miles 1 in. = 1900 ft.

SEE B MAP

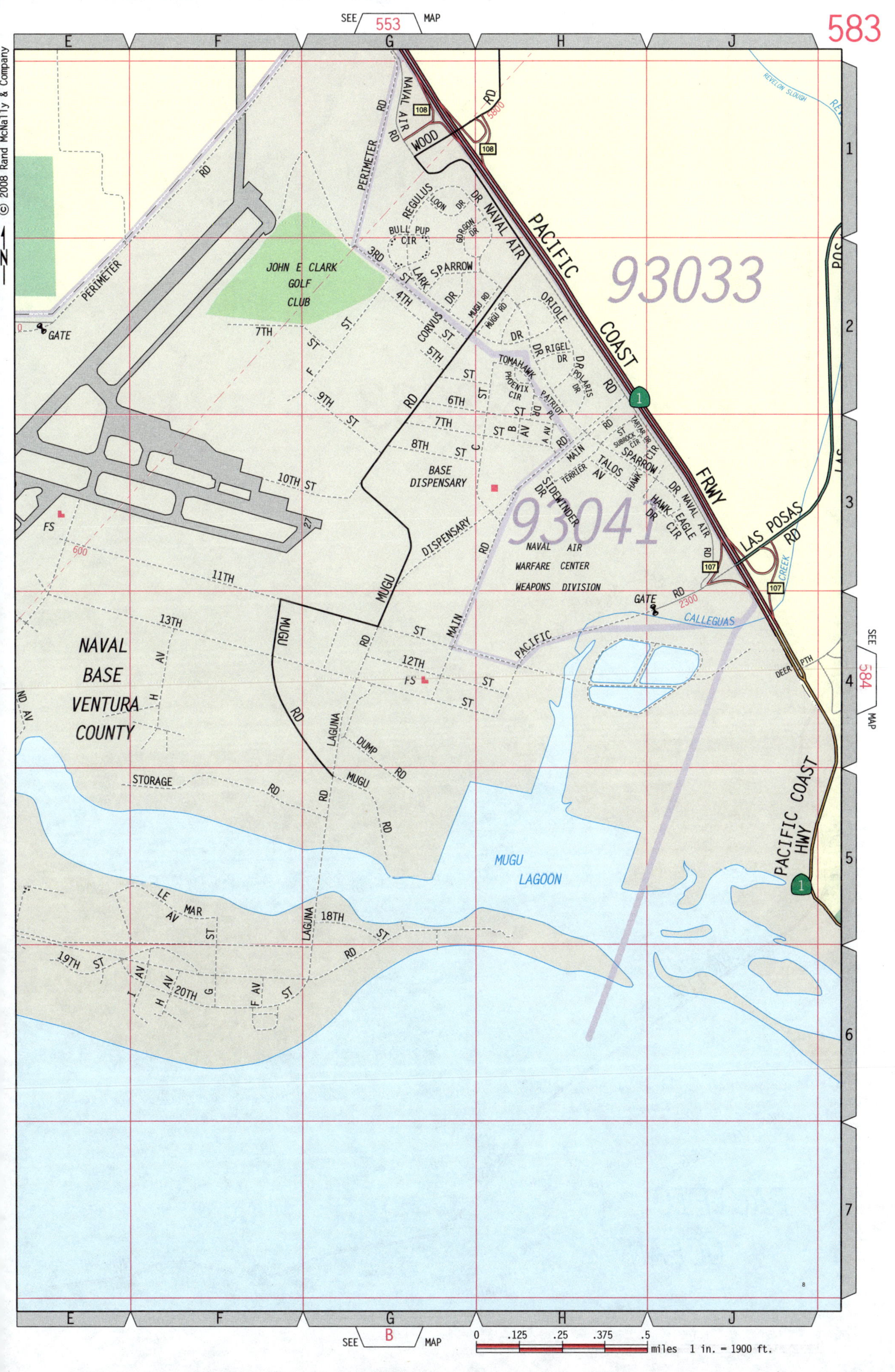
SEE 553 MAP
E
F
G
H
J
1
2
3
4
5
6
7
NAVAL BASE VENTURA COUNTY
JOHN E CLARK GOLF CLUB
93033
93041
NAVAL AIR WARFARE CENTER WEAPONS DIVISION
BASE DISPENSARY
PACIFIC COAST FRWY
PACIFIC COAST HWY
LAS POSAS RD
NAVAL AIR RD
PERIMETER RD
WOOD RD
MUGU RD
MAIN ST
DISPENSARY RD
LAGUNA RD
DUMP RD
STORAGE RD
PACIFIC RD
MUGU LAGOON
CALLEGUAS CREEK
REVELON SLOUGH
GATE
FS
SEE 584 MAP
SEE B MAP
miles 1 in. = 1900 ft.

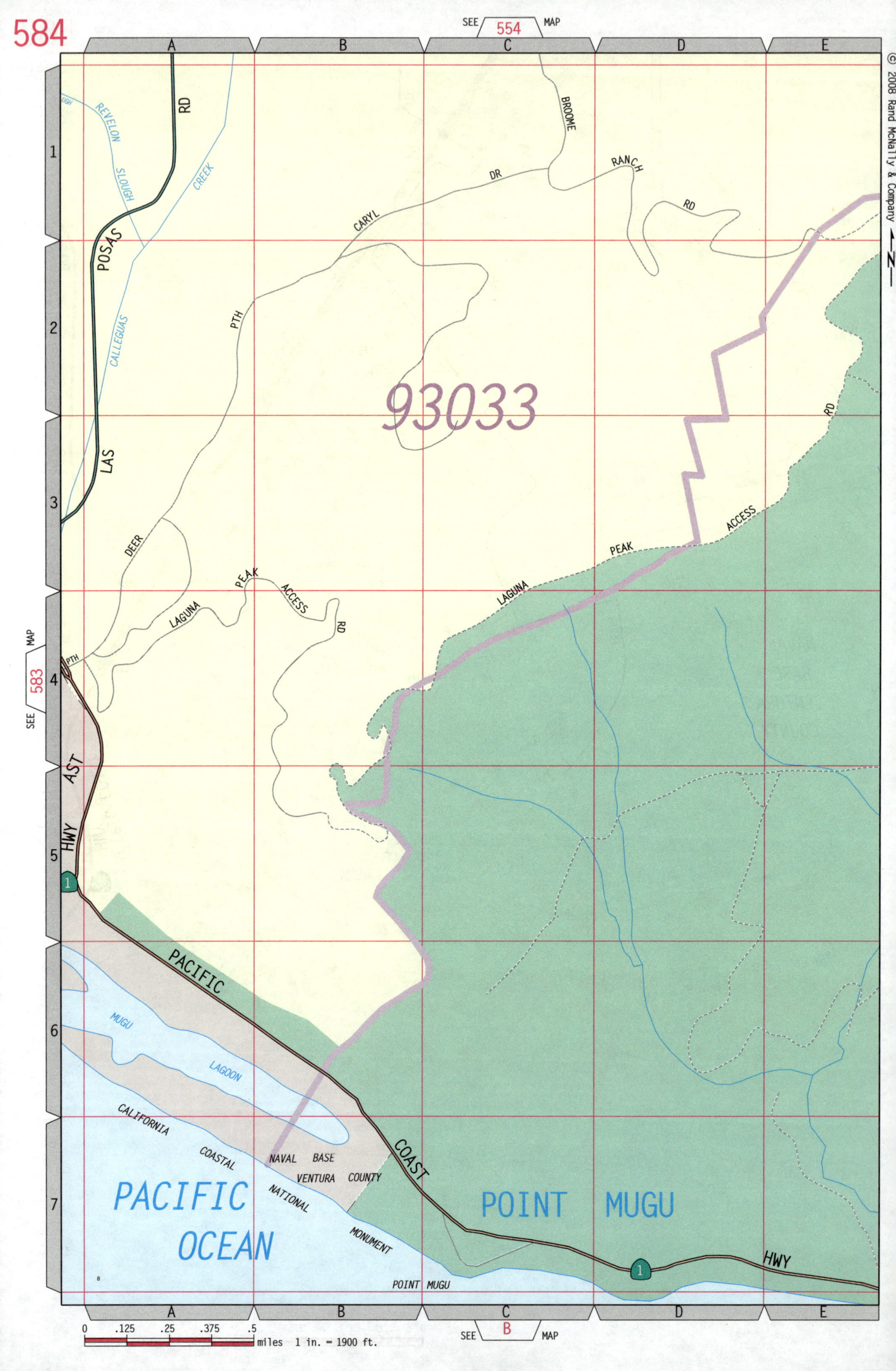
SEE 554 MAP
A
B
C
D
E
1
2
3
4
5
6
7
SEE 583 MAP
© 2008 Rand McNally & Company
N
RD
REVELON
SLOUGH
CREEK
POSAS
CALLEGUAS
LAS
BROOME
RANCH
DR
CARYL
RD
PTH
93033
RD
DEER
PEAK
ACCESS
LAGUNA
RD
ACCESS
PEAK
LAGUNA
PTH
AST
HWY
1
PACIFIC
MUGU
LAGOON
CALIFORNIA
COASTAL
NATIONAL
MONUMENT
NAVAL BASE
VENTURA COUNTY
COAST
PACIFIC
OCEAN
POINT MUGU
POINT MUGU
HWY
1
0 .125 .25 .375 .5
miles 1 in. = 1900 ft.
SEE B MAP

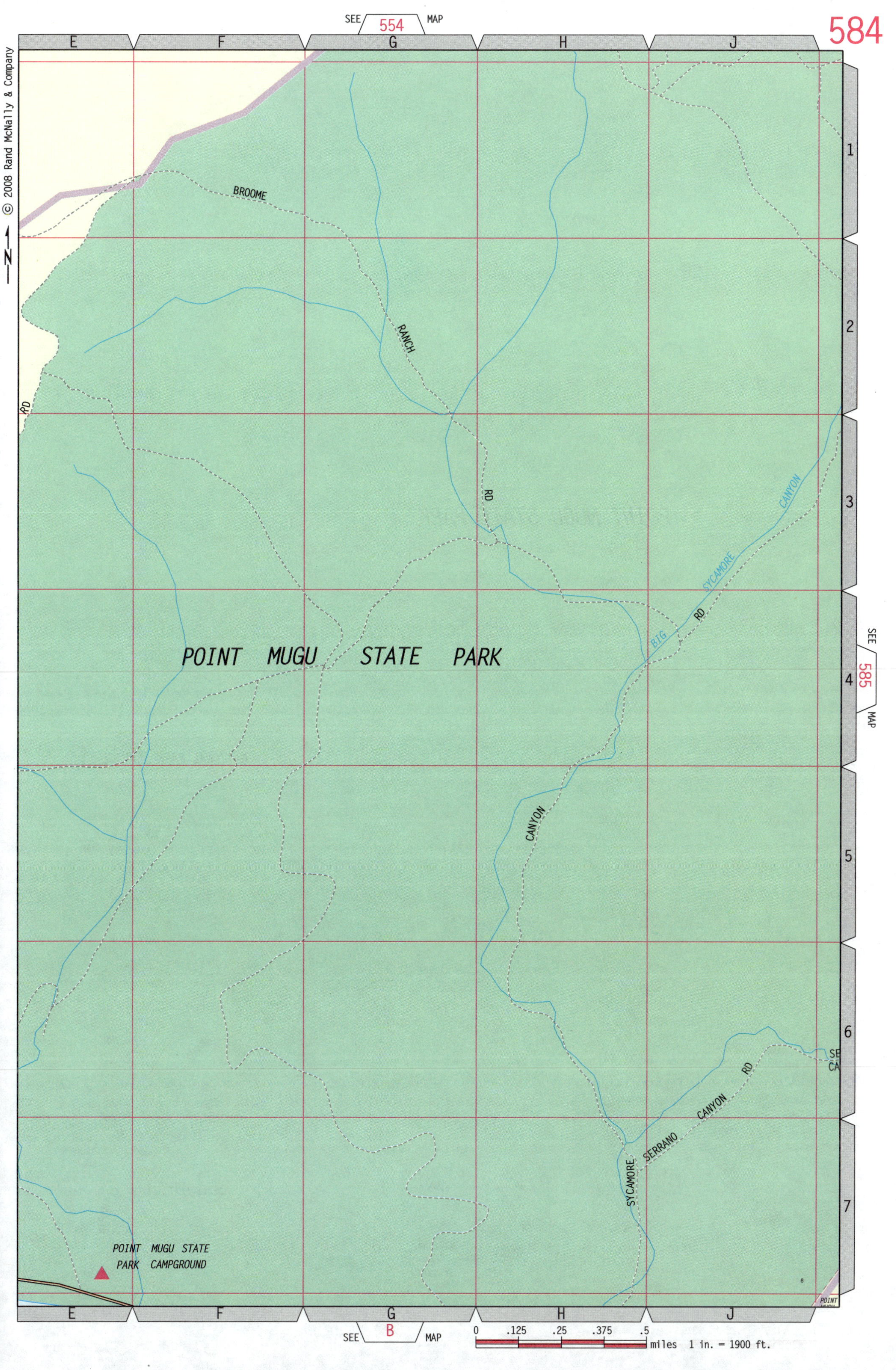
SEE 554 MAP
E
F
G
H
J
1
2
3
4
5
6
7
SEE 585 MAP
BROOME
RANCH
RD
RD
POINT MUGU STATE PARK
BIG SYCAMORE CANYON
RD
CANYON
SYCAMORE
SERRANO CANYON RD
POINT MUGU STATE
PARK CAMPGROUND
SEE B MAP
0 .125 .25 .375 .5
miles 1 in. = 1900 ft.

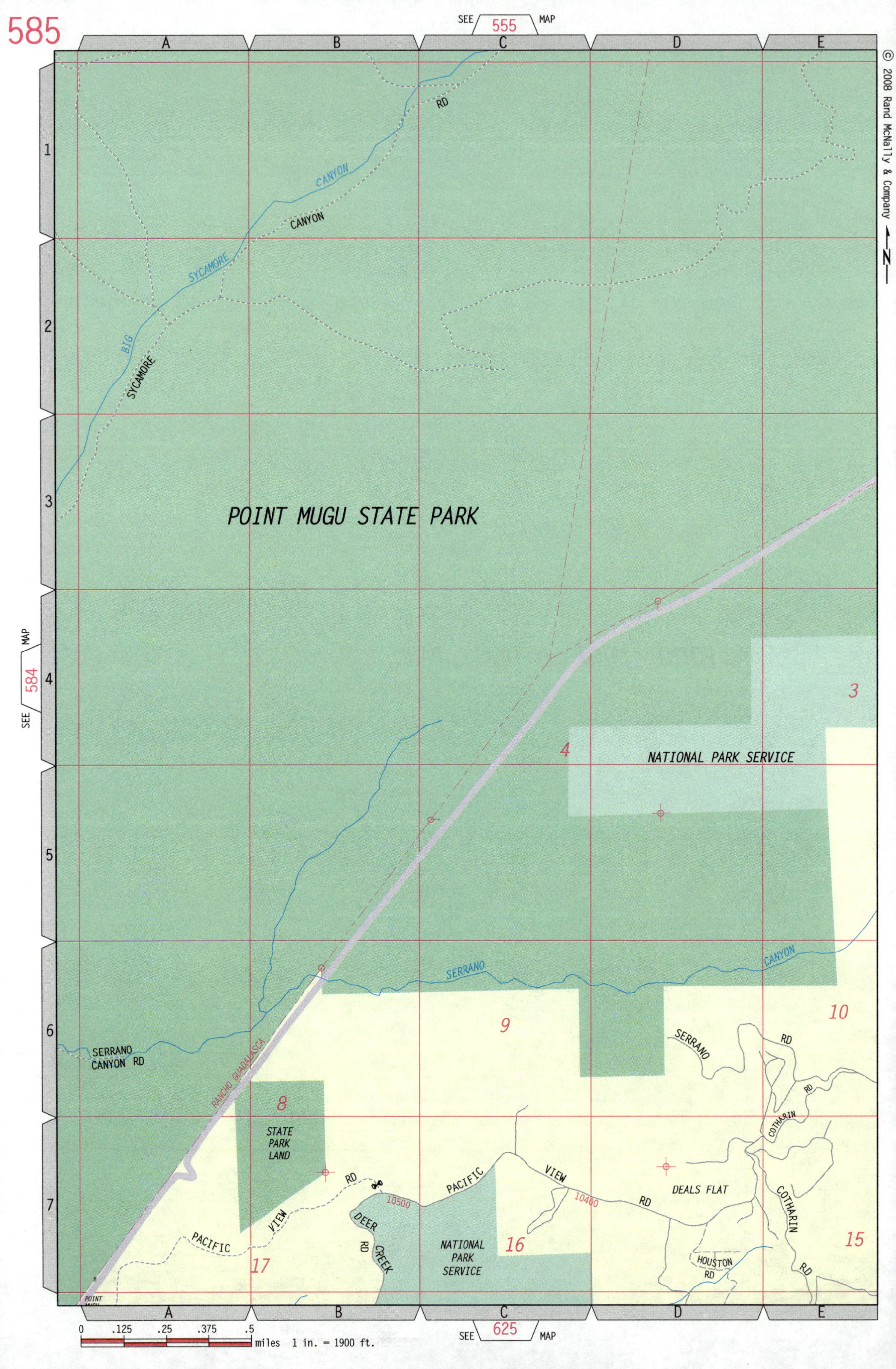

SEE 555 MAP
A
B
C
D
E
1
2
3
4
5
6
7
SEE 584 MAP
© 2008 Rand McNally & Company
N
RD
CANYON
CANYON
SYCAMORE
BIG
SYCAMORE
POINT MUGU STATE PARK
3
4
NATIONAL PARK SERVICE
SERRANO
CANYON
9
10
SERRANO
RD
RD
SERRANO
CANYON RD
RANCHO GUADALASCA
8
STATE
PARK
LAND
COTHARIN
RD
PACIFIC
VIEW
10500
10400
RD
DEALS FLAT
COTHARIN
PACIFIC
VIEW
DEER
CREEK
RD
NATIONAL
PARK
SERVICE
16
15
17
HOUSTON
RD
RD
SEE 625 MAP
0
.125
.25
.375
.5
miles 1 in. = 1900 ft.

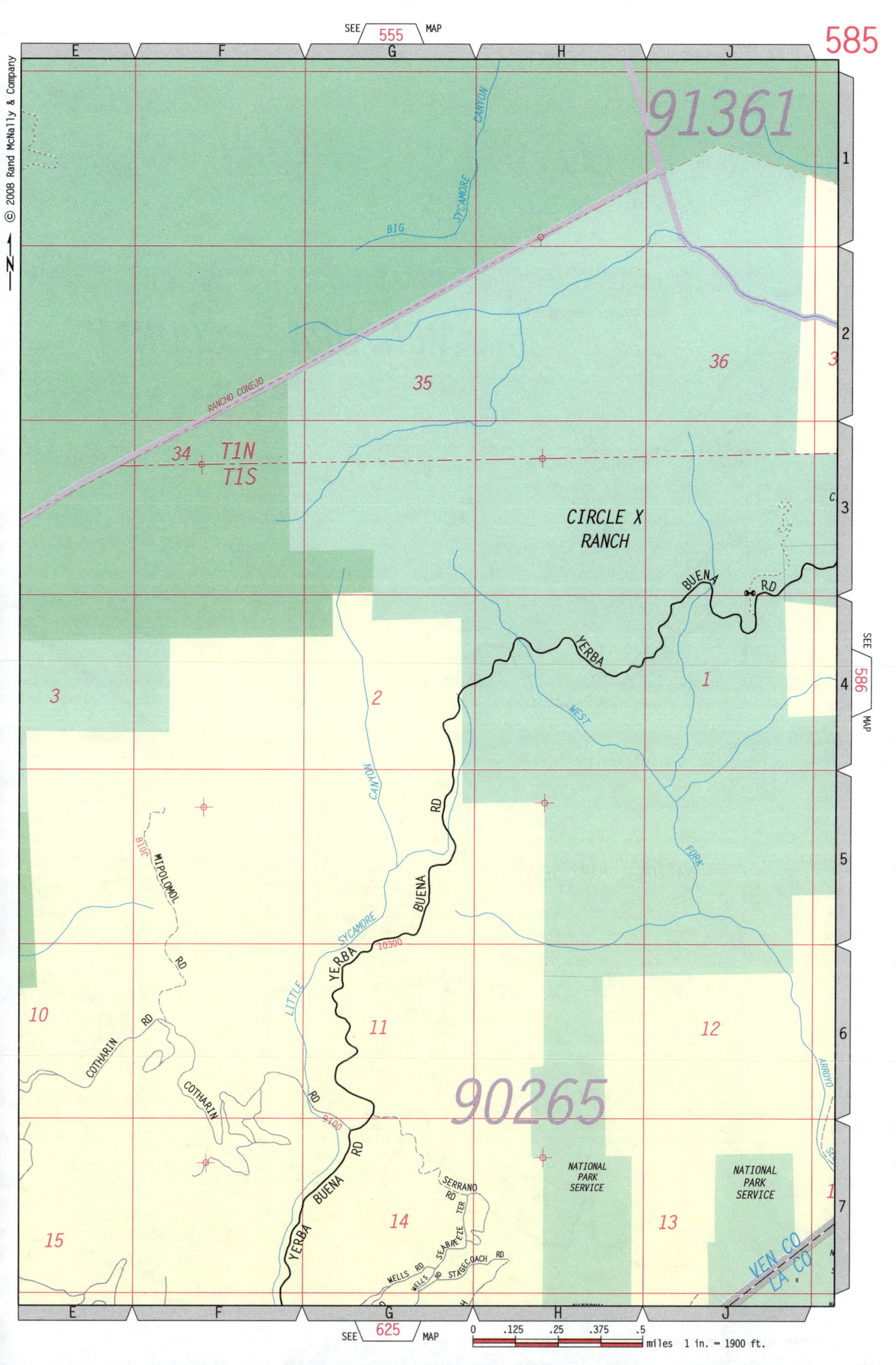
SEE 555 MAP
E
F
G
H
J
91361
BIG
SYCAMORE
CANYON
RANCHO CONEJO
35
36
34
T1N
T1S
CIRCLE X
RANCH
YERBA
BUENA
RD
1
2
3
WEST
FORK
CANYON
SYCAMORE
LITTLE
10300
YERBA
BUENA
RD
MIPOLOMOL
J018
RD
COTHARIN
RD
COTHARIN
RD
9100
10
11
12
90265
YERBA
BUENA
RD
SERRANO
RD
TER
SEABREEZE
WELLS
RD
STAGECOACH
RD
14
13
15
NATIONAL
PARK
SERVICE
NATIONAL
PARK
SERVICE
ARROYO
VEN CO
LA CO
SEE 586 MAP
SEE 625 MAP
0
.125
.25
.375
.5
miles 1 in. = 1900 ft.

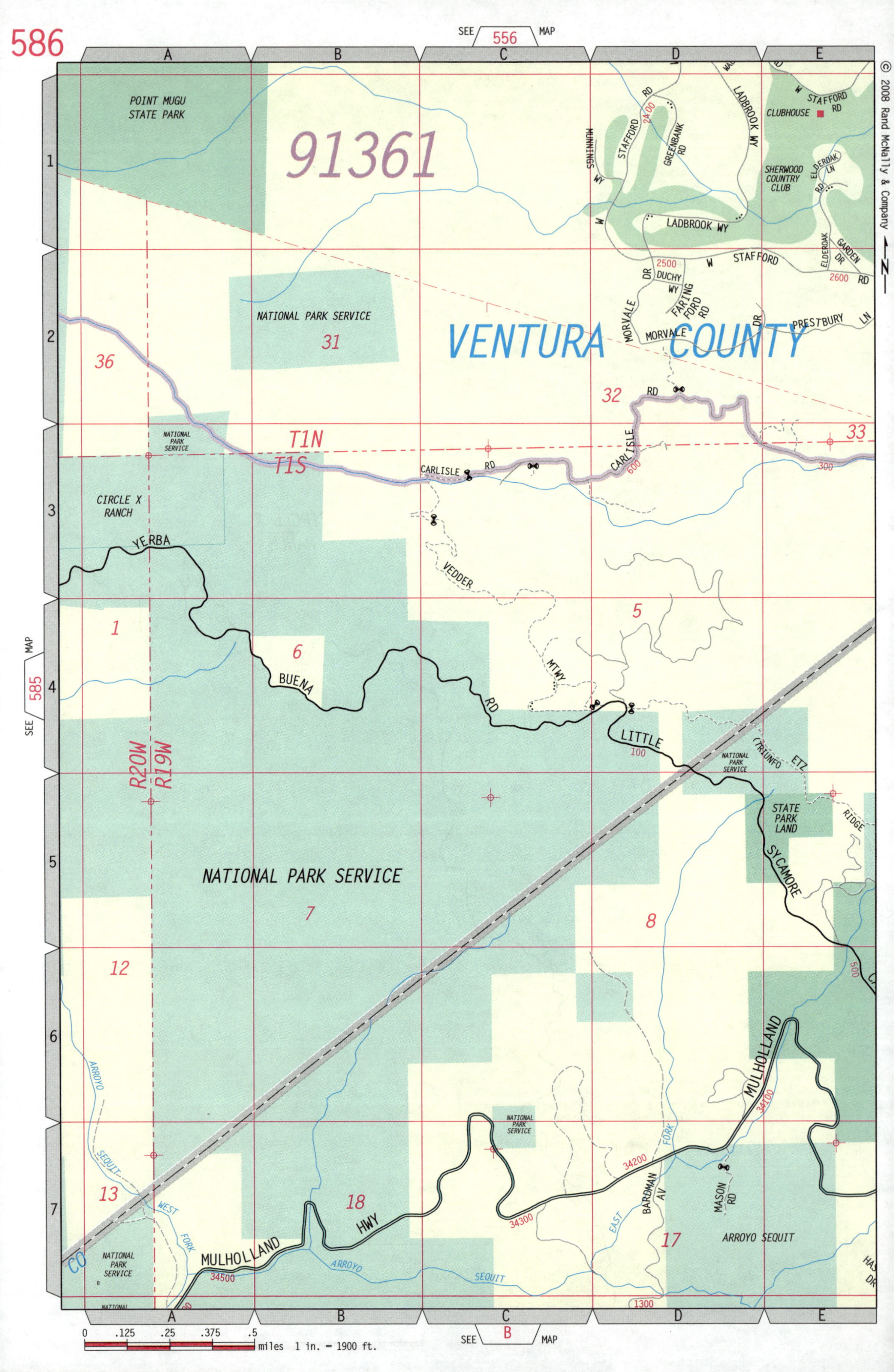
SEE 556 MAP
POINT MUGU STATE PARK
91361
STAFFORD RD
GREENBANK RD
LADBROOK WY
W STAFFORD RD
CLUBHOUSE
SHERWOOD COUNTRY CLUB
ELDEROAK LN
ELDEROAK RD
ELDEROAK DR
GARDEN DR
MUNNINGS WY
LADBROOK WY
W STAFFORD RD
2500
2600
MORVALE DR
DUCHY WY
FARINGFORD RD
NATIONAL PARK SERVICE
31
36
VENTURA COUNTY
MORVALE DR
PRESTBURY LN
32
CARLISLE RD
33
T1N
T1S
NATIONAL PARK SERVICE
CARLISLE RD
300
600
CIRCLE X RANCH
YERBA
VEDDER
5
1
6
MTWY
BUENA RD
LITTLE
100
NATIONAL PARK SERVICE
TRIUNFO
ETZ
R20W
R19W
STATE PARK LAND
RIDGE
SYCAMORE
NATIONAL PARK SERVICE
7
8
12
500
MULHOLLAND
34100
NATIONAL PARK SERVICE
34200
FORK
ARROYO
SEQUIT
13
WEST FORK
18
HWY
34300
BARDMAN AV
MASON RD
EAST
17
ARROYO SEQUIT
MULHOLLAND
34500
NATIONAL PARK SERVICE
ARROYO
SEQUIT
1300
SEE 585 MAP
SEE B MAP
0 .125 .25 .375 .5
miles 1 in. = 1900 ft.
© 2008 Rand McNally & Company

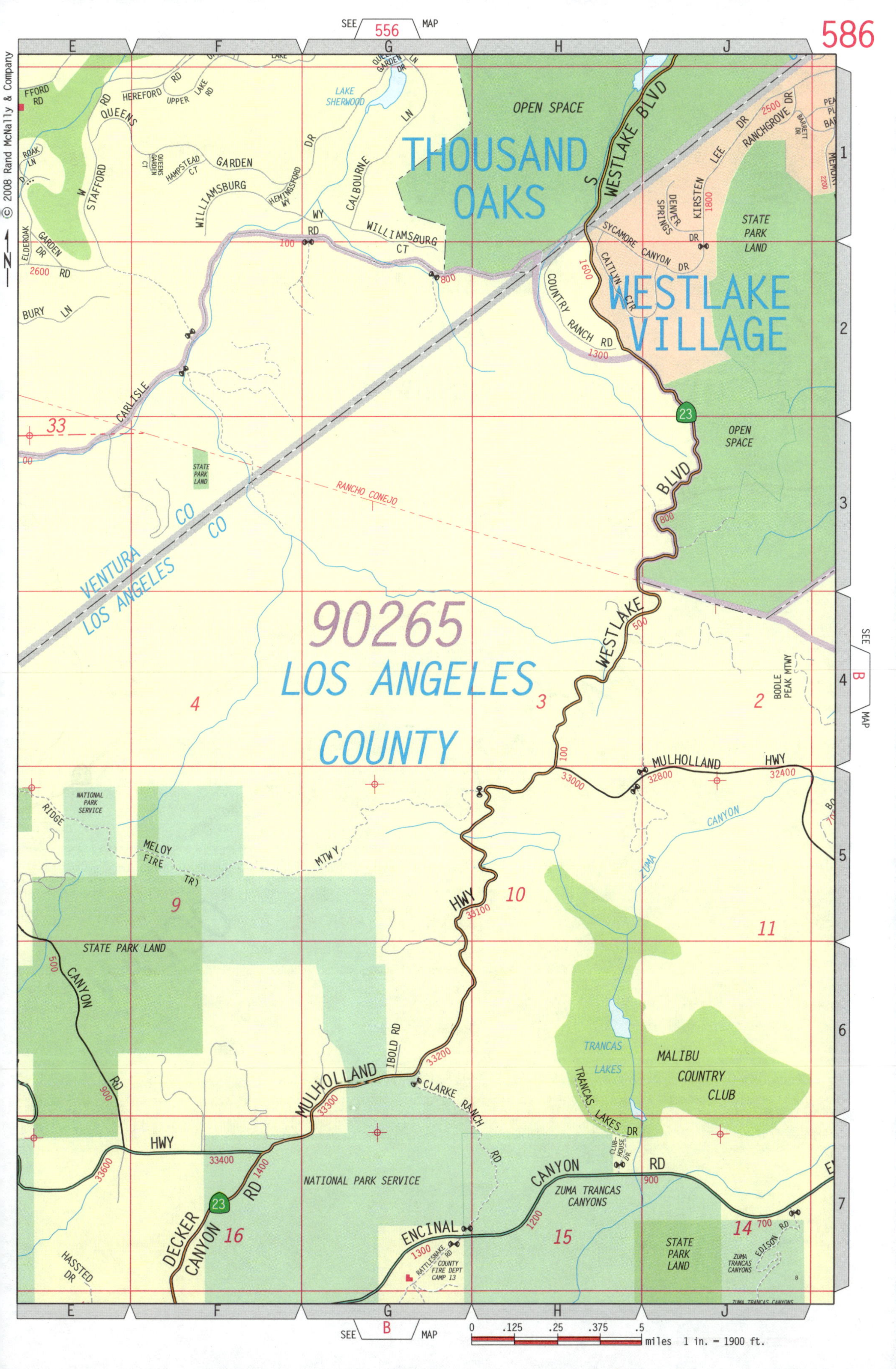

SEE 556 MAP
THOUSAND OAKS
WESTLAKE VILLAGE
OPEN SPACE
STATE PARK LAND
90265
LOS ANGELES COUNTY
VENTURA CO
LOS ANGELES CO
RANCHO CONEJO
WESTLAKE BLVD
MULHOLLAND HWY
NATIONAL PARK SERVICE
MELOY FIRE TR
STATE PARK LAND
MALIBU COUNTRY CLUB
TRANCAS LAKES
TRANCAS LAKES DR
ZUMA TRANCAS CANYONS
ENCINAL CANYON RD
DECKER CANYON RD
CLARKE RANCH RD
COUNTY FIRE DEPT CAMP 13
SEE B MAP
miles 1 in. = 1900 ft.

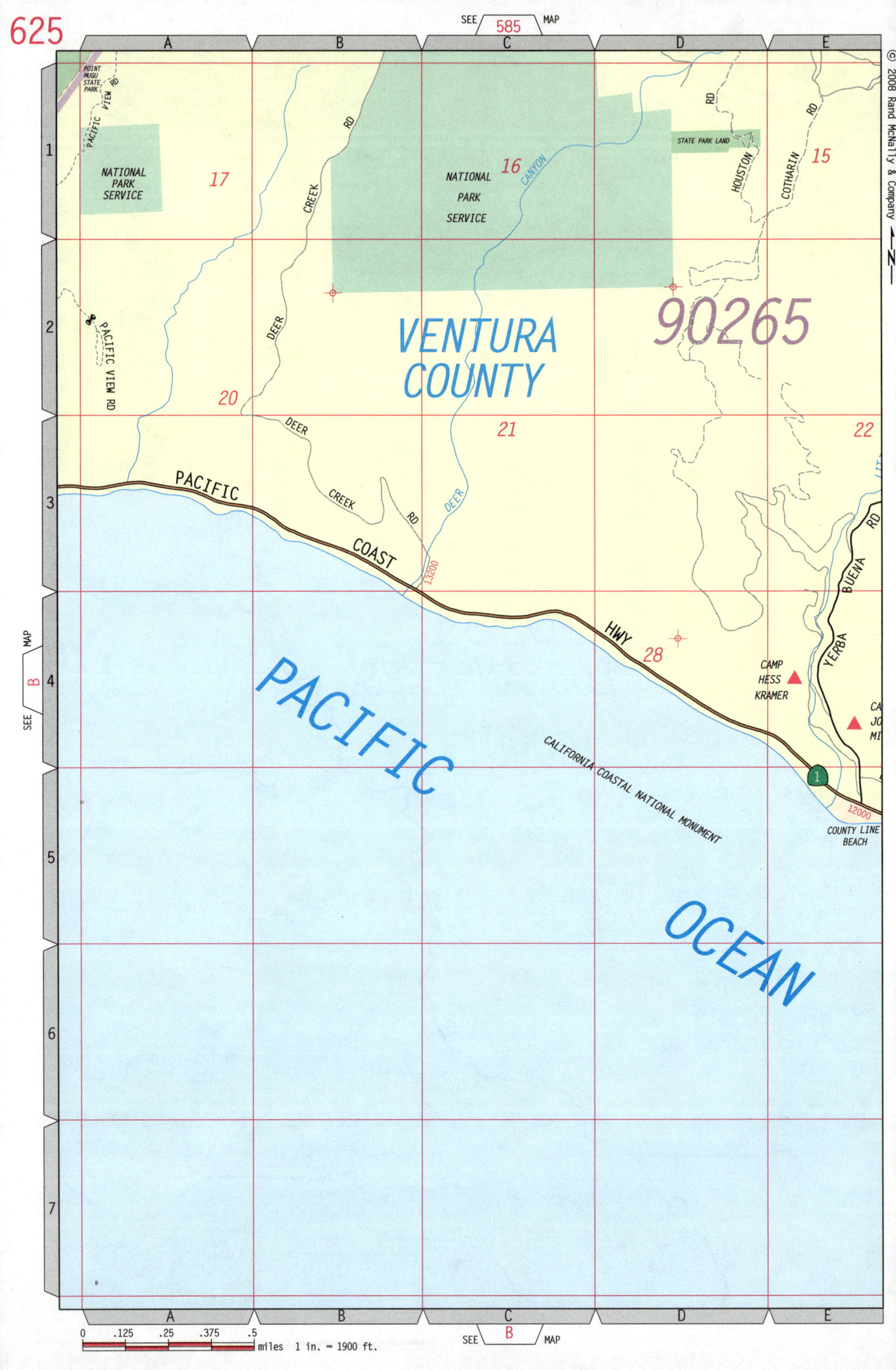
SEE 585 MAP
A
B
C
D
E
1
2
3
4
5
6
7
© 2008 Rand McNally & Company
POINT MUGU STATE PARK
PACIFIC VIEW RD
NATIONAL PARK SERVICE
17
DEER CREEK RD
NATIONAL PARK SERVICE
16
CANYON
STATE PARK LAND
RD
HOUSTON RD
COTHARIN RD
15
PACIFIC VIEW RD
VENTURA COUNTY
90265
20
DEER CREEK RD
21
22
PACIFIC COAST HWY
DEER
13200
28
YERBA BUENA RD
CAMP HESS KRAMER
PACIFIC OCEAN
CALIFORNIA COASTAL NATIONAL MONUMENT
1
12000
COUNTY LINE BEACH
SEE B MAP
0 .125 .25 .375 .5 miles 1 in. = 1900 ft.
SEE B MAP

SEE 585 MAP

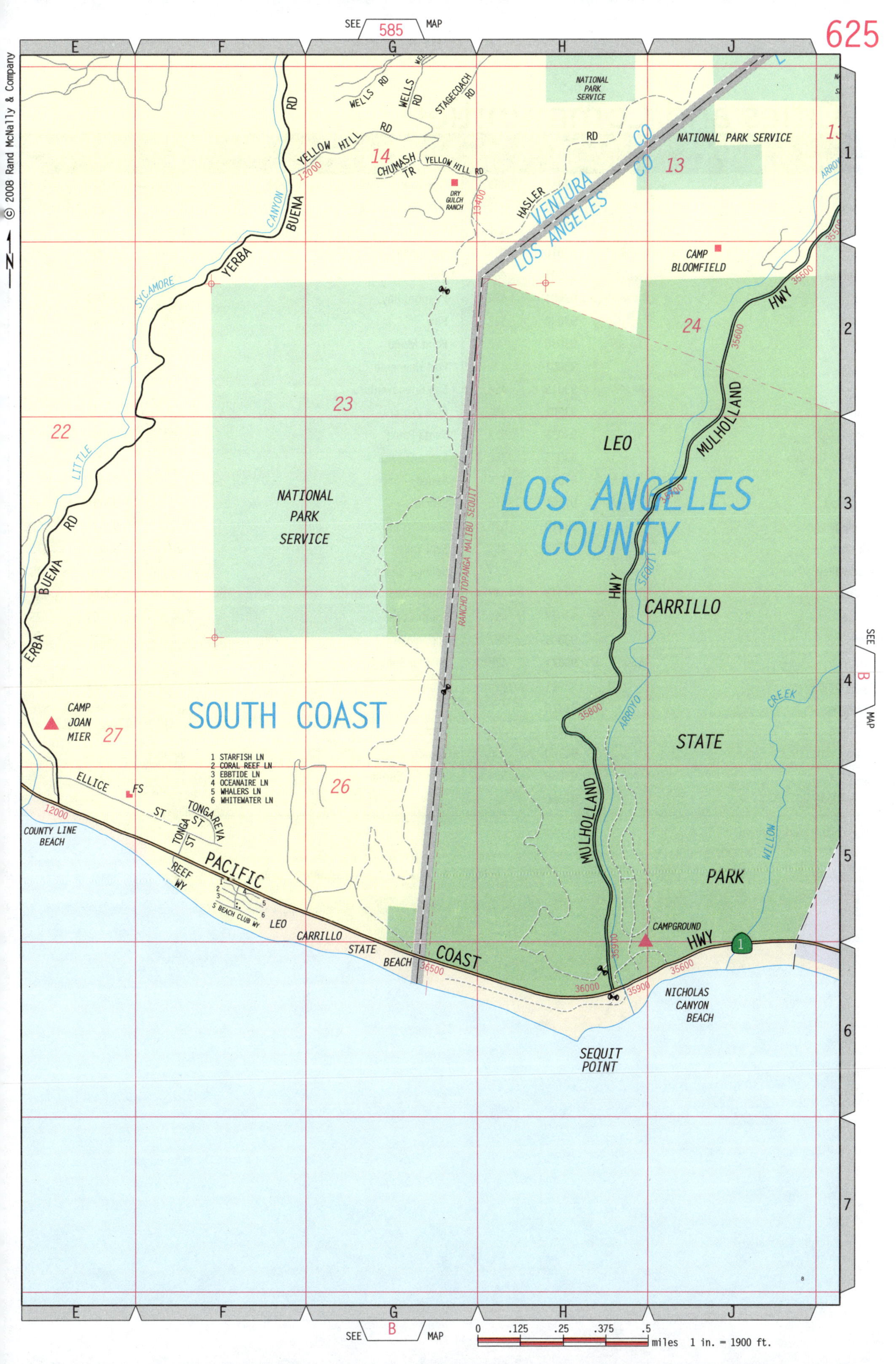

NATIONAL PARK SERVICE
WELLS RD
WELLS RD
STAGECOACH RD
YELLOW HILL RD
14
CHUMASH TR
YELLOW HILL RD
DRY GULCH RANCH
HASLER RD
VENTURA CO
LOS ANGELES CO
13
NATIONAL PARK SERVICE
CAMP BLOOMFIELD
YERBA BUENA RD
SYCAMORE CANYON
24
MULHOLLAND HWY
23
22
LITTLE
LEO
LOS ANGELES COUNTY
NATIONAL PARK SERVICE
RANCHO TOPANGA MALIBU SEQUIT
CARRILLO
SEQUIT
CAMP JOAN MIER
27
SOUTH COAST
STATE
ARROYO
CREEK
1 STARFISH LN
2 CORAL REEF LN
3 EBBTIDE LN
4 OCEANAIRE LN
5 WHALERS LN
6 WHITEWATER LN
26
ELLICE ST
FS
TONGAREVA ST
TONGA ST
COUNTY LINE BEACH
REEF WY
PACIFIC COAST HWY
BEACH CLUB WY
LEO CARRILLO STATE BEACH
MULHOLLAND HWY
WILLOW
PARK
CAMPGROUND
NICHOLAS CANYON BEACH
SEQUIT POINT

SEE B MAP

0 .125 .25 .375 .5 miles 1 in. = 1900 ft.

SEE B MAP

Cities and Communities

Community Name	Abbr.	ZIP Code	Map Page
Bardsdale		93015	465
Bell Canyon		91307	529
Buckhorn		93015	457
* Camarillo	CMRL	93010	524
Casitas Springs		93001	460
Chrisman		93001	471
Colonia		93030	522
El Rio		93030	522
Faria Beach		93001	470
* Fillmore	FILM	93015	456
Foster Park		93001	461
Hollywood Beach		93035	552
Hollywood-By-The-Sea		93035	552
La Conchita		93001	459
Lake Sherwood		91361	556
Leisure Village		93010	525
Live Oak Acres		93022	451
Lockwood Valley			367
Meiners Oaks		93023	441
Mira Monte		93023	451
Montalvo		93003	492
* Moorpark	MRPK	93021	476
Moorpark Home Acres		93021	496
Newbury Park		91320	525
North Fillmore		93015	455
Norwegian Grade		91360	496
Nyeland Acres		93030	523
Oakbrook Village		91360	527
Oak Park		91377	558
Oak View		93022	451
* Ojai	OJAI	93023	441
Ortonville		93001	471
* Oxnard	OXN	93030	522
Pierpont Bay		93003	491
Piru		93040	457
Point Mugu		93041	387
* Port Hueneme	PHME	93041	552
* San Buenaventura			
(See Ventura)			
* Santa Paula	SPLA	93060	464
Santa Susana		93063	499
Saticoy		93004	473
Seacliff		93001	459
Silver Strand		93030	552
* Simi Valley	SIMI	93065	478
Solimar Beach		93001	470
Somis		93066	495
South Coast		90265	625
Springville		93010	523
Sulphur Springs		93060	453
Summit		93023	453
* Thousand Oaks	THO	91360	526
* Ventura	VEN	93001	491
--Ventura County	VeCo		
Wheeler Springs		93023	366

*Indicates incorporated city

List of Abbreviations

PREFIXES AND SUFFIXES	
AL	ALLEY
ARC	ARCADE
AV, AVE	AVENUE
AVCT	AVENUE COURT
AVD	AVENIDA
AVD D LA	AVENIDA DE LA
AVD D LOS	AVENIDA DE LOS
AVD DE	AVENIDA DE
AVD DE LAS	AVENIDA DE LAS
AVD DEL	AVENIDA DEL
AVDR	AVENUE DRIVE
AVEX	AVENUE EXTENSION
AV OF	AVENUE OF
AV OF THE	AVENUE OF THE
AVPL	AVENUE PLACE
BAY	BAY
BEND	BEND
BL, BLVD	BOULEVARD
BLCT	BOULEVARD COURT
BLEX	BOULEVARD EXTENSION
BRCH	BRANCH
BRDG	BRIDGE
BYPS	BYPASS
BYWY	BYWAY
CIDR	CIRCLE DRIVE
CIR	CIRCLE
CL	CALLE
CL DE	CALLE DE
CL DL	CALLE DEL
CL D LA	CALLE DE LA
CL D LAS	CALLE DE LAS
CL D LOS	CALLE DE LOS
CL EL	CALLE EL
CLJ	CALLEJON
CL LA	CALLE LA
CL LAS	CALLE LAS
CL LOS	CALLE LOS
CLTR	CLUSTER
CM	CAMINO
CM DE	CAMINO DE
CM DL	CAMINO DEL
CM D LA	CAMINO DE LA
CM D LAS	CAMINO DE LAS
CM D LOS	CAMINO DE LOS
CMTO	CAMINITO
CMTO DEL	CAMINITO DEL
CMTO D LA	CAMINITO DE LA
CMTO D LAS	CAMINITO DE LAS
CMTO D LOS	CAMINITO DE LOS
CNDR	CENTER DRIVE
COM	COMMON
COMS	COMMONS
CORR	CORRIDOR
CRES	CRESCENT
CRLO	CIRCULO
CRSG	CROSSING
CST	CIRCLE STREET
CSWY	CAUSEWAY
CT	COURT
CTAV	COURT AVENUE
CTE	CORTE
CTE D	CORTE DE
CTE DEL	CORTE DEL
CTE D LAS	CORTE DE LAS
CTO	CUT OFF
CTR	CENTER
CTST	COURT STREET
CUR	CURVE
CV	COVE
DE	DE
DIAG	DIAGONAL
DR	DRIVE
DRAV	DRIVE AVENUE
DRCT	DRIVE COURT
DRLP	DRIVE LOOP
DVDR	DIVISION DR
EXAV	EXTENSION AVENUE
EXBL	EXTENSION BOULEVARD
EXRD	EXTENSION ROAD
EXST	EXTENSION STREET
EXT	EXTENSION
EXWY	EXPRESSWAY
FOREST RT	FOREST ROUTE
FRWY	FREEWAY
FRY	FERRY
GDNS	GARDENS
GN, GLN	GLEN
GRN	GREEN
GRV	GROVE
HTS	HEIGHTS
HWY	HIGHWAY
ISL	ISLE
JCT	JUNCTION
LN	LANE
LNCR	LANE CIRCLE
LNDG	LANDING
LNDR	LAND DRIVE
LNLP	LANE LOOP
LP	LOOP
MNR	MANOR
MT	MOUNT
MTWY	MOTORWAY
MWCR	MEWS COURT
MWLN	MEWS LANE
NFD	NAT'L FOREST DEV
NK	NOOK
OH	OUTER HIGHWAY
OVL	OVAL
OVLK	OVERLOOK
OVPS	OVERPASS
PAS	PASEO
PAS DE	PASEO DE
PAS DE LA	PASEO DE LA
PAS DE LAS	PASEO DE LAS
PAS DE LOS	PASEO DE LOS
PAS DL	PASEO DEL
PASG	PASSAGE
PAS LA	PASEO LA
PAS LOS	PASEO LOS
PASS	PASS
PIKE	PIKE
PK	PARK
PKDR	PARK DRIVE
PKWY, PKY	PARKWAY
PL	PLACE
PLWY	PLACE WAY
PLZ, PZ	PLAZA
PT	POINT
PTAV	POINT AVENUE
PTH	PATH
PZ DE	PLAZA DE
PZ DEL	PLAZA DEL
PZ D LA	PLAZA DE LA
PZ D LAS	PLAZA DE LAS
PZWY	PLAZA WAY
RAMP	RAMP
RD	ROAD
RDAV	ROAD AVENUE
RDBP	ROAD BYPASS
RDCT	ROAD COURT
RDEX	ROAD EXTENSION
RDG	RIDGE
RDSP	ROAD SPUR
RDWY	ROAD WAY
RR	RAILROAD
RUE	RUE
RUE D	RUE D
RW	ROW
RY	RAILWAY
SKWY	SKYWAY
SQ	SQUARE
ST	STREET
STAV	STREET AVENUE
STCT	STREET COURT
STDR	STREET DRIVE
STEX	STREET EXTENSION
STLN	STREET LANE
STLP	STREET LOOP
ST OF	STREET OF
ST OF THE	STREET OF THE
STOV	STREET OVERPASS
STPL	STREET PLACE
STPM	STREET PROMENADE
STWY	STREET WAY
STXP	STREET EXPRESSWAY
TER	TERRACE
TFWY	TRAFFICWAY
THWY	THROUGHWAY
TKTR	TRUCK TRAIL
TPKE	TURNPIKE
TRC	TRACE
TRCT	TERRACE COURT
TR, TRL	TRAIL
TRWY	TRAIL WAY
TTSP	TRUCK TRAIL SPUR
TUN	TUNNEL
UNPS	UNDERPASS
VIA D	VIA DE
VIA DL	VIA DEL
VIA D LA	VIA DE LA
VIA D LAS	VIA DE LAS
VIA D LOS	VIA DE LOS
VIA LA	VIA LA
VW	VIEW
VWY	VIEW WAY
VIS	VISTA
VIS D	VISTA DE
VIS D L	VISTA DE LA
VIS D LAS	VISTA DE LAS
VIS DEL	VISTA DEL
WK	WALK
WY	WAY
WYCR	WAY CIRCLE
WYDR	WAY DRIVE
WYLN	WAY LANE
WYPL	WAY PLACE

DIRECTIONS	
E	EAST
KPN	KEY PENINSULA NORTH
KPS	KEY PENINSULA SOUTH
N	NORTH
NE	NORTHEAST
NW	NORTHWEST
S	SOUTH
SE	SOUTHEAST
SW	SOUTHWEST
W	WEST

BUILDINGS	
CH	CITY HALL
CHP	CALIFORNIA HIGHWAY PATROL
COMM CTR	COMMUNITY CENTER
CON CTR	CONVENTION CENTER
CONT HS	CONTINUATION HIGH SCHOOL
CTH	COURTHOUSE
FAA	FEDERAL AVIATION ADMIN
FS	FIRE STATION
HOSP	HOSPITAL
HS	HIGH SCHOOL
INT	INTERMEDIATE SCHOOL
JR HS	JUNIOR HIGH SCHOOL
LIB	LIBRARY
MID	MIDDLE SCHOOL
MUS	MUSEUM
PO	POST OFFICE
PS	POLICE STATION
SR CIT CTR	SENIOR CITIZENS CENTER
STA	STATION
THTR	THEATER
VIS BUR	VISITORS BUREAU

OTHER ABBREVIATIONS	
BCH	BEACH
BLDG	BUILDING
CEM	CEMETERY
CK	CREEK
CO	COUNTY
COMM	COMMUNITY
CTR	CENTER
EST	ESTATE
HIST	HISTORIC
HTS	HEIGHTS
LK	LAKE
MDW	MEADOW
MED	MEDICAL
MEM	MEMORIAL
MT	MOUNT
MTN	MOUNTAIN
NATL	NATIONAL
PKG	PARKING
PLGD	PLAYGROUND
RCH	RANCH
RCHO	RANCHO
REC	RECREATION
RES	RESERVOIR
RIV	RIVER
RR	RAILROAD
SPG	SPRING
STA	SANTA
VLG	VILLAGE
VLY	VALLEY
VW	VIEW

City ZIP Pg-Grid
A
VeCo 93042 583-H3
OXN 93033 552-G3
OXN 93030 522-G5
FILM 93015 456-A6
FILM 93015 455-J4
OXN 93033 552-G3
#-23
FILM 93015 456-A6
FILM 93015 466-A1
PHME 93041 552-E5
OXN 93030 522-G5
PHME 93041 552-E5
NE CV
PHME 93041 552-C2
NE DR
OXN 93035 552-A2
CT
THO 91320 555-F4
VOOD CT
SIMI 93063 498-D1
VOOD DR
CanP 91307 529-D5
TON CT
WLKV 91361 557-D6
BURY ST
VeCo 91361 556-F6
AV
CMRL 93010 524-G1
CMRL 93010 494-G7
ST
OXN 93033 553-A5
ARE ST
VEN 93004 492-G3
E ST
SIMI 93063 478-H5
VEN 93004 492-H2
R
SIMI 93065 498-A4
AM ST
SIMI 93065 498-A3
DR
CMRL 93012 525-A3
AJ RD
VeCo 93060 453-D2
VeCo 93023 451-C3
LN
VEN 93004 493-A2
RD
VeCo 91320 556-C2
SPLA 93060 463-J7
SPLA 93060 473-J1
ST
OXN 93033 552-H2
CMRL 93012 524-F4
WY
SPLA 93060 473-J1
GLEN ST
AGRH 91301 558-B3
Y DR
THO 91320 525-H6
AV
AGRH 91301 558-B3
PL
VEN 93003 492-B4
ST
SIMI 93065 498-D3
T
CMRL 93010 524-G1
US CT
AGRH 91301 558-A3
CO AV
SIMI 93065 497-F4
CO CT
SIMI 93065 497-F3
OXN 93035 522-E7
T
SIMI 93063 498-E2
RD
PHME 93043 552-C5
ST
Chat 91311 499-J6
T
SIMI 93065 498-A1
PHME 93041 552-E4
D
SIMI 93063 478-F7
R RD
CALB 91302 558-H3
ST
VEN 93003 492-E1
CANYON RD
VeCo 93060 463-F3
VeCo 93060 453-E7
CIR
VEN 93003 492-F4
N CIR
THO 91360 526-F4
ST
PHME 93041 552-E5
PHME 93043 552-E3
E CT
OXN 93035 552-C1
THO 91360 526-D5
CT
AGRH 91301 557-H5
ACK AV
VEN 93003 472-B7
VEN 93003 492-B1
ACK CT
SIMI 93065 497-C6
NDACK CT
THO 91362 557-C2
NDACK CT
THO 91362 557-B2
PL
MRPK 93021 496-F2
CT
VeCo 91377 527-H7
WY
OXN 93035 522-A7
Y
CMRL 93012 525-C2
N
CMRL 93012 524-H5
CMRL 93012 525-A5
RD
CMRL 93010 524-G1
CMRL 93012 524-G1

STREET Block City ZIP Pg-Grid
ADOLFO RD
5200 CMRL 93012 525-A3
ADONIS PL
4600 MRPK 93021 496-F2
ADRIAN ST
1700 THO 91320 556-A1
1900 THO 91320 555-J1
ADRIATIC ST
- OXN 93035 522-B7
AFFIRMED PL
6300 MRPK 93021 476-A6
AGATE CT
2100 SIMI 93065 497-G2
7900 VEN 93004 492-F3
AGATE ST
3500 THO 91360 526-H1
8000 VEN 93004 492-F3
AGGEN RD
4000 VeCo 93066 494-F3
5100 VeCo 93066 474-E7
AGNEW ST
1100 SIMI 93065 497-H2
AGNUS DR
200 VEN 93003 491-H2
AGOURA CT
29900 AGRH 91301 557-H6
AGOURA RD
2600 THO 91361 557-B5
2900 WLKV 91361 557-D5
26400 CALB 91302 558-G7
26600 LACo 91302 558-G7
26800 CALB 91301 558-G7
27000 Ago 91301 558-D6
27400 AGRH 91301 558-A6
29200 AGRH 91301 557-G6
AGOURA GLEN DR
5500 AGRH 91301 558-B5
AGUSTA AV
1000 CMRL 93010 524-D1
AHART ST
1200 SIMI 93065 497-H2
AHOY LN
- OXN 93035 552-A1
AILEEN ST
500 CMRL 93010 524-B2
AIREDALE AV
2000 VEN 93003 492-F5
AIREDALE CT
7300 VEN 93003 492-F5
AIRPORT WY
100 CMRL 93010 524-A5
AKERS ST
700 FILM 93015 456-A5
AKRON AV
700 VEN 93004 492-J1
AL WY
6000 SIMI 93063 499-B2
ALAMAR ST
- THO 91360 526-F2
ALAMEDA AV
2000 VeCo 93003 492-D5
2000 VEN 93003 492-D5
ALAMO ST
1700 SIMI 93065 497-J1
1700 SIMI 93065 498-A1
1900 SIMI 93065 478-A7
3300 SIMI 93063 478-C7
5400 SIMI 93063 479-A7
ALAMOS DR
1100 THO 91362 556-H1
ALAMOS CANYON RD
23600 SIMI 93065 477-D7
23600 VeCo 93065 477-D7
ALAN CT
23600 SIMI 93063 498-H1
ALANDIA CT
4200 MRPK 93021 496-E3
ALASKA DR
5700 VEN 93003 492-C5
ALBACORE WY
200 OXN 93035 552-B4
ALBANY AV
700 VEN 93004 492-H2
ALBANY DR
2800 OXN 93033 552-H2
ALBATROSS ST
6400 VEN 93003 492-D4
ALBERTSON MTWY
- VeCo 93065 527-G4
23600 SIMI 93063 528-E2
23600 SIMI 93065 527-G4
23600 SIMI 93065 528-C2
23600 THO 91362 527-G4
23600 VeCo 93063 528-E2
23600 VeCo 93065 528-A3
ALBION AV
5700 VEN 93003 492-C1
ALBION DR
- OXN 93036 492-H5
ALBION PL
- THO 91320 556-A2
ALBORADA DR
23600 CMRL 93010 494-C7
ALCOVE ST
500 SIMI 93065 527-D1
E ALDEN ST
2300 SIMI 93065 498-B1
N ALDEN ST
2400 SIMI 93065 498-C1
ALDER CIR
- MRPK 93021 496-G3
ALDERBROOK ST
11700 MRPK 93021 496-C4
ALDERCREEK PL
1300 THO 91362 527-C6
ALDERDALE CT
23600 THO 91320 555-E4
ALDERGLEN ST
12300 MRPK 93021 496-D3
ALDERGROVE ST
12100 MRPK 93021 496-D4
ALDER SPRINGS DR
300 VeCo 91377 558-B1
ALDER VIEW LN
23600 CMRL 93012 525-A1
ALDER WOOD PL
1500 THO 91362 526-J2
ALDREN CT
5500 AGRH 91301 557-G5
ALDRICH CT
300 THO 91360 526-F4
A LEASE CANYON RD
23600 VeCo 93001 470-D3
ALEE LN
- OXN 93035 522-B7
ALELIA AV
1200 VeCo 93004 493-B1
ALEPPO CT
1700 THO 91362 526-J4

STREET Block City ZIP Pg-Grid
ALESSANDRO DR
1200 THO 91320 556-B1
1500 VEN 93001 491-D3
ALEUTIAN WY
- OXN 93035 552-B1
ALEX CT
- THO 91320 555-E2
ALEXANDER DR
4700 OXN 93033 553-A5
ALEXANDER ST
1100 SIMI 93065 497-H2
1700 OXN 93033 553-A2
ALEXANDRA CT
23600 VeCo 91377 528-A7
ALEXANDRIA ST
10200 VEN 93004 492-J2
ALFA RD
23600 VeCo 93063 498-H7
23600 VeCo 93063 528-H1
ALFONSO DR
5300 AGRH 91301 557-H5
ALFREDO CT
5500 AGRH 91301 557-H5
ALGONQUIAN ST
700 VEN 93001 471-D5
ALGONQUIN CT
2900 CMRL 93010 524-F1
ALGONQUIN DR
2100 SIMI 93065 497-D2
ALHAMBRA AV
- VEN 93004 492-F1
ALHAMBRA CT
- VeCo 93012 496-E7
ALIANO DR
4800 VeCo 91377 557-G1
ALICANTE CT
- VeCo 93012 496-E7
ALICE DR
3000 THO 91320 555-G1
3000 VeCo 91320 555-G1
ALICE ANN RD
2400 THO 91320 555-J2
2400 VeCo 91320 555-J2
ALIENTO WY
400 CMRL 93012 524-J2
ALISO LN
100 VEN 93001 491-E2
ALISO PL
300 OXN 93036 522-H3
1300 VEN 93001 491-D1
ALISO ST
100 OJAI 93023 441-H6
200 VEN 93001 491-D1
400 VEN 93001 471-D7
N ALISO ST
100 VEN 93001 491-E1
W ALISO ST
100 OJAI 93023 441-H6
ALISO CANYON RD
2900 VeCo 93060 462-H3
6200 VeCo 93060 472-J1
6700 VeCo 93060 473-A2
23600 VeCo 93060 452-G7
ALISON DR
12400 VeCo 93012 496-D7
ALIZIA CANYON DR
26000 CALB 91302 558-H3
26000 VeCo 91302 558-H3
N ALLEGHENY CT
200 THO 91362 557-B3
S ALLEGHENY CT
100 THO 91362 557-B3
ALLEGRO CT
200 SIMI 93065 527-D1
ALLEN ST
1100 THO 91320 556-B1
ALLENBY CT
32000 WLKV 91361 557-C6
ALLENVALE CT
500 SIMI 93065 497-D7
ALLMAN ST
28900 AGRH 91301 558-A3
ALLYSON CT
23600 THO 91362 527-B5
ALMADEN CT
2500 SIMI 93065 498-A1
ALMANOR ST
1800 OXN 93030 522-J3
1800 OXN 93036 522-J3
ALMAR ST
6300 SIMI 93063 499-C2
ALMENDRA PL
800 OXN 93036 522-H3
ALMENDRO CT
1500 CMRL 93010 524-G1
ALMENDRO WY
3500 CMRL 93010 524-G1
ALMON DR
200 THO 91362 557-A2
ALMOND AV
10400 VeCo 93022 451-C6
ALMOND DR
3400 VeCo 93036 523-D2
ALMOND TREE CT
23600 SIMI 93063 498-D4
ALOE LN
23600 SIMI 93065 497-E5
ALOHA LN
1800 OXN 93033 552-J1
1800 OXN 93033 553-A1
ALOHA ST
2600 CMRL 93010 494-F7
2600 VeCo 93010 494-F7
ALOMAR ST
600 VeCo 93023 451-C3
ALOSTA DR
100 VeCo 93010 494-F6
ALOSTA LN
1300 CMRL 93010 494-G6
1300 VeCo 93010 494-G6
ALOSTA PL
300 VeCo 93010 494-G6
600 CMRL 93010 494-G6
ALOSTA WY
600 VeCo 93010 494-G6
ALPINE AV
100 VEN 93004 472-H6
ALPINE CT
400 VEN 93004 472-H6
2800 THO 91362 557-C3
ALPINE ST
100 OXN 93030 522-J5
4400 SIMI 93063 498-G2
ALSACE DR
- Ago 91301 558-G3
- LACo 91302 558-G3
ALSCOT AV
1800 SIMI 93063 499-B1
ALTA ST
4800 SIMI 93063 478-H7

STREET Block City ZIP Pg-Grid
ALTA WY
23200 Chat 91311 499-F6
ALTA COLINA RD
4900 CMRL 93012 524-J2
5100 CMRL 93012 525-A2
ALTADENA ST
8300 VEN 93004 492-F1
E ALTA GREEN ST
100 PHME 93041 552-E2
W ALTA GREEN ST
100 PHME 93041 552-D2
ALTAIR AV
2700 THO 91360 526-F3
ALTA MIRA ST
400 VeCo 93065 497-G5
23600 SIMI 93065 497-G5
ALTAMONT WY
- VeCo 93010 494-C6
ALTA SAGUNA CT
23600 CMRL 93010 494-C7
ALTA VISTA PL
23600 CMRL 93012 494-J7
23600 CMRL 93012 524-H1
ALTA VISTA RD
600 VeCo 93063 499-B4
ALTA VISTA RIDGE RD
6300 VeCo 93063 499-C4
ALTHEA CT
1300 OXN 93036 522-E3
ALTO CT
300 VeCo 93022 451-C5
ALTO DR
- VeCo 93022 451-C5
ALTUNA CT
3300 THO 91360 526-H2
ALTURAS ST
1300 OXN 93035 552-D1
ALTUS WY
2700 OXN 93035 552-D1
ALUMNI WY
7300 MRPK 93021 477-A4
ALVA CIR
1500 SIMI 93065 498-B3
N ALVARADO AV
100 VeCo 93023 441-D6
S ALVARADO AV
100 VeCo 93023 441-D7
ALVARADO ST
2400 OXN 93036 522-J2
2400 VeCo 93036 522-J2
3000 VeCo 93036 523-A1
ALVERSTONE AV
600 VEN 93003 492-B1
600 VEN 93003 472-B7
ALVIRIA DR
1100 VeCo 93023 451-B1
ALVISO DR
1200 VeCo 93010 494-A7
ALVISO ST
1500 SIMI 93065 497-J2
1700 SIMI 93065 498-A2
ALYSHEBA DR
10600 MRPK 93021 476-A7
ALYSSAS CT
23600 MRPK 93021 476-J6
ALYSSUM LN
- VEN 93004 493-A2
AMADOR AV
300 VEN 93004 472-H6
400 VeCo 93004 472-H6
AMADOR LN
1500 THO 91320 526-A7
AMAGRO WY
100 OXN 93033 552-G5
AMALFI DR
1300 SIMI 93063 499-C3
AMALFI WY
5000 OXN 93035 551-J1
5000 OXN 93035 552-A1
AMAPOLA AV
1200 VeCo 93004 493-B1
AMARELLE ST
1000 THO 91320 526-A6
AMARILLO AV
3000 SIMI 93063 478-G7
AMARYLLIS AV
23600 SIMI 93065 497-G5
AMAZON RIVER CT
- OXN 93036 492-G7
- OXN 93036 522-H1
AMBER AV
1100 OXN 93030 522-D4
AMBER DR
1000 SPLA 93060 464-A2
2600 CMRL 93010 494-E7
2600 VeCo 93010 494-E7
AMBER LN
800 OJAI 93023 451-G1
800 VeCo 93023 451-G1
AMBERCREST PL
4000 THO 91362 557-D1
AMBER GROVE CT
2300 SIMI 93065 478-B7
AMBERLEAF LN
23600 SIMI 93065 497-A1
AMBERLY PL
2300 SIMI 93065 498-B1
AMBERMEADOW ST
12500 MRPK 93021 496-D3
AMBERRIDGE CT
11500 MRPK 93021 496-B4
AMBERTON LN
1100 THO 91320 556-B1
AMBERWICK LN
4300 MRPK 93021 496-F3
AMBER WOOD PL
2600 THO 91362 526-J3
AMBRIDGE DR
5000 CALB 91301 558-F6
AMBROSE AV
1400 OXN 93035 552-D1
AMBROSIA ST
- OXN 93030 522-G4
AMELIA CT
100 OXN 93030 522-J5
AMELIA DR
30100 AGRH 91301 557-H5
AMERICAN ST
400 SIMI 93065 477-G7
AMERICAN WY
1800 VEN 93004 492-G4
AMERICAN OAKS AV
400 THO 91320 555-H3
AMERITE WY
2800 SIMI 93065 477-G7
AMETHYST AV
- VEN 93004 492-F3
1400 OXN 93030 522-D4
AMGEN CT
600 THO 91320 526-A7

STREET Block City ZIP Pg-Grid
AMGEN CENTER DR
2000 THO 91320 525-J7
2000 THO 91320 526-A7
AMHERST ST
5500 VEN 93003 492-B2
E AMHERST ST
14300 MRPK 93021 476-G6
N AMHERST ST
6400 MRPK 93021 476-H6
AMIGO RD
100 Chat 91311 499-F6
AMOND LN
8300 LA 91304 529-F2
AMONDO CIR
5900 SIMI 93063 499-A1
AMPHITHEATER RD
23600 VeCo 93001 470-E4
AMY PL
2600 PHME 93041 552-D2
ANACAPA AV
100 VeCo 93035 552-B5
ANACAPA CIR
400 THO 91320 555-F1
ANACAPA DR
100 CMRL 93010 524-E1
100 VeCo 93010 494-D6
100 VeCo 93010 524-E1
100 CMRL 93010 494-D6
ANACAPA ST
- VEN 93001 491-E3
ANACAPA TER
400 SPLA 93060 463-J6
400 VeCo 93060 463-J6
ANACAPA ISLAND DR
- VeCo 93012 554-E4
ANASAZI CT
23600 SIMI 93063 479-A6
ANASTASIA AV
6200 SIMI 93063 499-B2
ANCHOR AV
2500 PHME 93041 552-B2
2700 PHME 93035 552-B2
ANCHOR CT
2200 THO 91320 525-J6
2200 THO 91320 526-A6
ANCHORAGE AV
2900 SIMI 93063 478-F7
ANCHORAGE ST
3700 OXN 93033 552-J4
ANCHORS WY
1200 VEN 93001 491-F6
ANDALUSIA DR
- VeCo 93012 496-F6
ANDANTE CT
800 CMRL 93012 525-B2
ANDERSON DR
3100 VeCo 93065 478-B7
3100 SIMI 93065 478-B7
3300 SIMI 93063 478-B7
ANDERSON ST
1400 SIMI 93065 497-J2
ANDORA AV
9600 Chat 91311 499-J4
ANDORA PL
9800 Chat 91311 499-H5
ANDREA CIR
1500 SIMI 93065 498-B3
ANDREA CT
700 OXN 93033 552-H5
ANDREA DR
400 OXN 93033 552-H5
ANDREW DR
400 OJAI 93023 441-J5
ANDRUS ST
- VeCo 93022 451-B6
ANGEL CIR
2700 SIMI 93063 478-J7
ANGELA AV
7200 CanP 91307 529-F5
ANGELA ST
2400 SIMI 93065 498-B1
4000 SIMI 93063 498-F1
ANGELINE ST
- THO 91320 555-E3
ANGLER CT
23600 VEN 93001 491-G7
ANGUILA PL
100 CMRL 93012 524-J3
ANGUS AV
1800 SIMI 93063 498-G2
ANITA AV
200 OXN 93030 522-H5
1100 OJAI 93023 442-A6
ANLAUF RD
- VeCo 93060 453-J4
ANLAUF CANYON
- VeCo - 454-A2
- VeCo 93060 453-J4
- VeCo 93060 454-A2
ANN AV
100 PHME 93041 552-F6
N ANN ST
- VEN 93001 491-D2
S ANN ST
- VEN 93001 491-D2
ANNA WY
1400 OXN 93030 522-E3
ANNANDALE LN
2600 SIMI 93063 478-J7
ANNAPOLIS CT
5300 VEN 93003 492-B3
ANN ARBOR AV
700 VEN 93004 492-H2
ANNE CT
200 THO 91320 555-G2
ANNEPE WY
- Chat 91311 479-J7
E ANNETTE ST
13000 MRPK 93021 496-E3
ANSON ST
600 SIMI 93065 497-G4
ANTELOPE AV
1100 VEN 93003 492-E4
ANTELOPE PL
1100 THO 91320 555-G4
ANTHONY DR
2000 VEN 93003 492-E5
ANTIGUA PL
6400 CanP 91307 529-C7
ANTIGUA WY
2300 OXN 93035 552-A2
E ANTIOCH ST
3400 SIMI 93063 498-E2
ANTLER AV
2300 VEN 93003 492-F5
ANTONIO AV
2100 CMRL 93010 494-G6
2400 VeCo 93010 494-G6
ANZA CT
1300 OXN 93035 552-E1

STREET Block City ZIP Pg-Grid
ANZA LN
200 FILM 93015 456-C6
ANZIO WY
600 VeCo 91377 557-H1
APACHE AV
- THO 91362 557-A2
2800 VEN 93001 471-C5
APACHE CIR
3000 THO 91360 526-C2
APACHE CT
1400 CMRL 93010 524-F1
APACHE CANYON RD
- VeCo 93252 366-G1
APERSON RD
- VeCo 93015 367-B7
- VeCo 93015 455-F1
APOLLO CT
2000 SIMI 93065 497-G2
APOLLO DR
500 OXN 93035 521-J6
E APPALACHIAN CT
2800 THO 91362 557-C3
W APPALACHIAN CT
2700 THO 91362 557-B3
N APPALOOSA LN
- VeCo 91307 529-B3
APPIAN WY
300 VEN 93003 491-J2
3400 CMRL 93010 494-G7
APPLE AV
200 VEN 93004 473-A6
APPLE LN
2300 OXN 93036 522-G1
APPLEFIELD ST
1500 THO 91320 526-A6
APPLEGATE TER
9200 Chat 91311 499-F7
APPLEGLEN CT
4400 MRPK 93021 496-D2
APPLETON RD
400 SIMI 93065 498-C4
APPLETREE AV
200 CMRL 93012 524-H4
APPLETREE CT
400 CMRL 93012 524-H5
APPLEWOOD LN
2000 VeCo 93012 496-B7
2000 VeCo 93012 526-B1
APRICOT LN
1400 OXN 93033 553-B5
23600 VeCo 93063 499-B4
APRICOT RD
4000 SIMI 93063 498-F1
APRICOT ST
- VeCo 93022 451-B7
APRIL LN
1000 SPLA 93060 464-A2
AQUAMARINE AV
- VEN 93004 492-G2
AQUARIUS AV
6300 AGRH 91301 558-B3
AQUA VERDE CT
4700 CMRL 93012 524-J2
AQUEDUCT CT
600 SIMI 93065 497-G6
ARABIAN PL
6000 CMRL 93012 525-B1
ARABIAN ST
1400 SIMI 93065 497-J3
ARAGON WY
- OXN 93036 522-H1
ARANMOOR AV
900 THO 91361 557-A5
ARAPAHO AV
2300 THO 91362 556-J2
2300 THO 91362 557-A2
ARAPAHO ST
200 VEN 93001 471-C5
ARBELLA LN
- THO 91362 527-B3
ARBOL LN
6400 VeCo 93063 499-C4
ARBOLITA RANCH RD
2100 VeCo 93066 465-A6
ARBOR AV
600 VEN 93003 491-H4
ARBOR CT
- SIMI 93065 497-G7
ARBOR ST
- CMRL 93012 524-G5
ARBORHILL ST
12100 MRPK 93021 496-D4
ARBOR LANE CT
200 THO 91360 526-D7
ARBORWOOD ST
- FILM 93015 456-B6
ARCADE DR
- VEN 93003 491-F3
ARCADIA ST
1700 OXN 93033 552-H1
ARCADIAN SHORES TR
2400 OXN 93036 522-C2
ARCANE ST
1100 SIMI 93065 497-H4
1700 SIMI 93065 498-A4
ARCATA RD
1100 VeCo 93023 451-B4
ARCH PT
- VeCo 93012 554-F3
ARCH ST
4500 VeCo 93066 494-H4
ARCHBRIAR WY
300 SIMI 93065 497-F3
ARCHWOOD LN
2300 SIMI 93063 498-J1
ARCHWOOD ST
22100 CanP 91303 529-J6
22600 CanP 91307 529-D6
ARCO OIL CO RD
- VeCo 93023 453-B2
- VeCo 93060 453-B2
ARCTURUS AV
5500 OXN 93033 552-H6
ARCTURUS ST
100 THO 91360 526-F3
ARDENWOOD AV
1800 SIMI 93063 499-D2
E ARDENWOOD AV
6500 SIMI 93063 499-C2
N ARDENWOOD CIR
6600 SIMI 93063 499-D2
ARDMORE LN
- OXN 93036 522-C3
AREA I RD
23600 VeCo 93063 499-A7
23600 VeCo 93063 529-A1
ARENAS CT
3000 SIMI 93063 478-F7
ARGAL PL
2200 VEN 93003 492-E5

STREET Block City ZIP Pg-Grid
ARGOS ST
5300 AGRH 91301 558-B5
ARIANNA LN
2600 THO 91362 527-C3
ARIELLE LN
- Chat 91311 499-J3
23600 SIMI 93065 498-A5
ARIES ST
28700 AGRH 91301 558-B3
ARISTOTLE ST
100 SIMI 93065 497-F2
ARIZONA DR
1900 VEN 93003 492-C5
ARLENE AV
1700 OXN 93036 522-E3
ARLENE CT
2600 SIMI 93065 498-C3
ARLETTA LN
2200 VeCo 93012 496-B7
N ARLINGTON AV
3000 SIMI 93063 478-G6
ARMACOST CT
- SIMI 93065 527-E1
ARMADA DR
3100 VEN 93003 491-G4
ARMINTA ST
22900 LA 91304 529-E3
ARMITOS DR
5900 CMRL 93012 495-B6
ARMSTRONG AV
- VEN 93003 491-J3
ARMSTRONG RD
3700 VeCo 93066 465-B6
N ARNAZ AV
100 VeCo 93023 441-D6
S ARNAZ AV
100 VeCo 93023 441-D6
ARNAZ DR
- VeCo 93022 451-B6
ARNAZ RD
- VeCo 93001 460-J5
ARNEILL RD
100 CMRL 93010 524-E3
1500 CMRL 93010 494-E7
ARNESS FIRE RD
23600 VeCo 93063 498-E7
23600 VeCo 93063 528-E1
23600 VeCo 93064 498-E7
ARNETT AV
300 VEN 93003 492-B1
ARNOLD RD
6000 OXN 93033 583-A2
6000 VeCo 93033 553-A7
6000 VeCo 93033 583-A2
ARRASMITH LN
- FILM 93015 455-H5
ARROWHEAD AV
1200 VEN 93004 492-J2
ARROWHEAD CIR
100 OXN 93033 553-C3
3900 THO 91362 557-C1
ARROWHEAD LN
2200 OXN 93033 553-B5
ARROWOOD LN
5300 VeCo 91377 527-G7
ARROYO DR
900 MRPK 93021 477-A7
900 MRPK 93065 477-A7
900 SIMI 93065 477-A7
900 SIMI 93021 477-A7
15400 MRPK 93021 476-J6
ARROYO LN
- SIMI 93063 498-H2
ARROYO DEL MAR
200 CMRL 93010 524-B2
ARROYO OAKS DR
500 THO 91362 557-C2
ARROYO SECO DR
1700 VEN 93004 492-J4
ARROYO VIEW ST
1000 THO 91320 526-A6
ARROYO VISTA RD
4000 SIMI 93063 498-F3
ARROYO WILLOW LN
4100 CALB 91301 558-G7
ARTEMISIA AV
200 VEN 93001 491-E1
ARTHUR AV
100 SPLA 93060 464-A6
ARTHUR RONDO
7200 VEN 93003 492-E2
ARTISAN RD
400 THO 91320 526-A7
ARUNDELL AV
500 VEN 93003 491-H5
ARUNDELL CIR
300 FILM 93015 456-A4
3400 VEN 93003 491-H5
ARUNDELL RD
700 VeCo 93015 456-C3
ARVADA CT
800 SIMI 93065 527-C1
ASCOLI CT
11800 MRPK 93021 496-C5
ASCOT PL
2100 CMRL 93010 524-E2
ASH CIR
500 FILM 93015 455-J4
ASH CT
3000 THO 91360 526-H2
ASH LN
- VeCo 93023 441-E6
ASH ST
- VeCo 93063 499-B4
100 OXN 93033 552-G1
N ASH ST
- VEN 93001 491-C2
S ASH ST
- VEN 93001 491-C2
ASHBOURNE LN
3900 MRPK 93021 496-F4
ASHBROOK LN
13500 MRPK 93021 496-F4
ASHBURY CT
1000 CMRL 93010 524-E2
ASHBY CT
100 VeCo 93022 461-B1
ASHDALE CT
400 CMRL 93010 523-J1
ASHFORD CT
900 THO 91361 557-B5
ASHFORD ST
800 SIMI 93065 498-B5
ASHKELON CIR
- SIMI 93063 499-B1
ASHLAND AV
700 SIMI 93065 497-G3
ASHLAND ST
10000 VEN 93004 492-H2

STREET Block City ZIP Pg-Grid

ASHLEY DR
800 SIMI 93065 497-G4
ASHMORE CIR
2800 THO 91362 527-C3
ASHTON CT
7500 LA 91304 529-E4
23600 SIMI 93065 497-F7
23600 SIMI 93065 527-F1
ASHTON ST
200 OXN 93033 552-G5
N ASHTREE ST
4300 MRPK 93021 496-E3
ASH VIEW LN
5600 CMRL 93012 525-A2
N ASHWOOD AV
- VEN 93003 491-J2
S ASHWOOD AV
- VEN 93003 491-J3
ASHWOOD CT
500 THO 91320 555-G3
4000 VEN 93003 491-J2
5300 CMRL 93012 495-A7
5300 CMRL 93012 525-A1
ASIA CT
23600 SIMI 93065 498-A5
ASMAN AV
7100 CanP 91307 529-H5
ASPEN CIR
800 OXN 93030 522-D4
ASPEN CT
700 VEN 93004 492-G2
ASPEN GN
5100 OXN 93033 552-J5
ASPEN LN
4200 VeCo 93066 495-B3
ASPEN HILLS DR
6000 MRPK 93021 476-B7
ASPEN KNOLL DR
6100 VeCo 91377 558-A1
ASPEN OAK CT
700 VeCo 91377 558-B1
ASPENPARK CT
2100 THO 91362 527-A4
ASPEN RIDGE CT
500 VeCo 91377 558-B1
ASPEN TREE CT
4400 MRPK 93021 496-E3
ASPEN VIEW CT
500 VeCo 91377 558-B1
ASPENVIEW CT
32500 WLKV 91361 557-A7
ASPENWALL RD
1500 THO 91361 556-J6
ASPENWOOD PL
5900 VeCo 91377 558-A2
ASTA AV
200 THO 91320 556-A2
ASTA CT
2000 THO 91320 556-A2
ASTER ST
600 OXN 93036 522-F3
1200 VeCo 93063 499-B4
11000 VeCo 93004 493-A1
ASTERA CT
- THO 91320 555-F3
ASTORIA PL
1000 OXN 93030 522-E4
ASTORIAN DR
500 SIMI 93065 498-A5
ATHELING WY
7100 CanP 91307 529-G5
ATHENS AV
2000 SIMI 93065 497-F2
ATHERTON AV
200 VEN 93004 492-F1
ATHERTON CT
2400 SIMI 93065 498-A1
ATHERTON LN
7400 LA 91304 529-D4
ATHERWOOD AV
2600 SIMI 93065 498-B1
2600 SIMI 93065 478-B7
ATLANTA LN
600 VEN 93004 492-H2
ATLANTIS CT
5400 MRPK 93021 496-C1
ATLAS AV
2700 THO 91360 526-F3
ATMORE DR
200 SPLA 93060 463-J6
N ATMORE RD
100 VeCo 93015 465-E1
S ATMORE RD
100 VeCo 93015 465-E1
ATRON AV
7600 LA 91304 529-F3
N ATWATER AV
2000 SIMI 93063 498-D2
ATWOOD CT
14000 MRPK 93021 496-G3
AUBER LN
800 VEN 93003 492-B7
AUBURN AV
- THO 91362 557-B3
N AUBURN CIR
6600 MRPK 93021 476-H6
AUBURN CT
- THO 91362 557-B3
N AUBURN CT
3000 SIMI 93063 478-F6
AUBURY PL
- CMRL 93010 494-E7
AUGUSTA CT
1900 OXN 93036 522-D3
AUGUSTINE WY
300 SIMI 93065 497-D6
AURELIA ST
5300 SIMI 93063 498-J3
5400 SIMI 93063 499-A3
AURORA CT
100 VEN 93003 492-B2
AURORA DR
- OXN 93036 522-H3
4400 VEN 93003 492-B2
AURORA LN
- SIMI 93063 498-H1
AUSTIN AV
3000 SIMI 93063 478-G7
AUSTIN LN
800 VEN 93004 492-H2
AUTO CENTER DR
1100 SIMI 93065 497-H1
1500 OXN 93036 523-A2
6300 VEN 93003 492-D6
23600 OXN 93036 522-J2
AUTO MALL DR
3000 THO 91362 557-B3
AUTUMN PL
23600 SIMI 93065 497-D3

AUTUMNBREEZE PL
1800 SIMI 93065 497-E2
AUTUMNGLEN CT
4400 MRPK 93021 496-D3
AUTUMN LEAF DR
- THO 91360 526-F1
AUTUMN MEADOW CIR
4300 MRPK 93021 496-E3
AUTUMN RIDGE DR
2500 THO 91362 527-D3
AUTUMNWOOD ST
200 THO 91360 526-F2
AVALON PL
200 OXN 93033 552-H4
AVALON ST
10400 VEN 93004 492-J2
AVALON WY
700 OXN 93033 552-H4
AVEDON RD
4700 MRPK 93021 496-C2
AVENAL ST
2800 VeCo 93001 450-E3
AVENIDA ACASO
600 CMRL 93012 524-H1
AVENIDA AMARANTO
3100 THO 91362 527-A2
AVENIDA AMELGADO
4300 THO 91360 496-H7
AVENIDA CAFE
- CMRL 93012 524-H1
AVENIDA CAMPANA
4400 THO 91360 496-J7
AVENIDA CLASSICA
23600 OXN 93030 523-B4
AVENIDA COLONIA
14300 MRPK 93021 476-G7
AVENIDA DE APRISA
1900 CMRL 93010 523-G1
AVENIDA DE AUTLAN
- CMRL 93010 493-H6
- CMRL 93010 523-H1
- VeCo 93010 523-H1
AVENIDA DE LA CRUZADA
2000 VeCo 93023 442-B7
AVENIDA DE LA ENTRADA
100 VeCo 93023 442-B7
AVENIDA DE LA PLATA
400 THO 91320 526-A7
400 THO 91320 556-A1
AVENIDA DE LA ROSA
- CMRL 93012 495-A7
AVENIDA DE LAS FLORES
- THO 91360 526-F4
1600 THO 91362 526-J4
2000 THO 91362 527-A4
W AVENIDA DE LAS FLORES
- THO 91360 526-D4
AVENIDA DE LAS PLANTAS
2200 THO 91360 526-H4
AVENIDA DE LA VEREDA
100 VeCo 93023 442-B7
AVENIDA DEL DIA
23600 OXN 93030 523-B5
AVENIDA DEL MANZANO
1300 CMRL 93010 524-B1
E AVENIDA DE LOS ARBOLES
- THO 91360 526-H3
1700 THO 91362 526-H3
1800 THO 91362 527-B3
W AVENIDA DE LOS ARBOLES
- THO 91360 526-C3
AVENIDA DE LOS LOBOS
700 VeCo 91377 557-J2
AVENIDA DEL PLATINO
400 THO 91320 526-B7
400 THO 91320 556-B1
AVENIDA DEL RECREO
100 VeCo 93023 442-B7
AVENIDA DE MARGARITA
1300 CMRL 93010 523-F2
AVENIDA DE ROYALE
200 THO 91362 557-B2
AVENIDA ENCANTO
4900 CMRL 93012 525-A3
AVENIDA GAVIOTA
200 CMRL 93012 524-H3
AVENIDA LADERA
3200 THO 91362 527-A2
AVENIDA LOMA PORTAL
700 THO 91320 525-F7
AVENIDA MAGDALENA
600 CMRL 93010 524-B3
N AVENIDA MONTUOSO
3300 THO 91362 527-B2
AVENIDA NAVIDAD
- CMRL 93012 524-J1
E AVENIDA OTONO
2200 THO 91362 527-B2
AVENIDA PLACIDA
2000 SIMI 93063 499-B2
AVENIDA PRADO
4200 THO 91360 496-H7
N AVENIDA REFUGIO
2000 SIMI 93063 499-B2
AVENIDA SAN ANTERO
2200 CMRL 93010 494-H7
AVENIDA SIMI
2400 SIMI 93065 478-D7
2500 VeCo 93065 478-D7
2900 SIMI 93063 478-D7
2900 VeCo 93063 478-D7
AVENIDA SOLEDAD
700 VeCo 91377 557-J1
AVENIDA SOLTURA
1400 CMRL 93010 524-C1
1600 CMRL 93010 494-C7
AVENIDA VALENCIA
23600 CMRL 93012 524-H3
AVENIDA VERANO
3600 THO 91360 526-H1
N AVENIDA VISTA DEL MONTE
2000 SIMI 93063 499-B2
N AVIADOR ST
200 CMRL 93010 523-H3
AVIANO DR
6600 CMRL 93012 495-C7
AVIARA LN
- OXN 93036 522-C3

AVIARY RD
- VeCo 93060 453-J5
AVIATION DR
300 CMRL 93010 523-G4
600 VeCo 93010 523-G4
AVIGNON CT
5400 WLKV 91362 557-F5
AVILA DR
1100 VeCo 93023 451-B1
AVILA PL
2000 OXN 93036 522-G3
AVOCADO AV
3600 OXN 93033 553-B5
AVOCADO CT
3000 THO 91320 555-G3
AVOCADO PL
- CMRL 93010 524-A1
100 CMRL 93010 523-J1
100 VeCo 93010 493-J7
100 VeCo 93010 523-J1
100 VeCo 93010 524-A1
400 VeCo 93010 494-A7
AVOCADO HILL RD
23600 VeCo 93001 366-G9
23600 VeCo 93001 459-B1
AVON CIR
1000 THO 91360 526-F6
AVON ST
5300 VEN 93003 492-B2
AVONDALE LN
- OXN 93036 522-B3
AWENITA CT
11400 Chat 91311 499-H1
AYALA ST
2000 VEN 93001 491-E3
AYERS AV
800 OJAI 93023 441-J6
900 OJAI 93023 442-A5
AYERS CT
700 OJAI 93023 441-J5
700 OJAI 93023 442-A5
AYHENS ST
700 SIMI 93065 497-G3
AZAHAR ST
10900 VeCo 93004 493-B1
10900 VEN 93004 493-A1
AZALEA CT
300 VeCo 93010 494-C7
300 VeCo 93010 524-C1
AZALEA ST
400 THO 91360 526-C3
800 OXN 93036 522-E3
AZALEA WY
- SIMI 93065 497-H3
- VEN 93004 493-A2
AZTEC AV
2200 VEN 93001 471-D6
AZTEC CT
2500 VEN 93001 471-D5
3800 SIMI 93063 498-E2
AZUL CIR
8800 LA 91304 529-E1
AZUL DR
8700 WHil 91304 529-D1
8700 LA 91304 529-D1
AZURE CT
600 VeCo 93022 451-C6
AZURE HILLS DR
500 SIMI 93065 497-H5
AZURITE CIR
2500 THO 91320 525-H6
AZUSA AV
100 VEN 93004 492-E1

B

B AV
- VeCo 93042 583-H3
B ST
100 OXN 93030 522-G5
100 FILM 93015 455-J5
1500 OXN 93033 552-G1
E B ST
100 PHME 93041 552-E5
N B ST
100 OXN 93030 522-G5
W B ST
100 PHME 93041 552-E5
BACCARAT ST
3200 THO 91362 526-J2
BACH RD
500 VEN 93003 492-B3
BADEN AV
9500 Chat 91311 499-H5
BADGER CIR
7200 VEN 93003 492-F4
BAHAMA ST
22000 LA 91304 529-J1
BAHIA CIR
- SPLA 93060 463-J7
BAHIA DR
2000 OXN 93036 522-G3
W BAILEY CT
3600 THO 91320 555-F4
BAINBRIDGE CT
- THO 91360 526-E1
5900 AGRH 91301 558-A4
BAINBROOK CT
31700 WLKV 91361 557-D6
BAJA CT
400 CMRL 93010 524-D3
BAJA VISTA WY
1700 CMRL 93010 494-C7
BAJO AGUA AV
100 CMRL 93010 523-H3
BAKER AV
- THO 91360 556-F1
200 VEN 93004 492-F2
BAKERSFIELD AV
6900 VeCo 93001 459-C4
BALASIANO AV
- LA 91304 529-G4
BALBOA CIR
- CMRL 93012 525-A4
BALBOA ST
2400 OXN 93036 522-H2
2400 VeCo 93036 522-H2
2600 PHME 93041 552-E2
3200 VeCo 93036 492-J7
3300 VeCo 93036 493-A7
8000 VEN 93004 492-F2
BALCOM CANYON RD
1700 VeCo 93060 465-C6
4000 VeCo 93021 495-E1
4000 VeCo 93066 495-E1
5500 VeCo 93021 475-E6
5500 VeCo 93066 475-C1
8400 VeCo 93066 465-C6
BALD ST
100 OJAI 93023 441-J7

BALDEN LN
700 FILM 93015 455-J6
700 FILM 93015 456-A6
BALDWIN AV
200 VEN 93004 492-F2
BALDWIN RD Rt#-150
- VeCo 93001 450-H3
- VeCo 93023 450-H3
600 VeCo 93023 451-A3
BALEWIN DR
1800 VeCo 93015 455-F5
BALFE ST
700 VEN 93003 492-B3
BALI LN
1800 OXN 93033 552-J1
1800 OXN 93033 553-A1
BALKINS DR
28000 AGRH 91301 558-C4
BALLANTINE PL
7000 VeCo 91377 528-B6
BALLARD ST
1600 SIMI 93065 497-J2
W BALLINA CT
900 THO 91320 556-C1
BALLINGER ST
22000 Chat 91311 499-H6
BALMORAL CT
2400 CMRL 93010 524-E1
BALMORAL LN
23300 CanP 91307 529-F5
BALSAM ST
100 OXN 93030 522-J5
BALSAMO AV
1000 SIMI 93065 497-G4
BALTAR ST
22100 LA 91304 529-E3
BALTIC ST
- OXN 93035 552-B1
BAMBI CT
15300 MRPK 93021 476-J6
BAMBOO CT
2100 THO 91362 526-J4
BAMFIELD DR
28500 AGRH 91301 558-B3
BANCAL WY
- OXN 93036 522-H3
BANCOCK ST
2600 SIMI 93065 498-A1
2600 SIMI 93065 478-A7
BANCROFT ST
1800 CMRL 93010 524-D2
BANDERA DR
500 CMRL 93010 524-D2
BANG RD
- WHil 91304 499-C7
- WHil 91304 529-C1
BANGOR LN
1000 VEN 93001 491-E4
BANNER AV
- VEN 93004 492-F2
BANNISTER WY
- SIMI 93065 527-E1
BANTA CT
1300 OXN 93035 522-E7
1300 OXN 93035 552-E1
BARBADOS CT
4900 VeCo 91377 557-G2
BARBARA DR
1800 VeCo 93012 495-J7
BARBARA ST
- VeCo 93022 451-B4
BARBER LN
800 VEN 93003 492-A7
E BARCA ST
3400 CMRL 93010 524-G1
N BARCA ST
1400 CMRL 93010 524-G1
BARCELONA PL
3900 THO 91320 555-E1
BARCELONA ST
1500 CMRL 93010 524-D4
BARCELONA WY
- OXN 93036 492-H7
- OXN 93036 522-H1
BARCLAY CT
1900 THO 91361 557-A5
BARD LN
- PHME 93041 552-E4
- VeCo 93001 471-C2
BARD RD
400 PHME 93041 552-E4
700 OXN 93033 553-A4
1800 OXN 93033 552-E4
E BARD RD
- OXN 93033 552-G4
W BARD RD
- OXN 93033 552-G4
800 PHME 93033 552-G4
800 PHME 93041 552-G4
BARD ST
300 FILM 93015 456-A5
300 MRPK 93021 496-E1
600 MRPK 93021 476-E7
BARDELL DR
28900 AGRH 91301 558-B4
BARDET PL
1900 SIMI 93065 498-A1
BARDMAN AV
1300 LACo 90265 586-D7
BARDSDALE AV
100 VeCo 93035 552-B5
100 VeCo 93015 465-F3
BARLETTA PL
11800 MRPK 93021 496-C3
BARNACLE CV
2600 PHME 93041 552-C1
BARNARD ST
4400 SIMI 93063 498-G1
5400 SIMI 93063 499-A1
BARNARD WY
1600 VEN 93001 491-E2
BARNARO RD
300 VeCo 93015 455-B7
BARNES DR
- VeCo 93001 471-C3
BARNES ST
1500 SIMI 93063 498-E3
E BARNES ST
2700 SIMI 93065 498-C3
3200 SIMI 93063 498-D3
BARNETT ST
2000 OXN 93033 553-A4
E BARNETT ST
- VEN 93001 471-C7
W BARNETT ST
- VEN 93001 471-B7
BARODA DR
- CMRL 93012 525-A3
BARONS WY
23600 VeCo 91377 528-A7

BARONSGATE RD
4200 WLKV 91361 557-E6
BARR DR
500 VEN 93003 491-J4
BARRACUDA WY
200 OXN 93035 552-A3
BARRAGAN ST
28800 AGRH 91301 558-B3
BARRANCA AV
- VEN 93003 492-E2
200 VeCo 93003 492-E2
BARRANCA DR
- Cstc 91384 458-H4
BARRANCA RD
200 THO 91320 556-A2
200 VeCo 91320 556-A2
11200 VeCo 93012 496-B6
BARRETT DR
32700 WLKV 91361 586-J1
BARR HIGHLAND RD
- VeCo 93060 472-J5
BARRINGTON CT
500 THO 91320 555-H3
BARROW AV
4200 SIMI 93063 478-F7
BARROW CT
1000 THO 91361 557-A5
BARRY DR
- VEN 93001 471-C6
BARRY ST
2300 CMRL 93010 524-E3
BARRYMORE DR
5200 OXN 93033 552-G5
BARSTOW ST
7700 VEN 93004 492-F1
BART CIR
1000 THO 91360 526-F6
BARTON AV
800 CMRL 93010 524-B2
BARVO DR
- OXN 93030 522-G5
BASALT ST
1000 OXN 93030 522-D4
BASCOM CT
2300 THO 91362 527-A7
BASELBRIER LN
23600 SIMI 93065 497-A1
BASIE ST
- VEN 93003 492-B4
BASOLO TEXICO RD
- VeCo 93015 466-C2
- VeCo 93021 466-C2
BASS CT
2600 OXN 93035 552-A2
BASSET LN
1600 VEN 93003 492-F4
BASSETT ST
22000 CanP 91303 529-H6
22400 CanP 91307 529-F6
BASSWOOD AV
- VeCo 91377 558-B3
BASSWOOD CT
1100 VEN 93004 492-J2
2100 THO 91361 557-A4
BATES CT
1700 THO 91362 526-J6
BATES RANCH RD
23600 VeCo 93001 366-G9
23600 VeCo 93001 459-A2
BATH CT
5000 VeCo 91377 557-H1
BATH LN
1000 VEN 93001 491-E4
BATTEN LN
500 OXN 93033 552-G5
BAXTER ST
3300 THO 91320 555-F2
BAXTER WY
4200 THO 91362 557-C4
E BAY BLVD
100 PHME 93041 552-E2
300 OXN 93033 552-E2
300 PHME 93033 552-E2
BAY DR
2200 THO 91361 557-A5
BAYBERRY ST
6300 VeCo 91377 558-B2
BAYBRIDGE CT
2500 PHME 93041 552-C2
BAYBROOK CT
- VeCo 91361 556-F6
BAYHAM CIR
2800 THO 91362 527-B3
BAYHILL CT
2300 OXN 93036 522-D2
E BAYLOR CIR
14400 MRPK 93021 476-G6
BAYLOR DR
- VEN 93003 491-J2
- VEN 93003 492-A3
E BAYMARE RD
- VeCo 91307 529-A4
BAYONNE CT
30800 WLKV 91362 557-F5
BAYPORT WY
300 VeCo 91377 557-G2
BAYS ST
5700 VEN 93003 492-C2
BAYSHORE AV
2400 VEN 93001 491-F5
BAYSHORE DR
32000 WLKV 91361 557-C7
BAYSIDE CIR
- OXN 93035 522-A7
BAYSIDE CT
2300 THO 91361 557-B6
BAYSIDE LN
- OXN 93035 522-A7
BAYSIDE ST
3800 SIMI 93063 498-E1
BAYVIEW AV
300 VEN 93003 492-A1
BAYVIEW DR
1300 OXN 93035 522-B7
1400 OXN 93035 552-B1
BAYWATER PL
2600 THO 91362 527-B3
BAYWOOD AV
1100 CMRL 93010 524-C2
BAYWOOD CT
1100 CMRL 93010 524-C1
BAYWOOD LN
400 SIMI 93065 497-D5
BEACH RD
- VeCo 93042 583-B4
BEACH WY
5000 OXN 93035 551-J1
5000 OXN 93035 552-A1
S BEACH CLUB WY
11800 VeCo 90265 625-F5

BEACHCOMBER ST
5000 OXN 93035 521-J7
BEACHFRONT LN
32100 WLKV 91361 557-C6
BEACH HAVEN WY
600 PHME 93041 552-F6
BEACHLAKE LN
32100 WLKV 91361 557-C6
BEACHMEADOW LN
4100 WLKV 91361 557-C6
BEACHMONT ST
1200 VeCo 93001 491-F5
1200 VEN 93001 491-F5
BEACHNUT AV
700 SIMI 93065 498-D5
BEACHPORT DR
500 PHME 93041 552-F6
BEACHSIDE CT
- VEN 93001 491-A2
BEACHSIDE PL
- VEN 93001 491-A2
BEACHVIEW LN
32100 WLKV 91361 557-C6
BEACON AV
2600 VEN 93003 491-G4
BEACON PL
1100 OXN 93033 552-J1
BEACONSFIELD CT
4400 WLKV 91361 557-D6
BEAGLE CT
7200 VEN 93003 492-F4
BEALL ST
500 THO 91360 526-G7
BEAR CIR
2600 SIMI 93063 478-J7
BEARCLAW CT
900 THO 91320 555-G5
BEAR CREEK CT
3400 THO 91320 555-F2
BEAR CREEK DR
3200 THO 91320 555-F2
BEARDEN CT
1800 OXN 93035 552-C1
BEARDSLEY RD
5600 VeCo 93010 493-G7
5600 VeCo 93010 523-F1
6100 CMRL 93010 493-H6
BEAR FENCE CT
- MRPK 93021 476-F6
BEAR RIVER CIR
3400 THO 91362 557-C2
BEAR VALLEY RD
13500 MRPK 93021 496-F3
BEATTY PL
- THO 91320 556-A2
BEAUCROFT CT
4200 WLKV 91361 557-D6
BEAUFORT DR
1800 OXN 93033 553-A2
BEAUMONT AV
4300 OXN 93033 553-A5
5000 VeCo 93033 553-A5
BEAUMONT ST
4600 SIMI 93063 478-G7
BEAVER AV
2700 SIMI 93065 498-C5
BEAVER ST
1800 VEN 93003 492-F4
BECKETT CT
2700 THO 91360 526-E3
BECKFORD ST
4900 VEN 93003 492-B1
BECKWITH RD
100 SPLA 93060 473-H1
400 SPLA 93060 463-G7
BECKY ST
3900 SIMI 93063 498-F2
BEDFORD CT
700 SPLA 93060 464-B4
1700 CMRL 93010 524-D1
BEDFORD DR
1000 CMRL 93010 524-D2
BEDFORD PL
100 THO 91360 526-F6
BEDFORD ST
1100 SPLA 93060 464-B4
BEDFORDHURST CT
31700 WLKV 91361 557-D6
BEE AV
6200 AGRH 91301 558-B3
BEE CANYON
10800 Chat 91311 499-J2
E BEECH CT
4900 SIMI 93063 478-H7
BEECH DR
1000 SPLA 93060 464-A2
BEECH RD
- THO 91320 556-B2
BEECHGROVE CT
12400 MRPK 93021 496-D4
BEECH VIEW CIR
1100 CMRL 93012 525-B2
BEECHWOOD ST
1000 CMRL 93010 524-C1
BEEDY AV
23600 VeCo 93036 492-J5
23600 VeCo 93036 493-A5
BEEDY ST
100 VeCo 93036 492-J5
100 VeCo 93036 493-A5
BEENE RD
2600 VEN 93003 492-E6
BEER SHEBA
- SIMI 93063 499-C1
BEETHOVEN AV
900 VEN 93003 492-B4
BEGONIA PL
- VEN 93004 473-C7
BEL CIR
2700 SIMI 93063 478-J7
BELAIR CT E
3100 CMRL 93010 524-F1
BELAIR CT N
1300 CMRL 93010 524-F1
BELBERT CIR
5800 CALB 91302 558-H3
BELBROOK PL
2700 SIMI 93065 478-B7
2700 SIMI 93065 498-B1
BELBURN PL
2600 SIMI 93065 498-A1
BELCARO WY
500 VeCo 91377 557-G1
BELDEN AV
400 CMRL 93010 524-F3
BELEN PL
10500 VEN 93004 492-J1
BELFAST LN
1000 VEN 93001 491-E4

BELFORD CT
24000 LA 91304
N BELGRAVE CT
2000 SIMI 93063
BELHAM CT
4500 WLKV 91361
N BELHAVEN AV
1800 SIMI 93063
BELINDA ST
4000 SIMI 93063
BELL PL
6200 VeCo 93003
6200 VEN 93003
BELL ST
5300 VeCo 93066
6200 VeCo 93003
6200 VEN 93003
BELL WY
- VEN 93001
BELLA DR
400 VeCo 91320
400 VeCo 91320
600 THO 91320
BELLAFONTE CT
- CMRL 93012
BELLAGIO CT
1100 VeCo 91377
BELLA VISTA DR
4400 MRPK 93021
BELL CANYON RD
- CanP 91307
- VeCo 91307
E BELL CANYON RD
- VeCo 91307
- VeCo 91307
BELL CANYON FIRE R
23600 VeCo 91302
23600 VeCo 91307
BELLEMEADE CT
- SIMI 93063
BELLERIVE CT
2600 OXN 93036
BELLEVUE AV
100 VeCo 93015
BELLEVUE AV Rt#-23
700 VeCo 93015
700 VeCo 93015
BELLEZA DR
- OXN 93030
BELLEZA ST
1000 CMRL 93012
BELLFLOWER CT
- SIMI 93063
BELLINI LN
900 VEN 93003
BELL RANCH RD
4500 VeCo 93010
4500 VeCo 93066
BELLSHIRE CT
4800 THO 91362
N BELMAR CT
2000 SIMI 93063
BELMONT AV
900 CMRL 93010
BELMONT CT
27300 AGRH 91301
BELMONT LN
- OXN 93036
BELSIZE PL
5800 AGRH 91301
BELTRAMO RANCH R
4600 MRPK 93021
BELVEDERE CT
2500 SIMI 93065
BEN CT
400 VeCo 91320
BENCHLEY CT
30900 WLKV 91361
BENDING BRANCH W
23600 SIMI 93065
BENDING OAK CT
11600 MRPK 93021
BENECIA WY
100 OXN 93033
BENEDICT CT
5300 VeCo 91377
BENITO DR
2100 CMRL 93010
BENJAMIN CT
- VEN 93003
BENNETT AV
- VEN 93003
BENNETT RD
4400 SIMI 93063
4400 VeCo 93063
4600 VeCo -
23600 VeCo -
BENNETT ST
500 SIMI 93065
BENNINGTON CT
2000 THO 91360
BENSON WY
600 THO 91360
600 THO 91360
BENTCREEK RD
4100 MRPK 93021
BENT GRASS PL
- MRPK 93021
BENTLEY PL
300 SIMI 93065
BENTON WY
1300 OXN 93033
BENT TWIG AV
300 CMRL 93012
BENWOOD DR
15300 MRPK 93021
15300 MRPK 93021
BERAGAN ST
23600 MRPK 93021
BEREA CIR
1400 THO 91362
BERG LN
4600 VEN 93003
BERGAMO CT
11800 MRPK 93021
BERING ST
100 OXN 93033
BERKELEY AV
- VEN 93004
N BERKELEY CIR
6400 MRPK 93021
BERKSHIRE CT
4300 OXN 93033
BERKSHIRE DR
1600 THO 91362
1800 THO 91362
BERKSHIRE PL
600 OXN 93033
BERKSHIRE ST
1000 OXN 93033

STREET
City ZIP Pg-Grid
RE ST
OXN 93033 553-A4
ST
VEN 93003 492-B7
A CT
VEN 93003 491-J3
A DUNES DR
OXN 93036 522-D2
A DUNES PL
OXN 93036 522-D2
ETTE ST
OXN 93030 522-D3
NE AV
CanP 91307 529-F5
LA 91304 529-F5
OINE ST
THO 91320 555-G2
ST
SIMI 93063 499-C2
A CT
OXN 93030 522-J5
DR
WHil 91304 499-E6
CT
VeCo 91377 557-G1
LI CIR
OXN 93030 523-A5
IN LN
VEN 93003 492-A7
AV
WdHl 91367 529-F7
CanP 91307 529-F7
ST
SIMI 93063 478-F7
OOK CT
MRPK 93021 496-C3
SA AV
VEN 93004 492-J3
LL CIR
THO 91362 527-F6
RD
THO 91320 555-H2
ID DR
AGRH 91301 557-J3
AGRH 91301 558-A3
PL
THO 91361 556-J6
ST
CMRL 93010 494-F7
V
OXN 93030 522-D3
OXN 93036 522-D3
OOD RD
VeCo 93066 494-F1
RD
VeCo 93023 441-E7
VeCo 93023 451-D1
R ST
VEN 93003 491-J4
VEN 93003 492-A4
SIMI 93063 478-H5
SIMI 93065 478-B7
SIMI 93065 498-B1
CT
THO 91360 526-E5
ST
THO 91360 526-D5
V
VEN 93003 491-J2
T
SIMI 93065 498-A5
VEN 93003 491-J2
CT
CMRL 93010 524-C1
CIR
VeCo 93010 494-F6
DR
CMRL 93010 494-F7
VeCo 93010 494-F6
LY DR
OXN 93030 522-F5
V
OXN 93036 522-E2
N
THO 91362 557-A2
CIR
SIMI 93063 478-D6
ST
SIMI 93063 498-G1
LE WK
OXN 93033 552-G5
R WY
OXN 93033 553-C3
CT
MRPK 93021 496-E2
YON RD
VeCo 93023 452-J3
VeCo 93023 453-A1
UD CIR
THO 91360 526-C2
NTRY CT
MRPK 93021 496-G2
OW AV
SIMI 93065 498-A2
N CT
CMRL 93010 524-C2
N ST
VEN 93004 492-J3
K TR
LA 91304 529-E1
WHil 91304 529-E1
KY CIR
THO 91360 526-B2
DR
THO 91360 526-C2
PL
SIMI 93065 478-A7
NGS AV
SIMI 93063 478-G6
IE LN
VEN 93004 492-H3
RIVER PL
OXN 93036 492-H7
OXN 93036 522-H1
IL CIR
MRPK 93021 496-F2
T
SIMI 93063 478-D7
S ST
OXN 93033 552-J4
D
THO 91320 555-H2
VeCo 91320 555-H2
LE ST
OXN 93035 522-D6
I CT
THO 91320 526-A7

STREET
Block City ZIP Pg-Grid
BIRCH ST
1200 SPLA 93060 464-B2
1500 OXN 93035 552-D1
3700 VEN 93003 491-J3
6000 VeCo 93063 499-B4
E BIRCH ST
100 OXN 93033 552-G1
W BIRCH ST
100 OXN 93033 552-F1
BIRCHCREEK PL
2900 THO 91360 526-E3
BIRCHCROFT ST
5200 SIMI 93063 498-J2
BIRCHDALE CT
2000 THO 91362 527-A4
BIRCHDALE DR
1800 THO 91362 527-A4
BIRCHFIELD ST
2200 SIMI 93065 498-B2
BIRCH GLEN AV
2200 SIMI 93063 498-J2
BIRCH HILL ST
800 THO 91320 556-C2
BIRCHPARK CIR
500 THO 91360 526-E7
BIRCHSPRING WK
- CMRL 93012 524-H2
BIRCHTON AV
6600 CanP 91307 529-F6
BIRCH VIEW LN
5600 CMRL 93012 525-A2
BIRCHWOOD AV
- VeCo 91377 558-A2
BIRDSONG AV
3300 THO 91360 526-G2
BISCAYNE CT
800 CMRL 93010 524-D2
BISCAYNE PALM PL
23600 SIMI 93065 498-D5
BISHOP LN
1600 SIMI 93063 498-F3
BISHOP ST
8200 VEN 93004 492-F1
BISHOP WY
- OXN 93033 552-G5
BISMARK AV
600 VEN 93004 492-J1
BISMARK WY
800 OXN 93033 552-H3
BITNER PL
15300 MRPK 93021 476-J5
BITTERN CT
6900 VEN 93003 492-E4
BITTERNUT CIR
2600 SIMI 93065 498-D1
2700 SIMI 93065 478-C7
BIXBY RD
8400 VeCo 93066 465-C6
8400 VeCo 93066 475-D1
BIZET LN
4600 VEN 93003 492-A7
BLACK AV
3200 VeCo 93063 478-E6
BLACK PT
- VeCo 93012 554-F3
BLACKBERRY CIR
2000 OXN 93036 522-G3
BLACKBERRY LN
4200 VeCo 93066 495-B3
BLACKBIRD AV
100 THO 91362 557-G2
BLACKBOURNE
23600 VeCo 91377 528-A7
BLACKBURN PL
- VEN 93004 472-J7
- VEN 93004 492-J1
BLACKBURN RD
7700 VEN 93004 492-F2
9200 VeCo 93004 492-H1
10600 VEN 93004 472-J7
BLACK CANYON RD
- VeCo 93063 499-B4
BLACKFOOT LN
200 VEN 93001 471-C5
BLACKHAWK DR
300 THO 91320 555-E2
BLACKHAWK ST
- Chat 91311 499-J4
E BLACK HILLS CT
3300 THO 91362 557-C2
W BLACK HILLS CT
3000 THO 91362 557-B2
BLACK MOUNTAIN FIRE RD
24400 CanP 91307 529-D5
23600 VeCo 93023 451-J2
23600 VeCo 93023 452-A2
BLACK OAK ST
2800 THO 91362 557-B2
BLACKPOOL AV
800 VeCo 91377 557-H1
BLACK ROCK CIR
- MRPK 93021 476-F6
BLACKSMITH CT
13600 MRPK 93021 496-F3
BLACKSTOCK AV
1400 SIMI 93065 498-D3
BLACKWALL DR
1500 SIMI 93063 498-E3
BLACKWOOD ST
3700 THO 91320 555-E4
BLAINE AV
200 FILM 93015 456-A5
700 FILM 93015 455-J5
BLAIR CT
- THO 91320 556-A1
BLAIR PL
4800 AGRH 91301 558-B6
BLAIRWOOD DR
3900 MRPK 93021 496-E3
BLAKE CT
6800 VEN 93003 492-E3
BLAKE RIDGE CT
- THO 91361 556-H2
BLANCA PL
800 OXN 93036 522-H3
BLANCHARD AV
200 SPLA 93060 464-A5
BLANCHARD PL
10600 VeCo 93012 495-J7
10600 VeCo 93012 496-A7
BLANCHARD RD
2200 VeCo 93012 496-A7
BLANCHARD CANYON RD
23600 VeCo 93040 367-D7
BLANCHE ST
100 OJAI 93023 441-H6
S BLANCHE ST
100 OJAI 93023 441-H7
BLANCO CT
300 CMRL 93012 525-A2

STREET
Block City ZIP Pg-Grid
BLAZE AV
1400 SIMI 93065 497-J3
BLAZEWOOD ST
- SIMI 93063 499-B2
BLAZING STAR DR
3000 THO 91362 527-C3
BLISS CT
400 SIMI 93065 497-H6
BLONDELL PL
3000 THO 91320 555-G3
BLOOM ST
- SIMI 93063 479-B7
- SIMI 93063 499-B1
BLOOMFIELD PL
- CMRL 93012 524-G5
BLOOMFIELD ST
5600 SIMI 93063 499-A2
BLOSSOM CT
1600 THO 91320 526-A6
BLOSSOM ST
4700 SIMI 93063 478-H7
BLOSSOMWOOD CT
11700 MRPK 93021 496-C4
BLUEBELL PL
300 OXN 93036 522-F3
4300 THO 91362 527-D6
BLUEBELL ST
900 OXN 93036 522-E3
BLUEBERRY DR
2400 OXN 93036 522-G1
E BLUEBERRY LN
200 THO 91360 526-F7
BLUEBIRD AV
1300 VEN 93003 492-C4
BLUEBIRD CIR
3200 SIMI 93063 478-J6
BLUEBIRD LN
3900 OXN 93033 553-B5
BLUEBONNET AV
1200 VEN 93004 492-J2
1200 VEN 93004 493-A2
BLUEBONNET CT
600 THO 91360 526-D2
BLUE CANYON ST
1500 THO 91320 526-A6
BLUE DOLPHIN DR
400 PHME 93041 552-F7
BLUEFIELD AV
- THO 91320 555-F2
BLUEFIN CIR
200 OXN 93035 552-B4
BLUEGRASS ST
600 SIMI 93065 497-G6
BLUE HERON CIR
12500 VeCo 93023 451-A1
BLUE HILL CT
1700 THO 91362 527-D6
BLUEJAY AV
1900 VEN 93003 492-E5
2100 OXN 93033 553-B5
BLUE JAY ST
1400 FILM 93015 455-H6
BLUE LAKE CT
400 SIMI 93065 497-E6
BLUE MEADOW LN
31600 WLKV 91361 557-D7
BLUE MESA ST
2900 THO 91362 557-C2
BLUE MOUNTAIN CIR
700 THO 91362 557-F1
BLUE OAK AV
600 THO 91320 556-D2
BLUE OAK ST
1100 CMRL 93010 524-C1
BLUE RIDGE CIR
2500 VeCo 93065 478-C6
BLUE RIDGE CT
- MRPK 93021 476-F6
N BLUE RIDGE CT
200 THO 91362 557-B2
S BLUE RIDGE CT
100 THO 91362 557-B3
BLUE RIDGE WY
- MRPK 93021 476-F6
BLUE ROCK RDG
32300 WLKV 91361 557-B7
BLUESAGE CT
- SIMI 93065 477-J7
BLUESAIL CIR
1300 THO 91361 557-B6
BLUE SKY CIR
400 SIMI 93065 527-D1
BLUE SKY CT
23600 SIMI 93065 527-F1
BLUESPRING DR
800 THO 91361 557-A5
BLUE SPRUCE CIR
2900 THO 91360 526-H2
BLUESTONE AV
1600 SIMI 93063 499-C3
BLUEWATER WY
600 PHME 93041 552-F7
BLUEWOOD CT
- MRPK 93021 496-G2
BLUFFSIDE LN
23600 SIMI 93065 497-E4
BLYTHE ST
22100 LA 91304 529-E3
BLYTHEDALE RD
27800 AGRH 91301 558-D3
BOALT AV
2300 SIMI 93063 498-E1
BOARDMAN RD
100 OJAI 93023 442-B7
100 VeCo 93023 442-B7
BOARDWALK AV
100 THO 91360 556-F1
BOB CT
400 VeCo 91320 555-G1
BOBBYBOYAR AV
6400 CanP 91307 529-G4
7500 LA 91304 529-G3
BOBOLINK LN
1100 VEN 93003 492-E4
BOBWHITE CT
3800 WLKV 91361 557-B6
BODEGA PL
13200 MRPK 93021 496-E2
BODIE AV
1500 SIMI 93065 497-J4
BODLE PEAK MTWY
600 LACo 90265 586-J4
BOE CIR
2100 THO 91362 527-A2
BOGART ST
2500 CMRL 93010 524-E2
BOGOTA CT
1100 OXN 93035 522-D7
BOISE ST
8300 VEN 93004 492-G2

STREET
Block City ZIP Pg-Grid
BOLAM CT
23600 SIMI 93065 497-F7
BOLERO LN
200 OXN 93036 522-G3
N BOLIVAR CT
2000 SIMI 93063 498-E2
BOLKER DR
2500 PHME 93041 552-D1
2700 PHME 93035 552-D1
BOLKER WY
2600 PHME 93041 552-D2
BOLLIN AV
1000 CMRL 93010 524-E2
BOLSA WY
300 OXN 93036 522-H3
BO-MERRITT RD
23600 VeCo 93023 452-J1
BONANZA ST
1700 SIMI 93063 499-C3
BONHAM ST
4700 SIMI 93063 478-H7
BONITA AV
100 OXN 93030 522-H6
N BONITA AV
100 OXN 93030 522-H5
BONITA CT
1100 VEN 93001 491-G5
BONITA DR
300 VeCo 93023 441-F7
E BONITA DR
100 SIMI 93065 497-F3
W BONITA DR
- SIMI 93065 497-E3
BONITA HEIGHTS ST
13300 MRPK 93021 496-F2
BONMARK DR
1100 VeCo 93023 451-B4
N BONNIE CT
1600 SIMI 93065 497-E3
BONNIE VIEW ST
300 MRPK 93021 476-F7
BONSAI AV
200 MRPK 93021 496-D1
BONWIT PL
600 SIMI 93065 497-G5
BOOSEY RD
800 VeCo 93060 464-F3
BOOTH ST
2000 SIMI 93065 478-A7
S BORCHARD DR
- VEN 93003 491-G3
BORCHARD RD
2200 THO 91320 555-E1
2900 VeCo 91320 555-F1
BORDEAUX AV
1000 CMRL 93010 524-E2
BORDEN AV
1000 SIMI 93065 497-J4
BORDERO LN
3100 THO 91362 527-A2
BORDERS ST
- SIMI 93063 498-H1
BORGES CT
15700 MRPK 93021 477-A5
BORGES DR
15300 MRPK 93021 477-A4
BORREGO AV
3900 OXN 93033 552-G4
BORREGO CT
200 OXN 93033 552-H4
BORREGO WY
700 OXN 93033 552-H4
BOSTON AV
- VEN 93004 492-J1
BOSTON DR
3500 OXN 93033 552-J4
BOSTON WY
4400 OXN 93033 552-J5
BOTTENS CT
- MRPK 93021 476-F5
BOTTLEBRUSH CIR
100 OXN 93030 522-E5
BOTTLEBRUSH CT
100 OXN 93030 522-E5
BOTTLEBRUSH PL
1000 OXN 93030 522-E5
BOULDER CT
10400 VEN 93004 492-J2
BOULDER ST
600 FILM 93015 455-J5
BOULDER CREEK RD
300 VeCo 93015 455-C5
23600 SIMI 93065 527-F1
BOULDER RIDGE TER
10500 Chat 91311 499-H3
BOUNDS RD
- VeCo 93001 471-C1
BOUNDS RD W
- VeCo 93001 471-C1
BOUQUET CIR
1200 THO 91362 527-A6
BOUQUET DR
7200 CanP 91307 529-F5
BOWCLIFF TER
1600 THO 91361 557-B6
BOWER WY
200 THO 91360 556-G1
BOWFIELD ST
4800 THO 91362 557-F1
4900 VeCo 91362 557-F1
5000 VeCo 91377 557-F1
BOWIE CT
4900 SIMI 93063 478-H6
BOWL RD
23600 VeCo 93063 529-A1
BOWLINE PL
5100 OXN 93033 552-G5
E BOWLING GREEN ST
100 PHME 93041 552-E2
W BOWLING GREEN ST
100 PHME 93041 552-D2
BOWMAN KNOLL DR
32500 WLKV 91361 557-A7
BOWSPRIT CIR
3800 WLKV 91361 557-B6
BOX CANYON RD
1000 VeCo 93063 499-E5
1000 WHil 91304 499-E5
23600 Chat 91311 499-E6
23700 LA 91304 499-E6
23700 WHil 91304 499-E6
BOX ELDER CT
23600 SIMI 93065 498-D4
BOXTHORN AV
600 THO 91320 555-F4
BOXWOOD CIR
3100 THO 91360 526-H2
BOY SCOUT CAMP RD
- VeCo - 366-L1

STREET
Block City ZIP Pg-Grid
BRADBURY CT
1000 THO 91361 557-A5
BRADEMAS CT
600 SIMI 93065 527-C1
BRADFIELD DR
3700 OXN 93033 552-G4
BRADFIELD PL
4700 OXN 93033 552-H5
BRADFORD AV
- CMRL 93010 524-A1
BRADLEY RD
3900 VeCo 93066 494-H1
5300 VeCo 93066 474-J7
5300 VeCo 93066 475-B5
BRADLEY ST
200 SPLA 93060 464-A5
BRAEMAR CT
6100 AGRH 91301 557-J3
BRAKEY RD
100 VEN 93001 491-C1
BRAMBLE CT
- CMRL 93010 524-A2
BRAMWELL PL
1200 THO 91361 557-C6
N BRANCH AV
1400 SIMI 93065 497-E3
BRANDON AV
900 SIMI 93065 498-B4
BRANDT AV
- VeCo 93022 451-C4
BRANDT WY
- OXN 93030 522-E5
BRANDYWINE CT
5700 CMRL 93012 495-B7
BRANNAN ST
3500 SIMI 93063 498-E3
7700 VEN 93004 492-F2
BRAUN CT
15300 MRPK 93021 476-J4
15300 MRPK 93021 477-A5
BRAVO LN
26300 CALB 91302 558-H4
BRAVO RD
23600 VeCo 93063 528-H1
BRAXFIELD CT
23600 VeCo 91361 556-G6
E BRAZIL ST
- THO 91360 556-F1
W BRAZIL ST
- THO 91360 556-F1
BRAZOS CT
10000 VEN 93004 492-J3
BREA CT
400 CMRL 93010 524-B1
BREA CANYON RD
2600 SIMI 93065 477-F7
2600 VeCo 93065 477-F7
BREAKER CT
3100 VEN 93003 491-G1
BREAKER DR
300 VEN 93003 491-G1
BREAKERS WY
5100 OXN 93035 521-J7
23600 VeCo 93001 459-D5
BREAKWATER WY
5100 OXN 93035 521-J7
BRECKENRIDGE PL
500 SIMI 93065 497-D7
500 SIMI 93065 527-D1
BRECKFORD CT
1300 THO 91361 557-A5
BREESE DR
2500 VeCo 93012 496-A7
BREEZEPORT DR
3300 WLKV 91361 557-C7
BREEZEWATER CT
2500 PHME 93041 552-C2
BREEZY DR
- CMRL 93012 524-G5
BREEZY GLEN DR
- MRPK 93021 476-E6
BRENDA CT
3000 THO 91320 555-G2
BRENNAN
- PHME 93041 552-E4
BRENNAN AV
6600 CanP 91307 529-F6
BRENNAN RD
3900 VeCo 93021 496-H3
N BRENT ST
100 VEN 93003 491-G2
S BRENT ST
100 VEN 93003 491-G4
BRENTFORD AV
1500 THO 91361 556-J6
E BRENTFORD AV
1600 THO 91361 556-J6
BRENTFORD CT
100 VeCo 93010 494-E7
BRENTLY AV
100 CMRL 93010 524-D2
BRENTWOOD AV
- VEN 93003 491-J3
N BRENTWOOD AV
2000 SIMI 93063 498-D2
BRETON AV
800 SIMI 93065 498-D5
BRETT WY
200 SPLA 93060 464-B6
BREVARD AV
300 VEN 93003 492-C1
BREVARD CT
5600 VEN 93003 492-B1
BRIAN CIR
- CMRL 93010 524-C3
BRIAN CT
1900 THO 91362 527-A6
BRIANA CIR
- OXN 93030 522-G4
S BRIAR AV
800 THO 91320 555-E4
BRIAR BLUFF CIR
3800 THO 91360 526-E1
BRIARCLIFF CIR
7200 VEN 93003 472-D7
BRIARCLIFF RD
600 THO 91360 526-G6
BRIARFIELD ST
2100 CMRL 93010 524-E1
BRIARGATE CT
1200 VeCo 91377 528-A7
BRIARGLEN AV
1400 THO 91361 556-J5
BRIAR HILL CIR
700 SIMI 93065 498-D5
BRIARHURST CT
2400 SIMI 93063 498-D1
BRIARPATCH DR
2600 SIMI 93065 498-C4

STREET
Block City ZIP Pg-Grid
BRIAR RIDGE CT
23600 THO 91320 555-E4
BRIARSTONE LN
7100 CanP 91307 529-D5
BRIARWOOD LN
- VeCo 91377 558-A2
BRIARWOOD PL
2600 THO 91362 526-J3
BRIARWOOD TER
300 VEN 93001 491-G1
BRICKFIELD CT
23600 THO 91362 527-B5
BRIDGE RD
16800 VeCo 93060 454-A7
16900 VeCo 93060 464-B1
BRIDGEGATE CT
2000 THO 91361 557-A6
BRIDGEGATE ST
1700 THO 91361 556-H5
1800 THO 91361 557-A5
BRIDGEHAMPTON WY
- CMRL 93012 524-F4
BRIDGEPORT LN
1500 CMRL 93010 524-D3
BRIDGES CT
23600 VeCo 93060 464-D5
BRIDGET AV
1500 SIMI 93065 498-B3
BRIDGETON WY
- CMRL 93012 524-G4
BRIDGETOWN PL
4900 THO 91362 527-F6
BRIDGEVIEW DR
5800 VEN 93003 472-C6
BRIDGEVIEW LN
- THO 91320 555-E3
BRIDGEWATER CT
5900 AGRH 91301 557-H4
BRIDGEWOOD LN
3400 THO 91362 557-C2
N BRIDLE LN
- VeCo 91307 529-A5
BRIDLE CREST AV
- SIMI 93063 478-H5
BRIDLE GLEN ST
5500 AGRH 91301 558-A5
BRIDLE OAKS CT
1600 THO 91362 527-A5
BRIDLEWOOD LN
100 FILM 93015 456-A7
BRIER ST
600 VeCo 93023 451-C4
BRIGANTINE CIR
3700 WLKV 91361 557-C7
BRIGGS RD
100 VeCo 93060 473-F1
700 VeCo 93060 463-E7
S BRIGGS RD
100 VeCo 93060 473-G3
BRIGHAM ST
2000 OXN 93033 553-A4
BRIGHT GLEN CIR
2800 THO 91361 557-C5
BRIGHTON CT
4700 THO 91362 527-E6
BRIGHT STAR CIR
800 THO 91360 526-B2
BRIGHT STAR ST
700 THO 91360 526-C2
BRIGHTSTONE CT
900 THO 91361 557-A5
BRINDISI PL
4000 MRPK 93021 496-C4
BRINDLE CT
2600 SIMI 93063 498-D1
BRISBAINE AV
300 THO 91320 555-F3
BRISTLECONE CIR
- MRPK 93021 496-G3
BRISTOL AV
400 SIMI 93065 497-G5
BRISTOL RD
- OJAI 93023 441-G7
6000 VeCo 93003 492-D5
6300 VEN 93003 492-D5
7600 VEN 93004 492-G5
7600 VeCo 93004 492-G5
BRISTOL PARK CT
- CMRL 93012 524-G4
BRITTANY CT
- LACo 91302 558-G4
BRITTANY PARK RD
1800 VeCo 93012 526-A1
2000 VeCo 93012 496-A7
BRITTEN LN
900 VEN 93003 492-A7
BROADBECK DR
- THO 91320 525-H6
BROADHAVEN ST
- VeCo 91361 556-C7
BROADMOOR AV
2600 SIMI 93065 498-A1
2700 SIMI 93065 478-A7
BROADMOOR CT
2300 OXN 93036 522-D2
BROADVIEW DR
11100 MRPK 93021 496-B3
BROADWAY
13000 VeCo 93021 476-B4
23100 VeCo 93021 475-J4
BROADWAY Rt#-23
14900 VeCo 93021 476-D4
BROCK LN
- VeCo 93001 461-A3
BROCKTON LN
800 VEN 93001 491-E4
BROCKTON RD
23600 SIMI 93065 497-F7
BRODERICK AV
200 VEN 93003 492-B3
BRODERICK WY
400 PHME 93041 552-C2
BRODIEA AV
1300 VEN 93001 491-E1
BRODIEA PL
300 VEN 93001 491-E1
BROKEN ARROW ST
6000 SIMI 93063 479-B7
BROKENHILL ST
3400 THO 91320 555-F4
BROMELY DR
5400 VeCo 91377 527-H6
BROMFIELD ST
2100 SIMI 93065 498-A1
N BRONCO LN
- VeCo 91307 528-J5
BRONSON ST
1700 CMRL 93010 524-D2
BRONZE PL
3300 SIMI 93063 478-D7

STREET
Block City ZIP Pg-Grid
BRONZEWOOD CT
1700 THO 91320 556-A2
BROOK RD
200 VeCo 91320 556-B2
BROOKBERRY LN
23600 SIMI 93065 497-A1
BROOKCREST CT
4100 MRPK 93021 496-B2
BROOKDALE LN
4300 MRPK 93021 496-E3
BROOKE AV
10100 Chat 91311 499-J4
BROOKFIELD DR
2000 THO 91362 527-A3
BROOKGLEN ST
4300 MRPK 93021 496-D3
BROOKHAVEN AV
1200 CMRL 93010 524-F1
BROOKHILL DR
2600 CMRL 93010 494-E7
BROOK HOLLOW CT
2000 OXN 93036 522-E3
BROOKHURST CT
3900 MRPK 93021 496-E4
BROOK MEADOW CT
800 THO 91362 557-E1
BROOKMONT PL
7600 LA 91304 529-E4
BROOKMONT TERRACE CT
5100 THO 91362 527-G6
BROOKPEBBLE LN
23600 SIMI 93065 497-A1
BROOKS RD
23400 Chat 91311 499-F7
23600 SIMI 93065 497-G7
BROOKSFALL CT
1700 THO 91361 557-A6
N BROOKSHIRE AV
- VEN 93003 492-C1
S BROOKSHIRE AV
- VEN 93003 492-C2
BROOKSHIRE CT
- CMRL 93012 524-G4
BROOKSIDE AV
1400 OXN 93035 552-D1
BROOKSIDE PL
100 THO 91320 556-D1
BROOKTREE CT
1800 THO 91362 526-J3
BROOKTREE DR
1300 SIMI 93063 499-C3
BROOKVIEW AV
900 THO 91361 556-J5
BROOKWOOD LN
- OXN 93036 522-C3
BROOME RANCH RD
- VeCo - 584-F1
- VeCo 93033 554-A6
200 VeCo 93033 553-H6
23600 VeCo 93033 584-C1
BROOMFIRTH CT
2000 THO 91361 557-A5
BROSSARD DR
500 THO 91360 556-G1
E BROWER ST
2100 SIMI 93065 498-B2
N BROWER ST
2000 SIMI 93065 498-A2
BROWNING AV
600 VEN 93003 492-E3
BROWNING DR
4200 OXN 93033 552-J4
4400 OXN 93033 553-A4
BROWNS CANYON RD
- StvR 91381 479-G1
2500 Nor 91326 479-J4
2500 Chat 91311 479-H3
BROWNSTONE CREEK AV
2100 SIMI 93063 499-A2
BRUBECK ST
- VEN 93003 492-C4
BRUCE CIR
900 THO 91362 526-H7
BRUCE DR
1200 SPLA 93060 464-B3
BRUCKER RD
200 OXN 93033 552-F4
BRUNSTON CT
2900 THO 91362 527-C5
BRUNSWICK LN
800 VEN 93001 491-E5
BRUSH HILL RD
700 THO 91360 526-G5
BRUSH OAK CT
1800 THO 91320 526-A5
BRYAN AV
3200 SIMI 93063 478-H6
BRYANT CIR
400 OJAI 93023 441-J7
BRYANT DR
500 WHil 91304 499-D5
BRYANT PL
800 OJAI 93023 441-J7
BRYANT ST
100 OJAI 93023 441-J7
22100 LA 91304 529-J1
BRYCE WY
1100 VEN 93003 492-B4
BRYCE CANYON AV
100 OXN 93033 552-F3
700 PHME 93033 552-F3
700 PHME 93041 552-F3
BRYNDALE AV
23600 VeCo 91377 528-A7
N BRYN MAWR ST
5300 VEN 93003 492-B2
S BRYN MAWR ST
- VEN 93003 492-B2
BRYSON AV
1100 SIMI 93065 497-G4
E BRYSON PL
2300 SIMI 93065 498-B4
BUBBLING BROOK ST
11900 MRPK 93021 496-C3
BUCHANAN AV
- VEN 93003 492-E2
BUCKAROO AV
2600 OXN 93036 492-F7
2600 OXN 93036 522-F1
BUCKBOARD CIR
300 SIMI 93065 497-F6
BUCKBOARD LN
200 OJAI 93023 441-H7
500 OJAI 93023 451-J1
BUCKEYE PL
3300 THO 91320 555-G4
BUCKEYE ST
- SIMI 93063 499-A4

STREET
Block City ZIP Pg-Grid

BUCKINGHAM DR
1000 THO 91360 526-G6
BUCKLIN PL
3900 THO 91360 526-F1
BUCKNELL AV
100 VEN 93003 492-B3
BUCKSGLEN CT
1600 THO 91361 556-J5
BUCKSKIN AV
1400 SIMI 93065 497-H3
N BUCKSKIN RD
- VeCo 91307 528-J4
BUCKSMOORE CT
1300 THO 91361 556-J5
BUCKTHORN CT
3800 THO 91320 555-E2
BUELL CT
1900 SIMI 93065 498-A4
BUENA MESA CT
5200 CMRL 93012 525-A2
BUENA VISTA AV
500 OXN 93030 522-J6
BUENA VISTA DR
- VeCo 93010 494-D6
400 OJAI 93023 441-J6
BUENA VISTA ST
600 VEN 93001 491-C1
8200 VeCo 93021 476-D3
BUENOS TIEMPOS DR
500 CMRL 93012 524-J3
BUFF CIR
2800 SIMI 93065 498-C5
BUFFALO AV
2200 VEN 93003 492-E5
BUFFALO ST
6100 SIMI 93063 479-B6
BUFFUM ST
3500 SIMI 93063 498-E2
BUFFWOOD PL
5500 AGRH 91301 558-A5
BUGGY LN
10300 VeCo 93012 495-J6
BULL PUP CIR
- VeCo 93041 583-G1
BUMBLEBEE AV
1000 THO 91320 526-A6
BUNDREN ST
- VeCo 93022 451-B6
BUNSEN AV
2800 VEN 93001 492-D7
2800 VEN 93003 492-D7
BUNTING AV
2500 VEN 93003 492-E5
BURANO CT
700 VeCo 91377 557-H1
BURBANK AV
100 VeCo 93035 552-C6
BURCH AV
1800 SIMI 93063 498-E2
N BURKE CT
2200 SIMI 93063 498-E2
BURL AV
200 VEN 93003 492-C2
BURLESON AV
1800 THO 91360 526-G5
BURLESON ST
28900 AGRH 91301 558-A3
N BURLINGHAM PL
2400 SIMI 93063 498-E1
BURLINGTON AV
700 VEN 93004 492-H2
BURLINGTON ST
- FILM 93015 455-J7
- FILM 93015 456-A7
BURNETT AV
200 VEN 93003 492-C1
BURNETT CIR
6300 VEN 93003 492-C1
BURNETT CT
6300 VEN 93003 492-C1
BURNHAM RD
- VeCo 93001 450-J6
- VeCo 93022 450-J6
100 VeCo 93022 451-A5
700 VeCo 93001 451-A5
700 VeCo 93023 451-A5
BURNING TREE DR
1700 THO 91362 526-J3
BURNLEY ST
1400 CMRL 93010 524-C2
BURNS ST
4900 VEN 93003 492-A2
BURNSIDE DR
1500 VEN 93004 492-J3
E BURNSIDE ST
2200 SIMI 93065 498-B2
BURR CIR
2300 THO 91360 526-F4
N BURREL AV
2000 SIMI 93063 498-E2
BURSON LN
200 FILM 93015 455-J6
BURSON WY
4700 VeCo 93036 493-A5
BURSON RANCH RD
- VeCo 93015 455-J3
- VeCo 93015 456-A3
BURTON CT
300 THO 91360 526-F4
BURTON ST
300 THO 91360 526-G4
22100 LA 91304 529-E2
BURTONWOOD AV
1000 THO 91360 526-G7
BURY CIR
800 THO 91360 526-G6
BUSH ST
23600 VEN 93003 492-E2
BUSHELL RD
4700 VeCo 93066 495-B2
BUSHGROVE CT
23600 VeCo 91361 556-F6
BUSINESS CENTER CIR
1000 THO 91320 525-G6
BUSTER ST
1400 SIMI 93065 497-G3
BUTLER RD
2200 OXN 93033 553-A3
BUTTE ST
8400 VEN 93004 492-F1
BUTTER CREEK RD
4900 MRPK 93021 496-B2
BUTTERCUP LN
- CMRL 93012 524-F5
BUTTERFIELD LN
4300 MRPK 93021 496-F3
BUTTERFIELD ST
5300 CMRL 93012 525-A1
BUTTERFLY CT
1600 THO 91320 526-A6
BUTTONWOOD AV
6600 VeCo 91377 558-B2
BUYERS ST
1600 SIMI 93063 498-F3
BYRD DR
2100 OXN 93033 552-J2
BYRON AV
200 VEN 93003 492-B1

C

C ST
- VeCo 93042 583-H3
- FILM 93015 455-J6
100 OXN 93030 522-G7
1000 OXN 93033 522-G7
1200 OXN 93033 552-G2
E C ST
100 PHME 93041 552-E5
N C ST
100 OXN 93030 522-G4
1600 OXN 93036 522-G3
W C ST
- PHME 93041 552-E5
CABALLERO ST
1700 SIMI 93065 497-J4
1700 SIMI 93065 498-A4
CABEZONE WY
200 OXN 93035 552-A3
CABIN CV
2500 PHME 93041 552-C3
CABLE CANYON
- VeCo 93001 471-A3
CABLE RACK RD
- VeCo 93042 583-D4
CABOT CT
2700 THO 91360 526-E3
CABOT PL
2000 OXN 93030 523-A6
CABRILLO AV
- THO 91320 555-F1
CABRILLO CIR
- THO 91320 555-E1
CABRILLO CT
100 SPLA 93060 463-J6
CABRILLO DR
2700 VEN 93003 491-G3
CABRILLO LN
300 FILM 93015 456-C6
CABRILLO WY
1000 VeCo 93010 494-D6
1600 OXN 93030 522-D4
CABRILLO MESA CT
23600 CMRL 93010 494-C7
CACHUMA AV
500 VEN 93004 492-H1
CACTUS AV
9600 Chat 91311 499-H5
CACTUS CT
800 THO 91320 526-A6
CACTUS DR
300 OXN 93036 492-F7
CACTUS TR
26800 CALB 91301 558-G7
CADIZ CT
1100 OXN 93035 522-D7
CADIZ DR
1000 VeCo 93065 497-G4
E CADMAN ST
3800 SIMI 93063 498-E2
CADWAY ST
1000 SPLA 93060 464-B3
CAHUENGA DR
200 VeCo 93035 552-B5
CAITLYN CIR
- WLKV 91361 586-H2
CAJON CIR
10600 VeCo 93012 496-A5
CAJUN CT
- CanP 91303 529-J5
CALABASAS HILLS RD
- CALB 91301 558-G7
CALABRIA
28800 AGRH 91301 558-B4
CALABRIA CT
800 CMRL 93010 524-C1
CALAIS CT
- Ago 91301 558-G3
CALAISE CT
30800 WLKV 91362 557-F5
CALAMAR CT
23600 CMRL 93010 494-C7
CALAMINE DR
26900 CALB 91301 558-F6
CALAROSA RANCH RD
- CMRL 93012 495-A7
CALAVERAS DR
2300 CMRL 93010 494-E7
CALAVERAS ST
8000 VEN 93004 472-F7
8000 VEN 93004 492-E1
S CALAVO ST
100 SPLA 93060 463-H7
CALBOURNE LN
- VeCo 91361 556-G7
- VeCo 91361 586-G1
CALCITE CIR
2500 THO 91320 525-H7
CALDWELL AV
2100 SIMI 93065 497-H1
CALEDONIA CT
23600 VeCo 91377 528-A7
CALENDULA CT
2800 THO 91360 526-D3
CALETA CT
- CMRL 93012 524-J2
CALETA DR
- CMRL 93012 524-H2
CALETA RD
4300 Ago 91301 558-B7
CALGARY AV
800 VEN 93004 492-H2
CALIENTE LN
800 VEN 93001 491-C1
CALIENTE WY
600 OXN 93036 522-H3
CALIFORNIA AV
700 SIMI 93065 497-G2
2100 VeCo 93015 465-F4
CALIFORNIA ST
200 SPLA 93060 464-B6
1300 OXN 93033 552-H1
N CALIFORNIA ST
- VEN 93001 491-C2
S CALIFORNIA ST
- VEN 93001 491-C2
CALIFORNIA OAK ST
- SIMI 93063 499-A3
CALLADO ST
700 VeCo 93010 494-B5
CALLAHAN AV
2100 SIMI 93065 497-J2
CALLA LILY CT
- SIMI 93063 498-H1
CALLAS CT
1700 OXN 93035 522-E7
CALLAS DR
1100 OXN 93035 522-E7
1200 OXN 93035 552-E1
CALLE ABEDUL
2500 THO 91360 526-G3
CALLE ABETO
2600 THO 91360 526-H4
CALLE ACOPADA
600 VeCo 93010 493-J6
CALLE AGRADO
600 CMRL 93012 525-C5
CALLE AGUILA
3900 CMRL 93012 524-H4
CALLE ALAMO
1500 THO 91360 526-H3
CALLE ALBERCA
1700 CMRL 93010 494-B7
1700 CMRL 93010 524-B1
CALLE ALMENDRO
800 THO 91360 526-H3
CALLE ALTA VISTA
3700 THO 91320 525-E7
CALLE ALTO
4500 CMRL 93012 524-J5
CALLE ALUCEMA
2300 THO 91360 526-J4
CALLE AMAPOLA
500 THO 91360 526-G4
CALLE AMOROSA
- CMRL 93012 525-B4
CALLE ANAPOL
23600 CMRL 93010 523-F2
CALLE ANGOSTA
1800 VeCo 91360 526-C5
CALLE ARAGON
600 VeCo 91377 557-J1
CALLE ARENA
5900 CMRL 93012 525-B2
CALLE ARGOLLA
4200 CMRL 93012 524-H3
CALLE ARINO
2900 THO 91360 526-G3
CALLE ARROYO
600 VeCo 91360 526-C7
CALLE ARTIGAS
1300 THO 91360 496-J7
CALLE AURORA
1200 VeCo 93010 494-A6
CALLE AVELLANO
1300 THO 91360 526-H3
CALLE BALSA
1200 THO 91360 526-H3
CALLE BELLA VISTA
1400 CMRL 93010 524-A1
CALLE BELLOTA
3500 CMRL 93010 494-G7
CALLE BIENVENIDO
2600 THO 91360 526-G3
CALLE BODEGA
5900 CMRL 93012 525-C2
CALLE BOLERO
4500 CMRL 93012 524-H6
CALLE BONITA
1200 CMRL 93012 525-A1
CALLE BORREGO
1900 VeCo 91360 526-B5
CALLE BOUGANVILLA
2400 THO 91360 526-H4
CALLE BRISA
- CMRL 93012 524-H1
CALLE BRUSCA
900 VeCo 91360 526-B6
CALLE BUENA VISTA
3800 THO 91320 525-E7
CALLE CAMELIA
1100 THO 91360 526-H4
CALLE CAMELLIA
800 CMRL 93010 524-B2
CALLE CANCUN
23600 CMRL 93012 494-H7
23600 CMRL 93012 524-J1
CALLE CANON
600 CMRL 93012 525-B2
CALLE CAPISTRANO
23600 OXN 93030 523-C7
CALLE CARDO
500 THO 91360 526-G4
CALLE CARGA
4500 CMRL 93012 524-H6
CALLE CASTANO
2700 THO 91360 526-G2
CALLE CATALPA
600 THO 91360 526-G2
CALLE CATALUNA
- CMRL 93012 525-B5
CALLE CEDRO
2800 THO 91360 526-G3
CALLE CIELITO
23600 OXN 93030 523-C7
CALLE CINCO DE MAYO
- VeCo 93022 451-B5
E CALLE CIRCULO
300 CMRL 93010 524-B2
N CALLE CIRCULO
800 CMRL 93010 524-B2
CALLE CIRUELO
600 THO 91360 526-G4
CALLE CITA
3500 CMRL 93010 494-G7
CALLE CLARA VISTA
3700 THO 91320 525-F7
CALLE CLAVEL
600 THO 91360 526-G4
CALLE COLINA
1200 THO 91360 496-H7
CALLE COLLADO
900 VeCo 91360 526-B6
CALLE COMPO
1400 VeCo 91360 526-C5
CALLE CONTENTO
700 THO 91360 526-H1
CALLE CONVERSE
100 CMRL 93010 524-B1
400 CMRL 93010 494-B7
CALLE CORTA
600 VeCo 91360 526-C6
CALLE CORVA
1700 VeCo 93010 493-J6
CALLE COVINA
- CMRL 93012 524-H1
CALLE CRISANTEMO
1300 THO 91360 526-H4
CALLE CUESTA
600 THO 91360 526-G2
4900 CMRL 93012 524-J4
4900 CMRL 93012 525-A4
CALLE DALIA
2300 THO 91360 526-G4
CALLE DAMASCO
2700 THO 91360 526-G3
CALLE DE DEBESA
3000 CMRL 93010 493-J6
CALLE DE LA ROSA
- CMRL 93012 524-H4
CALLE DE LAS OVEJAS
500 VeCo 91377 557-J2
CALLE DEL NORTE
800 VeCo 93010 494-A6
CALLE DEL PRADO
23600 THO 91320 555-D2
CALLE DEL SOL
3700 THO 91360 526-J1
CALLE DEL SUR
500 THO 91360 526-G3
CALLE DE MAREJADA
3000 CMRL 93010 493-J6
CALLE DE ORO
1200 THO 91360 526-J1
CALLE DE ORO CT
3300 THO 91360 526-H1
CALLE DESCANSO
- CMRL 93012 524-H1
CALLE DIA
2000 CMRL 93012 495-D7
CALLE DIAMONTE
1500 THO 91320 526-B7
CALLE DURAZNO
1300 THO 91360 526-H4
CALLE ELAINA
1000 VeCo 91360 526-C6
CALLE EL AVION
300 CMRL 93010 524-B1
CALLE EL CAMERON
1200 VeCo 91360 526-B7
CALLE ELEGANTE
2500 THO 91360 526-G3
CALLE EL HALCON
1000 CMRL 93010 524-B2
W CALLE EL PRADO
- VeCo 93022 451-B5
CALLE EL VOLADOR
300 CMRL 93010 524-B2
CALLE ENTRAR
500 THO 91360 526-G3
CALLE ESCALON
1400 CMRL 93010 524-A1
CALLE ESCORIAL
- CMRL 93012 524-G4
CALLE ESTEPA
2900 THO 91360 526-G3
CALLE FAMILLIA
200 VeCo 91377 558-A2
CALLE FIDELIDAD
1200 THO 91360 496-H7
CALLE FLORENCIA
1600 THO 91360 526-J1
CALLE FRESNO
500 THO 91360 526-G3
CALLE FRONTE
- CMRL 93012 524-H2
CALLE FUEGO
3500 THO 91360 526-C1
CALLE GALVEZ
5900 CMRL 93012 525-B5
CALLE GLADIOLO
2400 THO 91360 526-H4
CALLE GLICINA
2100 THO 91360 526-H4
CALLE GOMERO
2800 THO 91360 526-H3
CALLE HAYA
2600 THO 91360 526-G3
CALLE HERMOSA
2500 THO 91360 526-G3
CALLE HIGUERA
200 CMRL 93010 524-B1
800 CMRL 93010 494-C7
CALLE HONDANADA
1400 THO 91360 496-H7
CALLE JAZMIN
700 THO 91360 526-G4
CALLE JON
800 VeCo 91360 526-D6
CALLEJON DE ROSAS
900 VeCo 91360 526-C7
CALLE LACOTA
800 THO 91360 526-G3
CALLE LA CUMBRE
900 CMRL 93010 524-B1
CALLE LA FIESTA
- CMRL 93010 524-B2
CALLE LA GRANADA
- CMRL 93010 524-B2
E CALLE LA GUERRA
- CMRL 93010 524-B2
W CALLE LA GUERRA
- CMRL 93010 524-A2
CALLE LAGUNA
23600 OXN 93030 523-C7
CALLE LA PALMERA
800 CMRL 93010 524-B2
CALLE LA PAZ
1100 CMRL 93010 524-B1
CALLE LA PRADA
800 CMRL 93010 524-B2
CALLE LAREDO
500 THO 91360 526-C7
500 VeCo 91360 526-C7
CALLE LARIOS
- CMRL 93010 524-B1
CALLE LA ROCHA
800 CMRL 93010 524-B2
CALLE LA RODA
600 CMRL 93010 524-B2
CALLE LAS CASAS
1300 VeCo 91360 526-B7
CALLE LAS COLINAS
800 THO 91320 525-E7
CALLE LA SOMBRA
2000 SIMI 93063 499-B2
E CALLE LA SOMBRA
- CMRL 93010 524-B2
N CALLE LA SOMBRA
800 CMRL 93010 524-B2
W CALLE LA SOMBRA
- CMRL 93010 524-A2
CALLE LAS TRANCAS
900 VeCo 91360 526-C6
CALLE LILA
2100 THO 91360 526-G4
CALLE LIMONERO
2600 THO 91360 526-J3
CALLE LINDA VISTA
3700 THO 91320 525-E7
CALLE LIRIO
2300 THO 91360 526-H4
CALLE LOMA VISTA
3800 THO 91320 525-E7
CALLE LOS ACEITUNOS
600 VeCo 93010 493-J6
CALLE LOS GATOS
800 CMRL 93010 524-A2
CALLE LOZANO
1100 CMRL 93012 525-A1
CALLE LUMINOSO
- CMRL 93012 525-C1
CALLE LYS
2100 THO 91360 526-G4
CALLE MADRESELVA
1300 THO 91360 526-H4
CALLE MADURO
- CMRL 93010 523-J1
- VeCo 93010 523-J1
CALLE MALVON
2300 THO 91360 526-H4
CALLE MANDARINAS
600 VeCo 91360 526-C6
CALLE MANZANO
2500 THO 91360 526-H3
CALLE MAPACHE
4600 CMRL 93012 524-H2
CALLE MARGARITA
500 THO 91360 526-G4
27800 AGRH 91301 558-D7
CALLE MARLENA
600 VeCo 91377 557-J1
CALLE MAR VISTA
23600 OXN 93030 523-C7
CALLE MAZATLAN
3700 THO 91320 525-F7
CALLE MENDOTA
23600 CMRL 93012 524-J2
CALLE MIGUEL
23600 CMRL 93010 524-B2
CALLE MILAGROS
22000 Chat 91311 499-J3
CALLE MIMOSA
2300 THO 91360 526-H4
CALLE MIRADO
600 VeCo 91377 557-J2
CALLE MIRA MONTE
900 THO 91320 525-E7
CALLE MIRASOL
23600 CMRL 93010 524-B2
CALLE MONTECILLO
4900 AGRH 91301 558-D7
CALLE MORENO
3400 VeCo 93023 442-D5
CALLE MORERA
1500 THO 91360 526-H3
CALLE NARANJO
600 THO 91360 526-G3
CALLE NARCISO
2400 THO 91360 526-H4
CALLE NARDO
2100 THO 91360 526-H4
CALLE NAVARRO
- CMRL 93010 524-B1
CALLE NOGAL
500 THO 91360 526-G3
CALLE NORTE
23600 THO 91320 555-D2
CALLENS RD
500 VEN 93003 491-J5
CALLE OLIVO
2600 THO 91360 526-H3
CALLE OLMO
2800 THO 91360 526-H3
CALLE ORINDA
1400 VeCo 93010 494-A6
CALLE OROVISTA
100 CMRL 93012 524-H3
CALLE PAMARO
5800 CMRL 93012 525-B4
CALLE PARADORA
3900 CMRL 93012 524-H3
CALLE PECOS
700 VeCo 91360 526-C6
CALLE PENSAMIENTO
500 THO 91360 526-G4
CALLE PERA
2500 THO 91360 526-H3
CALLE PETALUMA
1800 VeCo 91360 526-C5
CALLE PIMIENTO
1200 THO 91360 526-H3
CALLE PINATA
800 THO 91360 526-G1
CALLE PINO
2400 THO 91360 526-G4
CALLE PLANO
700 CMRL 93012 524-J5
CALLE PLANTADOR
1800 VeCo 91360 526-C5
CALLE PORTADA
1400 VeCo 93010 493-J6
1400 VeCo 93010 494-A6
CALLE PORTILLA
100 CMRL 93010 524-B1
CALLE POSADAS
3700 THO 91320 525-F7
CALLE PUNTA
600 THO 91360 526-G1
CALLE QUEBRACHO
2700 THO 91360 526-G1
CALLE QUETZAL
4500 CMRL 93012 524-J6
CALLE RETAMA
2400 THO 91360 526-H4
CALLE REY
900 VeCo 91360 526-C6
CALLE RIO VISTA
5600 VeCo 91377 557-J1
E CALLE RISCOSO
2000 THO 91362 527-A2
CALLE ROBLE
2400 THO 91360 526-G4
CALLE ROBLEDA
4900 AGRH 91301 558-D7
CALLE ROCAS
1700 VeCo 93010 493-J6
CALLE ROCHELLE
3600 THO 91360 526-J1
CALLE ROSA
2200 THO 91360 526-G4
CALLE RUIZ
800 THO 91360 526-G1
CALLE SALTO
1700 VeCo 91360 526-B5
CALLE SAN JUAN
23600 THO 91320 555-D3
CALLE SAN PABLO
500 CMRL 93012 524-E5
CALLE SANTIAGO
23600 THO 91320 555-D3
CALLE SEGUNDA
23600 CMRL 93010 524-C4
CALLE SEGURO
600 VeCo 91377 557-J2
CALLE SENCILLO
5700 CMRL 93012 525-B3
CALLE SEQUOIA
400 THO 91360 526-D7
400 VeCo 91360 526-D7
CALLE SERRA
23600 CMRL 93012 494-J7
CALLE SUERTE
900 CMRL 93012 524-H2
CALLE TAMEGA
- CMRL 93012 525-A3
CALLE TANIA
6700 CMRL 93012 495-C7
CALLE TECATE
3600 CMRL 93012 524-G2
CALLE TESORO
4100 CMRL 93012 524-H1
CALLE TIERRA VISTA
1300 CMRL 93010 523-H1
1700 VeCo 93010 523-H1
CALLE TILO
1500 THO 91360 526-H3
CALLE TULIPAN
1000 THO 91360 526-G3
CALLE TURQUESA
1500 THO 91320 526-A7
CALLE VALLE VISTA
3800 THO 91320 525-E7
CALLE VERACRUZ
23600 THO 91320 555-D3
CALLE VERBENA
2300 THO 91360 526-H4
CALLE VIEJO
3900 CMRL 93012 524-H4
CALLE VIOLETA
1300 THO 91360 526-H4
CALLE VISTA
1200 CMRL 93010 524-A2
CALLE VISTA CALMA
23600 OXN 93030 523-C6
CALLE VISTA DEL MONTE
- VeCo 93022 451-B5
CALLE VISTA VERDE
23600 OXN 93030 523-C7
CALLE YUCCA
400 THO 91360 526-C6
400 VeCo 91360 526-C5
CALLE ZAFIRO
1700 THO 91320 556-A1
CALLE ZOCALO
1500 THO 91360 496-J7
CALLICOTT AV
6200 WdHl 91367 529-F7
6600 CanP 91307 529-F6
CALMFIELD AV
5800 AGRH 91301 558-B3
CALUMET CANYON
- VeCo 93015 466-F2
- VeCo 93021 466-F2
CALUMET CANYON RD
23600 VeCo 93015 466-G1
CALUSA AV
3000 SIMI 93063 479-B6
CALVADOS DR
- CMRL 93012 525-A3
CALVERT CT
3000 VeCo 93012 496-E6
CALVERT ST
23800 WdHl 91367 529-C7
CALZONA CT
1500 SIMI 93065 497-F3
CAMARILLO AV
100 VeCo 93035 552-C6
CAMARILLO DR
- CMRL 93010 494-C7
- VeCo 93010 494-C7
CAMARILLO RD
- VeCo 93012 554-C3
CAMARILLO ST
- VeCo 93012 554-E4
- CMRL 93012 524-F4
CAMARILLO CENTER DR
300 CMRL 93010 524-B4
CAMARILLO RANCH RD
23600 CMRL 93012 524-G3
CAMARILLO SPRINGS RD
600 CMRL 93012 525-B6
600 VeCo 93012 525-C5
CAMBERWELL PL
1500 THO 91361 556-J6
CAMBON AV
2100 CMRL 93010 494-H7
CAMBON CIR
1100 VeCo 93023 451-C1
CAMBRIA AV
- VEN 93004 492-G1
CAMBRIA CT
1100 CMRL 93010 524-E1
3600 THO 91360 526-F1
CAMBRIDGE CT
29300 AGRH 91301 558-A4
29400 AGRH 91301 557-J4
E CAMBRIDGE ST
14300 MRPK 93021 476-G6
CAMDEN CT
12900 MRPK 93021 496-E4
CAMDEN LN
1300 VEN 93001 491-F5
CAMDEN VISTA CT
23600 SIMI 93065 498-B5
CAMELIA DR
800 PHME 93041 552-F5
CAMELIA LN
200 VeCo 91377 557-J2
CAMELIA WY
100 VEN 93004 473-A7
CAMELLIA ST
900 OXN 93036 522-E3
CAMELOT WY
1000 OXN 93030 522-G4
2000 OXN 93036 522-G4
CAMEO CT
1100 CMRL 93010 524-F2
CAMERON CT
- VEN 93001 471-C6
CAMERON ST
100 SPLA 93060 463-H6
800 VEN 93001 471-C6
CAMERTON CT
2000 VeCo 91361 556-H6
CAMILAR DR
2200 CMRL 93010
S CAMILLE CT
800 VeCo 93023
CAMILLE DR
1100 VeCo 93023
CAMINITO LUISA
- CMRL 93012
CAMINITO MIRADOR
- CMRL 93012
CAMINITO POSADA
- CMRL 93012
CAMINO AV
3400 OXN 93030
CAMINO AGUA DULCE
500 THO 91320
CAMINO ALGARVE
3900 CMRL 93012
CAMINO ALVAREZ
2200 CMRL 93010
CAMINO AVELLANA
- CMRL 93012
CAMINO CALANDRIA
2800 THO 91360
CAMINO CARILLO
- CMRL 93012
CAMINO CASTENADA
1300 CMRL 93010
CAMINO CIELO
- VeCo -
- VeCo -
- VeCo 93023
15400 VeCo 93023
CAMINO COMPRADE
5600 CMRL 93012
CAMINO CONCORDIA
500 VeCo 93010
600 VeCo 93010
CAMINO CORTINA
200 CMRL 93010
CAMINO CRISTOBAL
1300 VeCo 91360
CAMINO DE CELESTE
400 THO 91360
CAMINO DE LA LUNA
600 THO 91320
23600 OXN 93030
CAMINO DE LA LUZ
600 THO 91320
CAMINO DEL ARBOL
6200 CMRL 93012
CAMINO DE LA ROSA
4300 THO 91320
CAMINO DEL ARROYO
2000 VeCo 93023
CAMINO DE LAS ESTRELLAS
4300 THO 91320
CAMINO DEL CIELO
500 THO 91320
CAMINO DEL LAGO
500 THO 91320
CAMINO DEL MAR
600 THO 91320
CAMINO DEL RIO
23600 VeCo 93040
CAMINO DEL SOL
- CALB 91302
300 OXN 93030
600 THO 91320
1800 OXN 93030
1800 VeCo 93030
1800 VeCo 93030
CAMINO DEL ZURO
2900 THO 91360
CAMINO DEVILLE
5600 CMRL 93012
CAMINO DOS PALOS
300 THO 91360
CAMINO DOS RIOS
600 VeCo 91360
CAMINO DOS RIOS RD
2800 THO 91320
CAMINO DURANGO
600 VeCo 91360
CAMINO EL CARRIZO
700 VeCo 91360
CAMINO EL RINCON
- CMRL 93012
CAMINO ESPLENDIDO
- CMRL 93010
CAMINO ESTRADA
1300 CMRL 93010
CAMINO FLORES
700 VeCo 91360
CAMINO GRACIOSA
2900 THO 91360
CAMINO LA MADERA
900 CMRL 93010
CAMINO LA MAIDA
500 THO 91360
CAMINO LA POSADA
500 VeCo 93010
CAMINO LAS CONCHAS
700 VeCo 91360
CAMINO LAS RAMBLAS
700 CMRL 93012
CAMINO LEON
- CMRL 93012
CAMINO MADERO
800 VeCo 91360
CAMINO MAGENTA
1000 VeCo 91360
CAMINO MANZANAS
200 THO 91360
400 VeCo 91360
CAMINO OLMO
23600 THO 91320
CAMINO RANCHERO
23600 CMRL 93012
CAMINO ROBERTO
500 VeCo 91360
CAMINO ROJO
500 VeCo 91360
CAMINO RUIZ
100 CMRL 93012
1300 CMRL 93012
CAMINO SANTO REYES
600 VeCo 91360
CAMINO TIERRA SANTA
300 CMRL 93010
CAMINO TOLUCA
200 CMRL 93010
CAMINO VALLES
600 VeCo 91360
CAMINO VALVERDE
3900 CMRL 93012
CAMINO VERA CRUZ
1700 CMRL 93010
1700 CMRL 93010

City ZIP Pg-Grid
) VERDE
VeCo 91360 526-D6
NULA AV
VeCo 93004 473-B7
VeCo 93004 493-B1
ELL AV
THO 91360 526-D5
ELL WY
OXN 93033 552-G5
:HAFFEE RD
VeCo 93001 460-J5
OR AV
THO 91320 555-E4
OR CIR
THO 91320 555-E4
OR ST
SIMI 93063 499-A4
VERDE CT
VeCo 91377 557-J2
RAMAH RD
VeCo 93023 441-F5
ON DR
OXN 93030 522-J6
S DR
THO 91360 526-E1
PUS DR
OXN 93033 552-J3
OXN 93033 553-A3
PUS DR
OXN 93033 552-J4
OXN 93033 553-A4
THO 91360 526-E2
S RD
MRPK 93021 477-A6
VeCo 93021 477-B5
S ST
VEN 93003 492-A3
PUS WY
VEN 93003 492-A2
PUS WY
VEN 93003 492-A2
PUS WY
VEN 93003 492-A2
PUS WY
VEN 93003 491-J2
VEN 93003 492-A2
S PARK DR
MRPK 93021 476-H6
MRPK 93021 477-A6
WILLETT RD
VeCo 93001 451-D7
VeCo 93022 451-C7
OS ST
VeCo 93015 457-D5
VeCo 93040 457-E4
A ST
OJAI 93023 441-H6
A DE ALISOS
VeCo 93001 461-F4
A LARGA RD
VeCo 93001 461-G5
ST
OXN 93035 522-A7
IO CT
MRPK 93021 496-E3
Y LN
OXN 93033 553-A4
Y ST
VEN 93003 492-D5
N ST
SIMI 93065 497-F4
LARIA LN
FILM 93015 455-J4
LARIA RD
OXN 93030 523-B6
A CT
SIMI 93065 498-A1
CE CT
SIMI 93063 478-E7
ECREST DR
THO 91362 557-D1
THO 91362 527-D7
E PINE LN
SIMI 93065 497-A1
EWOOD CT
MRPK 93021 496-F3
EWOOD WY
CanP 91307 529-E5
TUFT ST
VEN 93004 493-A2
RD
VeCo 93001 461-B6
LD CT
THO 91360 526-F2
S DR
CALB 91301 558-G6
ORE ST
AGRH 91301 558-A3
A ST
THO 91360 526-D3
WY
VEN 93004 473-A7
S DR
THO 91362 526-J2
S SQ
OXN 93035 552-A2
GA PL
CMRL 93010 524-G1
CT
VEN 93003 472-C7
ST
VEN 93003 472-B7
Y DR
CMRL 93012 524-F5
RA ST
LA 91304 529-J2
R AV
CMRL 93010 524-D1
RA ST
THO 91360 526-F1
RBURY CT
VeCo 93023 441-E7
RBURY DR
AGRH 91301 558-A3
RBURY LN
SIMI 93063 498-H1
RBURY ST
THO 91362 527-D6
RBURY WY
OXN 93033 552-G5
RFORD CIR
THO 91361 557-C5
RHILL PL
WLKV 91361 557-C7
AY ST
CanP 91303 529-J5
CanP 91307 529-G5
ICE ST
SIMI 93065 527-D1

STREET Block City ZIP Pg-Grid
CANWOOD ST
26800 Ago 91301 558-F6
26800 CALB 91301 558-F6
28000 AGRH 91301 558-A6
29300 AGRH 91301 557-G6
CANYON RD
200 VeCo 91320 556-B2
23600 VeCo 93063 529-A1
CANYON WY
4800 AGRH 91301 558-C7
CANYON BREEZE CT
- SIMI 93065 497-G7
CANYON CLUB CIR
1800 SIMI 93065 497-J1
1800 SIMI 93065 478-A7
1800 SIMI 93065 498-A1
CANYON CREST CT
3500 THO 91360 526-H2
32100 WLKV 91361 557-C7
CANYON CREST DR
300 SIMI 93065 497-F7
300 SIMI 93065 527-F1
N CANYONLANDS RD
4500 MRPK 93021 496-E2
CANYON OAKS DR
6500 SIMI 93063 499-C1
CANYON RIDGE DR
32100 WLKV 91361 557-C7
CANYON RIM CIR
1300 THO 91362 527-G7
CANYON VIEW
800 FILM 93015 456-A5
CANYON VIEW DR
23600 SIMI 93065 497-F7
23600 SIMI 93065 527-F1
CANYON VISTA DR
1100 THO 91320 526-B7
CANYONWOOD CT
13400 MRPK 93021 496-F4
CANYONWOOD DR
24600 CanP 91307 529-C5
CANYON WREN CT
- MRPK 93021 476-E6
CAPE HORN DR
5800 AGRH 91301 557-G4
CAPELLA WY
2600 THO 91362 527-C3
CAPELLO WY
1100 VeCo 93023 451-C1
CAPEWOOD LN
23600 SIMI 93065 497-A2
CAPISTRANO AV
6100 WdHl 91367 529-J7
6500 CanP 91307 529-H5
7600 LA 91304 529-H2
9500 Chat 91311 499-H6
CAPISTRANO CT
300 CMRL 93010 524-D3
CAPITAN ST
100 THO 91320 556-C1
CAPRI AV
2700 VEN 93003 492-E6
CAPRI DR
100 VeCo 93065 497-F4
400 SIMI 93065 497-F4
CAPRI WY
1000 OXN 93035 521-J7
1200 OXN 93035 551-J1
CAPRICORN AV
6300 AGRH 91301 558-B3
CAPSTAN CIR
3700 WLKV 91361 557-C7
CAPSTAN DR
1700 OXN 93035 552-C1
CAPTAINS AV
2500 PHME 93041 552-D2
CAPTAINS PL
5300 AGRH 91301 557-G6
CARAWAY CT
3000 THO 91360 526-H2
CARDIFF CIR
1100 THO 91362 527-A6
CARDIGAN AV
1100 VEN 93004 492-G3
CARDINAL AV
2100 OXN 93033 553-B5
CARDINAL ST
5900 VEN 93003 492-C4
CARDINAL WY
5300 VeCo 91377 527-G7
CARDINAL RIDGE LN
23600 SIMI 93065 527-D1
CARDOZA DR
5800 WLKV 91362 557-F4
CAREFREE DR
900 SIMI 93065 497-G5
CARELL AV
5700 AGRH 91301 558-B4
CAREYBROOK DR
5900 AGRH 91301 558-A4
5900 AGRH 91301 557-J4
CARGO RD
- PHME 93043 552-C5
CARIBBEAN ST
- OXN 93035 552-B1
CARILLO RD
200 OJAI 93023 441-F7
200 OJAI 93023 451-F1
CARINA DR
- OXN 93030 522-G4
CARISSA CT
800 CMRL 93012 525-B2
CARISSA DR
- VEN 93004 493-A2
CARL CT
3400 VeCo 91320 555-F1
CARLA DR
200 SIMI 93065 497-F3
CARLA LN
8400 LA 91304 529-G2
CARLISLE CT
100 OXN 93033 552-G6
CARLISLE RD
100 VeCo 90265 586-C3
100 VeCo 91361 586-C3
600 THO 90265 586-E3
600 THO 91361 586-E3
CARLMONT PL
2700 SIMI 93065 478-A7
2700 SIMI 93065 498-A1
CARLOS ST
11000 VEN 93004 472-J7
11000 VEN 93004 473-A7
CARLOTTA ST
4000 SIMI 93063 498-F2
CARLSBAD CT
2200 SIMI 93063 498-E2
CARLSBAD PL
1100 VEN 93003 492-B4

STREET Block City ZIP Pg-Grid
CARLSON CIR
22200 CanP 91303 529-J5
22200 CanP 91307 529-J5
CARLTON DR
3200 THO 91360 526-G2
CARLYLE ST
10000 VEN 93004 492-J3
CARMEL CT
200 OXN 93033 553-C4
CARMEL DR
- FILM 93015 456-C6
1000 VeCo 93065 497-F4
CARMEL ST
8400 VEN 93004 492-G1
E CARMEL GREEN ST
100 PHME 93041 552-E2
W CARMEL GREEN ST
100 PHME 93041 552-D2
CARMELITA CT
100 OXN 93030 522-J5
CARMEN CT
2900 VeCo 91320 555-G1
CARMEN DR
1400 SIMI 93065 497-F3
23600 CMRL 93010 524-D4
N CARMEN DR
100 CMRL 93010 524-D2
CARMEN WY
1500 OXN 93036 522-E2
CARMENITA LN
7500 LA 91304 529-D4
CARMENTO DR
5300 VeCo 91377 557-H1
CARNATION AV
1500 VEN 93004 493-A2
CARNATION CT
23600 SIMI 93065 497-G5
CARNATION PL
300 OXN 93036 522-F3
CARNE RD
500 VeCo 93023 442-D6
CARNEGIE CT
1800 OXN 93033 553-A2
CARNEGIE ST
100 OXN 93036 492-J6
100 VeCo 93036 492-J6
CARNELLON CT
200 SIMI 93065 497-D7
CAROB DR
- THO 91320 555-J1
CAROB ST
1900 OXN 93035 552-D1
CAROL DR
200 VEN 93003 491-H2
CAROLINE AV
6200 SIMI 93063 499-B3
CARPENTER ST
1400 THO 91362 527-A6
CARPENTERIA AV
7100 VeCo 93001 459-C4
CARR DR
- VEN 93001 471-C7
CARRIAGE PL
100 FILM 93015 456-A7
CARRIAGE SQ
- OXN 93030 522-G3
CARRIE PL
32500 WLKV 91361 557-B7
CARRILLO CT
- FILM 93015 455-J4
CARRINGTON PT
- VeCo 93012 554-F2
CARRIZO ST
200 VeCo 93023 441-D6
CARSON ST
1400 SIMI 93065 497-J3
CARSON WY
1500 VEN 93004 492-H3
CARTAGENA WY
- OXN 93036 492-H7
CARTEGENA ST
100 CMRL 93010 524-D4
CARTHAGE WY
4900 VeCo 91377 557-H1
CARTPATH PL
- SIMI 93065 497-D5
CARTY DR
400 OXN 93030 522-G5
CARVER CT
2200 SIMI 93063 498-D2
CARVER SUMMIT RD
23600 VeCo 93001 459-D3
CARY CT
3400 VeCo 91320 525-F7
CARYL DR
23600 VeCo 93033 584-B1
CASA ST
11100 VEN 93004 472-J6
11200 VEN 93004 473-A6
CASABELLA CT
500 SPLA 93060 463-J7
CASA GRANDE RD
1000 VeCo 93063 499-C4
CASARIN AV
1500 SIMI 93065 497-J4
CASARIN ST
1700 SIMI 93065 497-J4
CASA SAN CARLOS
1300 OXN 93033 552-E2
CASCADE AV
100 THO 91362 557-C3
200 OXN 93033 552-G4
CASCADES CT
1900 OXN 93036 522-D3
CASCARA CT
- SIMI 93065 478-A5
CASE ST
4200 VEN 93003 491-J1
CASEY RD
100 MRPK 93021 476-D7
CASINO DR
2900 THO 91362 526-J2
2900 THO 91362 527-A2
CASITAS CT
1100 VEN 93004 492-J2
CASITAS PASS RD Rt#-150
2000 VeCo 93001 450-D5
3500 VeCo 93001 460-B1
4000 VeCo 93001 366-G8
4000 VeCo 93001 459-G1
7100 StBC 93013 459-G1
CASITAS PASS RD Rt#-192
6800 StBC 93013 459-A1
CASITAS VISTA RD
500 VeCo 93001 460-G4
7200 VeCo 93001 461-A5
CASMALIA CT
1300 SIMI 93065 497-H1

STREET Block City ZIP Pg-Grid
CASMALIA LN
800 VEN 93001 491-C1
CASNER WY
100 FILM 93015 456-B5
CASPER CT
4300 OXN 93033 553-A4
CASPER RD
2900 VeCo 93033 583-B2
2900 VeCo 93042 583-C2
4700 VeCo 93033 553-B7
CASPIAN CT
- AGRH 91301 557-G4
CASPIAN WY
- OXN 93035 522-B7
- OXN 93035 552-B1
CASTANO DR
3500 CMRL 93010 524-G1
CASTANO ST
1600 CMRL 93010 524-G1
CASTELLO WY
4800 VeCo 91377 557-G2
CASTILLIAN AV
100 THO 91320 556-C1
CASTILLIAN CT
- THO 91320 556-C1
CASTILLO CIR
2600 THO 91360 526-C4
CASTILLO DE ROSA
- CMRL 93012 495-A6
CASTLE CT
2200 SIMI 93063 499-B1
CASTLEBRIDGE CT
1600 THO 91362 527-E6
CASTLE CREEK LN
- OXN 93036 522-C3
CASTLEHILL CT
1600 THO 91361 556-J5
CASTLEHILL DR
29300 AGRH 91301 558-A4
29300 AGRH 91301 557-J4
CASTLEMERE CT
1100 SIMI 93065 498-C4
N CASTLEMONT CT
2400 SIMI 93063 498-E1
CASTLE PEAK DR
6900 CanP 91307 529-C5
CASTLETON ST
- CMRL 93012 524-F4
CASTLEVIEW CT
1500 THO 91361 556-J5
CASTLEWOOD LN
- SIMI 93065 478-B4
CASUAL CT
1900 SIMI 93065 498-A7
CATALANO CT
- FILM 93015 455-J4
CATALINA DR
- VeCo 93010 494-D7
10500 VeCo 93022 451-B4
W CATALINA DR
- VeCo 93010 494-D7
10500 VeCo 93022 451-B5
CATALINA PL
- OXN 93035 522-D7
N CATALINA ST
- VEN 93001 491-F2
S CATALINA ST
- VEN 93001 491-F2
CATAMARAN ST
900 OXN 93035 521-J7
CATANIA CT
11800 MRPK 93021 496-C5
CATARINA DR
30800 WLKV 91362 557-F4
CATHEDRAL CV
- VeCo 93012 554-E3
CATHERWOOD CT
29000 AGRH 91301 558-A3
CATHY DR
100 VeCo 91320 555-G1
CATLIN CIR
800 SIMI 93065 497-H4
CATLIN CT
1100 SIMI 93065 497-H4
CATLIN ST
700 SIMI 93065 497-G4
CAVALIER AV
1000 SIMI 93065 498-C4
CAVENWAY LN
3000 THO 91361 557-C5
CAVIN RD
300 VeCo 93015 456-H7
CAWELTI RD
- VeCo 93012 524-C7
CAY CT
200 VeCo 91320 555-G1
CAYMAN CT
- THO 91320 555-E3
CAYO GRANDE CT
500 THO 91320 525-E7
500 THO 91320 555-F1
N CAYTON AV
1600 SIMI 93065 497-E3
N CAYTON PL
1500 SIMI 93065 497-E3
CAYUGA DR
1500 SIMI 93065 497-F3
8300 VEN 93004 492-G4
CAYUSE LN
2200 VEN 93001 471-D6
CEANOTHUS LN
700 VeCo 93023 442-F5
CEANOTHUS PL
3900 CALB 91302 558-G7
CEBOLLA DR
23600 CMRL 93012 524-J3
CEDAR
5100 OXN 93033 552-J5
CEDAR CT
800 OXN 93033 552-F1
CEDAR DR
- CMRL 93010 524-D4
CEDAR PL
200 VEN 93001 491-C1
CEDAR ST
- VEN 93001 491-B1
800 VEN 93001 471-D6
1400 SPLA 93060 464-A2
6000 VeCo 93063 499-B4
E CEDAR ST
100 OXN 93033 552-G1
W CEDAR ST
200 OXN 93033 552-E1
CEDARBARK CT
6600 VeCo 91377 528-B7
CEDAR BLUFF DR
900 MRPK 93021 476-E7
CEDAR BRANCH CT
4400 MRPK 93021 496-E3

STREET Block City ZIP Pg-Grid
CEDARBROOK WK
- CMRL 93012 524-H1
CEDARCLIFF CT
600 THO 91362 557-F1
CEDAR CREST CT
- THO 91320 556-C1
CEDARDALE RD
4300 MRPK 93021 496-C3
CEDARGLEN CT
4400 MRPK 93021 496-D3
CEDAR GROVE LN
4200 MRPK 93021 496-F3
CEDARHAVEN DR
5300 AGRH 91301 557-H5
CEDAR HEIGHTS DR
100 THO 91360 526-E3
CEDAR MEADOW CT
4300 MRPK 93021 496-D3
CEDARPINE LN
3900 MRPK 93021 496-F3
CEDAR POINT PL
300 THO 91362 557-G2
CEDAR RIDGE CT
2200 OXN 93036 522-D2
CEDAR SPRINGS ST
3900 MRPK 93021 496-C3
CEDARVALLEY DR
31200 WLKV 91362 557-E5
N CEDARWOOD CIR
2400 SIMI 93063 498-E1
CEDAR WOOD PL
2600 THO 91362 526-J3
CELESTIAL PL
- CMRL 93012 524-F5
E CELIA CT
3900 SIMI 93063 498-F2
CELSIUS AV
2200 OXN 93030 523-B5
CEMETERY RD
100 SPLA 93060 463-J6
CENTENNIAL AV
1000 CMRL 93010 524-E2
CENTER LN
400 SPLA 93060 463-H6
CENTER RD
- VeCo 93066 493-G3
900 VeCo 93066 494-B1
1000 VeCo 93066 474-B7
CENTER ST
3400 VeCo 93040 457-E4
E CENTER ST
- VEN 93001 491-B1
W CENTER ST
- VEN 93001 491-B1
CENTER COURT DR
2300 THO 91361 557-A6
CENTER SCHOOL RD
3100 VeCo 93010 494-B5
3400 VeCo 93066 494-B5
CENTINELLA ST
6100 SIMI 93063 499-B2
CENTRAL AV
100 FILM 93015 456-A5
100 VeCo 93036 492-J4
100 VeCo 93036 493-A4
500 CMRL 93010 523-E1
2500 VeCo 93010 493-D7
2500 VeCo 93010 523-E1
3000 VEN 93003 491-G3
CENTRAL CAMPUS WY
100 VEN 93003 492-A2
CENTURY AV
2200 SIMI 93063 498-E2
CENTURY PL
2100 SIMI 93063 498-E2
CERCIS WY
1400 VEN 93004 493-A2
CERES ST
100 SIMI 93065 497-F2
CERRO CREST DR
- VeCo 93010 494-B7
CERRO VISTA WY
1300 CMRL 93010 524-C1
1700 CMRL 93010 494-C7
CERVANTES CT
600 VeCo 91377 557-J2
CERVATO CT
- CMRL 93012 525-C1
CERVATO DR
1700 CMRL 93012 525-C1
1800 CMRL 93012 495-C7
CESAR CHAVEZ DR
- OXN 93030 523-A4
- VeCo 93030 522-H4
- VeCo 93030 523-A4
400 OXN 93030 522-H4
CHADWICK CT
3500 THO 91320 555-F3
CHADWICK PL
23600 VEN 93003 492-B7
CHAFFEE ST
6300 VEN 93003 492-C1
CHAGALL DR
6000 VeCo 93021 475-H6
N CHAIN DR
2400 SIMI 93065 497-F1
CHALET CIR
1000 THO 91362 527-B7
CHALLENGE PL
23600 OXN 93030 523-C6
CHALLENGER CT
11900 MRPK 93021 496-C1
CHALMERS PL
25800 LACo 91302 558-J3
CHALMETTE AV
1100 VEN 93003 492-B4
W CHALON CT
- THO 91320 556-A2
W CHALON ST
1900 THO 91320 556-A2
1900 THO 91320 555-J2
CHAMBERLAIN ST
- VEN 93004 492-J3
CHAMBERS LN
500 SIMI 93065 497-G1
CHAMBERSBURG RD Rt#-23
300 FILM 93015 466-A2
300 VeCo 93015 466-A2
CHAMINADE AV
7400 LA 91304 529-F4
CHAMISE CT
- SIMI 93063 498-J2
CHAMOIS ST
7100 VEN 93003 492-E5
CHAMPAGNE CT
30800 WLKV 91362 557-F5
CHAMPIONSHIP DR
- MRPK 93021 476-C5

STREET Block City ZIP Pg-Grid
CHAMPLAIN AV
1400 VEN 93004 492-H3
CHANCERY PL
2800 THO 91362 527-B3
CHANDLER AV
2400 SIMI 93065 497-H1
CHANDLER ST
2100 CMRL 93010 524-E2
CHANNEL DR
1800 VEN 93001 491-E3
2300 VEN 93003 491-F3
CHANNEL WY
900 SPLA 93060 473-J1
5200 OXN 93035 521-H6
CHANNELFORD RD
1900 THO 91361 557-A6
CHANNEL HEIGHTS CT
6200 VEN 93003 472-C6
CHANNEL ISLANDS BLVD
1800 OXN 93033 553-A2
2200 VeCo 93033 553-A2
E CHANNEL ISLANDS BLVD
100 OXN 93033 552-H2
100 PHME 93041 552-H2
300 PHME 93033 552-H2
300 PHME 93043 552-H2
W CHANNEL ISLANDS BLVD
100 OXN 93033 552-F2
100 PHME 93041 552-C2
300 PHME 93043 552-E2
500 PHME 93035 552-C2
3800 OXN 93035 552-A2
4500 VeCo 93035 552-A2
CHANNEL ISLANDS DR
- VeCo 93012 554-E2
CHANTILLY CIR
23600 SIMI 93065 497-F7
CHANTRY CIR
700 SIMI 93065 497-H5
CHAPALA DR
1300 CMRL 93010 524-D2
CHAPALA ST
400 CMRL 93010 524-D2
CHAPARRAL CT
700 THO 91320 556-C2
CHAPARRAL RD
500 VeCo 93022 451-A6
3800 VeCo 93023 442-E4
9200 Chat 91311 499-E7
9200 LA 91304 499-E7
9200 WHil 91304 499-E7
CHAPARRAL ST
600 FILM 93015 455-J5
CHAPEL AV
1600 CMRL 93010 524-D3
CHAPEL DR
- VeCo 93012 554-E4
300 VEN 93003 491-J3
1300 CMRL 93010 524-D3
CHAPMAN PL
6700 MRPK 93021 476-H6
CHAPS CT
1700 SIMI 93063 499-C3
CHARI LN
6600 VeCo 93066 495-C3
CHARING CT
1800 SIMI 93063 499-D2
CHARING ST
6500 SIMI 93063 499-C2
CHARISMA CT
11200 VeCo 93012 496-C7
CHARLA CT
- THO 91320 556-B1
CHARLES ST
100 MRPK 93021 476-E7
5100 OXN 93033 552-G5
CHARLESTON PL
- VEN 93004 492-H2
CHARLOTTE ST
300 THO 91320 555-G2
N CHARRO AV
100 THO 91320 556-C1
CHARTER OAK DR
2000 CMRL 93010 494-E7
CHARTERWOOD CT
1300 THO 91362 556-J1
CHARTHOUSE CIR
3800 WLKV 91361 557-B6
CHASE PL
22700 LA 91304 529-H2
CHASE ST
8400 LA 91304 529-F2
CHATEAU CT
5900 VEN 93003 492-C2
CHATHAM CT
1000 THO 91360 526-H2
CHATLAKE DR
8700 LA 91304 529-E1
CHATSWORTH ST
22000 Chat 91311 499-J3
CHAUCER
9400 VeCo 93012 495-G4
9400 VeCo 93021 495-G4
CHAUCER LN
6800 VEN 93003 492-E3
CHAUCER PL
2500 THO 91362 527-B3
CHAUTAUGUA DR
1300 SIMI 93063 499-C3
N CHEAM AV
2000 SIMI 93063 499-C2
CHEERFUL CT
200 SIMI 93065 497-J6
CHELAN CT
300 SIMI 93065 497-F6
CHELAN LN
1100 VEN 93004 492-H3
CHELMAS CT
23600 SIMI 93063 478-E6
CHELSEA CT
800 SIMI 93065 498-D5
6300 AGRH 91301 557-H3
CHELSEA LN
- LA 91304 529-J2
CHELSEY CT
2200 CMRL 93010 494-D7
CHELTERHAM CIR
800 THO 91360 526-G6
CHENAULT PL
2000 SIMI 93065 497-D2
CHERBOURG CT
30800 WLKV 91362 557-F5
CHEROKEE CIR
5700 SIMI 93063 479-A6
CHEROKEE CT
1300 CMRL 93010 524-F1

STREET Block City ZIP Pg-Grid
CHERRY AV
1200 SIMI 93065 498-B4
1500 OXN 93033 553-B5
CHERRY ST
3700 VEN 93003 491-J3
CHERRY CREEK CIR
800 THO 91362 557-G1
CHERRYGROVE ST
12100 MRPK 93021 496-D4
CHERRY HILL RD
1600 SPLA 93060 464-A1
CHERRY HILLS CT
- THO 91320 556-D1
CHERRY HILLS LN
400 THO 91320 556-D1
CHERRY RIDGE DR
5500 CMRL 93012 525-A2
CHERRY VALLEY CIR
4500 THO 91362 527-D6
CHERRYWOOD DR
3000 THO 91360 526-F2
CHERRYWOOD PL
900 OXN 93030 522-H3
CHERRYWOOD ST
- FILM 93015 456-B6
CHERYL CT
2700 SIMI 93063 478-D7
CHESAPEAKE CT
- THO 91320 555-E3
CHESAPEAKE DR
- OXN 93035 522-A7
- OXN 93035 552-A1
CHESAPEAKE PL
- VEN 93004 492-H2
CHESEBRO RD
5000 AGRH 91301 558-D3
5300 Ago 91301 558-D3
6300 VeCo 91377 528-C7
6300 VeCo 91377 558-D3
CHESEBRO CANYON RD
- VeCo 91377 528-D5
- VeCo 91377 558-E1
5800 Ago 91301 558-E5
CHESHIRE ST
8100 VEN 93004 492-F4
CHESHIRE HILLS CT
- THO 91361 556-H5
CHESSHIRE CT
100 VeCo 93023 441-E7
CHESTER WY
200 OXN 93033 552-G5
CHESTERFIELD DR
13600 MRPK 93021 496-F2
CHESTERTON ST
2000 SIMI 93065 498-A1
CHESTNUT LN
3300 VeCo 93012 495-J5
CHESTNUT PL
5800 CMRL 93012 495-B7
CHESTNUT ST
- SIMI 93063 498-J1
700 THO 91320 556-C2
N CHESTNUT ST
- VEN 93001 491-C2
S CHESTNUT ST
- VEN 93001 491-C2
CHESTNUT HILL CT
300 THO 91360 526-E7
CHESTNUT RIDGE ST
11600 MRPK 93021 496-B4
CHESWICK PL
1500 THO 91361 556-J6
CHEVIOT HILLS CT
- THO 91361 556-J6
CHEYENNE AV
- THO 91362 557-A2
11200 Chat 91311 499-J1
CHEYENNE CIR
9900 VEN 93004 492-J3
CHEYENNE ST
9800 VEN 93004 492-H3
CHEYENNE WY
900 OXN 93033 552-J3
N CHICKADEE LN
1100 VEN 93003 492-F3
S CHICKADEE LN
1300 VEN 93003 492-F4
CHICO CT
2300 VeCo 93035 552-B5
CHICO DR
9200 VEN 93004 492-G2
CHICO RD
100 OJAI 93023 441-G7
CHICO LARSON WY
- VeCo - 366-L2
CHICORY LEAF PL
23600 SIMI 93063 498-D4
CHIEF CIR
3400 THO 91360 526-C2
CHILCO CT
1600 THO 91360 526-C5
CHINA FIR PL
23600 SIMI 93065 498-D4
CHINA FLATS RD
1000 VeCo 91361 556-F5
CHINOOK DR
600 VEN 93001 471-D6
CHIPMUNK CIR
7000 VEN 93003 492-F4
CHIPPENDALE AV
- SIMI 93065 497-D6
CHIPPENHAM RD
10600 VeCo 93012 495-J7
10600 VeCo 93012 496-A7
CHIPPEWA AV
2800 SIMI 93063 479-A7
CHIPPEWA LN
2300 VEN 93001 471-C6
CHIQUITA LN
2200 THO 91362 556-J2
2200 THO 91362 557-A2
CHISHOLM TR
- THO 91320 555-H2
CHISMAHOO RD
23600 VeCo - 366-G8
23600 VeCo 93001 366-G8
CHISMAHOO FIRE RD
23600 VeCo 93001 460-C2
CHOCTAW AV
2900 SIMI 93063 479-A7
CHOCTAW LN
400 VEN 93001 471-C6
CHRISMAN AV
- VEN 93001 491-E2
CHRISTIAN CT
5300 AGRH 91301 557-H5
CHRISTIAN BARRETT DR
13300 MRPK 93021 496-F3

STREET Block City ZIP Pg-Grid

CHRISTINA AV
5600 CMRL 93012 525-B6
CHRISTINA CT
1200 CMRL 93010 524-C2
CHRISTINE AV
1400 SIMI 93063 499-B2
CHRISTOPHER LN
100 VeCo 93023 441-E7
CHUKAR LN
200 VeCo 93010 494-F7
CHULA VISTA CT
4700 CMRL 93012 524-J2
CHUMASH AV
2900 SIMI 93063 478-J7
CHUMASH RD
12000 VeCo 93023 453-B1
CHUMASH TR
23600 VeCo 90265 625-G1
CHURCH DR
2000 VEN 93003 492-C5
CHURCH RD
400 OJAI 93023 441-F7
1500 THO 91362 526-J5
CHURCH ST
500 VeCo 93040 457-F4
700 VEN 93001 491-C1
N CHURCH ST
1400 SIMI 93065 498-D3
CHURCHILL DR
2100 OXN 93033 553-A2
4000 THO 91320 555-E3
CHURCHMAN LN
10200 VeCo 93012 495-J7
CHURCHWOOD DR
5100 VeCo 91377 557-H1
N CICERO CT
3000 SIMI 93063 478-F7
CID ST
11300 VEN 93004 473-A7
CIELO CIR
- CALB 91302 558-H6
CIELO VISTA CT
5800 CMRL 93012 495-B7
CIMA DE LAGO ST
9200 Chat 91311 499-E7
CIMARRON AV
1200 VEN 93004 492-J3
CIMMARON AV
2600 SIMI 93065 478-C7
2600 SIMI 93065 498-C1
N CINCH RD
- VeCo 91307 529-A4
CINCO DE MAYO
10200 VEN 93004 492-J3
10200 VEN 93004 493-A2
CINDY AV
- THO 91320 555-H1
CINDY PL
2600 PHME 93041 552-D2
CINERARIA ST
- VEN 93004 493-A2
CINNABAR PL
700 SIMI 93065 498-D5
CINNAMON OAK AV
- VEN 93004 473-A6
CIPRES CT
1400 CMRL 93010 524-D2
CIPRIAN AV
1700 CMRL 93010 494-G7
1700 CMRL 93010 524-G1
CIRCLE DR
2900 OXN 93033 552-H3
CIRCLE KNOLL DR
- SIMI 93065 527-C1
CIRCLE VIEW DR
2700 SIMI 93063 478-D7
CIRCULO JARDIN
23600 CMRL 93010 523-F2
CIRO AV
2400 THO 91360 526-E3
CIRO CIR
300 THO 91360 526-E4
CIRRUS WY
7200 CanP 91307 529-F5
CISCO CT
2900 SIMI 93063 478-G7
CITADEL AV
300 VEN 93003 492-A3
CITATION WY
400 THO 91320 526-B7
CITRONELLA CT
2600 SIMI 93063 498-E1
CITRONELLA ST
3600 SIMI 93063 498-E1
CITRUS DR
4000 VeCo 93021 496-A3
10700 VeCo 93021 495-J4
11000 VEN 93004 472-J7
11000 VEN 93004 473-A7
11100 VeCo 93004 473-A7
CITRUS ST
300 SPLA 93060 464-C4
3000 VeCo 93036 492-J7
CITRUS GROVE LN
- OXN 93036 522-G3
CITRUS VIEW DR
4000 VeCo 93040 457-F4
CIVIC ARTS PLAZA DR
1600 THO 91362 556-J2
CIVIC CENTER WY
23600 THO 91360 526-E7
CLAIRE CT
- THO 91320 555-F2
CLANCY CT
- SIMI 93065 497-E2
CLARA ST
6200 VeCo 93003 492-D5
E CLARA ST
100 OXN 93033 552-G6
100 PHME 93041 552-E5
800 PHME 93033 552-E5
W CLARA ST
100 OXN 93033 552-F5
100 PHME 93041 552-E5
CLAREMONT DR
1500 OXN 93035 552-D1
CLAREMONT WY
- VEN 93003 492-A2
CLARENDON PL
3300 THO 91360 526-H2
CLARETON DR
5100 AGRH 91301 558-B6
CLARIDGE CT
3500 SIMI 93063 478-G5
CLARINGTON DR
23900 LA 91304 529-D4
CLARITA CT
2500 THO 91362 527-C3
CLARK CT
200 OXN 93033 552-G6

CLARKE RANCH RD
- LACo 90265 586-G6
CLARKIA ST
- SIMI 93065 477-J5
- SIMI 93065 478-A5
CLARK RANCH RD
23600 VeCo 93022 451-E4
23600 VeCo 93023 451-E4
CLASSIC ROSE CT
1700 THO 91362 527-C6
CLAUDIA AV
1600 SIMI 93065 498-B3
CLAVEL AV
1200 VeCo 93004 493-B1
1200 VEN 93004 493-B1
CLAVELE AV
4300 MRPK 93021 496-E3
CLAVELE CT
4300 MRPK 93021 496-E3
CLAY AV
1100 VEN 93004 492-J2
CLAY BLVD
23600 VeCo 93060 453-G2
CLAY CT
- THO 91360 556-G1
CLAY ST
200 FILM 93015 456-A5
CLAYBOURNE CT
3500 THO 91320 555-F3
CLAYFORD AV
1100 THO 91361 557-A5
CLAYTON CT
1200 CMRL 93010 524-D1
CLAYTON WY
1400 SIMI 93065 497-H3
CLEAR DR
8600 VEN 93004 492-G4
CLEARCREEK CT
4400 MRPK 93021 496-B3
CLEARFIELD PL
2500 SIMI 93065 497-J1
CLEARFORD CT
3900 WLKV 91361 557-D6
CLEAR HAVEN DR
700 VeCo 91377 558-B1
CLEAR SKY PL
23600 SIMI 93065 497-E4
CLEAR SPRINGS RD
6400 VeCo 93063 499-C4
CLEARVIEW AV
2500 VEN 93001 491-F4
CLEARVIEW ST
100 THO 91360 526-F3
CLEARWATER DR
1700 CMRL 93012 495-B7
1700 CMRL 93012 525-B1
CLEARWATER ST
2500 THO 91362 557-B3
CLEARWATER CREEK DR
- THO 91320 555-F3
CLEARWOOD RD
4300 MRPK 93021 496-C3
CLEE CT
5500 AGRH 91301 558-A5
CLEMENS AV
8000 LA 91304 529-F3
CLEMENS ST
6300 VEN 93003 492-C1
CLEMSON ST
5200 VEN 93003 492-B2
14100 MRPK 93021 476-G6
CLEOMOORE AV
6500 CanP 91307 529-E6
CLERMONT CT
5400 WLKV 91362 557-F5
CLEVELAND CT
100 VEN 93003 492-E1
CLEVELAND DR
2800 OXN 93036 492-H7
28600 AGRH 91301 558-B6
CLEVENGER PL
100 SIMI 93065 497-E7
100 SIMI 93065 527-E1
CLIFF AV
700 VeCo 93015 455-G4
CLIFF DR
900 SPLA 93060 464-C3
CLIFFHOLLOW CT
500 SIMI 93065 527-C1
CLIFFROSE AV
4000 MRPK 93021 496-E4
CLIFFSIDE CIR
5300 VEN 93003 492-B1
CLIFFSIDE CT
- LA 91304 529-E4
CLIFFWOOD DR
200 SIMI 93065 497-E2
CLIFTON CT
700 SIMI 93065 497-J5
CLINTON AV
1000 VEN 93004 492-H3
CLINTON CIR
3100 OXN 93033 552-H3
8800 VEN 93004 492-G3
CLINTON CT
8800 VEN 93004 492-G3
CLINTON ST
3000 OXN 93033 552-H3
11800 VeCo 93021 476-C2
CLIPPER DR
500 OXN 93033 552-G5
CLIPPERS CIR
2300 THO 91361 557-B6
CLOUD CT
1800 SIMI 93065 498-A2
CLOUDCREST CT
200 THO 91320 555-G2
CLOUDPEAK ST
- THO 91360 526-F2
CLOVER DR
4300 OXN 93033 552-H5
CLOVER LN
- VEN 93004 493-A2
CLOVER ST
2000 SIMI 93065 498-C2
E CLOVERDALE ST
4300 MRPK 93021 496-E3
N CLOVERDALE ST
12800 MRPK 93021 496-E3
CLOVERLEAF LN
- SIMI 93063 498-H1
CLOVERLEAF ST
3900 THO 91362 527-C6
CLOVERLY ST
5900 VEN 93003 492-C2
CLOVERWOOD AV
100 THO 91320 555-J2
CLOW RD
200 VeCo 93060 473-G2

S CLOW RD
100 VeCo 93060 473-H2
CLOYNE ST
2900 OXN 93033 552-H3
CLUB CT
- CMRL 93010 493-H7
CLUBHOUSE DR
- LACo 90265 586-H7
200 SIMI 93065 497-E2
3900 VeCo 93066 493-F2
CLUB VIEW DR
4500 THO 91362 527-D6
CLYDESDALE CIR
4100 THO 91362 527-C6
CMWD TANK RD
- VeCo 93023 442-G7
- VeCo 93023 452-G1
COACHMAN CIR
4200 THO 91362 527-D7
COACHMAN DR
1700 CMRL 93012 495-A7
1700 CMRL 93012 525-A1
COALFAX CT
2200 THO 91362 527-A4
COASTAL OAK DR
23600 SIMI 93063 498-D4
23600 SIMI 93065 498-D4
COATI PL
7300 VEN 93003 492-F5
COATS ST
- PHME 93041 552-E4
- PHME 93043 552-E4
COBALT AV
- VEN 93004 492-F3
COBB CIR
3000 SIMI 93065 498-D4
COBBLECREEK CT
2500 THO 91362 527-D3
COBBLER HILL CT
700 SIMI 93065 498-D5
COBBLESTONE DR
6000 AGRH 91301 557-J3
6000 VEN 93003 492-C1
COCHE CANYON
23600 VeCo 93001 451-G7
23600 VeCo 93001 461-G1
COCHISE ST
5400 SIMI 93063 478-J7
COCHRAN ST
- SIMI 93063 479-B7
- SIMI 93065 497-G1
200 SIMI 93065 477-E7
1700 SIMI 93065 498-B1
3100 SIMI 93063 498-D1
5400 SIMI 93063 499-A1
COCOS CT
4000 VEN 93003 491-J3
CODY AV
1600 SIMI 93063 499-C3
COE ST
700 CMRL 93010 524-C2
COFFEETREE LN
- MRPK 93021 496-G2
COHASSET ST
22000 CanP 91303 529-J4
22600 CanP 91307 529-G4
23200 LA 91304 529-F4
COLBY CIR
300 VEN 93003 492-A3
1000 THO 91362 526-J6
COLCHESTER PL
1500 VeCo 91377 527-H6
COLDBROOK PL
600 SIMI 93065 497-H5
COLD SPRINGS ST
26800 CALB 91301 558-G7
COLD STREAM CT
2000 OXN 93036 522-E3
COLE AV
3200 VeCo 93063 478-E6
COLEMAN CT
2000 SIMI 93063 499-A2
COLETTE CT
3100 SIMI 93063 478-D6
COLGATE DR
1700 THO 91360 526-G5
COLGATE ST
300 SPLA 93060 463-J7
300 SPLA 93060 464-A7
COLIBRI CT
4200 MRPK 93021 496-E3
COLINA RD
23600 VeCo 93063 499-F3
COLINA VISTA
400 VEN 93003 472-C6
400 VEN 93003 492-D1
COLINA VISTA ST
28700 AGRH 91301 558-B3
COLISEUM ST
4100 VEN 93003 491-J2
COLLEEN AV
1700 SIMI 93063 498-J3
COLLEGE DR
- VEN 93003 491-J3
COLLEGE ST
2400 SIMI 93065 498-B5
COLLEGE HEIGHTS DR
6400 MRPK 93021 476-G6
COLLEGE VIEW AV
6400 MRPK 93021 477-A6
COLLEGIATE CIR
15200 MRPK 93021 476-J5
COLLIER CT
2200 SIMI 93065 498-A2
COLLINGSWOOD CT
1700 THO 91362 527-E6
COLLINGSWOOD PL
4800 THO 91362 527-E6
COLLINS DR
6400 MRPK 93021 476-J6
6500 MRPK 93021 477-A5
E COLLINS ST
200 VeCo 93036 492-H7
200 VeCo 93036 522-J1
700 VeCo 93036 523-A1
1000 OXN 93036 523-A1
W COLLINS ST
100 OXN 93036 492-H7
COLODNY DR
5200 AGRH 91301 558-D5
COLOMA CIR
5500 SIMI 93063 479-A7
COLONETT PL
3900 THO 91320 555-E1
COLONIA AV
2400 OXN 93036 522-H1
2700 OXN 93036 492-H7
COLONIA PL
1700 CMRL 93010 524-D3

COLONIA RD
1300 OXN 93030 522-G5
COLONY DR
4600 CMRL 93012 524-J2
5100 CMRL 93012 525-A2
COLORADO RIVER PL
- OXN 93036 492-G7
COLT LN
100 VeCo 91361 556-G3
E COLT LN
- VeCo 91307 528-J4
- VeCo 91307 529-A4
COLT ST
4800 VEN 93003 492-B6
COLTON ST
7700 VEN 93004 492-F2
23600 VEN 93003 492-E2
COLTRANE ST
- VEN 93003 492-C4
N COLUMBIA AV
6500 MRPK 93021 476-H6
COLUMBIA CT
800 OXN 93033 552-H4
COLUMBIA DR
700 OXN 93033 552-H4
1800 VEN 93004 492-G4
COLUMBIA PL
100 OXN 93033 552-H4
COLUMBIA RD
- THO 91360 526-F5
COLUMBINE CT
2800 THO 91360 526-D3
COLUMBUS PL
5100 OXN 93033 552-G5
COLUSA AV
300 VEN 93004 472-F7
300 VEN 93004 492-F1
COMANCHE AV
2700 THO 91362 557-A2
COMANCHE CT
900 CMRL 93010 524-C2
2500 VEN 93001 471-D5
COMBES AV
500 THO 91360 526-G7
COMBS RD
1100 VeCo 91320 556-B2
1200 THO 91320 556-B2
COMET AV
600 SIMI 93065 498-C5
COMMERCE AV
23600 MRPK 93021 496-C1
COMMERCIAL AV
100 OXN 93030 522-H6
1200 OXN 93030 552-H1
COMMONS PARK DR
- CMRL 93012 524-F5
COMMONWEALTH CIR
- THO 91361 556-H5
COMMUNITY ST
23200 LA 91304 529-E2
COMPASS WY
- PHME 93041 552-E5
COMSTOCK DR
- VEN 93001 471-C6
COMSTOCK PL
1200 THO 91320 555-G5
CONCERTO DR
200 VeCo 91377 557-G2
CONCHA ST
- OXN 93030 522-J4
N CONCHO LN
- VeCo 91307 529-B3
CONCORD AV
700 VEN 93004 492-H2
CONCORD CT
3700 OXN 93033 552-J3
E CONCORD CT
1900 SIMI 93065 498-A5
CONCORD DR
2900 OXN 93033 552-J3
CONCORD WY
4400 OXN 93033 552-J4
CONDOR CT
300 FILM 93015 455-H6
6300 VEN 93003 492-D5
CONDOR DR
5700 MRPK 93021 476-H7
CONEFLOWER ST
2800 THO 91360 526-D3
CONEJO BLVD
- THO 91360 556-F1
CONEJO CANYON CT
2600 THO 91362 527-B4
CONEJO CENTER DR
- THO 91320 525-H5
CONEJO MESA ST
4000 MRPK 93021 496-E4
CONEJO RIDGE AV
200 THO 91361 556-J3
CONEJO SCHOOL RD
100 THO 91361 556-J2
100 THO 91362 556-J2
200 THO 91362 557-A1
600 THO 91362 527-A7
CONEJO SPECTRUM ST
- THO 91320 525-H5
CONEJO VIEW DR
28500 AGRH 91301 558-B5
CONESTOGA CIR
800 THO 91320 555-G6
CONGRESSIONAL RD
600 SIMI 93065 497-C6
CONIFER CIR
5600 VeCo 91377 557-J2
CONIFER ST
5700 VeCo 91377 557-J2
5700 VeCo 91377 558-A2
N CONNELL AV
2100 SIMI 93063 499-A2
CONNER CT
- THO 91320 555-E3
CONNER DR
- OXN 93033 552-G6
CONSTITUTION AV
400 CMRL 93012 524-F5
CONSUELO AV
3600 THO 91360 526-F1
CONTAINER WY
- PHME 93043 552-C6
CONTINENTAL CT
300 THO 91320 555-G3
CONTRA COSTA AV
200 VEN 93004 492-F1
200 VEN 93004 472-F7
CONVAIR ST
400 CMRL 93010 523-J4
CONVERSE RD
23600 VeCo 93066 473-J2
23600 VeCo 93066 474-A2

CONWAY AV
1300 VEN 93004 492-H3
COOK CIR
2100 THO 91360 526-F4
COOK DR
100 FILM 93015 456-B5
COOLHAVEN CT
4500 WLKV 91361 557-D6
COOLIDGE ST
7200 VEN 93003 492-E2
N COOLWATER RD
- VeCo 91307 529-A3
COOPER RD
100 OXN 93030 522-H5
COOPER CANYON RD
- VeCo 93023 450-G1
COOSA ST
9600 VEN 93004 492-H3
COPA DE ORO CT
1600 THO 91362 556-J1
COPLAND CIR
- VEN 93003 492-A4
- VeCo 93003 492-A4
COPLAND DR
4500 VEN 93003 492-A7
E COPLEY ST
3100 SIMI 93063 498-D2
N COPLEY ST
2100 SIMI 93063 498-D2
2100 SIMI 93065 498-D2
COPPER CREEK PL
- MRPK 93021 476-D6
COPPERFIELD ST
3500 SIMI 93063 498-D1
COPPER RIDGE CT
- SIMI 93063 478-H5
COPPERSTONE LN
- SIMI 93065 478-C4
COPPERTREE CT
23600 SIMI 93065 498-B5
CORAL LN
1800 OXN 93033 552-J3
1800 OXN 93033 553-A2
CORAL ST
1100 VEN 93001 491-F5
CORAL WY
4900 OXN 93035 521-J7
CORALBELL LN
22200 WdHl 91367 529-J7
CORALBERRY CT
11500 MRPK 93021 496-B2
CORALCREST CT
12600 MRPK 93021 496-D4
CORAL GUM LN
- SIMI 93065 478-C7
CORAL PINK CIR
6100 WdHl 91367 529-J7
CORAL REEF LN
11800 VeCo 90265 625-F5
CORAL TREE LN
5300 VeCo 91377 527-G7
CORBETT LN
1100 SIMI 93065 497-H4
CORBINA WY
5000 OXN 93035 551-J1
5000 OXN 93035 552-A1
CORBY AV
3000 CMRL 93010 524-F1
3400 CMRL 93010 494-G7
CORD AV
- THO 91362 557-B4
CORDERO AV
2100 SIMI 93065 497-J2
2100 SIMI 93065 498-A2
CORDOVA CT
3500 THO 91320 525-F7
3500 VeCo 91320 525-F7
CORDOVA DR
- FILM 93015 456-C6
CORDOVA ST
100 OXN 93030 523-A5
500 CMRL 93010 524-C1
500 VeCo 93010 524-C1
CORDUA CT
3000 SIMI 93063 478-E7
CORIE LN
6700 LACo 91307 529-D6
CORINNE DR
- THO 91320 555-J1
CORINTH WEIGH
1900 OXN 93035 552-B1
CORKWOOD DR
- MRPK 93021 496-H3
CORLSON AV
2200 SIMI 93063 498-E2
CORLSON PL
2200 SIMI 93063 498-E2
CORNELL CIR
6400 MRPK 93021 476-H6
CORNELL DR
500 SPLA 93060 473-J1
500 SPLA 93060 474-A1
CORNELL PL
300 VEN 93003 492-A3
CORNELL RD
3900 Ago 91301 558-A7
4400 AGRH 91301 558-A6
CORNELL WY
4600 AGRH 91301 558-A6
CORNETT AV
300 MRPK 93021 496-E1
CORNING ST
3300 THO 91320 555-G3
CORNWALL DR
600 OXN 93035 522-D6
CORNWALL LN
1100 VEN 93001 491-E4
CORONA CIR
500 VEN 93003 472-E7
CORONA ST
3300 CMRL 93010 524-G1
CORONADO CIR
- SPLA 93060 464-B3
3700 THO 91320 555-E1
CORONADO CT
1600 CMRL 93010 524-D3
CORONADO DR
100 FILM 93015 456-C6
CORONADO PL
500 OXN 93030 522-E4
CORONADO ST
- VEN 93001 491-F3
CORPORATE CENTER DR
2000 THO 91320 525-J6
CORPORATION ST
600 SPLA 93060 473-J1
CORPUS CHRISTI AV
2800 SIMI 93063 478-H6
N CORRAL RD
- VeCo 91307 528-H4

CORRAL ST
- SIMI 93063 478-H5
CORRIENTE CT
1100 VeCo 93010 494-C7
CORRINE HILL CT
200 THO 91320 556-D2
CORSA AV
5700 WLKV 91362 557-F4
CORSICANA DR
- VeCo 93036 492-J7
600 VeCo 93036 522-J1
700 VeCo 93036 523-A1
CORTA ST
300 VeCo 93023 451-D2
CORTE AGUACATE
600 CMRL 93010 524-B1
CORTE AMIGOS
2600 CMRL 93010 494-F7
CORTE ANTIGUA
6000 CMRL 93012 525-B5
CORTE ARBUSTO
- CMRL 93012 494-H7
CORTE AUGUSTA
- CMRL 93010 523-H1
CORTE AZAL
800 CMRL 93010 524-C1
CORTE BARATA
6100 CMRL 93012 525-C5
CORTE BARROSO
900 CMRL 93010 523-G2
CORTE BAYA VISTA
23600 OXN 93030 523-C7
CORTE BOCINA
- CMRL 93012 524-J1
- CMRL 93012 525-A1
CORTE BREVE
1400 THO 91360 526-H1
CORTE CABALLOS
2700 CMRL 93010 494-F7
CORTE CAMPANERO
1200 CMRL 93010 493-J6
CORTE CAMPINA
6300 CMRL 93012 525-C5
CORTE CANCION
3600 THO 91360 526-J1
CORTE CASTANO
600 CMRL 93010 524-B1
CORTE CERRITOS
- CMRL 93010 524-B1
CORTE CIMA
1600 THO 91360 526-J1
CORTE COLINA
600 CMRL 93010 524-B1
CORTE CORRIDA
300 CMRL 93010 523-J1
CORTE DE ACERO
3600 THO 91360 526-J2
CORTE DE CHARCO
6500 VEN 93003 472-D7
CORTE DE ENCINITAS
1500 CMRL 93010 493-H6
CORTE DE LOS REYES
3600 THO 91360 526-H1
CORTE DEL REY
3600 THO 91360 526-J1
CORTE DE PRIMAVERA
1200 THO 91360 526-H1
CORTE DE QUINTERO
600 CMRL 93010 493-J5
CORTE DESCANSO
1000 SPLA 93060 473-F1
CORTE DE TAJO
1000 THO 91360 526-H1
CORTE ELEGANTE
- CMRL 93010 523-J2
- CMRL 93010 524-A2
CORTE ENTRADA
1300 THO 91360 526-H1
CORTE ESPALDERA
- CMRL 93012 525-A1
CORTE ESTIMA
- CMRL 93012 524-J1
- CMRL 93012 525-A1
CORTE ESTRELLA
- CMRL 93010 523-J2
- CMRL 93010 524-A2
CORTE FRESCA
23600 CMRL 93012 524-H3
CORTE FRONDOSA
600 CMRL 93010 523-H1
CORTE GOLONDRINA
600 CMRL 93010 524-B1
CORTE GRANADA
1000 SPLA 93060 473-F1
CORTE JANA
23600 OXN 93030 523-C7
CORTE JUBILO
- CMRL 93012 525-C1
CORTE LA BRISA
15500 SPLA 93060 463-H7
CORTE LA CIENAGA
600 CMRL 93010 523-H2
CORTE LAS HOLAS
23600 OXN 93030 523-B4
CORTE LEJOS
23600 CMRL 93010 524-C4
CORTE LINDA
200 SPLA 93060 473-F1
CORTE LUCINDA
6100 CMRL 93012 525-C5
CORTE MALPASO
3200 CMRL 93012 524-G2
CORTE MIRA FLORES
1000 SPLA 93060 463-H7
1000 SPLA 93060 473-H1
CORTE MONARCA
- CMRL 93012 524-J1
CORTE OLIVAS
23600 CMRL 93012 524-J1
CORTE OLMO
2600 CMRL 93010 494-E7
CORTE PALOMA
1000 SPLA 93060 473-F1
CORTE PASTORAL
600 CMRL 93010 523-H2
CORTE PICADO
6000 CMRL 93012 525-B5
CORTE PICO VERDE
5300 CMRL 93012 525-A2
CORTE PINATA
6900 CMRL 93012 495-D7
CORTE PRIMAVERA
23600 OXN 93030 523-C6
CORTE REGALO
- CMRL 93010 523-J2
- CMRL 93010 524-A2
CORTE RIVIERA
23600 CMRL 93010 523-H2
CORTE ROSELINDA
700 CMRL 93010 524-C1

CORTE SAFIRO
800 CMRL 93012
CORTE SOL
- CMRL 93010
CORTE TELA
2600 CMRL 93010
CORTE TIARA
- CMRL 93012
CORTE TULAROSA
1000 CMRL 93010
CORTE TUNITAS
700 CMRL 93012
CORTE VALDEZ
23600 OXN 93030
CORTE VERANO
1400 THO 91360
CORTE VIENTO
- CMRL 93010
CORTE VINA
700 CMRL 93010
CORTE VISTORA
23600 CMRL 93012
CORTEZ CIR
- CMRL 93012
CORTEZ ST
2400 VeCo 93036
3000 VeCo 93036
3500 VeCo 93036
CORTO DR
6000 VeCo 93063
CORTO ST
300 SPLA 93060
2700 SIMI 93065
14600 SIMI 93063
CORTO TR
1900 OXN 93036
CORVALLIS CT
1100 VEN 93004
CORVETTE ST
400 PHME 93041
CORVUS DR
- VeCo 93041
CORY ST
6200 SIMI 93063
COSMOS AV
- VEN 93004
COSMOS CT
400 THO 91360
COSTA DE ORO
4400 OXN 93035
COSTA MESA ST
7800 VEN 93004
COTA CIR
3000 OXN 93033
COTHARIN RD
9100 VeCo 90265
11700 VeCo 90265
COTTAGE CT
1100 VEN 93001
COTTAGE GROVE AV
100 CMRL 93012
COTTAGES CT
- CMRL 93012
COTTONTAIL AV
- SIMI 93063
COTTONTAIL RD
23600 MRPK 93021
COTTONTAIL ST
7000 VEN 93003
COTTONWOOD AV
900 VeCo 93023
COTTONWOOD CT
2800 THO 91320
COTTONWOOD DR
- SIMI 93063
COTTONWOOD LN
1400 FILM 93015
COTTONWOOD GROVE
3800 CALB 91301
COULTER CT
1000 SIMI 93065
COUNTRY CT
600 FILM 93015
600 FILM 93015
COUNTRY DR
500 VeCo 93023
COUNTRY LN
2600 WLKV 91361
3000 SIMI 93063
3000 VeCo 93063
COUNTRY PL
1800 VeCo 93023
COUNTRY CLUB DR
400 OJAI 93023
400 SIMI 93065
500 OJAI 93023
900 VeCo 93023
23600 VeCo 93065
COUNTRY CLUB RD
400 OJAI 93023
1800 THO 91360
COUNTRY CREEK CT
11500 MRPK 93021
COUNTRY CREEK LN
- CALB 91302
COUNTRY GLEN RD
27200 AGRH 91301
COUNTRY HAVEN CIR
3400 THO 91362
COUNTRY HILL RD
4100 MRPK 93021
COUNTRY HOME CT
- THO 91362
COUNTRY MEADOW ST
4200 MRPK 93021
COUNTRY OAKS LN
1700 THO 91362
COUNTRY PARK CT
2300 THO 91362
COUNTRY RANCH RD
1300 LACo 91361
1300 THO 91361
COUNTRYSIDE RD
300 VeCo 91377
COUNTRY SPRINGS CT
11600 MRPK 93021
COUNTRY VALLEY RD
100 THO 91362
COUNTRY VIEW CT
100 SPLA 93060
COUNTRY VIEW PL
500 VeCo 93010
COUNTRY VISTA ST
- THO 91362
COUNTRYWALK CT
- SIMI 93065
COUNTRY WIDE WY
400 SIMI 93065
400 SIMI 93065
400 VeCo 93065

City ZIP Pg-Grid
YWOOD DR
MRPK 93021 496-B3
LINE RD
Chat 91311 499-F6
OAK RD
WdHl 91367 529-C7
CanP 91307 529-C7
SQUARE DR
VEN 93003 492-C3
AV
VEN 93003 491-J2
ST
SIMI 93065 498-D3
AND ST
OXN 93033 552-G6
EY CT
THO 91320 525-H7
EY LN
MRPK 93021 496-C2
ARD DR
PHME 93041 552-F6
PHME 93033 552-F6
ARD WY
PHME 93041 552-F6
R
PHME 93041 552-C1
VEN 93001 491-F4
REEK CT
THO 91362 527-C2
O ST
CanP 91303 529-J4
CanP 91307 529-G4
LA 91304 529-F4
GARDEN CT
THO 91362 527-B4
RY AV
VEN 93004 492-G3
RY CT
THO 91362 526-J5
RY DR
THO 91360 526-F6
OOD ST
VeCo 91377 527-H7
TON AV
THO 91361 556-J6
SIMI 93065 498-A5
Y CT
SIMI 93063 499-D3
Y ST
SIMI 93063 499-D3
L CT
SIMI 93063 499-D3
AV
LA 91304 529-E3
CANYON RD
VeCo 93066 474-J3
VeCo 93066 475-A5
WELLS CIR
THO 91362 527-E6
EL PL
SIMI 93065 497-E4
PLE CT
MRPK 93021 496-H3
CanP 91307 529-D5
CT
SIMI 93065 498-A4
Y VIEW ST
Chat 91311 499-J4
VIEW ST
Chat 91311 499-J4
ONT CT
SIMI 93065 498-A1
R
SPLA 93060 464-A6
OXN 93036 522-G2
T
VeCo 93022 451-B6
RRY DR
OXN 93036 522-G1
OOK ST
CMRL 93010 494-D7
ST
VEN 93003 492-C4
ONT CT
SIMI 93065 527-C1
MYRTLE CT
WdHl 91367 529-J7
DR
VEN 93004 492-G4
ST
SIMI 93063 498-D3
ORD ST
OXN 93030 522-J6
HORSE DR
SIMI 93063 479-A6
VEN 93001 471-C6
LN
VeCo 93001 461-B1
VeCo 93022 461-B1
RD
VeCo 93012 554-E1
VeCo 93001 461-B1
VeCo 93022 451-E4
VeCo 93022 461-B1
VeCo 93023 451-H2
OJAI 93023 451-H2
ONT CT
VEN 93003 472-D7
IDGE AV
SIMI 93065 497-E2
IDE CIR
CMRL 93012 525-A2
IDE LN
OXN 93036 522-C3
IDE RD
CMRL 93012 524-J2
CMRL 93012 525-A2
IDE WY
OJAI 93023 441-F7
VOOD ST
THO 91361 557-A6
HTON CIR
MRPK 93021 476-H6
NA WY
VeCo 91377 557-H2
NT ST
VEN 93003 492-E6
NT WY
THO 91362 557-A2
NT MEADOW CT
MRPK 93021 496-D3
DR
FILM 93015 456-C6
OXN 93033 552-J3
LN
THO 91361 557-A5
CT
OXN 93035 552-B1

STREET Block City ZIP Pg-Grid
CREST CT
23600 SIMI 93065 497-G7
CRESTA CT
3800 THO 91360 526-F1
CRESTHAVEN CT
29400 AGRH 91301 557-J3
CRESTHAVEN DR
3600 THO 91362 527-D7
3600 THO 91362 557-C1
CRESTHILL DR
400 VeCo 91377 558-A1
CRESTLAKE AV
1200 VEN 93004 492-H3
CRESTLINE DR
13500 VeCo 93012 496-F5
CRESTMONT DR
2100 VEN 93003 492-D5
CRESTON CT
- SIMI 93065 477-J7
CRESTON LN
5100 VeCo 93066 495-A1
CRESTONE CT
5500 VEN 93003 472-B7
CRESTRIDGE DR
400 VeCo 91377 558-A1
CRESTVIEW AV
- CMRL 93010 524-A1
- VeCo 93010 524-A1
300 CMRL 93010 523-G2
300 VeCo 93010 523-J1
CRESTVIEW CIR
3900 THO 91362 557-C1
CRESTVIEW DR
300 OJAI 93023 441-H7
700 SPLA 93060 464-B4
CRESTWOOD AV
300 VEN 93003 492-B1
CRESTWOOD CT
400 THO 91320 555-F3
CRETE LN
- OXN 93035 552-B1
CRICKETFIELD CT
400 VeCo 91361 556-G6
N CRIMEA ST
100 VEN 93001 491-D1
S CRIMEA ST
- VEN 93001 491-D2
CRIMEA ST FIRE RD
300 VeCo 93001 471-E6
CRINKLAW LN
5600 SIMI 93063 499-A3
5600 VeCo 93063 499-A3
CRISWELL ST
22200 CanP 91303 529-J6
22400 CanP 91307 529-H6
N CROCKER AV
- VEN 93004 492-F1
S CROCKER AV
- VEN 93004 492-F2
CROCKER ST
1300 SIMI 93065 497-J3
CROMBIE CT
- VeCo 91361 556-D7
CROMWELL PL
1500 THO 91361 556-H6
CROOKED PALM RD
4200 VeCo 93001 471-C2
CROOKED TRAIL PL
1700 THO 91362 527-F6
CROSBY AV
700 SIMI 93065 498-B5
CROSS AV
2600 OXN 93036 522-G1
CROSS LN
6900 VeCo 93003 492-D2
7000 VEN 93003 492-D2
CROSSBILL ST
- VEN 93003 492-D5
CROSS BRIDGE PL
1600 THO 91362 526-J7
CROSS CREEK AV
2000 SIMI 93063 498-J2
CROSSJACK ST
400 PHME 93041 552-B2
CROSSLAND ST
3200 THO 91362 527-D3
CROSSPOINTE CT
- SIMI 93065 478-A6
CROSSRIDGE CT
3800 THO 91360 526-G1
CROTHERS CT
8000 LA 91304 529-E3
CROWLEY AV
6300 VEN 93003 492-D5
CROWN CT
23600 SIMI 93065 497-G7
W CROWN ST
- VeCo 93023 451-B4
CROWNE OAK LN
23600 SIMI 93065 497-A1
CROWNFIELD CT
4200 WLKV 91361 557-D6
CROWN HAVEN CT
3700 THO 91320 555-E2
CROWNHILL CT
6200 VEN 93003 472-C6
CROWN HILL DR
800 VeCo 93063 499-B4
CROWN POINT CT
2300 OXN 93036 522-C2
CROWN RIDGE CT
1500 THO 91362 527-F6
CROWN VIEW CT
2300 THO 91362 527-A7
E CROYDON AV
4100 CMRL 93010 494-H7
N CROYDON AV
1800 CMRL 93010 494-H7
CRUSOE CIR
800 THO 91362 526-J7
CRUZERO ST
200 VeCo 93023 451-C2
CRYSTAL CIR
3300 SIMI 93063 478-D6
CRYSTAL PL
8000 VEN 93004 492-F3
CRYSTAL DOWNS CT
2300 OXN 93036 522-D2
CRYSTAL RANCH RD
12400 MRPK 93021 496-D3
CRYSTAL VIEW CIR
1600 THO 91320 556-A2
CTL II RD
23600 VeCo 93063 498-H7
CTL III RD
23600 VeCo 93063 528-J1
23600 VeCo 93063 529-A1
CTL IV RD
23600 VeCo 91307 528-G2
23600 VeCo 93063 528-G2

STREET Block City ZIP Pg-Grid
CUESTA DEL MAR DR
200 OXN 93033 552-F6
CULLEN CT
3600 THO 91320 555-F4
CULVER LN
100 THO 91320 556-B2
100 VeCo 91320 556-B2
CULVIEW CT
23600 SIMI 93065 497-F7
E CUMBERLAND CT
3300 THO 91362 557-C2
W CUMBERLAND CT
3000 THO 91362 557-B2
CUMMINGS RD
300 VeCo 93060 473-E1
CUMMINGS WY
- OXN 93033 552-G5
CUMULUS CT
1900 THO 91362 526-J1
CUNNINGHAM RD
- THO 91362 556-H1
CURLEW PL
6300 VEN 93003 492-D5
CURLEW WY
3800 OXN 93035 552-B3
CURRAN ST
2000 OXN 93033 553-A4
CURRANT AV
1200 SIMI 93065 498-B4
E CURRIER AV
2700 SIMI 93065 498-C4
N CURRIER AV
1000 SIMI 93065 498-C4
CURT DR
3100 CMRL 93010 524-F2
CUSHMAN CT
2000 SIMI 93063 499-A2
CUTLER ST
2000 SIMI 93065 498-A4
CUTTER DR
900 OXN 93035 522-D7
CUTTING RD
400 PHME 93041 552-C3
400 PHME 93043 552-C3
CUYAMA RD
400 OJAI 93023 441-F7
400 VeCo 93023 441-F7
CUYLER HARBOR
- VeCo 93012 554-F3
CYNTHIA ST
6200 SIMI 93063 499-B2
CYPRESS LN
5000 VeCo 93001 471-C1
CYPRESS PL
1300 THO 91360 526-H2
CYPRESS RD
5100 OXN 93033 552-H6
CYPRESS ST
600 THO 91320 556-C1
1500 OXN 93030 552-H1
6000 VeCo 93063 499-B4
CYPRESS POINT LN
1100 VEN 93003 492-C4

D

D ST
- FILM 93015 455-H6
- VeCo 93015 455-H6
100 OXN 93030 522-G6
1200 OXN 93033 522-G7
1500 OXN 93033 552-G1
N D ST
100 OXN 93030 522-G5
DAFFODIL AV
1500 VEN 93004 493-A2
DAFFODIL CT
2700 OXN 93030 522-D4
23600 SIMI 93065 497-G5
DAFFODIL WY
500 OXN 93030 522-D4
DAHL AV
400 PHME 93041 552-F5
DAHLIA ST
900 OXN 93036 522-E3
DAHLIA WY
100 VEN 93004 473-A7
E DAILY DR
- CMRL 93010 524-B3
W DAILY DR
- CMRL 93010 524-A3
200 CMRL 93010 523-J3
DAISY CT
4400 MRPK 93021 496-B3
DAISY DR
- VEN 93004 493-A2
DAISY ST
- SIMI 93063 499-A2
DAKIN AV
1400 SIMI 93065 497-J4
DAKOTA DR
- MRPK 93021 496-G3
- VEN 93001 471-C5
DALAWAY DR
3800 MRPK 93021 496-A4
3800 VeCo 93021 496-A4
DALBY DR
- VeCo 91361 556-D7
DALE AV
100 THO 91320 555-E2
N DALE AV
10400 VeCo 93022 451-C7
DALE CT
100 SPLA 93060 463-J6
22700 Chat 91311 499-H5
DALECREST AV
6100 WdHl 91367 529-F7
DALENHURST PL
2700 SIMI 93065 478-A7
2700 SIMI 93065 498-A1
DALEWOOD CIR
4200 THO 91320 555-D4
DALHART AV
2700 SIMI 93063 478-H6
DALLAS DR
500 THO 91360 526-G7
500 THO 91360 556-G1
1000 OXN 93033 552-J2
DALLAS ST
2600 OXN 93033 552-J3
DALTON ST
- VEN 93003 491-G2
DALY RD
700 OJAI 93023 441-J5
DAMIANA DR
100 THO 91320 555-E1
DAMON ST
5700 SIMI 93063 499-A3
DANA AV
6200 SIMI 93063 499-C3

STREET Block City ZIP Pg-Grid
DANA DR
300 SPLA 93060 464-A5
300 FILM 93015 456-C6
DANA POINT AV
- VEN 93004 492-F2
DANBROOK AV
2300 CMRL 93010 494-E7
DANBURY CT
800 VEN 93004 492-H2
DANBURY DR
1700 CMRL 93012 495-A7
1700 CMRL 93012 525-A1
DANDELION CT
- THO 91320 555-J2
DANETTE ST
6400 SIMI 93063 499-C2
DANIEL ST
3300 THO 91320 555-F2
DANIELSON FIRE RD
- VeCo - 555-E6
- VeCo 91320 555-E5
DANMONT CT
3600 THO 91320 555-F4
DANNYBOYAR AV
6300 CanP 91307 529-G6
DANTE WY
500 VeCo 91377 557-G1
DANTES VIEW DR
5000 CALB 91301 558-F6
N DANTON PL
2600 SIMI 93065 498-B1
DANUBE WY
- OXN 93036 522-H1
DANVERS CIR
700 THO 91320 555-F4
DANVERS RIVER ST
- OXN 93036 492-H7
DANVILLE AV
300 THO 91320 555-E3
DANWOOD DR
4100 THO 91362 527-C5
DAPHNE AV
1500 VEN 93004 493-A2
DAPHNE ST
1600 CMRL 93010 494-D7
DAPHNEY CT
3000 SIMI 93063 478-D7
DAPPER CT
4300 OXN 93033 553-A4
DAPPLE AV
1500 CMRL 93010 524-D1
N DAPPLEGRAY RD
- VeCo 91307 529-B4
DARA ST
800 CMRL 93010 524-G2
DARBY ST
3100 SIMI 93063 498-D1
3100 SIMI 93065 498-D1
DARCY AV
1500 SIMI 93065 498-B3
DARGAN ST
28900 AGRH 91301 558-A3
DARKWOOD CIR
1900 THO 91360 526-D4
DARLENE LN
6000 MRPK 93021 476-C7
8400 LA 91304 529-G2
DARLING RD
9400 VEN 93004 492-H2
10600 VeCo 93004 493-A1
10600 VEN 93004 493-A1
10900 VEN 93004 473-B7
10900 VeCo 93004 473-B7
DARLINGTON DR
2900 THO 91360 526-G2
DARMONT CIR
700 SIMI 93065 497-J5
DARNELL CT
1600 CMRL 93010 524-D2
DARNOCH WY
6900 CanP 91307 529-E4
DARRAH AV
1500 SIMI 93063 498-E3
DART CT
5500 AGRH 91301 557-G5
DARTMOOR CT
- MRPK 93021 496-E2
E DARTMOUTH CIR
14300 MRPK 93021 476-G6
DARTMOUTH RD
100 SPLA 93060 463-J7
400 SPLA 93060 473-J1
400 SPLA 93060 474-A1
13600 MRPK 93021 496-F3
DARTMOUTH ST
5200 VEN 93003 492-B3
DARYN DR
6600 LACo 91307 529-D6
DATE AV
- VEN 93004 473-A6
DATE ST
100 OXN 93033 552-G1
600 OXN 93030 552-H1
W DATE ST
100 OXN 93033 552-E1
DAUNET AV
2500 SIMI 93065 498-C4
DAVENPORT ST
- CMRL 93012 524-G4
DAVEY JONES DR
30700 AGRH 91301 557-G5
DAVIDS LN
200 VeCo 91361 556-F6
DAVIDSON DR
- OXN 93033 552-G5
DAVIDSON LN
1600 SIMI 93063 499-B2
DAVIS CT
4300 OXN 93033 552-H4
DAVIS DR
300 VEN 93003 492-A3
DAVIS RD
23600 VeCo 93060 453-G2
DAVIS ST
100 SPLA 93060 464-B5
DAVIS WY
23300 Chat 91311 499-F7
DAWN CIR
1700 SIMI 93063 498-J2
DAWN CT
2100 THO 91362 526-J4
DAWN MEADOW ST
1700 THO 91362 527-E6
DAWSON AV
2600 VEN 93003 491-G3
N DAWSON DR
- CMRL 93012 524-F3
S DAWSON DR
- CMRL 93012 524-E4
DAWSON PL
2500 CMRL 93012 524-E4

STREET Block City ZIP Pg-Grid
DAY CT
2200 SIMI 93065 497-H2
DAY RD
- VEN 93003 492-B2
DAYBREAK CIR
- THO 91320 556-A1
DAYLIGHT CT
1900 THO 91362 526-J1
DAYLIGHT DR
6300 AGRH 91301 558-A3
DAY LILY LN
23600 SIMI 93065 497-A1
DAYLOMA AV
200 VEN 93003 492-A1
DEACON ST
2900 SIMI 93065 498-C3
DEAN CT
100 VEN 93003 492-A3
DEAN DR
100 SPLA 93060 463-J6
100 SPLA 93060 464-A6
3500 VEN 93003 491-H3
4300 VEN 93003 492-A3
DEANNA AV
1600 SIMI 93063 499-A3
DE ANZA DR
- VEN 93001 471-C6
DE ANZA WY
200 OXN 93033 552-H3
DEARBORN AV
700 THO 91320 555-G3
DEBBIE ST
500 VeCo 91320 525-G7
500 VeCo 91320 555-H1
DE BERRY DR
26000 CALB 91301 558-F6
DEBORAH ST
4000 SIMI 93063 498-F2
DEBS AV
6100 WdHl 91367 529-E7
6500 CanP 91307 529-E7
DEBUSSY LN
- VEN 93003 492-B4
DECATUR AV
700 VEN 93004 492-G3
DECKER CANYON RD
Rt#-23
1400 LACo 90265 586-F7
DECKSIDE CT
1400 OXN 93035 552-C1
DECKSIDE DR
900 OXN 93035 522-C7
DEEP SHADOW DR
29200 AGRH 91301 558-A5
DEEP WATERS CT
- SIMI 93065 478-B6
DEEPWELL LN
4300 MRPK 93021 496-F3
DEEPWOOD DR
800 THO 91362 557-C1
1000 THO 91362 527-C7
DEER PTH
- VeCo 93033 583-J4
- VeCo 93033 584-A3
DEERBROOK RD
6700 VeCo 91377 528-A7
DEER CREEK AV
2000 SIMI 93063 498-J2
DEER CREEK RD
14700 VeCo 90265 585-B7
14700 VeCo 90265 625-B2
DEERFIELD CT
2400 CMRL 93010 524-E1
DEERFIELD DR
100 FILM 93015 455-J7
DEERFIELD ST
2100 THO 91362 526-J4
2100 THO 91362 527-A4
DEERFOOT PL
800 THO 91320 555-G5
DEER GRASS CT
- MRPK 93021 476-D6
DEER HAVEN CT
- THO 91362 527-D7
DEERHILL RD
800 VeCo 91377 528-A6
800 VeCo 91377 558-A1
DEER HUNTER LN
600 CMRL 93010 524-F2
DEERHURST AV
400 CMRL 93012 524-H5
DEERING LN
13600 MRPK 93021 496-F3
DEER LICK DR
23900 LA 91304 529-E2
DEER MEADOW ST
12600 MRPK 93021 496-D3
DEERPARK CT
4300 WLKV 91361 557-D6
DEERPATH LN
- THO 91320 555-H2
DEER RUN LN
1200 VeCo 91377 527-G7
DEER SPRING PL
900 THO 91320 555-G5
DEER TRAIL CT
26900 CALB 91301 558-G7
DEER VALLEY AV
3100 THO 91320 555-G4
DEERVIEW CT
29400 AGRH 91301 557-J4
DEERWALK PL
300 THO 91320 555-J1
DEERWEED TR
20900 CALB 91301 558-G7
DEER WILLOW CT
700 THO 91320 555-G4
DEERWOOD AV
2600 SIMI 93065 478-C7
2600 SIMI 93065 498-C1
DEFENDER DR
4000 AGRH 91301 558-E7
DEKOVEN ST
4900 VEN 93003 492-B7
DELACODO AV
3000 THO 91320 555-G2
DE LA GARRIGUE RD
23600 VeCo 93023 450-G1
DEL AMO WY
2000 OXN 93036 522-H3
DELANO CT
3800 SIMI 93063 498-E1
DELAWARE DR
- MRPK 93021 496-G3
200 VEN 93001 471-C4
DEL CERRO CIR
23600 LA 91304 529-E4
DEL CIERVO PL
- CMRL 93012 494-H7
- CMRL 93012 524-H1

STREET Block City ZIP Pg-Grid
DELFEN ST
6500 MRPK 93021 477-A6
DELGADA CT
1900 CMRL 93010 524-D2
DELGADA ST
1000 CMRL 93012 525-B6
E DELILAH ST
3500 SIMI 93063 498-E2
DELIUS ST
4900 VEN 93003 492-A4
DEL MAR PL
4000 OXN 93033 552-G4
DEL MAR TR
6800 VeCo 93063 499-D4
DELMONICO AV
8600 LA 91304 529-J1
DEL NIDO CT
1100 OJAI 93023 442-A6
DEL NORTE BLVD
100 OXN 93030 523-D5
22200 OXN 93010 523-D5
DEL NORTE RD
100 OJAI 93023 441-G7
300 VeCo 93023 441-F6
1300 CMRL 93010 523-F3
DEL NORTE ST
10800 VEN 93004 472-J6
DELORES CT
- VEN 93004 492-J3
DEL ORO DR
800 OJAI 93023 441-G5
DEL ORO PL
4800 OXN 93033 552-G5
DELOZ DR
- CMRL 93012 525-A3
DELPHA CT
2100 THO 91362 527-A3
DELPHINIUM PL
200 OXN 93036 522-F3
DEL PRADO CT
1100 OJAI 93023 442-A6
DEL PRADO DR
1700 CMRL 93010 524-D2
DEL RAY CIR
- THO 91360 526-F2
DEL RAYO CT
- CMRL 93012 494-H7
DEL REY PL
- OXN 93030 523-A5
DEL RIO ST
4600 SIMI 93063 478-H7
DEL ROBLES DR
6300 VeCo 93063 499-C4
DEL ROBLES PL
1000 VeCo 93063 499-C4
DEL SUR WY
300 OXN 93033 552-H3
DELTA DR
8600 VEN 93004 492-G4
DELTA RD
23600 VeCo 93063 528-G2
DELTA CC RD
23600 VeCo 93063 528-G2
W DELTA GREEN ST
100 PHME 93041 552-D2
DEL TIO CT
- CMRL 93010 493-G7
DEL VALLE DR
200 FILM 93015 455-J6
500 FILM 93015 456-A6
DEL VALLE ST
- VeCo 93022 451-C4
DEL VERDE CT
1000 THO 91320 526-B6
DELWOOD CT
400 THO 91320 555-E2
DENA DR
100 VeCo 91320 555-G1
500 VeCo 91320 525-G7
DENALI CT
- MRPK 93021 496-D1
DENBY CT
6500 SIMI 93063 499-C2
DENHAM CT
1800 SIMI 93065 498-A2
DENISE CT
500 THO 91320 525-H7
DENISE LN
8300 LA 91304 529-G2
DENISE ST
2600 THO 91320 525-H7
DENNIS AV
700 SIMI 93065 497-G3
DENNIS LN
7200 CanP 91307 529-F5
DENNIS WY
9300 Chat 91311 499-F6
DENNISON RD
- VeCo 93023 452-D1
DENNY ST
2000 SIMI 93065 498-A3
DENTON AV
3500 SIMI 93063 478-G5
DENVER PL
900 OXN 93033 552-J3
900 VEN 93004 492-G3
DENVER ST
8000 VEN 93004 492-F3
DENVER SPRINGS DR
1400 WLKV 91361 586-J1
W DEODAR AV
100 OXN 93030 522-F5
N DEODORA ST
1400 SIMI 93065 498-C3
DE PAUL ST
4200 VEN 93003 491-J3
DE QUINCY CT
24100 LA 91304 529-D3
DERBY ST
2100 CMRL 93010 524-E1
DERRY AV
5300 AGRH 91301 558-B6
DESCANSO AV
100 OJAI 93023 441-F7
200 OJAI 93023 451-F1
DESCANSO CT
1300 OXN 93035 552-E1
DESCHUTES DR
1500 VEN 93004 492-J3
DESEO AV
400 VeCo 93010 494-A6
DESERT CREEK AV
2100 SIMI 93063 499-B2
DESERT FOREST CT
2200 OXN 93036 522-D2
DESERT SAGE CT
23600 SIMI 93065 498-D5
DESMOND AV
- VEN 93003 492-C4

STREET Block City ZIP Pg-Grid
DETROIT DR
2800 OXN 93036 522-H1
2800 OXN 93036 492-H7
DEVEREUX DR
900 VeCo 93023 441-D6
DEVERON RIDGE RD
6900 CanP 91307 529-E5
DEVIA DR
- VeCo 91320 555-G1
DEVILFISH DR
800 OXN 93035 522-D7
DEVILS CANYON MTWY
- Chat 91311 479-G2
- Chat 91311 499-J1
DEVILS CANYON RD
- VeCo 93001 471-B5
DEVON CT
800 SIMI 93065 498-D5
DEVON LN
1200 VEN 93001 491-F5
DEVONSHIRE AV
1500 THO 91361 556-J6
DEVONSHIRE CT
1600 THO 91361 556-J6
DEVONSHIRE DR
800 OXN 93030 522-D4
W DEVONSHIRE DR
300 OXN 93030 522-F4
DEVONSHIRE ST
10300 Chat 91311 499-J4
DEVORE AV
700 SIMI 93065 497-H5
DEVORE CT
5500 AGRH 91301 558-C5
DEWAYNE AV
1600 CMRL 93010 524-G1
1700 CMRL 93010 494-G7
DEWBERRY CT
2000 THO 91361 557-A5
DEWBERRY LN
400 OXN 93036 522-G1
DEWDROP PL
23600 THO 91362 527-C4
N DEWEY AV
- THO 91320 555-G2
S DEWEY AV
100 THO 91320 555-G2
DEXTER ST
2100 CMRL 93010 524-E2
DIABLO AV
600 MRPK 93021 496-D1
DIABLO PT
- VeCo 93012 554-F2
DIABLO WY
100 OXN 93033 553-C3
DIAMOND AL
200 VEN 93001 491-C1
DIAMOND CT
3700 SIMI 93063 498-E1
DIAMOND DR
- CMRL 93010 493-H7
DIAMOND HEAD WY
2300 OXN 93036 522-D2
DIANA CT
2900 VeCo 91320 555-G1
30100 AGRH 91301 557-H5
DIANE ST
5300 SIMI 93063 498-J2
DIAZ AV
500 OXN 93030 522-H6
DICHA DR
- OXN 93030 522-H4
DICKENS CIR
6900 VEN 93003 492-E3
DICKENS DR
5300 OXN 93033 552-G5
DICKENSON AV
- THO 91320 555-F2
DICKENSON DR
- SPLA 93060 463-J5
- VeCo 93060 463-J5
DICKENSON RD
23600 SPLA 93060 463-J5
23600 VeCo 93060 463-J5
DICKINSON LN
6600 VEN 93003 492-D3
DICKINSON PL
2100 OXN 93033 553-A1
DIEGO WY
1600 OXN 93030 522-E4
DIKE RD
- VeCo 93060 464-D5
DILLER CT
3800 SIMI 93063 498-E2
DILLON CT
2300 THO 91360 526-D4
DINSMORE AV
100 THO 91362 556-H2
DINSMORE ST
1300 SIMI 93065 497-H4
DISCOVERY CT
11900 MRPK 93021 496-C1
DISCOVERY CV
2600 PHME 93041 552-C2
DISCOVERY DR
23600 OXN 93030 523-C6
DISPENSARY RD
- VeCo 93041 583-G3
- VeCo 93042 583-G3
DITCH RD
- VeCo 93042 583-C4
2800 VeCo 93063 478-D6
2800 VeCo 93065 478-D6
2900 SIMI 93063 478-D6
N DIVERNON AV
3000 SIMI 93063 478-F7
DIVIDE TER
8300 LA 91304 529-E2
E DIXON CT
3800 SIMI 93063 498-E2
DOANE ST
4000 VEN 93003 491-J2
W DOBKIN PL
- SIMI 93065 497-F3
DOCK RD
- PHME 93043 552-D5
DOCKSIDE LN
1500 CMRL 93010 524-D3
DOCKSON PL
2500 PHME 93041 552-D2
DODD ST
500 SIMI 93065 497-G4
DODGE RD
23600 OXN 93033 553-C3
23600 VeCo 93033 553-C4
DODSON ST
- PHME 93041 552-E4
- PHME 93043 552-E3
5000 VeCo 93066 494-J4
5000 VeCo 93066 495-A4

STREET — Block City ZIP Pg-Grid

DOE CREEK CIR
500 THO 91320 555-E3
DOGWOOD CIR
2900 THO 91360 526-H3
DOGWOOD DR
2500 OXN 93036 522-G1
DOGWOOD ST
2200 SIMI 93065 498-B2
DOHENEY CT
- SIMI 93063 478-H5
DOLE DR
- WLKV 91362 557-E5
DOLLIE ST
100 OXN 93033 552-G5
W DOLLIE ST
- OXN 93033 552-G5
DOLORES CT
100 OXN 93030 522-J5
DOLPHIN CT
1000 VEN 93001 491-G5
DOLPHIN WY
5000 OXN 93035 551-J1
DOMAR PL
2100 OXN 93036 522-H3
DOMBEY CIR
- THO 91360 526-F6
DOMINGO PL
- OXN 93030 522-H4
DOMINGUEZ CANYON RD
- VeCo - 367-D7
- VeCo 93040 367-D7
DOMINICA CTE
1400 CMRL 93010 523-J1
DOMINICA DR
- OXN 93035 522-D7
- OXN 93035 552-D1
DOMINION DR
1000 VeCo 93023 441-D6
N DONALD AV
- THO 91320 555-G2
DON ANTONIO WY
800 VeCo 93023 451-C3
DON CARLOS
800 VeCo 93023 451-C2
DON CARLOS ST
300 VEN 93001 491-D2
DONEGAL AV
100 THO 91320 556-A1
DONEGAL WY
- OXN 93035 522-B7
- OXN 93035 552-B1
DONEVA RD
4000 MRPK 93021 496-D3
DON FELIPE
800 VeCo 93023 451-C2
DONIZETTI AV
600 VEN 93003 492-A3
DONLIN LN
200 VeCo 91320 556-B3
DONLIN RD
300 VeCo 91320 556-B2
DONLON AV
800 OXN 93030 522-G7
DONLON RD
2900 VeCo 93066 495-B1
5300 VeCo 93066 475-B7
DONLON ST
100 VEN 93003 492-A5
600 VEN 93003 491-J5
DONNA ST
100 VeCo 93022 451-B7
DONNER AV
100 VEN 93003 492-C1
1100 SIMI 93065 498-A4
DONNER ST
600 OXN 93033 552-H4
W DONNICK AV
100 THO 91360 526-E5
DONNINGTON CT
700 SIMI 93065 497-C6
DONNYBROOK LN
13600 MRPK 93021 496-F3
DON RICARDO
800 VeCo 93023 451-C2
DONVILLE AV
2000 SIMI 93065 497-J2
DOONE ST
- THO 91360 526-F6
DORA CT
2200 SIMI 93063 499-B1
DORADO CT
500 VeCo 91377 558-A1
2400 THO 91362 527-C3
DORAL CIR
1400 THO 91362 527-E7
DORAL CT
2600 OXN 93036 522-D2
DORCHESTER ST
800 THO 91360 526-G6
DOREEN WY
3100 VEN 93003 491-H3
DORENA DR
100 VeCo 91320 555-G1
400 VeCo 91320 525-G7
DORHAM CT
2900 SIMI 93065 498-C3
DORIE DR
7400 LA 91304 529-E4
DORIS AV
1400 OXN 93030 522-D5
1400 VeCo 93030 522-B5
W DORIS AV
200 OXN 93030 522-F5
DORIS CT
15400 MRPK 93021 477-A5
DORMAN ST
2700 CMRL 93010 494-F7
DOROTHY AV
200 MRPK 93021 496-E1
200 VEN 93003 491-J2
400 VeCo 93003 491-J2
1400 SIMI 93063 499-C3
DOROTHY DR
28000 AGRH 91301 558-C6
DORRIT CT
- THO 91320 556-A1
DORRIT ST
1800 THO 91320 556-A1
DORSET AV
1400 THO 91360 526-F6
DORSEY ST
- VEN 93003 492-C4
DORY LN
5100 OXN 93033 552-G5
N DOS CAMINOS AV
- VEN 93003 491-G2
S DOS CAMINOS AV
- VEN 93003 491-G3
DOUBLE EAGLE DR
600 SIMI 93065 497-D5
DOUBLETREE RD
800 VeCo 91377 558-A1
900 VeCo 91377 528-A7
W DOUGLAS AV
200 OXN 93030 522-F4
DOUGLAS ST
300 OJAI 93023 441-H5
DOVE CT
300 FILM 93015 455-H6
300 SPLA 93060 464-D5
DOVE ST
6800 VEN 93003 492-E4
DOVE CANYON DR
- OXN 93036 522-C2
DOVER AV
1100 THO 91360 526-E6
DOVER LN
- SIMI 93063 498-H1
1000 VEN 93001 491-E4
DOVER ST
1500 OXN 93030 522-G3
DOVERWOOD CT
31900 WLKV 91361 557-C6
DOVETAIL CT
- THO 91360 526-F3
DOVETAIL DR
5800 AGRH 91301 557-G4
DOWEL DR
6400 SIMI 93063 499-C2
DOWELL DR
1400 VEN 93003 492-B5
DOWNEY CT
3900 SIMI 93063 498-F2
E DOWNING ST
1400 SIMI 93065 497-J1
DOWNWIND WY
500 OXN 93033 552-G5
DOYLE LN
500 VEN 93003 492-D1
DRACENA AV
15400 MRPK 93021 477-A6
DRACO WY
23600 CanP 91307 529-F5
DRAKE DR
1200 SIMI 93065 497-G4
2300 THO 91362 527-B6
4200 OXN 93033 553-A4
DRAPER CT
2000 SIMI 93065 497-J2
DRAYTON AV
2200 THO 91360 526-F4
DRESDEN CT
- VEN 93003 492-B3
DREXEL AV
200 VEN 93003 492-C1
DREXEL CIR
1000 THO 91360 526-F6
DRIFFILL BLVD
200 OXN 93030 522-G7
DRIFT DR
5900 WLKV 91362 557-F4
DRIFTWOOD AV
1200 SIMI 93065 497-H3
DRIFTWOOD CIR
900 THO 91320 555-E4
DRIFTWOOD LN
1000 VEN 93001 491-E4
DRIFTWOOD ST
- FILM 93015 456-B6
5100 OXN 93035 521-J6
DRISKILL ST
100 OXN 93030 523-A5
DRIVER AV
5200 Ago 91301 558-G6
5200 CALB 91301 558-G6
28100 AGRH 91301 558-B5
DROWN AV
100 OJAI 93023 441-J6
DRUMCLIFF CT
1700 THO 91361 556-J5
DRUMMOND LN
6700 VEN 93003 492-D3
DRUMMOND PL
2700 THO 91360 526-E3
DRY CANYON RD
4500 SIMI 93063 478-E3
4500 SIMI 93065 478-E3
4500 VeCo 93063 478-E3
DRY CREEK LN
- OXN 93036 522-B3
DRYDEN ST
100 THO 91360 526-F7
DUARTE CIR
1400 SIMI 93065 498-A3
DUBBERS ST
100 VEN 93001 491-B1
DUBONNET CT
1400 VeCo 91377 527-H6
DUCHY WY
2500 VeCo 91361 586-D2
DUCOR AV
7600 LA 91304 529-G2
DUDLEY AV
1200 VEN 93004 492-H3
DUDLEY DR
1600 VeCo 93015 455-G5
DUESENBERG DR
2500 THO 91362 557-B3
DUFAU RD
3600 VeCo 93033 553-E5
DUKE AV
100 VEN 93003 492-B2
DUKE ST
6400 MRPK 93021 476-H6
DULCE DR
600 OXN 93036 522-H3
DULCIE CIR
1700 SIMI 93063 498-J2
DUMAINE AV
1400 VeCo 91377 527-G6
DUMETZ ST
2500 CMRL 93010 524-F3
DUMP RD
- VeCo 93042 583-G4
DUNAWAY DR
- THO 91320 555-E3
DUNBAR DR
- OXN 93033 552-H6
N DUNBAR LN
400 THO 91360 526-D7
DUNCAN ST
1700 SIMI 93065 497-J3
DUNEGAL CT
5900 AGRH 91301 557-G3
DUNES CIR
900 OXN 93035 521-J7
DUNES ST
800 OXN 93035 521-J7
4800 OXN 93035 522-A7
DUNHAM CIR
1600 THO 91360 526-D5
N DUNHAM RD
5600 VeCo 93066 475-C7
5600 VeCo 93066 495-C1
DUNKIRK DR
600 OXN 93035 522-C6
DUNLIN CT
800 THO 91361 557-A5
DUNLO PL
6400 CanP 91307 529-D7
DUNN CT
2100 THO 91360 526-F4
DUNNIGAN ST
1600 CMRL 93010 524-D2
N DUNNING ST
- VEN 93003 491-H2
S DUNNING ST
- VEN 93003 491-H3
DUNRAVEN CT
31700 WLKV 91361 557-D6
DUNSMUIR AV
200 VEN 93004 492-F2
DUNSMUIR CT
2500 OXN 93035 552-D1
DUNSMUIR ST
1600 OXN 93035 552-D1
DUNTON LN
100 FILM 93015 455-J7
DUPONT CT
4400 VEN 93003 492-A5
DUPONT ST
1800 OXN 93033 553-A1
4500 VEN 93003 492-A5
DURAND DR
6900 VeCo 93021 475-J5
DURANGO CT
1600 CMRL 93010 524-D2
DURANT CT
5400 VeCo 91377 527-H7
DURHAM LN
9800 VEN 93004 492-H2
DURHAM ST
1200 SIMI 93065 497-H4
DURKIN ST
700 CMRL 93010 524-F2
DURLEY AV
100 CMRL 93010 524-A4
200 CMRL 93010 523-J4
E DUSAN ST
2300 SIMI 93065 498-B4
DUSK DR
- CMRL 93012 524-G4
DUSKWOOD WY
1600 SIMI 93065 497-F2
DUSTY LN
7800 VeCo 93066 475-C4
DUSTY ROSE CT
200 SIMI 93065 497-E7
DUTCH ELM CIR
1200 THO 91360 526-H2
DUVAL DR
2200 VeCo 93012 496-A7
DUVAL RD
2300 VeCo 93012 496-A7
DUVALI DR
100 VEN 93003 492-B2
DUVALL AV
700 CMRL 93010 524-D2
N DWIGHT AV
1500 CMRL 93010 524-G1
1700 CMRL 93010 494-G7
DWIGHT AV S
3000 CMRL 93010 524-F1
DYER CT
200 THO 91360 526-F4

E

E ST
- FILM 93015 455-H7
- VeCo 93015 455-H7
100 OXN 93030 522-F7
1300 OXN 93033 552-G3
23600 OXN 93033 522-F7
N E ST
100 OXN 93030 522-F5
EAGLE CIR
- VeCo 93041 583-J3
EAGLE CT
600 FILM 93015 455-H5
EAGLE DR
6800 VEN 93003 492-E4
EAGLE ST
6500 VEN 93003 492-D4
EAGLE BEND LN
- OXN 93036 522-C3
EAGLEBROOK DR
30300 AGRH 91301 557-G5
EAGLE CREEK LN
2300 OXN 93036 522-D2
EAGLE FLIGHT DR
- SIMI 93065 478-A5
EAGLEHAVEN LN
6800 VeCo 91377 528-B7
EAGLE HEIGHTS CT
2800 THO 91360 526-E3
EAGLE MOUNTAIN RD
24000 LA 91304 529-D2
EAGLE MOUNTAIN ST
24000 LA 91304 529-D1
EAGLEPEAK AV
1600 SIMI 93063 498-E3
EAGLE POINT CIR
4800 THO 91362 557-F1
EAGLE RIDGE ST
100 THO 91320 555-G2
EAGLE ROCK AV
100 VeCo 93035 552-C6
EAGLES CLAW AV
2800 THO 91362 527-B2
EAGLESNEST PL
3400 THO 91320 555-F4
EAGLETON ST
28600 AGRH 91301 558-B3
EAGLEVIEW PL
300 THO 91320 555-J1
EAGLEWOOD AV
- THO 91362 527-B2
EAKINS LN
500 VEN 93003 492-D1
EARHART CT
1800 OXN 93033 553-A1
EARL AV
1500 SIMI 93065 498-B3
EARLHAM CT
1400 VeCo 91377 527-G6
EARL JOSEPH DR
- CMRL 93010 524-A2
EARLY DAWN LN
23600 SIMI 93065 497-A1
EAST DR
1100 VEN 93003 492-D4
EAST PK
- CMRL 93012 524-G4
EAST RD
- VeCo 93001 470-E4
6300 VeCo 93021 475-F6
6300 VeCo 93066 475-F6
EAST ST
3000 SIMI 93065 498-C3
3400 VeCo 93066 495-A5
EASTBOURNE BAY
4400 OXN 93035 552-A1
EASTERLY RD
5500 AGRH 91301 558-C5
EAST FORK HALL CANYON RD
2800 VeCo 93001 471-H5
EASTHAVEN LN
- CanP 91307 529-E5
EASTMAN AV
1500 VEN 93003 492-A5
1800 OXN 93030 522-J6
1800 OXN 93030 523-A6
EASTRIDGE CT
2200 OXN 93036 522-D3
EASTRIDGE LP
2100 OXN 93036 522-E2
EASTRIDGE TR
2000 OXN 93036 522-E2
EASTVALE CT
29900 AGRH 91301 557-H4
EASTWARD ST
23600 Chat 91311 499-F6
EASTWIND CIR
1300 THO 91361 557-B6
EASTWOOD DR
400 OXN 93030 522-F4
EASY ST
100 SPLA 93060 464-A7
E EASY ST
100 SIMI 93065 497-F1
W EASY ST
- SIMI 93065 497-E1
EASY WY
2000 SIMI 93065 497-H2
EATON HOLLOW AV
- MRPK 93021 476-F6
EATON HOLLOW CT
- MRPK 93021 476-F5
EATOUGH AV
8500 LA 91304 529-J1
EATOUGH PL
8500 LA 91304 529-J2
EBB CT
1400 OXN 93035 552-C1
EBB TIDE CIR
600 PHME 93041 552-F7
EBBTIDE LN
11800 VeCo 90265 625-F5
EBONY DR
600 OXN 93030 522-D4
ECCLES ST
22100 LA 91304 529-H2
ECHIDNA PL
7000 VEN 93003 492-E4
ECHO AV
700 OXN 93036 522-H2
ECHO CT
4900 VEN 93003 492-A2
ECHO ST
1300 OXN 93036 522-J2
N ECROYD AV
2100 SIMI 93063 499-A2
EDDINGHAM WY
- LA 91304 529-E4
EDDY CT
5500 VEN 93003 492-C3
EDELWEISS ST
2000 OXN 93036 522-G2
EDEN ST
3000 OXN 93033 553-A3
EDENPARK DR
26000 CALB 91302 558-J3
EDGAR CT
- THO 91320 555-F2
EDGAR ST
- OXN 93033 552-H5
EDGEBROOK PL
5100 THO 91362 527-F7
EDGECLIFF CIR
1800 THO 91362 527-F6
EDGEHILL CIR
5300 VEN 93003 492-B1
EDGEMIRE LN
23600 SIMI 93065 497-A1
EDGEMONT DR
1400 CMRL 93010 524-D1
EDGERTON PL
2500 PHME 93041 552-C2
EDGEVIEW CT
- THO 91320 555-H3
EDGEWARE DR
5200 CALB 91301 558-G6
EDGEWATER LN
1500 CMRL 93010 524-D2
EDGEWOOD DR
- FILM 93015 456-A7
1700 SIMI 93063 499-B2
EDGEWOOD WY
1300 OXN 93030 522-E4
EDINBURGH CT
6100 AGRH 91301 557-J3
EDISON DR
5500 OXN 93033 552-H7
6100 VeCo 93033 552-H7
8200 VeCo 93001 461-A4
EDISON LN
700 FILM 93015 455-J5
EDISON RD
- LACo 90265 586-J7
- VeCo 93001 461-A5
23600 SIMI 93063 498-E7
23600 SIMI 93063 528-E1
23600 THO 91320 554-G4
23600 THO 91320 555-A3
23600 VeCo 93012 554-G4
23600 VeCo 93063 498-E7
23600 VeCo 93066 528-E1
EDISON WY
800 FILM 93015 455-J5
EDMUND ST
1500 SIMI 93065 497-J4
EDWARD RD
200 THO 91320 556-A2
200 VeCo 91320 556-A2
EDWARDS RD
23600 VeCo 93060 464-J1
EDWARDS CANYON RD
23600 VeCo 93015 457-D5
23600 VeCo 93040 457-D5
EDWARDS RANCH RD
100 VeCo 93060 473-C4
EGRET AV
1300 VEN 93003 492-D4
EGRET CT
6300 VEN 93003 492-D4
EHLERS DR
9300 Chat 91311 499-F6
23500 Chat 91311 499-F6
EILAT CIR
- SIMI 93063 479-B7
- SIMI 93063 499-B1
EILEEN ST
4000 SIMI 93063 498-F2
EISENHOWER CIR
600 OXN 93033 552-H6
EISENHOWER ST
7200 VEN 93003 492-E2
EISENHOWER WY
- SIMI 93065 497-D5
ELAINE ST
3400 VeCo 93036 492-J7
3400 VeCo 93036 493-A7
ELAND LN
7000 VEN 93003 492-E4
EL AZUL CIR
500 VeCo 91377 557-J1
ELBA CT
11800 MRPK 93021 496-C5
ELBA PL
6100 WdHl 91367 529-E7
ELBA ST
2800 VEN 93003 492-E6
ELBERTA AV
1600 SIMI 93063 498-J3
ELBURY CT
- VeCo 91361 556-E7
EL CAJON CIR
1900 OXN 93035 522-E7
EL CAJON CT
1200 OXN 93035 522-E7
1200 OXN 93035 552-E1
EL CAJON DR
1400 THO 91362 526-J5
EL CAJON ST
9200 VEN 93004 492-G2
EL CAJON WY
1600 OXN 93035 522-D7
EL CAMINO
100 OJAI 93023 441-G6
EL CAMINO DR
100 VeCo 93023 441-E7
EL CAMINO CORTO
800 VeCo 93023 441-C7
EL CAMINO REAL
1000 VeCo 93063 499-B4
EL CAMINO REAL U.S.-101
- VeCo - 366-E8
- VeCo - 459-C5
- VeCo - 469-H1
- VeCo - 470-E5
- VeCo - 490-H1
- VEN - 490-H1
- VEN - 491-G4
EL CAMPO ST
600 VeCo 93015 455-D6
EL CANON AV
6100 WdHl 91367 529-D7
EL CAPITAN PL
4200 CMRL 93012 524-J3
EL CENTRO DR
1400 THO 91362 526-J6
EL CENTRO ST
1000 VeCo 93023 451-D1
EL CERRITO CIR
10100 VEN 93004 492-G1
EL CERRITO DR
1300 THO 91362 526-H6
EL CIELO
100 THO 91320 525-E6
EL CINO DR
1300 SIMI 93065 497-G4
EL CONEJO DR
100 VeCo 93023 441-D6
EL CORAZON CT
4900 CMRL 93012 524-H3
EL CORTIJO PL
5100 CMRL 93012 524-J1
ELDER ST
900 OXN 93036 522-E2
ELDERBERRY AV
4700 MRPK 93021 496-C2
ELDERBERRY CT
1000 SPLA 93060 464-A1
ELDERBERRY DR
2400 OXN 93036 522-F1
ELDEROAK LN
2600 VeCo 91361 586-E1
ELDEROAK RD
2700 VeCo 91361 586-E2
ELDER VIEW LN
1100 CMRL 93012 525-A2
EL DORADO AV
1800 OXN 93033 553-B2
EL DORADO CT
300 VEN 93004 492-E1
EL DORADO DR
100 FILM 93015 456-C6
1400 THO 91362 526-J6
EL DORADO ST
7600 VEN 93004 492-E1
ELECTRA AV
2000 SIMI 93065 497-F2
ELEGANTE DR
- OXN 93030 523-C7
ELENA WY
200 OXN 93036 522-G3
ELEPHANT SEAL CV
- VeCo 93012 554-E3
EL ESCORPION RD
6000 WdHl 91367 529-E7
ELEVAR CT
700 SIMI 93065 527-C1
ELEVAR ST
- OXN 93030 523-C6
E ELFIN GRN
100 PHME 93041 552-E2
W ELFIN GRN
100 PHME 93041 552-D2
ELFSTONE CT
1000 THO 91361 557-A5
EL GALLARDO
200 THO 91320 525-E7
EL GRECO DR
1900 OXN 93035 522-E7
ELIAS DR
- OXN 93033 552-H6
ELINOR CT
2900 THO 91320 525-H7
ELIOT DR
4200 OXN 93033 553-A4
E ELIOT ST
100 SPLA 93060 464-A6
W ELIOT ST
100 SPLA 93060 463-J6
100 SPLA 93060 464-A6
ELIZA CT
100 OXN 93030 522-J5
ELIZABETH CT
- SPLA 93060 463-J7
30100 AGRH 91301 557-H5
ELIZABETH DR
2000 VEN 93003 492-E5
ELIZABETH RD
500 VeCo 93003 472-G6
500 VeCo 93060 472-G6
ELIZABETH WY
- OXN 93033 552-H5
ELIZONDO AV
2500 SIMI 93065 498-C3
ELIZONDO ST
1900 SIMI 93065 498-A3
EL JARDIN AV
2100 VEN 93001 491-F2
EL JINA LN
400 VeCo 93023 442-E6
ELKHORN CT
- SIMI 93063 478-H5
ELKINS LN
600 FILM 93015 456-B5
ELKINS RD
100 VeCo 93015 466-B3
ELKO AV
700 VEN 93004 492-G2
ELK RIVER ST
- OXN 93036 492-H7
ELK RUN LP
- MRPK 93021 476-F5
ELK RUN WY
- MRPK 93021 476-F5
ELKTON CT
- MRPK 93021 476-F6
ELKWOOD AV
3700 THO 91320 555-E4
ELKWOOD CT
- FILM 93015 456-B6
ELKWOOD ST
22000 LA 91304 529-E3
EL LADO DR
500 SIMI 93065 497-G3
EL LAZO CT
1300 CMRL 93012 525-B1
ELLEN CT
3000 THO 91320 555-G2
ELLENVIEW AV
5900 WdHl 91367 529-D7
6200 CanP 91307 529-D7
ELLESMERE WY
1300 VeCo 91377 528-A7
ELLFRED CT
600 SPLA 93060 463-J7
ELLICE ST
11700 VeCo 90265 625-E5
ELLINGTON CT
2400 SIMI 93063 498-D1
ELLINGTON ST
23600 VEN 93003 492-A3
ELLIOT CT
1200 SIMI 93065 497-D7
ELLIOTT CT
6800 VEN 93003 492-D3
N ELLIS PL
- THO 91320 556-A1
S ELLIS PL
- THO 91320 556-A2
ELLISTON CT
- SIMI 93065 477-J7
ELLSWORTH CIR
400 THO 91360 526-D6
ELM
700 VeCo 93023 451-C3
ELM CT
800 OXN 93033 552-F1
21300 SIMI 93063 499-B3
ELM DR
- CMRL 93010 524-E4
5100 OXN 93033 552-J5
ELM RD
100 THO 91320 556-B2
100 VeCo 91320 556-B2
ELM ST
200 SPLA 93060 463-J7
E ELM ST
100 OXN 93033 552-G1
W ELM ST
100 OXN 93033 552-E1
ELMA ST
3300 CMRL 93010 524-G1
EL MALABAR ST
7000 VEN 93003 472-D7
ELM COTTAGE CT
- CMRL 93012 524-G5
N ELMDALE AV
2000 SIMI 93065 498-B2
EL MEDIO ST
- VEN 93001 471-C7
ELMHURST LN
900 FILM 93015 455-J7
ELMHURST ST
4900 VEN 93003 492-B3
ELMIRA ST
2600 THO 91320 555-H1
EL MONTE AV
100 VEN 93004 492-G2
EL MONTE DR
900 SIMI 93065 497-G5
1100 THO 91362 526-J5
2000 THO 91362 527-A5
ELMORE ST
3200 SIMI 93063 498-D2
ELMROCK AV
13200 MRPK 93021 496-E3
ELMSBURY LN
7000 CanP 91307 529-D5
ELMSBURY RD
1900 THO 91361 557-A7
ELMSFORD PL
1500 THO 91361 556-H6
ELM VIEW DR
5400 CMRL 93012 525-A2
ELMWOOD ST
2900 THO 91320 555-G6
EL NIDO CT
2200 CMRL 93010 494-G7
EL NIDO ST
3200 CMRL 93010
ELOISE CIR
1600 SIMI 93063
EL PAJARO
100 THO 91320
EL PASEO RD
300 OJAI 93023
EL PASEO ST
1000 FILM 93015
EL PASILLO
100 THO 91320
EL PASO AV
2800 SIMI 93063
EL PLANO DR
100 VeCo 93023
EL PORTAL CT
9500 VEN 93004
EL PORTAL WY
1200 OXN 93035
1300 OXN 93035
EL PRADO ST
4600 SIMI 93063
EL RANCHO DR
1900 CMRL 93010
EL REPOSO DR
2200 CMRL 93012
EL RETIRO CT
900 VeCo 91377
EL RIO DR
100 VeCo 93023
300 OXN 93036
300 OXN 93036
EL ROBLAR DR
100 VeCo 93023
EL SEGUNDO DR
800 THO 91362
ELSINOR AV
1200 VEN 93004
1200 VEN 93004
ELSINOR CT
1100 VEN 93004
ELSINORE AV
1300 OXN 93035
ELSINORE CIR
2600 OXN 93035
ELSINORE CT
1900 OXN 93035
EL SOL AV
500 VeCo 93023
EL SONETO CT
23600 CMRL 93010
ELSTOW CT
1600 THO 91361
EL TORO RD
700 OJAI 93023
900 VeCo 93023
EL TORO FIRE TRUCK TR
- Nwhl 91382
EL TUACA CT
300 VeCo 93010
300 VeCo 93010
ELVADO DR
1400 SIMI 93065
EL VERANO DR
1400 THO 91362
ELWIN ST
11800 MRPK 93021
ELY WY
2700 SIMI 93065
EMBER CT
5500 AGRH 91301
EMERALD AV
3000 SIMI 93063
EMERALD CT
900 VEN 93004
EMERALD ST
1300 OXN 93036
7800 VEN 93004
EMERALD ISLE WY
1600 OXN 93035
EMERIC AV
1400 SIMI 93065
EMERSON AV
1100 OXN 93033
1600 OXN 93033
1600 VeCo 93033
EMERSON CT
5700 AGRH 91301
EMERSON ST
700 THO 91362
900 THO 91362
EMILIO CT
11800 MRPK 93021
EMILY LN
2800 SIMI 93063
EMILY ST
600 OJAI 93023
EMMA AV
- VEN 93003
EMMA CT
2000 THO 91362
N EMMETT AV
2100 SIMI 93063
EMORY AV
1700 SIMI 93063
EMPIRE AV
600 VEN 93003
EMPRESA LN
2100 OXN 93036
EMPRESS AV
700 CMRL 93010
EMPTY SADDLE AV
1700 SIMI 93063
ENADIA WY
22500 CanP 91307
ENCANTO AV
2600 VEN 93003
ENCHANTED WY
900 SIMI 93065
N ENCINAL AV
100 VeCo 93023
S ENCINAL AV
100 VeCo 93023
ENCINAL PL
- VEN 93001
ENCINAL WY
- VEN 93001
ENCINAL CANYON RD
600 LACo 90265
ENCINAS CANYON
300 VeCo 93001
ENCINO AV
100 VeCo 93010
300 CMRL 93010
ENCINO DR
- VeCo 93022
ENCINO LN
4200 VeCo 93001

STREET Block City ZIP Pg-Grid

PL
SPLA 93060 464-C3
OXN 93033 552-G4
VISTA CT
THO 91362 556-H1
VISTA DR
THO 91362 556-H1
THO 91362 526-H7
ST
VeCo 93022 461-B1
VeCo 93063 499-B3
OR ST
AGRH 91301 558-E7
OUR CT
MRPK 93021 496-C1
T ST
PHME 93041 552-E4
CIR
THO 91360 526-F6
OAKS CT
SIMI 93063 499-C1
VEN 93004 492-J2
D
VeCo 93015 455-D4
OA AV
THO 91320 556-C1
PL
OXN 93035 522-D6
A DR
OXN 93030 522-G3
OXN 93036 522-H3
VEN 93003 491-G4
IAN AV
THO 91360 526-G6
O
THO 91362 556-J1
THO 91362 526-J1
THO 91362 527-A1
THO 91362 497-A7
THO 91360 497-A7
THO 91360 496-J7
AV
VEN 93001 491-F1
THO 91362 557-A2
IR
CanP 91307 529-F5
L
OXN 93036 522-F2
T
SIMI 93065 498-B2
ON PL
SIMI 93065 498-B1
VEN 93004 492-J2
SIMI 93065 498-A5
LA 91304 529-E3
AV
THO 91320 555-F4
AV
VEN 93003 492-F5
DR
SPLA 93060 464-C3
ER RD
SIMI 93065 477-J7
SIMI 93065 478-A6
SIMI 93065 497-J5
SIMI 93065 498-A3
LN
FILM 93015 455-J6
T
THO 91360 526-E4
T
WdHl 91367 529-F7
N DR
OXN 93035 522-E7
OXN 93035 552-E1
A RD
VeCo 93012 496-B5
RA AV
VeCo 93012 496-A6
RA CIR
VeCo 93012 496-A6
IDO CT
CMRL 93010 524-D3
LN
VEN 93001 471-C6
LN
THO 91362 527-C3
NCE DR
VeCo 93065 497-B3
VeCo 93021 497-B3
NADE DR
OXN 93036 522-H2
NADE DR
OXN 93036 522-G1
Y
THO 91360 526-G6
UNCTION CT
THO 91362 527-C2
N DR
VeCo 93010 494-C7
IA PL
CMRL 93012 524-G3
AV
VEN 93003 492-A2
DR
THO 91320 525-G6
AV
MRPK 93021 496-E1
T
CMRL 93010 524-F2
A DR
CALB 91302 558-H6
A ST
VEN 93003 491-G2
ITA LN
VeCo 91377 558-A2
CT
SPLA 93060 463-J6
WY
OXN 93035 522-B7
OXN 93035 552-A1
DR
CALB 91301 558-F6
T
VeCo 91320 525-F7
VEN 93003 472-D6
Y
THO 91360 526-G6
V
SIMI 93065 497-H5
RD
OXN 93033 553-B4
VeCo 93033 553-E4

ETTING RD
21200 VeCo 93012 553-E4
ETZ MELOY MTWY
- LACo 90265 586-E4
- VeCo 90265 586-E4
EUBANKS ST
400 CMRL 93010 523-J5
EUCALYPTUS CIR
1500 THO 91360 526-H3
EUCALYPTUS DR
2500 VeCo 93036 523-C2
N EUCALYPTUS DR
- VeCo 93015 465-E1
- VeCo 93015 455-E7
S EUCALYPTUS DR
100 VeCo 93015 465-E1
EUCALYPTUS ST
100 OJAI 93023 441-H6
3700 SIMI 93063 478-E7
W EUCALYPTUS ST
400 OJAI 93023 441-G6
EUCLID AV
900 CMRL 93010 524-C1
EUCLID CIR
1900 CMRL 93010 524-E1
EUGENE AV
700 VEN 93004 492-H2
EUGENIA DR
- VEN 93003 491-G2
EUNICE AV
5600 SIMI 93063 499-A3
EUREKA ST
400 PHME 93041 552-E5
8300 VEN 93004 492-G2
EUREKA CANYON RD
- VeCo 93040 457-G7
- VeCo 93040 458-A7
- VeCo 93040 467-H1
EVA ST
100 VEN 93003 491-G4
EVANGELINE PL
1500 OXN 93030 522-D4
EVANS AV
1700 VEN 93001 491-E2
EVANS DR
3500 SIMI 93063 498-E3
EVANSTON PL
900 OXN 93033 552-J3
EVANWOOD AV
5000 VeCo 91377 557-G1
EVE RD
4200 SIMI 93063 498-F1
EVELYN AV
3000 SIMI 93063 478-D7
EVENING SIDE DR
2900 THO 91362 526-J2
EVENING SKY DR
5300 SIMI 93063 478-J6
5300 SIMI 93063 479-A6
EVENSTAR AV
800 THO 91361 557-B5
EVEREST AV
700 MRPK 93021 496-D1
EVEREST ST
100 OXN 93030 523-A5
EVERETT ST
- MRPK 93021 476-E7
EVERGLADES ST
5300 VEN 93003 492-C5
EVERGREEN AV
500 THO 91320 555-G3
EVERGREEN CT
23600 SIMI 93065 497-F7
EVERGREEN DR
2100 SIMI 93065 497-E2
N EVERGREEN DR
- VEN 93003 491-F2
- VEN 93001 491-F2
S EVERGREEN DR
- VEN 93003 491-F3
EVERGREEN LN
400 PHME 93041 552-E5
1100 OXN 93033 552-F5
1100 PHME 93033 552-F5
EVERGREEN SQ
400 PHME 93041 552-F5
EVESHAM AV
2800 THO 91362 527-A3
EVITA CT
5500 AGRH 91301 557-H5
EVITA PL
- OXN 93030 522-H4
EWANA PL
- Chat 91311 479-J7
EXETER AV
1300 VEN 93004 492-H3
EXETER CT
2500 CMRL 93010 524-F1
EXPLORER CV
2500 PHME 93041 552-C3

F

F AV
- VeCo 93042 583-F6
F ST
- VeCo 93041 583-G2
- VeCo 93042 583-G2
100 OXN 93030 522-F6
1300 OXN 93033 552-F1
23600 VeCo 93063 498-H7
23600 VeCo 93063 528-F1
N F ST
100 OXN 93030 522-F4
FABLE AV
8300 LA 91304 529-F2
FACILITY RD
23600 VeCo 93063 499-B7
FACTORY AV
500 OXN 93030 522-G6
FACTORY LN
300 OXN 93030 522-H7
FACTORY STORES DR
- CMRL 93010 524-B4
FACULTY CT
- THO 91360 526-F2
FACULTY ST
- THO 91360 526-E3
FAIR AV
1500 SIMI 93063 498-E3
FAIRBANKS AV
2800 SIMI 93063 478-F7
FAIRBOURNE PL
300 OXN 93033 552-G5
FAIRBREEZE CIR
3900 WLKV 91361 557-C6
FAIRBROOK LN
4300 MRPK 93021 496-E3
FAIRCHILD AV
900 CMRL 93010 524-E2

FAIRCREST LN
5100 VeCo 93066 495-A1
FAIRFAX AV
200 VEN 93003 492-B1
FAIRFIELD CIR
- VEN 93003 492-A3
FAIRFIELD RD
500 SIMI 93065 497-E5
FAIRFORD ST
8500 VEN 93004 492-G4
FAIRGRANGE DR
5400 AGRH 91301 557-H5
FAIRGROVE CIR
1000 VeCo 93010 494-F6
FAIRHAVEN CT
300 THO 91320 555-G2
6100 AGRH 91301 558-A3
FAIRMONT DR
3300 VEN 93003 491-H2
FAIRMONT LN
- OXN 93036 522-C2
FAIRMOUNT RD
1400 THO 91362 527-D6
FAIR OAKS
8000 VeCo 93021 476-D3
FAIRPOINT AV
6500 VEN 93003 492-D5
FAIRVIEW CT
1200 OJAI 93023 441-G5
1200 VeCo 93023 441-G5
FAIRVIEW DR
100 VEN 93001 491-F2
FAIRVIEW PL
5400 AGRH 91301 558-C4
FAIRVIEW RD
- THO 91362 557-A3
100 OJAI 93023 441-E5
100 VeCo 93023 441-D5
200 THO 91361 557-A3
E FAIRVIEW RD
100 OJAI 93023 441-G5
100 VeCo 93023 441-G5
FAIRVIEW CANYON RD
23600 VeCo 93015 456-G6
FAIRVIEW FIRE RD
400 THO 91361 556-J3
400 THO 91361 557-A3
FAIRWAY CT
1300 CMRL 93010 494-A5
1300 VeCo 93010 494-A5
1600 THO 91362 527-D6
2300 OXN 93036 522-C2
FAIRWAY DR
500 VeCo 93010 494-A5
FAIRWAY LN
100 OJAI 93023 442-A7
FAIRWAY PARK LN
2600 SIMI 93063 478-J7
FAIR WEATHER CRSG
23600 SPLA 93060 464-B1
23600 VeCo 93060 454-C7
23600 VeCo 93060 464-B1
FAITH CT
6400 SIMI 93063 499-C3
FALCON ST
- SIMI 93065 477-J7
- SIMI 93065 478-A7
6000 VEN 93003 492-C4
FALCON WY
1000 FILM 93015 455-J5
FALCONROCK LN
400 VeCo 91377 558-A1
FALCONVIEW LN
6800 VeCo 91377 528-B7
FALKIRK AV
1500 OXN 93035 552-A1
FALKIRK BAY
4400 OXN 93035 552-A1
FALKNER PL
1900 OXN 93033 553-A1
FALLBROOK AV
- THO 91320 555-F2
6100 WdHl 91367 529-H7
6400 CanP 91307 529-H3
7400 LA 91304 529-H3
FALLCREEK CT
- SIMI 93063 479-B7
- SIMI 93063 499-B1
FALLEN LEAF AV
300 CMRL 93012 524-H5
1100 VEN 93004 492-J2
FALLEN LEAF CT
- SIMI 93063 479-B7
- SIMI 93063 499-A1
10100 VEN 93004 492-J2
FALLEN OAKS DR
- THO 91360 526-F1
FALLING STAR AV
1200 THO 91362 527-F6
FALLING WATER CT
3300 SIMI 93063 478-J6
FALLON CIR
2500 SIMI 93065 498-B3
FALL RIVER CIR
3400 THO 91362 557-C3
FALLVIEW RD
1800 THO 91361 557-A6
1800 WLKV 91361 557-A6
FALMOUTH ST
800 THO 91362 526-J7
900 THO 91362 527-A6
FALON CT
1900 THO 91362 527-A5
FANNIN DR
4600 SIMI 93063 478-G6
FANSHELL WK
1100 OXN 93035 522-D7
FAR COUNTRY CT
- MRPK 93021 496-F2
FARGO ST
400 THO 91360 526-D4
FARIA RD
4000 VeCo 93001 470-A3
FARIA ST
3300 CMRL 93010 524-G1
FARING FORD RD
2900 VeCo 91361 586-D2
FARLAND ST
100 THO 91320 556-B2
FARLEY ST
- PHME 93043 552-E4
FARM RD
- VeCo 93012 554-D3
FARMFIELD RD
26000 CALB 91302 558-H3
FARNHAM RD
30800 WLKV 91362 557-G7
FARNSWORTH ST
2100 CMRL 93010 524-E1

FARRAGUT CT
1900 OXN 93033 553-A1
FARRAGUT DR
2600 OXN 93033 553-A2
FARRALON WY
- OXN 93035 552-B1
FARRALONE AV
6400 CanP 91303 529-J6
7600 LA 91304 529-J1
8900 LA 91304 499-J7
9000 Chat 91311 499-J3
FARRELL CIR
3500 THO 91320 555-F2
FARWELL ST
2000 SIMI 93065 497-J2
FASHION PARK PL
100 OXN 93033 552-G4
E FASLEY AV
5800 SIMI 93063 499-A1
FASTWATER CT
32400 WLKV 91361 557-B7
FATHOM CT
1000 OXN 93035 522-C7
FATHOM DR
1300 OXN 93035 522-C7
1300 OXN 93035 552-C1
FAULKNER CT
6800 VEN 93003 492-E3
FAULKNER RD
14900 VeCo 93060 473-G2
23600 SPLA 93060 473-H1
FAUNA DR
2000 OXN 93036 522-G3
FAUST AV
6700 CanP 91307 529-H4
7600 LA 91304 529-H2
FAWN AV
2300 VEN 93003 492-E5
FAWN PL
2100 VEN 93003 492-E5
FAWN CHASE LN
23600 SIMI 93065 497-A2
FAWNGLEN PL
900 THO 91320 555-G5
FAWNRIDGE AV
23600 THO 91362 527-B4
FAWN VALLEY CT
200 SIMI 93065 497-E6
FAXTON CT
3200 VeCo 93063 478-E6
FAYANCE PL
3300 THO 91362 526-J2
FAYTON CT
2000 CMRL 93010 494-D7
E FEARING ST
5600 SIMI 93063 499-A2
FEATHER AV
1300 THO 91360 526-E6
FEATHER ST
9000 VEN 93004 492-H4
FEATHERFALL WY
23600 SIMI 93065 497-A2
FEATHER HILL CT
1100 THO 91320 526-A6
FEATHER RIVER PL
- OXN 93036 492-H7
FEATHERSTONE ST
100 OXN 93030 523-A5
FEATHERWOOD ST
2400 THO 91362 527-B5
FELICIA CT
1200 OXN 93030 522-J5
FELICIA ST
5200 CMRL 93012 525-A3
FELIX AV
3200 VeCo 93063 478-E6
FELIX DR
100 VeCo 93023 441-E7
FELIZ DR
- VeCo 93022 451-C4
FELKINS RD
200 SPLA 93060 463-J7
200 SPLA 93060 473-J1
FELTON ST
2700 THO 91320 555-G3
FENMORE AV
1700 CMRL 93010 524-G1
1700 CMRL 93010 494-G7
FENMORE CT
1700 CMRL 93010 524-G1
FENMORE ST
14600 MRPK 93021 476-J6
FENWICK WY
- SIMI 93065 527-E1
FENWOOD AV
6100 WdHl 91367 529-G7
FENWORTH CT
6300 AGRH 91301 558-A3
FERAL AV
6200 AGRH 91301 558-B3
FERNANDO DR
100 VeCo 93023 441-D6
FERN ANN FALLS RD
- Chat 91311 479-H7
FERNBROOK RD
8600 LA 91304 529-E1
FERNCREST PL
3000 THO 91362 527-C3
FERNDALE PL
300 THO 91360 526-D5
FERNDALE ST
6000 VEN 93003 492-C3
FERNGLEN CIR
600 FILM 93015 456-A5
FERNHILL AV
800 THO 91320 555-E4
FERNHILL CT
800 THO 91320 555-D4
FERNLEAF CT
2100 THO 91362 527-A1
FERN OAK DR
1100 SPLA 93060 464-B3
FERNRIDGE CT
5200 CMRL 93012 524-J1
5200 CMRL 93012 525-A1
FERN VALLEY CT
4500 MRPK 93021 496-F2
FERNVIEW ST
2100 SIMI 93065 498-A1
N FERNWOOD CT
2000 SIMI 93065 498-A2
FERNWOOD DR
400 OXN 93030 522-F4
2400 VEN 93001 491-F2
FERRARA CT
30800 WLKV 91362 557-G7
FERRARA DR
1100 VeCo 93023 451-B1
FERRARA WY
1800 OXN 93030 522-J6

FERRARA WY
1800 OXN 93030 523-A6
FERRIS DR
4000 VeCo 93060 464-D5
FERRO DR
200 VEN 93001 491-B1
FESTIVAL CT
3600 THO 91360 526-G1
FESTIVO ST
- OXN 93030 523-A5
FICUS WY
- VEN 93004 493-A2
FIELD ST
- OXN 93033 552-H5
FIELDCREST CT
3600 THO 91360 526-G1
FIELDCREST DR
5300 CMRL 93012 525-A1
FIELDFLOWER LN
23600 SIMI 93065 497-A2
FIELDGATE DR
2300 CMRL 93010 494-H7
FIELDMONT PL
24400 CanP 91307 529-D5
FIELDSTONE WY
300 SIMI 93065 497-D6
FIERRO DR
1100 VeCo 93023 451-B1
FIESTA AV
2300 CMRL 93010 524-E2
E FIESTA GRN
100 PHME 93041 552-E2
W FIESTA GRN
100 PHME 93041 552-D2
FIESTA ST
5900 VEN 93003 492-C2
FIG ST
2100 SIMI 93063 498-G1
FIGUEROA ST
- VEN 93001 491-B2
FILLMORE AV
100 VeCo 93035 552-B5
100 VeCo 93043 552-B5
6900 VeCo 93001 459-C4
FILLMORE ST
200 FILM 93015 456-A5
700 SPLA 93060 463-H7
FINANCIAL SQ
2400 OXN 93036 522-H1
FINCH AV
1300 VEN 93003 492-D4
FINCH CT
500 FILM 93015 455-H5
2000 SIMI 93063 499-C2
FINCHLEY CT
3500 SIMI 93063 478-E7
FINE RD
700 VeCo 93015 456-G6
FINE ST
700 FILM 93015 456-A5
FINO AV
6500 CMRL 93012 525-C6
FINROD CT
1000 THO 91361 557-A5
E FIR AV
200 OXN 93033 552-G1
W FIR AV
100 OXN 93033 552-E1
FIR CT
1600 OXN 93033 552-H1
FIR ST
- CMRL 93010 524-E3
N FIR ST
- VEN 93001 491-C1
S FIR ST
- VEN 93001 491-C2
FIREBIRD CT
5700 CMRL 93012 495-B7
FIRECREST CT
500 THO 91320 555-G3
FIRENZE ST
300 OXN 93036 522-H3
FIRESIDE LN
4300 MRPK 93021 496-F3
FIRESTONE CIR
900 SIMI 93065 497-C6
FIRESTONE CT
2100 OXN 93036 522-D2
FIRETHORNE PL
1600 OXN 93030 522-E4
FIRWOOD CT
2900 THO 91320 555-G3
FISHER CT
3600 OXN 93035 552-C1
FISHER DR
1700 OXN 93035 552-C1
FISHERS CT
- MRPK 93021 476-F6
FISH HATCHERY RD
100 FILM 93015 456-D6
FISK CT
1700 THO 91362 526-J6
FISKE PL
1200 OXN 93033 552-J1
FITCH AV
600 MRPK 93021 496-F1
FITZGERALD AV
- VEN 93003 492-C3
FITZGERALD RD
1000 SIMI 93065 497-H4
1700 SIMI 93065 498-A4
FITZGERALD ST
23600 LA 91304 529-E3
FIVE OAK CT
5600 SIMI 93063 499-A1
FIX WY
- VEN 93001 491-B1
FLAGSTAFF CT
700 VEN 93004 492-H2
FLAGSTONE LN
- SIMI 93063 498-H1
N FLAMINGO WY
1100 VEN 93003 492-F4
S FLAMINGO WY
1300 VEN 93003 492-F4
FLAMING STAR AV
600 THO 91360 526-D4
FLANAGAN DR
5700 SIMI 93063 479-A7
FLATHEAD RIVER ST
- OXN 93036 492-G6
FLATTOP CT
- MRPK 93021 476-F6
FLAX PL
- OXN 93036 522-B2
FLEET AV
700 VEN 93003 491-J4
FLEET ST
- VeCo 93042 583-D4
400 PHME 93041 552-D2

FLEISCHER REDMAND RD
23600 VeCo 93060 464-H3
FLETCHER CT
2100 THO 91362 556-H2
FLETCHER ST
2700 SIMI 93065 498-C4
FLEURY LN
6100 WdHl 91367 529-J7
FLICKER CT
6900 VEN 93003 492-E4
FLINN AV
500 MRPK 93021 496-F1
W FLINT ST
- VEN 93001 471-B7
FLINTLOCK LN
4200 WLKV 91361 557-F6
4200 AGRH 91301 557-F6
N FLINTLOCK LN
- VeCo 91307 529-A5
FLINTON CT
1400 THO 91361 557-A6
FLINTRIDGE CT
2200 THO 91362 527-A4
FLITTNER CIR
100 THO 91360 556-G1
FLOATING CLOUD ST
3600 THO 91360 526-G1
FLOOD ST
3600 VeCo 93063 478-E6
FLORA LN
- OXN 93030 523-A4
FLORADALE CT
3600 THO 91360 526-H1
FLORAL DR
4000 VeCo 93001 471-C1
4700 VeCo 93001 461-C7
FLORA VISTA AV
- CMRL 93012 524-H4
FLORENCE AV
200 PHME 93041 552-F5
FLORENCE ST
4000 SIMI 93063 498-F2
FLORENTINA DR
23600 OXN 93030 522-J5
FLORENTINE CT
- THO 91362 527-B3
FLORESTA CT
4800 THO 91362 527-E7
FLORY AV
- MRPK 93021 496-E1
FLOTOW LN
4600 VEN 93003 492-A7
FLOWER ST
3900 VEN 93003 491-J3
FLOWERCREEK DR
11500 MRPK 93021 496-B3
FLOWERDALE ST
1600 SIMI 93063 499-C3
FLOWER GLEN ST
900 SIMI 93065 477-G7
900 SIMI 93065 497-H1
FLOWERVIEW CT
4200 MRPK 93021 496-B2
FLOWERWOOD CT
11600 MRPK 93021 496-B4
FLOYD DR
300 SPLA 93060 464-A7
FLOYD ST
- VEN 93003 492-C3
FLYING HILLS LN
700 THO 91360 526-G1
FLYNN RD
- CMRL 93012 524-G2
18300 CMRL 93012 494-H7
FOGHORN CV
2600 PHME 93041 552-C1
FOLKESTONE TERRACE RD
1600 THO 91361 557-A6
FONT LN
1500 THO 91361 557-A6
FONTANA DR
100 OXN 93033 553-C4
FOOTHILL DR
400 FILM 93015 456-A4
1200 VeCo 93063 499-B3
1900 THO 91361 557-A3
5500 AGRH 91301 558-C5
FOOTHILL LN
100 OJAI 93023 441-G6
FOOTHILL RD
100 OJAI 93023 441-G5
500 SPLA 93060 463-H6
700 VeCo 93060 463-E7
1100 VeCo 93023 441-G4
2700 VEN 93003 491-H1
2800 VeCo 93003 491-H1
3800 VeCo 93003 492-A1
3800 VEN 93003 492-A1
7600 VeCo 93004 472-J6
7600 VEN 93004 472-J6
7600 VEN 93004 492-D1
7600 VeCo 93004 492-D1
8300 VeCo 93003 472-F7
8300 VEN 93003 472-F7
9500 VeCo 93060 472-J6
10600 VEN 93060 472-J6
11400 VeCo 93060 473-C1
FOOTHILL TR
- VeCo - 441-F3
- VeCo 93023 441-D4
FORAR CIR
1700 CMRL 93010 524-H1
FORBES LN
- VEN 93001 471-B6
FORD AV
23600 VEN 93003 492-E2
FORDHAM AV
300 VEN 93003 492-B3
1200 THO 91360 526-D5
N FORDHAM ST
14300 MRPK 93021 476-G6
FORDYCE RD
700 VeCo 93023 442-C5
FORELOCK CT
700 SIMI 93065 497-G6
FOREST AV
1100 VeCo 93023 451-B3
1200 SIMI 93065 498-D4
FOREST DR
1200 SPLA 93060 464-B3
FOREST COVE LN
5300 AGRH 91301 557-H4
FORESTGLEN CT
4400 MRPK 93021 496-D3
FOREST GROVE LN
- SIMI 93065 478-C4
FOREST HILLS RD
7100 CanP 91307 529-F5

FOREST KNOLL DR
1400 VeCo 91377 527-G6
FOREST LOOP DR
600 PHME 93041 552-F5
FOREST OAKS DR
4100 THO 91360 496-J7
FOREST PARK BLVD
- OXN 93036 492-G6
FOREST RIDGE DR
5400 AGRH 91301 557-G5
FORNEY LN
6400 VeCo 93063 499-C4
FORRESTER CIR
23600 SIMI 93065 497-G7
FORT COURAGE AV
3000 THO 91360 526-D2
FORT DAVIS ST
4600 SIMI 93063 478-G6
FORTUNA AV
3900 CMRL 93010 494-H7
FORTUNA LN
4100 OXN 93033 553-C4
FORT WORTH DR
4400 SIMI 93063 478-G7
FOSTER AV
1800 VEN 93001 491-E2
FOSTER PARK DR
- VeCo 93001 460-J5
- VeCo 93001 461-A6
FOSTER PARK WY
- VeCo 93001 460-J5
FOUNTAIN PL
28500 AGRH 91301 558-C5
FOUNTAIN ST
- CMRL 93012 524-G4
FOUNTAIN CREST LN
2300 THO 91362 527-C4
FOUNTAINWOOD ST
28900 AGRH 91301 558-A3
29300 AGRH 91301 557-J3
FOURNIER ST
2900 OXN 93033 552-H3
FOUR OAK CT
5600 SIMI 93063 499-A1
FOURSITE LN
1800 THO 91362 556-J1
FOWLER AV
600 THO 91320 555-G4
FOWLER RD
6600 SIMI 93063 499-C3
FOX ST
100 OJAI 93023 441-J7
FOXBORO LN
7600 LA 91304 529-E4
FOX CANYON RD
23600 VeCo 93066 474-G5
FOXDALE CT
23600 THO 91320 555-E4
FOX DEN CT
2600 OXN 93036 522-D2
FOXFIELD DR
31500 WLKV 91361 557-D7
FOXGLOVE CT
3900 THO 91362 557-C1
FOXGLOVE PL
300 OXN 93036 522-F2
FOX HILL LN
9400 Chat 91311 499-H6
FOX HILLS DR
200 THO 91361 556-F2
FOXMOOR CT
31900 WLKV 91361 557-C6
FOX RIDGE DR
200 THO 91361 556-F2
FOX SPRINGS CIR
1500 THO 91320 526-A6
FOXTAIL CT
3100 THO 91362 527-C3
FOXTAIL ST
23600 SIMI 93065 497-F7
FOXWOOD CT
3600 THO 91360 526-H1
FOXWOOD DR
5600 VeCo 91377 557-J1
FRAGRANS WY
6100 WdHl 91367 529-J7
FRANCE AV
700 SIMI 93065 497-J5
FRANCE CIR
200 OJAI 93023 441-H6
FRANCES ST
100 VEN 93003 491-G3
FRANCIS AV
3900 CMRL 93010 494-H7
FRANCISCA WY
5300 AGRH 91301 557-J5
FRANCISCO PL
4000 OXN 93033 552-G4
E FRANDON CT
3900 SIMI 93063 498-F2
FRANK AV
100 OXN 93033 552-G3
FRANKFORT CT
3200 OXN 93033 552-J3
FRANKIE DR
3200 VeCo 91320 525-F7
FRANKLIN CT
900 SIMI 93065 497-H4
FRANKLIN DR
400 OJAI 93023 441-J6
FRANKLIN LN
- VEN 93001 471-C6
FRANKLIN ST
9200 Chat 91311 499-F7
FRANRIVERS AV
6400 CanP 91307 529-D7
FRASER LN
- VeCo 93001 471-C2
FRASER PT
- VeCo 93012 554-F3
FRASER ST
23600 VeCo 93022 451-D6
FRAZIER ST
1400 CMRL 93012 525-B1
FRAZIER MOUNTAIN RD
- VeCo - 367-B1
FRED AV
1700 SIMI 93065 498-B3
FREEBIRD LN
- VeCo 91377 527-J7
FREEBORN WY
2100 VeCo 93012 496-B7
2100 VeCo 93012 526-B1
FREEDOM PARK DR
500 VeCo 93010 523-J5
500 CMRL 93010 523-J5
FREEPORT CT
1000 THO 91361 557-B5
FREEPORT LN
2800 OXN 93035 522-D6

STREET Block City ZIP Pg-Grid
FREESIA AV
- SIMI 93063 499-A2
FREETOWN LN
27400 AGRH 91301 558-E7
FRWY Rt#-23
- MRPK - 496-G1
- THO - 496-J7
- THO - 497-A7
- THO - 526-J1
- THO - 556-H1
- VeCo - 496-H3
- VeCo - 497-A4
FREMLIN DR
- FILM 93015 456-A4
FREMONT AV
1500 SIMI 93065 497-J4
FREMONT CIR
5900 CMRL 93012 525-B1
5900 CMRL 93012 495-B7
FREMONT DR
1800 THO 91362 526-J5
FREMONT ST
- MRPK 93021 496-E2
5900 VEN 93003 492-C2
FREMONT WY
1300 OXN 93030 522-E4
FREMONTIA ST
1200 SPLA 93060 464-B3
FRENCH CT
2600 SIMI 93065 498-C3
FRENCHYS CV
- VeCo 93012 554-F3
FRESCA DR
- OXN 93030 522-H4
FRESHMAN CT
15700 MRPK 93021 477-A5
FRESH MEADOWS RD
300 SIMI 93065 497-C6
FRESHWATER DR
29000 AGRH 91301 558-A4
FRESHWIND CIR
3900 WLKV 91361 557-C6
FRESNO CT
10700 VEN 93004 472-H7
FREY CANYON RD
- VeCo 93015 466-H2
- VeCo 93021 466-G4
FRIANT AV
1300 SIMI 93065 498-A3
FRIAR ST
22400 WdHl 91367 529-D7
FRIEDRICH LN
1300 OXN 93033 552-E2
FRIEDRICH RD
2500 VeCo 93036 523-C2
E FRONT ST
800 VEN 93001 491-D2
W FRONT ST
200 VEN 93001 491-A2
FRONTAGE RD
300 VEN 93004 472-J7
FRONTIER AV
2900 THO 91360 526-C3
FRONTIER PL
11300 Chat 91311 499-J2
FROST AV
2500 THO 91360 526-F3
FROST CIR
6900 VEN 93003 492-E3
FROST DR
4200 OXN 93033 552-H4
FRUITVALE AV
8000 VeCo 93021 476-D3
FRYS HARBOR
- VeCo 93012 554-F3
FUCHSIA LN
1100 SPLA 93060 464-B3
FUCHSIA PL
- VEN 93004 473-A7
FUCHSIA ST
900 OXN 93036 522-E2
FUELBREAK RD
5300 VeCo - 366-L7
5300 VeCo - 442-H4
5300 VeCo 93023 366-L7
5300 VeCo 93023 442-H4
FUENTE DR
- OXN 93030 522-H4
FUJI ST
- MRPK 93021 496-D1
FULLBROKE DR
1900 THO 91362 527-A4
FULLER AV
1200 SIMI 93065 498-A4
FULMAR AV
1800 VEN 93003 492-E4
FULTON ST
100 OJAI 93023 441-J6
100 CMRL 93010 524-E3
S FULTON ST
100 OJAI 93023 441-J7
FURMAN AV
100 VEN 93003 492-B2
FUTURA PT
3100 THO 91362 527-A2

G

G ST
- VeCo 93042 583-F6
100 OXN 93030 522-F6
1200 OXN 93033 522-F7
1200 OXN 93033 552-F1
23600 VeCo 93063 498-G7
23600 VeCo 93063 528-F1
N G ST
300 OXN 93030 522-F5
GABBERT RD
5000 MRPK 93021 496-C1
5200 MRPK 93021 476-B6
GABRIELA CT
2400 CMRL 93012 495-B6
GABRIELLA DR
23600 OXN 93030 522-J5
GADSHILL LN
4100 AGRH 91301 558-F7
GAGE AV
2700 SIMI 93065 478-B7
GAIL CT
2900 THO 91320 555-H2
E GAINES CT
3800 SIMI 93063 498-E2
E GAINSBOROUGH RD
- THO 91360 526-F6
W GAINSBOROUGH RD
- THO 91360 526-F6
GALANO DR
4900 CMRL 93012 524-J3
GALANTE WY
200 OXN 93036 522-G3
GALAPAGOS WY
- OXN 93035 552-B1
GALAXY PL
3400 OXN 93030 523-D5
GALE WY
3300 VEN 93003 491-H2
GALENA AV
2100 SIMI 93063 498-D1
2100 SIMI 93065 498-D1
2700 SIMI 93065 478-D7
E GALENA AV
2700 SIMI 93065 498-C2
2800 SIMI 93063 498-C2
GALENA PL
- OXN 93030 522-H4
GALERITA ST
- OXN 93030 523-A5
GALESMOORE CT
1000 THO 91361 557-A5
GALINDO AV
2500 SIMI 93065 498-C4
GALLATIN PL
1100 OXN 93030 522-D4
1800 OXN 93036 522-D4
GALLEON AV
2600 PHME 93041 552-D1
GALLILEE WY
- SIMI 93063 499-B1
GALLOP CT
1800 SIMI 93065 497-J6
1800 SIMI 93065 498-A5
GALLOPING HILL RD
400 SIMI 93065 497-E6
GALSWORTHY ST
100 THO 91360 526-F7
GALT ST
1700 SIMI 93065 497-J3
GALVESTON AV
3000 SIMI 93063 478-G7
GALVIN CIR
400 VEN 93004 472-H6
GALVIN LN
700 FILM 93015 456-A5
GALVIN ST
10500 VEN 93004 472-H6
GALWAY LN
- SIMI 93065 497-E2
1800 THO 91320 556-A1
GAMEBIRD CT
29300 AGRH 91301 558-A5
GAMMON CT
1800 THO 91362 526-J2
GANTLIN AV
1100 SIMI 93065 497-H4
GARCES AV
4400 CMRL 93010 494-H7
GARCIA ST
100 SPLA 93060 464-C5
GARDEN DR
200 VeCo 91361 586-E1
E GARDEN GRN
100 PHME 93041 552-E1
W GARDEN GRN
100 PHME 93041 552-D1
GARDEN ST
- SIMI 93063 499-B1
N GARDEN ST
- VEN 93001 491-B1
S GARDEN ST
- VEN 93001 491-B2
GARDENIA AV
1400 CMRL 93010 494-D7
1600 VeCo 93010 494-C7
1600 VeCo 93010 524-C1
GARDENIA LN
- SIMI 93065 497-H3
GARDENIA ST
1100 OXN 93036 522-E2
GARDEN OAKS CT
29000 AGRH 91301 558-A3
GARDENSTONE CT
2000 THO 91361 557-A5
GARDENSTONE LN
24500 CanP 91307 529-C5
GARDNER AV
700 VEN 93004 492-H2
GARDNER ST
2800 SIMI 93065 498-C5
GARFIELD AV
- OXN 93030 522-H6
N GARFIELD AV
100 OXN 93030 522-H5
GARFIELD RONDO
300 VEN 93003 492-E2
GARLAND CT
2800 THO 91360 526-D3
GARLAND ST
- VeCo 93001 471-C1
GARNET AV
700 VEN 93004 492-F3
GARNET PL
3200 SIMI 93063 478-D7
GARNET HILL CT
28800 AGRH 91301 558-B4
GARONNE ST
- OXN 93036 492-G6
GARRET DR
26900 CALB 91301 558-G6
GARRIDO CT
1000 VeCo 93010 494-B6
GARRIDO DR
900 VeCo 93010 494-B6
GARRISON WY
8900 VEN 93004 492-H3
23600 VeCo 93060 453-G2
GARST LN
1500 VeCo 93023 442-E4
GARVIN AV
1700 SIMI 93065 498-B3
GARY CT
3400 SIMI 93063 498-D2
GARY DR
1000 OXN 93033 552-J3
1800 OXN 93033 553-A3
GASTON RD
1000 VeCo 93063 499-B4
GASWAY DR
- FILM 93015 456-A7
- VeCo 93015 456-A7
GATEHOUSE LN
- SIMI 93063 498-J1
GATES PL
2600 SIMI 93065 498-B1
GATESHEAD BAY
4400 OXN 93035 552-A1
GATESHEAD WY
7100 CanP 91307 529-F5
GATEWAY DR
6400 SIMI 93063 499-C3
GATEWOOD LN
1200 SPLA 93060 464-B2
GAUCHO WY
1800 OXN 93030 522-J6
1800 OXN 93030 523-A6
GAULT ST
22000 CanP 91303 529-J5
22700 CanP 91307 529-G5
GAVIN ST
- SIMI 93063 498-H1
GAVIOTA CT
1800 SIMI 93065 498-A2
GAVIOTA LN
1300 VEN 93003 492-C4
GAVIOTA PL
100 OXN 93033 552-G4
GAVIOTA WY
700 OXN 93033 552-H4
GAY DR
- VEN 93003 492-B4
GAYLE PL
2400 SIMI 93065 498-A1
E GAYTHORNE RD
12600 VeCo 93060 473-E5
GAZANIA CT
200 THO 91362 556-H1
GAZEBO LN
- CMRL 93012 524-G5
GAZENIA CT
- OXN 93030 523-A4
GEM CIR
3200 SIMI 93063 478-D7
GEMINI AV
1000 CMRL 93010 524-F2
GEMINI CT
2600 CMRL 93010 524-F1
GENE AV
1500 SIMI 93065 498-B3
GENEIVE CIR
200 CMRL 93010 524-D4
GENEIVE ST
- CMRL 93010 524-D4
GENEVA ST
6000 VeCo 93003 492-D6
GENEVA WY
2000 OXN 93035 552-D1
GENIAL CT
300 SIMI 93065 497-J6
GENOA DR
200 SIMI 93065 497-F3
GENOA LN
- OXN 93035 522-D6
GENOVA CT
30800 WLKV 91362 557-G6
GENTILLY PL
1400 VeCo 91377 527-H6
GENTLE BROOK LN
- SIMI 93063 498-G2
GENTLE CREEK CIR
500 THO 91320 555-E3
GENTLEWOOD DR
11500 MRPK 93021 496-B3
GEOFFREY AV
1800 SIMI 93063 498-J3
1800 SIMI 93063 499-A2
GEORGE ST
3300 VeCo 93036 523-A1
3400 VeCo 93036 493-A7
GEORGETOWN AV
400 VEN 93003 492-A1
GEORGETTE ST
2600 SIMI 93063 498-D1
2700 SIMI 93063 478-D7
GEORGIA ST
3900 VEN 93003 491-J3
GEORGIA WY
9200 Chat 91311 499-E7
GERALD DR
3100 VeCo 91320 555-G1
GERANIUM LN
600 SIMI 93065 497-D5
GERANIUM PL
200 OXN 93036 522-F2
GERANIUM WY
100 VEN 93004 473-A7
GERMAIN ST
3400 CMRL 93010 524-G1
22100 Chat 91311 499-J3
GERMAINE LN
31500 WLKV 91361 557-D7
GERMANIA CT
6300 AGRH 91301 558-A3
GERONIMO AV
2900 SIMI 93063 479-A6
GERONIMO DR
2300 OXN 93033 553-A2
GERRAD WY
23600 CanP 91307 529-E4
GERRY RD
1800 VeCo 93012 495-G7
1800 VeCo 93012 525-G1
GERSHWIN LN
600 VEN 93003 492-B3
GERSHWIN PL
2100 OXN 93033 553-A1
GERST DR
600 VeCo 91320 525-G7
GERTRUDE ST
4000 SIMI 93063 498-F2
GETMAN ST
1400 CMRL 93010 524-C1
GETTYSBURG ST
4000 VEN 93003 491-J2
GETZ AV
- VEN 93003 492-B4
GEYSER CT
1300 THO 91320 526-A6
GIANT OAK AV
- THO 91320 556-A1
GIBRALTAR ST
100 OXN 93030 523-A5
GIBRALTER ST
- OXN 93030 523-A4
- VeCo 93030 523-A4
GIBSON AV
800 SIMI 93065 497-J5
GIBSON PL
- OXN 93033 552-H5
GIERSON AV
9400 Chat 91311 499-J5
GIFFORD ST
22200 CanP 91303 529-J4
W GILA CT
1900 THO 91320 555-J2
1900 THO 91320 556-A2
GILBERT CT
4700 VEN 93003 492-A7
GILBERT LN
900 VEN 93003 492-A7
GILBERT ST
500 THO 91320 525-H7
GILDA CIR
1700 SIMI 93065 498-A3
GILES RD
100 VeCo 91361 556-F7
GILL AV
400 PHME 93041 552-F5
GILLESPIE ST
- VEN 93003 492-B4
GILLIARD LN
200 VEN 93001 491-D1
GILLINGHAM CIR
2300 THO 91362 527-A2
GILMORE ST
22000 CanP 91303 529-J7
22300 CanP 91307 529-C7
GINA DR
1200 OXN 93030 522-E4
1800 OXN 93036 522-E4
GINA ST
1200 THO 91320 556-B1
GINGER CIR
2300 THO 91320 555-J1
GINGER DR
1700 OXN 93033 552-J2
GINGER ST
1900 OXN 93036 522-F3
GINGERWOOD CT
3600 THO 91360 526-H1
GINKO CT
3200 THO 91360 526-F2
GISLER AV
1600 OXN 93033 552-H2
GISLER RD
- MRPK 93021 496-D1
GITANA AV
5600 CMRL 93012 525-B6
GITANO DR
- OXN 93030 522-H4
GLACIER AV
800 PHME 93041 552-F4
800 OXN 93033 552-F4
800 OXN 93041 552-F4
1300 VEN 93003 492-B5
W GLACIER AV
100 OXN 93033 552-G4
GLACIER ST
1400 SIMI 93063 498-D3
GLADE AV
6400 CanP 91303 529-J5
7600 LA 91304 529-J4
9200 Chat 91311 499-J4
GLADE DR
500 SPLA 93060 464-A5
GLADEHOLLOW CT
5500 AGRH 91301 558-A5
GLADE SPRINGS CT
2100 OXN 93036 522-D2
GLADHILL ST
4000 THO 91320 555-E4
GLADIOLA ST
800 OXN 93036 522-F2
GLADSTONE DR
500 THO 91360 526-G6
GLAMOUR TER
- LA 91304 529-D2
GLANVILLE RD
23600 VeCo 93060 464-J4
23600 VeCo 93060 465-A4
N GLASSELL AV
1500 SIMI 93065 498-C3
GLASTONBURY RD
1900 THO 91361 557-A6
GLEAM CT
5900 AGRH 91301 558-B4
GLEDHILL ST
22000 Chat 91311 499-J6
GLEN ST
2800 VEN 93003 491-G3
GLEN WY
200 FILM 93015 455-J6
GLEN ABBEY LN
- OXN 93036 522-C2
GLENBRIDGE CIR
1100 THO 91361 557-B5
GLENBRIDGE RD
31400 WLKV 91361 557-D7
GLENBROCK LN
1500 THO 91320 526-A7
GLENBROOK AV
- CMRL 93010 524-D1
700 CMRL 93010 494-C7
GLENCOE AV
2600 SIMI 93063 478-D7
GLENCREST CIR
6300 VEN 93003 472-C6
GLENDALE AV
100 VeCo 93035 552-B5
GLENDIVE CT
- SIMI 93065 478-A6
GLENDON CT
23600 SIMI 93065 497-G7
GLEN EAGLES CT
2600 OXN 93036 522-D2
GLEN EAGLES WY
500 SIMI 93065 497-E5
GLEN ELLEN DR
- VEN 93003 491-H2
GLENHAVEN CIR
4800 THO 91362 557-G1
GLENHAVEN CT
7200 CanP 91307 529-E5
GLEN HOLLOW ST
2000 THO 91361 557-A5
GLENHURST CT
2400 SIMI 93063 498-D1
GLENLOCH LN
23600 SIMI 93065 497-A1
GLENMARE CT
1300 THO 91361 557-A6
GLENMONT CT
4000 THO 91320 555-E4
GLENN DR
- CMRL 93010 524-E3
S GLENN DR
- CMRL 93010 524-E4
GLENNCLIFF CIR
3100 THO 91360 526-C2
GLENNON CT
1600 THO 91361 556-J5
GLEN OAKS RD
600 THO 91360 556-G1
GLENSIDE LN
2300 VeCo 93012 496-B7
GLENTANA ST
- SIMI 93065 478-A6
GLENVIEW AV
1700 SIMI 93063 498-E3
GLENWAY ST
700 SPLA 93060 464-B5
GLENWOOD AV
200 VEN 93003 492-C2
GLENWOOD DR
100 OXN 93030 522-F4
GLENWOOD PL
300 THO 91362 556-J1
GLIDE AV
6100 WdHl 91367 529-F7
GLIDER CT
1900 THO 91320 526-A6
GLOBE AV
2800 THO 91360 526-F3
GLORIA CT
1000 OXN 93030 522-H5
GLORIA DR
3200 VeCo 91320 525-F7
GLORIA LN
1500 SIMI 93063 499-B3
GLORIOSA CT
- OXN 93030 523-A3
GLORYETTE AV
2100 SIMI 93063 498-G1
GLOUCESTER LN
700 THO 91362 526-J7
GLOVER DR
2100 VEN 93003 492-C5
GOBELS PASTURE RD
1700 THO 91362 527-A7
GODDARD AV
2000 SIMI 93063 498-F2
GOLD CIR
- VEN 93004 492-G3
GOLD CV
2500 PHME 93041 552-C3
GOLD DUST CT
1600 SIMI 93063 499-C3
GOLDEN AMBER LN
- SIMI 93065 497-H3
GOLDEN BEAR CT
800 SIMI 93065 497-E6
GOLDEN CANYON CIR
11200 Chat 91311 499-H2
GOLDEN CREST AV
3200 THO 91320 555-G4
GOLDEN EAGLE DR
1200 VeCo 91377 527-G7
GOLDENEYE ST
- VEN 93003 492-D5
GOLDEN FERN CT
200 SIMI 93065 497-E6
GOLDEN GLEN DR
- SIMI 93065 497-D6
GOLDEN GROVE CT
800 SIMI 93065 497-E6
GOLDEN KNOLL CT
4900 THO 91362 557-F3
GOLDENLEAF DR
3600 WLKV 91361 557-C7
GOLDEN MOSS CT
700 SIMI 93065 497-E6
GOLDEN NUGGET WY
5300 VeCo 91377 527-H7
GOLDEN OAK ST
- THO 91320 526-A6
GOLDEN PARK PL
400 SIMI 93065 497-E6
GOLDEN POND DR
- CMRL 93012 524-G4
GOLDENRIDGE CT
5200 CMRL 93012 524-J1
5200 CMRL 93012 525-A1
GOLDEN ROD CT
1900 THO 91361 557-A6
GOLDENROD PL
26600 CALB 91302 558-G7
GOLDEN SKY CIR
1900 THO 91362 527-G5
GOLDENSPUR DR
3000 VeCo 93010 494-C6
GOLDEN VINE CT
400 SIMI 93065 497-E6
GOLDEN WEST AV
200 OJAI 93023 442-A6
200 VeCo 93023 442-A6
GOLDENWOOD CIR
500 SIMI 93065 497-E6
GOLDFIELD PL
2700 SIMI 93063 478-E7
2700 SIMI 93063 498-D1
GOLDFINCH DR
6800 VEN 93003 492-E4
GOLD HILL CIR
3100 THO 91360 526-D2
GOLD HILL RD
- VeCo - 367-C1
GOLDIN AV
2400 SIMI 93065 498-B1
GOLDMAN AV
- MRPK 93021 496-D1
GOLDSMITH AV
2200 THO 91360 526-F4
GOLD SPRING PL
800 THO 91361 557-A5
GOLDSTONE LN
- SIMI 93065 478-B4
GOLD STRIKE AV
2300 THO 91360 526-D4
GOLF COURSE CT
1800 THO 91362 527-D6
GOLF COURSE DR
2800 VEN 93003 492-D7
2900 VEN 93001 492-D7
4300 THO 91362 527-D6
GOLF MEADOWS CT
2600 SIMI 93063 478-H7
GOLF VILLA WY
- CMRL 93010 493-H7
GOLIAD CIR
4800 SIMI 93063 478-H7
GOLONDRINA ST
13100 MRPK 93021 496-E3
GONDOLA DR
4800 VeCo 91377 557-G2
GONZAGA ST
5200 VEN 93003 492-B3
GONZALES RD
- OXN 93030 522-H3
100 OXN 93036 522-F3
1100 VeCo 93063 499-A3
1800 OXN 93030 523-A3
2100 OXN 93036 523-A3
2700 VeCo 93030 522-A3
2900 VeCo 93036 522-A3
3900 VeCo 93030 521-H3
3900 VeCo 93036 521-H3
5000 VeCo 93035 521-H3
GONZALES SERVICE RD
500 OXN 93030 522-F3
GOODENOUGH RD
700 FILM 93015 455-J5
1100 VeCo 93015 455-J3
2100 VeCo 93015 367-B7
GOODHOPE ST
500 VeCo 93022 451-A7
GOODMAN ST
800 VEN 93003 492-A4
GOODSPEED ST
1000 PHME 93041 552-E5
GOODSPRING DR
30300 AGRH 91301 557-G5
E GOODWIN CT
3900 SIMI 93063 498-F2
GOODYEAR AV
1700 VEN 93003 492-A5
GORGON DR
- VeCo 93041 583-G2
GORHAM RD
100 VeCo 93023 442-B6
GORMAN ST
2100 CMRL 93010 524-E2
GORRION AV
- VEN 93004 472-J6
- VEN 93004 473-A6
GOSHEN ST
6100 SIMI 93063 499-B2
GOTITA WY
1200 OXN 93030 522-H5
E GOULD ST
2600 SIMI 93065 498-C5
GRABLE PL
700 THO 91320 555-G3
GRACE CT
- CMRL 93010 494-D7
- CMRL 93010 524-D1
E GRACELAND ST
2200 SIMI 93065 498-B2
GRACIA DR
- OXN 93030 522-H4
GRACIA ST
800 CMRL 93010 524-G2
GRADA AV
600 VeCo 93010 494-B6
GRADUATE CIR
15800 MRPK 93021 477-A4
E GRAFTON ST
3100 SIMI 93063 498-D2
N GRAFTON ST
2200 SIMI 93063 498-D2
GRAHAM AV
400 CMRL 93010 524-F3
GRAHAM CT
10100 VEN 93004 492-J2
GRAHAM ST
1100 SIMI 93065 497-H2
GRANADA LN
- FILM 93015 456-C6
GRANADA ST
- CMRL 93010 524-D4
GRANADILLA DR
4200 MRPK 93021 496-E3
N GRANBY AV
800 SIMI 93065 498-C4
GRAND AV
200 OJAI 93023 441-H6
900 VeCo 93015 455-H2
900 OJAI 93023 442-A6
1100 VeCo 93023 442-D5
1900 VEN 93003 492-D5
2000 VeCo 93003 492-D5
GRANDE ST
200 OXN 93036 522-H2
GRANDE VISTA DR
3000 THO 91320 525-G6
GRANDE VISTA ST
100 VeCo 93022 461-A1
GRAND ISLE DR
13600 MRPK 93021 496-F2
GRAND OAK LN
300 THO 91360 526-D6
GRANDOAKS DR
2600 WLKV 91361 557-A7
GRAND RIDGE CT
6200 VEN 93003 472-C6
GRANDSEN CT
6400 MRPK 93021 477-A6
GRANDVIEW AV
700 OJAI 93023 441-J6
GRANDVIEW CIR
100 CMRL 93010 524-D4
GRANDVIEW CT
5300 VEN 93003 492-B1
GRANDVIEW DR
- VeCo 93010 494-E6
2000 CMRL 93010 524-E4
GRANDVIEW TER
23200 Chat 91311 499-G6
GRANGER ST
1800 CMRL 93010 524-D2
GRANITE ST
100 SIMI 93065 497-F6
GRANITE HILLS ST
500 SIMI 93065 527-D1
GRANITE PEAK AV
- SIMI 93065 478-A6
GRANITO DR
1000 VeCo 93023 451-C1
GRANT AV
100 OXN 93030 522-H6
N GRANT AV
100 OXN 93030 522-H5
GRANT LN
500 SPLA 93060 464-C3
GRANT ST
7300 VEN 93003 492-E2
GRANT WY
600 OXN 93033 552-F4
GRANT LINE ST
300 SPLA 93060 464-B3
GRANT PARK FUEL BREAK
500 VeCo 93001 471-D7
500 VEN 93001 471-D7
500 VEN 93001 491-C1
N GRANVIA PL
2600 THO 91360 526-C3
GRANVILLE AV
3000 SIMI 93063 478-G7
GRAPE HILL RD
300 VeCo 93023 453-B1
GRAPEVINE CT
- SIMI 93063 499-B1
GRAPEVINE DR
2400 OXN 93036 522-F1
GRAPEVINE RD
- VeCo 93001 450-J6
- VeCo 93001 451-A6
- VeCo 93022 450-J6
- VeCo 93022 451-A6
GRASS VALLEY ST
500 SIMI 93065
GRAVES AV
300 OXN 93030
GRAVES CT
1000 CMRL 93010
GRAY CT
800 THO 91362
GRAYROCK ST
900 THO 91320
GRAYSON CT
2600 SIMI 93065
GRAYSTONE DR
7600 LA 91304
GRAYSTONE PL
2500 SIMI 93065
E GREAT SMOKEY CT
2800 THO 91362
W GREAT SMOKEY CT
2700 THO 91362
GREELY CT
2000 OXN 93033
GREEN LN
600 SIMI 93065
GREEN ST
100 SPLA 93060
8000 VEN 93004
GREENBANK RD
2400 VeCo 91361
GREEN BAY CT
10400 VEN 93004
N GREENBRIAR AV
700 SIMI 93065
GREENBRIAR CT
5900 AGRH 91301
GREENBROOK DR
2100 OXN 93033
2600 OXN 93033
GREENBUSH LN
4100 MRPK 93021
GREENCASTLE CT
2500 OXN 93035
GREENCASTLE LN
2200 OXN 93035
GREENCASTLE WY
2000 OXN 93035
GREENDALE AV
800 THO 91320
GREENDALE CIR
700 THO 91320
GREENFIELD ST
100 THO 91360
GREENGATE CT
4500 WLKV 91361
GREEN GLADE CT
- CMRL 93010
GREEN GRASS CT
29400 AGRH 91301
29400 AGRH 91301
GREEN HEATH PL
200 THO 91361
GREENHILL AV
6500 VEN 93003
GREEN LAWN AV
800 CMRL 93010
GREEN LEA PL
200 THO 91361
GREENLEAF AV
2600 SIMI 93063
2700 SIMI 93063
GREENMEADOW AV
- THO 91320
300 THO 91361
N GREENMEADOW AV
- THO 91320
GREEN MEADOW DR
5700 AGRH 91301
GREENMEADOW DR
- THO 91320
GREENMEADOW LN
600 THO 91320
GREEN MOOR PL
200 THO 91361
GREEN MOUNTAIN ST
500 SIMI 93065
GREEN OAK CT
2300 THO 91362
GREENOCK LN
1300 VEN 93001
GREENPARK CT
2100 THO 91362
GREEN PASTURE LN
- SIMI 93063
GREEN PINE PL
23600 SIMI 93063
GREENRIDGE DR
5200 VeCo 93021
5200 VeCo 93021
GREENRIDGE ST
100 THO 91360
GREEN RIVER ST
- OXN 93036
GREENSBORO RD
800 VEN 93004
GREEN SHADOWS LN
- SIMI 93065
GREENSWARD ST
2200 SIMI 93065
N GREENTREE DR
5400 VeCo 93066
5400 VeCo 93066
5700 VeCo 93066
W GREENTREE DR
5400 VeCo 93066
5400 VeCo 93066
GREENVALE DR
- CMRL 93010
GREEN VALLEY DR
800 THO 91320
GREENVIEW CIR
6300 VEN 93003
GREENVIEW RD
5800 CALB 91302
GREENVILLE DR
3200 SIMI 93063
GREEN VISTA CIR
7000 CanP 91307
GREENWAY AV
200 THO 91320
GREENWICH DR
500 THO 91360
GREENWOOD RD
900 SPLA 93060
GREENWOOD ST
3700 THO 91320
GREGORY ST
1200 OJAI 93023
GRENOBLE CT
30800 WLKV 91362

City ZIP Pg-Grid
LE CT
WLKV 91361 557-C6
M ST
LA 91304 529-J1
T
THO 91360 526-F4
ATHER CT
THO 91362 527-F6
CK RD
AGRH 91301 558-A4
AGRH 91301 557-J3
RD
OJAI 93023 442-A6
VeCo 93023 442-B3
VeCo - 442-B3
DR
FILM 93015 455-J3
VeCo 93015 455-J3
LN
MRPK 93021 477-A4
CT
SIMI 93065 478-A6
CANYON RD
MRPK 93021 476-A6
VeCo 93021 475-H7
VeCo 93021 476-A6
VeCo 93021 495-H1
CANYON RD
VeCo 93015 465-J4
VeCo 93015 466-A5
VeCo 93021 466-A5
VeCo 93021 476-B2
TONE CT
MRPK 93021 476-F6
CT
SIMI 93065 497-F6
M ST
THO 91362 527-A6
M WY
OXN 93033 552-G6
AV
CanP 91307 529-F7
ES WY
MRPK 93021 476-F6
DBRIER AV
SIMI 93065 497-A2
WY
VEN 93003 492-E4
LN
VEN 93001 491-G1
VEN 93003 491-G1
ST
VEN 93003 491-G2
WY
SIMI 93065 497-E2
ALE LN
MRPK 93021 496-F3
CIR
SIMI 93063 499-A2
PL
VeCo 93066 494-H4
EASE RD
VeCo 93001 470-G4
LN
Chat 91311 499-E7
LCANAL ST
PHME 93041 552-E5
DR
PHME 93041 552-E5
DR
PHME 93041 552-E5
AN ST
SIMI 93063 498-F3
CT
OXN 93033 552-F1
A ST
OXN 93033 552-G1
A ST
OXN 93033 552-F1
NE AV
SIMI 93063 498-E2
SON RD
VeCo 93040 457-F7
VeCo 93015 466-G1
VeCo 93015 467-B1
VeCo 93015 457-E7
SON ST
SPLA 93060 464-C4
ALL CT
WLKV 91361 557-E6
RD CIR
THO 91360 526-F5
CT
VeCo 93010 494-C5
VEN 93003 492-E4
R
SIMI 93065 478-C7
EE ST
OXN 93036 522-B2
R LN
SIMI 93063 499-B3
OKE RD
MRPK 93021 496-F3
LN
LA 91304 529-F2
REZ LN
OXN 93033 552-H6
RDISON
VeCo 93015 465-A1
VeCo 93060 465-A1
VeCo 93060 455-A7
T
SIMI 93063 498-H1
CT
THO 91362 556-H2
LN
VeCo 93010 494-F6

H

PHME 93035 552-B3
PHME 93043 552-B3
VeCo 93042 583-F4
OXN 93030 522-F5
OXN 93036 522-F1
OXN 93030 522-F6
OXN 93033 522-F7
OXN 93033 552-F1
Y
OXN 93030 522-J5
OXN 93030 523-A5
CT
CMRL 93010 524-D1

STREET Block City ZIP Pg-Grid
HACIENDA CIR
800 CMRL 93012 524-J2
HACIENDA DR
- OXN 93030 522-H4
500 CMRL 93012 524-J2
900 VeCo 93065 497-F4
N HACIENDA RD
- VeCo 91307 528-J3
N HACKAMORE LN
- VeCo 91307 529-A4
HACKAMORE ST
800 VeCo 93023 451-C3
HACKBERRY DR
- VeCo 93001 471-C3
HACKERS LN
6000 AGRH 91301 557-G3
E HACKNEY RD
6000 VeCo 93066 495-C1
HACKNEY ST
22000 LA 91304 529-J2
HADJIAN LN
22100 CanP 91303 529-J5
HADLEY DR
300 VEN 93003 492-B3
HAGEN CT
1000 SIMI 93065 497-H4
HAIFA RD
- SIMI 93063 479-B7
- SIMI 93063 499-B1
HAIGH RD
100 THO 91320 556-C1
HAILES RD
3100 VeCo 93033 553-D3
HAILEY CT
23600 SIMI 93065 498-B5
HAINES CANYON
23600 VeCo 93015 456-F6
HALCON ST
100 OXN 93030 523-A5
HALESIA LN
- OXN 93030 523-A4
HALEVY ST
600 VEN 93003 492-B7
HALEY RANCH RD
100 VeCo 93001 450-H7
100 VeCo 93001 451-A5
HALIFAX CT
1200 VEN 93004 492-H3
HALIFAX LN
- OXN 93035 522-C6
HALIFAX ST
8800 VEN 93004 492-H3
HALL RD
100 VeCo 93060 465-A2
300 VeCo 93060 455-A7
HALL CANYON RD
100 VEN 93001 491-G2
500 VeCo 93001 471-G6
500 VEN 93001 471-G6
HALLOCK DR
100 SPLA 93060 464-D5
S HALLOCK DR
200 SPLA 93060 464-E5
HALSBURY CT
23600 VeCo 91361 556-F6
HALSEY WY
4800 OXN 93033 552-H5
HALSTED ST
22100 Chat 91311 499-J6
HALYARD ST
600 PHME 93041 552-B1
HAMILTON AV
300 VEN 93003 491-J2
4200 OXN 93033 552-J5
HAMILTON ST
1500 SIMI 93065 497-J4
1700 SIMI 93065 498-A4
HAMLIN AV
3200 SIMI 93063 478-G6
HAMLIN ST
22200 CanP 91303 529-J6
22600 CanP 91307 529-F6
HAMMIL CT
2600 SIMI 93065 498-C4
HAMPSHIRE RD
- THO 91362 557-A3
100 THO 91361 557-A3
HAMPSTEAD CT
- VeCo 91361 586-F1
HAMPTON AV
2300 SIMI 93063 498-J1
HAMPTON CT
- THO 91362 527-C2
HAMPTON CANYON RD
3600 VeCo 93060 463-A4
3900 VeCo 93060 462-J3
HANCOCK PL
2100 OXN 93033 553-A2
HANDEL CT
4700 VEN 93003 492-A7
HANFORD ST
9300 VEN 93004 492-G2
HANLEY AV
1700 SIMI 93065 498-B3
HANNA AV
8500 LA 91304 529-J1
9300 Chat 91311 499-J4
HANNAH CIR
1700 SIMI 93063 499-A3
HANOVER AV
500 THO 91320 555-G3
HANOVER CT
3200 THO 91320 555-G3
HANOVER LN
1200 VEN 93001 491-F5
HANSEN CT
2400 SIMI 93065 498-B4
HANSON RD
4900 VEN 93003 492-B3
HAPPY LN
1500 VeCo 93023 442-D4
2900 VeCo 93063 478-C6
HAPPY ST
300 SPLA 93060 464-A7
HAPPY CAMP RD
7900 VeCo 93021 476-F1
9400 VeCo 93021 466-F5
HAPPY CAMP CANYON RD
- MRPK 93021 476-G4
- VeCo 93021 466-G7
- VeCo 93021 476-F1
23600 VeCo - 367-E9
23600 VeCo - 467-E4
23600 VeCo 93021 467-A6
HAPPY TALK RANCH RD
14800 VeCo 93060 463-F6
HAPPY VALLEY RD
23600 VeCo 93063 499-A7
23600 VeCo 93063 529-B1

STREET Block City ZIP Pg-Grid
HAPPY VALLEY SCHOOL RD
23600 VeCo 93023 442-F7
23600 VeCo 93023 452-F1
HARBOR BLVD
100 OXN 93035 521-G2
100 VeCo 93030 521-H4
100 VeCo 93035 521-H4
1200 OXN 93035 552-A1
1900 OXN 93036 521-G2
1900 VeCo 93036 521-G2
2500 VeCo 93001 521-G2
2500 VEN 93001 521-G2
3000 VeCo 93035 552-B4
E HARBOR BLVD
- VEN 93001 491-B2
2500 VeCo 93001 491-D3
3300 VEN 93001 521-G1
HARBOR RD
4600 PHME 93043 552-D6
HARBOR LIGHTS LN
400 PHME 93041 552-C2
HARBORVIEW CT
6100 VEN 93003 472-C5
HARBORVIEW LN
32100 WLKV 91361 557-C6
HARBOUR ISLAND LN
4200 OXN 93035 552-A1
HARDING AV
- VEN 93003 492-E2
100 OXN 93030 522-H6
N HARDING AV
- VEN 93003 492-E1
HARDISON ST
300 SPLA 93060 463-H6
HARDISON TER
23600 VeCo 93060 453-G2
HARDNEGO RD
1800 VeCo 93060 465-B6
2100 VeCo 93066 465-B6
HARGROVE CT
14000 MRPK 93021 496-G4
HARMON DR
6800 VEN 93003 492-E5
HARMON CANYON RD
23600 VeCo 93003 472-B2
23600 VeCo 93003 492-E1
23600 VeCo 93060 472-D1
23600 VEN 93003 492-E1
HARMONY CT
1400 THO 91362 527-A6
HAROLD AV
1200 SIMI 93065 498-B4
HARPER DR
1700 VEN 93004 492-H4
E HARPER ST
600 SIMI 93065 497-G5
HARPSTONE LN
23600 SIMI 93065 497-A1
HARRIER CT
- THO 91320 525-J5
- THO 91320 526-A5
HARRIET ST
300 VEN 93001 491-A1
HARRINGTON RD
2700 SIMI 93065 498-C4
HARRIS AV
1000 CMRL 93010 524-C1
HARRIS CT
900 THO 91362 526-J7
HARRIS ST
- PHME 93043 552-E4
HARRISON AV
100 OXN 93030 522-G6
E HARRISON AV
- VEN 93001 491-B1
N HARRISON AV
100 OXN 93030 522-G5
W HARRISON AV
- VEN 93001 491-B1
HARRY ST
- MRPK 93021 496-F1
HART ST
22000 CanP 91303 529-J5
HARTE AV
200 VEN 93003 492-B2
HARTE LN
15500 MRPK 93021 477-A4
HARTFIELD CT
4200 WLKV 91361 557-D6
HARTFORD ST
14600 MRPK 93021 476-H6
HARTGLEN AV
800 THO 91361 557-A4
HARTGLEN PL
5500 AGRH 91301 557-H5
HARTHORN LN
- FILM 93015 455-H5
HARTLAND CIR
2600 THO 91361 557-B5
HARTLAND ST
22200 CanP 91303 529-H6
22400 CanP 91307 529-E6
HARTLEY AV
1200 SIMI 93065 498-C4
HARTMAN DR
- VeCo 93012 525-C5
- VEN 93003 491-G3
HARTMAN WY
9300 WHil 91304 499-E7
HARTMAN TURNOFF
- VeCo 93001 471-C3
HARTNELL ST
2500 CMRL 93010 524-E2
HARTUNG CT
3600 THO 91320 555-F4
HARTWICK CIR
2000 THO 91360 526-D4
E HARVARD BLVD
100 SPLA 93060 464-C5
1300 VeCo 93060 464-C5
W HARVARD BLVD
100 SPLA 93060 464-A7
200 SPLA 93060 463-J7
HARVARD ST
300 OXN 93036 522-H2
5200 VEN 93003 492-B3
N HARVARD ST
6400 MRPK 93021 476-H6
HARVEST LN
1700 CMRL 93012 525-A1
1800 CMRL 93012 495-A7
HARVESTER ST
11800 MRPK 93021 496-C2
HARVEY DR
1000 SPLA 93060 464-B3
HARWICH PL
23700 CanP 91307 529-E5
HARWOOD LN
500 THO 91360 526-D7

STREET Block City ZIP Pg-Grid
HASLER RD
- VeCo 90265 625-H1
HASSETT AV
23600 VeCo 91361 556-G6
HASSTED DR
33100 LACo 90265 586-E7
HASTINGS AV
- VEN 93003 492-C2
HASTINGS CT
5000 VeCo 91377 557-H1
HASTINGS ST
6700 MRPK 93021 476-G5
HATFIELD CT
13700 MRPK 93021 496-F4
HATHAWAY AV
23600 THO 91362 527-B5
HATMOR DR
26100 CALB 91302 558-H4
HAUSER CIR
1500 THO 91362 526-J7
HAVASU ST
9000 VEN 93004 492-H4
HAVEN AV
1000 SIMI 93065 498-A4
HAVENCREST ST
12000 MRPK 93021 496-C4
HAVENRIDGE CT
4000 MRPK 93021 496-B4
HAVENSIDE AV
300 THO 91320 555-E2
HAVENWOOD DR
1800 THO 91362 526-J4
HAVILAND ST
800 SIMI 93065 498-C4
HAWK CIR
- VeCo 93041 583-H3
HAWK DR
- VeCo 93041 583-J3
HAWK ST
2100 SIMI 93065 498-A1
N HAWK ST
2400 SIMI 93065 498-B1
HAWK WY
6800 VEN 93003 492-E4
HAWKEYE PL
3600 THO 91320 555-F4
HAWKS BILL PL
500 SIMI 93065 527-D1
HAWKSWAY CT
1600 THO 91361 556-J5
HAWTHORN ST
1200 SPLA 93060 464-B3
HAWTHORNE DR
5000 VeCo 91377 557-G1
HAWTHORNE LN
900 VEN 93003 492-D3
HAYDEN ST
1700 CMRL 93010 524-D2
HAYES AV
- VEN 93003 492-E2
100 OXN 93030 522-G5
N HAYES AV
100 OXN 93030 522-G5
HAYMARKET ST
2400 THO 91362 527-B3
HAYNES ST
22200 CanP 91303 529-J6
22400 CanP 91307 529-E6
HAYNIE CT
- MRPK 93021 476-B5
HAYS DR
1700 THO 91320 556-A1
HAYWARD ST
7600 VEN 93004 492-E1
HAZEL CIR
6400 SIMI 93063 499-C2
HAZEL ST
9200 Chat 91311 499-G7
HAZEL WY
9200 Chat 91311 499-G7
HAZELCREST CIR
4800 THO 91362 557-F2
HAZELNUT CT
3400 SIMI 93065 498-D5
HAZEL RIDGE CT
200 SIMI 93065 498-A6
HAZELTINE DR
- OXN 93036 522-C3
HAZEL TOP CT
- MRPK 93021 476-F6
HAZELWOOD DR
400 OXN 93030 522-F4
HAZELWOOD WY
400 SIMI 93065 497-D5
HEALY TER
9300 Chat 91311 499-E6
9300 Chat 91311 499-F7
HEARON DR
6900 MRPK 93021 476-J5
7200 MRPK 93021 477-A5
HEARST DR
300 OXN 93030 523-A6
3500 SIMI 93063 498-E3
HEARTLAND AV
- SIMI 93065 478-A6
HEATHER CT
4800 MRPK 93021 496-C2
29600 AGRH 91301 557-J3
HEATHER ST
100 OXN 93036 522-F2
600 VeCo 93023 451-C3
2000 SIMI 93065 498-B2
5300 CMRL 93012 525-A3
HEATHER WY
- VEN 93004 473-C7
HEATHERBANK CT
- VeCo 91361 556-D7
HEATHERDALE CT
4200 MRPK 93021 496-B3
HEATHERFIELD CT
3200 THO 91320 555-G2
HEATHERGLEN CT
4500 MRPK 93021 496-B2
HEATHERGLOW ST
3200 THO 91360 526-F2
HEATHER OAKS LN
1400 THO 91361 556-H5
HEATHER RIDGE AV
100 THO 91320 556-A1
HEATHERTON DR
5200 VeCo 93066 475-A7
5200 VeCo 93066 495-A1
HEATHERVIEW DR
1100 VeCo 91377 528-A7
HEATHERWISP LN
23600 SIMI 93065 497-A1
HEATHERWOOD HOLLOW AV
3900 MRPK 93021 496-D4

STREET Block City ZIP Pg-Grid
HEATH MEADOW CT
100 SIMI 93065 497-D6
HEATH MEADOW PL
100 SIMI 93065 497-D7
HEAVENLY CT
3000 SIMI 93065 478-C7
24500 CanP 91307 529-D4
HEAVENLY RIDGE ST
- THO 91362 527-B2
HEAVENLY VALLEY RD
- VeCo 91320 556-C2
HEBERT DR
100 CMRL 93010 524-C4
HEBRIDES CIR
7000 CanP 91307 529-F5
HEDERA LN
- OXN 93030 523-A3
HEDGE LN
- CMRL 93012 524-G4
HEDGE ROW LN
600 SIMI 93065 527-D1
HEDGEWALL DR
6000 WLKV 91362 557-F3
HEDON CIR
1700 CMRL 93010 524-H1
HEDYLAND CT
600 MRPK 93021 476-F7
HEIDELBERG AV
300 VEN 93003 492-B1
HEIDEMARIE ST
22100 Chat 91311 499-J6
HELECHO CT
- THO 91362 556-J1
HELEN CT
2900 VeCo 91320 555-G1
HELEN ST
600 PHME 93041 552-F4
HELENA CT
700 OXN 93033 552-H5
3900 VEN 93003 491-J3
HELENA WY
400 OXN 93033 552-H5
HELENE ST
4000 SIMI 93063 498-F2
HELGA CT
400 THO 91320 555-H2
HELLBENDER LN
7000 VEN 93003 492-F3
HELM DR
1200 OXN 93035 522-D7
1400 OXN 93035 552-D1
HELM ST
2800 SIMI 93065 498-C4
HELMA CT
3500 CMRL 93010 524-G1
HELMOND DR
26900 CALB 91301 558-F6
HELMSDALE CIR
7100 CanP 91307 529-F5
HELMSDALE RD
7000 CanP 91307 529-E5
HELSAM AV
200 VeCo 93036 492-J7
700 VeCo 93036 493-A7
700 VeCo 93036 523-A1
HEMINGSFORD WY
- VeCo 91361 586-F1
HEMINGWAY LN
6600 VEN 93003 492-D3
HEMLOCK LN
100 VEN 93001 491-D2
1100 VeCo 91320 556-C2
E HEMLOCK ST
200 OXN 93033 552-H1
N HEMLOCK ST
- VEN 93001 491-D2
S HEMLOCK ST
- VEN 93001 491-D2
W HEMLOCK ST
400 OXN 93033 552-F1
1500 OXN 93035 552-B1
2300 PHME 93035 552-B1
23600 PHME 93041 552-D1
HEMLOCK RIDGE CT
- SIMI 93065 497-H5
HEMMINGWAY ST
22100 LA 91304 529-J3
HEMPSTEAD DR
5700 AGRH 91301 557-H4
HEMPSTEAD ST
4400 SIMI 93063 478-G5
HEMWAY CT
3900 SIMI 93063 498-F2
HENDERSON PL
10900 VEN 93004 493-A1
HENDERSON RD
7500 VEN 93004 492-J1
10800 VEN 93004 493-A1
HENDRICKSON RD
700 VeCo 93023 442-E5
HENDRIX AV
900 THO 91360 526-F4
HENLEY CT
4400 WLKV 91361 557-D6
HENNESSY AV
300 SIMI 93065 527-D1
HENRIETTA AV
200 THO 91320 555-F2
HENRY DR
200 VeCo 91320 555-F1
HENRY PL
- OXN 93033 552-H5
HENRY MAYO DR Rt#-126
31100 Cstc 91384 458-H5
31800 VeCo 93040 458-H5
HERBERT DR
- CMRL 93010 524-C3
HERCULES CT
2000 SIMI 93065 497-G2
HEREFORD CT
3200 SIMI 93063 478-G6
HEREFORD RD
- VeCo 91361 586-E1
2400 VeCo 91361 556-F7
HERITAGE DR
6100 AGRH 91301 557-J3
6100 AGRH 91301 558-A3
HERITAGE PL
1200 THO 91362 527-D7
5900 CMRL 93012 525-B1
HERITAGE TR
1500 CMRL 93012 525-B1
HERITAGE OAK CT
3800 SIMI 93063 498-F3
HERITAGE PASS PL
22300 Chat 91311 499-H2
HERMANO TR
200 OXN 93036 522-G2

STREET Block City ZIP Pg-Grid
HERMES ST
100 SIMI 93065 497-F2
HERMITAGE LN
- VeCo - 442-C3
- VeCo 93023 442-C3
HERMITAGE RD
2600 VeCo - 442-C3
2600 VeCo 93023 442-C3
HERMOSA RD
23600 OJAI 93023 451-F1
23600 VeCo 93023 451-F1
HERMOSA ST
7600 VEN 93004 492-E1
HERMOSA WY
200 OXN 93036 522-H2
HERON ST
6900 VEN 93003 492-E5
HERRINGBONE CT
- THO 91320 555-H2
HERRON CT
2000 CMRL 93010 494-D7
HERTZ ST
12000 MRPK 93021 496-C1
HEWITT PL
1700 SIMI 93065 497-J5
HEWITT ST
10400 VEN 93004 492-J2
HEYNEMAN LN
2100 SIMI 93065 498-A5
HEYWOOD ST
1600 SIMI 93065 497-J3
1700 SIMI 93065 498-B3
HI DR
4000 SIMI 93063 498-F3
HIAWATHA ST
22000 Chat 91311 499-J4
HIBBERT CT
3900 SIMI 93063 498-F2
HIBISCUS ST
1100 OXN 93036 522-E2
HIBISCUS WY
- VEN 93004 473-C7
HICKORY DR
5800 VeCo 91377 558-A1
HICKORY GROVE DR
200 THO 91320 556-C2
HICKORY KNOLL CT
2800 THO 91362 527-C4
HICKORY VIEW CIR
900 CMRL 93012 525-A2
HICKORY WOOD LN
2800 THO 91362 527-C4
HIDALGO CT
300 CMRL 93010 524-D3
HIDALGO ST
5200 CMRL 93012 525-A3
HIDDEN BROOK CT
1600 THO 91362 527-G6
HIDDEN CREEK AV
3100 THO 91360 526-C1
HIDDEN GLEN CT
5100 THO 91362 527-G6
HIDDEN HOLLOW CT
- SIMI 93063 498-H2
HIDDEN MEADOW CT
- THO 91320 526-A6
HIDDEN OAK CT
1800 THO 91320 526-A5
HIDDEN PARK CT
- SIMI 93063 498-J2
HIDDEN PINES CT
3800 MRPK 93021 496-F4
HIDDEN RANCH DR
- SIMI 93063 498-H2
- SIMI 93063 499-A3
HIDDEN SPRINGS AV
1400 VeCo 91377 527-H7
HIDDEN VALLEY CT
2100 OXN 93036 522-D2
HIDDEN VALLEY RD
1100 VeCo 91361 556-A6
1400 VeCo 91361 555-J6
HIDDEN VISTA CT
- SIMI 93063 498-J3
HIETTER AV
2000 SIMI 93063 498-E2
HIGH RD
- VeCo 93001 470-D4
HIGH ST
100 MRPK 93021 496-E1
100 VeCo 93022 451-B7
1100 SPLA 93060 464-B4
HIGHBRUSH LN
23600 SIMI 93065 497-A2
HIGHBURY CT
3500 SIMI 93063 478-G5
HIGHCLIFF CT
5800 THO 91362 527-G6
HIGH COUNTRY PL
- MRPK 93021 476-E6
HIGHCREST CT
400 THO 91320 555-G3
HIGHGATE PL
2700 SIMI 93065 478-B7
2700 SIMI 93065 498-B1
HIGHGATE RD
2100 THO 91361 557-A7
2100 WLKV 91361 557-A7
HIGHGROVE PL
- MRPK 93021 476-D5
HIGH KNOLL CIR
1900 THO 91362 527-D5
HIGH KNOLL CT
23600 SIMI 93065 527-F1
HIGHLAND AV
4200 OXN 93033 552-J5
HIGHLAND DR
100 VeCo 93035 552-B5
200 VeCo 93023 451-C3
E HIGHLAND DR
- VeCo 93010 494-E6
W HIGHLAND DR
600 VeCo 93010 494-C6
HIGHLAND RD
100 SIMI 93065 497-F5
HIGHLAND TER
- VeCo 93010 494-D6
HIGHLANDER RD
23700 CanP 91307 529-D5
HIGHLAND HILLS DR
200 VeCo 93010 494-E5
HIGH MEADOW ST
100 SIMI 93065 497-E7
HIGH PEAK PL
5600 AGRH 91301 557-J5
HIGH PLAINS LN
600 SIMI 93065 527-D1
HIGH POINT DR
500 VEN 93003 472-D7
500 VEN 93003 492-E1

STREET Block City ZIP Pg-Grid
HIGHPOINT PL
3300 SIMI 93065 498-D5
HIGHRIDGE CT
11200 VeCo 93012 496-B7
HIGHTOP ST
- MRPK 93021 476-F5
HIGH TREE RD
1300 SIMI 93063 499-C3
HIGHVIEW ST
300 THO 91320 555-G2
HIGHWAY Rt#-33
- VeCo 93023 366-J6
- VeCo 93252 366-G1
HIGHWINDS RD
12600 VeCo 93023 442-J7
12600 VeCo 93023 452-J1
HIGHWOOD CT
3500 SIMI 93063 498-D1
HIGUERA DR
1100 OXN 93030 522-J5
HILA LN
4900 OXN 93033 552-J5
HILARIA ST
23600 OXN 93030 522-J5
HILARY CT
2700 THO 91362 527-A3
HILBURN CT
13600 MRPK 93021 496-F3
HILDRETH CT
11000 VeCo 93012 526-A1
N HILGARD AV
1400 SIMI 93065 498-D3
HILL DR
10600 VeCo 93021 495-J3
10600 VeCo 93021 496-A3
HILL RD
2000 VEN 93003 492-D5
N HILL RD
100 VEN 93003 492-D2
100 VeCo 93003 492-D2
S HILL RD
- VeCo 93003 492-D2
- VEN 93003 492-D2
500 VEN 93009 492-D3
HILL ST
- VeCo 93022 451-B6
100 OXN 93033 552-F1
1400 OXN 93035 552-D1
HILLARY CT
1800 SIMI 93065 498-A2
HILLARY DR
7800 LA 91304 529-F2
HILLBROOK CT
4200 MRPK 93021 496-B2
HILL CANYON AV
3300 THO 91360 526-C1
HILL CANYON RD
1800 VeCo 93012 525-J3
23600 THO 91320 525-J3
23600 THO 91360 525-J3
HILL CANYON FIRE RD
23600 THO 91320 525-H4
HILLCREST DR
500 CMRL 93012 524-J2
1700 VEN 93001 491-E1
2400 THO 91362 557-A2
E HILLCREST DR
- THO 91360 556-F1
1000 THO 91362 556-H1
2000 THO 91362 557-A1
W HILLCREST DR
- THO 91360 556-E1
300 THO 91360 526-C7
600 THO 91320 526-A7
600 VeCo 91360 526-C7
1000 THO 91320 556-E1
2000 THO 91320 525-H7
HILLCREST LN
400 VEN 93001 491-F1
HILLCROFT DR
8200 LA 91304 529-D1
HILLDALE AV
2000 SIMI 93063 498-D2
HILLGATE WY
1900 SIMI 93065 497-E2
HILLHAVEN CT
6300 VEN 93003 472-C6
HILLHURST DR
- CanP 91307 529-D5
- LA 91304 529-D5
HILLIARD AV
1700 SIMI 93063 499-A3
HILLIARD LN
2600 THO 91320 525-H6
HILLMAN ST
2800 THO 91360 526-H3
HILLMONT AV
200 VEN 93003 491-G2
HILLPARK CT
4100 MRPK 93021 496-B2
HILL RANCH DR
200 THO 91362 556-H1
HILLRIDGE DR
1600 CMRL 93012 525-A1
2300 CMRL 93012 494-J7
2300 CMRL 93012 495-A7
HILLRISE DR
29100 AGRH 91301 558-A5
29400 AGRH 91301 557-J5
HILLROSE CT
300 THO 91320 555-E2
HILLROSE PL
2400 OXN 93036 522-F1
HILLSBOROUGH ST
400 THO 91361 556-F2
HILLSBURY RD
2200 THO 91361 557-A6
HILLSHIRE CT
3800 MRPK 93021 496-E4
HILLSIDE DR
1000 SPLA 93060 464-B3
12400 MRPK 93021 496-D3
HILLSVIEW CT
7300 LA 91304 529-E4
HILLTOP DR
3000 VEN 93003 491-G1
HILLTOP LN
1900 VeCo 93012 495-E7
HILLTOP RD
1100 VeCo 93063 499-B3
HILLTOP WY
- THO 91362 557-A2
HILL VALLEY CT
23600 SIMI 93065 497-F7
23600 SIMI 93065 527-F1
HILLVIEW AV
- VEN 93003 492-C2
HILLVIEW CIR
800 SIMI 93065 497-G4

STREET / Block City ZIP Pg-Grid

HILLVIEW LN
1100 SIMI 93065 497-H4
HILLWAY CIR
6100 VEN 93003 472-C6
HINCKLEY LN
- FILM 93015 455-J5
HINGHAM LN
1000 VEN 93001 491-E4
HIRAM AV
100 THO 91320 555-H1
HITCH BLVD
3800 VeCo 93021 496-A3
4000 VeCo 93021 495-J2
HITCHING POST LN
- VeCo 91307 529-A5
HOBART DR
1400 CMRL 93010 524-D1
HOBBIT CT
1200 SIMI 93065 498-C4
HOBBS CIR
- SPLA 93060 464-A5
HOBSON RD
5200 VeCo 93001 469-H2
5200 VeCo 93001 470-A3
5200 VeCo 93001 459-G7
23600 VeCo 93060 464-G4
23600 VeCo 93060 474-B1
HOBSON WY
500 OXN 93030 522-F7
HODENCAMP RD
- THO 91360 556-G1
500 THO 91360 526-G7
HOFER DR
3100 VEN 93003 492-D6
HOGAN ST
- MRPK 93021 476-B6
HOLBERTSON CT
700 SIMI 93065 527-C1
N HOLBROOK AV
700 SIMI 93065 498-A5
HOLIDAY AV
- VEN 93003 492-B4
HOLIDAY PINES LN
2100 VeCo 93012 496-A7
2100 VeCo 93012 526-A1
HOLLEY AV
1400 SIMI 93063 498-E3
HOLLINGS ST
- VEN 93003 492-B2
HOLLISTER ST
2500 SIMI 93065 498-C3
8100 VEN 93004 492-G2
HOLLOWAY CT
3100 THO 91320 555-G6
HOLLOWAY ST
3300 THO 91320 555-F3
HOLLOW BROOK AV
28900 AGRH 91301 558-B4
HOLLOW OAK CT
29000 AGRH 91301 558-A3
HOLLOWPARK CT
2200 THO 91362 527-A4
HOLLY AV
400 OXN 93036 522-E2
HOLLY CT
1500 THO 91360 526-H3
HOLLY DR
100 CMRL 93010 524-E4
HOLLY RD
900 SPLA 93060 464-B3
HOLLY ST
600 VeCo 93023 451-C3
HOLLYBURNE LN
500 THO 91360 526-D7
HOLLYCREST AV
2800 THO 91362 527-C3
HOLLYGLEN CT
4900 MRPK 93021 496-B2
HOLLY GROVE ST
3300 THO 91362 557-B3
HOLLYHOCK AV
- VEN 93004 493-A1
HOLLYHOCK CT
900 THO 91362 557-C1
HOLLY KNOLL DR
900 VeCo 93022 461-A1
HOLLY OAK CT
- SIMI 93063 498-J3
HOLLY RIDGE DR
5500 CMRL 93012 525-A1
HOLLYTREE DR
5600 VeCo 91377 557-J1
5600 VeCo 91377 558-A1
HOLLYVIEW PL
2400 THO 91362 527-B3
HOLLYWOOD AV
100 VeCo 93035 552-C6
HOLLYWOOD BLVD
200 VeCo 93035 552-B4
400 PHME 93035 552-B4
400 PHME 93043 552-B4
HOLMES AV
500 VEN 93003 492-D2
HOLSER WK
1800 OXN 93036 523-A3
HOLSER CANYON RD
23600 VeCo 93040 367-E7
N HOLSTER LN
- VeCo 91307 529-B4
HOLT ST
- VeCo 93001 471-C2
HOMER AV
200 VEN 93003 491-G2
HOMER ST
100 OXN 93033 552-G3
HOMESTAKE PL
1200 THO 91320 555-F5
HOMEWOOD AV
2200 SIMI 93063 499-C1
HOMEWOOD CT
6400 SIMI 93063 499-C1
HOMEZELL DR
23900 LA 91304 529-E1
HOMEZELL TR
24000 LA 91304 529-C1
HOMOJA CIR
- PHME 93041 552-E4
HOMOJA DR
1100 PHME 93041 552-D4
HONDO BARRANCA
23600 VeCo 93066 474-E7
HONDO RANCH RD
1400 VeCo 93066 494-C1
HONEY DR
3100 SIMI 93063 478-E6
E HONEYBEE ST
13100 MRPK 93021 496-E3
HONEYBROOK CT
11900 MRPK 93021 496-C3

HONEY CREEK CT
- THO 91320 526-B6
HONEYGLEN CT
4400 MRPK 93021 496-D2
HONEY HILL DR
2100 VeCo 93012 496-A7
2100 VeCo 93012 526-A1
HONEYMAN ST
5400 SIMI 93063 498-J2
5400 SIMI 93063 499-A2
HONEY PINE CT
23600 SIMI 93063 498-D4
HONEYSUCKLE AV
- VEN 93004 493-A2
HONEYSUCKLE CT
3500 THO 91360 526-H2
HONEYSUCKLE DR
2600 OXN 93036 492-F7
2600 OXN 93036 522-F1
HONEYWOOD CT
1000 SPLA 93060 464-A1
HOOD DR
2000 THO 91362 526-J6
2000 THO 91362 527-A6
HOOD WY
- OXN 93033 552-G6
HOOPER AV
- SIMI 93065 527-E1
HOOP PINE PL
23600 SIMI 93065 498-D4
HOOVER AV
- VEN 93003 492-E2
HOPE RD
100 THO 91320 556-B2
HOPE ST
4300 VEN 93003 491-J2
4300 VEN 93003 492-A2
6100 SIMI 93063 499-B3
HOPEWELL CT
2000 THO 91360 526-C4
HOPI CT
- MRPK 93021 496-H3
HOPI LN
2300 VEN 93001 471-C6
HOPPER CANYON RD
500 VeCo 93015 457-A5
1600 VeCo - 457-A3
HORIZON CIR
100 CMRL 93010 524-A4
HORIZON DR
1000 VEN 93003 472-D6
HORIZON LN
600 THO 91320 526-B7
HORIZON PL
22200 Chat 91311 499-J2
HORIZON RIDGE CT
- SIMI 93063 478-G5
HORN CT
2800 SIMI 93065 498-C3
HORNBLEND CT
400 SIMI 93065 527-C1
HORN CANYON RD
- VeCo - 442-J2
5100 VeCo 93023 442-G4
E HORSESHOE RD
- VeCo 91307 529-A4
HORSHOE CIR
- CALB 91302 558-H4
HOSPITAL RD
23600 VEN 93003 491-G2
HOT SPRINGS PL
26800 CALB 91301 558-G7
HOUCK ST
500 CMRL 93010 523-J5
HOUSTON DR
- THO 91360 556-G1
400 THO 91360 526-G7
HOUSTON PL
1500 OXN 93033 552-J3
HOUSTON RD
9500 VeCo 90265 585-D7
9500 VeCo 90265 625-D1
HOWARD AV
- VeCo 93022 451-D4
HOWARD RD
- CMRL 93012 524-J6
600 VeCo 93012 524-J7
1400 VeCo 93012 525-A7
1400 VeCo 93012 555-A1
HOWARD ST
- VEN 93003 491-F3
1000 FILM 93015 455-J6
HOWE RD
2700 VeCo 93065 478-C7
3400 VeCo 93015 457-E6
3700 VeCo 93040 457-E6
HOWE ST
23600 VEN 93003 492-D6
HOWELL RD
300 OXN 93033 552-H5
HOWIE CT
400 SPLA 93060 463-J5
400 SPLA 93060 464-A5
HOYT CT
1300 SIMI 93065 498-C3
HUBBARD ST
1800 SIMI 93065 497-J3
HUBBELL CT
- VEN 93003 492-B3
HUCKLEBERRY OAK ST
- SIMI 93063 498-J3
HUDSON CT
1100 SIMI 93065 497-H4
HUDSON LN
400 PHME 93041 552-D2
HUDSPETH AV
500 SIMI 93065 497-J5
HUENEME AV
100 PHME 93035 552-B5
100 VeCo 93035 552-B5
HUENEME RD
- PHME 93041 552-D6
- PHME 93043 552-D6
500 VeCo 93012 553-H6
500 VeCo 93012 554-A5
E HUENEME RD
100 OXN 93033 552-H6
1100 VeCo 93033 552-H6
1100 VeCo 93033 553-B6
W HUENEME RD
- OXN 93033 552-G6
HUENEME ST
1000 VeCo 93015 465-F3
HUERTA ST
- OXN 93030 522-G4
3500 CMRL 93010 494-G7
HUGHES DR
100 OXN 93033 552-G3
1000 CMRL 93010 524-C3

HUGO CT
10100 VEN 93004 493-A2
HULA DR
23600 OXN 93033 553-A2
HULL CT
2100 SIMI 93063 499-B2
HULL PL
1000 OXN 93030 522-E6
HUMBOLDT ST
100 SIMI 93065 497-F6
8300 VEN 93004 492-F1
HUME DR
400 FILM 93015 455-J6
HUMMINGBIRD ST
3200 SIMI 93063 478-J6
6300 VEN 93003 492-D5
HUNT CIR
100 THO 91360 526-F4
600 CMRL 93012 524-J2
HUNT CLUB LN
4200 WLKV 91361 557-E6
9500 Chat 91311 499-H6
HUNTER CT
- VEN 93003 492-B2
HUNTER DR
500 FILM 93015 456-A4
HUNTER ST
5400 VEN 93003 492-B2
HUNTER CREST CT
3800 MRPK 93021 496-D4
HUNTERS GROVE CT
3800 MRPK 93021 496-E4
HUNTERS POINT DR
200 THO 91361 556-F2
HUNTER VALLEY LN
4900 THO 91362 557-E1
HUNTINGTON AV
200 VEN 93004 492-F2
HUNTLEY ST
5200 SIMI 93063 498-J2
HUNTSDALE CT
23600 THO 91320 555-F3
HUNTSWOOD WY
900 OXN 93030 522-E4
HUPA ST
300 VEN 93001 471-C5
HURFORD CT
5600 AGRH 91301 557-H4
N HURLES AV
1900 SIMI 93063 498-E2
HURON CT
- MRPK 93021 496-G3
HURON DR
1800 VEN 93004 492-G4
HURRICANE CV
2600 PHME 93041 552-C3
HURST AV
- VEN 93001 491-E3
HUSTON RD
9100 Chat 91311 499-E7
9300 Chat 91311 499-E7
HUYLER LN
900 SIMI 93065 497-E6
HYACINTH CT
2900 THO 91360 526-D3
HYACINTH DR
2000 OXN 93036 522-F2
HYACINTH ST
800 CMRL 93010 494-C7
800 VeCo 93010 494-C7
HYANNIS DR
7200 CanP 91307 529-F4
HYLAND AV
2100 VEN 93001 491-F1
HYSSOP CT
2200 THO 91362 497-A7

I

I AV
- VeCo 93042 583-F6
I ST
100 OXN 93030 522-F5
1100 OXN 93033 522-F6
23600 VeCo 93063 528-F1
S I ST
1200 OXN 93033 522-F7
1200 OXN 93033 552-F1
IAN LN
2700 SIMI 93063 478-D7
IBEX SQ
1100 VEN 93003 492-E3
IBIZA LN
- OXN 93035 522-C6
IBOLD RD
600 LACo 90265 586-G6
IBSEN PL
100 OXN 93033 552-G4
ICELAND ST
2900 THO 91320 555-H2
IDA PL
23200 Chat 91311 499-F7
IDA ST
1700 CMRL 93010 524-D3
IDA WY
23600 WHil 91304 499-E6
IDAHO DR
1900 VEN 93003 492-C5
IDE CT
1700 THO 91362 526-J7
IDLE DR
28900 AGRH 91301 558-B4
IDYLLWILD ST
8300 VEN 93004 492-G2
IGUANA CIR
1300 VEN 93003 492-F4
ILENA ST
900 OXN 93030 522-F7
ILEX DR
- THO 91320 555-J1
2000 OXN 93036 522-G3
ILLINOIS CT
- MRPK 93021 496-H3
IMATION DR
2600 CMRL 93012 524-F4
IMBACH PL
7100 MRPK 93021 477-A5
IMBLER CT
6300 AGRH 91301 557-J3
IMPALA DR
7100 VEN 93003 492-E5
IMPATIENS DR
- OXN 93030 523-A3
IMPERIAL AV
- VEN 93004 492-F1
300 VEN 93004 472-E7
400 VeCo 93004 472-E7
IMPERIAL CIR
3000 THO 91320 555-H2
IMPERIAL ST
200 OXN 93030 523-A5

INCA CT
2500 VEN 93001 471-C5
INCA DR
- OXN 93030 522-H4
INDEPENDENCE CT
3200 THO 91360 526-F2
INDIAN DR
22000 Chat 91311 499-J1
INDIANA DR
2000 OXN 93036 522-H3
INDIANBROOM CT
6600 VeCo 91377 528-A7
INDIAN CREEK PL
3200 SIMI 93063 478-J6
INDIAN CREST CIR
1700 THO 91362 527-G6
INDIAN HILL LN
24400 CanP 91307 529-D4
INDIAN HILLS DR
5100 SIMI 93063 478-J7
5400 SIMI 93063 479-A7
INDIAN HILLS RD
- Chat 91311 479-H7
INDIAN MESA DR
3100 THO 91360 526-C2
INDIAN OAK LN
- VeCo 91377 527-J7
- VeCo 91377 528-A7
- VeCo 91377 557-J1
- VeCo 91377 558-A1
INDIAN POINTE DR
5700 SIMI 93063 479-A7
INDIAN PONY CIR
4200 THO 91362 527-D6
INDIAN RIDGE CIR
3200 THO 91362 527-D3
INDIAN RIDGE CT
29000 AGRH 91301 558-A3
INDIAN SKY LN
2100 THO 91360 555-J3
INDIAN TERRACE DR
5700 SIMI 93063 479-A7
INDIAN TRAIL CT
5000 THO 91362 527-F7
INDIAN WELLS CT
2700 OXN 93036 522-C2
INDIAN WELLS LN
600 THO 91320 556-D1
INDIGO PL
800 OXN 93036 522-F2
INDIO DR
- OXN 93030 522-H4
INDUS PL
- OXN 93036 492-H7
INDUSTRIAL AV
600 PHME 93041 552-F7
900 OXN 93030 522-H7
E INDUSTRIAL ST
4400 SIMI 93063 498-G2
INEZ DR
- OXN 93030 523-A4
INEZ ST
1000 CMRL 93012 525-A6
6000 VeCo 93003 492-D6
6000 VEN 93003 492-D6
INFINIDAD ST
- OXN 93030 522-G4
INGELOW CT
300 THO 91360 526-F4
INGLEWOOD ST
12800 MRPK 93021 496-E3
INGOMAR ST
22100 LA 91304 529-D3
INGRAM PL
4900 THO 91362 557-G1
INLET DR
900 OXN 93030 522-F7
INMAN CIR
1000 SIMI 93065 497-J4
INNESS CIR
6900 VEN 93003 492-E3
INNWOOD RD
100 SIMI 93065 497-C6
INSPIRATION PT
- VeCo 93012 554-F2
INSPIRATION WY
100 VEN 93001 491-D1
INSTONE CT
2900 THO 91361 557-C5
INVAR CT
2400 SIMI 93065 498-B4
INVERNESS CT
2100 OXN 93036 522-E2
INVERNESS ST
- THO 91361 556-F2
INYO CIR
2800 SIMI 93063 478-J7
INYO ST
10600 VEN 93004 472-H6
IOLITE ST
- SIMI 93065 478-A6
IOWA PL
200 OXN 93036 492-H7
IRENA AV
5400 CMRL 93012 525-A6
IRENE CT
1500 SIMI 93065 497-J3
IRIS ST
1200 VeCo 93063 499-B4
E IRIS ST
100 OXN 93033 552-G2
W IRIS ST
100 OXN 93033 552-E1
IRIS WY
200 VEN 93004 473-A7
IRONBARK CT
1700 OXN 93030 522-F3
IRONBARK DR
2000 OXN 93036 522-F3
IRONGATE PL
2600 THO 91362 527-A2
IRON RIDGE LN
300 SIMI 93065 497-E6
IRONSIDE CV
2600 PHME 93041 552-C3
IRONSTONE CT
2500 OXN 93036 522-F1
IRONWOOD CIR
200 THO 91360 526-F2
IRONWOOD DR
5700 AGRH 91301 557-J4
IROQUOIS CT
1500 CMRL 93010 524-F1
5500 SIMI 93063 479-A7
IROQUOIS LN
2300 VEN 93001 471-D6
IRVINE RD
700 SIMI 93065 497-F5
IRVING DR
300 OXN 93030 523-A6

IRVING DR
500 THO 91360 556-G1
IRVING BERLIN DR
- VEN 93003 492-A4
IRWIN WY
- OXN 93033 552-G6
ISABEL AV
5600 CMRL 93012 525-B6
ISABELLA CT
1700 VEN 93004 492-H4
5300 AGRH 91301 557-H5
ISABELLA ST
1900 OXN 93036 522-J3
ISCHIA DR
4000 OXN 93035 552-B2
ISELA ST
- OXN 93030 523-A5
ISH DR
4100 SIMI 93063 498-F3
ISLA CT
1300 CMRL 93010 524-G1
ISLAND AV
- VeCo 93042 583-E4
ISLAND FOREST PL
4900 THO 91362 527-F7
ISLAND OAK ST
- SIMI 93063 498-J3
- SIMI 93063 499-A3
ISLAND VIEW AV
100 PHME 93043 552-B5
100 VeCo 93035 552-B5
900 VeCo 93043 552-B5
1700 PHME 93035 552-B5
ISLAND VIEW CIR
400 PHME 93041 552-E6
ISLAND VIEW DR
3000 VEN 93003 491-G1
3200 VeCo 93003 491-G1
ISLAND VIEW ST
600 FILM 93015 456-B5
1300 OXN 93035 552-A1
1600 OXN 93035 551-J1
ISLE WY
2900 OXN 93035 552-C1
N ISLE ROYALE DR
4500 MRPK 93021 496-E2
ISLETON PL
1000 OXN 93030 522-E6
ITAMO ST
1100 CMRL 93012 525-C6
ITASCA ST
22100 Chat 91311 499-H6
IVAN DR
4800 OXN 93033 552-H5
IVANHOE AV
1500 OXN 93030 522-D4
IVAR PL
- OXN 93030 522-H4
IVERSON LN
11100 Chat 91311 499-J2
IVERSON RD
11300 Chat 91311 499-H2
11400 Chat 91311 499-H2
IVES AV
1100 OXN 93033 552-J1
1800 OXN 93033 553-A2
IVES CT
2000 OXN 93033 553-A1
IVES PL
1900 OXN 93033 553-A2
IVORY AV
2800 SIMI 93063 478-D7
IVORY WY
2300 OXN 93036 522-F1
IVY ST
4000 VEN 93003 491-J3
IVYWOOD DR
400 OXN 93030 522-F3
IVYWOOD LN
400 SIMI 93065 497-D5

J

J CT
500 OXN 93030 522-F6
J ST
- VeCo 93042 583-E5
100 OXN 93030 522-F5
1100 OXN 93033 522-F7
1100 OXN 93033 552-F1
4300 PHME 93033 552-F5
23600 VeCo 93063 528-F1
JACARANDA AV
- THO 91320 556-C1
JACARANDA DR
2400 OXN 93036 522-F1
JACINTO CIR
3000 SIMI 93063 478-G7
JACINTO DR
- OXN 93030 523-A4
JACINTO WY
10000 VeCo 93004 493-B2
JACKIE AV
6200 WdHl 91367 529-F7
JACKLIGHT CV
2600 PHME 93041 552-C3
JACKPINE LN
11400 VeCo 93012 496-C7
JACKSON ST
2200 OXN 93033 552-F2
3400 PHME 93033 552-F3
3400 PHME 93041 552-F3
7300 VEN 93003 492-E1
7400 VEN 93004 492-E1
JACKTAR AV
2900 OXN 93035 552-C1
JACOBS CT
5300 VeCo 91377 527-H6
JACOBSON PL
- MRPK 93021 476-B5
JADE CT
3300 SIMI 93063 478-D6
JADE DR
900 VEN 93004 492-G3
JADESTONE AV
2800 SIMI 93063 478-D7
JAFFA RD
- SIMI 93063 479-C7
JAKE CT
- THO 91320 555-E3
JAKE LN
- LA 91304 529-J2
JALISCO CT
1600 CMRL 93010 524-D3
JAMAICA LN
1100 OXN 93030 522-E6
JAMES AV
100 OXN 93033 552-G3
2100 VeCo 93003 492-D5

JAMES CT
2000 THO 91362 556-H2
JAMES DR
- VEN 93001 471-C6
JAMES WY
5900 SIMI 93063 499-B3
JAMES ALAN CIR
22100 Chat 91311 499-J4
JAMESTOWN CT
2300 OXN 93035 552-A2
JAMESTOWN LN
2200 OXN 93035 552-A2
JAMESTOWN ST
9800 VEN 93004 492-H2
JAMESTOWN WY
2000 OXN 93035 552-A1
JAMES WEAK AV
12400 MRPK 93021 496-D2
JAMISON CT
100 SIMI 93065 497-D7
JANE CT
700 OXN 93033 552-F6
2900 THO 91320 555-H2
JANE DR
700 OXN 93033 552-F6
700 PHME 93033 552-F6
700 PHME 93041 552-F6
JANET LN
1500 SIMI 93063 499-B3
JANET WY
5900 SIMI 93063 499-B3
JANETWOOD DR
500 OXN 93030 522-F3
JANIS LN
1500 SIMI 93063 499-B3
JANIS WY
6000 SIMI 93063 499-B3
JANLOR DR
30600 AGRH 91301 557-G4
30800 WLKV 91362 557-F4
JANSS CIR
1800 THO 91360 526-E5
E JANSS RD
- THO 91360 526-G5
1000 THO 91362 526-G5
1800 THO 91362 527-A6
W JANSS RD
- THO 91360 526-E4
JANSS FIRE RD
500 THO 91361 556-F3
700 VeCo 91361 556-F6
JAPONICA AV
100 CMRL 93012 524-H4
JAPONICA CT
4300 CMRL 93012 524-H4
JAPONICA PL
4300 CMRL 93012 524-H4
JARDIN DR
2200 OXN 93036 522-H2
JARED CT
6100 WdHl 91367 529-D7
JASMINE ST
2000 OXN 93036 522-F3
JASMINE GLEN AV
2700 SIMI 93065 478-B7
JASON AV
7400 CanP 91307 529-F4
7700 LA 91304 529-F2
JASON CT
2700 THO 91362 527-A3
JASON LN
23200 CanP 91307 529-F4
JASON PL
1000 OXN 93033 552-J3
JASPER AV
500 VEN 93004 492-H2
JAVA PL
- OXN 93036 492-H6
JAVELIN CT
1600 THO 91320 526-A6
JAY AV
800 CMRL 93010 524-B2
2400 SIMI 93065 498-B1
JAYCROFT CT
23600 VeCo 91361 556-F6
JAZMIN AV
600 VEN 93004 492-J1
JEAN LN
2000 WLKV 91361 557-A7
JEANETTE AV
800 THO 91362 526-J7
JEANETTE DR
1500 OXN 93030 522-E3
JEANINE CT
- THO 91320 556-B1
JEANNE AV
10300 VeCo 93022 451-C7
JEANNE CT
400 VeCo 91320 555-G1
JEAUNINE DR
100 THO 91360 526-E6
JEFFERSON AV
100 VEN 93003 492-E1
JEFFERSON SQ
5100 OXN 93033 552-H5
JEFFERSON WY
- SIMI 93065 497-J1
JEFFREY RD
2300 CMRL 93012 495-B7
JEFFREY MARK CT
22400 Chat 91311 499-H4
JEFFREYS PL
1900 OXN 93033 553-A4
JELLEY DR
- PHME 93041 552-D4
JENNIFER CT
6200 SIMI 93063 499-B2
JENNIFER LN
- LA 91304 529-J2
JENNIFER PL
2000 VeCo 93012 496-A7
2000 VeCo 93012 526-A1
JENNY DR
300 VeCo 91320 555-F1
500 VeCo 91320 525-F7
JENSEN CT
100 THO 91360 556-G1
JENSEN DR
23900 LA 91304 529-E2
JEPSON ST
1500 VeCo 93015 455-G4
JERANIOS CT
1100 THO 91362 556-J1
JEREMIAH DR
400 SIMI 93065 497-D2
JEROME AV
- THO 91320 556-A2
JERRY DR
400 PHME 93041 552-F5

JERSEY PL
1100 THO 91362
JERUSALEM RD
- SIMI 93063
JESSICA ST
3000 THO 91320
JETTY ST
1800 OXN 93035
2000 PHME 93035
2000 PHME 93041
JEWEL CT
- CMRL 93010
JILL CT
2000 SIMI 93063
JILL PL
2700 PHME 93041
JIM BOWIE RD
3900 Ago 91301
3900 AGRH 91301
JIMILYN ST
6400 SIMI 93063
JIMS CANYON RD
23600 VeCo 93040
JOAN DR
800 PHME 93041
JOAN LN
8300 LA 91304
JOAN WY
4700 VeCo 93036
N JOANNE AV
- VEN 93003
S JOANNE AV
100 VEN 93003
JOANNE CT
1500 OXN 93030
JOANNE WY
1600 OXN 93030
JODY LN
- VeCo 93010
100 VEN 93001
JOELTON DR
4000 AGRH 91301
JOHN WY
6000 SIMI 93063
JOHN COX DR
400 VeCo 93015
JOHNELL RD
9200 Chat 91311
JOHNSON DR
500 VEN 93003
3000 VeCo 93003
JOHNSON MTWY
- Chat 91311
23600 VeCo 93063
JOHNSON PL
9300 Chat 91311
JOHNSON RD
100 OXN 93033
JOIE CT
4700 SIMI 93063
JOLIET PL
700 OXN 93030
JONATHAN ST
23100 LA 91304
JON DODSON DR
5300 AGRH 91301
JONES ST
300 VEN 93003
JONES WY
2100 OXN 93033
23600 SIMI 93065
JONESBORO AV
2200 SIMI 93063
JONNA CIR
- CMRL 93010
JONQUIL FIELD RD
3300 WLKV 91361
JONQUILL AV
- VEN 93004
JOPLIN WY
10100 VEN 93004
JORDAN AV
- VEN 93001
JOSE AV
1600 CMRL 93010
1700 CMRL 93010
JOSE DR
800 VeCo 93023
JOSHUA CT
2500 OXN 93036
JOSHUA PL
1500 CMRL 93012
JOSHUA ST
6400 VeCo 91377
JOSHUA TR
5900 CMRL 93012
JOSHUA TREE CT
23600 SIMI 93063
JOURDAN ST
2800 VeCo 93036
2800 VeCo 93036
JOYA ST
- OXN 93030
JOYCE DR
500 PHME 93041
JOYCE PL
2100 OXN 93033
JUANITA AV
100 OXN 93030
N JUANITA AV
100 OXN 93030
JUAREZ AV
4800 MRPK 93021
JUBILEE LN
500 SIMI 93065
JUDSON AV
200 VEN 93003
JUDY CIR
300 THO 91360
JUDY LN
1300 VeCo 93023
JUEGO ST
- OXN 93030
JULIA CT
1400 CMRL 93010
JULIAN ST
- VEN 93001
100 OXN 93030
JULIANA ST
- SIMI 93063
JULIE CIR
1700 SIMI 93065
JULIE LN
6600 LACo 91307
JULLIARD AV
6600 MRPK 93021
JUNE CIR
1500 VEN 93004
JUNE CT
- THO 91360

ty ZIP Pg-Grid
SPLA 93060 464-B3
IR
SIMI 93063 478-F7
OXN 93036 492-H7
Y PL
OXN 93036 522-E2
D CT
OXN 93030 522-F3
D WY
OXN 93030 522-E3
CT
VEN 93003 492-B1
ST
VEN 93003 492-B2
T
SIMI 93063 499-B3
THO 91320 555-G3
N
VeCo 93023 441-E6
T
OXN 93033 552-H2
R ST
OXN 93033 552-E2
ST
VEN 93001 491-B2
VeCo 93063 499-B4
OXN 93036 522-H3
T
OXN 93030 523-D4
T DR
OXN 93030 522-F7
T
LA 91304 529-F3
LN
OXN 93030 523-A4
AV
SIMI 93065 498-B2
MRPK 93021 496-C2
LA 91304 529-G4
Y
OXN 93033 552-H4

K

OXN 93030 522-F6
OXN 93033 522-F7
OXN 93033 552-F1
OXN 93030 522-F5
WY
SIMI 93063 479-B7
ST
SIMI 93063 498-H1
SIMI 93063 478-G6
VEN 93003 472-B7
PHME 93043 552-D3
PL
THO 91320 526-C7
CT
OXN 93030 523-A4
IA DR
VEN 93001 491-D1
AMA ST
VEN 93001 491-D2
AMA ST
VEN 93001 491-D2
ST
OXN 93033 552-H2
A ST
OXN 93033 552-F2
RD
VeCo 93060 465-B4
VEN 93003 492-B1
CT
Chat 91311 499-J1
D
VeCo 91377 558-A1
VeCo 91377 557-H1
VeCo 91377 527-E6
THO 91362 527-C6
VeCo 91362 527-E6
AGRH 91301 558-A5
D Rt#-N9
Ago 91301 558-A7
AGRH 91301 558-A7
SIMI 93065 498-B3
DR
OXN 93036 522-E2
V
VeCo 93022 451-C6
THO 91320 556-A1
CT
CMRL 93010 524-G2
T
SIMI 93063 479-A7
ST
SIMI 93065 498-A3
V
VEN 93001 471-D5
NE AV
VeCo 93003 492-D5
VEN 93003 492-D5
RINE AV
VeCo 93022 451-C6
RINE DR
VEN 93003 491-G2
RINE DR
VEN 93003 491-G3
NE LN
SIMI 93063 499-B3
NE RD
VeCo 93063 499-B4
SIMI 93063 499-B3
NE ST
SIMI 93063 498-J3
SIMI 93063 499-A3
NE WY
SIMI 93063 499-B3
N DR
VeCo 91320 556-B3
THO 91320 556-B3
WY
OXN 93030 522-H4
VeCo 93063 499-B4
T
SIMI 93063 478-J6
SIMI 93063 499-C3

STREET
Block City ZIP Pg-Grid
KAYAK CV
2600 PHME 93041 552-C3
KAZUKO CT
200 MRPK 93021 496-D1
KEARNEY AV
1400 SIMI 93065 497-J4
1700 SIMI 93065 498-A4
KEARNY ST
6200 VEN 93003 492-C1
KEATS AV
2400 THO 91360 526-E3
KEATS CIR
100 VEN 93003 492-E3
KEATS PL
1800 OXN 93033 552-J4
1800 OXN 93033 553-A4
KEEL AV
3400 OXN 93035 552-B1
KEEL WY
2900 OXN 93035 552-C1
KEHALA AV
- VEN 93001 471-B5
KEISHA DR
13900 MRPK 93021 496-G4
KEITH RD
2400 VeCo 93015 455-E7
KELLEY AV
400 CMRL 93010 524-F3
KELLOGG ST
- VEN 93001 471-B7
100 FILM 93015 456-B6
KELLWOOD CT
900 VeCo 91377 557-H1
E KELLY RD
- THO 91320 556-A1
W KELLY RD
- THO 91320 555-H2
- VeCo 91320 555-H2
KELLY KNOLL LN
2700 THO 91320 555-H2
2700 VeCo 91320 555-H2
KELMSCOTT CT
2200 THO 91361 557-A6
KELP LN
2800 OXN 93035 522-C7
KELP ST
1100 OXN 93035 522-C7
1300 OXN 93035 552-C1
KELSEY ST
2200 SIMI 93063 498-G2
KELSFORD CT
1100 THO 91361 557-A5
KELTIC LODGE DR
- OXN 93036 522-C3
KELTON CT
23600 SIMI 93065 497-F7
KEMPER LAKES CT
1900 OXN 93036 522-E2
KENDALE LN
600 THO 91360 526-D6
KENDALL AV
1300 CMRL 93010 524-F1
1700 CMRL 93010 494-F7
KENEWA ST
1600 VeCo 93022 451-E5
KENMORE CIR
700 THO 91320 555-F4
KENNEBEC ST
8800 VEN 93004 492-H4
KENNEDY AV
23600 VEN 93003 492-E2
KENNEDY LN
1500 VeCo 93023 442-D4
KENNEDY PL
1800 OXN 93033 552-J2
1800 OXN 93033 553-A2
KENNERICK LN
900 SIMI 93065 497-D6
KENNETH ST
- CMRL 93010 524-D3
KENNY ST
900 VeCo 93036 522-J1
KENROSE CIR
26100 CALB 91302 558-H4
KENS WY
- LA 91304 529-G4
KENSINGTON AV
2400 THO 91362 527-B3
KENSINGTON CT
7400 CanP 91307 529-E4
KENSINGTON DR
500 FILM 93015 456-A6
KENSINGTON LN
1700 OXN 93030 522-E4
KENT CT
1500 OXN 93030 522-E4
KENT DR
1500 VEN 93004 492-H3
KENT PL
1000 THO 91362 527-B7
KENTFIELD CT
31700 WLKV 91361 557-D6
E KENTFIELD ST
2200 SIMI 93065 478-B7
KENTIA ST
2200 OXN 93036 522-F1
KENTLAND AV
6100 WdHl 91367 529-H7
6500 CanP 91307 529-H5
7600 LA 91304 529-H2
9600 Chat 91311 499-H6
KENTON CT
3000 SIMI 93065 498-D5
KENTWOOD DR
500 OXN 93030 522-F3
KENWATER AV
6100 WdHl 91367 529-E7
6400 CanP 91307 529-E7
KENWATER PL
6400 CanP 91307 529-E7
KENWOOD CT
600 THO 91320 556-D2
KENWOOD ST
500 THO 91320 556-D2
KEPLER DR
1800 OXN 93033 553-A2
KERN ST
300 VEN 93003 492-B3
1700 OXN 93033 552-F3
1700 PHME 93033 552-F3
1700 PHME 93041 552-F3
KERNVALE AV
15500 MRPK 93021 477-A6
KERRIA CT
- OXN 93030 523-A4
KERRMOOR DR
6000 WLKV 91362 557-F3
KERRY DR
2700 SIMI 93063 478-E7

STREET
Block City ZIP Pg-Grid
KERRYGLEN ST
1500 THO 91361 556-J6
KERRYHILL CT
6300 AGRH 91301 558-A3
KESWICK CT
2400 SIMI 93063 498-D1
KESWICK ST
22200 LA 91304 529-F4
KETCH AV
3300 OXN 93035 552-B1
KETCH PL
2900 OXN 93035 552-C1
KEVIN ST
100 THO 91360 526-F5
KEY LARGO CT
4800 VeCo 91377 557-G2
KEYSER RONDO
700 CMRL 93010 524-F2
KEYSTONE ST
2200 SIMI 93063 499-C1
KEY WEST CT
1100 OXN 93030 522-F6
KHYBER DR
700 VEN 93001 491-C1
KIAWAH RIVER DR
- OXN 93036 492-G6
KICKAPOO DR
600 VEN 93001 471-D6
KILAINE DR
2900 SIMI 93063 478-E7
KILBURN CT
5300 VeCo 91377 527-G6
KILLDALE CT
600 SIMI 93065 497-D7
KILTY AV
7100 CanP 91307 529-F5
KILTY PL
23400 CanP 91307 529-F5
KIMBALL CT
2000 SIMI 93065 498-A2
N KIMBALL RD
- VEN 93004 492-E1
S KIMBALL RD
- VEN 93004 492-E2
KIMBER DR
3300 THO 91320 555-F2
W KIMBER DR
3700 THO 91320 555-F2
KIMBERLY AV
2400 CMRL 93010 524-E1
KIMBERLY DR
- VeCo 93001 471-C2
29600 AGRH 91301 557-H3
KIMBERWICK LN
4300 MRPK 93021 496-F3
KINETIC DR
200 OXN 93030 523-C5
KING CT
400 SPLA 93060 463-H6
KING DR
6000 VEN 93003 492-D6
KING PL
3500 SIMI 93063 498-E3
KING ST
400 FILM 93015 455-H6
900 OXN 93030 522-F7
KING CANYON RD
700 VeCo 93015 465-J3
700 VeCo 93015 466-A3
KINGFISHER PL
6300 VEN 93003 492-D5
KINGFISHER WY
700 OXN 93030 522-F7
KINGHAM CT
5900 AGRH 91301 558-A4
KING JAMES CT
1500 VeCo 91377 527-H6
KINGLET ST
6800 VEN 93003 492-E5
KINGMAN AV
2000 SIMI 93063 498-J2
KING PALM DR
23600 SIMI 93063 498-D4
23600 SIMI 93065 498-D4
KINGS RD
10800 VEN 93004 472-H6
KINGSBORO CT
1400 THO 91362 527-E7
KINGSBRIDGE LN
2200 OXN 93035 552-A2
KINGSBRIDGE WY
2000 OXN 93035 552-A1
KINGS CANYON CT
2200 OXN 93033 553-B5
KINGS CANYON DR
- OXN 93036 492-H6
KINGSGROVE DR
5000 VeCo 93066 495-A1
5200 VeCo 93066 474-J7
5200 VeCo 93066 494-J1
KINGSLEY CIR
400 THO 91360 526-F7
KINGSPARK CT
31900 WLKV 91361 557-C6
KINGSTON CIR
1300 THO 91362 527-D7
KINGSTON LN
1100 VEN 93001 491-E4
KINGSVIEW RD
4100 MRPK 93021 496-B3
KINGSWOOD LN
400 SIMI 93065 497-D5
KINGSWOOD WY
1300 OXN 93030 522-E3
KINO ST
1900 CMRL 93010 524-D3
KINROSS CT
2200 THO 91361 557-A6
KINZIE ST
22000 Chat 91311 499-J5
KIOWA CT
1600 VeCo 93022 451-E4
KIPANA AV
- VEN 93001 471-C5
KIPLING CT
1500 OXN 93033 552-J4
KIPLING LN
500 VEN 93003 492-D1
KIPLING PL
1000 OXN 93033 552-J4
KIRK AV
600 VEN 93003 491-H4
1400 THO 91360 526-F6
KIRKCALDY CIR
24000 CanP 91307 529-E5
KIRKFORD WY
1200 THO 91361 557-C5
KIRKSIDE PL
- SIMI 93065 527-E1

STREET
Block City ZIP Pg-Grid
KIRKWOOD CT
2600 SIMI 93063 498-E1
KIRSTEN AV
1600 SIMI 93063 498-J3
KIRSTEN LEE DR
1800 WLKV 91361 586-J1
KIRTLAND CIR
2000 THO 91360 526-D4
KITE DR
2000 OXN 93035 522-D6
KITETAIL ST
100 SIMI 93065 527-E1
KITSY LN
1500 SIMI 93063 499-B3
KITTRIDGE ST
22000 CanP 91303 529-H6
22300 CanP 91307 529-G6
24500 LACo 91307 529-C6
KITTY ST
500 VeCo 91320 525-G7
500 VeCo 91320 555-G1
KIVA CT
29100 AGRH 91301 558-A5
KIWI WY
6900 VEN 93003 492-E4
KLAMATH AV
2800 SIMI 93063 479-B7
KLAMATH DR
1900 CMRL 93010 494-E7
KLEBERG ST
4600 SIMI 93063 478-G7
KNAPP RD
7600 Chat 91311 499-F6
KNAPP WY
9300 Chat 91311 499-F7
KNAPP RANCH RD
- WHil 91304 499-C7
- WHil 91304 529-C1
KNIGHT CT
2200 SIMI 93065 497-H2
KNIGHT DR
28200 AGRH 91301 558-C7
KNIGHT RONDO
2900 CMRL 93010 524-F3
KNIGHTSBRIDGE AV
2600 THO 91362 527-A3
KNIGHTSBRIDGE PL
2100 OXN 93030 522-D4
KNIGHTSGATE RD
4500 WLKV 91361 557-D6
N KNIGHTWOOD CIR
2500 SIMI 93063 498-E1
N KNIGHTWOOD PL
2400 SIMI 93063 498-E1
KNOB LN
13500 VeCo 93012 496-F4
KNOLL DR
1800 VEN 93003 492-B5
KNOLL CREST PL
2200 THO 91361 557-A4
E KNOLLHAVEN ST
2200 SIMI 93065 498-B2
KNOLL RIDGE RD
23600 SIMI 93065 497-F7
KNOLLVIEW CT
23600 SIMI 93065 527-F1
KNOLLVIEW LN
400 THO 91360 526-D7
KNOLLWOOD CIR
23600 SIMI 93065 497-F7
KNOLLWOOD CT
- CanP 91307 529-E5
KNOLLWOOD DR
700 THO 91320 555-E3
KNOTTINGHAM ST
1100 SIMI 93065 498-C4
KNOTTY PINE ST
12900 MRPK 93021 496-E3
KNOWLES ST
100 THO 91360 526-E6
KNOX AV
- VEN 93003 492-B2
KOALA DR
2000 OXN 93036 522-F3
KOALA WY
2000 VEN 93003 492-F5
KODIAK CIR
2700 SIMI 93063 478-G7
KODIAK ST
7100 VEN 93003 492-F5
KOENIGSTEIN RD
12400 VeCo 93060 366-L7
12400 VeCo 93060 453-D1
KOHALA ST
100 OXN 93030 523-A5
KONA DR
23600 OXN 93033 552-J1
KONA LN
4800 OXN 93033 552-J5
KOREAN WAR VET MEM HWY Rt#-126
2300 VeCo 93015 455-F6
2500 VeCo 93015 455-E7
2700 VeCo 93015 465-B2
17900 VeCo 93060 464-F3
18400 SPLA 93060 464-F3
20100 VeCo 93060 465-B2
KRENWINKLE CT
100 SIMI 93065 527-E1
KROTONA RD
- OJAI 93023 451-E1
KUDU PL
2300 VEN 93003 492-F5
KUEHNER DR
1300 SIMI 93063 499-C1
2500 SIMI 93063 479-D7
KUMQUAT PL
800 OXN 93036 522-E2
KUNKLE ST
- VeCo 93022 451-B7
KYLE CT
7400 CanP 91307 529-G4
KYLE LN
2800 SIMI 93063 478-E7

L

L AV
- VeCo 93042 583-D5
L CT
500 OXN 93030 522-E6
L ST
100 OXN 93030 522-E5
1100 OXN 93033 522-F7
1100 OXN 93033 552-F1
LA BAYA DR
5600 WLKV 91362 557-E4
LA BREA DR
1200 THO 91362 526-H7

STREET
Block City ZIP Pg-Grid
LA BREA ST
100 VeCo 93035 552-A3
4500 OXN 93035 552-A3
LA BROCHE CANYON RD
- VeCo - 453-G1
- VeCo 93060 453-G1
23600 VeCo - 366-L7
LA CAM RD
2200 THO 91320 555-H2
2200 VeCo 91320 555-H2
N LA CAMPANA RD
800 VeCo 93015 455-F5
LA CANADA AV
100 OXN 93033 552-G3
LA CASA CT
3100 THO 91362 527-C3
LA CORONA CT
600 VeCo 91377 557-J2
LA COSTA PL
3500 OXN 93033 552-G3
LA CRESCENTA DR
- VeCo 93010 493-J7
LA CRESCENTA ST
- VeCo 93035 552-A3
LA CRESTA DR
800 THO 91362 526-H7
23600 VeCo 93023 451-D2
LA CROSSE DR
- VeCo 93022 451-B6
LA CUESTA CT
6500 VEN 93003 472-D6
LA CULEBRA CIR
1200 CMRL 93012 524-J1
LA CUMBRA ST
- VeCo 93022 451-C4
LA CUMBRE CIR
7200 VEN 93003 472-D7
LA CUMBRE RD
5800 VeCo 93066 495-A3
LADA AV
6300 CMRL 93012 525-C6
LADBROOK WY
2500 VeCo 91361 556-D7
2500 VeCo 91361 586-D1
LADERA RD
1500 VeCo 93023 442-D4
2600 VeCo - 442-D4
LADERA VISTA DR
4900 CMRL 93012 524-J3
LADONIA ST
4800 SIMI 93063 478-H6
LADYCLIFF CIR
2000 THO 91360 526-C4
LADYFACE CT
29800 AGRH 91301 557-H6
LA ENCINA
- THO 91320 525-E6
E LA FALDA WY
23600 VeCo 93040 458-D5
LAFAYETTE CT
6500 MRPK 93021 476-G6
LAFAYETTE DR
200 OXN 93036 522-H2
LAFAYETTE ST
4700 VEN 93003 492-A3
6700 MRPK 93021 476-G6
LAFITTE DR
1500 VeCo 91377 527-H6
LA FONDA CT
7000 VEN 93003 492-D1
LA FONDA DR
400 VEN 93003 492-D1
LA FONDA DR E
400 VEN 93003 472-D7
400 VEN 93003 492-D1
LA FORTUNA
100 THO 91320 525-E7
LAGO LN
- OXN 93036 522-H3
LAGOON LN
- OXN 93035 522-E6
LA GRANADA DR
700 THO 91362 527-A6
1100 THO 91362 526-H6
LA GRANADA ST
100 VeCo 93035 552-A4
LA GRANGE AV
500 THO 91320 555-F4
LAGROSS WY
9400 Chat 91311 499-F6
LAGUNA DR
600 SIMI 93065 497-G5
600 VeCo 93065 497-G5
LAGUNA RD
- VeCo 93042 583-G4
- VeCo 93012 553-F2
- VeCo 93012 554-A2
1600 VeCo 93033 553-F2
LAGUNA TER
300 VeCo 93065 497-F5
LAGUNA WY
300 VeCo 93065 497-G4
LAGUNA PEAK ACCESS RD
- VeCo - 584-C4
23600 VeCo 93033 583-J4
23600 VeCo 93033 584-A4
LAGUNA RIDGE FIRE RD
- VeCo - 366-G8
- VeCo - 450-B6
- VeCo 93001 450-B6
LA JOLLA DR
1100 THO 91362 526-H7
LA JOLLA ST
100 VEN 93004 472-H7
100 VEN 93004 492-H1
LAKE AV
1100 VeCo 93023 451-C3
LAKE CT
300 SIMI 93065 497-F5
LAKE DR
2500 OXN 93036 522-F1
LAKE BREEZE PL
500 SIMI 93065 497-E6
LAKE CANYON
- VeCo 93003 472-C4
LAKE CASITAS FIRE RD
23600 VeCo 93001 460-A3
LAKE CREST CT
3300 WLKV 91361 557-C7
LAKE CREST DR
5300 AGRH 91301 557-F6
LAKEFIELD RD
100 THO 91361 557-B4
LAKEFRONT DR
30600 AGRH 91301 557-G5
LAKE HARBOR LN
3800 WLKV 91361 557-C6

STREET
Block City ZIP Pg-Grid
LAKEHURST AV
1700 CMRL 93010 524-G1
1700 CMRL 93010 494-G7
LAKEHURST ST
1400 OXN 93030 522-F4
LAKELAND TER
24000 LA 91304 529-C1
LAKE LINDERO DR
5300 AGRH 91301 557-G3
LAKE MANOR DR
23200 Chat 91311 499-F7
23400 Chat 91311 499-F7
LAKEMEADOW LN
32100 WLKV 91361 557-C6
LAKE NADINE PL
6000 AGRH 91301 557-G3
LAKE PARK DR
500 SIMI 93065 497-D6
LAKE PLEASANT DR
32300 WLKV 91361 557-B7
LAKEPORT DR
3300 WLKV 91361 557-C7
LAKERIDGE LN
1300 THO 91361 557-B5
LAKE SHERWOOD DR
- VeCo 91361 556-F7
900 THO 91361 556-F7
LAKE SHORE DR
200 VeCo 93035 552-B4
200 VeCo 93043 552-B4
200 PHME 93035 552-B4
200 PHME 93043 552-B4
LAKESIDE AV
300 CMRL 93010 524-D2
LAKEVIEW CT
- OXN 93036 492-H6
LAKEVIEW TER
9200 Chat 91311 499-F7
LAKEVIEW CANYON RD
- THO 91362 557-G1
100 THO 91361 557-C5
300 WLKV 91361 557-C5
1100 THO 91362 527-E7
5200 VeCo 91362 557-G1
LAKEVISTA ST
9900 VEN 93004 492-J3
LAKEWOOD AV
100 VEN 93004 492-G2
LAKEWOOD CIR
8300 VEN 93004 492-F2
LAKEWOOD CT
1300 THO 91361 557-C5
LAKEWOOD PL
2700 THO 91361 557-B5
LAKOTA ST
- SIMI 93065 477-J6
- SIMI 93065 478-A5
LA LOMA AV
- VeCo 93066 493-H2
500 VeCo 93066 494-A1
600 VeCo 93066 474-B7
LA LOMITA
100 THO 91320 525-E6
N LA LUNA AV
100 VeCo 93023 441-D6
S LA LUNA AV
100 VeCo 93023 441-D7
600 VeCo 93023 451-C2
LA MARINA DR
300 CMRL 93010 523-J2
LAMBERT ST
100 VeCo 93036 492-J5
LAMBOURNE PL
7000 VeCo 91377 528-B7
LA MESA AV
3400 SIMI 93063 478-G5
LAMINGTON ST
- VeCo 91361 556-D7
LAMONT AV
1200 THO 91362 527-A6
LAMPLIGHTER ST
2900 SIMI 93065 498-D4
LAMP POST CIR
400 SIMI 93065 497-F6
LANA CT
2200 SIMI 93063 499-C1
LA NARANJA ST E
600 VeCo 93015 455-E5
LANARK ST
22100 LA 91304 529-G3
LANCASTER CIR
1400 THO 91360 526-A4
LANCE PL
24000 CanP 91307 529-E5
E LANDEN ST
2600 CMRL 93010 494-F7
N LANDEN ST
1700 CMRL 93010 494-F7
1700 CMRL 93010 524-F1
LANDER CT
2600 THO 91320 555-H1
LANDING CV
- VeCo 93012 554-E4
LANDINO DR
6100 WLKV 91362 557-F3
LANDSBURN CIR
1100 THO 91361 557-C5
LANG ST
100 VEN 93003 491-H3
LANGDON WY
1700 VEN 93001 491-E2
LANGFORD DR
1500 OXN 93030 522-E4
LANGHALL CT
6300 AGRH 91301 557-J3
LANGLEY ST
2000 OXN 93033 553-A4
LANG RANCH PKWY
3000 THO 91362 527-C4
LANGSPUR CT
31800 WLKV 91361 557-D6
LANGUID LN
600 SIMI 93065 497-G5
LANIER PL
3200 THO 91360 526-G2
E LANSDALE CT
2200 SIMI 93065 498-B2
E LANSING PL
2300 SIMI 93065 498-B4
LANTANA ST
100 CMRL 93010 524-C2
1400 VeCo 93010 524-C1
1600 VeCo 93010 494-C7
1800 OXN 93030 522-F3
1900 OXN 93036 522-F3
LANTANA WY
100 VEN 93004 473-A7
LANTERN AV
- SIMI 93063 498-H1

STREET
Block City ZIP Pg-Grid
LANTERN LN
4300 MRPK 93021 496-F3
LANYARD WY
2000 OXN 93035 522-D6
LA PALMA
100 THO 91320 525-E6
LA PALOMA CIR
2500 THO 91360 526-D3
LA PATERA CT
- VeCo 93010 493-J7
- VeCo 93010 494-A7
LA PATERA DR
- VeCo 93010 494-A7
- VeCo 93010 493-J7
W LA PAZ CT
- SIMI 93065 497-E4
LA PAZ DR
1100 OJAI 93023 451-F1
LA PERESA DR
1200 THO 91362 526-H7
LAPEYRE RD
23600 VeCo 93021 497-A3
LA PLATA DR
- CMRL 93010 493-H7
LA PLAZA
1400 VeCo 93023 451-C2
LA PORTE ST
600 CMRL 93012 525-A2
LA PUENTE DR
23600 FILM 93015 456-C6
LA PUERTA AV
1800 OXN 93030 522-J6
1800 OXN 93030 523-A6
LA PUMA CT
- CMRL 93012 494-J7
- CMRL 93012 524-J1
LAPWORTH DR
5800 AGRH 91301 558-C4
LA QUILLA DR
22300 Chat 91311 479-J7
22400 Chat 91311 499-H1
LA QUINTA LN
1600 OXN 93036 522-E2
LA RAMADA DR
1800 CMRL 93012 495-B7
1800 CMRL 93012 525-C1
LARAMIE CT
700 THO 91320 555-G5
LARAMIE ST
9600 VEN 93004 492-H2
LARBOARD LN
5800 AGRH 91301 557-G4
LARCH ST
1800 SIMI 93065 498-A2
E LARCH ST
2000 SIMI 93065 498-A2
LARCH CREST CT
200 THO 91320 556-D2
LARCHMONT ST
1200 SIMI 93065 497-D6
LARCHWOOD CIR
6900 CanP 91307 529-F6
LARCOM ST
2700 THO 91360 526-E3
LAREDO LN
200 OJAI 93023 451-F1
LA REINA
100 THO 91320 525-E6
S LARGO LN
800 VeCo 93015 465-B2
LARIAT LN
23600 SIMI 93065 527-D1
LARK AV
1100 VEN 93003 492-D4
LARK DR
- VeCo 93041 583-G2
LARK ST
100 OXN 93033 552-G3
600 VeCo 93023 451-C4
1600 SIMI 93063 498-F3
LARKDALE CT
600 SIMI 93065 497-G6
LARK ELLEN AV
200 OJAI 93023 442-A6
LARKELLEN CT
6000 VeCo 91377 558-A2
LARKFIELD AV
1300 THO 91362 527-C6
LARKHAVEN CT
3300 THO 91360 526-H2
LARKHAVEN LN
2400 OXN 93036 522-F2
LARKHILL ST
100 THO 91360 526-F2
LARKIN CT
4700 SIMI 93063 498-H1
LARKIN ST
5400 VEN 93003 492-B3
LARKSBERRY LN
23600 SIMI 93065 497-A2
LARKSPUR DR
5000 VeCo 93001 471-C1
5200 VeCo 93001 461-C7
LARKSPUR ST
1200 VeCo 93063 499-B4
1400 SPLA 93060 464-B2
LARMIER AV
100 VeCo 93022 451-A7
600 VeCo 93022 461-A1
LARO DR
28900 AGRH 91301 558-A3
29300 AGRH 91301 557-J4
LA ROSA DR
4800 VeCo 91377 557-G1
LARRY CT
23600 THO 91320 556-C1
LARSON WY
9300 Chat 91311 499-F6
9300 Chat 91311 499-F6
LARWIN AV
10000 Chat 91311 499-H4
LA SALLE AV
300 VEN 93003 492-A1
LAS BRISAS DR
2700 VeCo 93012 496-A6
LAS CRUCES ST
9500 VEN 93004 492-H3
LA SENDA CT
6400 CMRL 93012 495-C7
LAS ESTRELLAS CT
- CMRL 93012 494-J7
LA SIERRA CT
- CMRL 93012 495-A6
LAS LLAJAS CANYON RD
- Nwhl 91382 479-E2
- StvR 91381 479-E2
5100 VeCo 93063 478-J5
5100 VeCo 93063 479-A5
5500 Chat 91311 479-E2

STREET
Block City ZIP Pg-Grid

LAS LLAJAS CANYON RD
5500 VeCo - 479-E2
LAS PALMAS ST
100 VeCo 93035 552-A4
LAS PALOMAS DR
400 PHME 93041 552-C2
LAS POSAS CIR
2500 VeCo 93012 496-B6
LAS POSAS RD
- CMRL 93010 524-B2
900 VeCo 93010 524-B2
2100 CMRL 93010 494-F7
2400 VeCo 93012 554-A4
3200 VeCo 93010 494-F7
3600 VeCo 93033 554-A7
5400 VeCo 93033 583-J3
5400 VeCo 93033 584-A3
E LAS POSAS RD
10800 VeCo 93012 496-A6
N LAS POSAS RD
300 CMRL 93010 524-B2
S LAS POSAS RD
100 CMRL 93010 524-B6
700 VeCo 93010 524-B6
1100 VeCo 93012 524-B6
1500 VeCo 93012 554-B1
LAS POSAS ST
300 VeCo 93015 465-J3
LASSEN AV
300 MRPK 93021 496-D1
LASSEN CT
10700 VEN 93004 472-H7
23600 MRPK 93021 496-D1
LASSEN DR
600 SPLA 93060 463-H6
LASSEN ST
2200 OXN 93033 552-F2
22000 Chat 91311 499-H5
LAS TUERO CT
300 VeCo 93010 493-J7
300 VeCo 93010 494-A7
LAS TUNAS PL
3500 OXN 93033 552-H3
LA SUEN DR
100 CMRL 93010 494-E7
100 VeCo 93010 494-E7
LAS VEREDAS PL
- CMRL 93012 494-H7
LAS VIRGENES RD
5100 CALB 91302 558-H3
5100 LACo 91302 558-H3
5700 VeCo 91302 558-H3
LAS VIRGENES RD Rt#-N1
3700 CALB 91302 558-H7
4800 LACo 91302 558-H7
E LAS VIRGENES CANYON RD
23600 VeCo 91302 528-J7
23600 VeCo 91302 529-A7
23600 VeCo 91302 558-H2
LATHAM ST
2000 SIMI 93065 478-A7
LATHAN AV
1700 CMRL 93010 494-D7
1700 CMRL 93010 524-D1
LATHROP AV
3300 SIMI 93063 478-F6
LA TIENDA RD
31600 THO 91362 557-D5
31600 WLKV 91362 557-D5
LATIGO AV
2200 OXN 93030 523-B4
LATIMER RD
6300 SIMI 93063 499-C3
LA TUNA LN
- CMRL 93012 494-H6
LAURA ST
1100 VeCo 93023 451-B2
LAURA LA PLANTE DR
28100 AGRH 91301 558-C6
LAUREL CT
200 VeCo 93035 552-B4
LAUREL LN
- MRPK 93021 496-G3
LAUREL RD
900 SPLA 93060 464-B2
LAUREL ST
100 OXN 93033 552-H2
N LAUREL ST
- VEN 93001 491-D2
S LAUREL ST
- VEN 93001 491-D2
W LAUREL ST
100 OXN 93033 552-F2
LAUREL BLUFF PL
5600 AGRH 91301 557-J5
LAUREL FIG DR
23600 SIMI 93063 498-D4
23600 SIMI 93065 498-D4
LAUREL GLEN DR
4200 MRPK 93021 496-E3
LAURELHURST RD
13200 MRPK 93021 496-F3
LAUREL PARK CIR
800 CMRL 93012 524-J2
LAUREL PARK CT
2100 THO 91362 527-B4
LAUREL PARK DR
5000 CMRL 93012 524-J2
5000 CMRL 93012 525-A2
LAUREL RIDGE DR
23600 SIMI 93065 497-F7
E LAUREL RIDGE LN
5600 CMRL 93012 525-A1
LAUREL VALLEY PL
1900 OXN 93036 522-D2
LAURELVIEW DR
4100 MRPK 93021 496-B3
LAURELWOOD AV
- SIMI 93063 499-A2
LAUREL WOOD CT
23600 SIMI 93065 497-G7
LAURELWOOD CT
1800 THO 91362 526-J3
1800 THO 91362 527-A3
LAURELWOOD DR
1900 THO 91362 527-A3
LAUREN LN
- LA 91304 529-G4
LAUREN ST
3300 SIMI 93063 498-D1
LAURIE LN
100 SPLA 93060 463-J7
300 THO 91360 526-F7
300 THO 91360 556-F1
400 SPLA 93060 473-J1
400 SPLA 93060 474-A1

LAUTREC CT
400 THO 91360 526-D5
LAVA PL
8700 LA 91304 529-E1
LAVANDA DR
2200 OXN 93036 522-H2
LA VELLA DR
4800 VeCo 91377 557-G1
LAVENDER AV
1900 SIMI 93065 498-A2
LAVENDER ST
10700 VEN 93004 493-A2
LAVENDER BELL LN
22300 WdHl 91367 529-J7
LA VENTA DR
1200 THO 91361 557-B6
LA VERADA CT
23600 CMRL 93010 524-C4
LA VERNE AV
- VEN 93003 492-C2
LAVERY CT
2600 THO 91320 525-J6
LA VETA DR
5000 CMRL 93012 524-G3
LA VISTA AV
4000 VeCo 93066 493-H3
LA VUELTA PL
900 SPLA 93060 464-B4
LAWNVIEW CT
2300 SIMI 93065 498-B2
LAWNWOOD WY
500 OXN 93030 522-F3
LAWRENCE CIR
1200 SIMI 93065 498-A3
LAWRENCE DR
800 THO 91320 525-J7
800 THO 91320 526-A5
LAWRENCE WY
1100 OXN 93035 522-D7
1200 OXN 93035 552-D1
LAWSON AV
1700 SIMI 93065 498-B3
LAWTON RANCH RD
23600 VeCo 93015 456-G6
LAYTON CIR
1000 SIMI 93065 497-J4
LAYTON ST
100 VeCo 93023 441-G5
2000 THO 91362 526-J5
LAZARO LN
- OXN 93035 522-C6
LAZIO WY
4900 VeCo 91377 557-G2
LAZY BROOK CT
500 SIMI 93065 497-E6
LAZY OAK PL
29600 AGRH 91301 557-J5
LEADWELL ST
22000 CanP 91303 529-J4
22500 CanP 91307 529-H4
LEAFLOCK AV
2400 THO 91361 557-B5
LEAFWOOD DR
2500 CMRL 93010 494-F6
LEAR CIR
100 THO 91360 526-F7
LEAR CT
1600 OXN 93030 522-E4
LEATHERWOOD CT
4300 CMRL 93012 524-H4
LEAVENS CT
400 SPLA 93060 463-H6
E LECONT CT
3500 SIMI 93063 498-F2
LEDERER AV
6100 WdHl 91367 529-F7
6400 CanP 91307 529-F7
LEE PL
2800 OXN 93035 552-C1
LEE ST
1600 SIMI 93065 498-B2
LEEDS ST
4800 SIMI 93063 498-H2
LEEWARD CIR
2300 THO 91361 557-B6
LEEWARD WY
2900 OXN 93035 552-B1
LEGACY DR
- SIMI 93065 477-J7
- SIMI 93065 478-A6
LEGAN
23600 VeCo 93015 456-G6
LEGENDS DR
- SIMI 93065 478-A5
LEHIGH ST
5300 VEN 93003 492-B2
LEHMAN RD
- PHME 93043 552-C4
LEI DR
1000 OXN 93033 552-J5
LEI LN
1800 OXN 93033 552-J1
1800 OXN 93033 553-A1
LEIGHTON DR
- VEN 93001 471-C7
LEIGHTON POINT RD
3800 CALB 91301 558-G7
LEISURE LN
900 SIMI 93065 497-H5
1300 THO 91320 556-B1
LEISURE VILLAGE DR
5600 CMRL 93012 525-B2
LEISURE VILLAGE DR W
5100 CMRL 93012 525-A3
LELAND CIR
5300 SIMI 93063 498-J3
LELAND ST
6000 VEN 93003 492-D6
LE MAR AV
- VeCo 93042 583-F5
LEMAR AV
300 VeCo 93036 492-J7
700 VeCo 93036 493-A7
LEMARSH ST
22000 Chat 91311 499-J4
LEMAY ST
24000 CanP 91307 529-D6
LEMBERT ST
2600 SIMI 93065 498-C4
LEMON AV
3600 OXN 93033 553-B3
LEMON DR
2600 SIMI 93065 498-E1
2700 SIMI 93063 478-E7
2800 VeCo 93010 494-E7
3200 VeCo 93063 478-E7
E LEMON DR
800 VeCo 93010 494-F7
2900 CMRL 93010 494-F7

LEMON WY
600 FILM 93015 455-J5
LEMONBERRY PL
3900 THO 91362 497-A7
3900 THO 91362 527-A1
LEMON GROVE AV
500 VEN 93003 491-H4
LEMONWOOD DR
1700 SPLA 93060 464-D5
10400 VeCo 93021 495-J1
LEMONWOOD ST
700 THO 91320 555-G4
LEMUR CT
6900 VEN 93003 492-E5
LEMUR ST
7000 VEN 93003 492-E4
LENA AV
6200 WdHl 91367 529-G7
6800 CanP 91307 529-G4
7600 LA 91304 529-G3
LENNOX CT
1800 OXN 93030 522-E4
LEON DR
1900 OXN 93036 522-H3
LEONARD ST
500 CMRL 93010 524-F2
LEORA ST
3400 SIMI 93063 478-D6
LEOTA LN
7100 WHil 91304 499-E7
22700 WHil 91304 499-E7
LE SAGE AV
6100 WdHl 91367 529-F7
LESLIE CT
3100 SIMI 93063 478-D6
LESSER DR
3200 VeCo 91320 525-F7
3500 THO 91320 525-F7
LESTER LN
8300 LA 91304 529-F2
LETA YANCY RD
- MRPK 93021 496-D2
LETICIA CT
30100 AGRH 91301 557-H5
LEVEN AV
2000 CMRL 93010 494-H7
LEVI CT
3400 SIMI 93063 478-F6
LEVI WY
1600 OXN 93033 552-J3
LEWIS LN
900 FILM 93015 455-J6
5500 AGRH 91301 558-C5
LEWIS PL
28400 AGRH 91301 558-C6
LEWIS RD
600 VeCo 93012 524-F5
1800 VeCo 93012 554-D2
4900 AGRH 91301 558-C5
N LEWIS RD Rt#-34
- CMRL 93010 524-G2
1700 CMRL 93010 494-H7
S LEWIS RD Rt#-34
- CMRL 93010 524-F4
200 CMRL 93012 524-F4
E LEWIS ST
- VEN 93001 471-C7
W LEWIS ST
200 VEN 93001 471-B6
LEXINGTON CT
1400 CMRL 93010 524-E1
LEXINGTON DR
2300 VEN 93001 491-G2
2400 VEN 93003 491-G2
LEXINGTON WY
30900 AGRH 91301 557-F6
30900 WLKV 91361 557-F6
LEXINGTON HILLS LN
13000 VeCo 93012 496-F5
LEYTE ST
- PHME 93041 552-E4
LIADA WY
- OXN 93030 522-H4
LIBBEY AV
700 OJAI 93023 441-H6
LIBERTY CV
2600 PHME 93041 552-C3
LIBERTY CANYON RD
3900 AGRH 91301 558-E7
4000 Ago 91301 558-E7
LIBRARY VIEW RD
23600 VeCo 93021 497-B3
LIBRE ST
- OXN 93030 522-G4
LICHO WY
- OXN 93030 522-J4
LICIA PL
2700 SIMI 93065 478-B7
2700 SIMI 93065 498-B1
LIDO BLVD
2500 PHME 93041 552-D2
2700 OXN 93035 552-E2
2700 OXN 93041 552-E2
LIDO CT
300 CMRL 93010 524-D3
LIDO DR
2600 PHME 93041 552-D2
2700 OXN 93035 552-D2
2700 OXN 93041 552-D2
LIGGETT ST
22000 Chat 91311 499-J6
LIGHTHOUSE LN
700 OXN 93030 522-F7
LIGHTHOUSE WY
500 PHME 93041 552-F7
LIGHTNING RIDGE WY
- SIMI 93063 478-E6
LILAC LN
200 SPLA 93060 464-A5
10200 VeCo 93063 499-F3
10200 SIMI 93063 499-F3
LILAC WK
2500 OXN 93030 522-D4
LILAC WY
- VEN 93004 473-A7
LILLA PL
7500 LA 91304 529-E4
LILLIAN DR
400 PHME 93041 552-F5
LILY CT
3400 VeCo 91320 525-F7
LILY PL
200 VEN 93004 473-A7
LILYWOOD LN
1800 OXN 93030 522-H4
LIMCO RD
600 VeCo 93015 457-A6
LIME AV
1600 OXN 93033 553-B5

LIME CANYON RD
23600 VeCo 93040 367-D7
LIMEROCK TR
8600 LA 91304 529-E1
LIMESTONE DR
- THO 91362 527-B3
LIMOGES CT
- LACo 91302 558-G3
LIMONEIRA AV
- VeCo 93003 492-D2
- VEN 93003 492-D2
LIMONERO PL
- OXN 93030 522-H4
LINCOLN CT
- SIMI 93065 497-D5
1800 OXN 93033 553-A4
1900 OXN 93033 552-J5
LINCOLN DR
- VEN 93001 491-E1
LINDA CT
1500 SIMI 93065 497-J3
LINDA FLORA DR
12000 VeCo 93023 451-A2
LINDALE AV
2000 SIMI 93065 498-C2
LINDAMERE CT
- SIMI 93065 497-H5
LINDA VISTA AV
200 VEN 93001 491-E1
LINDAWOOD ST
800 THO 91320 556-C1
LINDBERGH DR
1800 OXN 93033 553-A1
LINDEN CIR
800 THO 91360 526-F7
LINDEN DR
400 OXN 93033 552-F2
N LINDEN DR
- VEN 93004 472-H7
S LINDEN DR
- VEN 93004 472-J7
LINDENGROVE ST
2000 THO 91361 557-A4
LINDERO CANYON RD
100 THO 91362 557-G3
100 WLKV 91362 557-G3
5400 WLKV 91361 557-E5
5500 VeCo 91377 527-G7
5900 VeCo 91362 527-G7
5900 VeCo 91362 557-G3
6000 VeCo 91377 557-G3
W LINDERO CANYON RD
5300 WLKV 91362 557-C7
5400 WLKV 91361 557-C7
LINDSAY CT
- THO 91320 555-E2
LINDSAY LN
100 SPLA 93060 463-H7
100 SPLA 93060 473-H1
LINDSAY PL
1000 OXN 93033 552-J4
LINFIELD DR
300 VEN 93003 492-A3
LINGDOLY RANCH RD
- VeCo 93060 463-E4
LINKS VIEW DR
- SIMI 93065 497-C6
LINLEY LN
7500 LA 91304 529-E4
LINVILLE CT
6400 MRPK 93021 477-A6
LION ST
300 OJAI 93023 441-H6
LION CANYON FIRE RD
23600 VeCo 93023 451-H3
23600 VeCo 93023 452-C3
LIONS CIR
- SIMI 93065 477-C7
LIONS GATE DR
600 OXN 93030 522-D4
LIRIO AV
1400 VeCo 93004 493-B2
LISA CT
700 VeCo 91320 525-G7
LISBON LN
- OXN 93036 492-G6
N LITA PL
2500 SIMI 93063 498-E1
LITTLE CREEK CIR
2300 THO 91320 555-J2
LITTLE FARMS RD
1500 OXN 93030 522-E5
LITTLE FAWN CT
1400 THO 91362 527-F6
LITTLE FEATHER AV
3200 SIMI 93063 479-A6
LITTLEFIELD CT
2500 THO 91362 527-D3
LITTLE HOLLOW PL
4000 MRPK 93021 496-D3
LITTLE OAK LN
6000 WdHl 91367 529-C7
LITTLER CT
- MRPK 93021 476-D5
LITTLE SYCAMORE CANYON RD
100 VeCo 90265 586-D4
200 LACo 90265 586-D4
LIVELY CIR
- VeCo 93023 452-D1
LIVEOAK AV
7300 VeCo 93060 453-B7
7300 VeCo 93060 463-B1
LIVE OAK CT
26800 CALB 91301 558-G7
LIVE OAK DR
- VEN 93001 491-E2
LIVE OAK RD
1500 THO 91320 556-A2
LIVE OAK ST
2500 THO 91362 557-A2
LIVE OAK TER
22600 Chat 91311 499-H5
LIVE OAK TR
6700 VeCo 93063 499-D4
LIVERMORE AV
100 VEN 93004 492-F1
LIVERPOOL CT
5500 VeCo 91377 527-J6
LIVINGSTON AV
- VEN 93003 492-B3
LIVORNO CT
30800 WLKV 91362 557-G6
LIZ CT
7400 LA 91304 529-E4
LLAMA CT
1200 VEN 93003 492-E4
LLANERCH LN
600 SIMI 93065 497-D5

LLEVARANCHO RD
2100 SIMI 93065 497-D2
LLOYD CT
- THO 91320 555-F2
LLOYD BUTLER RD
23600 VeCo 93036 493-D3
23600 VeCo 93066 493-D3
LLOYD TURN-OFF
- VeCo 93001 471-C4
LOBELIA AV
1500 VEN 93004 493-A2
LOBELIA DR
1900 OXN 93030 522-F3
1900 OXN 93036 522-F1
LOCKE AV
1100 SIMI 93065 497-H4
LOCKFORD CT
3600 THO 91360 526-H1
LOCKHART LN
600 FILM 93015 456-A5
LOCKHURST DR
6000 WdHl 91367 529-E7
6300 CanP 91307 529-E7
LOCKWOOD CT
3400 SIMI 93063 498-D1
LOCKWOOD ST
700 OXN 93036 523-A3
1700 OXN 93036 522-J3
LOCKWOOD VALLEY RD
900 VeCo - 367-A1
15900 VeCo - 366-H2
LOCUST AV
- VeCo 91377 558-A2
LOCUST ST
- SIMI 93063 499-B2
LODESTONE CT
900 THO 91320 555-G5
LODGEWOOD ST
2800 THO 91320 555-G3
LODGEWOOD WY
900 OXN 93030 522-E3
LOEWE LN
900 VEN 93003 492-A4
LOFTUS CANYON RD
- VeCo 93066 465-A7
- VeCo 93066 474-J1
23600 VeCo 93060 464-J5
23600 VeCo 93066 464-J7
LOGAN AV
800 VEN 93004 492-G3
LOGAN LN
- SIMI 93065 497-E2
LOGWOOD RD
5800 WLKV 91362 557-G4
LOIRE CT
30800 WLKV 91362 557-F5
LOIRE VALLEY DR
- SIMI 93065 497-G7
- SIMI 93065 527-G1
N LOIS AV
600 THO 91320 525-G7
600 VeCo 91320 525-G7
LOIS LN
1100 CMRL 93010 524-C4
LOISE ST
300 SPLA 93060 464-A7
LOLA WY
- OXN 93030 522-J4
LOMA DR
- CMRL 93010 494-F7
- VeCo 93010 494-F7
800 VeCo 93023 451-D1
1400 CMRL 93010 524-F1
LOMA LN
1000 VeCo 93063 499-B4
LOMA VERDE MTWY
- Cstc 91384 458-F1
- VeCo 93040 367-E7
- VeCo 93040 458-F1
LOMA VISTA PL
600 SPLA 93060 464-A4
LOMA VISTA RD
2600 VEN 93003 491-G2
4300 VEN 93003 492-C1
7500 VEN 93004 492-E1
10100 VeCo 93004 472-H7
10100 VEN 93004 472-H6
10900 VEN 93060 472-H6
LOMBARD ST
100 OXN 93030 523-A4
200 THO 91360 556-F1
LOMITA AV
600 VeCo 93023 441-C7
N LOMITA AV
100 VeCo 93023 441-E6
S LOMITA AV
100 VeCo 93023 441-E7
LOMITA ST
2300 CMRL 93010 524-E3
LONDELIUS ST
21900 LA 91304 529-J1
LONDON CIR
700 THO 91360 526-G7
LONDON LN
- OXN 93036 492-H6
LONDON GROVE CT
12100 MRPK 93021 496-D3
LONE OAK DR
400 THO 91362 556-J1
400 THO 91362 557-A1
400 THO 91362 526-J7
LONESTAR WY
2000 THO 91362 556-J1
2000 THO 91362 557-A1
LONE TRAIL CT
- MRPK 93021 476-D6
LONE TREE CT
2400 THO 91362 526-J4
LONG CT
- THO 91360 556-G1
LONGBRANCH RD
100 SIMI 93065 497-F5
LONG CANYON DR
100 VeCo 93004 492-G1
100 VEN 93004 492-G1
LONG CANYON RD
1300 VeCo 93003 472-F5
1300 VeCo 93060 472-F5
23600 SIMI 93065 497-G7
23600 SIMI 93065 527-F1
LONG COVE DR
- OXN 93036 522-C3
LONGFELLOW CT
100 THO 91360 526-E3
LONGFELLOW ST
100 THO 91360 526-E3
LONGFELLOW WY
5100 OXN 93033 552-H5
S LONGFORD AV
600 THO 91320 555-F4

LONGHORN LN
100 OJAI 93023 441-H7
100 OJAI 93023 451-H1
LONG RIDGE CT
1500 THO 91360 526-E6
LONGRIDGE CT
6300 VEN 93003 472-D6
LONG SHADOW CT
5000 THO 91362 527-F7
LONGVIEW DR
9200 VEN 93004 492-H3
LONGVIEW PL
300 THO 91360 526-E5
LONGWOOD CT
200 THO 91320 555-E2
LONSDALE ST
2100 CMRL 93010 524-E1
LOOKOUT DR
1100 OXN 93035 522-C7
1500 OXN 93035 552-C1
LOOKOUT ROCK TR
1000 VeCo 93063 499-C4
LOON DR
- VeCo 93041 583-G1
E LOOP DR
300 CMRL 93010 494-F6
300 VeCo 93010 494-F6
N LOOP DR
100 VeCo 93010 494-E6
W LOOP DR
- CMRL 93010 494-E6
- CMRL 93010 524-E1
100 VeCo 93010 494-E6
LOOP LN
18000 VeCo 93060 464-D4
LOOP RD
3000 VEN 93003 492-E6
LOPACO CT
300 VeCo 93010 494-A7
LOPEZ CT
- MRPK 93021 476-B5
LORA LN
100 FILM 93015 456-B6
LORABEL WY
- SIMI 93065 527-E1
LORAINE PL
2700 SIMI 93065 478-B7
2700 SIMI 93065 498-B1
LORD CREEK RD
600 VeCo 93015 455-D4
LORENA DR
- OXN 93030 522-J4
LORENZO DR
500 VeCo 91377 557-G1
LORETA CT
3300 CMRL 93010 524-G2
LORETO CIR
3800 THO 91320 555-E1
N LORETTA CIR
2500 SIMI 93065 498-B1
LORETTA DR
11900 MRPK 93021 496-C2
LORI CIR
3000 SIMI 93063 478-E7
LORI LN
- VeCo 93010 494-E6
LORRAINE LN
- MRPK 93021 496-F2
LOS ALAMOS DR
400 OJAI 93023 442-A6
LOS ALISOS CT
23600 CMRL 93010 524-C4
LOS ALTOS ST
- VeCo 93035 552-A3
LOS AMIGOS AV
- SIMI 93065 497-E3
LOS ANGELES AV
- VeCo 93012 554-D4
- VEN 93004 493-A1
- VeCo 93035 552-C6
1000 VeCo 93004 493-A1
1300 VeCo 93015 465-E3
LOS ANGELES AV Rt#-118
- MRPK 93021 496-F1
900 VeCo 93066 493-H4
900 VeCo 93066 494-A4
1200 VeCo 93004 493-B2
2000 VeCo 93036 493-B2
4500 VeCo 93066 495-A4
8000 VeCo 93021 495-H3
10000 VeCo 93021 496-A2
E LOS ANGELES AV
100 SIMI 93065 497-G2
1700 SIMI 93065 498-A2
3200 SIMI 93063 498-A2
5400 SIMI 93063 499-A2
W LOS ANGELES AV
100 SIMI 93065 477-D7
100 SIMI 93065 497-E1
LOS ARCOS CIR
2500 THO 91360 526-G3
LOS ARCOS DR
5300 VeCo 91377 557-H1
LOS CABOS LN
- VeCo 93001 471-C2
LOS CEDROS CIR
2800 VeCo 93012 496-C6
LOS COYOTES PL
6800 CMRL 93012 495-D6
LOS DAMASCOS PL
- CMRL 93012 494-H6
LOS ENCINOS RD
2000 VeCo 93023 451-A4
LOS FELIZ DR
1600 THO 91362 556-J1
2000 THO 91362 557-A2
LOS FELIZ ST
100 VeCo 93035 552-A3
200 OXN 93035 552-A3
LOS FRESNOS CIR
2800 VeCo 93012 496-C6
LOS NOGALES AV
2700 CMRL 93010 524-F1
LOS NOGALES RD
3300 SIMI 93063 478-F6
LOS OLIVOS
2900 OXN 93036 523-B2
LOS PADRES CT
6600 VEN 93003 472-D6
LOS PADRES DR
- THO 91361 556-F2
LOS PINOS CIR
2700 VeCo 93012 496-C6
LOS PRIETOS CT
1300 OXN 93035 552-E1
LOS PUEBLOS DR
100 CMRL 93012 525-A3
600 CMRL 93012 524-J2

LOS ROBLES DR
1200 SPLA 93060
LOS ROBLES RD
2700 THO 91362
LOS ROBLES ST
100 VeCo 93035
LOS ROSAS ST
23900 LA 91304
LOS SANTOS CT
23600 CMRL 93010
LOS SERENOS DR
200 FILM 93015
LOST CANYONS DR
- SIMI 93063
- SIMI 93065
- SIMI 93065
LOST HILLS RD
4100 CALB 91302
4100 CALB 91301
4800 Ago 91301
5000 LACo 91302
LOST OAK CT
26900 CALB 91301
LOST POINT LN
1200 OXN 93030
LOST SPRINGS DR
3800 CALB 91301
N LOS VIENTOS DR
- THO 91320
500 THO 91320
S LOS VIENTOS DR
- THO 91320
LOTA LN
- AGRH 91301
LOT DYLAN DR
- OXN 93033
LOTUS AV
500 THO 91360
LOU DR
4100 SIMI 93063
LOUIS DR
400 VeCo 91320
400 VeCo 91320
LOUISE ST
3200 SIMI 93063
LOUISIANA PL
200 OXN 93036
LOVE CIR
1700 SIMI 93063
LOVEDAY AV
1000 SIMI 93065
LOWELL CT
2500 SIMI 93065
LOWELL PL
300 OXN 93033
LOWER LAKE RD
- VeCo 91361
LOWERY ST
1300 SIMI 93065
LOYOLA AV
- VEN 93003
LOYOLA PL
6600 MRPK 93021
LOYOLA ST
14500 MRPK 93021
E LOYOLA ST
14300 MRPK 93021
LUBBOCK CT
23600 SIMI 93063
LUBBOCK DR
4400 SIMI 93063
LUCADA ST
100 SPLA 93060
400 SPLA 93060
400 SPLA 93060
LUCAS CT
- THO 91320
3800 SIMI 93063
LUCERNE CT
1300 VEN 93004
LUCERNE ST
9500 VEN 93004
LUCERO CT
1100 CMRL 93010
LUCERO ST
- OXN 93030
- THO 91360
1100 CMRL 93010
LUCIA CT
3900 MRPK 93021
LUCILLE CIR
600 MRPK 93021
LUCILLE CT
700 MRPK 93021
LUCKY LN
1800 SIMI 93063
LUCY CIR
400 SIMI 93065
LUDGATE DR
5000 CALB 91301
LUFF CT
2900 OXN 93035
LUGANO WY
400 VeCo 91377
LUIS DR
5400 AGRH 91301
LUKENS LN
2500 SIMI 93065
LULL ST
7600 LA 91304
LUNA CT
- CALB 91302
LUNA DR
- CMRL 93010
2900 VEN 93003
LUNAR CT
3400 OXN 93030
LUNDY DR
1100 SIMI 93065
LUPE AV
- THO 91320
LUPIN ST
2000 SIMI 93065
LUPINE LN
4600 VeCo 93023
LUPINE WY
300 VEN 93001
LUPITA ST
100 OXN 93030
LURAY CIR
2500 VeCo 93065
LUSTRE DR
- OXN 93030
LUTHER AV
3200 THO 91360
LUTHER CIR
6800 MRPK 93021
LUXENBERG DR
9200 VeCo 93021

STREET / Block City ZIP Pg-Grid

R
SIMI 93065 498-A3
Y
OXN 93035 552-A2
OOK CT
WLKV 91361 557-C6
RST AV
CMRL 93010 494-D7
CMRL 93010 524-D1
URST AV
CMRL 93010 524-D1
ST
SIMI 93063 498-D1
VeCo 91320 525-G7
VeCo 91320 555-G1
VEN 93003 491-H2
VEN 93003 491-H2
THO 91360 526-D3
THO 91360 556-C2
VeCo 91360 526-D7
THO 91320 556-A2
VeCo 91320 556-C2
THO 91320 555-H2
RD
THO 91320 555-D4
OOK AV
VEN 93003 492-B1
RE DR
THO 91360 526-B4
KS AV
THO 91320 556-C2
KS CT
THO 91320 556-C2
W ST
THO 91320 555-H3
OD DR
CMRL 93012 525-A1
CMRL 93012 524-J1
D ST
THO 91360 526-C5
SIMI 93065 498-B1
LACo 91302 558-G3
VeCo 93063 499-B4
LN
OXN 93030 523-A4
T
SIMI 93065 497-G4
T
PHME 93043 552-D3
ER AV
SIMI 93065 497-F2

M

OXN 93030 522-E7
VeCo 93042 583-D4
OXN 93030 522-E6
OXN 93033 522-E7
OXN 93033 552-F2
PHME 93041 552-F3
OXN 93030 522-E4
N DR
VeCo 93021 475-J7
VeCo 93021 495-H1
CT
THO 91360 526-H2
M CT
AGRH 91301 558-A3
MIA LN
SIMI 93065 497-E5
HUR PL
OXN 93033 552-J2
OXN 93033 553-A2
AV
VEN 93003 492-E5
ALD LN
PHME 93041 552-D2
O ST
SIMI 93065 498-C3
AV
VEN 93004 492-F2
LAN AV
VEN 93001 491-E2
LN
Chat 91311 479-J7
VeCo 93042 583-D4
AV
VEN 93003 492-C2
CIR
PHME 93041 552-E2
PL
OXN 93033 553-B3
RD
SIMI 93065 497-F4
VeCo 93065 497-F4
SIMI 93065 477-F7
N ST
VEN 93003 491-J3
NA LN
THO 91320 556-B2
ELVA CT
CMRL 93012 525-A2
AV
THO 91320 555-J1
A PL
OXN 93030 522-H5
E ST
SIMI 93065 498-B2
PL
THO 91362 556-H1
O AV
LA 91304 529-F3
O PL
LA 91304 529-F4
CIR
THO 91360 526-E4
AN AV
OXN 93033 552-G6
AN ST
THO 91360 526-F1
IA AV
OXN 93030 522-E5
IA DR
VeCo 93001 471-C2
SPLA 93060 464-B2
IA ST
MRPK 93021 476-E7
MRPK 93021 496-E1
SIMI 93065 498-B2
CMRL 93012 524-F4

MAGPIE CT
- THO 91320 525-J5
MAHAN CT
15300 MRPK 93021 476-J5
MAHAN RD
- VeCo 93021 476-G3
MAHOGANY LN
23600 SIMI 93065 497-E5
MAHONEY AV
- VeCo 93022 451-B6
600 VeCo 93001 451-B6
MAIDSTONE LN
400 THO 91320 556-D1
MAIDU CT
5900 SIMI 93063 479-B7
MAIN RD
- VeCo 93041 583-H3
- VeCo 93042 583-G4
MAIN ST
100 FILM 93015 456-A6
100 VeCo 93040 457-F3
700 SPLA 93060 463-J7
E MAIN ST
- VEN 93001 491-C2
100 SPLA 93060 464-B6
1300 VeCo 93060 464-B6
2300 VEN 93003 491-H4
3900 VEN 93003 492-A4
N MAIN ST
- VeCo 93015 465-E1
- VeCo 93015 455-E7
S MAIN ST
100 VeCo 93015 465-E1
W MAIN ST
- VEN 93001 491-A1
100 SPLA 93060 463-J6
100 SPLA 93060 464-A6
MAINMAST DR
30500 AGRH 91301 557-G5
MAINMAST PL
5600 AGRH 91301 557-G5
MAINSAIL CIR
3800 WLKV 91361 557-B6
MAINSAIL CT
100 PHME 93041 552-E6
MAINSAIL LN
- OXN 93035 522-E7
MAJESTIC CT
- MRPK 93021 496-E2
MAJORCA CT
800 THO 91360 526-C3
MAJORCA DR
1900 OXN 93035 552-A1
MAKENZIE CT
- THO 91362 557-A1
MALAGA CT
600 THO 91320 525-F7
MALAT DR
600 VeCo 91320 525-G7
MALCOLM ST
2000 SIMI 93065 498-A3
MALDEN ST
22300 LA 91304 529-H1
MALIBU AV
100 VeCo 93035 552-B5
200 VEN 93004 492-E1
MALIBU HILLS RD
26700 CALB 91301 558-G7
26700 CALB 91302 558-G7
MALLARD AV
1600 VEN 93003 492-E4
2900 THO 91360 526-F3
MALLARD ST
400 FILM 93015 455-H6
MALLARD WY
100 OXN 93030 522-E5
100 VeCo 93030 522-E5
MALLATT WY
1000 CMRL 93010 524-C3
MALLORY CT
15300 MRPK 93021 477-A4
MALLORY WY
300 OJAI 93022 441-H6
MALO CT
700 SIMI 93065 497-G4
MALONE ST
- PHME 93043 552-D3
E MALTON AV
5800 SIMI 93063 499-A1
N MALTON AV
2100 SIMI 93063 499-B2
MAMMOTH ST
10100 VEN 93004 492-J3
10300 VEN 93004 493-A2
MAMMOTH PEAK DR
- MRPK 93021 476-D6
MANASSAS AV
1400 VEN 93003 492-B4
MANCHESTER CT
2500 THO 91362 527-B3
MANCINI CT
5600 VEN 93003 492-C4
MANDALAY CT
1400 CMRL 93010 524-D1
MANDALAY BEACH RD
500 OXN 93035 521-H6
1200 OXN 93035 551-J1
1900 OXN 93035 552-A2
MANDAN CT
2500 VEN 93001 471-C5
MANDAN PL
400 SIMI 93065 497-D2
MANDELL ST
22300 LA 91304 529-J2
MANDEVILLE PL
23600 VeCo 91377 528-A7
MANDOLIN CIR
- SIMI 93063 478-G5
MANDRILL AV
2000 VEN 93003 492-F5
MANET LN
2400 SIMI 93063 499-B1
MANGO LN
6100 SIMI 93063 499-B3
MANGROVE ST
- MRPK 93021 496-G3
MANLEY CT
25900 LACo 91302 558-J3
MANN CT
- MRPK 93021 476-B5
MANORGATE PL
3200 SIMI 93065 498-D5
MANOR RIDGE RD
600 SPLA 93060 464-A4
MANORVIEW CT
4200 MRPK 93021 496-B3
MANSFIELD LN
100 CMRL 93010 494-E7
100 VeCo 93010 494-E7

MANTON AV
6100 WdHl 91367 529-F7
MANUEL CANYON
23600 VeCo 93001 471-D1
MANZANILLO DR
5200 VeCo 93021 475-G7
5200 VeCo 93021 495-G1
MANZANITA AV
200 VEN 93001 491-E1
MANZANITA CT
400 VEN 93001 491-E1
MANZANITA DR
600 FILM 93015 455-J5
1200 SPLA 93060 464-B3
2200 OXN 93033 552-F2
MANZANITA LN
- THO 91362 557-A3
200 THO 91361 557-A3
200 THO 91361 556-J3
MANZANITA ST
300 CMRL 93012 524-J3
300 CMRL 93012 525-A3
MAPLE CT
200 VEN 93003 491-H3
500 FILM 93015 455-J4
23600 SIMI 93063 499-B3
MAPLE RD
100 THO 91320 556-B2
200 VeCo 91320 556-B2
MAPLE ST
200 OXN 93033 552-G2
1200 SPLA 93060 464-B2
3500 VEN 93003 491-J3
MAPLECREEK WK
- CMRL 93012 524-H2
MAPLECREST ST
11800 MRPK 93021 496-C4
MAPLEGROVE ST
6400 VeCo 91377 558-B2
MAPLEKNOLL PL
3400 THO 91362 527-A1
MAPLELEAF AV
100 THO 91320 555-J2
MAPLERIDGE CT
11400 MRPK 93021 496-B4
MAPLE VIEW CIR
5300 CMRL 93012 525-A2
MAPLEWOOD AV
700 THO 91320 555-G4
MAPLEWOOD CT
700 THO 91320 555-G4
MAPLEWOOD WY
800 PHME 93041 552-F5
MARA AV
- VEN 93004 492-F2
MARBELLA CT
- OXN 93035 522-C6
MARBLEHEAD AV
300 SIMI 93065 497-D7
MARCELLA ST
1700 SIMI 93065 498-C3
MARCELLO AV
100 THO 91320 556-C1
MARCH AV
7500 LA 91304 529-F3
MARCH ST
200 SPLA 93060 463-J6
200 SPLA 93060 464-A6
MARCO DR
1800 CMRL 93010 494-H7
1800 CMRL 93010 524-H1
MARCUS CT
- THO 91320 555-E2
MARCY CT
3300 SIMI 93063 498-D1
MARDIGRAS CT
700 CMRL 93010 524-D2
MARETO WY
700 VeCo 91377 557-H1
MARGARITA AV
400 CMRL 93012 525-A5
MARGATE PL
1500 THO 91361 556-H6
MARGO DR
700 SIMI 93065 497-G3
MARIA DR
6200 VeCo 93021 475-J5
MARIA LN
- VeCo 93010 494-E6
MARIA WY
23600 OXN 93030 522-H4
MARIA HERRERA LN
- OXN 93033 552-H6
MARIAN AV
1500 THO 91360 526-D5
1500 VeCo 91360 526-D5
MARIANO DR
1100 VeCo 93023 451-B1
MARIANO ST
1600 CMRL 93010 493-J5
MARICIO CIR
1900 THO 91360 526-F5
MARICOPA DR
5300 SIMI 93063 478-J7
5400 SIMI 93063 479-A7
MARICOPA HWY Rt#-33
1000 OJAI 93023 441-E6
1000 OJAI 93023 451-F1
1700 VeCo 93023 441-B2
10000 VeCo 93023 366-J6
E MARIE ST
2300 SIMI 93065 498-B1
MARIETTA CIR
2800 THO 91360 526-H3
MARIGOLD AV
1500 VEN 93004 493-A2
MARIGOLD CT
26600 CALB 91302 558-G7
MARIGOLD LN
- SIMI 93065 497-H3
1100 SPLA 93060 464-B3
MARIGOLD PL
1200 THO 91360 526-H2
MARILLA ST
22200 Chat 91311 499-H5
MARILYN CT
3000 THO 91320 555-G2
MARILYN ST
2200 SIMI 93065 498-B1
MARIMAR ST
- THO 91360 526-F5
MARIN LN
7800 VEN 93004 492-E1
MARIN RD
100 SPLA 93060 464-A6
MARIN ST
100 THO 91360 556-E1
MARIN WY
2100 OXN 93033 553-A2

MARINA CIR E
- VeCo 93040 457-F4
MARINA CIR W
300 VeCo 93040 457-F4
MARINA VILLAGE
700 PHME 93041 552-B2
MARINE WY
1400 OXN 93035 551-J1
MARINER CIR
4000 WLKV 91361 557-C6
MARINER CV
2600 PHME 93041 552-C3
MARINER DR
1300 OXN 93033 522-H7
1300 OXN 93033 552-H1
MARINERO PL
- OXN 93030 522-H4
MARINE VIEW DR
- CMRL 93010 494-B7
- VeCo 93010 494-B7
MARINO WY
2000 VEN 93003 492-E5
MARION ST
1000 THO 91320 525-H7
MARIPOSA CT
- LA 91304 529-E2
MARIPOSA DR
100 CMRL 93012 525-A3
200 THO 91320 555-E1
300 VEN 93001 491-E1
400 CMRL 93012 524-J3
1100 SPLA 93060 464-B2
2200 OXN 93036 522-E2
MARIPOSA PL
5100 CMRL 93012 525-A3
MARIPOSA ST
2000 OXN 93036 522-E3
MARISA PL
2400 SIMI 93065 498-A1
MARISOL DR
1600 VEN 93001 491-E2
MARISSA LN
- VeCo 93010 494-D6
MARJORI AV
100 THO 91320 556-C2
MARK CT
700 SIMI 93065 497-G4
5300 AGRH 91301 557-H5
MARK DR
400 SIMI 93065 497-G4
MARK LN
1500 SIMI 93063 499-B3
MARKER ST
100 CMRL 93010 524-D4
MARKET ST
100 PHME 93041 552-E6
300 FILM 93015 456-B6
3400 VEN 93003 491-H4
3800 VeCo 93040 457-E4
4200 VEN 93003 492-A5
4700 VeCo 93003 492-A5
MARKHAM AV
2100 THO 91360 526-F4
MARKS RD
3800 Ago 91301 558-F7
MARK TWAIN LN
600 VEN 93003 492-D3
MARLA AV
8300 LA 91304 529-E2
N MARLBORO LN
- VeCo 91307 528-J4
- VeCo 91307 529-A3
MARLBOROUGH CT
7600 LA 91304 529-F4
E MARLIES AV
5800 SIMI 93063 499-A1
N MARLIES AV
2100 SIMI 93063 499-A2
MARLIES ST
28900 AGRH 91301 558-A3
MARLIN PL
22200 CanP 91303 529-J5
22400 CanP 91307 529-H5
MARLIN WY
5000 OXN 93035 551-J1
5000 OXN 93035 552-A1
MARLOWE ST
1800 THO 91360 526-E5
MARMON AV
1800 THO 91362 557-B3
MARMOTA CT
7400 VEN 93003 492-F4
MARMOTA ST
7000 VEN 93003 492-E4
MARQUAND AV
7700 LA 91304 529-E3
MARQUETTE CIR
14800 MRPK 93021 476-H5
MARQUETTE ST
14700 MRPK 93021 476-J6
N MARQUETTE ST
6400 MRPK 93021 476-J6
MARQUIS CT
7000 VeCo 91377 528-B7
MARQUITA ST
100 OXN 93030 522-J6
N MARQUITA ST
100 OXN 93030 522-H5
MARRISA WY
- CMRL 93012 524-H1
MARSALA WY
- CMRL 93012 524-J1
MARSALIS AV
- VEN 93003 492-C3
MARSDEN CT
25900 LACo 91302 558-J3
MARSEILLE WY
30800 WLKV 91362 557-F5
MARSELLA DR
- OXN 93030 522-J4
MARSHA AV
6200 SIMI 93063 499-B3
MARSHALL AV
2100 SIMI 93063 498-G1
MARSHALL ST
3900 VEN 93003 491-J3
MARSH BROOK RD
2100 VeCo 91361 556-E7
MARSH RONDO
700 CMRL 93010 524-F2
MARTER AV
2200 SIMI 93065 498-A2
N MARTER CT
2200 SIMI 93065 498-A2
MARTHA DR
500 VeCo 91320 525-G7
3000 VEN 93003 491-G2
N MARTHA MORRISON DR
- SIMI 93065 497-D7

S MARTHA MORRISON DR
- SIMI 93065 497-D7
100 SIMI 93065 527-D1
MARTHAS VINEYARD CT
1100 VEN 93001 491-E5
MARTIN CT
6300 VEN 93003 492-D5
MARTIN ST
800 VeCo 93023 451-C3
MARTINDALE AV
200 OJAI 93023 442-A6
MARTINIQUE DR
9500 VeCo 93021 475-H6
MARTINIQUE LN
2100 OXN 93035 552-A2
MARTINIQUE PL
400 THO 91320 525-F7
400 THO 91320 555-F1
MARTIN LUTHER KING JR DR
1400 OXN 93030 522-H4
MARTONA DR
4900 VeCo 91377 557-G1
MARTY CT
- THO 91320 555-G2
MARTZ ST
3600 SIMI 93063 478-E6
N MARVEL AV
2000 SIMI 93065 498-A2
MARVELLA CT
12400 VeCo 93012 496-G6
MARVIEW DR
1600 THO 91362 526-J5
1700 THO 91362 527-A5
MARVIN CT
- SIMI 93065 497-E3
MAR VISTA DR
2300 CMRL 93010 494-G6
2300 VeCo 93010 494-G6
MARY CT
2900 THO 91320 555-H2
MARYGOLD AV
2500 OXN 93033 552-H2
MARYMOUNT CT
400 VeCo 93003 492-B1
400 VEN 93003 492-B1
MARYMOUNT ST
14500 MRPK 93021 476-H5
MARYVILLE AV
400 VEN 93003 492-A1
MASADA WY
- SIMI 93063 479-C7
MASCAGNI ST
4900 VEN 93003 492-A4
MASEFIELD CT
8000 LA 91304 529-E3
MASON CT
3400 SIMI 93063 478-F5
MASON RD
- LACo 90265 586-D7
MASSEY ST
300 THO 91360 526-E5
MASTERSON DR
600 THO 91360 526-G7
MASTHEAD DR
1100 OXN 93035 522-C7
1600 OXN 93035 552-C1
MATILIJA RD
200 VeCo - 366-H6
200 VeCo - 441-A1
200 VeCo 93023 366-H6
200 VeCo 93023 441-A1
MATILIJA RD N
200 VeCo - 441-A1
200 VeCo 93023 441-A1
MATILIJA RD S
- VeCo - 441-A2
700 VeCo 93023 441-A2
MATILIJA ST
100 OJAI 93023 441-H6
W MATILIJA ST
100 OJAI 93023 441-H7
MATTEO ST
4800 VeCo 91377 557-G2
MATTHEWS DR
1500 VEN 93004 492-J3
MAUI LN
1800 OXN 93033 552-J5
1800 OXN 93033 553-A1
MAULHARDT AV
500 OXN 93030 523-B4
MAULHARDT RD
4000 OXN 93033 553-B4
4000 VeCo 93033 553-B4
MAUREEN LN
4700 MRPK 93021 496-C1
MAURICE DR
3900 THO 91320 555-E3
MAURY AV
5900 WdHl 91367 529-C7
E MAVERICK LN
- VeCo 91307 528-G3
MAX CT
23600 SIMI 93065 498-A6
MAXANA DR
400 VeCo 93023 451-D1
MAXINE AV
- VeCo 93022 451-B7
800 OXN 93033 552-F5
800 PHME 93041 552-F5
MAXINE DR
- VeCo 93010 494-E7
MAY CT
2100 SIMI 93063 499-C2
MAYA CIR
- MRPK 93021 496-G3
MAYA LINDA
3300 CMRL 93012 524-G2
MAYALL ST
21900 Chat 91311 499-J4
MAYANS LN
200 VEN 93001 471-C5
MAYA PRADERA LN
- THO 93021 497-A6
MAYBROOK AV
2200 CMRL 93010 494-E7
MAYBROOK WY
1700 SIMI 93065 497-F2
MAYENNE CT
30800 WLKV 91362 557-F5
E MAYFAIR ST
1300 SIMI 93065 497-J1
MAYFIELD CT
200 THO 91320 555-E2
MAYFIELD ST
3500 THO 91320 555-E2
MAYFLOWER ST
- THO 91360 526-F6

E MAYLAND PL
1900 SIMI 93065 498-A5
MAYNARD AV
- THO 91320 555-F2
6800 CanP 91307 529-H4
7600 LA 91304 529-H2
MAYSVILLE CIR
1700 THO 91360 526-C5
MAYWIND LN
23600 SIMI 93065 497-A1
MAYWOOD CT
300 THO 91362 557-G2
MAYWOOD WY
2500 OXN 93033 552-G2
MCAFEE CT
- THO 91360 526-F2
MCANDREW RD
- VeCo 93023 442-F6
MCBEAN RD
5800 VeCo 93066 495-B2
MCBETH CT
4500 MRPK 93021 496-F2
MCCAMPBELL ST
200 FILM 93015 455-J6
MCCLOUD AV
400 THO 91360 526-E7
MCCLOUD RD
8900 VEN 93004 492-H4
MCCOY PL
- SIMI 93065 497-F3
MCCREA RD
2600 THO 91362 527-A1
3500 THO 91362 526-J1
MCCULLOCH ST
2600 CMRL 93010 524-F2
MCDONALD DR
11900 VeCo 93023 451-A1
MC DONALD ST
2200 SIMI 93065 498-A2
MCEDDON PL
100 VEN 93001 491-D1
MCFADDEN AV
300 MRPK 93021 496-E1
W MCFARLANE DR
- VEN 93001 471-B6
E MCFARLANE ST
- VEN 93001 471-C6
MCGILL AV
300 VEN 93003 491-J2
MCGRATH ST
4400 VEN 93003 492-A5
MCGREGER RD
- VeCo 93015 466-J1
- VeCo 93021 466-J1
MCHUGH CT
900 VEN 93003 492-C4
MCKEE ST
- VeCo 93001 471-C2
200 OJAI 93023 441-H6
MCKEEHAN DR
700 PHME 93041 552-F4
MCKENZIE ST
- FILM 93015 456-B6
MCKEVETT HTS
400 SPLA 93060 464-B5
MCKEVETT RD
800 SPLA 93060 464-B5
MCKINLEY AV
100 OXN 93030 522-H6
N MCKINLEY AV
100 OXN 93030 522-H5
MCKINLEY DR
2300 VEN 93003 491-G2
MCKNIGHT RD
1200 VeCo 91320 556-B2
1200 THO 91320 556-B2
S MCKNIGHT RD
100 VeCo 91320 556-B2
MCLAREN AV
6200 WdHl 91367 529-H7
6800 CanP 91307 529-H5
7500 LA 91304 529-H3
MCLEOD RONDO
700 CMRL 93010 524-F2
MCLOUGHLIN AV
1300 OXN 93035 552-D1
MCMILLAN AV
100 OXN 93033 552-G3
MCNAB CT
200 FILM 93015 455-H6
MCNELL RD
100 VeCo 93023 442-E5
MCPHERSON WY
10900 VeCo 93001 450-H5
MCWANE BLVD
400 OXN 93033 552-H7
W MCWANE BLVD
500 OXN 93033 552-G7
MEAD AV
1000 SIMI 93065 497-J4
1200 VEN 93004 492-J2
MEADOW CT
11600 MRPK 93021 496-B2
MEADOW ST
4600 MRPK 93021 496-B2
MEADOW TR
2500 OXN 93036 522-E1
MEADOWBLUFF CT
5300 CMRL 93012 525-A1
MEADOW BROOK CT
1900 THO 91362 526-J3
1900 THO 91362 527-A3
MEADOWBROOK RD
1100 OJAI 93023 441-J5
MEADOWCREST ST
700 THO 91320 555-F4
MEADOW GATE ST
3900 THO 91362 557-C3
MEADOWGLADE DR
6000 VeCo 93021 475-G7
MEADOWGLEN CT
1500 THO 91320 556-A1
MEADOW GROVE LN
200 THO 91362 557-E3
MEADOW HAVEN DR
6300 AGRH 91301 558-A3
MEADOWLAND CT
2300 THO 91361 557-B5
MEADOWLARK DR
- FILM 93015 455-J6
MEADOW LARK LN
1200 OXN 93036 522-E2
MEADOWLARK LN
100 VeCo 91377 557-J3
MEADOWLARK ST
6800 VEN 93003 492-E4
MEADOW MIST CT
200 SIMI 93065 498-A6
MEADOWMIST WY
29500 AGRH 91301 557-J4

MEADOW OAK DR
3200 WLKV 91361 557-C7
MEADOWRIDGE CT
5200 CMRL 93012 524-J1
5200 CMRL 93012 525-A1
MEADOWRUN ST
500 THO 91360 526-G1
MEADOWSIDE DR
2500 THO 91362 527-A3
MEADOWSTONE DR
2900 SIMI 93063 478-C7
MEADOW VIEW CT
1900 THO 91362 526-J5
MEADOWVIEW CT
6700 VEN 93003 472-D6
MEADOW VIEW DR
5100 CMRL 93012 524-J2
5200 CMRL 93012 525-A2
MEADOW VISTA WY
5400 AGRH 91301 557-J5
MEADOWWOOD AV
2900 THO 91360 526-F3
MEANDER DR
1400 SIMI 93065 497-J7
MEDEA LN
- AGRH 91301 558-A5
MEDEABROOK PL
5600 AGRH 91301 557-J5
MEDEA CREEK LN
- VeCo 91377 558-A1
MEDEA VALLEY DR
5500 AGRH 91301 558-A5
MEDFIELD ST
28500 AGRH 91301 558-B5
MEDFORD PL
800 VEN 93004 492-G3
MEDFORD ST
8300 VEN 93004 492-F3
MEDICAL CENTER DR
7100 CanP 91307 529-G5
N MEDICINE BOW CT
200 THO 91362 557-B3
S MEDICINE BOW CT
100 THO 91362 557-B3
N MEDINA AV
2000 SIMI 93063 498-C2
MEEHAM WY
13800 MRPK 93021 496-F3
MEG CT
3300 SIMI 93063 478-D7
MEINERS RD
1800 VeCo 93023 441-E6
MELBA AV
6200 WdHl 91367 529-G7
6600 CanP 91307 529-F4
7500 LA 91304 529-F2
MELBOURNE CT
3600 THO 91320 555-F3
MELFORD CT
2200 VeCo 91361 556-E7
MELIA ST
500 VeCo 93010 524-C1
6200 SIMI 93063 499-B3
MELITO DR
- OXN 93030 522-H4
MELLISA CT
3900 SIMI 93063 478-E6
MELLOW LN
800 SIMI 93065 497-H6
MELODY LN
3000 SIMI 93063 478-E7
MELRAY ST
6400 MRPK 93021 477-A6
MELROSE DR
200 VeCo 93035 552-B4
MELVILLE LN
500 VEN 93003 492-D1
MELVIN CT
3400 VeCo 91320 525-F7
E MELVINA PL
800 SIMI 93065 498-A5
MEMORIAL PKWY
- THO 91360 526-E2
MEMPHIS CT
600 VEN 93004 492-H1
MENCKEN AV
7900 LA 91304 529-E3
MENDOCINO CT
10100 VEN 93004 472-H7
MENDOCINO LN
1500 THO 91320 526-A7
MENDOCINO PL
3000 OXN 93033 553-B3
MENLO ST
6300 SIMI 93063 499-C2
MENLO PARK AV
- VEN 93004 492-G2
MENOTTI LN
4700 VEN 93003 492-B7
MENTA LN
1500 CMRL 93010 524-A1
MERALDA AV
2400 SIMI 93063 499-A1
MERCANTILE ST
700 OXN 93030 522-H7
MERCED DR
800 CMRL 93010 494-F7
MERCED PL
3000 OXN 93033 553-B3
MERCED ST
10500 VEN 93004 472-H7
MERCER AV
600 OJAI 93023 442-A6
600 VEN 93004 492-J1
MERCURY PL
3800 SIMI 93063 498-E2
MEREDITH AV
300 VEN 93003 491-J1
MEREDITH CT
23900 LA 91304 529-E3
MERIDIAN AV
4200 OXN 93035 552-A2
MERIDIAN HILLS DR
- MRPK 93021 476-E6
MERION WY
- OXN 93036 522-C3
MERLIN ST
- VEN 93003 492-D5
E MERRILL CT
3800 SIMI 93063 498-E2
MERRITT AV
300 CMRL 93010 524-F3
MESA AV
- THO 91320 556-A2
MESA CIR
7200 VEN 93003 472-D7
MESA DR
- VeCo 93010 494-E6
100 VeCo 93023 441-D7
200 CMRL 93010 494-E6

VENTURA COUNTY STREET INDEX

STREET — Block City ZIP Pg-Grid

- **MESA DR** — 800 FILM 93015 456-A5; 7800 VeCo 93063 499-F4
- **MESA RD** — 100 WHil 91304 499-D6
- **MESA MINT CT** — - SIMI 93063 498-J3
- **MESA RIDGE AV** — 1600 THO 91362 527-G6
- **MESA SCHOOL RD** — - VeCo 93066 493-H4
- **MESA VERDE AV** — 1400 VEN 93003 492-C5
- **MESA VERDE DR** — 12800 MRPK 93021 496-E2
- **MESCALLERO PL** — 6100 SIMI 93063 479-B6
- **MESQUITE ST** — 500 CMRL 93012 524-J3
- **MESSINA PL** — 600 VeCo 91377 557-G1
- **META ST** — 400 OXN 93030 522-G6; 1000 VEN 93001 491-D2
- **METZ CT** — 1900 SIMI 93065 498-A4
- **MEYER RD** — 1100 VeCo 93023 441-C5
- **MIAMI LN** — 800 VEN 93004 492-J2
- **MICAELA DR** — 5400 AGRH 91301 557-H5
- **MICHAEL DR** — 2200 THO 91320 555-H1; 2900 VeCo 91320 555-G1
- **MICHALE ST** — 22100 LA 91304 529-H1
- **MICHELLE CT** — 3300 SIMI 93063 478-D6
- **MICHELLE DR** — 28800 AGRH 91301 558-B4
- **MICOMA CT** — 5500 SIMI 93063 479-A7
- **MIDBURY HILL RD** — - VeCo 91320 556-B2
- **MIDDLE CREST DR** — 5600 AGRH 91301 557-H4
- **MIDDLE FORK CIR** — 4700 THO 91362 557-D1
- **MIDDLEGATE RD** — 3900 WLKV 91361 557-D6
- **MIDDLE RANCH RD** — - VeCo 93021 476-G3
- **MIDDLE RANGE FIRE RD** — 23600 VeCo - 467-D7; 23600 VeCo - 477-E1; 23600 VeCo - 478-A1; 23600 VeCo 93021 466-J7; 23600 VeCo 93021 467-A7; 23600 VeCo 93021 476-G1; 23600 VeCo 93021 477-E1; 23600 VeCo 93063 478-D2; 23600 VeCo 93065 478-D2
- **MIDDLESBURY RIDGE CIR** — 7000 CanP 91307 529-E5
- **MIDNIGHT MOON LN** — 23600 SIMI 93065 497-A1
- **MIDWAY DR** — 4500 PHME 93041 552-E5
- **MIGUEL LN** — 400 OXN 93030 522-H4
- **MIKA WY** — - OXN 93030 522-H4
- **MILAGRO PL** — - OXN 93030 523-A4
- **MILAN DR** — 1400 SIMI 93065 497-G3
- **MILANO PL** — 4000 MRPK 93021 496-C4
- **MILBURN ST** — 1900 CMRL 93010 524-E3
- **MILDRED ST** — 5200 SIMI 93063 498-J3
- **MILESTONE AV** — - SIMI 93065 477-J7
- **MILL CT** — 23600 SIMI 93065 497-F7
- **MILL DR** — - VeCo 93001 471-C3
- **MILL PL** — 1000 SPLA 93060 464-B4
- **N MILL ST** — 100 SPLA 93060 464-B4
- **S MILL ST** — 100 SPLA 93060 464-B6
- **MILLARD ST** — - MRPK 93021 496-E1
- **MILLBRAE CT** — 200 VEN 93004 492-G2
- **MILL CANYON RD** — 23600 VeCo 93001 460-G7; 23600 VeCo 93001 470-H1; 23600 VeCo 93001 471-A1
- **MILL CREEK CT** — 3500 THO 91360 526-H2
- **MILLCROFT CT** — 700 SIMI 93065 498-D5
- **MILLER CT** — 800 VEN 93003 492-C3
- **MILLER PKWY** — 100 MRPK 93021 496-F2
- **MILLER PL** — - THO 91362 527-C3; 100 SPLA 93060 464-C5
- **E MILLERTON RD** — 13100 MRPK 93021 496-E2
- **N MILLERTON RD** — 4400 MRPK 93021 496-E2
- **MILLIGAN DR** — 1000 CMRL 93010 524-G2
- **MILLIGAN BARRANCA RD** — 4000 VeCo 93066 494-C2; 4600 VeCo 93066 474-C7
- **MILLPARK LN** — 23600 SIMI 93065 497-A2
- **MILLS RD** — - PHME 93043 552-C3
- **N MILLS RD** — - VEN 93003 491-H2
- **S MILLS RD** — - VEN 93003 491-H3
- **MILLTRACE WY** — - SIMI 93065 497-F3
- **MILL VALLEY RD** — 4300 MRPK 93021 496-F2
- **MILLVILLE CT** — 1900 THO 91360 526-D5
- **MILLWOOD CT** — 9900 VEN 93004 492-J3
- **MILLWOOD ST** — 9800 VEN 93004 492-J3
- **MILNE CT** — 15800 MRPK 93021 477-A5
- **MILPAS ST** — 4200 CMRL 93012 524-H4
- **MILTON AV** — 700 VEN 93003 491-H4
- **MILTON ST** — - VeCo 93022 451-B7
- **MIMOSA CT** — 5600 VeCo 91377 557-J2
- **MINDENVALE CT** — 400 SIMI 93065 527-D1
- **MINE RD** — - VeCo - 478-G2
- **MINERAL WELLS DR** — 3000 SIMI 93063 478-G7
- **MINERS CANDLE CT** — - SIMI 93063 498-J2
- **MINGUS DR** — 30800 WLKV 91362 557-F3
- **MINNA ST** — 3300 VeCo 93036 492-J7
- **MINNECOTA DR** — 4100 THO 91360 496-J7
- **MINOR ST** — 300 MRPK 93021 496-F1
- **MINSTREL AV** — 6900 CanP 91307 529-G4; 7600 LA 91304 529-G3
- **MINT LN** — 400 VEN 93001 491-E1
- **MINT WY** — 2400 OXN 93036 522-F2
- **MINUET PL** — 400 VeCo 93022 451-B7
- **MINUTEMAN WY** — 30900 AGRH 91301 557-F6; 30900 WLKV 91361 557-F6
- **MIPOLOMOL RD** — 8100 VeCo 90265 585-F5
- **MIRABELLA ST** — 23600 MRPK 93021 496-C4
- **MIRADA LN** — - OXN 93033 553-C4
- **MIRA FLORES CT** — 300 CMRL 93012 525-A2
- **MIRAGE CT** — 700 THO 91320 555-G6
- **MIRA LOMA CIR** — 500 OXN 93030 522-E6; 500 OXN 93035 522-E6
- **MIRAMAR CT** — 2900 OXN 93035 522-C7
- **MIRAMAR DR** — 1700 VEN 93001 491-E1
- **MIRAMAR PL** — 2400 OXN 93035 522-D7
- **MIRAMAR ST** — - CMRL 93010 524-D4
- **MIRAMAR WK** — 2000 OXN 93035 552-D1; 2100 OXN 93035 522-D7
- **MIRAMAR WY** — 3300 OXN 93035 522-B7
- **MIRAMONTE DR** — 200 OXN 93036 522-J2
- **MIRA MONTES** — 7800 VeCo 93063 499-F3
- **MIRA SOL DR** — 4700 MRPK 93021 496-B2
- **MIRASOL LN** — - OXN 93036 522-H3
- **MIRROR LAKE AV** — 1900 VeCo 93023 451-C3
- **MISSILE WY** — - PHME 93043 552-C5
- **W MISSION AV** — - VEN 93001 491-B1
- **MISSION CIR** — 11300 Chat 91311 499-H1
- **MISSION DR** — - CMRL 93010 494-D7; - CMRL 93010 524-D1; 100 VeCo 93010 494-D6
- **MISSION PZ** — - VEN 93001 491-B2
- **MISSION TER** — 900 VeCo 93010 494-D6
- **MISSION HILLS DR** — - OXN 93036 522-C3
- **MISSION OAKS BLVD** — 3000 CMRL 93012 524-F3; 5100 CMRL 93012 525-A2; 6200 CMRL 93012 495-B7
- **MISSION ROCK RD** — 100 VeCo 93060 473-F3
- **MISSION VERDE DR** — 5400 CMRL 93012 525-A1
- **MISTLETOE RD** — 8000 VeCo 93060 453-J5
- **MISTRAL PL** — 2000 OXN 93035 522-D6
- **MISTY CT** — 5900 AGRH 91301 558-B4
- **MISTY CANYON AV** — 600 THO 91362 557-G1
- **MISTY CREEK RD** — 1600 THO 91362 527-G6
- **MISTY FALLS CT** — 300 SIMI 93065 497-E6
- **MISTY GROVE ST** — 12400 MRPK 93021 496-D4
- **MISTY HOLLOW CT** — 4100 MRPK 93021 496-D3
- **MISTY LAKE CT** — 500 SIMI 93065 497-E6
- **MISTYMEADOW ST** — 4300 MRPK 93021 496-D3
- **MISTY TRAILS PL** — 400 SIMI 93065 497-E6
- **MITCHELL RD** — 800 THO 91320 525-J7
- **MOBERLY CT** — 2300 THO 91360 526-B4
- **MOBIL AV** — - CMRL 93010 524-E2
- **MOBIL LN** — 100 VeCo 93001 461-A3
- **MOBILE ST** — 22300 CanP 91303 529-J7; 22600 CanP 91307 529-E7
- **MOBIL PIER RD** — 23600 VeCo 93001 459-E6
- **MOBY DICK LN** — 700 OXN 93030 522-E7
- **MOCKINGBIRD CT** — - VeCo 91377 557-J2
- **MOCKINGBIRD LN** — 400 FILM 93015 455-H6; 2100 OXN 93033 553-A4
- **MOCKINGBIRD ST** — 6200 VEN 93003 492-D4
- **MODELLO CANYON RD** — 23600 VeCo 93040 367-D7; 23600 VeCo 93040 457-G1
- **MODENA PL** — 5500 AGRH 91301 557-G5
- **MODESTO AV** — 200 VEN 93004 492-E1; 1000 CMRL 93010 524-D2
- **MODOC CT** — - VEN 93004 472-J7
- **MODOC DR** — 3300 OXN 93033 553-B3
- **MODOC ST** — 10500 VEN 93004 472-J7
- **MOFFATT CIR** — 700 SIMI 93065 497-J5
- **MOHAVE DR** — 5100 SIMI 93063 478-J7
- **MOHAWK AV** — - THO 91362 557-A2; 2800 VEN 93001 471-C5
- **MOHICAN LN** — 2300 VEN 93001 471-C6
- **MOHICAN ST** — 6100 SIMI 93063 479-B6
- **MOJAVE DR** — 1600 VEN 93004 492-H4
- **E MOLINE ST** — 4100 SIMI 93063 478-F6
- **MOLLISON DR** — 300 SIMI 93065 497-F6
- **MOLLY CT** — 2900 VeCo 91320 555-G1
- **MONACO CT** — 30800 WLKV 91362 557-G6
- **MONACO DR** — 2300 OXN 93035 552-B2
- **MONARCH CT** — 2400 SIMI 93063 498-H1
- **MONDEGO PL** — 700 THO 91360 526-C3
- **MONDOVI CT** — 3900 MRPK 93021 496-C4
- **MONET CT** — 1500 OXN 93033 552-J4
- **MONET DR** — 9900 VeCo 93021 475-J6
- **MONET PL** — 1000 OXN 93033 552-J4
- **MONICA CIR** — 100 THO 91320 555-G2
- **MONITA DR** — 1700 VEN 93001 491-E1
- **MONMOUTH DR** — 2100 VEN 93001 491-E4
- **MONMOUTH WY** — 600 VEN 93001 491-E4
- **MONO CT** — 4900 VEN 93003 492-A1
- **MONO ST** — 1900 OXN 93036 522-J3
- **MONROE AV** — 15300 MRPK 93021 476-J5
- **MONROE ST** — 3900 VEN 93003 491-J3
- **MONTAGNE WY** — 3100 THO 91362 526-J2
- **MONTAIR DR** — 23600 MRPK 93021 496-A1
- **MONTALVO DR** — 6000 VeCo 93003 492-D6; 6000 VEN 93003 492-D6
- **MONTANA CIR** — 300 VeCo 93023 441-F6
- **MONTANA DR** — 1900 VEN 93003 492-C5
- **MONTANA RD** — 100 OJAI 93023 441-E7; 100 VeCo 93023 441-E7
- **MONTAUK LN** — 1000 VEN 93001 491-E4
- **MONT BLANC DR** — 700 VEN 93001 491-D1
- **MONT CALABASAS DR** — - Ago 91301 558-G3; - LACo 91302 558-G3
- **MONTCLAIR DR** — 700 SPLA 93060 464-A4; 6200 VEN 93003 472-C7
- **MONTE CT** — 500 VeCo 93022 451-A6
- **MONTEBELLO AV** — 200 VEN 93004 492-F2
- **MONTEBELLO ST** — 1100 SPLA 93060 464-C6
- **MONTE CARLO DR** — 3000 THO 91362 527-A2; 3100 THO 91362 526-J2
- **MONTE CARLO ST** — 600 OXN 93035 522-B6
- **MONTECITO AV** — 23600 THO 91362 527-B5
- **MONTELEONE AV** — 800 VeCo 91377 557-H1
- **MONTENEGRO CIR** — - THO 91320 555-F1
- **MONTEREY CT** — 3900 THO 91320 555-E1
- **MONTEREY DR** — - VeCo 93022 451-D4
- **MONTEREY PL** — 23600 SPLA 93060 464-B4
- **MONTEREY ST** — 3000 OXN 93033 552-F3
- **MONTE SERENO DR** — 900 THO 91360 526-D6
- **MONTESSA DR** — 5800 CMRL 93012 525-B1
- **MONTE VIA** — - VeCo 93022 451-A6
- **MONTEVINA CIR** — - OXN 93030 523-B4
- **MONTE VISTA** — - THO 91320 525-E6
- **MONTE VISTA AV** — 500 VEN 93003 472-D7
- **MONTE VISTA CT** — 6900 VEN 93003 472-D7
- **MONTE VISTA DR** — 800 SPLA 93060 464-B4; 1700 CMRL 93010 524-D3
- **MONTE VISTA PL** — 400 SPLA 93060 464-A4
- **MONTGOMERY AV** — 100 VeCo 93036 492-J5; 500 VEN 93004 492-G2; 1300 VeCo 93004 492-G4
- **MONTGOMERY CT** — 900 THO 91360 526-G5; 8300 VEN 93004 492-G3
- **MONTGOMERY PL** — 700 VEN 93004 492-G3
- **MONTGOMERY RD** — 1400 THO 91360 526-G5; 9200 Chat 91311 499-F7
- **MONTGOMERY ST** — 100 OJAI 93023 441-J5
- **S MONTGOMERY ST** — 100 OJAI 93023 441-H7
- **MONTGOMERY FIRE RD** — 23600 SIMI 93065 498-A7; 23600 SIMI 93065 528-B1
- **MONTICELLO AV** — 3300 SIMI 93063 478-F6
- **MONTILLA CIR** — 800 THO 91360 526-C3
- **MONTROSE DR** — 2000 THO 91362 527-A6
- **MONTROSE ST** — 1700 OXN 93033 552-H1
- **MONTSALAS CT** — - CMRL 93012 524-H1
- **MONTVIEW CT** — 2700 WLKV 91361 557-A7
- **MONUMENT ST** — - SIMI 93063 498-H1
- **MOODY CT** — - THO 91360 556-G1
- **MOON DR** — 5700 VEN 93003 492-C5; 5900 VeCo 93003 492-C5
- **MOONCREST CT** — 3300 THO 91320 555-G2
- **MOONDANCE ST** — 400 THO 91360 526-D2
- **MOONFLOWER CIR** — 2800 THO 91360 526-H3
- **MOONLIGHT CT** — 3500 THO 91362 527-D3
- **MOONLIGHT PARK AV** — - OXN 93036 492-G7
- **MOONRIDGE AV** — 300 THO 91320 555-J2; 400 VeCo 91320 555-J2
- **MOONSEED LN** — 23600 SIMI 93065 497-A2
- **MOONSHADOW CIR** — 1700 CMRL 93012 495-B7; 1700 CMRL 93012 525-A1
- **MOONSHADOW ST** — 5300 SIMI 93063 478-J6; 5500 SIMI 93063 479-A6
- **MOONSONG CT** — - MRPK 93021 496-E1
- **MOONSTONE AV** — - SIMI 93065 478-A7
- **MOONSTONE WY** — 5000 OXN 93035 521-J7
- **MOORCROFT AV** — 6500 CanP 91303 529-J4; 7600 LA 91304 529-J3; 8800 LA 91304 499-J7
- **MOORCROFT PL** — 8700 LA 91304 529-J1
- **MOORE ST** — 1700 SIMI 93065 497-J4; 1700 SIMI 93065 498-A4
- **MOORE CANYON RD** — - CanP 91307 529-C7; 23600 VeCo 91302 529-C7; 23600 VeCo 91307 529-C7
- **MOORING WK** — 1100 OXN 93030 522-F7
- **MOORPARK AV** — 100 MRPK 93021 496-E2; 100 VeCo 93035 552-B5; 100 VeCo 93043 552-B5
- **MOORPARK AV Rt#-23** — - MRPK 93021 476-E7; 500 MRPK 93021 496-E1
- **N MOORPARK AV Rt# 23** — - MRPK 93021 496-E1
- **MOORPARK RD** — - VeCo 93012 496-G4; - VeCo 93021 496-G4
- **N MOORPARK RD** — 200 THO 91360 556-F1; 500 THO 91360 526-F1; 3100 THO 91360 496-G6; 3100 THO 93012 496-G6; 3100 VeCo 93012 496-G6
- **S MOORPARK RD** — - THO 91360 556-E2; - THO 91361 556-E2
- **MORADO PL** — - OXN 93030 522-H4
- **MORAGA CT** — 2400 SIMI 93065 498-A1
- **MORAINE WY** — 2500 OXN 93030 522-D4
- **MORANDA PKWY** — 100 PHME 93041 552-F6
- **MORELAND RD** — - SIMI 93065 497-E2
- **MORELIA CT** — 600 VeCo 91360 526-C6
- **MORENA LN** — 4100 OXN 93033 553-C4
- **MORENO DR** — 800 VeCo 93023 451-B1; 1400 SIMI 93063 498-D3
- **MORGAN CIR** — 2800 CMRL 93010 494-E7
- **E MORGAN RD** — - VeCo 91307 528-H4
- **MORGAN ST** — 1700 VeCo 93023 451-C3
- **MORGAN CANYON RD** — - VeCo 93066 464-D7
- **MORGAN HILL ST** — 200 SIMI 93065 527-E1
- **MORLEY ST** — 1600 SIMI 93065 498-A3
- **MORNING ARBOR WY** — 1600 SIMI 93065 497-F2
- **MORNING GLORY ST** — 2000 SIMI 93065 498-A2
- **MORNING RIDGE AV** — - THO 91362 527-D2
- **MORNINGSIDE DR** — 2800 THO 91362 526-J3; 2800 THO 91362 527-A2
- **MORNINGSTAR AV** — 23600 THO 91360 526-E2
- **MORNING VIEW CT** — 1900 THO 91362 526-J1
- **MORNINGWOOD WY** — 3600 SIMI 93065 497-A1
- **MOROCCO LN** — 9300 WHil 91304 499-E7
- **MORONGO DR** — 1600 CMRL 93012 525-D1; 1700 CMRL 93012 495-D7
- **MORRIS DR** — 500 FILM 93015 456-A4
- **MORRIS ST** — 1300 OXN 93030 522-J5
- **MORRISON LN** — 400 SPLA 93060 463-H6
- **MORRISON RANCH RD** — - Ago 91301 558-F4; 26400 CALB 91302 558-F4; 26400 LACo 91302 558-F4
- **MORRO WY** — 700 OXN 93033 552-H3
- **MORRO BAY LN** — 5600 VEN 93003 492-C4
- **MORROW CIR** — 1300 THO 91362 527-A6
- **MORSE AV** — 800 VEN 93003 491-J5
- **MORVALE DR** — 2900 VeCo 91361 586-D2
- **MOSER RD** — 1300 VeCo 91320 555-J3; 2100 THO 91320 555-J3
- **MOSES LN** — 500 VEN 93003 492-D1
- **MOSS CT** — 2100 THO 91362 526-J4
- **MOSS LANDING BLVD** — - OXN 93036 492-H7
- **MOTT CT** — 11000 VeCo 93012 526-B1
- **MOTT PL** — 23600 VeCo 93060 453-G2
- **MOULTRIE PL** — 200 SPLA 93060 464-A7; 200 SPLA 93060 463-J7
- **MOUND AV** — 3500 VEN 93003 491-H2
- **MOUNTAIN CREEK DR** — 3900 THO 91320 555-E3
- **MOUNTAIN CREST CIR** — - THO 91362 557-A1
- **MOUNTAIN LION RD** — 11900 VeCo 93023 452-H1
- **MOUNTAIN LOOKOUT RD** — - VeCo 93066 474-C1
- **S MOUNTAIN LOOKOUT RD** — 23600 VeCo 93066 474-H2; 23600 VeCo 93066 475-A2
- **MOUNTAIN MEADOW DR** — 4200 MRPK 93021 496-C3
- **MOUNTAIN OAK PL** — 1000 THO 91320 556-C1
- **MOUNTAIN PARK CT** — 4100 MRPK 93021 496-B2
- **MOUNTAIN SHADOW CT** — 2900 THO 91360 526-B2
- **MOUNTAIN TRAIL AV** — 3300 THO 91320 555-G4
- **MOUNTAIN TRAIL ST** — 11200 MRPK 93021 496-B3
- **MOUNTAIN VIEW AV** — 500 OXN 93030 522-H6; 800 OJAI 93023 441-J5; 900 OJAI 93023 442-A5
- **MOUNTAIN VIEW DR** — - LACo 91302 558-J3; 5500 CMRL 93012 525-A3
- **MOUNTAIN VIEW RD** — 1200 VeCo 91320 556-B3
- **MOUNTAIN VIEW ST** — - VeCo 93022 451-B7; 100 FILM 93015 456-B5
- **MOUNTAIN VISTA LN** — - SIMI 93065 498-A6
- **MOUNTCLEF BLVD** — 2800 THO 91360 526-F3
- **MOUNT PINOS RD** — 23600 VeCo - 367-A1
- **MOUNT SINAI DR** — 23600 SIMI 93063 479-B7; 23600 SIMI 93063 499-C1
- **MOUNT WHITNEY CT** — 100 VEN 93003 492-C2
- **MOWER CT** — 900 THO 91362 526-J7
- **MOZART LN** — 5000 VEN 93003 492-B4
- **MUD CREEK RD** — - VeCo 93060 453-J5; - VeCo 93060 454-A5
- **MUGU RD** — 1300 VeCo 93041 583-G2; 1300 VeCo 93042 583-F4
- **MUIR ST** — 1200 VeCo 93015 455-G4; 5800 SIMI 93063 499-A2
- **N MUIRFIELD AV** — 800 SIMI 93065 498-A5
- **MUIRFIELD DR** — 1600 OXN 93036 522-E2
- **E MUIRWOOD CT** — 2800 SIMI 93063 478-H7
- **N MUIRWOOD CT** — 2700 SIMI 93063 478-H7
- **MULBERRY CIR** — 3000 THO 91360 526-H2
- **MULBERRY DR** — - VeCo 93001 471-C3
- **MULBERRY LN** — - VeCo 93023 441-E6
- **MULBERRY PL** — 23600 SIMI 93063 499-B3
- **MULBERRY RIDGE DR** — 5600 CMRL 93012 525-B2
- **MULCAHEY DR** — 1700 VeCo 93033 553-F7
- **MULHOLLAND HWY** — 32400 LACo 90265 586-J5; 35500 LACo 90265 625-J3
- **MULHOLLAND HWY Rt#-23** — 33000 LACo 90265 586-G6
- **MUNDA DR** — 1100 PHME 93041 552-E4
- **MUNGER DR** — 500 SPLA 93060 463-H6
- **MUNNINGS WY** — 2700 VeCo 91361 586-C1
- **MUNSON ST** — 1800 CMRL 93010 524-F1; 1800 CMRL 93010 494-F7
- **MUPU AV** — 100 SPLA 93060 464-A5
- **MUPU RD** — - VeCo 93060 453-J4
- **MURDOCH LN** — 700 VEN 93003 492-D3
- **MUREAU RD** — 25400 CALB 91302 558-J5; 25400 LACo 91302 558-J5
- **MURPHY LN** — 1800 OXN 93033 553-B4
- **MURRAY AV** — - CMRL 93010 524-D3
- **MURRE WY** — 3800 OXN 93035 552-B4
- **MURRIETA ST** — 5400 VEN 93003 492-B3
- **MUSTANG CT** — 1700 VeCo 93023 451-C3
- **MUSTANG DR** — 5700 SIMI 93063 479-A6
- **N MUSTANG LN** — - VeCo 91307 528-H4
- **MUTAU CIR** — 200 FILM 93015 455-J6
- **MUTAU FLAT RD** — - VeCo - 366-L2
- **MYRNA DR** — 500 PHME 93041 552-F6
- **MYRNA-JOYCE DR** — 800 OXN 93033 552-F5; 800 PHME 93033 552-F5; 800 PHME 93041 552-F5
- **MYRTLE CT** — - SIMI 93063 499-B2; 5100 VeCo 91377 557-H1
- **MYRTLE ST** — - OXN 93036 522-H1
- **MYSTIC LN** — 7300 CanP 91307 529-E5

N

- **N ST** — 400 OXN 93030 522-E5; 1100 OXN 93033 522-E7; 1100 OXN 93033 552-E1
- **NACIMIENTO AV** — - VEN 93004 492-J3
- **NADADOR PL** — - OXN 93030 522-J4
- **NADINE CT** — - THO 91320 555-G2
- **NADIR ST** — 23600 LA 91304 529-E2
- **NAHUA LN** — 2300 VEN 93001 471-D6
- **NANCHARO RD** — 2100 VeCo 93012 496-A7; 2100 VeCo 93012 526-A1
- **NANCY CIR** — 1800 THO 91362 526-J6
- **NANCY ST** — - VeCo 93010 494-D7
- **NANDINA CIR** — 2400 OXN 93036 522-G2
- **NANDINA CT** — 2300 OXN 93036 522-F2
- **NANDINA PL** — 300 OXN 93036 522-F2
- **NANNYBERRY CT** — - MRPK 93021 496-F2
- **NANTUCKET PKWY** — 3600 OXN 93035 522-B6
- **NAPA CT** — 23600 SIMI 93065 497-G7
- **NAPA ST** — 3000 OXN 93033 552-E3; 22100 LA 91304 529-H1
- **NAPLES CT** — 1300 SIMI 93065 497-F3
- **NAPLES DR** — 2900 OXN 93035 522-C6
- **NAPOLEON AV** — 1800 OXN 93033 552-J2; 1800 OXN 93033 553-A2; 5500 VeCo 91377 527-H6
- **NAPOLI DR** — 2000 OXN 93035 552-B2
- **NAPOLI PL** — 4000 MRPK 93021 496-C4
- **NARANJA** — 700 VeCo 93015 455-D5
- **NARANJA LN** — - OXN 93036 522-J3
- **NARDO ST** — 10900 VeCo 93004 493-A2
- **NARROWS CT** — 1700 OXN 93035 552-C1
- **NASH LN** — 1800 OXN 93033 553-B4
- **NASHVILLE PL** — 1900 OXN 93033 553-A5
- **NASSAU DR** — 2100 OXN 93036 522-E2
- **NATALIE LN** — 8300 LA 91304 529-F2
- **NATALIE PL** — 1600 OXN 93030 522-D4
- **NATALIE WY** — - VeCo 93010 494-E7
- **NATASHA CT** — 5300 AGRH 91301 557-H5
- **NATHAN LN** — 1300 VEN 93001 491-F5
- **NAUMAN RD** — 5600 VeCo 93033 553-E5
- **NAUTICAL WY** — 1200 OXN 93030 522-E7
- **NAUTILUS ST** — 4900 OXN 93035 521-J7; 4900 OXN 93035 551-J1
- **NAVAJO AV** — 2700 THO 91362 557-A2
- **NAVAL AIR RD** — 7800 VeCo 93041 583-G1; 15100 VeCo 93041 553-F6; 15100 VeCo 93042 553-F6; 18500 VeCo 93033 553-F6
- **NAVARRO ST** — 300 OXN 93030 522-J6
- **NAVIGATOR DR** — 1100 VEN 93001 491-G6
- **NAVIGATOR WY** — - OXN 93035 522-E7
- **NAVITO WY** — - OXN 93030
- **NAVY LN** — 1000 OXN 93035
- **NEAL CT** — 1100 SIMI 93065
- **NEAP CT** — 3100 OXN 93035
- **NEAP PL** — 3000 OXN 93035
- **NEATH ST** — 8400 VEN 93004
- **NEBULA ST** — 2800 OXN 93030
- **NECTARINE ST** — 200 OXN 93033
- **NEDDY AV** — 6100 WdHl 91367; 6400 CanP 91307
- **NEEDLES ST** — 22100 Chat 91311
- **NEISH ST** — 100 VeCo 93010
- **E NELDA ST** — 5900 SIMI 93063
- **NELLIE CT** — 200 THO 91320
- **NELLORA ST** — - CMRL 93010
- **NELSON PL** — 1000 OXN 93033
- **NELSON RD** — - MRPK 93021
- **NEMESIS CT** — - PHME 93043
- **NEPTUNE PL** — 2500 PHME 93041
- **NEPTUNE SQ** — 5100 OXN 93035; 5100 OXN 93035
- **NET CT** — 2900 OXN 93035
- **NET PL** — 3100 OXN 93035
- **NETTLEBROOK ST** — 1900 THO 91361
- **NEVA CIR** — 3400 THO 91320
- **NEVADA AV** — - VEN 93004; 3000 OXN 93033; 6100 WdHl 91367; 6500 CanP 91303; 7700 LA 91304; 8900 LA 91304; 9600 Chat 91311
- **NEVELSON LN** — 5900 SIMI 93063
- **NEVIN AV** — 1400 VEN 93004
- **NEW ST** — 1000 SPLA 93060
- **NEWARK WY** — 10000 VEN 93004
- **NEW BEDFORD CT** — 1100 VEN 93001
- **NEWBOLT LN** — 500 VEN 93003
- **NEWBURY LN** — - VeCo 91320
- **NEWBURY RD** — 800 THO 91320; 1900 THO 91320
- **NEWCASTLE DR** — - OXN 93036
- **NEWCASTLE ST** — 400 THO 91361
- **NEWCOMB DR** — 300 VEN 93003
- **NEWGATE RD** — 6900 CanP 91307
- **NEW HAVEN PL** — 2200 OXN 93035
- **NEW HAVEN ST** — - VEN 93004
- **NEWHAVEN ST** — 4900 VeCo 91377
- **NEWMAN ST** — - VEN 93003; 1200 SIMI 93065
- **NEWMAN RANCH RD** — 23600 VeCo 93001; 23600 VeCo 93001
- **NEWPORT AV** — 200 VEN 93004
- **NEWPORT CIR** — 1300 THO 91360; 7000 CanP 91307
- **NEWPORT WEIGH** — 23600 OXN 93035
- **NEWQUIST CT** — 2200 CMRL 93010
- **NEWTOWN ST** — 8400 VEN 93004
- **NEY CT** — 1000 SIMI 93065
- **NICE CT** — 4000 OXN 93035
- **NICHOLAS ST** — 2500 SIMI 93065
- **NICOLE DR** — 500 THO 91320
- **NICOLLE ST** — 5700 VEN 93003
- **NIDIA WY** — - OXN 93030
- **NIELSEN ST** — - VEN 93003
- **NIGHTFALL PL** — 3200 SIMI 93063
- **NIGHTINGALE PL** — 800 OXN 93036
- **NIGHTINGALE ST** — 6300 VEN 93003; 11800 MRPK 93021
- **NIGHT JASMINE DR** — - SIMI 93065; - SIMI 93065
- **NIGHT RAIN LN** — 23600 SIMI 93065
- **NIGHTSKY DR** — 13200 VeCo 93012
- **NIGHTWIND LN** — 23600 SIMI 93065
- **NIKE ZEUS RD** — - VeCo 93042
- **NILE RIVER DR** — - OXN 93036
- **NILES ST** — 2700 SIMI 93065

VENTURA COUNTY STREET INDEX

STREET
Block City ZIP Pg-Grid

PL
VEN 93003 492-F4
N
OXN 93036 492-H7
DR
OXN 93033 552-H4
R
OXN 93030 522-J4
WdHl 91367 529-J7
CanP 91303 529-J4
LA 91304 529-J3
Chat 91311 499-J5
N
OXN 93030 522-H4
T
VEN 93003 492-E1
L LN
VEN 93003 472-C7
RD
SIMI 93065 497-F5
REE CT
VeCo 91377 557-H1
DR
OXN 93030 522-H4
ST
VEN 93001 471-D5
R
SIMI 93065 498-B3
S AV
MRPK 93021 476-G7
A AV
VeCo 93001 450-E3
CT
THO 91362 527-A6
WY
OXN 93030 522-G4
IR
SIMI 93063 478-F7
LANT DR
SIMI 93065 497-H6
DE WY
OXN 93035 522-E7
VK
OXN 93030 522-J5
O ST
VEN 93004 492-J1
FF RD
VeCo 93023 442-E7
VeCo 93023 452-E1
FF ST
Chat 91311 499-J7
AN DR
CMRL 93010 524-C2
D CT
VeCo 91361 556-E7
ET LN
SIMI 93065 497-D6
K CT
MRPK 93021 496-E2
PL
OXN 93030 522-D4
CT
VeCo 93010 494-E7
OXN 93036 522-E2
ST
OXN 93036 522-E3
WY
SIMI 93063 499-B3
N AV
THO 91360 526-F6
AN AV
THO 91360 526-F6
NDY DR
LACo 91302 558-G3
NDY TER
VeCo 91377 528-B7
AN CT
OXN 93030 522-E6
ST
VeCo 93066 494-J4
VeCo 93066 495-A4
M AV
THO 91320 555-J1
AMERICAN CUT
VeCo 93063 499-C5
BANK DR
VEN 93003 492-E6
VEN 93004 492-J3
VeCo 93004 493-A2
VEN 93004 493-A2
ROOK DR
OXN 93036 522-E1
REST CT
SIMI 93063 478-E7
DALE DR
MRPK 93021 496-C3
AKE CIR
THO 91361 557-B5
AND ST
THO 91320 555-E2
ARK ST
THO 91362 527-A4
ORT LN
OXN 93035 522-C6
IDGE DR
VeCo 93066 493-F3
HORE LN
THO 91361 557-B5
TAR CV
PHME 93041 552-C3
TAR LN
OXN 93036 522-E1
VALLEY DR
THO 91362 557-C2
VIEW DR
THO 91362 527-D6
WIND CT
VEN 93003 492-B4
WOOD PKWY
THO 91360 526-H2
WOODS VIEW RD
CanP 91307 529-E5
N AV
VEN 93003 492-E5
N ST
OXN 93033 552-J2
K ST
VEN 93004 492-H2
Y DR
VeCo 93001 471-C1
VeCo 93001 461-C7
CH AV
THO 91360 526-F6
CH LN
VEN 93001 491-E5
OD CT
VEN 93004 492-J2

STREET
Block City ZIP Pg-Grid

NOTRE DAME AV
9200 Chat 91311 499-F7
9200 Chat 91311 499-F7
9200 Chat 91311 499-F6
NOTTINGHAM DR
700 OXN 93030 522-E4
NOTTINGWOOD CIR
1200 THO 91361 557-B5
NOVA CT
4900 VEN 93003 492-A1
NOVA LN
1300 VeCo 93023 451-E2
NOVARA WY
500 VeCo 91377 557-G1
NOVATO DR
600 OXN 93035 522-D7
1300 OXN 93035 552-D1
NOVINA PL
500 CMRL 93012 524-J3
N NOWAK AV
1800 THO 91360 526-E5
NUEVE CT
300 CMRL 93012 525-A3
NUEVO CANYON RD
- VeCo 93040 367-E7
- VeCo 93040 458-C1
NO 2 CANYON FIRE RD
23600 MRPK 93021 477-B3
23600 VeCo - 477-B3
23600 VeCo 93021 477-B3
23600 VeCo 93065 477-B3
NUMBER TEN CANYON RD
- VeCo - 367-E9
23600 VeCo 93040 367-E9
23600 VeCo 93040 458-D7
NUTCRACKER CT
- THO 91320 526-A5
NUTMEG CIR
2600 SIMI 93065 498-C1
NUTWOOD CIR
5700 SIMI 93063 499-A2
NYE RD
8600 VeCo 93001 461-A3
NYELAND AV
3200 VeCo 93036 523-C2
NYE RANCH FIRE RD
23600 VeCo 93001 460-J2

O

OAHU LN
4900 OXN 93033 552-J5
OAK
2000 VeCo 93023 451-C3
OAK AV
700 VeCo 93015 455-G4
OAK BEND
- VeCo 91377 527-J7
- VeCo 91377 528-A7
OAK CT
800 PHME 93041 552-F5
OAK DR
- VeCo 93022 451-B6
- VeCo 93023 451-G1
5100 OXN 93033 552-J5
OAK LN
100 THO 91362 556-H1
OAK RD
1400 SIMI 93063 499-B3
OAK ST
- CMRL 93010 524-E3
100 OJAI 93023 441-J6
100 VeCo 93015 465-E1
600 VeCo 93022 451-B7
600 VeCo 93022 461-B1
N OAK ST
- VEN 93001 491-C2
100 SPLA 93060 464-B4
S OAK ST
- VEN 93001 491-C2
100 SPLA 93060 464-C5
W OAK ST
100 OJAI 93023 441-H6
OAK BANK
- VeCo 91377 557-J1
OAK BLUFF DR
900 MRPK 93021 476-E7
OAK BRANCH DR
700 VeCo 91377 558-B1
OAK BROOK DR
2400 THO 91362 526-J4
OAKBURY CT
2700 THO 91360 526-D3
OAK CANYON RD
900 CMRL 93012 525-B1
OAKCLIFF DR
4100 MRPK 93021 496-G3
OAKCOTTAGE CT
23600 VeCo 91361 556-F6
OAK CREEK DR
400 THO 91361 556-E2
OAK CREEK LN
- AGRH 91301 558-A5
200 OJAI 93023 441-H7
N OAKCREST AV
10900 VeCo 93022 451-C4
10900 VeCo 93023 451-B4
OAK CREST DR
31200 WLKV 91361 557-E6
OAKDALE CIR
2100 SIMI 93063 498-J2
OAKDALE LN
100 FILM 93015 455-J7
OAKDALE PL
1000 SPLA 93060 464-B3
OAKFEN CT
5500 AGRH 91301 557-G5
OAK FERN CT
- SIMI 93063 499-A3
OAK FOREST DR
6500 VeCo 91377 558-A1
OAK GLEN AV
100 OJAI 93023 442-A7
OAK GLEN CT
4000 MRPK 93021 496-E3
OAK GLEN DR
200 THO 91320 555-E1
OAK GLEN ST
4300 CALB 91302 558-H7
OAK GROVE CT
700 VeCo 93023 451-A3
OAK GROVE PL
1200 THO 91362 527-C7
OAK GROVE FIRE RD
7400 VeCo 93012 525-D5
OAKHAMPTON ST
400 THO 91361 556-F3
OAK HAVEN AV
2200 SIMI 93063 498-J1

STREET
Block City ZIP Pg-Grid

OAK HAVEN CT
400 VeCo 91377 558-B1
OAKHILL CIR
2100 OXN 93036 522-E2
OAK HILLS DR
300 VeCo 91377 558-A2
500 VeCo 91377 557-J1
OAK HOLLOW CIR
900 THO 91362 557-C1
OAKHURST CT
1300 CMRL 93010 524-E1
OAK KNOLL RD
10700 VeCo 93022 451-D6
OAK KNOLLS RD
5800 VeCo 93063 499-A3
OAKLAWN DR
100 VeCo 93022 461-A1
OAKLEAF AV
- VeCo 91377 558-B2
OAK LEAF DR
100 THO 91360 526-E7
9400 Chat 91311 499-J6
OAK MEADOW PL
5900 VeCo 91377 558-A2
OAK MIRAGE PL
1000 THO 91362 527-D7
1000 THO 91362 557-D1
OAKMONT CT
800 SIMI 93065 497-G5
OAKMONT PL
23900 LA 91304 529-E1
OAKMORE ST
1200 OJAI 93023 441-F7
OAKMOUND AV
800 THO 91320 555-E4
OAK PARK LN
4900 VeCo 91377 557-G1
4900 VeCo 91377 527-G7
OAK PATH CT
700 VeCo 91377 558-B1
OAKPATH DR
28800 AGRH 91301 558-A4
OAK PLACE DR
4100 THO 91362 527-C6
OAK POINT DR
600 VeCo 91377 558-A1
OAK RANCH CT
31800 WLKV 91361 557-D7
OAKRIDGE CT
1600 THO 91362 526-J6
OAKRIDGE PL
9500 Chat 91311 499-H6
OAKRIDGE RD
- LA 91304 529-C1
23600 VeCo - 367-E9
OAKRIM DR
30800 WLKV 91362 557-F4
OAK RUN TR
- VeCo 91377 527-J7
- VeCo 91377 557-J1
OAK SHADOW VIEW PL
600 THO 91320 556-D1
OAKSHORE DR
2400 THO 91361 557-B6
2600 WLKV 91361 557-B6
OAK SPRINGS DR
6500 VeCo 91377 558-B1
OAKSTAFF CT
2000 THO 91361 557-A6
OAK TERRACE LN
1800 THO 91320 526-A7
OAK TRAIL RD
23600 SIMI 93065 527-F1
OAK TRAIL ST
- THO 91320 526-A6
OAK TREE CT
23600 SIMI 93065 527-F1
OAK TREE LN
400 THO 91360 526-F7
400 THO 91360 556-F1
OAK VALLEY LN
2500 THO 91362 527-C3
OAK VIEW AV
- VeCo 93022 451-A7
E OAK VIEW AV
- VeCo 93022 451-B7
OAK VIEW CT
23600 SIMI 93065 527-F1
OAK VIEW DR
- THO 91362 557-A2
OAK VILLAGE RD
300 VeCo 93015 455-E7
OAKVISTA CT
29900 AGRH 91301 557-H4
OAKWOOD DR
1600 THO 91362 556-J2
OAKWOOD ST
200 VEN 93001 471-B7
700 VeCo 93023 451-C1
OARFISH CT
800 OXN 93035 522-D7
OARFISH LN
1000 OXN 93035 522-B7
OATFIELD WY
10300 VeCo 93012 495-J6
OAT MOUNTAIN MTWY
- Nor 91326 479-J2
- StvR 91381 479-J2
OBERLIN AV
200 VEN 93003 491-J2
1300 THO 91360 526-E6
OBERS PL
2500 PHME 93041 552-C2
OBRIEN CIR
2500 CMRL 93010 524-F3
OBSIDIAN CT
- SIMI 93063 479-A7
OCASO PL
- OXN 93030 523-A4
OCATILLO AV
- THO 91320 555-J2
OCATILLO CT
- THO 91320 555-J2
- THO 91320 556-A2
OCCIDENTAL DR
200 OXN 93036 522-H2
OCEAN AV
1500 VEN 93001 491-E3
2200 VEN 93003 491-F3
23600 VeCo 93001 459-D6
OCEAN DR
- PHME 93043 552-B5
100 VeCo 93035 552-A2
2900 OXN 93035 552-B5
OCEANAIRE LN
11900 VeCo 90265 625-F5
OCEANAIRE ST
5000 OXN 93035 551-J1
5000 OXN 93035 552-A1

STREET
Block City ZIP Pg-Grid

OCEAN BLUFF AV
23600 THO 91362 527-B2
OCEANMIST CT
2500 PHME 93041 552-C2
OCEAN VIEW DR
400 PHME 93041 552-F7
600 VeCo 93010 494-F6
E OCEAN VIEW DR
1200 VeCo 93010 494-F6
OCEAN VIEW RD
8000 VeCo 93001 459-C3
23600 VeCo 93001 366-G9
OCEAN WALK CT
- PHME 93041 552-D6
OCHO RIOS WY
300 VeCo 91377 557-G2
OCIE AV
2700 SIMI 93065 478-B7
OCOTLAN WY
- OXN 93030 522-H4
ODEBOLT DR
100 THO 91360 526-E3
OFELIA WY
- OXN 93030 522-J4
OFFSHORE ST
900 OXN 93035 522-C7
1300 OXN 93035 552-C1
OGDEN ST
8800 VEN 93004 492-G3
OHARA CANYON RD
1900 VeCo 93060 463-E4
OJAI AV
100 VeCo 93035 552-B5
6700 VeCo 93001 459-C5
E OJAI AV Rt#-150
200 OJAI 93023 441-H7
1100 OJAI 93023 442-B7
1600 VeCo 93023 442-B7
W OJAI AV Rt#-150
100 OJAI 93023 441-G7
1000 OJAI 93023 451-G1
OJAI DR
- VeCo 93022 451-B6
OJAI FRWY Rt#-33
- VeCo - 461-B6
- VeCo - 471-C3
- VEN - 471-B7
- VEN - 491-A1
N OJAI RD Rt#-150
100 SPLA 93060 464-B3
300 VeCo 93060 464-B3
OJAI ST
600 VeCo 93015 465-J3
N OJAI ST
100 SPLA 93060 464-B5
S OJAI ST
100 SPLA 93060 464-C6
OJAI SANTA PAULA RD Rt#-150
3100 VeCo 93023 442-D7
7000 VeCo 93023 452-E1
11900 VeCo 93023 453-A1
OJAI VALLEY SCHOOL
23600 VeCo 93023 442-J7
23600 VeCo 93023 453-A1
OKAPI LN
1100 VEN 93004 492-E4
OLD BALCOM CANYON RD
6200 VeCo 93066 475-D7
OLD BALDWIN RD
1200 VeCo 93023 451-B3
OLD BURY PL
1300 THO 91361 556-J6
OLD BUTTERFIELD RD
- VeCo 93012 496-F7
OLD CARRIAGE CT
29000 AGRH 91301 558-A3
OLDCASTLE PL
1500 THO 91361 556-H6
OLD COACH DR
3000 VeCo 93010 494-C6
3300 VeCo 93066 494-C6
OLD COLONY WY
30900 AGRH 91301 557-F6
30900 WLKV 91361 557-F6
OLD CONEJO RD
3000 THO 91320 525-E6
3000 VeCo 91320 525-F7
E OLD CREEK RD
200 VeCo 93001 461-B2
200 VeCo 93022 461-B2
W OLD CREEK RD
9500 VeCo 93001 461-A2
OLD DAIRY RD
- VeCo 93012 554-E1
OLD DUMP RD
2400 THO 91361 556-J3
OLDENBERG WY
6000 SIMI 93063 499-B1
OLD FARM CT
- THO 91360 526-G5
OLD FARM RD
600 THO 91360 526-G5
OLD GRADE RD
200 VeCo 93022 451-B7
1800 VeCo 93023 451-C3
OLDHAM CIR
2400 OXN 93035 552-A2
OLD HWY 150
9100 VeCo 93023 452-G1
OLD OAK AV
1200 THO 91320 526-A6
OLD ORCHARD RD
2100 VeCo 93015 455-E5
OLD PACIFIC COAST HWY
6200 VeCo 93001 459-D5
OLD RANCH CIR
11300 Chat 91311 499-J1
OLD RANCH RD
1100 CMRL 93012 525-B1
1700 CMRL 93012 495-B7
OLD RINCON HWY Rt#-1
2900 VeCo 93001 470-F6
4200 VeCo 93001 366-G9
4200 VeCo 93001 459-F7
4200 VeCo 93001 469-H1
23600 VeCo 93001 490-G1
OLDS RD
3000 OXN 93033 553-A3
4300 VeCo 93033 553-B6
OLD SALT LN
5500 AGRH 91301 557-G5
OLDSTONE CT
300 SIMI 93065 497-G6
OLDSTONE PL
400 SIMI 93065 497-F5

STREET
Block City ZIP Pg-Grid

OLD TELEGRAPH RD
700 FILM 93015 456-A6
700 FILM 93015 455-H5
1100 VeCo 93015 455-H5
OLD TELEGRAPH RD Rt#-126
2500 VeCo 93015 455-E7
2700 VeCo 93015 465-E1
OLD VENTURA AV
300 VeCo 93022 451-B7
OLD WALNUT RD
23600 VeCo 93023 452-G1
OLEANDER CT
100 THO 91320 555-J2
600 OXN 93033 552-G2
OLEANDER DR
500 OXN 93033 552-F2
OLEANDER WY
- SIMI 93065 497-H3
OLEARY CT
1700 THO 91320 556-A1
OLGA ST
1900 OXN 93036 522-E3
OLIN DR
9200 Chat 91311 499-F7
OLIVAS PARK DR
1100 VEN 93001 491-H7
3300 VeCo 93001 491-H7
4500 VeCo 93001 492-B7
4500 VeCo 93003 492-B7
4500 VeCo 93003 491-H7
4800 VEN 93003 492-D7
5800 VEN 93001 492-B7
OLIVE RD
300 VeCo 93060 473-C3
OLIVE ST
- MRPK 93021 496-G2
- OXN 93036 522-H1
- VeCo 93022 451-B7
200 FILM 93015 456-A6
200 OXN 93033 552-G2
700 OJAI 93023 441-H6
800 VeCo 93040 457-F3
1700 VeCo 93023 442-B5
N OLIVE ST
- VeCo 93022 451-B6
- VEN 93001 491-B1
100 SPLA 93060 464-A5
600 VEN 93001 471-B7
S OLIVE ST
- VEN 93001 491-B2
100 SPLA 93060 464-B6
W OLIVE ST
800 OXN 93033 552-F2
OLIVEBROOK WK
- CMRL 93012 524-H2
OLIVEGROVE PL
2500 THO 91362 527-D3
N OLIVE HILL RD
5100 VeCo 93066 495-B1
5600 VeCo 93066 475-C7
OLIVE MILL LN
- OJAI 93023 441-J7
OLIVER ST
800 FILM 93015 455-J6
OLIVEWOOD CT
1900 THO 91362 526-J4
1900 THO 91362 527-A4
OLIVEWOOD DR
2200 THO 91362 527-A4
OLIVIA DR
23600 OXN 93030 522-J4
OLIVO CT
3800 CMRL 93010 524-H1
OLOROSO CIR
4200 MRPK 93021 496-E3
OLSEN RD
- THO 91360 526-G1
1100 THO 91360 496-H7
1900 SIMI 93065 497-A6
2700 THO 91360 497-A6
2500 THO 93021 497-A6
2500 THO 93065 497-A6
2500 VeCo 91360 497-A6
2500 VeCo 93021 497-A6
2500 VeCo 93065 497-A6
W OLSEN RD
- THO 91360 526-E2
OLYMPIA AV
800 VEN 93004 492-G3
OLYMPIC ST
1300 SIMI 93063 498-D3
OLYMPUS LN
23600 OXN 93035 522-C6
OLYMPUS ST
- MRPK 93021 496-D1
OMAHA AV
2800 VEN 93001 471-C4
OMAHA CT
300 VEN 93001 471-D5
OMEGA AV
3000 SIMI 93063 478-E7
3100 VeCo 93063 478-E7
ONA CIR
1600 SIMI 93063 498-J3
ONDA DR
1700 CMRL 93010 524-D2
ONEIDA CT
- MRPK 93021 496-G3
1000 OXN 93030 522-E4
ONEIDA PL
1500 OXN 93030 522-D4
ONEIDA ST
9500 VEN 93004 492-H3
ONEIDA WY
2300 OXN 93030 522-D4
ONEILL PL
1800 OXN 93033 552-J2
1800 OXN 93033 553-A2
ONE OAK LN
2400 SIMI 93063 499-A1
ONONDAGA LN
100 VEN 93001 471-C5
ONTARIO AV
1200 VEN 93004 492-G3
ONTARIO ST
900 OXN 93035 522-E7
1400 OXN 93035 552-E1
ONYX CIR
3300 SIMI 93063 478-D7
ONYX ST
- VEN 93004 492-F3
OPAL AV
500 VEN 93004 492-F3
OPAL CT
2800 SIMI 93063 478-C7
8000 VEN 93004 492-F3
OPALO DR
- OXN 93030 522-J4

STREET
Block City ZIP Pg-Grid

OPEN CIR
4700 SIMI 93063 478-H5
OPHELIA CT
2600 SIMI 93063 478-J7
OPTAR LN
400 OXN 93030 522-H4
W ORACLE CT
1900 THO 91320 555-J2
1900 THO 91320 556-A2
ORANGE CIR
10600 VEN 93004 472-H7
ORANGE CT
3600 SIMI 93063 478-E7
ORANGE DR
- VeCo 93036 492-J7
300 VeCo 93036 522-J1
900 VeCo 93036 523-A1
3200 OXN 93036 523-C2
ORANGE LN
1200 VeCo 93010 494-F7
ORANGE MALL
5100 OXN 93033 552-H5
ORANGE RD
600 OJAI 93023 442-B6
600 VeCo 93023 442-B6
ORANGE ST
200 VeCo 93015 465-E1
ORANGE BLOSSOM LN
100 FILM 93015 455-J6
ORANGE GROVE AV
200 FILM 93015 456-A6
3600 OXN 93033 553-B4
ORANGEWOOD AV
600 THO 91320 555-G3
N ORANGEWOOD PL
2400 SIMI 93065 498-A1
ORCHARD DR
- VeCo 93001 471-C3
1300 VeCo 93023 451-D2
ORCHARD LN
700 VeCo 93060 473-C2
ORCHARD PL
100 OXN 93036 522-F1
ORCHARD ST
400 FILM 93015 456-A6
600 VeCo 93040 457-F3
1000 SPLA 93060 464-B4
1500 VeCo 93060 464-B4
ORCHARD FARM RD
23600 VeCo 93060 473-D4
ORCHARD VIEW CIR
- CMRL 93010 524-D4
ORCHARDVIEW CT
4200 WLKV 91361 557-D6
ORCHID AV
1900 SIMI 93065 498-B2
ORCHID DR
1700 OXN 93033 553-A2
ORCHID PL
200 VEN 93004 473-C7
ORCUTT RD
200 VeCo 93060 464-E3
ORCUTT CANYON RD
200 VeCo 93060 454-E7
1000 VeCo 93060 464-E2
OREGON DR
2100 VEN 93003 492-C5
ORENA CT
400 CMRL 93010 524-B1
ORIENT ST
- FILM 93015 455-J7
ORILLA WK
300 OXN 93030 522-H4
ORINDA CT
1600 THO 91362 526-J4
ORIOLE CIR
1100 FILM 93015 455-H6
ORIOLE DR
- VeCo 93041 583-H2
ORIOLE LN
4000 OXN 93033 553-B4
ORIOLE ST
200 OJAI 93023 442-A6
6200 VEN 93003 492-D4
ORION WY
900 OXN 93036 522-F1
ORIONS FLIGHT WY
- VeCo 93012 496-F6
ORLEANS CT
30800 WLKV 91362 557-F4
ORLEANS LN
- OXN 93036 492-H7
ORLOP PL
2000 OXN 93035 522-E6
ORO ST
400 VeCo 93022 451-A7
ORR AV
1600 SIMI 93065 498-C3
ORR RD
100 VeCo 93060 473-G3
ORTEGA DR
- THO 91320 556-B1
ORTEGA ST
- OXN 93030 523-B4
900 FILM 93015 455-J6
4600 VEN 93003 492-A6
ORWELL LN
- VeCo 93033 552-J2
500 VEN 93003 492-D1
OSA CT
1100 OXN 93035 522-E7
OSAGE CIR
800 CMRL 93012 525-A2
OSAGE LN
1100 VEN 93004 492-H3
OSBORN RD
23600 VeCo 93060 453-D1
OSO RD
700 VeCo 93023 441-C5
OSPREY AV
- THO 91320 526-A5
N OSPREY LN
1100 VEN 93003 492-F4
S OSPREY LN
1300 VEN 93003 492-F4
OSTRICH HILL RD
1100 OXN 93036 522-E1
OTANO WY
- OXN 93030 522-H4
OTERO CT
500 VeCo 93010 494-B7
E OTONO CIR
2200 THO 91362 527-A2
OTONO CT
300 CMRL 93012 525-A2
OTTAWA DR
100 VEN 93001 471-C4
OTTER CREEK LN
2400 OXN 93035 522-E1

STREET
Block City ZIP Pg-Grid

OUTER DR
- SPLA 93060 464-A7
OUTLET CENTER DR
2000 OXN 93036 523-B3
21400 OXN 93030 523-B3
OUTLOOK CIR
1300 THO 91362 527-C7
OUTLOOK CV
2600 PHME 93041 552-C3
OUTRIGGER AV
3100 VEN 93001 491-G5
OUTRIGGER WY
5100 OXN 93035 521-J7
OUTSAIL LN
2000 OXN 93035 522-D7
OVERFALL DR
30800 WLKV 91362 557-F4
OVERLAND DR
24500 LA 91304 529-C4
OVERLOOK DR
700 VEN 93001 491-C1
OVERLOOK RD
600 SIMI 93065 497-E6
OVERLY ST
6400 MRPK 93021 477-A6
OWEN ST
1000 VeCo 93015 465-H3
OWENS AV
1200 VEN 93004 492-G3
OWENS RIVER DR
- OXN 93036 492-G6
OWL CT
6900 VEN 93003 492-E4
OWLS COVE LN
23600 SIMI 93065 497-G2
E OXFORD CIR
14400 MRPK 93021 476-G6
OXFORD DR
600 OXN 93030 522-E4
OXFORD ST
10400 VEN 93004 492-J1
11900 VeCo 93021 476-D3
OXLEY PL
4900 THO 91362 527-E6
OXNARD AV
100 VeCo 93035 552-B5
7000 VeCo 93001 459-C4
OXNARD BLVD
600 OXN 93036 492-H6
1000 OXN 93030 522-G3
2000 OXN 93036 522-G3
OXNARD BLVD Rt#-1
- OXN 93033 553-A2
- VeCo 93033 553-B3
100 OXN 93030 522-G7
1200 OXN 93030 552-H1
1200 OXN 93033 522-G7
1200 OXN 93033 552-H1
1500 OXN 93036 522-G1
19200 OXN 93036 492-G7
N OXNARD BLVD
- OXN 93036 492-H6
OXNARD CIR
- OXN 93036 492-H6
OXNARD SHORES DR
5100 OXN 93035 521-J6
OYSTER PL
1100 OXN 93030 522-E7
OYSTER ST
900 VeCo 93001 491-F5
900 VEN 93001 491-F5

P

PACIFIC AV
100 VeCo 93015 457-D5
500 OXN 93030 522-J7
700 SIMI 93065 497-G3
1100 OXN 93033 522-J7
1300 OXN 93033 552-J1
3500 VeCo 93040 457-D5
N PACIFIC AV
- VEN 93001 491-E2
S PACIFIC AV
- VEN 93001 491-E2
PACIFIC CIR
400 THO 91320 555-G3
PACIFIC RD
- PHME 93041 552-D4
- PHME 93043 552-D4
2800 VeCo 93041 583-H4
3400 VeCo 93042 583-H4
18600 VeCo 93033 583-H4
PACIFICA DR
100 OXN 93033 553-C4
PACIFIC BREEZE DR
- VeCo 93012 496-F6
PACIFIC COAST FRWY Rt#-1
- OXN - 553-C4
- VeCo - 553-C4
- VeCo - 583-H1
PACIFIC COAST HWY Rt#-1
2900 VeCo 93001 470-B3
4200 VeCo 93001 366-G9
4200 VeCo 93001 459-F6
4200 VeCo 93001 469-H1
9000 VeCo 90265 387-F4
9000 VeCo 90265 625-A3
9400 VeCo - 584-A6
12300 LACo 90265 625-F5
19900 VeCo 93033 583-J5
19900 VeCo 93033 584-A6
23600 VeCo 93001 490-G1
34100 MAL 90265 625-F5
PACIFIC COVE DR
500 PHME 93041 552-C2
N PACIFIC MILLING RD
6400 VeCo 93066 493-D2
13600 VeCo 93066 473-E7
S PACIFIC MILLING RD
100 OXN 93036 492-H6
PACIFIC OAK DR
22400 Chat 91311 499-H5
PACIFIC RIDGE RD
6300 VeCo 93063 499-C4
PACIFIC STRAND CT
- VEN 93003 492-B4
PACIFIC STRAND PL
- VEN 93003 492-B4
PACIFIC VIEW LN
900 VEN 93001 491-D1
PACIFIC VIEW RD
10300 VeCo 90265 585-A7
10700 VeCo 90265 387-A4
10700 VeCo 90265 625-A1

STREET
Block City ZIP Pg-Grid

PACKARD CIR
100 THO 91362 557-C4
PACKARD ST
23600 OXN 93033 553-B4
PACOS ST
- VEN 93001 471-B5
PADDINGTON PL
800 OXN 93030 522-E4
PADELFORD RD
900 FILM 93015 456-B4
PADOVA CT
30800 WLKV 91362 557-F5
PADRE LN
- CMRL 93012 524-H1
200 VeCo 93060 464-D3
N PADRE JUAN AV
100 VeCo 93023 441-D6
S PADRE JUAN AV
100 VeCo 93023 441-D7
PADRE JUAN CANYON RD
4000 VeCo 93001 470-A3
23600 VeCo 93001 460-C7
PADUA CIR
100 THO 91320 555-E1
PADUA LN
3700 THO 91320 555-E1
PAGENT CT
3200 THO 91360 526-F2
PAGENT ST
- THO 91360 526-F2
PAIGE AV
3000 SIMI 93063 478-E7
3100 VeCo 93063 478-E7
PAIGE LN
600 THO 91360 526-G7
900 THO 91362 526-H6
PAINE AV
300 VEN 93003 492-B3
PAINTED PONY CIR
5800 SIMI 93063 479-A6
PAINTED SKY ST
3800 MRPK 93021 496-E4
PAIUTE AV
11200 Chat 91311 499-J2
PAIUTE LN
200 VEN 93001 471-C5
PAJARO AV
- VEN 93004 472-J6
- VEN 93004 473-A7
PAJARO ST
- OXN 93030 523-B4
PALA DR
400 VeCo 93023 441-D7
PALA MESA DR
6800 VeCo 91377 528-B7
PALA VISTA
- CMRL 93012 494-J7
PALERMO CT
23600 SIMI 93063 478-G6
PALI DR
1000 OXN 93033 552-J5
PALISADES PARK DR
- OXN 93036 492-H7
N PALM AV
100 SPLA 93060 464-A6
S PALM AV
100 SPLA 93060 464-A6
PALM CT
1400 THO 91360 526-H2
E PALM CT
300 SPLA 93060 464-A5
N PALM CT
300 SPLA 93060 464-A5
PALM DR
- CMRL 93010 524-E4
23600 FILM 93015 456-C6
W PALM DR
100 OXN 93030 522-E5
PALM LN
5100 OXN 93033 552-H5
PALM ST
200 FILM 93015 456-A6
N PALM ST
- VEN 93001 491-C2
S PALM ST
- VEN 93001 491-C2
PALMA DR
1400 VEN 93003 492-A6
2900 VeCo 93003 492-A6
PALMER AV
900 CMRL 93010 524-E2
PALMER DR
- MRPK 93021 476-D4
- VeCo 93021 476-D4
PALMETTO LN
400 THO 91320 556-D1
PALMGROVE AV
- THO 91320 556-C2
PALMWOOD CIR
2500 THO 91362 527-D3
PALO ALTO
2100 VeCo 93023 451-C3
PALO COMADO DR
5900 AGRH 91301 558-D4
PALO COMADO CANYON RD
5000 AGRH 91301 558-D6
PALO COMADO FIRE RD
- VeCo 91377 527-J4
- VeCo 91377 528-A4
- VeCo 93065 528-A4
23600 SIMI 93065 527-J4
23600 VeCo 93065 527-J4
PALOMA CT
30800 WLKV 91362 557-F5
PALOMA DR
3600 VEN 93003 491-H2
PALOMAR AV
600 MRPK 93021 496-D1
2100 VEN 93001 491-F2
PALOMAR CIR
5800 CMRL 93012 495-B7
PALOMAR RD
200 OJAI 93023 441-G5
500 VeCo 93023 441-G6
PALOMAR WY
800 OXN 93033 552-F3
PALOMARES AV
- VEN 93003 491-H2
PALOMINO CIR
4100 THO 91362 527-C7
6000 VeCo 93066 495-B3
PALOMINO DR
4300 VeCo 93066 495-B3
PALOMITAS CIR
4200 MRPK 93021 496-D2
PALOS CT W
2100 THO 91320 555-J2

PALO VERDE CIR
11200 VeCo 93012 496-B6
PAMELA CT
100 SPLA 93060 463-J7
1800 SIMI 93065 497-J2
1800 SIMI 93065 498-A2
PAMELA LN
100 SPLA 93060 463-H6
PAMELA ST
1900 OXN 93036 522-E3
PAMELA WOOD ST
700 THO 91320 556-C1
PAMPAS LN
- VEN 93001 491-B1
PAN CT
23600 THO 91320 556-B1
PANAL CT
1200 OXN 93030 522-H4
PANAMA DR
2200 PHME 93035 552-B4
2200 PHME 93043 552-B4
2200 VeCo 93035 552-B4
2600 VeCo 93043 552-B4
E PANAMINT CT
2800 THO 91362 557-C3
W PANAMINT CT
2700 THO 91362 557-B3
PANCHO RD
100 VeCo 93012 524-H7
400 CMRL 93012 524-H7
1600 VeCo 93012 554-H1
S PANCHO RD
400 CMRL 93012 524-H4
PANDA PL
2300 VEN 93003 492-E5
PANORAMA CT
1300 THO 91360 526-H2
PANSY ST
- SIMI 93063 499-A2
PANSY WY
- VEN 93004 473-C7
PAPAGO TER
8400 LA 91304 529-D1
PAQUITA ST
1000 CMRL 93012 525-C6
PARADE AV
- SIMI 93063 498-H1
PARADISE CIR
300 VeCo 93010 494-F6
PARAKEET CT
1600 VEN 93003 492-F4
PAR FIVE CT
1900 THO 91362 527-D5
PAR FIVE DR
1800 THO 91362 527-C6
PARIS CT
30800 WLKV 91362 557-F5
PARK AV
- VeCo 93022 451-B7
400 PHME 93041 552-F4
PARK DR
1400 VeCo 93023 451-B2
2000 VEN 93003 492-C5
PARK LN
- MRPK 93021 496-E2
PARK PL
2200 THO 91362 527-A4
PARK RD
100 OJAI 93023 441-J5
PARK ST
- PHME 93041 552-E4
200 OJAI 93023 441-H6
700 VeCo 93040 457-F3
1000 SPLA 93060 464-B4
1600 SIMI 93063 498-G3
PARK AND RIDE DR
- CMRL 93010 524-B3
PARK CENTER DR
2600 SIMI 93065 477-F7
2600 SIMI 93065 497-F1
PARK COTTAGE PL
- CMRL 93012 524-G5
PARK CREST LN
- MRPK 93021 496-E2
N PARKDALE AV
2400 SIMI 93063 498-E1
PARKER AV
- THO 91360 556-F1
PARKER CT
2900 SIMI 93065 498-A2
N PARKER CT
2100 SIMI 93065 498-A2
PARKER LN
8400 VEN 93004 492-G4
PARKFRONT PL
400 SIMI 93065 497-E6
PARKHAVEN CT
200 FILM 93015 455-H7
PARKHEATH DR
28900 AGRH 91301 558-B5
PARKHILL CIR
6000 VEN 93003 472-C6
PARKHILL CT
1300 CMRL 93010 524-E1
PARK HILL RD
23600 SIMI 93065 497-F7
23600 SIMI 93065 527-F1
PARKHURST ST
1200 SIMI 93065 497-H4
PARKING LOT RD
23600 VeCo 93063 498-H7
PARK MEADOW CT
2500 SIMI 93065 497-H1
PARKMOR RD
5300 CALB 91302 558-H3
E PARK ROW AV
- VEN 93001 491-B1
W PARK ROW AV
- VEN 93001 491-B1
PARKSIDE CT
- VeCo 91377 527-J7
- VeCo 91377 528-A7
PARKSIDE DR
23600 SIMI 93065 527-F1
PARK SPRINGS CT
400 VeCo 91377 558-B1
PARK TERRACE DR
4300 WLKV 91361 557-E6
PARKVIEW AV
2300 THO 91362 527-A4
PARKVIEW CT
23600 SIMI 93065 527-F1
PARK VIEW DR
100 VeCo 91377 558-A2
PARKVIEW DR
2400 THO 91362 527-A3
8000 VeCo 93001 461-A4
PARKVILLE RD
5000 CALB 91301 558-G6
5100 Ago 91301 558-G6

PARKWAY DR
2300 CMRL 93010 494-E7
PARKWOOD CT
1900 THO 91362 526-J3
PARMA DR
4800 VeCo 91377 557-G1
PARMENTER CT
700 THO 91362 527-A7
PARRISH ST
- VEN 93003 492-A3
PARRON ST
3900 CMRL 93010 494-H7
PARROT CT
1600 VEN 93003 492-E4
PARSONS AV
300 VEN 93003 492-A2
PARSONS DR
900 PHME 93041 552-E4
PARTHENIA ST
22000 LA 91304 529-J1
PARTRIDGE CT
5100 THO 91362 527-F6
PARTRIDGE DR
800 OXN 93036 522-F1
1000 VEN 93003 492-D3
PARTRIDGE PL
1600 VEN 93003 492-D4
PASADENA AV
100 VeCo 93035 552-C6
100 VeCo 93043 552-C6
700 VeCo 93015 465-F2
700 VeCo 93015 466-A2
PASEO ARROYO
800 CMRL 93010 524-B2
PASEO BARONA
1300 CMRL 93010 524-C1
PASEO BRISAS LINDAS
23600 OXN 93030 523-C6
PASEO CAMARILLO
200 CMRL 93010 524-C3
PASEO CASTILLE
1000 CMRL 93010 524-C1
PASEO DE CORTAGA
600 CMRL 93010 524-B3
PASEO DE INVIERNO
3500 THO 91360 526-B1
PASEO DE LA PAZ
23600 THO 91320 555-D4
PASEO DEL CAMPO
5200 CMRL 93012 524-J1
5300 CMRL 93012 525-A1
PASEO DE LEON
500 THO 91320 555-F3
PASEO DEL ROBLEDO
800 VeCo 91360 526-C6
PASEO DEL ROBLES CT
1100 OJAI 93023 442-A6
PASEO DEL VALLE
200 CMRL 93010 524-B3
PASEO DE NUBLADO
3500 THO 91360 526-D1
PASEO DE PETALOS
23600 CMRL 93010 523-G2
PASEO DE PLAYA
300 VEN 93001 491-C2
PASEO ELEGANTE
- OXN 93030 523-A5
PASEO ENCANTADA
5900 CMRL 93012 525-B5
PASEO ESMERALDA
500 THO 91320 526-A7
PASEO ESPLENDIDO
- CMRL 93010 524-A2
PASEO GIRASOL
23600 CMRL 93012 494-H7
PASEO GRANDE
400 THO 91320 526-C7
PASEO HACIENDA
- OXN 93030 523-A5
PASEO ISLA
- OXN 93030 523-A4
PASEO LA PERLA
500 THO 91320 526-A7
PASEO LAS NUBES
23600 OXN 93030 523-B4
PASEO LA VIDA
23600 OXN 93030 523-C7
PASEO LA VISTA
6100 WdHl 91367 529-C7
PASEO LINDO
- OXN 93030 523-A4
PASEO LOMA
23600 CMRL 93010 524-D4
PASEO LUNAR
4400 CMRL 93010 524-B3
PASEO MARAVILLA
23600 CMRL 93012 494-H7
23600 CMRL 93012 524-H1
PASEO MARGARITA
- OXN 93030 523-A5
5400 CMRL 93012 525-A5
PASEO MERCADO
2800 OXN 93036 523-B2
PASEO MONTECITO
600 THO 91320 525-F7
PASEO MONTELENA
4600 CMRL 93012 524-J2
PASEO NOCHE
1800 CMRL 93012 495-C7
PASEO NOGALES
- OXN 93030 523-A5
PASEO ORTEGA
- OXN 93030 523-B5
PASEO RICOSO
5200 CMRL 93012 525-A2
PASEO SABANERO
100 CMRL 93012 524-H3
PASEO SANTA BARBARA
23600 THO 91320 555-D4
PASEO SANTA CATARINA
23600 THO 91320 555-D4
PASEO SANTA CRUZ
23600 THO 91320 555-D4
PASEO SANTA FE
23600 THO 91320 555-D4
PASEO SANTA MONICA
23600 THO 91320 555-D4
PASEO SANTA ROSA
23600 THO 91320 555-D4
PASEO SERENATA
800 CMRL 93012 525-C5
PASEO TESORO
23600 OXN 93030 523-C7
PASEO TOSAMAR
800 CMRL 93012 525-B5
PASEO VERDE
500 VeCo 93010 494-A6
PASEO VISTA
500 THO 91320 526-C7

PASEO YOLO
2600 CMRL 93010 494-F7
N PASO FLORES RD
5500 VeCo 93066 475-C7
5500 VeCo 93066 495-B1
PASO ROBLES
7700 VEN 93004 492-E1
PASO ROBLES CT
1500 CMRL 93012 524-J1
PASQUAL AV
100 VEN 93004 472-J7
100 VEN 93004 473-A7
PASSAGEWAY PL
30300 AGRH 91301 557-G5
PASTEUR DR
5800 VEN 93003 492-C6
PAT AV
5900 WdHl 91367 529-D7
6200 CanP 91307 529-D7
PATHELEN AV
- VeCo 93022 451-B7
PATHFINDER AV
1300 THO 91362 527-G6
4700 VeCo 91362 527-G6
4700 VeCo 91377 527-G6
PATHWAY AV
- SIMI 93063 498-H1
PATINA CT
- CMRL 93010 493-H6
PATRICIA AV
1200 SIMI 93065 497-H2
1700 SIMI 93065 498-A3
PATRICIA CT
900 OJAI 93023 441-J5
PATRICIA ST
1000 OXN 93030 522-E4
1800 SIMI 93065 497-H3
1800 OXN 93036 522-E3
PATRICK ST
3100 SIMI 93065 498-D3
PATRICK HENRY PL
3800 AGRH 91301 558-E7
PATRIOT PL
- VeCo 93041 583-H2
- VeCo 93042 583-H2
PATTERSON RD
2400 PHME 93043 552-D5
2500 PHME 93041 552-D5
2700 PHME 93035 552-D5
N PATTERSON RD
100 VeCo 93030 522-D4
500 OXN 93030 522-D4
1900 OXN 93036 522-C2
S PATTERSON RD
500 OXN 93030 522-D7
500 OXN 93035 522-D7
1200 OXN 93035 552-D1
PATTON CT
1600 OXN 93030 522-J7
PATTY CT
3100 SIMI 93063 478-E6
PAUL DR
800 PHME 93041 552-F5
PAUL ST
1400 SIMI 93065 497-G3
PAULA CIR
2900 OXN 93033 552-H3
PAULA ST
2900 OXN 93033 552-H3
PAULINE ST
100 OJAI 93023 441-H6
PAULING DR
600 THO 91320 526-A7
PAVAROTTI DR
500 VeCo 91377 557-G2
PAVIN DR
- OXN 93036 522-C3
PAVO CT
2000 THO 91362 556-H2
PAWNEE CT
2500 VEN 93001 471-C5
3100 SIMI 93063 478-J6
PAZ MORADA
1000 VEN 93003 472-D6
PEACEFUL CT
400 SIMI 93065 497-J6
PEACE PIPE CT
5700 SIMI 93063 479-A7
PEACH AV
200 VEN 93004 473-A7
300 VeCo 93004 473-A7
PEACH LN
1400 OXN 93033 553-B5
PEACH HILL RD
13000 MRPK 93021 496-F2
PEACH SLOPE RD
4200 MRPK 93021 496-E3
PEACHSPRING CT
4200 MRPK 93021 496-B2
PEACHWOOD PL
32700 WLKV 91361 586-J1
PEACOCK AV
2300 VEN 93003 492-D5
PEACOCK CT
3900 THO 91362 527-C6
PEACOCK RIDGE RD
3700 CALB 91301 558-F7
PEAK PL
2100 THO 91362 527-A2
PEAR AV
1200 OXN 93033 553-B4
PEARL CIR
3300 SIMI 93063 478-D6
PEARL CT
200 PHME 93043 552-E4
PEARL ST
100 PHME 93041 552-E6
600 OJAI 93023 441-J7
7900 VEN 93004 492-F3
PEARL WY
1600 OXN 93035 552-B1
PEARSON RD
400 PHME 93041 552-F3
PEBBLE PL
3500 THO 91320 555-F2
PEBBLE BEACH DR
100 THO 91320 556-D1
PEBBLE BEACH TR
2100 OXN 93036 522-D2
PEBBLESTONE PL
3100 SIMI 93063 478-D7
PECAN AV
6600 MRPK 93021 476-J5
PECAN VALLEY PL
2000 SIMI 93065 497-C6
PECIOLO CT
1600 THO 91362 556-J1
PECK PL
100 SPLA 93060 463-H7

PECK RD
400 SPLA 93060 473-J1
500 VeCo 93060 473-J1
N PECK RD
200 SPLA 93060 463-H6
200 VeCo 93060 463-H6
S PECK RD
200 SPLA 93060 463-J7
200 SPLA 93060 473-J1
PEDERSON RD
600 THO 91360 526-G2
1500 THO 91362 526-J3
19400 THO 91362 527-A3
PEGASUS ST
800 VeCo 93023 451-C3
PEGGY CT
3100 SIMI 93063 478-E6
PEKING ST
- VEN 93001 491-B1
PELICAN AV
1600 VEN 93003 492-D4
PELICAN WY
3700 OXN 93035 552-B4
PELLBURNE CT
200 SIMI 93065 527-E1
PEMBRIDGE ST
3300 THO 91360 526-G2
PEMBROKE CT
1700 THO 91362 527-E6
PEMBROKE ST
5600 VEN 93003 492-B1
E PENA CT
3400 SIMI 93063 498-D2
PENA RANCH RD
23600 Cstc 91384 458-H1
23600 VeCo 93040 458-G4
PENELOPE PL
2300 VeCo 93012 496-B7
PENGUIN ST
6800 VEN 93003 492-E6
PENINSULA RD
2000 OXN 93035 552-B2
PENINSULA ST
800 VEN 93001 491-F5
N PENLAN AV
2100 SIMI 93063 499-B2
PENN ST
6400 MRPK 93021 476-J6
PENNEY DR
3000 SIMI 93063 478-D7
PENNGROVE ST
1900 SIMI 93065 498-A1
PENNSFIELD PL
400 THO 91360 526-F7
400 THO 91360 556-F1
PENNY WY
- OXN 93030 522-E4
PENOBSCOT DR
- LA 91304 529-D4
PENROD DR
30400 AGRH 91301 557-G5
PENROSE AV
4700 MRPK 93021 496-C2
PENROSE CT
2000 THO 91362 527-A5
PENTLAND WY
23900 CanP 91307 529-E5
PENZANCE AV
- CMRL 93012 524-F4
PEONY ST
10500 VEN 93004 493-A2
PEOPLES AV
200 CMRL 93010 524-F3
PEORIA AV
1800 OXN 93033 553-A5
E PEORIA AV
4000 SIMI 93063 478-F6
N PEORIA AV
3000 SIMI 93063 478-F7
PEORIA PL
1900 OXN 93033 553-A5
PEPPER
2100 VeCo 93023 451-C3
PEPPER LN
- VEN 93001 491-B1
PEPPER RD
- THO 91320 556-B2
N PEPPERDINE CIR
6400 MRPK 93021 476-H6
PEPPER MILL ST
4600 MRPK 93021 496-B2
PEPPERMINT PL
3100 THO 91320 555-G3
PEPPERMINT ST
3200 THO 91320 555-G3
PEPPER TREE CT
1800 THO 91362 526-J4
PEPPER TREE LN
400 VeCo 93022 451-B7
PEPPERTREE LN
900 VeCo 93064 498-F4
1200 SIMI 93063 498-F4
1200 VeCo 93063 498-F4
6000 VeCo 93063 499-B3
6400 VeCo 93066 495-B3
PEPPERTREE CANYON RD
700 VeCo 93060 472-J3
700 VeCo 93060 473-A4
PEPPERWOOD CT
300 THO 91360 526-F2
PEPPERWOOD DR
2800 CMRL 93010 494-E6
PERALTA DR
300 SPLA 93060 463-J7
300 SPLA 93060 464-A7
PERCY ST
400 OXN 93033 552-H4
PEREGRINE CIR
- VeCo 91377 558-B3
PEREGRINE CT
- SIMI 93065 477-J6
- SIMI 93065 478-A6
PERELLO RANCH RD
- VeCo 93036 493-B4
PERES LN
300 VeCo 93060 464-E3
PERICLES PL
1800 OXN 93033 553-A2
PERIMETER RD
- OXN 93033 583-A2
- OXN 93042 583-A2
- VeCo 93041 583-A2
- VeCo 93042 553-G7
- VeCo 93042 583-G1
PERIWINKLE CT
400 THO 91360 526-D3
PERIWINKLE WY
- WdHl 91367 529-J7

PERKIN AV
3100 VEN 93003 492-D7
23600 VEN 93001 492-D7
PERKINS RD
5100 OXN 93033 552-G7
PERRY DR
- PHME 93041 552-D4
PERRY WY
4700 VeCo 93036 493-A5
PERSIMMON LN
1400 OXN 93033 553-B5
PERSIMMON ST
- MRPK 93021 496-G3
PERTH PL
600 OXN 93035 522-D6
PERTHSHIRE CIR
6900 CanP 91307 529-E6
PESARO ST
400 VeCo 91377 557-G1
PESCADOR WY
- OXN 93030 522-J3
PESTO WY
5300 VeCo 91377 557-H2
PETER PL
500 SIMI 93065 498-A5
PETERSON AV
6100 WdHl 91367 529-E7
6500 CanP 91307 529-E6
N PETIT AV
- VEN 93004 492-F1
300 VEN 93004 472-F7
S PETIT AV
- VEN 93004 492-G2
PETIT CIR
9500 VEN 93004 492-H3
PETIT CT
9400 VEN 93004 492-H2
PETIT DR
3700 OXN 93033 552-H4
PETIT RD
1800 VeCo 93060 465-C5
PETIT ST
2600 CMRL 93012 524-G3
PETIT RANCH RD
1700 VeCo 93060 465-D5
PETREL PL
1800 VEN 93003 492-D4
PETTICOAT LN
500 OXN 93036 522-F1
PETUNIA ST
- VEN 93004 493-A2
PETUNIA WY
- OXN 93030 522-G4
PHEASANT LN
6700 VeCo 91377 528-A7
N PHEASANT LN
1100 VEN 93003 492-F4
S PHEASANT LN
1300 VEN 93003 492-F4
PHEASANT HILL
2600 CMRL 93010 524-F2
PHEASANT RUN ST
3900 MRPK 93021 496-E4
PHELPS AV
1100 VEN 93004 492-J2
1200 VEN 93004 493-A2
PHELPS CT
1000 VEN 93004 492-J2
PHILRICH CIR
2600 CALB 91302 558-J4
E PHIPPS AV
2500 SIMI 93065 498-C3
PHLEGER RD
4900 VeCo 93066 495-B1
PHLOX CT
400 THO 91360 526-D3
PHOENIX AV
700 VEN 93004 492-G3
PHOENIX CIR
- VeCo 93042 583-H2
PHOENIX DR
4400 OXN 93033 553-A5
PHYLLIS CT
- THO 91320 556-B1
E PHYLLIS ST
2400 SIMI 93065 498-B1
N PHYLLIS ST
2500 SIMI 93065 498-B1
PICADO DR
5000 CMRL 93012 524-G3
PICASO LN
2400 SIMI 93063 499-B1
PICASSO LN
- OXN 93033 552-J2
PICCADILLY CIR
2800 THO 91362 527-B3
PICKET AV
- CMRL 93012 524-G4
PICKFORD CT
700 THO 91320 555-G3
PICKWICK CT
900 THO 91360 526-G5
PICKWICK DR
2100 CMRL 93010 524-E2
PICO AV
1300 SIMI 93065 497-H3
PICO PL
3000 OXN 93033 552-J3
PIDDUCK RD
2600 VeCo 93033 553-C4
PIEDMONT DR
4800 VeCo 91377 557-G2
PIEDMONT ST
900 OXN 93035 522-E7
1400 OXN 93035 552-E1
PIEDRA WY
- OXN 93030 522-H4
PIER WK
3400 OXN 93035 522-C7
PIERCE CT
600 THO 91360 556-G1
2400 SIMI 93065 498-B4
PIERCE ST
7300 VEN 93003 492-E1
PIERCE ARROW AV
- THO 91362 557-B4
PIERPONT BLVD
2000 VEN 93001 491-E3
PIERSIDE LN
1500 CMRL 93010 524-D3
PILOT WY
900 OXN 93035 522-C7
PIMA LN
2300 VEN 93001 471-C6
PIMLICO DR
10600 MRPK 93021 476-A6
PINATA DR
- OXN 93030 522-J4
PINE LN
- VEN 93001 491-B1

PINE RD
7400 VeCo 93060
PINE ST
1200 VeCo 93063
1400 OXN 93030
PINEBLUFF PL
32500 WLKV 91361
PINECLIFF PL
400 SIMI 93065
PINECONE CT
100 SIMI 93065
PINE CREEK CT
- THO 91320
PINECREST DR
- THO 91361
PINECREST ST
2200 SIMI 93065
PINEDALE RD
11600 MRPK 93021
PINEFIELD CT
- MRPK 93021
PINEGROVE RD
5600 VeCo 93060
5800 VeCo 93060
PINEHILL LN
400 SPLA 93060
PINEHILL RD
- VeCo 91320
PINEHILL ST
1000 THO 91320
PINE HOLLOW PL
4000 MRPK 93021
PINEHURST DR
2200 OXN 93036
PINEHURST PL
1000 CMRL 93010
PINELAKE DR
8400 LA 91304
PINEPLANK LN
23600 SIMI 93065
PINE RIDGE CT
4400 MRPK 93021
PINE ROSE CT
- SIMI 93063
PINESONG LN
23600 SIMI 93065
PINE TERRACE DR
2000 THO 91362
PINETREE CIR
500 THO 91360
PINE VALLEY PL
4500 THO 91362
PINE VIEW DR
23600 SIMI 93063
23600 SIMI 93065
PINEWOOD AV
- AGRH 91301
- VeCo 91377
N PINEWOOD PL
2000 SIMI 93065
PINION ST
6300 VeCo 91377
PINK CEDAR CT
3200 SIMI 93065
PINKERTON RD
13300 VeCo 93060
PINKERTON RANCH RD
500 VeCo 93060
PINNACLE CT
- MRPK 93021
PINNACLE WY
- MRPK 93021
PINO CT
1400 CMRL 93010
PINTO ST
1400 SIMI 93065
PIONEER AV
3200 THO 91360
PIRATE CV
2600 PHME 93041
PIRIE RD
200 OJAI 93023
PIROPO CT
600 VeCo 93010
PIRU AV
2200 VeCo 93035
PIRU SQ
600 VeCo 93040
PIRU CANYON RD
- VeCo -
- VeCo 93040
23600 VeCo 93040
23600 VeCo 93040
PISCES ST
28700 AGRH 91301
PISCO LN
1000 OXN 93035
PISTACHIO AV
- VEN 93004
E PITTMAN ST
5600 SIMI 93063
PITTSFIELD LN
1000 VEN 93001
PIUMA CT
5900 SIMI 93063
PIUTE AV
2700 THO 91362
PIVOT POINT WY
- OXN 93035
PIXTON ST
23600 VeCo 91361
PLACER AV
100 VEN 93004
PLACER CT
100 VEN 93004
PLACERITA DR
5200 SIMI 93063
5400 SIMI 93063
PLACERVILLE CT
2600 SIMI 93063
2600 SIMI 93063
PLACID AV
1100 VEN 93004
PLACID CT
1500 SIMI 93065
PLACITA BUENA ROSA
23600 CMRL 93012
PLACITA SAN DIMAS
2200 CMRL 93010
PLACITA SAN LEANDRO
2200 CMRL 93010
PLACITA SAN RUFINO
2200 CMRL 93010
PLAINFIELD PL
2100 OXN 93036
PLAINVIEW ST
5600 VEN 93003
N PLANETREE AV
700 SIMI 93065

City ZIP Pg-Grid
N
CALB 91302 558-H4
ROSA CT
CMRL 93012 495-A7
RM PL
OXN 93035 522-D7
JM ST
VEN 93004 492-F3
T
SIMI 93065 497-G2
V
WdHl 91367 529-F7
CanP 91307 529-F5
LA 91304 529-F3
AV
VEN 93004 492-G3
WY
OXN 93036 492-H5
HARBOR
VeCo 93012 554-F3
T
OXN 93035 552-B4
VeCo 93035 552-B4
VeCo 93035 552-A3
VeCo 93035 552-A3
MALL
OXN 93030 522-G6
A VISTA
CMRL 93010 524-C4
NT AV
OJAI 93023 441-J5
OJAI 93023 442-A5
VeCo 93023 442-A5
NT PL
VEN 93001 471-B6
NT ST
SPLA 93060 464-A5
NT WY
THO 91362 557-A2
NT DALE PL
THO 91362 557-G1
NT GROVE CIR
THO 91362 526-J4
NT OAKS PL
THO 91362 526-J6
NTON PL
SIMI 93065 497-G6
NT VALLEY RD
PHME 93043 552-D5
CMRL 93010 524-A5
VeCo 93010 524-A5
PHME 93041 552-D5
VeCo 93010 523-J5
CMRL 93010 523-J5
OXN 93033 552-D5
VeCo 93033 523-F7
VeCo 93033 553-C3
VeCo 93012 524-F5
CMRL 93012 524-H5
OXN 93033 553-C3
VeCo 93030 523-J5
NT VALLEY RD
VeCo 93012 524-F5
CMRL 93012 524-F5
SANT VALLEY
OXN 93033 552-J5
VeCo 93033 552-J5
OXN 93033 553-A4
SANT VALLEY
OXN 93033 552-G5
NT VALLEY
RD
PHME 93043 552-C5
V
SIMI 93065 498-B4
L
OXN 93036 522-G1
T
VEN 93004 473-A7
S AV
VEN 93004 472-H7
VeCo 93004 472-H7
AGO ST
VeCo 93010 524-C1
RIA CIR
THO 91360 526-H3
HOLLOW CIR
THO 91362 527-D6
HER ST
Chat 91311 499-H6
REE CT
CanP 91307 529-D5
UTH CIR
THO 91360 526-G6
O CT
THO 91362 527-A2
ELLO CT
SIMI 93065 497-J1
OKE CT
SIMI 93065 497-J1
VEN 93003 492-D1
PL
Chat 91311 479-J7
Chat 91311 499-J1
ST
CMRL 93010 524-C2
EXTER AV
MRPK 93021 496-C1
ETTIA AV
THO 91362 557-F1
ETTIA PL
VEN 93001 491-C2
ETTIA GARDENS
VEN 93004 473-B7
VEN 93004 493-A1
ED OAK PL
AGRH 91301 558-A5
N
SIMI 93065 498-A1
VeCo 93033 553-F6
IS DR
VeCo 93041 583-H2
IS WY
PHME 93041 552-F3
OXN 93033 552-F3
PHME 93033 552-F3
REEK ST
FILM 93015 456-C4
VeCo 93015 456-C4
AV
VeCo 93023 441-D6

STREET Block City ZIP Pg-Grid
S POLI AV
100 VeCo 93023 441-D7
POLI ST
100 VEN 93001 491-C1
2400 VEN 93003 491-E2
POLK ST
23600 VEN 93003 492-E2
POLLOCK LN
6800 VEN 93003 492-D3
POMELO DR
6900 CanP 91307 529-E5
7400 LA 91304 529-E4
POMO DR
200 VEN 93001 471-C5
POMONA ST
4000 VEN 93003 491-J2
4400 VEN 93003 492-A2
PONCE AV
6300 WdHl 91367 529-H7
6400 CanP 91307 529-H4
7600 LA 91304 529-H2
PONDERA CIR
7200 CanP 91307 529-E5
PONDEROSA CIR
2900 THO 91360 526-H3
PONDEROSA DR
- CMRL 93010 524-C2
3400 CMRL 93010 494-G7
W PONDEROSA DR
100 CMRL 93010 524-A2
300 CMRL 93010 523-G2
PONDEROSA DR N
3600 CMRL 93010 494-G7
3600 VeCo 93010 494-G7
PONDEROSA LP
2200 OXN 93033 553-B5
PONDEROSA RD
- VeCo 93066 494-H4
PONOMA ST
100 PHME 93041 552-E6
PONS CT
900 THO 91320 555-F4
PONTOON WY
- OXN 93035 522-E7
POPE AV
1700 SIMI 93065 498-C3
POPE LN
600 OJAI 93023 441-J7
POPLAR CT
1000 SIMI 93063 498-D4
POPLAR ST
200 OXN 93033 552-G2
W POPLAR ST
800 OXN 93033 552-F2
POPLAR CREST AV
- THO 91320 556-C2
POPPY CT
2900 THO 91360 526-D2
POPPY LN
1100 SPLA 93060 464-B3
POPPY ST
1500 VEN 93004 493-A2
POPPYGLEN CT
11500 MRPK 93021 496-B2
POPPYSEED PL
3900 CALB 91302 558-H7
POPPY TREE PL
23600 SIMI 93063 498-D4
POPPYVIEW DR
6600 VeCo 91377 528-B7
6600 VeCo 91377 558-A1
PORPOISE WY
4100 OXN 93035 552-B2
PORT CIR
1100 OXN 93035 522-C7
PORT DR
1300 OXN 93035 522-C7
1300 OXN 93035 552-C1
PORTAL ST
- VeCo 93022 451-B7
PORTER LN
2800 VEN 93003 491-G3
PORTHOLE CT
1100 OXN 93030 522-F7
E PORT HUENEME RD
800 PHME 93033 552-E6
800 PHME 93041 552-E6
PORTIA ST
5100 SIMI 93063 478-J7
PORTOFINO PL
- OXN 93030 522-C6
- OXN 93035 522-C6
500 THO 91360 526-D6
PORTOLA CT
- SPLA 93060 464-B4
5700 WLKV 91362 557-G6
PORTOLA LN
300 FILM 93015 456-C6
2100 THO 91361 557-A5
PORTOLA RD
700 VEN 93003 492-B4
1800 VeCo 93003 492-B5
PORTOLA WY
800 OXN 93033 552-F3
PORTSIDE PL
30500 AGRH 91301 557-G5
PORTSMOUTH CT
700 VeCo 91377 557-H1
PORTULACA PL
3900 THO 91362 557-C1
POSADA DR
- OXN 93030 523-A4
POSADA LILLIA
PETALOS
23600 CMRL 93010 523-F2
POSEY LN
23600 LA 91304 529-E4
POSITA RD
8000 VeCo 93066 475-E6
POST ST
400 CMRL 93010 523-J4
400 CMRL 93010 524-A4
POTAWATOMI ST
- VEN 93001 471-B5
POTEAU DR
- VeCo 93001 471-C3
POTOMAC AV
1700 VEN 93004 492-H4
POTRERO RD
- VeCo 91361 556-A5
1000 THO 91320 555-G5
1000 VeCo 91320 555-G5
1000 THO 91361 556-H6
1500 VeCo 91361 555-G5
W POTRERO RD
1600 VeCo 93012 554-C4
3100 VeCo 93012 555-B5
3900 VeCo 91320 555-B5
3900 THO 91320 555-D4

STREET Block City ZIP Pg-Grid
POTTER AV
1900 SIMI 93065 498-A2
2800 THO 91360 526-H2
N POTTER AV
2000 SIMI 93065 498-A2
POWDERHORN CT
1000 VeCo 91377 528-B7
POWELL DR
1700 VEN 93004 492-H4
POWELL RD
100 VeCo 93015 457-C6
E PRADERA RD
11500 VeCo 93012 496-C7
PRADO WY
- OXN 93030 523-A4
PRAIRIE CT
3300 THO 91320 555-G6
PRAIRIE ST
22000 Chat 91311 499-J7
PRAIRIE DOG PL
1300 VEN 93003 492-F4
PRAIRIE RIDGE CT
- SIMI 93063 478-H5
PRAIRIEVIEW ST
5100 CMRL 93012 524-J2
PRANCE CT
1800 SIMI 93065 498-A6
N PRATHER ST
2500 SIMI 93065 498-B3
PRATO CT
3900 MRPK 93021 496-C5
PREAKNESS PL
700 THO 91320 555-E4
PREBLE AV
2400 VEN 93003 491-F3
PRENTISS ST
- THO 91360 526-E4
PRESIDENTIAL DR
700 SIMI 93065 497-D5
700 VeCo 93065 497-D5
PRESIDIO DR
3400 SIMI 93063 478-F5
PRESILLA PL
2100 VeCo 93010 494-D7
PRESILLA RD
7500 VeCo 93012 495-G5
10600 VeCo 93012 496-A5
PRESTBURY LN
- VeCo 91361 586-E2
PRESTON WY
300 SIMI 93065 497-D6
PRICE RD
4000 VeCo 93066 494-D3
5100 VeCo 93066 474-D7
PRICE ST
400 FILM 93015 455-J6
PRIDE ST
1200 SIMI 93065 497-H4
PRIETO ST
1400 SPLA 93060 464-C4
PRIMA CT
1400 CMRL 93010 524-D1
PRIMPTON CT
300 SIMI 93065 497-D7
PRIMROSE DR
5000 VeCo 93001 471-C1
5200 VeCo 93001 461-C7
PRIMROSE ST
600 THO 91360 526-D3
PRINCE AL
1900 VEN 93001 491-E3
PRINCE RD
6000 VeCo 93063 499-B3
PRINCESSA DR
23600 OXN 93030 522-J5
PRINCETON AV
- OXN 93036 522-H2
200 VEN 93003 492-A3
500 MRPK 93021 476-H6
500 MRPK 93021 496-F1
PRINCETON RD
1000 THO 91360 526-H5
PRINCETON ST
300 SPLA 93060 463-J7
PRINCEVILLE LN
2200 OXN 93036 522-E2
PRINCIPE PL
10400 VeCo 93012 495-J7
PRINGLE CT
- THO 91320 556-B1
PROMENADE
- VEN 93001 491-B3
PROMENADE ST
- SIMI 93063 498-H1
PROMONTORY PL
29400 AGRH 91301 557-J5
PROPANE RD
23600 VeCo 93015 456-F7
PROSPECT ST
- VeCo 93022 451-A7
E PROSPECT ST
- VEN 93001 491-B1
W PROSPECT ST
- VEN 93001 491-B1
PROSPECTOR PL
900 THO 91320 555-G4
PROVENCE DR
- Ago 91301 558-G3
- LACo 91302 558-G3
PROVENCE PL
3100 THO 91362 526-J2
PROVIDENCE AV
600 VEN 93004 492-H2
PROVIDENT RD
27300 AGRH 91301 558-E7
PROVO LN
800 VEN 93004 492-J2
PUCCINI RD
4900 VEN 93003 492-B7
N PUEBLO AV
100 VeCo 93023 441-E6
S PUEBLO AV
100 VeCo 93023 441-D7
PUEBLO DR
500 THO 91362 526-H7
PUEBLO ST
9500 VEN 93004 492-H2
22100 Chat 91311 499-J2
PUEBLO VISTA
6900 CMRL 93012 525-C1
PUESTA DEL SOL
600 VeCo 91360 526-C7
10500 VeCo 93022 451-B4
10900 VeCo 93023 451-B4
PULLMAN AV
2000 SIMI 93063 499-A2
PURCELL LN
1000 VEN 93003 492-A7
PURDUE AV
300 VEN 93003 492-A2

STREET Block City ZIP Pg-Grid
PURDUE ST
100 OXN 93036 522-H2
E PURDUE ST
14300 MRPK 93021 476-G6
PYRAMID AV
1500 VEN 93004 492-J3
PYRITE PL
2500 OXN 93030 522-D4

Q

Q ST
1500 VEN 93004 493-A2
QUAIL CT
300 SPLA 93060 464-D5
1200 FILM 93015 455-H6
QUAIL ST
700 VeCo 93023 451-C1
6400 VeCo 93003 492-D5
N QUAIL CANYON RD
6000 VeCo 93066 495-C1
6200 VeCo 93066 475-D7
QUAILCREEK CT
11600 MRPK 93021 496-C3
QUAIL OAKS DR
400 OJAI 93023 441-G6
QUAIL PASS RD
300 SIMI 93065 527-D1
QUAILRIDGE DR
5300 CMRL 93012 525-A1
QUAIL RUN DR
29100 AGRH 91301 558-A5
29400 AGRH 91301 557-H5
QUAIL RUN WY
900 OXN 93036 522-F1
QUAILS TR
100 THO 91361 556-F2
QUAILSPRING CT
4200 MRPK 93021 496-B2
QUAIL SUMMIT
13200 MRPK 93021 496-E3
QUAIL VIEW CT
700 VeCo 91377 558-B1
QUAILWOOD ST
3900 MRPK 93021 496-C4
QUAINT ST
28600 AGRH 91301 558-B3
QUARTER HORSE LN
900 VeCo 91377 558-A1
QUARTERS A DR
- PHME 93041 552-E5
QUARTZ ST
- VEN 93004 492-F3
N QUARZO CIR
3200 THO 91362 527-A2
QUASAR CT
23600 SIMI 93065 497-H4
QUEENS CT
6800 MRPK 93021 476-H6
QUEENS ST
5300 VEN 93003 492-B3
QUEENS WY
2700 THO 91362 527-B3
29300 AGRH 91301 557-J4
29300 AGRH 91301 558-A4
QUEENSBURY ST
300 THO 91360 526-E5
QUEENS GARDEN CT
23600 VeCo 91361 586-F1
QUEENS GARDEN DR
- VeCo 91361 556-G7
23600 VeCo 91361 586-E1
QUEENSLAND CT
2100 THO 91360 526-B4
QUIET CT
200 SIMI 93065 497-J6
QUIET HILLS CT
8200 LA 91304 529-E3
QUILAN CT
- OXN 93035 522-C6
QUIMBY AV
7400 CanP 91307 529-G4
7600 LA 91304 529-G4
QUIMISA DR
23600 SIMI 93065 477-C7
QUINCY AV
3400 SIMI 93063 478-F6
QUINCY ST
- OXN 93033 552-J2
8100 VEN 93004 492-F2
QUINN ST
- VEN 93003 492-C3
QUINTA VISTA DR
- THO 91362 557-A2
QUITO CT
6900 CMRL 93012 525-D1
6900 CMRL 93012 495-D7

R

R ST
1500 VEN 93004 493-A2
RABBIT CREEK LN
4200 THO 91320 555-E3
RACCOON CT
7200 VEN 93003 492-F4
RACHAEL AV
3400 SIMI 93063 478-F6
RACHEL DR
1100 OXN 93030 522-E4
RACINE ST
2700 SIMI 93065 498-C1
RACQUET CLUB LN
500 THO 91360 526-D7
RADCLIFF ST
5100 VEN 93003 492-B2
RADCLIFFE RD
800 THO 91360 526-G2
RADFORD CT
2500 SIMI 93063 498-D1
RADNOR AV
1500 VEN 93004 492-G4
RAEMERE ST
2100 CMRL 93010 524-E3
RAFFERTY RD
4800 VeCo 93060 454-A7
RAFT LN
500 OXN 93035 522-D7
RAIDERS WY
1200 OXN 93033 552-J3
RAILROAD AV
800 SPLA 93060 464-B5
RAINBOW DR
100 OXN 93033 553-C3
RAINBOW CREEK CIR
3300 THO 91360 526-C2
N RAINBOW CREST DR
5500 AGRH 91301 557-G5
W RAINBOW CREST DR
29800 AGRH 91301 557-H5

STREET Block City ZIP Pg-Grid
RAINBOW HILL RD
5700 AGRH 91301 557-G3
RAINBOW VIEW DR
30300 AGRH 91301 557-G4
RAINCLOUD CT
3500 THO 91362 526-J1
RAINDANCE ST
300 THO 91360 526-D2
RAINEY RD
1200 VeCo 93063 499-A3
RAINFIELD AV
23600 THO 91362 527-B5
RAINIER ST
- MRPK 93021 496-D1
5400 VEN 93003 492-B1
RAINS CT
1000 OJAI 93023 441-J5
15300 MRPK 93021 476-J5
RAINTREE CT
800 THO 91361 557-A4
RAIN WOOD ST
5200 SIMI 93063 498-J2
RALEIGH PL
800 THO 91360 526-G2
RALLEY CT
2100 THO 91362 527-A2
RALPH WY
700 SPLA 93060 464-C3
RALSTON AV
2000 SIMI 93063 498-H1
RALSTON ST
4700 VEN 93003 492-D4
7300 VeCo 93003 492-E4
RAMA PL
5000 CMRL 93012 524-G3
RAMBLE RIDGE DR
100 THO 91360 526-F2
RAMBLING RD
1000 SIMI 93065 497-H6
1600 SIMI 93065 498-A6
RAMBLING ROSE DR
- CMRL 93012 495-A7
RAMELLI AV
1100 VeCo 93003 492-E4
1100 VEN 93003 492-F5
RAMELLI RANCH RD
- VeCo - 366-G8
- VeCo 93001 366-G8
23600 VeCo 93001 459-H1
RAMONA DR
1100 THO 91320 556-A1
1300 CMRL 93010 494-A6
1400 CMRL 93010 493-J6
1400 VeCo 93010 494-A6
RAMONA PL
- VeCo 93010 493-J7
- VeCo 93010 523-J1
RAMONA ST
1600 CMRL 93010 493-J7
1600 VeCo 93010 493-J7
E RAMONA ST
- VEN 93001 471-B7
- VEN 93001 491-C1
W RAMONA ST
- VEN 93001 471-B7
RAMONA CANYON RD
- VeCo 93040 458-D1
RAMROD CT
3500 THO 91320 555-F4
RAMSGATE CIR
1800 THO 91360 526-C5
N RAMUDA LN
- VeCo 91307 529-A5
RANCH RD
- VeCo 93001 461-A4
12400 VeCo 93060 473-C2
23600 VeCo 93001 366-G9
23600 VeCo 93001 459-D4
23600 VeCo 93023 450-J2
RANCH CREEK CT
23600 SIMI 93065 497-G7
RANCHERO PL
- OXN 93030 522-J3
E RANCHERO RD
- VeCo 91307 528-J4
RANCHGROVE DR
2400 WLKV 91361 586-J1
RANCH HOUSE RD
900 THO 91361 557-A5
RANCHITA LN
4100 OXN 93033 553-C4
RANCHO CT
1100 VeCo 93023 441-F6
RANCHO DR
100 OJAI 93023 441-E7
100 VeCo 93023 441-F6
200 VEN 93003 491-G4
S RANCHO DR
100 OJAI 93023 441-E7
100 VeCo 93023 441-E7
300 OJAI 93023 451-E1
300 VeCo 93023 451-E1
RANCHO LN
- THO 91362 526-J7
1300 THO 91362 556-H1
RANCHO RD
- THO 91362 556-H1
300 THO 91362 526-H7
23600 THO 91361 556-H1
23600 VeCo 93012 524-H7
S RANCHO RD
- THO 91361 556-H2
RANCHO ADOLFO CT
100 CMRL 93012 524-H2
RANCHO ADOLFO DR
- CMRL 93012 524-H2
RANCHO CALLEGUAS DR
100 CMRL 93012 524-H3
RANCHO CONEJO BLVD
600 THO 91320 525-H5
1000 THO 91320 526-A6
23600 THO 91320 555-H1
RANCHO DOS RIOS
23600 VeCo 93023 451-F3
RANCHO DOS VIENTOS
DR
1000 THO 91320 555-A3
RANCHO FILOSO
400 VeCo 93060 463-H5
RANCHO LA VISTA RD
1500 VeCo 93023 451-E2
RANCHO VISTA CT
13300 MRPK 93021 496-E6
RANCHO VISTA LN
500 VeCo 93060 472-J5
RANCH VIEW PL
600 THO 91362 557-A1
700 THO 91362 527-A7
RANCHWOOD ST
3200 THO 91320 555-G4

STREET Block City ZIP Pg-Grid
RAND ST
6400 MRPK 93021 476-J6
RANDI AV
6200 WdHl 91367 529-J7
6400 CanP 91303 529-J7
RANDIWOOD LN
6600 LACo 91307 529-C6
RANDY DR
500 VeCo 91320 525-G7
500 VeCo 91320 555-G1
RANGELY CT
200 SIMI 93065 497-F6
RANGER CT
3000 THO 91360 526-D2
RANGE VIEW CIR
- MRPK 93021 476-F5
RANGEWOOD CT
- MRPK 93021 476-E6
RANSOM RD
13800 MRPK 93021 496-F4
RASPBERRY PL
100 OXN 93036 522-G1
RATEL PL
7000 VEN 93003 492-E4
RATTLESNAKE RD
- LACo 90265 586-G7
RAVELLO CT
- THO 91362 527-C3
RAVEN AV
1300 VEN 93003 492-C4
RAVEN LN
4000 OXN 93033 553-B5
RAVENCREST CT
200 THO 91320 555-G2
RAVENNA ST
2100 SIMI 93065 498-C2
RAVENSBURY ST
500 VeCo 91361 556-G6
RAVENS POINT CT
23600 SIMI 93065 498-C5
RAVENWOOD AV
800 THO 91320 555-E4
RAVOLI DR
2000 OXN 93035 552-B1
RAWHIDE PL
900 THO 91320 555-G5
RAWLS RD
- MRPK 93021 476-B5
RAYBURN ST
1800 THO 91362 527-D5
RAYEN ST
22000 LA 91304 529-J1
23900 WHil 91304 529-E1
RAYLENE CT
6200 SIMI 93063 499-C2
RAYMOND ST
200 OJAI 93023 441-G6
23200 Chat 91311 499-F7
E RAYMOND ST
500 VeCo 93022 451-C6
RAYSHIRE ST
1900 THO 91362 526-J7
1900 THO 91362 527-A7
RAYTHEON RD
4100 VeCo 93033 553-F6
REA WY
200 VEN 93001 491-A1
READ RD
4900 THO 93021 496-J6
4900 THO 93021 497-A6
4900 VeCo 93021 496-G5
4900 VeCo 93021 497-A5
13100 VeCo 93012 496-G5
13100 THO 93012 496-G5
READING DR
4400 OXN 93033 553-A5
READING ST
- FILM 93015 455-J7
REAGAN CT
100 VEN 93003 492-E1
REAL CANYON RD
700 VeCo 93040 457-E3
REATA AV
- VEN 93004 473-A6
REBECCA RD
- SIMI 93063 479-C7
REBECCA ST
2000 SIMI 93063 498-F2
REBURTA LN
3500 SIMI 93063 478-E7
RECODO WY
5800 CMRL 93012 525-B1
RED BARN RD
11000 VeCo 93012 496-A7
RED BIRD CT
- MRPK 93021 476-E6
RED BLUFF CT
3400 SIMI 93063 479-A6
RED BLUFF DR
26000 CALB 91302 558-J4
REDCOAT LN
4200 WLKV 91361 557-F6
REDDINGTON CT
100 CMRL 93010 524-D1
100 CMRL 93010 494-D7
REDFIELD AV
- THO 91320 555-H1
RED HAWK CT
- SIMI 93063 478-G5
RED HILL RD
500 OJAI 93023 441-J5
RED LAKES PL
600 SIMI 93065 497-C5
REDMAN CT
2000 SIMI 93063 498-J2
REDMESA DR
10900 Chat 91311 499-J2
RED MOUNTAIN EAST
FIRE RD
23600 VeCo 93001 460-G6
RED MOUNTAIN FIRE
RD
23600 VeCo 93001 460-B2
RED OAK AV
100 THO 91320 556-D2
RED OAK PL
1000 CMRL 93010 524-C2
REDONDO AV
2700 VeCo 93012 496-C6
REDONDO CIR
2700 VeCo 93012 496-C7
REDONDO ST
7600 VEN 93004 492-E1
RED PINE DR
23600 SIMI 93065 498-D4
RED ROBIN PL
- THO 91320 526-A5
RED ROCK AV
- VEN 93004 492-J3

STREET Block City ZIP Pg-Grid
RED ROCK CT
5100 THO 91362 527-F6
RED SAIL CIR
1300 THO 91361 557-B6
REDWING LN
1200 OXN 93036 522-E1
REDWOOD AV
- VEN 93003 491-J3
REDWOOD CIR
- VEN 93003 491-J3
1500 THO 91360 526-H3
REDWOOD DR
1000 VeCo 93063 499-C4
REDWOOD LN
100 SPLA 93060 464-A5
REDWOOD ST
200 OXN 93033 552-E2
1500 OXN 93043 552-E2
REED WY
400 PHME 93041 552-D2
REEDER AV
4100 OXN 93033 553-B5
REEDLEY ST
14700 MRPK 93021 476-H6
REEF CIR
600 PHME 93041 552-F7
REEF ST
2900 VEN 93001 491-F5
REEF WY
5100 OXN 93035 521-J7
11800 VeCo 90265 625-F5
REEVES RD
3200 VeCo 93023 442-G6
REFLECTIONS LN
- SIMI 93065 478-B4
REFSING DR
3800 OXN 93033 552-G4
REFSING PL
4700 OXN 93033 552-G5
REGAL AV
100 THO 91320 555-J2
REGAL OAK CT
100 THO 91320 556-A2
REGAN CIR
1700 SIMI 93065 498-A3
REGATTA PL
3300 OXN 93035 522-C7
REGENT AV
3200 THO 91360 526-F2
REGENT CT
700 SPLA 93060 464-A4
REGENT ST
1500 CMRL 93010 524-D2
REGENTS CT
4400 WLKV 91361 557-D6
REGINA AV
2700 THO 91360 526-E3
REGIS AV
200 VEN 93003 492-C1
REGULUS DR
- VeCo 93041 583-G1
REIMER PETIT RD
1600 VeCo 93060 465-C5
REINA CIR
- OXN 93030 523-B4
REINHARDT AV
- VEN 93003 492-C3
N REINO RD
- THO 91320 555-F1
400 THO 91320 525-F7
S REINO RD
- THO 91320 555-F3
REMINGTON AV
600 VEN 93003 492-D3
REMINGTON PL
800 THO 91320 555-G4
REMONT CIR
1600 VeCo 91377 527-H6
RENAISSANCE PL
- WLKV 91362 557-G6
RENATA CT
2500 THO 91362 527-C4
RENE ST
3400 VeCo 93036 493-A7
RENEE CT
- SIMI 93065 478-B6
RENEE DR
28100 AGRH 91301 558-C7
REPOSO DR
- VeCo 93022 451-C4
RESEDA CT
3500 CMRL 93010 494-G7
RESERVOIR DR
2600 SIMI 93065 478-C7
2600 SIMI 93065 498-C1
2800 SIMI 93063 478-C7
3000 VeCo 93063 478-C7
3000 VeCo 93065 478-C7
RESPLANDOR WY
- OXN 93030 522-H4
RESTFUL CT
1700 SIMI 93065 497-J6
1700 SIMI 93065 498-A6
RETIRO CT
900 VeCo 93010 494-B5
REVELLO ST
4000 MRPK 93021 496-C3
REVERE AV
- VEN 93004 472-H6
REX ST
200 VEN 93001 491-B1
REXFORD PL
1100 THO 91360 526-F6
REXFORD ST
3400 VEN 93003 491-H4
REYES ST
- MRPK 93021 496-D1
REYES ADOBE RD
4900 AGRH 91301 557-G3
REYNOLDS CT
1300 THO 91362 526-H7
RHAME TER
100 SPLA 93060 464-A5
RHAPSODY DR
4800 VeCo 91377 557-G2
RHEINLAND CT
23600 SIMI 93065 498-A5
RHODA ST
2000 SIMI 93065 498-A3
RHODES CT
200 FILM 93015 455-H6
RHONA CT
5300 AGRH 91301 557-H5
RHONDA AV
1900 OXN 93036 522-E3
RHONDA ST
2000 OXN 93036 522-E3
RHONE ST
- VEN 93004 492-J3

STREET Block City ZIP Pg-Grid

RIALTO ST
700 OXN 93035 522-E7
1400 OXN 93035 552-E1
RIATA CT
2400 VeCo 93012 496-D6
RIAVE CT
2400 CMRL 93012 495-B6
RIBERA DR
- OXN 93030 522-J4
- OXN 93030 523-A4
RIBERA WY
- OXN 93030 523-A4
N RICE AV
200 OXN 93030 523-B5
1900 OXN 93036 523-B5
23600 OXN 93033 523-B5
S RICE AV
- OXN 93033 553-B3
100 OXN 93030 523-B7
900 VeCo 93030 523-B7
900 VeCo 93033 523-B7
1500 VeCo 93033 553-B3
RICE CT
100 THO 91362 556-J1
4500 VEN 93003 492-A2
RICE RD
- VeCo 93023 441-C2
N RICE RD
100 VeCo 93023 441-D5
S RICE RD
100 VeCo 93023 441-C7
600 VeCo 93023 451-C2
RICE ST
5300 VeCo 93066 495-A5
RICE CANYON RD
- VeCo 93023 441-B5
RICHARD RD
400 SPLA 93060 463-H6
RICHARDS AV
1000 VEN 93004 492-J2
RICHARDSON AV
900 SIMI 93065 497-G5
RICHARDSON CANYON RD
- VeCo 93066 464-D7
- VeCo 93066 474-E1
RICHFORD LN
400 VeCo 93022 451-A7
RICHGROVE CT
31900 WLKV 91361 557-C6
RICHMOND AV
500 OXN 93030 522-H7
RICHMOND CT
600 SPLA 93060 464-C4
25900 LACo 91302 558-J3
RICHMOND RD
1100 SPLA 93060 464-B4
RICKEY CT
3100 THO 91362 527-A2
RIDDEN ST
3400 CMRL 93010 494-G7
RIDGE DR
12200 VeCo 93012 496-D6
RIDGEBROOK DR
5700 AGRH 91301 557-H4
RIDGEBROOK PL
2100 THO 91362 527-A3
RIDGECREST CT
6900 VEN 93003 472-D7
RIDGE CREST DR
500 SPLA 93060 463-H6
RIDGECREST DR
- MRPK 93021 476-F6
RIDGECREST LN
6500 VeCo 93066 475-A6
RIDGECREST PL
900 THO 91362 527-C7
RIDGEFORD DR
3200 WLKV 91361 557-D7
RIDGEGATE LN
1700 SIMI 93065 497-E2
RIDGE LINE DR
400 VeCo 93022 451-C6
RIDGEMARK CT
- MRPK 93021 476-D6
RIDGEMARK DR
- MRPK 93021 476-D6
RIDGEMONT CT
300 THO 91320 555-E2
RIDGEMOOR DR
5200 VeCo 93021 475-H7
5200 VeCo 93021 495-J1
RIDGETON LN
900 SIMI 93065 497-E6
RIDGE VIEW CT
2400 SIMI 93065 497-H1
RIDGE VIEW DR
2200 SIMI 93065 497-E2
RIDGE VIEW ST
4200 CMRL 93012 524-H4
5200 CMRL 93012 525-A5
RIDGEWAY CT
4800 THO 91362 557-F1
RIDGEWAY DR
29500 AGRH 91301 557-J3
RIDGEWAY PL
300 VEN 93004 472-H6
RIDGEWOOD DR
1600 CMRL 93012 525-A1
1700 CMRL 93012 495-A7
RIDLEY CIR
900 SIMI 93065 498-C5
RIENTE ST
900 VeCo 93010 494-B5
RIESS RD
900 VeCo 93063 499-B4
RIFLEMAN RD
- VeCo 93021 475-J4
RIGEL DR
- VeCo 93041 583-H2
RIGGER RD
30500 AGRH 91301 557-G5
RIGGING PL
1100 OXN 93030 522-F7
RIKKARD DR
2400 THO 91362 527-A2
RILEY LN
500 VEN 93003 492-D1
RIM CREST CIR
2300 THO 91361 557-B4
RIM CREST DR
2200 THO 91361 557-B4
RIMROCK RD
200 VeCo 91361 556-G2
RINCON CT
300 SPLA 93060 463-J6
RINCON DR
- VeCo 93012 554-E3
RINCON RD Rt#-150
6600 StBC 93013 459-A1
23600 VeCo 93001 366-G9
23600 VeCo 93001 459-A1
RINCON ST
100 OJAI 93023 441-H6
100 VEN 93001 491-E2
1200 SIMI 93065 498-B4
RINCON WY
400 OXN 93033 552-G3
RINCON BEACH PARK DR
- VeCo 93001 459-G7
- VeCo 93001 469-G1
RING CIR
3200 SIMI 93063 478-D7
RINGO AV
- VEN 93003 492-C3
RINGWOOD ST
2700 SIMI 93063 478-H7
E RINGWOOD ST
4900 SIMI 93063 478-H7
RIO BRAVO CT
- MRPK 93021 496-G2
RIODOSA TR
5500 VeCo 91377 557-J1
RIO GRANDE CIR
500 THO 91360 526-D3
RIO GRANDE ST
- FILM 93015 455-J7
- VEN 93004 492-J4
RIO GRANDE WY
- OXN 93036 492-H5
RIO HATO CT
3500 CMRL 93010 494-G7
RIO LINDO ST
400 OXN 93036 522-H2
S RIOPELLE CT
900 THO 91320 555-F4
RIO SCHOOL LN
- VeCo 93036 522-H1
RIO VIA
200 VeCo 93022 451-B6
RIO VISTA CT
1300 SIMI 93065 497-H1
RIPLEY ST
- CMRL 93010 524-A2
RIPLEY WY
1700 OXN 93033 552-J3
RIPPLE DR
900 OXN 93035 522-C7
RIPPLE CREEK LN
13000 VeCo 93012 496-F5
RISING STAR AV
- SIMI 93063 479-A6
RISTA DR
5700 AGRH 91301 557-J4
RIVA CT
3900 MRPK 93021 496-C4
RIVAS LN
1100 OXN 93035 522-E7
RIVENDELL CIR
1800 THO 91320 556-A2
RIVER DR
3900 VeCo 93001 471-C3
RIVER ST
200 FILM 93015 456-A6
500 VeCo 93040 457-F4
700 FILM 93015 455-G7
RIVERA ST
800 SIMI 93065 497-G4
RIVERBIRCH DR
2000 SIMI 93063 498-J2
RIVERDALE CT
- CMRL 93012 524-G4
RIVER FARM DR
3700 WLKV 91361 557-C7
RIVERFIELD CT
200 SIMI 93065 497-F6
RIVERGLEN ST
4200 MRPK 93021 496-D3
RIVERGROVE CT
11900 MRPK 93021 496-C3
RIVERGROVE ST
12100 MRPK 93021 496-D3
RIVER HILLS CT
500 SIMI 93065 497-G6
RIVERMORE ST
3400 CMRL 93010 494-G7
RIVERPARK BLVD
- OXN 93036 492-H7
- OXN 93036 522-G1
RIVER RIDGE RD
2200 OXN 93036 522-E2
RIVERROCK CIR
400 THO 91362 557-G1
RIVERRUN LN
13200 VeCo 93012 496-E4
RIVERSIDE AV
700 VeCo 93015 465-H2
700 VeCo 93015 466-A2
RIVERSIDE RD
- VeCo 93022 451-A6
RIVERSIDE ST
700 VEN 93001 471-B7
RIVERSTONE LN
600 VeCo 91377 527-G7
RIVER WOOD CT
23600 SIMI 93063 499-B3
RIVIERA CT
- OXN 93035 522-C6
RIVOL RD
7000 CanP 91307 529-D5
ROADRUNNER AV
- THO 91320 525-J5
- THO 91320 526-A5
ROADRUNNER DR
6800 VEN 93003 492-E4
ROADRUNNER PL
- THO 91320 525-J5
ROADSIDE DR
28300 AGRH 91301 558-A6
29300 AGRH 91301 557-J6
ROAN ST
1400 SIMI 93065 497-J3
ROB CT
2800 THO 91362 527-A3
ROBBINS CT
- SIMI 93065 497-E3
ROBERT AV
100 OXN 93033 552-G3
W ROBERT AV
200 OXN 93030 522-F4
ROBERTA CT
- SIMI 93065 498-C4
ROBERTS AV
200 MRPK 93021 496-E1
ROBERT S HOLLAND DR
- THO 91361 556-G2
ROBERTSON RD
23600 VeCo 93063 499-D4
ROBERTSON WY
- THO 91320 556-B1
ROBIN AV
1100 VEN 93003 492-D4
1100 VEN 93009 492-D4
2100 OXN 93033 553-A4
ROBIN CT
400 FILM 93015 455-H6
ROBIN ST
- OJAI 93023 442-A6
ROBIN HILL ST
3500 THO 91360 526-G2
ROBINWOOD LN
4300 MRPK 93021 496-F3
ROBLE LN
23600 OXN 93036 522-H3
ROBLES LN
5300 AGRH 91301 557-H5
ROBYN WY
1100 CMRL 93010 524-C3
ROCA AV
2600 THO 91360 526-C3
ROCA RD
23600 VeCo 93063 528-H2
ROCHELLE PL
2600 SIMI 93063 478-D7
2600 SIMI 93063 498-D1
ROCHESTER CT
600 VEN 93004 492-H1
ROCK ST
2700 SIMI 93065 498-C3
ROCKAWAY RD
- VeCo 93022 451-A5
ROCK CASTLE CT
5300 VeCo 91377 527-G6
ROCK CREEK RD
5600 AGRH 91301 558-A4
N ROCKDALE AV
2000 SIMI 93063 499-B1
ROCKEDGE DR
300 VeCo 91377 558-A1
ROCKET ST
- VeCo 93042 583-D4
ROCKETDYNE RD
23700 LA 91304 499-D7
23900 WHil 91304 499-D7
24900 VeCo 93063 499-B7
ROCKFIELD ST
4800 THO 91362 557-G1
4900 VeCo 91362 557-G1
5000 VeCo 91377 557-H1
ROCKFORD CT
4700 VEN 93003 492-A2
ROCKGATE PL
3000 SIMI 93063 478-E7
ROCKHILL DR
23500 Chat 91311 499-F7
ROCKINGHAM DR
1300 SIMI 93063 499-C4
ROCKING HORSE DR
1700 SIMI 93065 497-J6
1700 SIMI 93065 498-A7
ROCKLITE RD
- VEN 93001 471-C6
- VeCo 93001 471-C6
ROCKLYN ST
2000 CMRL 93010 524-E1
ROCKMAN WY
400 PHME 93041 552-D2
ROCKRIDGE PL
2800 THO 91360 526-E3
ROCKRIDGE TER
7100 CanP 91307 529-E5
ROCKROSE LN
100 VeCo 91377 557-J2
ROCK SPRING ST
- THO 91320 526-A6
ROCK TREE DR
5500 AGRH 91301 558-A5
ROCK VISTA DR
29000 AGRH 91301 558-A5
ROCKY RD
1200 VeCo 93063 499-D4
ROCKY HIGH RD
- VeCo 93012 526-A1
ROCKY MESA PL
9200 WHil 91304 499-D7
ROCKY MOUNTAIN
- VeCo 93001 461-B6
ROCKY MOUNTAIN DR
- OXN 93036 492-H7
ROCKY PEAK FIRE RD
- Chat 91311 479-E3
- StvR 91381 479-E3
15900 SIMI 93063 499-F1
23600 VeCo 93063 479-D4
23600 VeCo 93063 499-F1
ROCKY POINT CT
2600 THO 91362 527-D3
ROCKYRIVER CT
1600 SIMI 93063 498-E3
ROCKYRIVER ST
3700 SIMI 93063 498-E3
ROCKY TOP CIR
- MRPK 93021 476-F5
ROD AV
6000 WdHl 91367 529-C7
RODAX ST
22700 LA 91304 529-H2
RODENE ST
- THO 91320 555-E3
RODEO CT
2000 THO 91362 556-H2
RODEO DR
200 VeCo 93022 451-C5
W RODERICK AV
- OXN 93030 522-F4
RODGERS ST
200 VEN 93003 492-B3
RODNEY ST
2600 THO 91320 525-H7
ROGER RD
800 SPLA 93060 464-C3
12400 VeCo 93060 473-E6
ROGUE RIVER CIR
1800 VEN 93004 492-G4
ROHDEA WY
- OXN 93030 523-A4
ROHNER AV
2000 SIMI 93063 499-C2
ROHNER CT
2200 SIMI 93063 499-C1
ROIA LN
- OXN 93036 492-H7
ROLAND WY
5400 OXN 93033 552-F6
ROLDAN AV
1100 SIMI 93065 498-A4
ROLLING KNOLL RD
4400 MRPK 93021 496-F3
ROLLING MEADOWS CT
500 THO 91320 526-B7
ROLLING OAKS DR
100 THO 91361 556-F2
500 VeCo 91361 556-G2
ROLLING RIDGE DR
29900 AGRH 91301 557-H4
ROLLING RIVER LN
- SIMI 93063 498-G2
ROLLINGS AV
2800 THO 91360 526-H2
ROLLINS RD
9300 Chat 91311 499-F6
ROMAN AV
1700 CMRL 93010 494-G7
1700 CMRL 93010 524-G1
ROMANO DR
800 VeCo 93023 451-C1
ROMANY DR
4000 OXN 93035 552-B2
ROMAR ST
22000 Chat 91311 499-J4
ROMBERG LN
800 VEN 93003 492-B7
ROMERO PL
- CMRL 93012 494-H7
RONALD REAGAN FRWY Rt#-118
- Chat - 499-E2
- MRPK - 476-H7
- MRPK - 477-B6
- MRPK - 496-G1
- SIMI - 477-B6
- SIMI - 497-G1
- SIMI - 498-F1
- SIMI - 499-E2
- VeCo - 477-B6
RONDELL ST
4100 AGRH 91301 558-E7
RONEL CT
400 THO 91320 556-C1
ROOSEVELT AV
100 OXN 93030 522-H6
200 VEN 93003 492-E1
N ROOSEVELT AV
100 OXN 93030 522-H5
ROOSEVELT BLVD
2300 VeCo 93035 552-B5
ROOSEVELT CT
- SIMI 93065 497-D5
- VEN 93003 492-E1
RORY LN
1600 SIMI 93063 499-B2
RORY WY
5900 SIMI 93063 499-B3
ROSA LN
100 THO 91320 555-H2
W ROSA ST
200 OXN 93033 552-G5
ROSADA CT
900 VeCo 93010 494-B5
ROSAL LN
10900 VeCo 93004 493-B1
ROSALIE ST
3500 SIMI 93063 498-D2
ROSALINDA DR
23600 OXN 93030 522-J5
ROSARIO CT
500 THO 91362 526-H7
ROSARIO DR
400 THO 91362 526-H7
ROSCOE BLVD
22000 LA 91304 529-D2
24000 WHil 91304 529-D2
ROSE AV
2900 VeCo 93036 523-A1
3300 VeCo 93036 493-C5
N ROSE AV
100 OXN 93030 522-J4
1900 OXN 93036 522-J4
2600 OXN 93036 523-A2
2600 VeCo 93036 523-A2
S ROSE AV
100 OXN 93030 522-J7
500 VeCo 93030 522-J7
1100 OXN 93033 522-J7
1100 VeCo 93033 522-J7
ROSE CIR
VEN 93004 493-A2
ROSE LN
2300 VeCo 93012 496-B7
ROSE ST
1200 VeCo 93063 499-B4
E ROSE ST
200 OXN 93033 552-G5
ROSE ARBOR LN
- SIMI 93065 497-H3
ROSEBAY ST
2000 THO 91361 557-A5
ROSEBUD DR
500 OXN 93036 522-F1
ROSECRANS ST
2100 SIMI 93065 498-A4
ROSECREEK DR
11400 MRPK 93021 496-B3
ROSEDALE CT
13100 VeCo 93012 496-E6
ROSE GARDEN CIR
- THO 91361 556-H5
ROSEHEDGE LN
200 VeCo 91377 557-J2
ROSEHILL CIR
3200 THO 91360 526-F2
ROSELAND AV
8200 VeCo 93021 476-E2
ROSELAWN AV
1300 THO 91362 527-A6
ROSEMARY ST
2100 SIMI 93065 498-A4
ROSEMONT CT
- VeCo 91361 556-F6
4700 VEN 93003 492-A2
ROSETTA WY
- CMRL 93012 524-H1
ROSETTE ST
2700 SIMI 93065 498-C5
ROSETTI LN
500 VEN 93003 492-D1
ROSE VALLEY RD
- VeCo - 366-K5
ROSE VISTA TER
- CMRL 93012 495-A7
ROSEWATER PL
23600 OXN 93035 522-C7
ROSEWOOD AV
100 CMRL 93010 524-C3
ROSEWOOD CT
1800 OXN 93030 522-F3
1900 THO 91362 526-J3
1900 THO 91362 527-A3
ROSEWOOD DR
900 OXN 93030 522-F3
ROSEWOOD ST
200 VEN 93001 471-B7
ROSITA DR
1500 SIMI 93065 497-F3
ROSITA RD
8900 VeCo 93012 495-G7
10600 VeCo 93012 496-A7
ROSS CIR
1700 SIMI 93065 498-C3
ROSSINI LN
4600 VEN 93003 492-A4
ROSSMORE DR
200 VeCo 93035 552-B5
ROSWELL CT
700 VEN 93004 492-G2
ROSWELL ST
8300 VEN 93004 492-G3
ROTELLA ST
1000 THO 91320 555-F4
ROTH CT
2600 THO 91320 525-H6
ROTHKO LN
6000 SIMI 93063 499-B1
ROULETTE CIR
1700 THO 91362 526-J2
ROUNDHOUSE RD
- PHME 93043 552-D2
ROUND MOUNTAIN RD
- VeCo 93012 554-D4
ROUNDTREE PL
4800 THO 91362 557-F1
ROUNDUP CIR
3000 THO 91360 526-C2
N ROUNDUP RD
- VeCo 91307 528-J5
- VeCo 91307 529-A5
ROUSSEAU ST
- PHME 93041 552-E4
ROWELL AV
9200 Chat 91311 499-F6
9200 Chat 91311 499-F7
ROWLAND AV
2100 SIMI 93063 498-G1
E ROWLAND AV
1600 CMRL 93010 524-D1
N ROWLAND AV
300 CMRL 93010 524-E2
ROXBURY PL
1100 THO 91360 526-F6
ROXBURY ST
4100 SIMI 93063 478-F5
ROXY ST
2400 SIMI 93065 478-B7
ROYAL AV
- SIMI 93065 497-G3
1600 SIMI 93065 498-D3
3200 SIMI 93063 498-E3
ROYAL GLEN RD
3900 WLKV 91361 557-C6
ROYAL HILLS CT
23600 SIMI 93065 478-B7
ROYAL LONDON CT
23600 VeCo 91361 556-F5
ROYAL OAK PL
1100 SPLA 93060 464-B3
ROYAL OAKS DR
3000 THO 91362 557-A3
ROYAL RIDGE CT
5000 THO 91362 527-F6
ROYAL SAINT GEORGE DR
1600 THO 91362 527-D6
ROYAL VISTA CT
5000 THO 91362 557-E1
ROYCE CT
1400 CMRL 93010 524-D1
ROYCETON CT
32000 WLKV 91361 557-C6
ROYER AV
6200 WdHl 91367 529-G7
6400 CanP 91307 529-G5
7500 LA 91304 529-G2
ROYMOR DR
26100 CALB 91302 558-H4
RUBENS PL
600 OXN 93033 552-H4
RUBICON AV
1100 VEN 93004 492-J2
RUBICON CT
10000 VEN 93004 492-J3
RUBIO AV
100 CMRL 93010 524-D4
RUBIO CIR
- OXN 93030 522-J4
RUBY AV
800 VEN 93004 492-F3
RUBY DR
200 THO 91320 525-H6
2500 OXN 93030 522-D4
RUDDER AV
2500 PHME 93041 552-C2
RUDMAN DR
600 VeCo 91320 525-G7
RUDNICK AV
6600 CanP 91303 529-J6
7600 LA 91304 529-J1
9500 Chat 91311 499-J5
RUDOLPH DR
300 VeCo 91320 556-B3
23600 SIMI 93065 498-B5
RUGBY AV
1100 VEN 93004 492-G3
RUGBY CIR
1500 THO 91360 526-F5
RUGBY RD
1100 VeCo 93023 442-F5
RUNKLE FIRE RD
23600 SIMI 93063 528-E1
23600 VeCo 93063 528-E1
RUNKLE HAUL RD
- SIMI 93063 498-D7
RUNNING CREEK CT
- SIMI 93065 497-G6
RUNNING TRAILS AV
3200 SIMI 93063 478-J6
RUNNYMEDE ST
22000 CanP 91303 529-J4
22700 CanP 91307 529-G4
RUNWAY ST
4400 SIMI 93063 498-G3
RUSCHIA WY
- OXN 93030 523-A4
RUSH CIR
2000 THO 91362 526-J6
2000 THO 91362 527-A6
RUSH HAVEN WY
1700 SIMI 93065 497-F3
RUSHING CREEK PL
500 THO 91360 526-G1
RUSHMORE ST
5400 VEN 93003 472-B7
RUSKIN AV
2100 THO 91360 526-G4
RUSS CT
3800 SIMI 93063 478-E6
RUSSELL CT
6800 VEN 93003 492-E3
RUSSELL RANCH RD
31300 WLKV 91362 557-E5
RUSSEL TEMPLE RD
300 VeCo 93060 455-B6
RUSSETWOOD LN
23600 SIMI 93065 497-A2
RUSTIC GLEN DR
2700 THO 91362 526-J3
RUSTIC HILLS DR
23600 SIMI 93065 527-F1
RUSTIC OAK DR
31500 WLKV 91361 557-D6
RUSTIC PARK CT
2100 THO 91362 527-A4
RUSTIC VIEW CT
4200 MRPK 93021 496-B2
RUSTLING HEIGHTS CT
- SIMI 93065 497-G7
RUSTLING OAKS DR
5900 AGRH 91301 558-A3
E RUTGER CIR
14400 MRPK 93021 476-G6
RUTGERS CT
700 THO 91360 526-G5
RUTGERS DR
1800 THO 91360 526-G5
RUTH AV
200 MRPK 93021 496-E1
RUTH DR
600 VeCo 91320 525-G7
RUTHERFORD HILL DR
- LA 91304 529-D4
RUTHWOOD DR
5400 CALB 91302 558-H3
RUTLAND PL
2300 THO 91362 527-A2
RYDER CUP DR
1600 THO 91362 527-D6
RYE CT
- THO 91362 557-A1
RYNERSON CT
2600 SIMI 93065 478-B7

S

S ST
1500 VEN 93004 493-A2
S & D RD
- VeCo 93015 455-G5
S S & J RD
23600 VeCo 93015 456-J7
S & J RANCH RD
23600 VeCo 93015 456-J5
23600 VeCo 93015 457-A5
SABET CT
1800 CMRL 93010 494-G7
SABINA CIR
1500 SIMI 93063 499-A3
SABINA ST
8900 VEN 93004 492-H4
SABLE ST
7500 VEN 93003 492-F5
SABLE RIDGE CT
- SIMI 93063 478-H5
SABRA AV
- VeCo 91377 558-A2
SABRINA ST
1300 OXN 93036 522-J3
SACRAMENTO DR
300 VEN 93004 472-H6
SACRAMENTO ST
- VeCo 93040 457-F4
SADDLE AV
2600 OXN 93036 522-G1
2600 OXN 93036 492-G7
SADDLE LN
200 OJAI 93023 441-J7
200 OJAI 93023 451-H1
SADDLE TR
200 VeCo 91361 556-G2
SADDLEBACK CIR
1100 CMRL 93012 525-B2
SADDLEBACK CT
3000 THO 91360 526-C2
SADDLEBACK DR
- MRPK 93021 476-F5
SADDLEBACK TR
1100 CMRL 93012 525-B1
SADDLEBACK WY
5900 CMRL 93012 525-B1
N SADDLEBOW RD
- VeCo 91307 528-G3
SADDLEBROOK DR
29000 AGRH 91301 558-A4
SADDLE CREST LN
4200 WLKV 91361 557-E6
SADDLEHORN PL
900 THO 91320 555-G5
SADDLE MOUNTAIN DR
32300 WLKV 91361 557-C7
SADDLERIDGE CT
12600 VeCo 93012 496-D6
SADDLERIDGE LN
- CALB 91302 558-H4
SADDLE TREE DR
31500 WLKV 91361 557-D7
SADRING AV
7800 LA 91304 529-F3
SAFED RD
- SIMI 93063 479-B7
- SIMI 93063 499-B1
SAFFRON CIR
3000 THO 91360 526-H2
SAGAMORE LN
1200 VEN 93001 491-E5
E SAGE LN
- VeCo 91307 528-J3
- VeCo 91307 529-A4
SAGE ST
11300 VEN 93004 473-A6
23600 SIMI 93065 497-F7
SAGEBROOK RD
- Chat 91311 499-J3
SAGEBRUSH AV
- Chat 91311 499-H6
SAGEBRUSH PL
800 THO 91320 555-G5
SAGEWOOD DR
11500 MRPK 93021 496-C3
SAILBOAT CIR
5300 AGRH 91301
SAILFISH WY
2600 OXN 93035
SAILOR AV
2700 VEN 93001
SAILVIEW LN
32100 WLKV 91361
SAILWIND CT
400 SIMI 93065
SAINT ANDREWS CT
1900 OXN 93036
SAINT ANDREWS PL
1700 THO 91362
SAINT CHARLES CT
- THO 91320
SAINT CHARLES DR
200 THO 91360
SAINT CHARLES PL
- THO 91360
SAINT CLAIR AV
2100 SIMI 93065
E SAINT CLAIR CT
2200 SIMI 93063
SAINT CLAIR ST
10100 VEN 93004
SAINT CROIX AV
1800 VEN 93004
SAINT CROIX CT
4800 VeCo 91377
SAINT EDENS CIR
24200 CanP 91307
SAINT JAMES CT
- THO 91320
SAINT JEAN CT
30800 WLKV 91362
SAINT JOHN CT
- THO 91320
SAINT LAURENT DR
5800 AGRH 91301
SAINT MARYS DR
100 OXN 93036
SAINT PAULS DR
- VEN 93003
SAINT STEPHEN CT
- THO 91320
SAINT THOMAS DR
100 VeCo 93023
4800 VeCo 91377
SAINT VINCENT DR
300 VeCo 91377
SAIPAN
- PHME 93041
SALAS ST
500 SPLA 93060
SALE AV
6100 WdHl 91367
6400 CanP 91307
7600 LA 91304
SALEM AV
300 VeCo 93036
700 VeCo 93036
700 VeCo 93036
SALERNO DR
5500 WLKV 91362
SALINAS CT
5400 SIMI 93063
5400 SIMI 93063
SALISBURY RD
7000 CanP 91307
SALLY ST
2300 SIMI 93065
SALMON RIVER CIR
3400 THO 91362
SALSA ST
- PHME 93043
SALT CANYON RD
- Nwhl 91382
SALT CREEK AV
- SIMI 93063
SALT CREEK RD
23600 Nwhl 91382
23600 VeCo 93040
SALTINO WY
4800 VeCo 91377
SALT MARSH RD
- VeCo 93060
SALT RIVER AV
- VEN 93004
SALVADOR DR
- OXN 93033
SAMANTHA CT
2600 SIMI 93063
SAMRA DR
8300 LA 91304
N SAMSON AV
2000 SIMI 93063
SAMUEL AV
2900 OXN 93033
SAMUEL DR
3800 OXN 93033
SAN ANDRES CIR
600 THO 91320
SAN ANGELO AV
2900 SIMI 93063
SAN ANTONIO ST
- THO 91320
400 OJAI 93023
SAN ARDO CT
6100 CMRL 93012
SAN BENITO AV
- VEN 93004
SAN BENITO ST
1900 OXN 93033
SAN BERNARDINO A
- VEN 93004
SAN CARLOS DR
600 THO 91320
SAN CAYETANO RD
1000 VeCo -
1000 VeCo 93015
SAN CAYETANO ST
900 VeCo 93015
SANCHEZ DR
2100 CMRL 93010
SAN CLEMENTE AV
100 VeCo 93035
SAN CLEMENTE CT
3700 THO 91320
SAN CLEMENTE ST
- VEN 93001
300 SPLA 93060
SAN CLEMENTE WY
900 VeCo 93010
SAN COMO CT
1000 CMRL 93012
SAN COMO LN
6300 CMRL 93012
SAND CT
900 VEN 93001

ity ZIP Pg-Grid
OOD DR
SIMI 93063 499-C3
OOD PL
FILM 93015 456-B6
THO 91362 526-J3
OOD ST
CanP 91307 529-E4
G AV
OXN 93033 553-A3
G LN
VEN 93003 492-D3
G ST
THO 91360 526-E3
NYON RD
VeCo 93066 495-C1
VeCo 93066 475-D7
FT ST
VeCo 91361 556-G6
LAR LN
PHME 93041 552-E5
NG ST
VEN 93003 492-D5
ST AV
THO 91362 527-A3
O AV
VEN 93004 492-F1
N ST
SIMI 93063 498-J2
SIMI 93063 499-A2
AS AV
CMRL 93012 525-B5
AL PL
THO 91360 526-C3
ER CIR
THO 91361 557-A5
ER CT
VEN 93001 491-F5
WLKV 91361 557-B7
ER WY
OXN 93035 521-J7
NT LN
VEN 93004 492-H3
CT
THO 91320 555-G2
NE
SIMI 93063 478-D7
P DR
AGRH 91301 557-G4
V
SIMI 93065 498-C5
R
VeCo 93036 492-J5
OLLOW CT
MRPK 93021 496-D3
CE CT
MRPK 93021 496-C5
PE AV
THO 91320 555-E1
MANDO AV
VeCo 93035 552-C6
VeCo 93001 459-C4
ST
OXN 93033 553-A5
OXN 93033 552-J5
VeCo 93033 553-A5
NCESCA DR
CMRL 93012 525-A2
NCISCO AV
VEN 93004 472-F7
VEN 93004 492-F1
RIEL AV
VEN 93004 492-H4
RIEL ST
OJAI 93023 442-A6
SIMI 93063 498-E1
GONIO AV
OXN 93030 522-J5
OXN 93030 523-A5
LERMO RD
VeCo - 366-L3
ON RD
CMRL 93012 524-J6
CMRL 93012 525-A6
NTO AV
SIMI 93063 498-E1
NTO ST
OXN 93030 523-A5
QUIN AV
VEN 93004 492-H4
QUIN ST
SIMI 93063 478-J7
SIMI 93063 479-A7
RD
VEN 93001 491-D3
BARRANCA RD
VeCo 93001 471-F5
VEN 93001 471-F7
VEN 93001 491-F1
E ST
OXN 93030 523-A5
Chat 91311 499-J4
N AV
OXN 93033 552-H4
N DR
FILM 93015 456-C6
N ST
SPLA 93060 463-H6
AS AV
THO 91320 555-E2
ST
OXN 93030 523-A5
VEN 93003 491-H3
THO 91320 555-E1
RCOS CT
THO 91320 555-E1
RCOS ST
VEN 93001 491-F3
VEN 93003 491-F3
RINO AV
VEN 93003 491-H2
RINO ST
OXN 93033 552-G2
RINO OIL
Y RD
VeCo 93015 465-J4
VeCo 93015 466-A4
RTIN PL
THO 91360 526-C3
RTINEZ
CYN RD
Cstc 91384 458-G1
ATEO AV
VEN 93004 492-F1
VEN 93004 472-F7
ATEO AV
VEN 93004 492-F2
TEO PL
OXN 93033 553-A2
UEL AL
VEN 93001 491-E2

STREET Block City ZIP Pg-Grid
SAN MIGUEL AV
- VeCo 93035 552-B4
SAN MIGUEL CIR
400 PHME 93041 552-E6
2600 THO 91360 526-C3
SAN MIGUEL DR
- VeCo 93010 494-D7
SAN MIGUEL WY
400 SPLA 93060 463-H5
SAN MIGUEL ISLAND DR
- VeCo 93012 554-F3
SAN NICHOLAS ST
1600 VEN 93001 491-E2
2300 VEN 93003 491-E2
SAN NICOLAS AV
- VeCo 93035 552-B5
300 SPLA 93060 463-J5
SAN NICOLAS CIR
100 PHME 93041 552-E6
SAN NICOLAS CT
3700 THO 91320 555-E1
SAN ONOFRE DR
1700 CMRL 93012 495-B7
1700 CMRL 93012 525-C1
SAN PABLO ST
3300 VEN 93003 491-H2
SAN PEDRO ST
400 PHME 93041 552-E5
600 VEN 93001 491-E3
SAN RAFAEL AV
6200 CMRL 93012 525-C1
SAN RAFAEL ST
1400 OJAI 93023 442-A6
SAN RAFAEL WY
1200 CMRL 93012 525-C1
SAN RAMON WY
1200 OJAI 93023 442-A6
SAN REMO DR
1300 SIMI 93063 499-C3
SAN ROQUE AV
1300 VEN 93003 491-H2
SAN SEBASTIAN CT
- VeCo 93012 496-D7
SAN SEBASTIAN DR
1900 OXN 93035 552-A1
SAN SIMEON AV
3500 OXN 93033 552-J4
SAN SIMEON CT
1300 VEN 93003 492-C4
SAN SIMEON DR
800 THO 91320 526-A7
4200 OXN 93033 552-J4
SANTA ANA AV
100 VeCo 93035 552-A4
SANTA ANA BLVD
- VeCo 93022 451-A6
800 VeCo 93001 450-J6
800 VeCo 93022 450-J6
SANTA ANA RD
7700 VeCo 93001 460-J1
8300 VeCo 93001 461-A2
10400 VeCo 93001 450-E3
11000 VeCo 93001 451-A6
SANTA ANA ST
100 OJAI 93023 441-H7
SANTA ANA WY
- VeCo 93022 451-B6
SANTA ANITA CT
2100 CMRL 93010 494-D7
SANTA ANNA ST
100 SPLA 93060 464-A7
W SANTA ANNA ST
200 SPLA 93060 463-J7
200 SPLA 93060 464-A7
SANTA BARBARA AV
- VeCo 93012 554-D3
6700 VeCo 93001 459-C5
SANTA BARBARA CIR
400 THO 91320 555-F1
SANTA BARBARA ST
1600 VEN 93001 491-E2
E SANTA BARBARA ST
100 SPLA 93060 464-A6
W SANTA BARBARA ST
100 SPLA 93060 463-H7
100 SPLA 93060 464-A6
SANTA BELLA PL
23600 THO 91362 527-B4
SANTA CLARA AV
3000 OXN 93030 523-C2
3000 OXN 93036 523-C2
3300 VeCo 93036 523-C2
3800 VeCo 93036 493-D7
4600 VeCo 93010 493-D7
4600 VeCo 93066 493-D7
SANTA CLARA ST
100 FILM 93015 456-A6
700 FILM 93015 455-J6
1200 SPLA 93060 464-C6
E SANTA CLARA ST
- VEN 93001 491-C2
W SANTA CLARA ST
- VEN 93001 491-B2
SANTA CREG LP
23600 SPLA 93060 473-J2
SANTA CRUZ AV
- VeCo 93035 552-B4
SANTA CRUZ CIR
400 PHME 93041 552-E6
SANTA CRUZ CT
3700 SIMI 93063 478-E7
SANTA CRUZ ST
500 SPLA 93060 464-A7
600 SPLA 93060 463-J7
700 SPLA 93060 473-J1
N SANTA CRUZ ST
- VEN 93001 491-E2
S SANTA CRUZ ST
- VEN 93001 491-E3
SANTA CRUZ WY
900 VeCo 93010 494-D6
SANTA CRUZ ISLAND DR
- VeCo 93012 554-E3
SANTA FE AV
900 VEN 93004 492-H2
SANTA FE ST
- FILM 93015 455-J7
- FILM 93015 456-A7
SANTA FELICIA CANYON FIRE RD
23600 VeCo 93040 367-E7
SANTA LUCIA AV
1800 OXN 93030 522-J5
1800 OXN 93030 523-A5
SANTA LUCIA CT
- VEN 93003 492-C1
SANTA LUCIA ST
3700 SIMI 93063 478-E7

STREET Block City ZIP Pg-Grid
SANTA MARGARITA RD
8900 VEN 93004 492-H4
SANTA MARIA ST
6200 VeCo 93063 499-B4
9300 VEN 93004 492-G2
E SANTA MARIA ST
100 SPLA 93060 464-C6
W SANTA MARIA ST
100 SPLA 93060 463-J7
100 SPLA 93060 464-A7
600 SPLA 93060 473-J1
SANTA MONICA AV
100 VeCo 93035 552-C6
SANTA MONICA CT
3800 THO 91320 555-E1
SANTA MONICA DR
200 VeCo 93035 552-B4
SANTA PAULA AV
- VeCo 93012 554-E4
100 VeCo 93035 552-B5
100 VeCo 93043 552-B5
7000 VeCo 93001 459-C4
SANTA PAULA FRWY Rt#-126
- SPLA - 463-J7
- SPLA - 464-D5
- SPLA - 473-F4
- VeCo - 473-B6
- VeCo - 492-D3
- VEN - 472-J7
- VEN - 473-B6
- VEN - 491-J4
- VEN - 492-D3
SANTA PAULA ST
700 VeCo 93015 465-G3
14600 VeCo 93060 463-G7
14900 VeCo 93060 473-E2
E SANTA PAULA ST
100 SPLA 93060 464-A5
W SANTA PAULA ST
100 SPLA 93060 463-J6
100 SPLA 93060 464-A6
SANTA PAULA CANYON RD
23600 VeCo 93040 458-A3
SANTA PAULA OJAI RD Rt#-150
4300 VeCo 93060 464-A1
4400 VeCo 93060 454-A7
4600 VeCo 93060 453-H4
12400 VeCo 93023 453-H4
SANTA ROSA AV
100 VeCo 93035 552-B5
SANTA ROSA DR
4100 VeCo 93021 496-A3
SANTA ROSA LP
400 SPLA 93060 473-J2
SANTA ROSA RD
4600 CMRL 93012 524-J3
5000 CMRL 93012 525-B2
6900 VeCo 93012 525-G1
7200 CMRL 93012 495-E7
7200 VeCo 93012 495-E7
10600 VeCo 93012 496-D7
N SANTA ROSA ST
- VEN 93001 491-E2
S SANTA ROSA ST
- VEN 93001 491-E2
SANTA ROSA ISLAND DR
- VeCo 93012 554-F2
SANTA SUSANA CT
- VEN 93003 492-C1
SANTA SUSANA TR
8600 VeCo 93063 499-C4
SANTA SUSANA FIRE RD
23600 VeCo 93063 499-E4
SANTA SUSANA PASS RD
6600 SIMI 93063 499-G2
6700 VeCo 93063 499-D4
7600 Chat 91311 499-G2
SANTA TOMAS PL
3900 THO 91320 555-E1
SANTA YNEZ AV
2200 SIMI 93063 478-E7
2300 SIMI 93063 498-F1
SANTA YNEZ ST
1600 VEN 93001 491-E2
SANTEE CT
10000 VEN 93004 492-J3
SAN TELMO CIR
500 THO 91320 525-E7
500 THO 91320 555-E1
SANTI ST
23600 THO 91320 556-C1
SANTIAGO CT
2300 OXN 93030 523-B4
SANTIAGO ST
2900 THO 91362 557-C3
SANTINA ST
23600 Chat 91311 499-F7
SANTO DR
4900 VeCo 91377 557-G1
SANTO DOMINGO
- CMRL 93012 494-H7
- CMRL 93012 524-H1
SAN TROPEZ CIR
1700 OXN 93035 552-A1
SAN TROPEZ PL
23600 MRPK 93021 496-C4
SAN VINCENT CT
3600 THO 91320 555-F1
SAN VINCENT PL
3600 THO 91320 555-F1
SAN VINCENTE CIR
200 THO 91320 555-F1
SAN VITO LN
- CMRL 93012 524-J1
SAN YSIDRO CT
1200 VEN 93003 472-D6
SAN YSIDRO ST
2200 CMRL 93010 494-G7
2300 VeCo 93010 494-G7
SAPPANWOOD AV
1400 THO 91320 526-A6
SAPPHIRE AV
500 VEN 93004 492-F3
2800 SIMI 93063 478-D7
SAPPHIRE CIR
900 VEN 93004 492-F3
SAPPHIRE DRAGON ST
1300 THO 91320 525-J5
1300 THO 91320 526-A5
SAPRA ST
1800 THO 91362 526-J5
1800 THO 91362 527-A5
SARA DR
23600 OXN 93030 522-J5

STREET Block City ZIP Pg-Grid
SARAH AV
200 MRPK 93021 496-E1
SARAH CT
2900 VeCo 91320 555-G1
SARALYNN DR
9100 Chat 91311 499-F7
SARALYNN LN
100 Chat 91311 499-E6
SARANAC ST
10200 VEN 93004 492-J2
SARATOGA AV
1100 VEN 93003 492-B4
SARATOGA ST
- FILM 93015 456-A5
700 OXN 93035 522-E7
1600 OXN 93035 552-E1
SARAZEN DR
- MRPK 93021 476-E5
SARELDA RD
23800 WHil 91304 499-E7
SARGENT AV
2000 SIMI 93063 498-D2
SARGENT LN
6600 VEN 93003 492-D3
SARITA DR
100 OXN 93030 522-J6
SARNO CT
3900 MRPK 93021 496-C4
SASHA CT
2600 SIMI 93063 498-D1
2700 SIMI 93063 478-D7
SASPARILLA ST
6600 SIMI 93063 499-D2
SASSAFRAS WY
1300 VeCo 91377 527-H7
SATICOY AV
200 VeCo 93004 492-J1
200 VEN 93004 492-J1
1200 VEN 93004 493-A2
N SATICOY AV
100 VEN 93004 472-H7
100 VeCo 93004 472-H7
S SATICOY AV
- VeCo 93004 472-H7
- VEN 93004 472-H7
- VeCo 93004 492-J1
SATICOY ST
1000 SPLA 93060 464-C4
22000 CanP 91303 529-G4
22200 CanP 91307 529-G4
22800 LA 91304 529-F4
SATINWOOD AV
100 VeCo 91377 558-B2
SATURN AV
1200 CMRL 93010 524-F1
SAUL PL
300 VEN 93004 472-H6
SAUSALITO AV
6500 CanP 91307 529-J5
7600 LA 91304 529-J2
SAUSALITO DR
700 CMRL 93010 524-C1
SAVANNAH AV
1700 VEN 93004 492-H4
SAVIERS RD
1100 OXN 93033 522-G7
1100 OXN 93033 552-G3
SAVONA WY
500 VeCo 91377 557-G1
SAVOY CT
400 VeCo 91377 557-H2
SAWMILL WY
- MRPK 93021 476-F6
SAWTELLE AV
100 VeCo 93035 552-C6
100 PHME 93043 552-C6
SAWTELLE CT
23600 SIMI 93065 497-F7
S SAWTOOTH CT
100 THO 91362 557-B2
SAWYER AV
1200 SIMI 93065 498-B4
SAXE CT
2100 THO 91360 526-F4
SAXON PL
1000 THO 91360 526-F6
SAY RD
1100 SPLA 93060 464-B3
SCANDIA AV
900 VEN 93004 492-J2
SCANNO DR
400 VeCo 91377 557-G2
SCARAB FIRE RD
23600 VeCo - 477-H3
23600 VeCo - 478-A2
23600 VeCo 93065 477-H3
SCARBOROUGH ST
200 THO 91361 556-F3
SCARBOROUGH PEAK DR
6900 CanP 91307 529-D5
SCARLET OAK AV
1200 THO 91360 526-H2
SCATTERWOOD LN
23600 SIMI 93065 497-G3
SCENIC DR
2200 SIMI 93065 497-E2
SCENICPARK ST
2200 THO 91362 527-A4
SCENIC WAY DR
800 VEN 93003 472-D6
SCHOENBORN ST
22200 LA 91304 529-E2
SCHOLARTREE CT
- MRPK 93021 496-H3
SCHOOL ST
2800 SIMI 93065 498-C2
SCHOOL CANYON RD
- VeCo 93001 471-C5
- VEN 93001 471-C5
SCHOOLCRAFT ST
22000 CanP 91303 529-J5
22300 CanP 91307 529-F6
SCHOOLHOUSE CIR
1600 THO 91362 527-C6
SCHOONER DR
1000 VeCo 93001 491-G6
1000 VEN 93001 491-G6
SCHOONER WK
3400 OXN 93035 522-B7
SCHUMAN PL
23600 VEN 93003 492-B7
SCHUMANN RD
23100 Chat 91311 499-G7
SCIENCE DR
- MRPK 93021 496-F1
SCIOTO CIR
1000 SIMI 93065 497-C5
SCOFIELD AV
3400 SIMI 93063 478-F6

STREET Block City ZIP Pg-Grid
SCOTER AV
2300 VEN 93003 492-E5
SCOTT AV
1800 VEN 93004 492-H4
SCOTT DR
3100 SIMI 93063 478-F6
SCOTT PL
2500 THO 91360 526-E4
SCOTT ST
100 PHME 93041 552-E6
SCOTTSDALE ST
9800 VEN 93004 492-H2
SCOTTYS TER
3100 SIMI 93063 478-F6
SCRIPPS CT
4700 VEN 93003 492-A1
SEABISCUIT PL
6000 MRPK 93021 476-A7
SEABORG AV
2800 VEN 93001 492-C7
2800 VEN 93003 492-C7
SEABREEZE CT
1700 THO 91320 526-A5
SEABREEZE ST
- THO 91320 525-J5
100 THO 91320 526-A5
SEABREEZE TER
- VeCo 90265 585-G7
SEABREEZE WY
5100 OXN 93035 521-J7
SEABRIDGE LN
- OXN 93035 522-B7
- OXN 93035 552-B1
SEABURY CT
100 THO 91320 555-J1
SEACLIFF CT
5700 VEN 93003 492-C4
SEACOVE CT
2500 PHME 93041 552-C2
SEACREST CT
23600 THO 91362 527-B2
SEADRIFT CT
2500 PHME 93041 552-C2
SEA ESTA PL
500 VEN 93003 491-J4
SEAFARER ST
1200 VEN 93001 491-F5
SEAFOAM CT
2500 PHME 93041 552-C2
SEAFOAM WY
2600 OXN 93035 552-A2
SEAGULL AV
2300 VEN 93003 492-E5
SEAHAWK ST
5900 VEN 93003 492-D5
6000 VeCo 93003 492-D5
SEAHORSE AV
2400 VEN 93001 491-F4
SEAHORSE CT
900 VEN 93001 491-F4
SEAHORSE WY
1000 OXN 93035 521-J7
SEAL CT
1100 VEN 93001 491-G5
SEALANE WY
4900 OXN 93035 521-J7
5100 OXN 93035 551-J1
SEAMIST CT
2500 PHME 93041 552-C2
SEAMIST PL
- VEN 93003 492-B4
SEAPORT DR
1100 OXN 93030 522-E7
SEASHELL AV
3100 VEN 93001 491-G5
SEASHORE CT
2500 PHME 93041 552-B2
SEASIDE CT
900 VEN 93001 491-F5
SEASIDE DR
2500 PHME 93041 552-C2
2700 OXN 93035 552-C2
2700 PHME 93035 552-C2
SEASONS ST
- SIMI 93065 478-A6
SEASPRAY WY
100 PHME 93041 552-E6
SEAVIEW AV
2900 VEN 93001 491-G5
SEAVIEW DR
5300 OXN 93035 521-H6
SEAVIEW ST
100 PHME 93041 552-E6
N SEAWARD AV
- VEN 93001 491-F2
- VEN 93003 491-F2
S SEAWARD AV
- VEN 93001 491-F3
- VEN 93003 491-F3
SEAWIND WY
600 PHME 93041 552-F7
SEBRING AV
2000 SIMI 93065 498-C2
SEBRING CT
2000 SIMI 93065 498-C2
SECKER DR
23600 WHil 91304 499-D6
SECO CT
2000 THO 91362 556-H2
SEDAN AV
6600 CanP 91307 529-G4
7600 LA 91304 529-G2
SEDGEWICK CT
7500 LA 91304 529-D4
SEDGEWORTH CT
600 SIMI 93065 527-C1
SEDGEWORTH PL
200 SIMI 93065 527-D1
SEEGER AV
- VEN 93003 492-B3
SEELY PL
1100 SIMI 93065 497-H5
SEINE CT
5400 WLKV 91362 557-F5
SEINE RIVER WY
- OXN 93036 492-H5
SEITZ CT
15300 MRPK 93021 476-J5
15300 MRPK 93021 477-A5
SELBY CIR
1800 CMRL 93010 494-H7
SELF DEFENSE RD
- PHME 93043 552-C5
SEMINARY RD
4700 CMRL 93012 494-J7
SEMINOLE CIR
4800 SIMI 93063 478-H6
SEMINOLE LN
2300 VEN 93001 471-C6

STREET Block City ZIP Pg-Grid
SEMPLE ST
3500 SIMI 93063 498-E2
SEMRAD RD
6900 CanP 91307 529-E5
SENAN ST
3700 CMRL 93010 494-G7
SENECA PL
5100 SIMI 93063 478-J7
5400 SIMI 93063 479-A6
SENECA ST
- VEN 93001 471-C5
SENNA WY
- OXN 93030 523-A4
SENTINEL CIR
900 VEN 93003 472-C7
SENTINEL CT
- SIMI 93065 478-B6
SEPTO ST
22000 Chat 91311 499-J5
SEQUAN CT
1400 CMRL 93010 524-D2
SEQUOIA AV
- VeCo 93003 492-D2
1400 SIMI 93063 498-D2
1400 SIMI 93065 498-D4
2400 SIMI 93063 478-D7
SEQUOIA CT
200 THO 91360 526-E7
SEQUOIA DR
1200 OXN 93033 553-B5
SEQUOIA ST
700 OXN 93033 552-H3
SERAPE PL
- CMRL 93010 494-F7
SERENA LN
- OXN 93033 553-C4
SERENA ST
5800 SIMI 93063 499-B1
SERENIDAD PL
- VeCo 93022 451-C5
SERENO AV
2600 VEN 93003 491-F4
SERENO PL
- CMRL 93010 523-J2
SERENTO CIR
400 THO 91360 526-D3
SERRA DR
- FILM 93015 456-C6
SERRANO RD
11600 VeCo 90265 585-D6
SERRANO CANYON RD
- VeCo - 584-H7
- VeCo - 585-A6
SERVICE RD
3600 OXN 93035 552-A2
SERVICE AREA RD
23600 VeCo 93063 498-J7
23600 VeCo 93063 499-A7
SESPE AV
- FILM 93015 456-A6
700 FILM 93015 455-H6
SESPE DR
1800 VEN 93004 492-H4
SESPE PL
700 FILM 93015 455-J6
700 FILM 93015 456-A6
SESPE ST
800 VeCo 93015 465-G2
S SESPE ST
1700 VeCo 93015 465-G4
SESPE LAND & WATER
100 FILM 93015 456-C6
100 VeCo 93015 456-C6
SESPE RIVER RD
- VeCo - 366-K6
- VeCo - 367-A5
SETON HALL AV
200 VEN 93003 492-A1
500 VeCo 93003 492-A1
SEVENOAKS CT
4400 WLKV 91361 557-D6
SEVILLA ST
1300 CMRL 93010 524-C4
SEVILLE CT
3500 THO 91320 525-F7
SEXTANT AV
2500 PHME 93041 552-C2
SEXTON CANYON RD
2900 VeCo 93003 472-A4
2900 VeCo 93003 492-C1
2900 VEN 93003 472-B6
2900 VEN 93003 492-C1
SEYBOLT AV
1000 CMRL 93010 524-C2
SEYMOUR CREEK RD
- VeCo - 366-L1
- VeCo - 367-A1
SHAD CT
3100 SIMI 93063 478-E6
SHADE TREE LN
7000 CanP 91307 529-D5
SHADOW LN
23600 SIMI 93065 527-E1
SHADOWBEND WY
23600 SIMI 93065 497-F3
SHADOW BROOK LN
2900 THO 91361 557-C5
SHADOW CANYON PL
4800 THO 91362 557-F1
SHADOW CREEK DR
- OXN 93036 522-B3
SHADOWGLEN CT
1400 THO 91361 556-J5
SHADOW HILL CIR
2900 THO 91360 526-B2
SHADOW HILLS RD
- CALB 91301 558-G7
SHADOW LAKE DR
500 THO 91360 526-D7
SHADOW MESA CIR
2900 THO 91360 526-B2
SHADOW OAK DR
10400 Chat 91311 499-J4
SHADOW OAKS PL
1400 THO 91362 526-J5
SHADOW RIDGE CT
7100 CanP 91307 529-D5
SHADOW SPRING PL
2200 THO 91361 557-B4
SHADOW VALLEY CIR
22200 Chat 91311 499-J1
SHADOW WOOD DR
- MRPK 93021 476-D6
SHADOW WOOD PL
- MRPK 93021 476-E5
SHADY LN
1100 FILM 93015 455-J4
N SHADY LN
100 OJAI 93023 442-A6

STREET Block City ZIP Pg-Grid
S SHADY LN
100 OJAI 93023 442-A7
SHADY BROOK CT
2400 THO 91362 527-A4
SHADY BROOK DR
1600 THO 91362 526-J4
1900 THO 91362 527-A4
SHADYCREEK DR
6000 AGRH 91301 558-A3
SHADY GROVE LN
100 THO 91361 556-F2
SHADY GROVE PL
25800 LACo 91302 558-J3
SHADY HILLS CT
200 SIMI 93065 497-E6
SHADY KNOLL CT
- MRPK 93021 496-F4
SHADY OAK LN
5500 SIMI 93063 499-A1
SHADY OAKS DR
400 THO 91320 526-A7
SHADY POINT DR
4100 MRPK 93021 496-F3
SHADYRIDGE DR
11100 MRPK 93021 496-B4
SHADY TRAIL ST
- SIMI 93063 478-H5
SHAKESPEARE DR
- OXN 93033 553-B3
SHAKESPEARE PL
6900 MRPK 93021 477-A5
SHAKESPEARE WY
6500 VEN 93003 492-D1
SHALIMAR ST
2500 CMRL 93010 524-F1
SHALLOWS DR
800 OXN 93035 522-B7
SHAMROCK CT
100 THO 91320 556-A1
SHAMROCK DR
- VEN 93003 491-H2
400 VeCo 93003 491-H2
SHANNON AV
1700 VEN 93004 492-H4
SHANNON DR
2800 SIMI 93063 478-E7
SHARON DR
600 CMRL 93010 524-F2
SHARON LN
200 PHME 93041 552-D2
900 VEN 93001 491-E4
SHARP RD
2700 SIMI 93065 478-C6
2700 VeCo 93065 478-C6
SHASTA AV
- MRPK 93021 496-D1
400 OXN 93033 552-G4
SHASTA DR
100 OXN 93033 553-B5
600 SPLA 93060 463-H6
SHASTA PL
6000 CMRL 93012 525-B1
SHASTA ST
8100 VEN 93004 492-F3
SHASTA WY
2200 SIMI 93065 497-G2
SHAVER CT
900 SIMI 93065 497-F5
900 VeCo 93065 497-F5
SHAVER ST
8100 VEN 93004 492-F3
SHAW CT
1900 THO 91362 527-A6
SHAW WY
6500 VEN 93003 492-D3
SHAWNEE CT
- MRPK 93021 496-G4
SHAWNEE DR
- Chat 91311 499-J1
SHAWNEE LN
2300 VEN 93001 471-C6
SHAWNEE ST
- MRPK 93021 496-G3
SHAWNESS CT
1700 THO 91362 527-E6
SHEARWATER ST
6300 VEN 93003 492-D5
SHEFFIELD LN
200 FILM 93015 455-J6
SHEFFIELD PL
800 THO 91360 526-F7
SHEFFIELD ST
700 SPLA 93060 463-H6
SHEKELL RD
8000 VeCo 93021 476-A2
SHELBURN LN
1100 VEN 93001 491-E4
SHELBURNE LN
1000 SIMI 93065 497-D6
SHELBY LN
2000 SIMI 93065 498-A2
SHELDON DR
3600 VEN 93003 491-H2
SHELL RD
200 VeCo 93001 471-B4
600 VeCo 93060 473-J2
E SHELL RD
- VeCo 93001 471-C4
W SHELL RD
- VeCo 93001 471-C4
SHELLCREEK PL
2800 WLKV 91361 557-A7
SHELLEY CIR
6900 VEN 93003 492-E3
SHELL HARBOR LN
- PHME 93041 552-E6
SHELL HARTMAN RD
- VeCo 93001 471-D3
SHELLY PL
- OXN 93033 553-B4
SHELTER WOOD CT
2800 THO 91362 526-J3
SHELTONDALE AV
6200 WdHl 91367 529-D6
6300 CanP 91307 529-D6
SHENANDOAH AV
3200 SIMI 93063 498-D3
SHENANDOAH DR
- OXN 93036 492-H7
SHENANDOAH ST
400 THO 91360 526-D3
4700 VEN 93003 492-B4
SHENANDOAH WY
- MRPK 93021 476-F6
SHEPHERD DR E
3100 CMRL 93010 524-F1
SHEPPARD RD
100 SPLA 93060 463-H7
SHERBORNE ST
2100 CMRL 93010 524-E1

STREET
Block City ZIP Pg-Grid

SHERGRA PL
3300 SIMI 93063 498-D1
SHERI DR
3100 SIMI 93063 478-E6
SHERIDAN CT
2000 SIMI 93065 498-A2
SHERIDAN WY
400 VEN 93001 491-B1
500 VEN 93001 471-B7
SHERMAN AV
200 MRPK 93021 496-E1
SHERMAN PL
23100 CanP 91307 529-G5
SHERMAN ST
2000 SIMI 93065 498-A2
SHERMAN WY
22000 CanP 91303 529-G5
22300 CanP 91307 529-F5
SHERWIN AV
2600 VEN 93003 492-E6
SHERWOOD CT
300 THO 91361 556-F2
SHERWOOD DR
2400 VEN 93001 491-F2
SHERWOOD RD NW
800 VeCo 93023 451-C3
SHERWOOD WY
500 OXN 93033 552-G5
SHETLAND PL
1500 THO 91362 527-D6
SHIELDS CT
2700 THO 91360 526-E3
SHIELLS DR
600 FILM 93015 456-A5
SHIELLS CANYON
- VeCo 93015 466-E2
- VeCo 93021 466-E2
SHILOH WY
5200 VEN 93003 492-B4
SHIPPEE LN
1100 VeCo 93023 442-D5
SHIPSIDE RD
- PHME 93043 552-D5
SHIRLEY DR
2800 THO 91320 525-H7
2900 VeCo 91320 525-H7
SHIRLEY ST
1700 CMRL 93010 524-D4
SHOAL CREEK CT
2100 SIMI 93065 497-C6
SHOEMAKER LN
1900 THO 91320 525-J7
1900 THO 91320 526-A7
SHOKAT DR
700 VeCo 93023 450-J2
700 VeCo 93023 451-A2
SHOOTINGSTAR LN
23600 SIMI 93065 497-A1
SHOPPING LN
4200 SIMI 93063 498-F2
SHORE DR
1000 VEN 93001 491-E4
SHORELINE DR
- VEN 93001 491-B3
SHORELINE ST
1500 CMRL 93010 524-D2
SHORELINE WY
5000 OXN 93035 551-J1
5000 OXN 93035 552-A1
SHOREVIEW CIR
2800 THO 91361 557-C6
SHOREVIEW DR
400 PHME 93041 552-E6
3300 WLKV 91361 557-C7
SHORT ST
- VeCo 93042 583-E4
- VeCo 93022 451-B7
SHOSHONE AV
11300 Chat 91311 499-J1
SHOSHONE ST
- VEN 93001 471-C6
5500 SIMI 93063 479-A7
W SHOSHONE ST
- VEN 93001 471-C6
SHOUP AV
6100 WdHl 91367 529-J7
6400 CanP 91307 529-J4
7600 LA 91304 529-J4
9300 Chat 91311 499-J6
SHREVE AV
2200 SIMI 93063 499-C1
SHREWSBURY CIR
24300 CanP 91307 529-D5
SHROPSHIRE CT
4100 WLKV 91361 557-D6
SHRUBWOOD CIR
2600 SIMI 93065 498-C1
2700 SIMI 93065 478-C7
SHUNK RD
1700 SIMI 93063 499-B2
E SIBLEY ST
6400 SIMI 93063 499-C2
SIDEWINDER DR
- VeCo 93041 583-H3
SIDLEE ST
- THO 91360 526-F5
E SIDLEE ST
- THO 91360 526-F4
W SIDLEE ST
- THO 91360 526-E4
SIDNEY LN
500 VEN 93003 492-D1
SIDONIA AV
700 VEN 93003 491-H4
SIENA CT
11800 MRPK 93021 496-C5
SIENNA LN
1000 SIMI 93065 478-A7
1000 SIMI 93065 498-A1
SIENNA WY
5500 WLKV 91362 557-F5
SIERRA AV
100 MRPK 93021 496-D1
SIERRA CT
1200 VeCo 93023 451-B1
SIERRA DR
300 VEN 93003 491-H2
E SIERRA DR
3300 THO 91362 557-C3
W SIERRA DR
2700 THO 91362 557-B2
SIERRA PL
1900 OXN 93033 553-A3
SIERRA RD
100 OJAI 93023 441-G7
200 VeCo 93023 441-G7
SIERRA WY
2100 OXN 93033 553-B2
SIERRA HEIGHTS CT
400 THO 91320 555-G3

SIERRA MADRE CT
3700 SIMI 93063 478-E7
SIERRA MADRE DR
1500 CMRL 93010 524-F1
SIERRA MESA DR
1800 CMRL 93010 494-C7
1800 CMRL 93010 524-C1
SIERRA PASS PL
11200 Chat 91311 499-J2
SIERRA VISTA AV
200 FILM 93015 455-H6
SIESTA AV
100 THO 91360 526-E4
SIESTA CIR
2300 THO 91360 526-E4
SIESTA WY
- VeCo 93033 553-D5
SIGNAL ST
100 OJAI 93023 441-H6
S SIGNAL ST
100 OJAI 93023 441-H7
SILAS AV
100 THO 91320 555-H2
100 VeCo 91320 555-H2
SILAS LN
200 THO 91320 555-H2
23600 THO 91320 555-H2
SILENTBROOK WY
1600 SIMI 93065 497-G3
SILKFIELD CT
- VeCo 91361 556-D7
SILK OAK AV
2800 THO 91362 527-C3
SILVER CIR
- VEN 93004 492-F3
SILVERADO DR
1700 THO 91360 496-J7
SILVERBELL CIR
- MRPK 93021 496-G2
SILVER CLOUD ST
700 THO 91360 526-C2
SILVER CREEK RD
28900 Ago 91301 558-B7
SILVER CREEK ST
12900 MRPK 93021 496-E3
SILVERCREST ST
11800 MRPK 93021 496-C4
SILVER FERN CT
400 SIMI 93065 497-E6
SILVER LAKE CT
400 SIMI 93065 497-E6
SILVER MAPLE CIR
3100 THO 91360 526-H2
SILVER MOSS CT
400 SIMI 93065 497-E6
SILVER OAK LN
- MRPK 93021 496-F2
SILVER SPRING DR
2100 THO 91361 557-A4
SILVER SPUR CT
1000 VeCo 93023 451-C3
3200 THO 91360 526-C2
SILVER SPUR LN
- VeCo 91307 529-A5
SILVER SPUR ST
1700 VeCo 93023 451-C3
SILVERSTAR AV
- SIMI 93065 478-A6
SILVERSTONE CT
- SIMI 93065 478-A5
SILVERSTONE ST
- SIMI 93065 478-A6
SILVERSTREAM CT
- SIMI 93063 499-A1
SILVER TREE LN
- SIMI 93065 497-H3
SILVER VALLEY AV
5600 AGRH 91301 557-J5
SILVERWHEEL PL
500 THO 91320 555-H3
SILVERWOOD ST
1300 SIMI 93065 497-H5
SIMI AV
100 VeCo 93035 552-B5
SIMI ST
1200 VeCo 93015 465-H3
SIMI HILLS LN
2600 SIMI 93063 478-H7
SIMI TOWN CENTER WY
- SIMI 93065 497-H1
- SIMI 93065 498-A1
SIMI VILLAGE DR
100 SIMI 93065 497-F3
SIMON WY
- VeCo 93036 492-J7
500 VeCo 93036 493-A7
700 VeCo 93036 523-A1
SIMPSON DR
4300 OXN 93033 553-A4
SIMPSON ST
200 VEN 93001 491-C1
E SIMPSON ST
- VEN 93001 491-B1
W SIMPSON ST
- VEN 93001 491-B1
200 VEN 93001 471-B7
SIMSBURY CT
1900 THO 91360 526-C5
SINALOA RD
300 SIMI 93065 497-G6
600 VeCo 93065 497-G5
SINALOA VILLA
400 SIMI 93065 497-G3
SINGLETREE LN
6700 VeCo 91377 528-A7
SIOUX AV
2800 VEN 93001 471-C5
SIOUX CT
3000 SIMI 93063 478-J7
SIOUX DR
22000 Chat 91311 499-J1
SIR GEORGE CT
700 MRPK 93021 476-F7
SIRIUS CIR
2600 THO 91360 526-F3
SIRIUS ST
2100 THO 91360 526-E3
SISAR RD
- VeCo - 366-L7
13000 VeCo 93023 453-C1
SI SE PUEDE ST
10200 VEN 93004 492-J3
10200 VEN 93004 493-A3
SISKIN CT
2000 SIMI 93065 497-D2
SISKIN PL
400 SIMI 93065 497-D2
SISKIYOU ST
8100 VEN 93004 472-F7
8100 VEN 93004 492-F1

SITKA AV
1500 SIMI 93065 498-D3
SITTING BULL PL
6000 SIMI 93063 479-A7
SIX OAK CT
2400 SIMI 93063 499-A1
SKAGWAY ST
3400 SIMI 93063 498-D2
SKEEL DR
800 CMRL 93010 524-C2
SKELTON CANYON CIR
3800 THO 91362 557-C1
SKIDMORE CT
4500 MRPK 93021 496-F2
SKINNER CT
2100 THO 91362 556-H2
SKUNK RANCH RD
23600 OJAI 93023 451-H1
23600 VeCo 93023 451-H1
SKY CT
3100 SIMI 93063 478-E6
SKYBROOK CT
4200 MRPK 93021 496-B2
SKYCREST CT
800 VEN 93003 472-C7
SKYFLOWER LN
23600 SIMI 93065 497-A1
SKYGLEN CT
4400 MRPK 93021 496-D2
SKY HIGH DR
300 VeCo 93001 460-J4
N SKYLARK CT
4300 MRPK 93021 496-E3
SKYLINE DR
700 SPLA 93060 463-H6
23600 VeCo 93063 498-J7
23600 VeCo 93063 528-H1
N SKYLINE DR
100 THO 91362 557-A2
S SKYLINE DR
- THO 91362 557-A3
100 THO 91361 557-A3
100 THO 91361 556-J3
SKYLINE RD
500 VEN 93003 492-B1
600 VEN 93003 472-B7
8900 VeCo 93021 476-C1
SKYRIDGE CT
1600 THO 91320 556-A2
SKY RIDGE LN
5300 VeCo 91377 527-G7
SKYVIEW TER
6200 VEN 93003 472-C7
SKYVIEW WY
5700 AGRH 91301 558-A4
SKYWALKER DR
4000 VeCo 93066 493-F3
SKYWAY DR
200 CMRL 93010 523-J5
200 CMRL 93010 524-A5
SLATE PL
- THO 91362 527-C3
SLATER TER
9200 Chat 91311 499-F7
SLEEPY HOLLOW ST
2900 SIMI 93065 498-D4
SLEEPY WIND ST
12900 MRPK 93021 496-E3
SLICERS CIR
5600 AGRH 91301 557-G5
SMETANA CT
600 VEN 93003 492-B7
SMETANA ST
600 VEN 93003 492-B7
SMITH RD
6500 SIMI 93063 499-C3
23100 Chat 91311 499-F7
SMITH ST
2400 OXN 93033 552-G5
5100 VEN 93003 492-B1
SMITH CANYON RD
900 VeCo 93015 457-F7
900 VeCo 93040 457-F7
SMOKETREE AV
- VeCo 91377 558-A2
SMOKETREE WY
23600 SIMI 93065 527-E1
SMOKEWOOD CT
1900 THO 91362 526-J3
1900 THO 91362 527-A3
SMOKEY RIDGE AV
1800 THO 91362 527-G6
SMOKY MOUNTAIN DR
- OXN 93036 492-H7
- OXN 93036 522-H1
SMUGGLERS CV
- VeCo 93012 554-E3
SNAPDRAGON ST
- VEN 93004 493-A1
SNEAD DR
- MRPK 93021 476-D4
SNIPE AV
1200 VEN 93003 492-C4
SNIPE WK
600 OXN 93035 522-E6
SNOW AV
- OXN 93030 522-J3
1900 OXN 93036 522-J3
SNOW CT
1800 VEN 93001 471-B7
SNOWBERRY CT
2000 SIMI 93063 498-J2
SNOW CREEK AV
5200 SIMI 93063 498-J2
SNOWGOOSE ST
- SIMI 93065 478-A5
SNOWPEAK DR
32400 WLKV 91361 557-B7
SOBRE COLINAS PL
400 CMRL 93012 524-J3
SOCORRO WY
1700 OXN 93030 522-J4
1700 OXN 93030 523-A4
SOCRATES AV
2000 SIMI 93065 497-F2
SOFT WHISPER CT
- SIMI 93065 478-A6
SOFTWIND WY
5400 AGRH 91301 557-J5
5400 AGRH 91301 558-A5
SOJKA DR
2800 SIMI 93065 498-C1
3000 SIMI 93063 498-C1
SOLANO DR
2000 CMRL 93012 495-D7
SOLANO ST
7800 VEN 93004 492-F1
SOLANO WY
2200 OXN 93033 553-B3

SOLANO VERDE DR
7000 VeCo 93066 475-A3
SOLAR DR
1800 OXN 93030 523-B3
1900 OXN 93036 523-B3
SOLIMAR BEACH RD
2800 VeCo 93001 470-D4
SOLWAY CT
2300 THO 91362 527-A3
SOMBRA WY
- OXN 93030 522-J4
SOMERA CT
- SIMI 93065 497-H5
SOMERSET CIR
200 CMRL 93012 524-H4
200 THO 91360 526-E6
SOMIS RD Rt#-34
2400 CMRL 93010 494-J6
2400 VeCo 93010 494-J6
2400 VeCo 93066 494-J6
2600 VeCo 93066 495-A5
SONATA DR
- OXN 93030 522-J4
SONATA WY
23600 SIMI 93065 527-D1
SONIA DR
- OXN 93030 522-J4
SONOMA CT
400 VEN 93004 492-E1
2100 THO 91362 526-J4
SONOMA LN
100 SPLA 93060 464-A6
SONOMA PL
22000 Chat 91311 499-J6
SONOMA ST
7800 VEN 93004 492-E1
SONOMA WY
500 OXN 93033 552-F5
SONORA CT
6700 VEN 93003 472-D6
SONORA DR
300 CMRL 93010 524-D3
SOPHIA CT
1500 OXN 93030 522-E4
SOPHIA DR
1600 OXN 93030 522-E3
SOPHOMORE CT
15700 MRPK 93021 477-A5
SORA ST
6500 VEN 93003 492-D4
SORORITY LN
23800 WHil 91304 499-E7
SORREL ST
1400 SIMI 93065 497-H3
1800 CMRL 93010 524-D1
SORRELWOOD CT
800 THO 91361 557-A4
SORTINO CT
11800 MRPK 93021 496-C4
SOSNA CT
15300 MRPK 93021 476-J5
SOULE PARK DR
1100 OJAI 93023 442-A7
1100 OJAI 93023 452-A1
SOUSA RD
5100 VEN 93003 492-B3
SOUTH DR
6400 VEN 93003 492-D4
N SOUTH BANK RD
3800 VeCo 93036 492-J5
SOUTHBY DR
7500 LA 91304 529-D4
SOUTHCREST PL
- SIMI 93065 497-E2
SOUTHERN CROSS CT
- VeCo 93012 496-F5
SOUTHERN HILLS DR
2200 OXN 93036 522-E2
SOUTHERN HILLS PL
1700 THO 91362 527-E6
SOUTHERN OAK AV
- SIMI 93063 499-A3
SOUTHERN PACIFIC ST
- FILM 93015 455-J7
SOUTHFIELD RD
500 CMRL 93010 524-D4
SOUTHFORK RD
- MRPK 93021 496-F2
SOUTHHAMPTON RD
3800 MRPK 93021 496-F3
SOUTH MOUNTAIN RD
400 SPLA 93060 464-D6
2100 VeCo 93015 465-A5
2400 VeCo 93060 465-A5
16500 VeCo 93066 474-A1
16500 VeCo 93060 474-A1
21000 VeCo 93066 464-G5
21000 VeCo 93060 464-G5
21700 VeCo 93066 465-A5
SOUTHPORT DR
1100 THO 91361 557-A5
SOUTHRIDGE DR
300 VeCo 91377 558-A1
SOUTH RIM ST
5000 THO 91362 527-F7
SOUTHSHORE PL
32500 WLKV 91361 557-B7
SOUTHVIEW CIR
6100 VEN 93003 472-C5
SOUTHWICK ST
600 SPLA 93060 463-H6
SOUTHWIND CIR
1300 THO 91361 557-B6
SOUTHWIND CT
- VEN 93003 492-B4
SPALDING DR
100 VeCo 93015 465-D1
SPALDING ST
600 THO 91360 526-G6
SPANISH GATE DR
3700 THO 91320 525-F7
SPANISH MOSS PL
- CMRL 93010 524-A2
SPANISH OAK LN
5400 VeCo 91377 557-J1
SPARKMAN AV
1200 CMRL 93010 524-D1
SPARKS CT
1900 SIMI 93065 498-A4
SPARROW DR
- VeCo 93041 583-G2
SPARROW ST
6000 VEN 93003 492-C4
SPARROWHAWK LN
100 VeCo 91377 557-J3
SPARTA CT
2100 SIMI 93065 497-F2
SPECK LN
2100 THO 91320 555-J2
2100 THO 91320 556-A2

SPECTRUM CIR
500 OXN 93030 523-D5
SPENCE ST
1600 SIMI 93065 497-J2
SPENCER CT
25900 LACo 91302 558-J3
SPENSER LN
700 VEN 93003 492-D2
SPERRY AV
1700 VEN 93003 492-C6
SPICEWOOD CT
23600 SIMI 93063 498-E4
SPINDLEWOOD AV
200 CMRL 93012 524-H4
SPINDLEWOOD CT
4300 CMRL 93012 524-H4
SPINDRIFT CT
5300 CMRL 93012 525-A1
SPINNAKER AV
2400 PHME 93041 552-C2
SPINNAKER DR
1100 VEN 93001 491-F7
SPINWOOD LN
23600 SIMI 93065 497-A2
SPIRES ST
23200 LA 91304 529-F3
SPIRITLAKE CT
5800 SIMI 93063 479-B6
SPLIT ROCK LN
5300 VeCo 91377 527-G7
S P MILLING RD
500 VeCo 93001 471-A7
500 VEN 93001 471-A7
500 VEN 93001 491-A1
SPRING CT
7200 CanP 91307 529-F5
SPRING RD
- MRPK 93021 476-F5
100 MRPK 93021 496-F2
SPRING ST
100 VeCo 93001 461-C7
500 VeCo 93022 451-B7
600 VeCo 93022 461-B1
7600 VeCo 93021 476-D4
SPRING BREEZE CT
700 SIMI 93065 497-E6
SPRINGBROOK CT
23600 THO 91362 527-B2
SPRINGBROOK ST
23600 THO 91362 527-B2
SPRING CANYON PL
3000 THO 91320 555-G4
SPRING CREEK CT
12500 MRPK 93021 496-D3
SPRING CREEK RD
12300 MRPK 93021 496-D3
SPRINGDALE CT
- THO 91360 526-F2
SPRINGFIELD AV
600 VEN 93004 492-G2
E SPRINGFIELD ST
4200 SIMI 93063 478-F6
N SPRINGFIELD ST
3000 SIMI 93063 478-F7
SPRING FOREST LN
4000 THO 91362 557-D1
SPRINGGATE LN
1700 SIMI 93065 497-F3
SPRINGHAVEN AV
- THO 91320 556-A1
SPRING HILL CT
4800 THO 91362 557-F1
SPRING MEADOW AV
3200 THO 91360 526-F2
SPRINGMIST LN
23600 SIMI 93065 497-A1
SPRING PARK RD
- CMRL 93012 524-G5
SPRINGTIME LN
3900 MRPK 93021 496-E4
SPRINGVILLE RD
3200 OXN 93030 523-E3
3200 VeCo 93030 523-E3
SPRING WOOD ST
600 THO 91320 556-C2
SPRUCE CIR
23600 SIMI 93065 497-F7
SPRUCE DR
100 OXN 93033 552-H5
SPRUCE ST
200 OXN 93033 552-F3
SPRUCE HILL CT
800 THO 91320 556-C2
SPRUCE MEADOW PL
400 THO 91362 557-D2
SPRUCEWOOD AV
300 VeCo 91377 558-A1
SPUR DR
100 OXN 93036 522-G1
SPURWOOD LN
23600 SIMI 93065 497-A2
SPYGLASS LN
500 THO 91320 556-D1
SPYGLASS TR
1800 OXN 93036 522-D3
SPYGLASS TR W
2400 OXN 93036 522-D2
SPYGLASS WY
1400 CMRL 93012 525-A1
SQUAW FLAT RD
- VeCo - 367-C5
SQUIRES DR
4500 OXN 93033 552-H5
SQUIRREL LN
1600 VEN 93003 492-E4
STABEN CT
100 SPLA 93060 464-A6
STABER RD
23600 VeCo 91361 555-J7
STACEY LN
- CMRL 93012 495-A7
STACY DR
2800 SIMI 93063 478-E7
STACY LN
- CMRL 93012 495-A7
STADIUM AV
- VEN 93003 492-A2
STADIUM WY
600 FILM 93015 456-A5
STAFFORD RD
2200 VeCo 91361 556-F7
W STAFFORD RD
2200 VeCo 91361 556-D7
2200 VeCo 91361 586-D1
STAGECOACH CT
- MRPK 93021 496-F2
STAGECOACH RD
- VeCo 90265 585-G7
- VeCo 90265 625-G1

E STAGECOACH RD
- VeCo 91307 528-J3
- VeCo 91307 529-A4
STAGECOACH TR
- MRPK 93021 496-F2
STAGG ST
22100 LA 91304 529-D3
STALLION CT
1000 VeCo 93010 494-C6
N STALLION RD
- VeCo 91307 528-J4
STANFORD AV
- OXN 93036 522-G2
STANFORD DR
900 SIMI 93065 498-A4
STANFORD ST
200 SPLA 93060 464-B6
5500 VEN 93003 492-B2
23600 OXN 93036 522-G2
E STANFORD ST
14600 MRPK 93021 476-H6
STANHOPE CT
23600 VeCo 91361 556-F6
STANISLAUS AV
- VEN 93004 492-F1
2700 SIMI 93063 478-J7
2700 SIMI 93063 498-J1
STANLEY AV
- VEN 93001 471-B6
STANLEY AV E
- VeCo 93001 471-C6
- VEN 93001 471-C6
STANLEY CT
15300 MRPK 93021 476-J5
STANTON CT
3600 SIMI 93063 478-E7
STANWOOD RD
23600 SIMI 93065 497-G7
STARBOARD LN
- PHME 93041 552-E5
STARBRIGHT CT
600 SIMI 93065 527-C2
STARDUST DR
100 SIMI 93065 497-E2
STARFIRE AV
3100 THO 91360 526-D2
STARFISH DR
4500 OXN 93035 552-A2
STARFISH LN
11800 VeCo 90265 625-F4
STARGAZE PL
400 SIMI 93065 497-E2
STARKLAND AV
8300 LA 91304 529-E2
STARLIGHT LN
24500 CanP 91307 529-D4
STARLING AV
2900 THO 91360 526-F3
STARPINE WY
1600 SIMI 93065 497-A2
STARR LN
2600 SIMI 93063 478-J7
2600 SIMI 93063 498-J1
STARSHINE ST
3500 THO 91360 526-H2
STARSTONE CT
100 SIMI 93065 497-J6
STARWOOD CT
1200 THO 91362 527-G7
STATHAM BLVD
1700 OXN 93033 552-J1
STATHAM PKWY
900 OXN 93033 552-H2
STAUNTON ST
400 CMRL 93010 524-F2
STEARMAN ST
500 CMRL 93010 524-A5
STEARNS ST
1700 SIMI 93063 498-J1
2600 SIMI 93063 478-J7
N STECKEL DR
100 SPLA 93060 463-J6
400 VeCo 93060 463-J6
S STECKEL DR
100 SPLA 93060 463-J6
200 SPLA 93060 464-A7
STEFFEN LN
800 VeCo 93063 499-B4
STEINBECK ST
6800 VEN 93003 492-D1
STELL DR
3800 SIMI 93063 478-F6
STELLAR DR
1100 OXN 93033 522-J7
1100 OXN 93033 552-J1
STEPHANIE WY
6000 SIMI 93063 499-B3
STEPHEN LN
8300 LA 91304 529-F2
STEPHENS ST
500 FILM 93015 456-A5
STEPHLY RD
1300 VeCo 93015 367-B7
1300 VeCo 93015 455-H1
STERLING AV
800 VEN 93004 492-F3
STERLING DR
1200 THO 91360 526-F6
STERLING CENTER DR
5300 WLKV 91361 557-E6
STERLING HILLS DR
- CMRL 93010 493-H6
STERLING OAKS CT
1300 VeCo 91377 527-G7
STERLINGVIEW DR
4100 MRPK 93021 496-B3
STERN CT
1000 OXN 93035 522-D7
STERN LN
900 OXN 93035 522-D7
STETSON CT
600 THO 91360 526-D4
STEVENS CIR
6900 VEN 93003 492-E3
STEVENS WY
9000 LA 91304 499-E7
9000 WHil 91304 499-E7
STILES AV
3100 CMRL 93010 524-F1
STILLWATER CT
10300 VEN 93004 492-J2
STILMAN CT
2100 SIMI 93063 498-J2
STINSON ST
500 CMRL 93010 524-A5
2100 SIMI 93065 498-A4
N STIRRUP LN
- VeCo 91307 529-B3
STOCK AV
1500 VEN 93004 493-A2

STOCKBRIDGE LN
100 VeCo 93023
STOCKTON AV
- VEN 93004
STOCKTON RD
7900 VeCo 93021
7900 VeCo 93066
STODDARD AV
1400 THO 91360
E STOKE CT
6100 SIMI 93063
STONE PL
8000 VEN 93004
STONE ST
900 VeCo 93015
7800 VEN 93004
STONEBROOK ST
100 SIMI 93065
STONECREEK CT
- VeCo 91361
STONE CREEK DR
1200 OXN 93036
STONECREST DR
5700 AGRH 91301
STONECROFT CT
2000 THO 91361
STONECUTTER ST
- THO 91362
STONEGATE DR
24500 LA 91304
STONEGATE RD
1000 SPLA 93060
STONEHAVEN LN
300 VeCo 91377
STONEHEDGE DR
500 FILM 93015
STONEHILL CIR
1900 THO 91360
STONEMAN ST
1800 SIMI 93065
STONE MEADOW DR
1300 CMRL 93010
STONE MOUNTAIN L
5200 THO 91362
STONEPINE CT
1400 THO 91360
STONERIVER CT
3400 THO 91362
STONESGATE ST
1700 THO 91361
1800 THO 91361
STONESHEAD CT
1000 THO 91361
STONETREE ST
4200 CMRL 93012
STONEWALL CIR
1200 THO 91361
STONEWOOD ST
2900 SIMI 93063
STONEYBROOK LN
1100 THO 91361
STONEYGLEN CT
4400 MRPK 93021
STONEY PEAK CT
500 SIMI 93065
STONEY RUN LN
23600 SIMI 93065
STONEYVIEW LN
6400 SIMI 93063
STORAGE RD
- VeCo 93042
STORK ST
6400 VEN 93003
STORM CLOUD ST
3200 THO 91360
STORMCROFT CT
2300 THO 91361
STOW ST
1500 SIMI 93063
STOWE DR
- OXN 93033
STRANDWAY CT
1600 THO 91361
STRATFORD AV
200 VEN 93003
STRATFORD ST
- THO 91360
STRATHEARN PL
- SIMI 93065
STRATHERN ST
22000 LA 91304
STRATHMORE DR
3100 VEN 93003
STRAUSS DR
500 THO 91320
500 THO 91320
800 VEN 93003
STRAVINSKY LN
1000 VEN 93003
STRAWBERRY LN
500 OXN 93036
STRAWBERRY HILL D
29600 AGRH 91301
STRAWBERRY HILL R
1300 THO 91360
STRICKLAND DR
4700 VeCo 93036
STRONG CT
400 VeCo 93003
400 VEN 93003
STROUBE ST
- VeCo 93036
100 OXN 93036
100 OXN 93036
1000 VeCo 93036
STUART CIR
900 THO 91362
STUART CT
400 OJAI 93023
STUART LN
600 VEN 93003
STUDENT ST
4600 VEN 93003
STUDIO RD
7100 VeCo 93063
STUMP RD
100 VeCo 93015
STURGIS RD
2200 OXN 93030
3400 VeCo 93030
STYLES ST
22500 WdHl 91367
SUBIDA CIR
3100 VeCo 93012
SUBROCK CIR
- VeCo 93041
SUDARIO CT
1000 VeCo 93010
SUE WY
200 VeCo 93036

ity ZIP Pg-Grid
AV
SIMI 93063 499-B2
VeCo 93010 494-B5
.N
CMRL 93010 524-C4
AV
THO 91360 526-F6
CT
VEN 93003 492-A1
APLE CT
MRPK 93021 496-E3
NE CT
THO 91320 556-D2
I ST
VEN 93003 492-A4
CANYON
VeCo 93001 451-H7
VeCo 93001 461-J1
CASCADE
VeCo 93060 453-G2
MOUNTAIN RD
VeCo 93001 461-B2
VeCo 93060 453-D3
VeCo 93023 452-J2
VeCo 93023 453-A4
VeCo 93060 452-J3
VeCo 93023 451-H6
VeCo 93060 451-H6
VeCo 93001 451-H6
VeCo 93022 451-E7
VeCo 93022 461-C2
SPRINGS ST
SIMI 93063 478-G7
R
VeCo 93023 451-C4
N
VeCo 93012 526-A1
VeCo 93012 496-B7
CT
Chat 91311 499-J3
ST
OJAI 93023 441-H6
MRPK 93021 496-D3
CLOUD DR
THO 91362 526-J2
THO 91362 527-A2
FIELD ST
THO 91360 526-F3
CMRL 93012 525-A1
CMRL 93012 495-A7
GLEN CT
MRPK 93021 496-C2
HILL CT
VeCo 91377 528-A7
PARK CT
THO 91362 527-A4
SHADE LN
MRPK 93021 496-F3
SHORE LN
WLKV 91361 557-C7
TIME AV
SIMI 93065 497-E3
TON CT
CMRL 93012 524-F4
TREE CT
SIMI 93065 498-A5
VIEW CIR
VeCo 93012 495-J7
VeCo 93012 496-A7
WOOD AV
SIMI 93063 498-H1
AV
SIMI 93063 478-H5
CIR
VeCo 93012 496-E6
DR
VEN 93001 491-C1
WHil 91304 499-E6
T DR
WHil 91304 499-E6
TR
VeCo 93060 453-C1
KNOLL CT
VeCo 91377 558-B1
T RIDGE CIR
Chat 91311 499-H6
T RIDGE CIR
Chat 91311 499-H6
RIDGE CT
THO 91362 557-C1
VIEW DR
THO 91362 557-E1
VUE DR
WdHl 91367 529-J7
VUE DR E
WdHl 91367 529-J7
VUE DR N
WdHl 91367 529-J7
CT
THO 91360 526-D5
I LN
SIMI 93065 497-A2
NET ST
SIMI 93065 527-D2
ST PL
THO 91360 526-H2
LE CT
SIMI 93065 497-E7
CE ST
THO 91360 526-D2
CE WY
CMRL 93012 525-A1
N RD
VeCo 91361 556-G2
R
CMRL 93010 494-H7
D CT
THO 91362 557-F2
WY
PHME 93041 552-F7
VER ST
SIMI 93063 499-A1
THO 91360 526-D3
VEN 93004 493-A2
W AV
SIMI 93063 478-F6
VE DR
CMRL 93010 524-C2
CIR
OXN 93033 552-H1
DR
OXN 93033 552-H1
ST
PHME 93041 552-E3
ND AV
VeCo 93001 459-C4
T ST
SIMI 93063 478-J6

STREET
Block City ZIP Pg-Grid
SUNLOFT LN
23600 SIMI 93065 497-A1
SUNNY LN
13300 VeCo 93012 496-E6
SUNNY ST
300 SPLA 93060 464-A7
SUNNY BROOK CT
400 VeCo 91377 558-B1
SUNNYCREST AV
1000 VEN 93003 472-C6
SUNNYCREST DR
6000 VeCo 91377 558-A1
SUNNYDALE AV
1500 SIMI 93065 497-J5
1700 SIMI 93065 498-A6
SUNNYDALE CT
1600 SIMI 93065 497-J5
SUNNYGLEN AV
1100 OJAI 93023 442-A6
SUNNYGLEN DR
12300 MRPK 93021 496-D3
SUNNYHILL CT
6300 VEN 93003 472-C7
SUNNYHILL ST
4400 THO 91362 527-D7
SUNNY POINT ST
23600 THO 91362 527-A2
SUNNYRIDGE DR
30000 AGRH 91301 557-H4
SUNNYSLOPE PL
13300 MRPK 93021 496-E4
SUNNYVISTA AV
- VeCo 91377 558-A3
SUNNYWAY DR
- VEN 93001 471-B7
SUNOAK PL
300 THO 91320 556-A2
SUN RANCH CT
22100 Chat 91311 499-J2
SUNRIDGE DR
1500 VEN 93003 492-D4
SUNRISE CT
1400 CMRL 93010 524-D1
7000 VEN 93003 472-D7
SUNRISE DR
2100 SIMI 93065 497-E2
SUNRISEMEADOW CIR
12800 MRPK 93021 496-E2
SUNROCK CT
200 SIMI 93065 527-E1
SUNSET
10800 VeCo 93021 496-A4
SUNSET AV
100 VeCo 93022 461-B1
300 VeCo 93022 451-A7
3400 SIMI 93063 478-J6
SUNSET CT
100 VeCo 93022 451-C6
SUNSET DR
- THO 91362 557-A3
100 THO 91361 557-A3
200 VeCo 93035 552-B4
1700 VEN 93001 491-F1
5200 OXN 93035 521-H6
SUNSET LN
3300 OXN 93035 552-A3
3300 VeCo 93035 552-A2
SUNSET PL
800 OJAI 93023 441-J6
3400 SIMI 93063 479-B6
SUNSET ST
- VeCo 93022 451-B6
SUNSET HILLS BLVD
1000 THO 91360 526-H1
1700 THO 91362 526-H1
1900 THO 91362 527-A2
SUNSET KNOLLS DR
3500 THO 91362 526-J1
SUNSETMEADOW CT
4400 MRPK 93021 496-D3
SUNSET OAK CIR
1000 THO 91320 556-C2
SUNSET RIDGE CT
6800 CanP 91307 529-D6
SUNSETRIDGE RD
3800 MRPK 93021 496-B4
SUNSET VALLEY RD
3200 VeCo 93021 496-H4
SUNSET VIEW CT
6100 VEN 93003 472-C7
SUNSHINE CT
1800 THO 91362 526-J2
SUNSHINE VALLEY CT
- SIMI 93063 479-B7
- SIMI 93063 499-B1
SUNSTONE ST
- VEN 93004 492-F3
4800 THO 91362 557-G1
SUNTREE LN
1600 SIMI 93063 498-J2
SUNVALE AV
500 VEN 93003 491-H4
SUN VALLEY CT
5400 AGRH 91301 557-J5
SUNWOOD LN
1000 VeCo 91377 528-A7
SUPERIOR AV
1100 VEN 93004 492-F3
SURFRIDER AV
2600 VEN 93001 491-F5
SURFRIDER WY
5100 OXN 93035 521-J7
SURFSIDE DR
500 OXN 93035 521-H6
600 PHME 93041 552-E6
W SURFSIDE ST
6900 VeCo 93001 459-C4
SURREY CIR
- OXN 93036 492-F7
- OXN 93036 522-F1
SURREY CT
2000 THO 91360 526-D4
SURREY WY
100 FILM 93015 456-A7
SURVEYOR AV
1600 SIMI 93063 498-F3
SUSAN AV
200 MRPK 93021 496-E1
10500 VeCo 93022 451-C6
SUSAN DR
1500 THO 91320 556-A2
SUSSEX CIR
800 THO 91360 526-G6
SUTTER AV
1100 SIMI 93065 497-H3
1700 SIMI 93065 498-A3
SUTTER DR
3300 OXN 93033 553-B3
SUTTER PL
1900 OXN 93033 553-A3

STREET
Block City ZIP Pg-Grid
SUTTER ST
6000 VEN 93003 492-C1
SUTTON CREST TR
- VeCo 91377 527-J7
SUZANNE CT
100 THO 91320 556-B1
SWALLOW ST
6300 VEN 93003 492-D4
SWAN ST
6500 VEN 93003 492-D5
SWANFIELD CT
- VeCo 91361 556-E7
SWANSEA AV
1100 VEN 93004 492-H3
SWANSEA PL
1600 THO 91361 556-J6
SWEET BRIAR PL
1500 THO 91362 526-J3
SWEET BRIAR ST
4300 VEN 93003 491-J2
4300 VEN 93003 492-A2
SWEET CLOVER ST
3200 THO 91362 527-D3
SWEETGRASS AV
- SIMI 93065 478-A6
SWEETLAND ST
2000 OXN 93033 553-A5
SWEETLEAF LN
23600 SIMI 93065 497-A2
SWEETSHADE WY
- SIMI 93065 478-C7
SWEETWATER AV
6000 SIMI 93063 499-B3
SWEETWATER LN
9800 VEN 93004 492-H3
SWEETWOOD ST
3500 SIMI 93063 498-D1
N SWEETWOOD ST
2400 SIMI 93063 498-D1
SWIFT AV
1500 VEN 93003 492-D4
SWIFT PL
15800 MRPK 93021 477-A5
SWIFT FOX CT
- SIMI 93065 478-A5
SWIFT RUN CT
- MRPK 93021 476-G6
SWIFT RUN ST
- MRPK 93021 476-F6
N SWINDON AV
2000 SIMI 93063 499-C2
SWISS PINE PL
23600 SIMI 93063 498-D4
SWITZAR LN
600 THO 91360 526-G7
SYCAMORE
2100 VeCo 93023 451-C4
SYCAMORE DR
- VeCo 93001 461-A4
600 PHME 93041 552-F5
700 OXN 93033 552-F5
1000 SIMI 93065 498-C2
2600 SIMI 93065 478-C7
SYCAMORE LN
- VeCo 93023 441-E6
SYCAMORE RD
600 VeCo 93022 451-A5
1400 VeCo 93015 455-F4
3600 VeCo 93015 465-B2
3800 VeCo 93060 465-B2
SYCAMORE ST
- OXN 93036 522-H1
300 SPLA 93060 464-C4
3200 OXN 93033 553-H3
SYCAMORE CANYON DR
1600 THO 91361 586-H1
1600 WLKV 91361 586-H1
SYCAMORE CANYON RD
3900 AGRH 91301 558-E7
- VeCo - 555-C7
- VeCo - 584-H7
- VeCo - 585-A2
- VeCo 91320 555-C7
SYCAMORE COTTAGE CT
- CMRL 93012 524-G4
SYCAMORE GROVE ST
100 SIMI 93065 527-E1
100 SIMI 93065 497-E7
SYCAMORE RIDGE ST
100 SIMI 93065 497-D7
200 SIMI 93065 527-D1
SYLVAN DR
6100 VeCo 93063 499-B3
SYLVAN ST
22200 WdHl 91367 529-E7
SYMPHONY LN
4800 VeCo 91377 557-G2
SYRACUSE DR
4300 OXN 93033 553-A5
SYRINGA ST
400 THO 91360 526-D3

T

T ST
1500 VEN 93004 493-A3
TABOR CIR
800 VeCo 93010 494-F6
TACKABERRY CT
29000 AGRH 91301 558-A3
TACOMA ST
8700 VEN 93004 492-G3
TAFFRAIL CT
900 OXN 93035 522-B7
TAFFRAIL DR
1000 OXN 93035 522-C7
TAFFRAIL LN
2400 OXN 93035 522-B7
TAFT AV
100 VEN 93003 492-E2
TAHOE DR
8600 VEN 93004 492-G4
TAHOE LN
2200 OXN 93033 553-B5
TAHOE PL
6000 CMRL 93012 525-B1
TAHQUITZ CT
- CMRL 93012 524-H2
TAHQUITZ DR
- CMRL 93012 524-H2
TALAL CT
1800 VeCo 93012 526-B1
TALBERT AV
400 SIMI 93065 498-C4
TALLOWBERRY LN
23600 SIMI 93065 497-A1
TALMADGE RD
4700 MRPK 93021 496-C2
TALOS AV
- VeCo 93041 583-H3

STREET
Block City ZIP Pg-Grid
TALOS RD
- PHME 93043 552-C5
TALUD TER
200 CMRL 93012 524-H2
TALUS ST
2800 OXN 93030 522-D3
TAM CT
2000 SIMI 93063 499-B2
TAMARAC ST
600 OXN 93033 552-H3
TAMARACK ST
1900 THO 91361 556-J4
1900 THO 91361 557-A4
TAMARIN AV
1700 VEN 93003 492-F4
TAMARIND ST
6000 VeCo 91377 558-A3
TAMARIX ST
1300 VeCo 93010 524-C1
1400 CMRL 93010 524-C1
TAMLEI AV
800 THO 91362 526-J7
TAM O SHANTER DR
4500 THO 91362 527-D6
TAMPA WY
10100 VEN 93004 492-J2
TANAGER ST
- VEN 93003 492-D5
TANBARK CT
1500 THO 91361 557-A6
TANGELO PL
6000 SIMI 93063 499-B3
TANGERINE PL
400 OXN 93033 552-G3
TANGLBRUSH LN
23600 SIMI 93065 497-A2
TANGLEWOOD CT
100 THO 91360 526-F2
TANGLEWOOD DR
2600 CMRL 93010 494-F6
TANISHA CT
23600 SIMI 93065 478-C7
TANNER RIDGE AV
400 THO 91362 557-G1
TANOAK LN
900 VeCo 91377 557-G1
TAORMINA LN
200 OJAI 93023 451-E1
TAOS AV
- VEN 93001 471-C5
TAPIES CT
900 THO 91320 555-F4
TAPIR CIR
1600 VEN 93003 492-E4
TAPLEY CT
1900 SIMI 93063 499-C2
TAPLEY ST
6500 SIMI 93063 499-C2
TAPO ST
3500 SIMI 93063 478-G7
13500 SIMI 93063 498-G2
TAPO CANYON RD
1400 SIMI 93063 498-F2
2600 SIMI 93063 478-F7
3400 VeCo 93063 478-F3
4800 VeCo - 478-F3
23600 VeCo 93040 367-E9
23600 VeCo 93040 458-E6
TARA ST
600 THO 91320 525-H7
TARANTO WY
4800 VeCo 91377 557-G2
TARKIO ST
100 THO 91360 526-E4
TARLOW AV
- VEN 93003 492-A3
TARRYTOWN LN
3900 AGRH 91301 558-E7
TARSIER LN
7200 VEN 93003 492-F4
TARTAR DR
- VeCo 93041 583-H3
TARTAR RD
- PHME 93043 552-C5
TASCOSA CT
- VeCo 91377 527-J7
TATU ST
3200 SIMI 93063 479-A6
TAXCO CT
1600 CMRL 93010 524-D2
W TAXCO CT
- SIMI 93065 497-F4
TAYLOR CT
- THO 91360 556-G1
- THO 91362 556-G1
TAYLOR LN
- FILM 93015 455-J4
TAYLOR ST
3800 VEN 93003 491-H2
TAYLOR RANCH RD
500 VeCo 93001 470-J4
500 VeCo 93001 471-A5
500 VeCo 93001 490-J1
500 VeCo 93001 491-A1
500 VEN 93001 490-J1
TEAGUE DR
600 SPLA 93060 464-B4
TEAGUE PL
23600 VeCo 93060 453-G2
TEAKWOOD CT
800 THO 91320 556-C2
TEAKWOOD ST
200 OXN 93033 552-F3
800 PHME 93041 552-F3
TEAL AV
1200 VEN 93003 492-D4
TEAL CT
2900 THO 91360 526-F3
TEAL CLUB RD
1500 OXN 93030 522-B5
1500 VeCo 93030 522-B5
TEARDROP CT
- THO 91320 555-F2
TEASDALE ST
- THO 91360 526-F4
TECH CIR
5400 MRPK 93021 496-D1
TECOLOTE CT
4200 MRPK 93021 496-E3
TECOPA SPRINGS LN
- SIMI 93063 479-A6
TEHAMA ST
1400 OXN 93035 552-E1
TEITSORT DR
- FILM 93015 456-A4
- VeCo 93015 456-A4
TEJEDA AV
12100 MRPK 93021 496-D1
TEJON CT
1600 CMRL 93010 524-D1

STREET
Block City ZIP Pg-Grid
TEJON CT
2800 SIMI 93063 479-A7
TELEGRAPH PL
- VEN 93003 491-J2
TELEGRAPH RD
6200 VEN 93003 492-D2
6400 VeCo 93003 492-D2
7500 VEN 93004 492-G1
9900 VEN 93004 472-H7
10600 VeCo 93004 472-H7
11000 VEN 93060 472-H7
11200 VEN 93004 473-A6
11200 VEN 93060 473-A6
11200 VeCo 93060 473-A6
15900 VEN 93004 491-H3
TELEGRAPH RD Rt#-126
- FILM 93015 456-E6
- VeCo 93015 456-E6
900 VeCo 93015 457-E5
1400 VeCo 93040 457-G4
2200 VeCo 93040 458-B5
2700 VeCo 93015 465-C1
17900 VeCo 93060 464-F3
18400 SPLA 93060 464-F3
20100 VeCo 93060 465-A2
E TELEGRAPH RD
17000 VeCo 93060 464-D5
17200 SPLA 93060 464-D5
E TELEGRAPH RD Rt#-126
100 FILM 93015 456-C6
300 VeCo 93015 456-C6
W TELEGRAPH RD
800 SPLA 93060 473-G1
800 SPLA 93060 463-H7
11000 VeCo 93004 473-B5
11000 VeCo 93060 473-G1
11000 VEN 93004 473-B5
TELEPHONE RD
4500 VeCo 93003 492-A5
4700 VEN 93003 492-B4
6800 VEN 93009 492-B4
7300 VEN 93004 492-H3
10500 VEN 93004 493-A1
23600 VeCo 93004 493-A1
TELEPHONE RELAY RD
23600 VeCo 93001 471-E7
TELLER RD
2200 THO 91320 525-J7
TELOMA DR
100 VEN 93003 492-B1
TELON CT
100 SIMI 93065 497-F6
TELSA ST
600 VeCo 93023 451-C3
TELSTAR DR
1100 OXN 93030 522-J7
1100 OXN 93033 522-J7
TEMESCAL ST
300 VeCo 93040 457-F4
TEMPE CT
4000 SIMI 93063 478-F6
TEMPE WY
32300 WLKV 91361 557-C7
TEMPLE AV
500 CMRL 93010 524-F1
700 VEN 93004 492-J1
1800 CMRL 93010 494-E6
TEMPLETON ST
- VEN 93003 492-A4
TENNEYSON DR
5700 AGRH 91301 557-J4
TENNYSON CT
2500 THO 91360 526-D3
TENNYSON LN
700 VEN 93003 492-D3
TENNYSON ST
100 THO 91360 526-D3
TERAZZA WY
- OXN 93030 523-A3
TERESA ST
23600 OXN 93030 522-J4
TERI CT
- LA 91304 529-J2
TERN CT
1500 VEN 93003 492-E4
TERNEZ DR
3800 VeCo 93021 496-A4
10400 VeCo 93021 495-J4
TERRA BELLA CT
5700 CMRL 93012 495-B7
TERRA BELLA LN
2200 CMRL 93012 495-A7
TERRACE AV
4200 OXN 93033 552-J5
TERRACE DR
200 SIMI 93065 497-E2
1800 VEN 93001 491-E1
3500 OXN 93033 552-J4
TERRACE HILL CIR
4900 THO 91362 557-G1
TERRACEMEADOW CT
4400 MRPK 93021 496-E3
TERRACERIDGE RD
3900 MRPK 93021 496-B4
TERRACE VIEW PL
400 PHME 93041 552-E6
TERRACINA DR
900 SPLA 93060 464-B4
TERRA GLEN WY
23600 SIMI 93065 497-A1
TERRAMAR WY
5000 OXN 93035 521-J7
TERRIER DR
- PHME 93043 552-C5
TERRIER ST
- VeCo 93041 583-H3
TERRONEZ PL
- OXN 93030 522-J4
TERRY DR
4900 VEN 93003 492-A1
TERRY RD
- VeCo 93012 554-C5
TEST AREA RD
23600 VeCo 93063 498-H7
23600 VeCo 93063 528-G1
TETLOW AV
1700 SIMI 93063 499-C2
TETON LN
4700 VEN 93003 492-B4
TEWA CT
1600 VeCo 93022 451-E4
TEXANIA TER
- LA 91304 529-D2
TEXAS AV
2700 SIMI 93063 478-H7
23600 FILM 93015 456-B6
23600 VeCo 93015 456-B6

STREET
Block City ZIP Pg-Grid
TEXAS LN
800 VeCo 93060 464-D4
THACHER RD
3000 VeCo 93023 442-E4
THACHER SCHOOL RD
5000 VeCo 93023 442-G4
THACKERY CT
6800 VEN 93003 492-E3
THAMES ST
100 THO 91360 526-E5
THAMES RIVER DR
100 OXN 93036 492-H7
THAYER LN
700 PHME 93041 552-F3
THELMA LN
11000 VeCo 93012 496-A7
THERESA DR
2900 THO 91320 555-G1
2900 VeCo 91320 555-G1
THERESA ST
2600 THO 91320 555-H1
THICKET PL
2700 SIMI 93065 478-C7
THILLE ST
4600 VEN 93003 492-B3
7800 VEN 93004 492-F3
THIONNET PL
15300 MRPK 93021 476-J5
THISTLEGATE RD
900 VeCo 91377 528-A7
900 VeCo 91377 558-A1
THISTLEWOOD ST
3000 THO 91360 526-F2
THOMAS AV
100 OXN 93033 552-G3
THOMAS CT
4200 SIMI 93063 478-F5
THOMAS DR
300 SPLA 93060 464-A7
THOMAS LN
1000 VEN 93003 492-A7
E THOMAS ST
500 VeCo 93022 451-C6
THOMASVILLE CT
13000 MRPK 93021 496-E4
THOMPSON AV
9400 Chat 91311 499-F6
E THOMPSON BLVD
- VEN 93001 491-C2
2300 VEN 93003 491-E2
W THOMPSON BLVD
- VEN 93001 491-B2
THOMPSON LN
200 Chat 91311 499-F6
500 VeCo 93063 499-F6
1400 SIMI 93065 497-J3
9200 Chat 91311 499-F7
THOMPSON RD
300 Chat 91311 499-F6
9200 Chat 91311 499-F6
9200 Chat 91311 499-F6
THOREAU CIR
100 THO 91360 526-F6
THOREAU LN
500 VEN 93003 492-D1
THORNCROFT CT
1300 THO 91361 556-J5
THORNHILL AV
1400 THO 91361 556-J5
THORN RIDGE CT
- SIMI 93063 478-H4
N THORNWOOD ST
800 SIMI 93065 498-A5
THORPE CIR
300 THO 91360 526-E5
THORSBY RD
2100 VeCo 91361 556-F7
THOUSAND OAKS BLVD
25800 LACo 91302 558-H4
26000 CALB 91302 558-H4
28700 AGRH 91301 558-A4
29400 AGRH 91301 557-G4
30700 WLKV 91301 557-G4
E THOUSAND OAKS BLVD
- THO 91360 556-F1
800 THO 91362 556-F1
2400 THO 91362 557-A3
30700 WLKV 91362 557-E4
W THOUSAND OAKS BLVD
- THO 91360 556-E1
THRASHER CT
1500 VEN 93003 492-F4
THREE OAK CT
2400 SIMI 93063 499-A1
THREE SPRINGS DR
2600 WLKV 91361 557-A7
THRUSH AV
1500 VEN 93003 492-E4
2200 OXN 93033 553-A4
THUNDERBIRD DR
2300 THO 91362 556-J2
2300 THO 91362 557-A2
THUNDERHEAD ST
300 THO 91360 526-D2
THURGOOD MARSHALL DR
- OXN 93030 522-D3
- OXN 93036 522-D3
TIARA DR
1800 VeCo 93023 451-D3
TIARA ST
8100 VEN 93004 492-F3
TIBER ST
8800 VEN 93004 492-H4
TIBERIAS WY
- SIMI 93063 479-C7
TIBER RIVER DR
- OXN 93036 492-H5
TIBURON CT
1600 THO 91362 526-J4
TICO AV
200 OJAI 93023 441-H6
TICO RD
100 VeCo 93023 441-D7
600 VeCo 93023 451-D2
N TICO RD
100 OJAI 93023 441-G6
TIERNEY AV
- VEN 93003 492-C3
TIERRA DR
1200 THO 91362 526-H7
TIERRA BUENA CT
23600 CMRL 93010 524-C4
TIERRA LINDA CT
700 CMRL 93010 524-C1
TIERRA REJADA RD
- SIMI 93065 497-A3
900 VeCo 93021 497-A3

STREET
Block City ZIP Pg-Grid
TIERRA REJADA RD
900 VeCo 93065 497-A3
2000 MRPK 93021 496-C2
9900 VeCo 93021 496-G4
TIESA DR
- OXN 93030 522-J3
TIFFANEY LN
2700 SIMI 93063 478-D7
TIFFANY CT
1600 CMRL 93010 494-D7
1600 CMRL 93010 524-D1
TIGHE LN
700 FILM 93015 456-A5
TIKI DR
1300 OXN 93033 552-J5
TIKI WK
1800 OXN 93033 552-J2
1800 OXN 93033 553-A1
TILBURY CT
2000 THO 91360 526-D4
TILDEN CT
- SIMI 93065 527-E1
TILLER AV
2500 PHME 93041 552-C2
2600 OXN 93035 552-C2
2600 PHME 93035 552-C2
TILLER DR
3600 OXN 93035 522-B7
TIMBER RD
- THO 91320 556-B2
- THO 91320 556-B2
TIMBER CANYON RD
1900 VeCo 93060 454-H4
3400 VeCo 93060 464-H2
TIMBERCREEK TR
800 OXN 93036 522-F1
TIMBERDALE RD
4200 MRPK 93021 496-C3
TIMBERHILL CT
1800 SIMI 93063 498-E2
TIMBER HOLLOW AV
- MRPK 93021 476-F6
TIMBERLANE AV
2100 SIMI 93063 499-A2
TIMBERLANE CT
2200 OXN 93036 522-E2
TIMBERLANE ST
6200 AGRH 91301 558-A3
TIMBERRIDGE CT
32400 WLKV 91361 557-B7
TIMBERRIDGE RD
3800 MRPK 93021 496-B4
TIMBERVIEW CT
3800 MRPK 93021 496-C4
TIMBERWOOD AV
400 THO 91360 526-D3
TINIAN
- PHME 93041 552-E5
TINKERMAN ST
5500 SIMI 93063 499-A2
TINSLEY MOUNTAIN RD
23600 VeCo 93060 453-F3
TIOGA DR
300 VEN 93001 491-C1
TIOGA PL
700 THO 91320 526-B7
22200 LA 91304 529-J1
TIPPERARY LN
1800 THO 91320 556-A1
TIRRE CT
300 SPLA 93060 464-A7
TITAN PL
1300 OXN 93033 522-J7
TITANIA PL
2600 SIMI 93063 478-J7
TIVERTON DR
- CMRL 93012 524-G4
TIVOLI LN
1100 SIMI 93065 497-H1
TOBAGA WY
- VeCo 91377 557-G2
N TOBY PL
2300 SIMI 93065 498-B1
TODD CT
300 OXN 93030 523-B5
TODD LN
100 SPLA 93060 473-H1
400 VeCo 93060 473-H2
TODD RD
100 VeCo 93060 473-E3
900 SPLA 93060 473-E3
TODD VIEW CT
8600 LA 91304 529-C1
TOLAND RD
100 VeCo 93060 454-J7
100 VeCo 93060 455-A6
100 VeCo 93060 464-J1
TOLAND PARK RD
- VeCo 93060 454-J7
- VeCo 93060 464-J1
TOLEDO CT
3500 THO 91320 525-F7
TOLSTOY PL
- OXN 93033 552-J2
TOLTECS CT
2500 VEN 93001 471-C5
TOMAHAWK DR
- PHME 93043 552-C5
- VeCo 93042 583-H2
TOMAHAWK TER
8400 LA 91304 529-D1
TONALE WY
400 VeCo 91377 557-G1
TONGA ST
11500 VeCo 90265 625-F5
TONGAREVA ST
11400 VeCo 90265 625-F5
TONOPAH CT
23600 SIMI 93063 479-A6
TONY AV
6100 WdHl 91367 529-E7
6400 CanP 91307 529-E6
TOP CIR
4800 SIMI 93063 478-H5
TOPA LN
100 VeCo 93060 453-C1
TOPANGA CANYON BLVD Rt#-27
9500 Chat 91311 499-J6
TOPANGA CANYON PL
9500 Chat 91311 499-J6
TOPA TOPA CT
700 VEN 93003 472-B7
TOPA TOPA DR
100 OJAI 93023 441-H7
5400 VEN 93003 472-B7
E TOPA TOPA ST
100 OJAI 93023 441-H7
W TOPA TOPA ST
100 OJAI 93023 441-H7

STREET Block City ZIP Pg-Grid

TOPA VIEW TR
1400 VeCo 91320 556-B3
TOPAZ AV
1700 VEN 93004 492-H4
2800 SIMI 93063 478-D7
TOPAZ CT
900 OJAI 93023 441-J5
2400 OXN 93030 522-D3
TOPEKA AV
600 VEN 93004 492-H2
TOPSAIL CIR
2300 THO 91361 557-B6
TOPSAIL CT
900 OXN 93035 522-B7
TORENA WY
- OXN 93030 523-A4
TORERO DR
- OXN 93030 522-H4
TORINO ST
23600 MRPK 93021 496-C3
E TORRANCE ST
2100 SIMI 93065 498-A4
TORREPINES PL
30000 AGRH 91301 557-H5
TORREY RD
100 VeCo 93015 457-F5
100 VeCo 93040 457-F5
TORREY CANYON RD
- VeCo - 467-F1
- VeCo 93040 467-F1
900 VeCo 93015 457-F7
900 VeCo 93015 467-F1
TORREY PINE CT
1500 THO 91360 526-H2
TORREY PINES CT
2200 OXN 93033 553-B5
TORRIDON CT
- MRPK 93021 496-E2
TORY WY
10100 VEN 93004 492-J2
TOTH PL
5700 AGRH 91301 558-C5
TOTTENHAM CT
1500 VeCo 91377 527-H6
TOUCAN WY
6900 VEN 93003 492-E4
TOULOUSE CIR
3100 THO 91362 526-J2
TOURMALINE DR
1000 THO 91320 525-H7
TOWER CT
- CMRL 93010 493-H7
TOWER DR
2500 VeCo 93023 442-C7
TOWER SQ
1300 VEN 93003 491-J4
TOWHEE CT
1400 VEN 93003 492-E4
TOWN CENTER DR
1000 OXN 93036 492-G7
TOWN FOREST CT
- CMRL 93012 524-G4
TOWNLEY CIR
1700 SIMI 93063 499-A3
TOWNS CT
300 SPLA 93060 463-H6
TOWNSGATE RD
2100 THO 91361 557-B4
TOWNSHIP AV
2900 SIMI 93063 478-D6
2900 VeCo 93063 478-D6
TRABAJO DR
1000 OXN 93030 523-E3
TRABUCO OAK DR
23600 SIMI 93063 498-D4
TRACT 13 RD
- PHME 93043 552-C6
TRACT 14 RD
- PHME 93043 552-C3
N TRACY AV
2000 SIMI 93063 498-E2
TRACY CT
100 THO 91320 555-G2
TRADEWINDS DR
3900 OXN 93035 522-A7
TRAFALGER PL
1500 THO 91361 556-H6
TRAIL CREEK DR
29900 AGRH 91301 557-H5
TRAILCREST DR
4000 MRPK 93021 496-F4
TRAILROCK CT
700 SIMI 93065 527-C1
TRAILS END DR
23600 Chat 91311 499-F6
TRAILSIDE CT
200 THO 91320 556-C1
TRAILVIEW CT
3400 THO 91360 526-H2
TRAILWAY LN
29200 AGRH 91301 558-A5
29400 AGRH 91301 557-J5
TRANA CIR
26000 CALB 91302 558-J3
TRANCAS LAKES DR
- LACo 90265 586-H6
TRANQUIL LN
300 VeCo 91377 558-A1
600 SIMI 93065 497-G5
TRANQUILA CIR
100 CMRL 93012 524-H2
TRANQUILA DR
- CMRL 93012 524-H2
TRANSOM WY
600 OXN 93035 522-E6
TRANSPORT ST
3700 VEN 93003 491-J5
4100 VEN 93003 492-A5
TRAPANI CT
11800 MRPK 93021 496-C5
TRAVIS AV
2900 SIMI 93063 478-H6
TREADWELL AV
1000 SIMI 93065 498-B4
TREE FERN CT
- CMRL 93010 524-A2
TREE HOLLOW CT
400 SIMI 93065 527-E1
TREE HOLLOW GN
29300 AGRH 91301 558-A5
TREELINE RD
- PHME 93043 552-C3
TREE RANCH RD
12300 VeCo 93023 453-B1
TREE TOP LN
500 THO 91360 526-D6
TREEVIEW CT
11500 MRPK 93021 496-B2
TREFOIL AV
6400 VeCo 91377 558-B1

TREGO CT
- SIMI 93065 477-J6
TRELLIS PL
- CMRL 93012 524-G4
N TREMONT AV
2000 SIMI 93063 499-C2
E TREMONT CIR
6600 SIMI 93063 499-C2
TRENLEY CT
2600 SIMI 93063 498-E1
TRENT LN
300 SPLA 93060 463-H6
TRENTHAM RD
1900 VeCo 91361 556-H7
TRENTON LN
9700 VEN 93004 492-H2
TRENTWOOD DR
23600 VeCo 91361 556-E7
TREVI PL
400 VeCo 91377 557-G2
TREVINO DR
- MRPK 93021 476-B5
TREVINO TER
800 OXN 93033 552-H5
TRIANGLE ST
- THO 91360 526-F5
TRICKLNG BROOK CT
200 SIMI 93065 498-A6
TRIGGER PL
9700 Chat 91311 499-H5
E TRIGGER RD
- VeCo 91307 528-H4
TRIGGER ST
22700 Chat 91311 499-G6
TRILLIUM ST
2800 THO 91360 526-D3
TRINIDAD WY
800 OXN 93033 552-H3
TRINITY DR
3100 VEN 93003 491-G4
TRINITY PL
2400 OXN 93033 553-A2
TRINWAY AV
2100 SIMI 93065 498-C2
TRITON ST
2500 PHME 93041 552-D2
2800 OXN 93041 552-D2
TRIUNFO CANYON RD
100 THO 91361 557-B4
1100 WLKV 91361 557-A5
TRIUNFO RIDGE FIRE TR
- LACo 90265 586-D4
- VeCo 90265 586-D4
TROJAN CT
6700 MRPK 93021 476-H6
TROLLOPE CT
15700 MRPK 93021 477-A5
TROUSDALE ST
5300 VeCo 91377 527-H7
TROWBRIDGE CT
3900 WLKV 91361 557-D6
TRUCKEE DR
8300 VEN 93004 492-G4
TRUCK HAUL RD
100 OXN 93036 492-H6
TRUENO AV
600 VeCo 93010 494-B5
TRUETT CIR
2000 THO 91360 526-D5
TRUMAN AV
- VEN 93004 492-E1
TRUMAN ST
2500 CMRL 93010 524-F1
TRUSTY LN
1300 VeCo 93023 451-B2
TUBA ST
22100 Chat 91311 499-J4
TUBBS ST
1600 THO 91362 526-J7
TUCKER ST
11900 VeCo 93021 476-D3
TUCSON ST
4100 SIMI 93063 478-F6
TUCSON WY
10100 VEN 93004 492-J2
TUDOR CIR
700 THO 91360 526-G6
TUDOR LN
1000 FILM 93015 455-J6
TUGBOAT WY
- PHME 93041 552-E5
TUJUNGA AV
100 VeCo 93035 552-B5
TULANE AV
200 VEN 93003 491-J2
N TULANE AV
6700 MRPK 93021 476-G6
TULARE LN
28400 AGRH 91301 558-C6
TULARE PL
2400 OXN 93033 553-A2
TULARE ST
10100 VEN 93004 492-J2
TULE LAKE ST
- VEN 93004 492-J3
TULIP AV
- SIMI 93063 499-A2
TULIP CT
200 VEN 93004 473-A7
TULIPAN CIR
- OXN 93030 523-A4
TULIPAN DR
- OXN 93030 523-A4
TULIP WOOD CT
- SIMI 93063 479-B7
- SIMI 93063 499-B1
TULL ST
- VEN 93003 492-C3
TULSA CIR
10400 VEN 93004 492-J1
TULSA DR
4700 OXN 93033 553-A5
4700 VeCo 93033 553-A5
TULSA ST
22000 Chat 91311 499-J3
TUMBLEWEED AV
2600 SIMI 93065 478-C7
2600 SIMI 93065 498-C1
TUOLUMNE AV
100 VEN 93004 472-H7
N TUOLUMNE AV
500 THO 91360 526-D7
TUPELO WOOD CT
800 THO 91320 556-C2
TURFWAY RD
6100 MRPK 93021 476-A6
TURIN ST
400 VeCo 91377 557-G1

TURLOCK AV
1300 VEN 93004 492-H3
TURNBERRY DR
- OXN 93036 522-B3
TURNBURY ST
1200 SIMI 93065 497-D7
TURNOUT PARK CRES
3300 OXN 93036 492-J7
TURNSTONE CIR
- MRPK 93021 476-E6
TURNSTONE ST
- VEN 93003 492-D5
TURQUOISE AV
- VEN 93004 492-F3
TURQUOISE CIR
2500 THO 91320 525-H6
TURTLE CREEK LN
- THO 91320 526-B6
TUSCANA CT
11800 MRPK 93021 496-C4
TUSCAN GROVE PL
- CMRL 93012 495-D7
TUSCANY DR
- VeCo 91377 557-G2
TUSCARORA AV
2300 VEN 93001 471-D6
TUTTLE AV
900 SIMI 93065 497-G5
TUXEDO RW
- OXN 93036 492-F7
TUXFORD PL
3300 THO 91360 526-G2
TWILIGHT CT
- CMRL 93012 524-F4
TWILIGHT CANYON TR
- VeCo 93063 499-E3
TWILIGHT GLEN LN
23600 SIMI 93065 497-A1
TWILIGHT RIDGE CIR
1600 THO 91362 527-F6
TWILLIN CT
700 SIMI 93065 497-D6
TWIN CIRCLE LN
6400 SIMI 93063 499-C3
TWIN FALLS CT
200 THO 91320 556-A1
TWINFOOT CT
1000 THO 91361 557-B5
TWIN HARBOR
- VeCo 93012 554-F3
TWINING LN
200 SIMI 93065 497-E6
TWIN LAKE RDG
3400 WLKV 91361 557-B7
TWIN OAK DR
1200 OXN 93036 522-E1
TWIN OAKS CT
400 THO 91362 557-A1
TWIN PEAKS ST
1300 SIMI 93065 497-D7
TWIN RIVER CIR
1800 VEN 93004 492-G4
TWIN SPRINGS AV
6300 VeCo 91377 558-A1
TWIN TIDES PL
- OXN 93035 522-A7
- OXN 93035 552-A1
TWISTED OAK DR
- CanP 91307 529-C7
23600 SIMI 93065 527-F1
TWO OAK CT
2400 SIMI 93063 499-A1
TYLER AV
200 VEN 93003 492-E1
TYLER CT
- VEN 93003 492-E1
2900 SIMI 93063 478-G7
TYNEBOURNE CT
31800 WLKV 91361 557-D6

U

U ST
1500 VEN 93004 493-A3
UKIAH ST
200 PHME 93041 552-E2
1300 OXN 93035 552-E1
2000 OXN 93041 552-E1
ULVERSTON ST
4900 VeCo 91377 557-H1
ULYSSES ST
100 SIMI 93065 497-F2
UNDERPASS ST
2600 OXN 93036 522-G1
UNICORN CIR
7200 VEN 93003 492-E4
UNIDAD WY
- OXN 93030 522-H3
UNIDOS AV
12400 MRPK 93021 496-D2
UNION PL
2100 SIMI 93065 497-F2
UNION PACIFIC ST
- FILM 93015 455-J7
- FILM 93015 456-A7
UNITED RD
3900 AGRH 91301 558-F7
UNIVERSE CIR
1500 OXN 93033 552-J1
UNIVERSITY AV
- VEN 93003 492-A2
UNIVERSITY DR
1900 VeCo 93012 554-E2
6900 MRPK 93021 477-A5
UNIVERSITY PL
200 SPLA 93060 464-B6
UPLAND RD
4500 CMRL 93010 494-J7
4500 VeCo 93010 494-J7
4600 CMRL 93012 494-J7
5100 CMRL 93012 495-A7
6600 CMRL 93012 525-D1
UPPER BAY DR
700 OXN 93036 522-F1
UPPER LAKE RD
- VeCo 91361 586-F1
- VeCo 91361 556-F7
UPPER RANCH RD
1400 THO 91362 527-C5
UPPINGHAM DR
700 THO 91360 526-G2
UPTON SINCLAIR DR
- OXN 93033 552-J2
URANIUM DR
2400 OXN 93030 522-D3
URBANA AV
100 THO 91320 555-H1
URBANA LN
- OXN 93030 522-J3

URSULA DR
23600 OXN 93030 522-J4
UTE LN
200 VEN 93001 471-C6
UTICA AV
700 VEN 93004 492-H2
UTIL CIR
- OXN 93030 522-J3

V

V ST
1500 VEN 93004 492-J2
1500 VEN 93004 493-A3
VALARIE AV
3200 SIMI 93063 478-E6
VALDEZ AL
- VEN 93001 491-B2
VALE PL
4000 THO 91362 527-C7
VALECROFT AV
900 THO 91361 556-J5
VALENCIA AV
2700 SIMI 93063 478-E7
2700 SIMI 93063 498-E1
VALENCIA CIR
2600 THO 91360 526-B3
VALENCIA CT
2600 SIMI 93063 498-E1
VALENCIA DR
1000 VeCo 93010 494-F6
VALENCIA PL
1400 OXN 93035 522-E7
VALENTINA DR
23600 OXN 93030 522-J5
VALENTINE RD
4400 VEN 93003 492-B4
VALERIO ST
22000 CanP 91303 529-H4
22300 CanP 91307 529-F4
23200 LA 91304 529-F4
VALERIO WY
- CMRL 93012 524-H1
VALERO CIR
4900 VeCo 91377 557-G2
VALEROSA WY
- OXN 93030 522-J3
VALEWOOD CIR
3200 THO 91360 526-F2
VALJEAN AV
1200 SIMI 93065 498-C4
VALLECITO DR
800 VEN 93001 491-D1
VALLEJO AV
800 SIMI 93065 498-A4
VALLE LINDO DR
700 CMRL 93010 524-C2
VALLERIO AV
100 OJAI 93023 441-F7
200 OJAI 93023 451-F1
VALLEY CIR
8300 LA 91304 529-E2
VALLEY RD
100 VeCo 93022 451-A7
700 MRPK 93021 476-F7
23600 VeCo 91361 556-A6
VALLEY CIRCLE BLVD
6000 WdHl 91367 529-D6
6300 CanP 91307 529-D5
6900 LACo 91307 529-D5
7100 LA 91304 529-E2
8600 LA 91304 499-G7
9000 Chat 91311 499-H5
9200 Chat 91311 499-G7
VALLEY CIRCLE TER
6300 CanP 91307 529-D7
VALLEY CREST
3600 VeCo 93021 495-H3
VALLEY CREST RD
300 SIMI 93065 497-E5
VALLEY FAIR ST
4000 SIMI 93063 498-F2
VALLEYFIELD AV
2100 THO 91360 526-A4
VALLEY FLORES DR
7800 LA 91304 529-E1
VALLEY GATE RD
- SIMI 93065 497-F6
VALLEY HEIGHTS DR
28900 AGRH 91301 558-A5
VALLEY HIGH AV
800 THO 91362 526-J7
1200 THO 91362 527-A6
VALLEY MEADOW CT
2300 VeCo 93022 451-C4
2300 VeCo 93023 451-C4
VALLEY MEADOW DR
2100 VeCo 93022 451-C4
2100 VeCo 93023 451-C4
VALLEY OAK LN
600 THO 91320 556-D2
VALLEY PARK DR
1400 OXN 93033 552-G1
W VALLEY RIDGE ST
- VeCo 93023 451-B4
VALLEY SPRING DR
4000 THO 91362 527-C7
VALLEY TERRACE DR
23600 SIMI 93065 478-B7
VALLEY VIEW DR
- VeCo 93022 451-B6
VALLEY VIEW RD
1400 OJAI 93023 441-H4
1400 VeCo 93023 441-H4
1400 VeCo 93023 442-A4
VALLEYVIEW WY
500 VEN 93003 492-B1
VALLEY VISTA
800 FILM 93015 456-A5
VALLEY VISTA DR
100 CMRL 93010 524-A1
100 VeCo 93010 524-A1
200 CMRL 93010 494-A7
200 VeCo 93010 494-B6
VALMORE AV
300 VEN 93003 491-G4
VAL VERDE DR
8400 LA 91304 529-D1
8500 WHil 91304 529-D1
VAN BUREN ST
7300 VEN 93003 492-E2
7400 VEN 93004 492-E2
VANCOUVER AV
2600 VEN 93003 491-G3
VANDA LN
- OXN 93036 522-B2
VANDERBILT CT
4500 VEN 93003 492-A1
VANDERBILT DR
200 OXN 93036 522-H2

VAN DYKE ST
- THO 91360 526-E4
VANESSA ST
2000 SIMI 93063 498-F2
VANETTA ST
2000 OXN 93033 553-A5
VAN GOUGH DR
- OXN 93033 552-J2
VANGUARD DR
1100 OXN 93033 522-J7
1100 OXN 93033 552-J1
2300 CMRL 93010 494-E7
VANILLA LN
- SIMI 93065 498-C1
VANITA PL
2100 VeCo 93010 494-E7
VAN NESS AV
300 OXN 93033 552-F5
VAN NUYS AV
100 VeCo 93035 552-C6
VANOWEN ST
21900 CanP 91303 529-G6
22200 CanP 91307 529-D6
24400 LACo 91307 529-D6
VAQUERO CIR
- OXN 93030 522-H3
VAQUERO DR
- OXN 93030 522-H3
1400 SIMI 93065 497-F3
VARE CT
- MRPK 93021 476-B5
VARSITY CT
- VEN 93003 492-A2
VARSITY ST
4200 VEN 93003 491-J3
4300 VEN 93003 492-A2
15000 MRPK 93021 476-J6
N VASSAR CIR
6400 MRPK 93021 476-H6
VASSAR ST
4300 VEN 93003 491-J1
4300 VEN 93003 492-A1
VAUGHN ST
23600 Chat 91311 499-G6
VEDDER MTWY
- VeCo 90265 586-C3
- VeCo 91361 586-C3
VEGA WY
800 VeCo 93023 451-C2
VEGAS DR
200 OXN 93030 522-J6
VEJAR DR
4900 AGRH 91301 558-B6
VELA CT
100 SPLA 93060 463-J6
VELARDE DR
600 THO 91360 526-C3
VELMA CT
2600 SIMI 93065 478-C7
VELVET OAK CT
- SIMI 93063 499-A4
VENADO AV E
100 THO 91320 556-C1
VENDELL RD
27400 AGRH 91301 558-E7
VENETIAN DR
5200 OXN 93035 521-J6
VENEZIA LN
- THO 91362 527-B3
VENICE RD
- PHME 93043 552-C6
VENICE ST
1300 SIMI 93065 497-G3
VENTANA CT
100 THO 91360 526-F1
VENTAVO DR
9400 VeCo 93012 495-J3
9400 VeCo 93021 495-J3
VENTOSO AV
6200 CMRL 93012 525-C1
N VENTU PARK RD
100 THO 91320 556-B1
400 THO 91320 526-A6
S VENTU PARK RD
- THO 91320 556-B1
- THO 91320 556-B2
VENTU PARK FIRE RD
1100 VeCo 91320 556-A3
1900 THO 91320 555-H2
1900 VeCo 91320 555-H3
2100 THO 91320 556-A3
23600 VeCo 91361 556-A3
VENTURA AV
100 VeCo 93035 552-C6
700 SIMI 93065 497-G3
2800 VeCo 93001 471-C1
2800 VEN 93001 471-C4
5500 VeCo 93001 461-B6
5900 VEN 93001 461-B6
VENTURA AV Rt#-33
- VeCo 93022 451-B5
4400 VeCo 93001 461-A2
4400 VeCo 93022 461-A2
11200 VeCo 93023 451-D2
11800 OJAI 93023 451-F1
N VENTURA AV
- VEN 93001 491-B1
600 VEN 93001 471-C6
2500 VeCo 93001 471-C6
S VENTURA AV
- VEN 93001 491-B2
VENTURA BLVD
- OXN 93036 522-H1
100 VeCo 93036 522-H1
800 CMRL 93010 523-F3
1000 VeCo 93010 523-F3
1100 OXN 93036 523-A2
1200 VeCo 93030 523-F3
1200 CMRL 93030 523-F3
1500 CMRL 93010 524-D3
2300 VEN 93003 492-D6
2300 VeCo 93003 492-D6
2500 VeCo 93036 523-C3
2900 OXN 93010 523-C3
E VENTURA BLVD
- CMRL 93010 524-B3
W VENTURA BLVD
- CMRL 93010 524-A3
100 CMRL 93010 523-J3
VENTURA FRWY U.S.-101
- Ago - 558-D6
- AGRH - 557-G6
- AGRH - 558-D6
- CALB - 558-D6
- CMRL - 523-A3
- CMRL - 524-A3
- CMRL - 525-C5
- LACo - 558-D6
- OXN - 492-F7

VENTURA FRWY U.S.-101
- OXN - 522-H2
- OXN - 523-A3
- THO - 525-C5
- THO - 526-D7
- THO - 555-J1
- THO - 556-E1
- THO - 557-B4
- VeCo - 366-F9
- VeCo - 459-A3
- VeCo - 469-J1
- VeCo - 470-B3
- VeCo - 490-H1
- VeCo - 492-F7
- VeCo - 523-A3
- VeCo - 525-C5
- VEN - 490-H1
- VEN - 491-A2
- VEN - 492-F7
- WLKV - 557-B4
VENTURA RD
100 OXN 93030 522-E4
100 PHME 93041 552-E6
900 OXN 93035 522-E7
1100 OXN 93033 522-E7
1100 OXN 93033 552-E2
1200 OXN 93035 552-E2
2000 OXN 93041 552-E2
3300 VEN 93003 492-E7
N VENTURA RD
100 OXN 93030 522-E1
100 PHME 93041 552-E5
1900 OXN 93036 522-E1
2100 PHME 93043 552-E5
2400 OXN 93033 552-E5
2500 VeCo 93036 492-F7
2500 VeCo 93036 522-E1
2700 OXN 93043 552-E5
2800 OXN 93036 492-G6
2800 PHME 93033 552-E5
S VENTURA RD
- OXN 93030 522-E6
1300 OXN 93033 552-E1
2300 PHME 93033 552-E1
13900 OXN 93033 522-E6
VENTURA ST
- VeCo 93012 554-D3
100 OJAI 93023 441-H6
100 SPLA 93060 464-A6
800 VeCo 93015 465-H3
VENTURA ST Rt#-126
100 FILM 93015 456-A6
400 FILM 93015 455-F7
800 VeCo 93015 455-F7
E VENTURA ST Rt#-126
- FILM 93015 456-B6
S VENTURA ST
100 OJAI 93023 441-H7
100 OJAI 93023 451-H1
100 VeCo 93023 451-H1
VENTURA WY
100 Chat 91311 499-F7
9200 Chat 91311 499-F7
VENUS AV
600 SPLA 93060 463-J6
VENUS CT
2700 THO 91360 526-F3
VENUS ST
- THO 91360 526-F3
VENWOOD AV
800 VEN 93001 471-B7
N VERA CT
2000 SIMI 93063 499-B2
E VERA ST
6000 SIMI 93063 499-B2
VERACRUZ LN
2000 OXN 93036 522-G3
VERA CRUZ ST
- SIMI 93065 497-E3
VERANO DR
300 VeCo 93023 441-F7
VERBENA ST
10500 VEN 93004 493-A2
VERCELLY CT
5600 WLKV 91362 557-G6
N VERDA CT
2400 SIMI 93065 490 D1
VERDEMONT CIR
1200 SIMI 93065 497-H5
VERDE OAK DR
100 VeCo 93022 461-A1
VERDE RIDGE LN
1000 THO 91361 556-H6
VERDE VISTA DR
- THO 91360 526-F1
VERDI RD
100 VEN 93003 492-B4
VERDUGO WY
4900 CMRL 93012 524-J3
5100 CMRL 93012 525-A4
W VERDULERA ST
600 CMRL 93010 523-H3
N VERNA AV
600 VeCo 91320 525-G7
VERNON PL
300 SPLA 93060 464-A7
VERNON ST
- VEN 93003 492-B3
VERNON WY
300 SPLA 93060 464-A7
VERONA CT
5500 WLKV 91362 557-G6
VERONICA LN
- VEN 93004 493-A2
VERSAILLE CT
3100 THO 91362 526-J2
VESSEL WY
- OXN 93035 522-D7
VETS CT
30600 AGRH 91301 557-G3
VEVA WY
26100 CALB 91302 558-H4
VIA ACIANDO
23600 CMRL 93012 494-H7
VIA ACORDE
1400 CMRL 93010 494-D7
VIA ACOSTA
1100 THO 91320 555-B4
VIA ADORNA
1000 THO 91320 555-D4
VIA ALAMITOS
- THO 91320 555-C2
VIA ALBA
6900 CMRL 93012 495-D7
6900 CMRL 93012 525-D1
VIA ALCAZAR
1100 CMRL 93010 494-C7

E VIA ALEGRE
5900 SIMI 93063
VIA ALISTA
1000 THO 91320
VIA ALLEGRA
23600 CMRL 93010
VIA ALONDRA
500 CMRL 93012
VIA AMISTOSA
27800 AGRH 91301
VIA ANDREA
4800 THO 91320
VIA ANITA
900 THO 91320
VIA ARABELLA
- THO 91320
VIA ARACENA
1400 CMRL 93010
VIA ARANDANA
23600 CMRL 93012
VIA ARROYO
200 VEN 93003
500 VEN 93003
VIA ARROYO CIR
6400 VEN 93003
VIA AURORA
4800 THO 91320
VIA AZUL
- THO 91320
VIA BAJA
100 VEN 93003
200 VEN 93003
VIA BAJADA
1500 THO 91360
VIA BARON
900 THO 91320
VIA BELLA
- THO 91320
VIA BENSA
4800 VeCo 91377
VIA BONITA
- THO 91320
VIA BONITO
- CMRL 93012
VIA BRAVA
- THO 91320
E VIA BREVE
5900 SIMI 93063
VIA BRISAS
23600 OXN 93030
VIA CALDERON
5000 CMRL 93012
5100 CMRL 93012
VIA CAMINO
- THO 91320
VIA CANADA
4500 THO 91320
VIA CANDELLA
4700 THO 91320
VIA CANTILENA
100 CMRL 93012
VIA CAPOTE
23600 THO 91320
VIA CARILLO
1100 THO 91320
VIA CARRANZA
1100 CMRL 93012
1100 CMRL 93012
VIA CARRO
600 THO 91320
VIA CERRITOS
- THO 91320
VIA CIELITO
500 VEN 93003
500 VEN 93003
VIA COLINAS
- THO 91362
- WLKV 91362
VIA CON DIOS
900 VeCo 93010
VIA CORONADO
- THO 91320
VIA CORZA
2600 CMRL 93010
VIA COZUMEL
6200 CMRL 93012
VIA CRESTA
- THO 91320
VIA CRISTAL
100 CMRL 93012
100 CMRL 93012
VIA CRISTINA
23600 THO 91320
VIA CUPERTINO
4600 CMRL 93012
VIA DE CANTO
- CMRL 93012
VIA DE CERRO
800 VeCo 93010
VIA DE COSTA
3500 THO 91360
VIA DE LA LUZ
- THO 91320
VIA DE LA MESA
- THO 91320
VIA DEL CABALLO
200 VeCo 91377
200 VeCo 91377
VIA DEL LAGO
- THO 91320
VIA DEL NOGAL
2700 CMRL 93010
VIA DEL PRADO
200 SPLA 93060
VIA DEL RANCHO
4500 THO 91320
VIA DEL REY
- THO 91320
VIA DEL SOL
- CMRL 93012
VIA DEL SUELO
2500 CMRL 93010
VIA DE TIERRA
600 THO 91320
VIA DOLORES
23600 THO 91320
VIA DON LUIS
4600 THO 91320
VIA DONTE
- THO 91320
VIA DULCE
- CMRL 93012
VIA EL CERRO
- THO 91320
VIA EL MOLINO
23600 THO 91320
VIA EL TORO
23600 THO 91320
VIA ENCANTO
- THO 91320

STREET Block City ZIP Pg-Grid

RADA
THO 91320 555-E2
ONDIDO
THO 91320 555-C2
NOSA
THO 91320 555-B2
RADA
OXN 93036 523-A2
RELLA
THO 91320 555-C2
ICIA
THO 91320 555-C2
TA
THO 91320 555-E2
SCO
CMRL 93012 524-J1
TERO
VeCo 93040 457-F4
BILAN
CMRL 93012 524-H4
BRIELLA
THO 91320 555-D2
O
THO 91320 555-B3
ETA
THO 91320 555-D4
NDE
THO 91320 555-D3
GORIO
THO 91320 555-C3
IENDA
THO 91320 555-D2
ENA
THO 91320 555-B3
ALDO
THO 91320 555-C4
PANO
THO 91320 555-C4
RESSO
THO 91320 555-C4
Z
THO 91320 555-D2
ARA
CMRL 93012 524-H2
INTO
THO 91320 555-B3
NITA
THO 91320 555-D2
REZ
THO 91320 555-B2
CIMA
THO 91320 555-B1
UNA
THO 91320 555-D2
OLLA
THO 91320 555-C3
PAZ
VEN 93003 492-D1
PRIMAVERA
THO 91360 526-C1
A
THO 91320 555-D2
BRISAS
THO 91320 555-D3
SILVA
CMRL 93010 524-C1
INA DR
CMRL 93012 525-B1
L
CMRL 93010 494-F7
DA
THO 91320 555-C3
BOA
CMRL 93012 524-H4
MA
CMRL 93012 495-B7
RENTE
CMRL 93012 525-B5
S ALTOS
THO 91320 555-B1
DERA
THO 91320 555-D3
GNOLIA
THO 91320 555-D2
NTILLA
CMRL 93010 494-H6
RIANO
THO 91320 555-D1
RINA AV
OXN 93035 522-C7
RINA CT
OXN 93035 522-D7
RIPOSA
THO 91320 555-D1
RISMA
CMRL 93012 524-H4
RQUESA
CMRL 93012 524-H2
DANOS
CMRL 93012 524-H3
RIDA
THO 91362 557-D4
RLA
THO 91320 555-B2
SITA
THO 91320 555-C2
RABELLA
THO 91320 555-C2
RA FLORES
THO 91320 555-A3
NTANEZ
CMRL 93012 525-C5
NTE
THO 91320 555-D1
NTECITO
CMRL 93012 525-D1
CMRL 93012 495-C7
NTEREY
THO 91320 555-D2
NTOYA
CMRL 93010 524-F2
OLA
THO 91320 555-B3
VELLA
VeCo 91377 557-J1
AS
THO 91320 555-B2
VERA
CMRL 93012 524-H3
DULANDO
VEN 93003 472-D7
IEDO
THO 91320 555-A3
CHECO
CMRL 93012 524-J2
CIFICA
SPLA 93060 463-H7
THO 91320 555-B2
CIFICA WK
OXN 93035 522-B7

VIA PAJARO
\- CMRL 93012 524-H1
VIA PALERMO
900 THO 91320 555-C4
VIA PALOMA
3900 CMRL 93012 524-H3
VIA PARQUE
1500 THO 91360 526-J1
VIA PASADA
1000 SPLA 93060 473-F1
VIA PASITO
6100 VEN 93003 472-D7
VIA PATRICIA
23600 THO 91320 555-B2
VIA PESCADOR
3500 CMRL 93012 524-G2
VIA PETIRROJO
23600 THO 91320 525-J5
VIA PISA
23600 THO 91320 555-B2
VIA PLAZA
500 VEN 93003 492-D1
VIA PLUMA
\- THO 91320 555-D2
VIA PRESIDIO
\- CMRL 93012 524-H1
VIA QUINTO
23600 THO 91320 555-B2
VIA RAFAEL
1100 THO 91320 555-C4
VIA REAL
\- CMRL 93012 524-H1
VIA REBECCA
\- THO 91320 555-D2
VIA RICARDO
23600 THO 91320 555-B3
VIA RINCON
23600 THO 91320 555-B2
VIA RIO
23500 THO 91320 555-D2
VIA RIVERA
900 THO 91320 555-D4
VIA ROBLE EXT
23600 VeCo 93040 458-F6
VIA ROCAS
5400 WLKV 91362 557-E5
VIA RODEO
500 FILM 93015 455-J5
4500 THO 91320 555-D3
VIA ROSAL
\- CMRL 93012 524-H4
VIA ROTA
900 CMRL 93012 525-B5
VIA SANDRA
23600 THO 91320 555-B2
VIA SAN JOSE
1000 THO 91320 555-C4
VIA SAN LUCAS
23600 THO 91320 555-B1
VIA SAN MARTIN
23600 THO 91320 555-C2
VIA SANTANA
23600 THO 91320 555-C1
VIA SECOYA
23600 CMRL 93012 494-J7
VIA SEDONA
\- THO 91320 555-A3
VIA SERENA
\- CMRL 93012 524-H1
VIA SIENA
\- THO 91320 555-H2
VIA SILVESTRE
23600 CMRL 93012 525-A2
VIA SINTRA
3900 CMRL 93012 524-H4
VIA SOLANA
100 SPLA 93060 463-H7
VIA SORRENTO
1000 THO 91320 555-B4
VIA TECA
23600 THO 91320 555-B2
VIA TERRADO
500 CMRL 93010 523-H1
VIA TERRASOL
2000 CMRL 93010 494-B7
2000 VeCo 93010 494-B7
VIA TOMAS
2300 CMRL 93010 494-F7
VIA VELA
2700 CMRL 93010 494-F7
VIA VENETO
1900 VeCo 93010 493-J7
1900 VeCo 93010 494-A7
VIA VERDE
3800 THO 91360 526-J1
VIA VISTA
23600 THO 91320 555-C3
VIA VISTOSA
23600 THO 91320 555-C1
VIA ZAMORA
400 CMRL 93010 523-J2
VIA ZURITA CT
2400 VeCo 93012 496-D6
VICKI CT
3400 SIMI 93063 478-D6
VICKIVIEW DR
6600 LACo 91307 529-C6
VICKSBURG LN
1400 VEN 93003 492-B4
VICKY AV
6500 CanP 91307 529-H5
7600 LA 91304 529-H4
VICTOR HERBERT DR
\- VEN 93003 492-A7
VICTORIA AV
\- VeCo 93003 492-C7
\- VEN 93003 492-C7
100 OXN 93030 522-B3
300 VeCo 93030 522-B3
500 OXN 93035 522-B7
1000 VeCo 93001 492-C7
1200 OXN 93036 522-B3
1200 VeCo 93036 522-B3
1400 OXN 93035 552-B3
1800 PHME 93035 552-B3
1800 VeCo 93001 522-B3
2100 PHME 93041 552-B3
4000 VeCo 93035 552-B3
N VICTORIA AV
\- VEN 93003 492-C1
600 VeCo 93003 472-C7
600 VeCo 93003 492-C1
600 VEN 93003 472-C7
S VICTORIA AV
\- VEN 93003 492-C2
700 VEN 93009 492-C3
2000 VeCo 93003 492-C3
VICTORIA ST
2400 SIMI 93065 498-B3

VICTORY BLVD
22000 WdHl 91367 529-C7
22000 CanP 91303 529-F7
22200 CanP 91307 529-C7
23600 VeCo 91302 529-C7
VIDA DR
\- OXN 93030 522-J4
VIEJO DR
300 CMRL 93010 524-D3
VIENTOS RD
400 VeCo 93010 494-B7
VIEW DR
100 SPLA 93060 464-A5
2100 SIMI 93065 497-E2
VIEWCREST CT
5900 VEN 93003 472-C7
VIEWCREST DR
600 VeCo 93003 472-C7
600 VEN 93003 472-C7
VIEWLAKE LN
32000 WLKV 91361 557-C7
VIEW LINE DR
\- SIMI 93065 477-F7
VIEW MESA ST
12900 MRPK 93021 496-E4
VIEW PARK CT
400 VeCo 91377 558-B1
VIEW POINT CIR
6100 VEN 93003 472-C5
VIEWPOINT DR
\- OXN 93035 522-A7
\- OXN 93035 552-A1
VIEW POINTE DR
3200 WLKV 91361 557-C7
VIKING DR
1900 CMRL 93010 494-E7
VILLA ADOBE
600 CMRL 93012 524-G3
VILLA CAMPESINA AV
12400 MRPK 93021 496-D2
VILLAGE CT
1200 SIMI 93065 497-H4
1700 THO 91362 527-A5
VILLAGE GN
900 THO 91361 557-C5
VILLAGE PKWY
2100 SIMI 93065 497-E2
VILLAGE RD
200 PHME 93041 552-E6
VILLAGE SQ
200 FILM 93015 455-J6
VILLAGE 1
\- CMRL 93012 525-A3
VILLAGE 11
500 CMRL 93012 525-B2
VILLAGE 13
5800 CMRL 93012 525-B2
VILLAGE 14
400 CMRL 93012 525-B2
VILLAGE 15
500 CMRL 93012 525-B2
VILLAGE 16
\- CMRL 93012 525-A3
VILLAGE 17
5600 CMRL 93012 525-B3
VILLAGE 18
\- CMRL 93012 525-A3
VILLAGE 19
\- CMRL 93012 525-B3
VILLAGE 2
100 CMRL 93012 525-A3
VILLAGE 20
\- CMRL 93012 525-B3
VILLAGE 22
5700 CMRL 93012 525-B3
VILLAGE 23
\- CMRL 93012 525-B3
VILLAGE 24
5700 CMRL 93012 525-B3
VILLAGE 25
\- CMRL 93012 525-B2
VILLAGE 26
5800 CMRL 93012 525-B3
VILLAGE 28
\- CMRL 93012 525-B3
VILLAGE 29
6000 CMRL 93012 525-B2
VILLAGE 3
200 CMRL 93012 525-A3
VILLAGE 30
6000 CMRL 93012 525-C2
VILLAGE 31
6100 CMRL 93012 525-C2
VILLAGE 32
6000 CMRL 93012 525-C2
VILLAGE 33
6200 CMRL 93012 525-C2
VILLAGE 34
6200 CMRL 93012 525-C2
VILLAGE 35
6300 CMRL 93012 525-C2
VILLAGE 37
900 CMRL 93012 525-C1
VILLAGE 38
\- CMRL 93012 525-C2
VILLAGE 39
900 CMRL 93012 525-C1
VILLAGE 4
100 CMRL 93012 525-A3
VILLAGE 40
6500 CMRL 93012 525-C2
VILLAGE 41
100 CMRL 93012 525-C1
VILLAGE 42
\- CMRL 93012 525-D1
VILLAGE 44
1000 CMRL 93012 525-D1
VILLAGE 5
300 CMRL 93012 525-A2
VILLAGE 6
\- CMRL 93012 525-A3
VILLAGE 7
5600 CMRL 93012 525-A2
VILLAGE 8
\- CMRL 93012 525-B2
VILLAGE 9
5700 CMRL 93012 525-B2
VILLAGE AT THE PARK DR
\- CMRL 93012 524-F4
VILLAGE BROOK RD
31800 WLKV 91361 557-D6
VILLAGE CENTER RD
31600 WLKV 91361 557-D6
VILLAGE COMMONS BLVD
\- CMRL 93012 524-G5
VILLAGE SCHOOL RD
31600 WLKV 91361 557-D6

VILLAGEVIEW CT
11700 MRPK 93021 496-B2
VILLA MALLORCA PL
5200 CMRL 93012 525-A2
VILLAMONTE CT
4300 CMRL 93010 494-G7
VILLANOVA AV
\- OXN 93030 522-H2
300 VEN 93003 492-B1
VILLANOVA RD
100 VeCo 93023 451-D3
E VILLANOVA RD
100 VeCo 93023 451-E2
800 OJAI 93023 451-E2
VINA DEL MAR
2100 OXN 93035 552-A2
VINCA LN
\- VEN 93004 493-A2
VINCA ST
\- SIMI 93063 499-A2
VINCA WY
\- OXN 93030 523-A3
E VINCE ST
\- VEN 93001 471-C7
W VINCE ST
\- VEN 93001 471-B7
VINCENNES ST
22000 Chat 91311 499-J6
VINCENTE AV
3800 CMRL 93010 494-G7
VINE PL
400 OXN 93033 552-G3
VINE ST
500 VeCo 93022 451-B7
500 VeCo 93022 461-B1
VINEWOOD
13300 MRPK 93021 496-F3
E VINEYARD AV
Rt#-232
500 OXN 93036 522-G2
2600 VeCo 93036 522-G2
2800 OXN 93036 492-H7
2800 VeCo 93036 492-H7
4100 VeCo 93036 493-A4
5100 VeCo 93066 493-A4
W VINEYARD AV
100 OXN 93036 522-D2
VINEYARD DR
\- SIMI 93065 497-G7
VINTAGE ST
22000 Chat 91311 499-J5
VINTAGE OAK ST
\- SIMI 93063 499-A3
VINTON CT
700 THO 91360 556-G1
VIOLA WY
\- OXN 93030 523-A4
VIOLET LN
\- SIMI 93065 497-H3
VIOLET WY
500 OXN 93036 522-F1
VIOLETA ST
11000 VeCo 93004 493-A1
VIRGINIA DR
\- VeCo 91320 555-H1
\- VEN 93003 491-G2
VIRGINIA TER
100 SPLA 93060 464-A5
VIRGINIA COLONY PL
5500 MRPK 93021 476-H7
VIRGO CT
200 THO 91360 526-E2
VISALIA CT
100 VEN 93004 492-F2
VISALIA ST
1300 OXN 93035 552-E1
8200 VEN 93004 492-F2
VISTA CIR
2600 CMRL 93010 524-F1
VISTA CT
1300 CMRL 93010 524-F1
VISTA LP
2600 OXN 93036 492-F7
2600 OXN 93036 522-F1
VISTA RD
5900 VeCo 93063 499-B4
VISTA ST
2600 CMRL 93010 524-F1
VISTA ALCEDO
1800 CMRL 93012 495-D7
1800 CMRL 93012 525-D1
VISTA ANACAPA RD
9000 VeCo 93021 475-F5
VISTA ARRIAGO
800 CMRL 93012 525-C5
VISTA ARROYO DR
2500 VeCo 93012 496-E6
VISTA BONITA
100 THO 91320 525-E6
VISTA CONEJO
\- THO 91320 525-E6
VISTA COTO VERDE
1100 CMRL 93010 494-C7
VISTA CREEK CIR
23600 SIMI 93065 497-D7
VISTA DEL CAMPO
800 VeCo 93010 494-A6
VISTA DEL CIMA
1100 VeCo 93010 494-B6
VISTA DEL MAR AV
1100 CMRL 93010 494-B7
1100 VeCo 93010 494-B7
VISTA DEL MAR DR
900 VEN 93001 491-E3
VISTA DEL MAR PL
1000 VEN 93001 491-D3
VISTA DEL MONTE
23600 FILM 93015 456-C6
VISTA DEL RINCON DR
6800 VeCo 93001 459-D5
VISTA DEL SOL
300 CMRL 93010 524-B3
VISTA DEL VALLE RD
4400 MRPK 93021 496-F2
VISTA DE VENTURA
500 VEN 93003 492-B1
VISTA DORADO LN
400 VeCo 91377 557-J2
VISTA GRANDE
2600 VeCo 93012 496-E6
VISTA GRANDE DR
23600 SPLA 93060 464-B4
VISTA HERMOSA DR
400 OJAI 93023 441-G5
VISTA HERMOSA ST
1100 SIMI 93065 497-E4
VISTA LAGO DR
\- SIMI 93065 497-F4
\- VeCo 93065 497-F4

VISTA LEVANA DR
13300 MRPK 93021 496-F2
VISTAMEADOW CT
4400 MRPK 93021 496-D3
VISTA MERCADO
3300 CMRL 93012 524-G2
VISTA MONTANA
400 VeCo 93010 494-A6
VISTA OAKS WY
1400 THO 91361 556-H6
VISTA PALACIO
700 CMRL 93012 524-H2
E VISTAPARK DR
12900 MRPK 93021 496-E2
VISTA POINTE PL
23600 SPLA 93060 464-B4
VISTA RIDGE LN
900 THO 91362 557-D1
VISTA WOOD CIR
2400 THO 91362 527-B4
VIVIAN CIR
800 THO 91320 526-C7
VIVIANA DR
\- OXN 93030 522-J4
VOLCANO CT
2600 OXN 93030 522-D3
VOLTAIRE DR
3000 OXN 93033 552-J3
VOLTAIRE WY
10400 VeCo 93012 495-J6
10400 VeCo 93012 496-A6
VORALE AV
400 SIMI 93065 497-G3
VOSE ST
22500 CanP 91307 529-G5
VOYAGER AV
1600 SIMI 93063 498-E3
VOYAGER PL
1000 OXN 93033 522-H7

W

W ST
1500 VEN 93004 492-J3
1500 VEN 93004 493-A3
WABASH ST
8200 VEN 93004 492-G3
WACO DR
2900 SIMI 93063 478-G6
WACO ST
8700 VEN 93004 492-G2
WADE CIR
1600 SIMI 93065 497-J5
WADES RD
600 VeCo 93015 455-J1
600 VeCo 93015 456-A1
WAGNER RD
5100 VEN 93003 492-B4
WAGNER WY
5300 VeCo 91377 527-H6
N WAGON LN
\- VeCo 91307 528-J3
WAGON WHEEL RD
900 OXN 93036 492-F7
2000 OXN 93036 522-G1
WAITE ST
100 OJAI 93023 441-J6
WAKE LN
\- OXN 93035 522-D7
WAKEFIELD AV
1500 THO 91360 526-F5
E WAKEFORD AV
900 SPLA 93060 464-A6
W WAKEFORD AV
100 SPLA 93060 463-J6
100 SPLA 93060 464-A6
WAKE FOREST AV
\- VEN 93003 492-C2
N WAKE FOREST AV
\- VEN 93003 492-B2
WALCOTT AV
\- VEN 93003 492-B3
WALDEMAR DR
23600 VeCo 91361 556-D7
WALDEN ST
100 SPLA 93060 463-H6
1900 OXN 93033 553-A5
WALDO AV
2100 SIMI 93065 498-C2
WALES DR
900 OXN 93035 522-E7
WALES ST
\- THO 91360 526-F6
WALHORD CT
30200 AGRH 91301 557-H4
WALKER AV
400 CMRL 93010 524-F2
WALKER LN
\- FILM 93015 456-A5
WALKER ST
4700 VEN 93003 492-B5
WALKER CUP CIR
1700 THO 91362 527-D6
WALKING HORSE LN
31500 WLKV 91361 557-E6
WALL ST
100 VEN 93001 491-B1
WALLABY CT
7400 VEN 93003 492-F4
WALLABY ST
7100 VEN 93003 492-E4
WALLACE ST
1500 SIMI 93065 497-J4
1700 SIMI 93065 498-A4
WALLBRIDGE WY
400 VeCo 93023 441-D7
WALLINGTON CT
31900 WLKV 91361 557-C6
WALNUT AV
4000 VeCo 93066 494-A3
WALNUT CT
700 THO 91320 556-C2
WALNUT DR
\- VeCo 93036 492-J7
300 VEN 93003 492-A1
500 VeCo 93036 522-J1
700 VeCo 93036 523-A1
WALNUT ST
300 SPLA 93060 464-B5
600 MRPK 93021 476-E7
600 MRPK 93021 496-E1
3400 VeCo 93063 478-E6
3400 SIMI 93063 478-E6
WALNUT CANYON RD
Rt#-23
800 MRPK 93021 476-E7
1100 VeCo 93021 476-E4
WALNUT CREEK RD
3900 MRPK 93021 496-D3

WALNUT GROVE LN
1300 SIMI 93065 497-H3
WALNUT RIDGE DR
5600 AGRH 91301 557-J5
WALSH RD
1100 VeCo 93063 499-G4
WALTER AV
100 THO 91320 555-F2
WALTER CIR
3600 THO 91320 555-F2
WALTER ST
600 VEN 93003 491-J5
WALTHAM CIR
1100 SIMI 93065 497-H4
WALTHAM RD
1000 SIMI 93065 497-H4
WALWORTH CT
1500 VeCo 91377 527-H6
WANDA AV
2600 SIMI 93065 498-B1
2600 SIMI 93065 478-B7
WANKEL WY
2300 OXN 93030 523-A3
WARBLE CT
\- THO 91320 525-J5
\- THO 91320 526-A5
WARBLER AV
2300 VEN 93003 492-E5
WARD AV
2100 SIMI 93065 497-G2
WARD WY
1700 VeCo 93023 451-A3
WAREHOUSE AV
500 OXN 93030 522-H7
WARFIELD CIR
1700 SIMI 93063 499-A3
WARING PL
28400 AGRH 91301 558-C6
WARMSPRINGS AV
1300 THO 91320 526-A6
E WARNER ST
\- VEN 93001 471-C7
W WARNER ST
\- VEN 93001 471-B7
WARREN AV
100 SPLA 93060 464-A6
WARREN CIR
700 MRPK 93021 476-F7
WARRENDALE ST
1400 SIMI 93065 497-D7
WARRING CANYON RD
700 VeCo 93040 457-E2
WARRINGTON WY
1000 OJAI 93023 451-F1
WARWICK AV
400 THO 91360 526-F6
400 THO 91360 556-F1
W WASATCH CT
2700 THO 91362 557-C3
WASHBURN ST
\- SIMI 93065 497-E3
WASHINGTON DR
1900 VEN 93003 492-C5
WATCH WY
\- OXN 93035 522-D7
WATERBURY LN
900 VEN 93001 491-E4
WATERBY ST
2100 THO 91361 557-A5
WATERFALL LN
23600 SIMI 93065 478-C7
WATERFORD LN
900 FILM 93015 455-H7
WATERGATE CT
31900 WLKV 91361 557-C6
WATERGATE RD
2700 THO 91361 557-B5
32000 WLKV 91361 557-C6
WATEROAK LN
500 VeCo 91377 557-J1
WATERS RD
7800 VeCo 93021 475-G3
WATERSIDE CIR
23600 THO 91362 527-B4
WATERSIDE LN
\- OXN 93035 522-A7
32000 WLKV 91361 557-C7
WATERTOWN CT
2100 THO 91360 526-B4
WATERTREE CT
6200 AGRH 91301 558-A3
WATERWHEEL PL
\- THO 91361 556-H5
WATKINS WY
\- VeCo 93022 451-B6
WATSON AV
600 SIMI 93065 498-C5
WATSON DR
\- MRPK 93021 476-B5
WATT DR
700 OXN 93030 552-H1
WATTS TREE FARM RD
100 VeCo 93023 453-B1
N WAUKEGAN AV
3000 SIMI 93063 478-F7
WAUNETA ST
3000 THO 91320 555-G2
WAVECREST WY
5000 OXN 93035 521-J7
WAVERLY AV
2600 CMRL 93010 524-F2
WAVERLY CT
500 OXN 93030 522-D4
2700 CMRL 93010 524-F2
WAVERLY DR
200 SIMI 93065 497-E2
WAVERLY HEIGHTS DR
600 THO 91360 526-G5
WAXWING AV
2300 VEN 93003 492-E5
WAYNE CIR
2300 SIMI 93065 498-A1
WAYSIDE CIR
1000 VeCo 93010 494-F6
WAYVIEW CT
6300 VEN 93003 472-D7
WEATHERFORD CT
3200 SIMI 93063 478-G6
WEATHERLY CIR
3800 WLKV 91361 557-B7
E WEAVER ST
600 SIMI 93065 497-G5
WEBB RD
23700 Chat 91311 499-E6
WEBER CIR
800 VEN 93003 492-A4
WEBER CT
4500 VEN 93003 492-A4
WEBSTER DR
4700 OXN 93033 553-A5

WEBSTER ST
5900 VEN 93003 492-C3
WEDGEWOOD CIR
100 THO 91360 526-F3
WEEPING WILLOW DR
3900 MRPK 93021 496-F4
29400 AGRH 91301 557-J4
WEINBERG ST
22400 Chat 91311 499-H4
WELAND
23600 VeCo 93015 456-F6
WELBY WY
2400 CanP 91307 529-D6
22100 CanP 91303 529-H6
24500 LACo 91307 529-C6
WELCOME CT
2300 SIMI 93063 499-B1
WELDON CANYON
23600 VeCo 93001 461-C5
WELLBROOK DR
32700 WLKV 91361 557-A7
32700 WLKV 91361 556-J7
WELLER CT
600 SIMI 93065 497-G4
WELLESLEY CT
700 THO 91360 526-G5
WELLESLEY DR
1700 THO 91360 526-G5
WELLINGTON CT
25900 LACo 91302 558-J3
WELLINGTON PL
1500 THO 91361 556-J6
WELLINGTON ST
8500 VEN 93004 492-G4
WELLS LN
200 WHil 91304 499-D6
WELLS RD
\- VeCo 90265 585-G7
\- VeCo 90265 625-G1
N WELLS RD
\- VEN 93004 472-J6
\- VeCo 93004 472-J6
\- VEN 93060 472-J6
200 VeCo 93060 472-J6
S WELLS RD
\- VEN 93004 472-J7
S WELLS RD Rt#-118
300 VEN 93004 472-J7
700 VEN 93004 473-A7
800 VEN 93004 493-A1
900 VeCo 93004 493-A1
WELLSTON CT
3500 SIMI 93063 478-F5
WELSH CT
1400 SIMI 93065 497-E3
WEMBLY AV
5500 VeCo 91377 527-H6
WENDELL ST
2700 CMRL 93010 524-F1
N WENDY DR
100 VeCo 91320 555-G1
400 VeCo 91320 525-G7
600 THO 91320 525-G7
S WENDY DR
\- THO 91320 555-G3
WENDY LN
400 SPLA 93060 464-A5
WENDY PL
2000 PHME 93041 552-D1
WESHAM ST
8400 VEN 93004 492-G4
WESLEY AV
200 VEN 93003 491-J3
WESLEYAN AV
300 VEN 93003 491-J1
WEST DR
1200 VEN 93003 492-D4
WEST RD
\- PHME 93043 552-B4
WEST ST
3500 VeCo 93066 495-A5
WESTAR DR
1100 OXN 93033 552-J1
WESTBEND RD
600 THO 91362 557-D1
800 THO 91362 527-D7
WESTBLUFF PL
23600 SIMI 93065 497-E4
WESTBURY CT
\- THO 91360 526-F6
WESTBURY ST
100 THO 91360 526-F6
WESTCHESTER CT
1900 OXN 93036 522-D3
WESTCHESTER LN
600 THO 91320 556-D1
WESTCLIFF DR
7300 LA 91304 529-D4
WESTCOTT CT
\- MRPK 93021 496-E2
WESTCREEK LN
900 THO 91362 557-G1
900 VeCo 91362 557-G1
1000 THO 91362 527-G7
WESTDALE RD
4200 MRPK 93021 496-B3
WESTFIELD CT
600 VEN 93004 492-H2
WEST FORK HALL CANYON RD
2800 VeCo 93001 471-G4
WESTGATE RD
13200 MRPK 93021 496-E3
WESTHAM CIR
2700 THO 91362 527-A3
WESTHILLS CT
2600 SIMI 93065 477-E7
2600 SIMI 93065 497-E1
WESTINGHOUSE ST
4400 VEN 93003 492-A5
WESTLAKE BLVD
700 THO 91361 556-J6
WESTLAKE BLVD Rt#-23
100 LACo 90265 586-H4
400 WLKV 90265 586-H4
400 WLKV 91361 586-H4
800 LACo 91361 586-H4
800 THO 91361 586-H4
N WESTLAKE BLVD
\- THO 91362 557-C3
1000 THO 91362 527-B4
S WESTLAKE BLVD
\- THO 91362 557-B5
S WESTLAKE BLVD Rt#-23
100 THO 91362 557-C4
100 THO 91361 557-C4
600 THO 91361 556-J7
800 THO 91361 586-H1

STREET Block City ZIP Pg-Grid

WESTLAKE EDISON RD
100 THO 91361 556-G4
100 VeCo 91361 556-G4
WESTLAKE VISTA LN
- THO 91362 557-A2
WESTLAND AV
23600 THO 91362 527-A1
WESTMINSTER AV
100 VEN 93003 492-B3
WESTMINSTER ST
500 THO 91360 526-G7
WESTMONT DR
12500 MRPK 93021 496-D3
WESTMONT ST
4400 VEN 93003 492-A3
WEST MOUNTAIN RD
20000 VeCo 93066 473-E7
20000 VeCo 93066 493-E1
WESTON CIR
1700 CMRL 93010 494-F7
1700 CMRL 93010 524-F1
WESTON CT
300 SPLA 93060 463-J6
WESTOVER PL
700 THO 91320 555-G3
WESTPARK CT
- CMRL 93012 524-F4
WEST POINT ST
5000 VEN 93003 492-B1
WESTPORT ST
12900 MRPK 93021 496-E4
WESTRANCH PL
23600 SIMI 93065 497-E4
WESTRIDGE CIR
2900 THO 91360 526-C3
WESTRIDGE DR
1000 VEN 93003 472-D6
WEST SHORE LN
1300 THO 91361 557-A6
WEST VAIL DR
23100 CanP 91307 529-F5
WESTVIEW CT
4800 THO 91362 557-F1
WESTWIND CIR
1300 THO 91361 557-B6
WESTWOOD DR
2100 CMRL 93010 494-E7
WESTWOOD ST
- SIMI 93063 478-G5
E WESTWOOD ST
6300 MRPK 93021 476-G6
N WESTWOOD ST
700 MRPK 93021 476-G6
WETHERBY ST
- SIMI 93065 497-H4
WETSTONE CT
2000 THO 91362 527-A4
WETSTONE DR
2100 THO 91362 527-A4
E WEXFORD CIR
1700 SIMI 93065 497-J5
1700 SIMI 93065 498-A5
WEYLAND CT
2600 SIMI 93065 478-B7
WEYMOUTH LN
1200 VEN 93001 491-F5
WHALEBOAT PL
30700 AGRH 91301 557-G5
WHALEN WY
- OXN 93036 492-H5
WHALERS LN
11900 VeCo 90265 625-F5
WHARF WY
- PHME 93041 552-E5
WHEATFIELD CIR
2600 SIMI 93063 498-D1
2600 SIMI 93063 478-D7
WHEATON CT
14600 MRPK 93021 476-H6
WHEATON DR
4500 VEN 93003 492-A3
WHEELER CANYON RD
2500 VeCo 93060 473-B1
2600 VeCo 93060 463-A3
7300 VeCo 93060 453-B6
WHEELHOUSE AV
2400 PHME 93041 552-C2
WHEELHOUSE LN
5800 AGRH 91301 557-G4
WHEELWRIGHT LN
1900 THO 91320 525-J7
1900 THO 91320 526-A7
WHIM DR
30800 WLKV 91362 557-F4
WHIPPLE RD
100 VeCo 93060 464-D5
WHIPPOORWILL ST
6300 VEN 93003 492-D6
WHISPERING GATES CT
- SIMI 93065 497-G7
WHISPERING GLEN CT
- SIMI 93065 478-B6
WHISPERING HILLS AV
23600 THO 91320 555-E4
WHISPERING OAKS PL
600 THO 91320 556-D1
WHISPERING PINES
4900 THO 91362 557-G1
WHISTLER WY
6500 VEN 93003 492-D1
WHITCOMB AV
1000 SIMI 93065 498-B4
WHITE ST
6300 SIMI 93063 499-C2
WHITE BIRCH CIR
3100 THO 91360 526-H2
WHITECAP CT
200 PHME 93041 552-E6
WHITE CAP DR
400 VEN 93003 491-H1
WHITECAP ST
5000 OXN 93035 521-J7
WHITE CEDAR PL
3100 THO 91362 527-C3
WHITECHAPEL PL
2400 THO 91362 527-B2
WHITECLIFF RD
900 THO 91360 526-G7
WHITE CLOUD CIR
5100 THO 91362 527-G7
WHITE DOVE CIR
1300 THO 91362 527-G7
WHITE FEATHER CT
1300 THO 91320 526-A6
WHITEGATE RD
400 THO 91320 555-H3
400 VeCo 91320 555-H3
E WHITEHALL CT
1900 SIMI 93065 498-A5

WHITEHALL LN
- CanP 91307 529-D5
WHITEHALL PL
1500 THO 91361 556-J6
WHITE HAWK LN
- SIMI 93065 478-B4
WHITEHEAD PL
23600 VEN 93003 492-C6
WHITE OAK CIR
500 OJAI 93023 441-J5
WHITE OAK LN
600 THO 91320 556-D2
WHITE PINE CT
1300 VeCo 91377 527-G7
WHITE RIDGE PL
2700 THO 91362 527-B3
WHITE RIVER PL
3400 WLKV 91361 557-B7
WHITE ROCK RD
- CMRL 93012 524-F4
WHITE SAGE RD
23600 MRPK 93021 496-G1
WHITESAIL CIR
4000 WLKV 91361 557-B6
WHITESIDE PL
200 THO 91362 557-A2
WHITE STALLION RD
- VeCo 91320 555-H4
- VeCo 91361 555-H4
WHITE SWAN CT
500 SIMI 93065 497-E6
WHITETAIL AV
3400 SIMI 93063 479-A6
WHITEWATER LN
11800 VeCo 90265 625-F5
WHITE WING CT
2600 VeCo 93012 496-A7
E WHITEWOOD ST
6500 SIMI 93063 499-C2
WHITFORD AV
23600 VeCo 91361 556-G6
WHITINGHAM CT
29300 AGRH 91301 558-A3
WHITMAN CT
500 THO 91360 526-G2
6800 VEN 93003 492-E3
WHITNEY AV
100 MRPK 93021 496-D1
WHITNEY CIR
100 OXN 93033 553-C3
WHITTIER CT
4300 VEN 93003 492-A3
WHITTIER ST
4400 VEN 93003 492-A3
WHITWORTH ST
100 THO 91360 526-E4
WICHITA FALLS AV
3200 SIMI 93063 478-H6
WICKFORD PL
- CMRL 93012 524-G4
WICKLOW CT
1600 THO 91361 556-J5
WICKS RD
- MRPK 93021 476-E7
WIGGIN ST
4800 VeCo 91377 557-G1
WILBUR CT
500 THO 91360 526-G7
WILBUR RD
- THO 91360 556-E1
E WILBUR RD
- THO 91360 526-F7
W WILBUR RD
- THO 91360 526-F7
100 THO 91360 556-F1
WILCOX ST
2100 CMRL 93010 524-E2
WILDCAT AV
2300 VEN 93003 492-E5
WILDCAT CT
- MRPK 93021 476-F5
WILD CLOVER WY
300 SIMI 93065 527-D1
WILDCREEK CIR
700 THO 91360 526-C2
WILDER ST
1200 THO 91362 527-A6
WILDFLOWER CT
11500 MRPK 93021 496-B2
WILD HORSE CT
3000 THO 91360 526-C2
WILDLIFE DR
- SIMI 93065 497-E5
W WILDOAK ST
- VeCo 93023 451-B4
WILDON RD
23600 CMRL 93010 524-C4
WILDRIDGE CT
- MRPK 93021 476-D5
WILD ROSE CT
- SIMI 93065 497-G7
WILD ROSE ST
2500 THO 91361 557-B5
WILDROSE WK
- OXN 93036 522-B3
WILD SAGE CT
3900 THO 91362 527-C6
WILDWEST CIR
13800 MRPK 93021 496-F3
WILDWOOD AV
300 THO 91360 526-B1
WILDWOOD LN
- FILM 93015 456-B6
WILDWOOD PL
22200 Chat 91311 499-J2
WILEMAN ST
300 FILM 93015 455-J6
WILEY CANYON RD
23600 VeCo - 467-B1
23600 VeCo 93015 467-B1
23600 VeCo 93021 467-B6
WILL AV
300 VeCo 93036 492-J7
700 VeCo 93036 493-A7
WILLAMETTE ST
10000 VEN 93004 492-J3
WILLARD RD
- VeCo 93060 464-F4
WILLDEN DR
- VeCo 93010 494-D7
W WILLEY ST
- VeCo 93023 451-B4
WILLIAM CT
600 SIMI 93065 497-G4
WILLIAM DR
3300 VeCo 91320 555-F1
WILLIAMS DR
1900 OXN 93030 523-A3
1900 OXN 93036 523-A3

WILLIAMS LN
1600 SIMI 93063 499-B3
WILLIAMS PL
700 OJAI 93023 441-J6
WILLIAMS ST
1800 SIMI 93065 497-H3
WILLIAMS WY
5900 SIMI 93063 499-B3
WILLIAMSBURG CT
- VeCo 91361 586-G1
WILLIAMSBURG WY
- VeCo 91361 586-F1
WILLIAMS CANYON RD
500 VeCo 93060 472-H5
500 VEN 93060 472-H5
WILLIAMS RANCH RD
12600 MRPK 93021 496-D3
WILLIS AV
200 CMRL 93010 523-J4
200 CMRL 93010 524-A4
WILLIS CANYON RD
- VeCo 93023 366-H7
- VeCo 93023 441-A6
WILLOUGHBY RD
- VeCo 93060 453-A6
23600 VeCo 93060 452-H7
WILLOW CT
- AGRH 91301 558-A5
2600 SIMI 93063 498-E1
WILLOW LN
100 SPLA 93060 464-A5
2400 THO 91361 556-J2
2400 THO 91361 557-A3
WILLOW ST
400 OXN 93033 552-G3
E WILLOW ST
400 OJAI 93023 441-J7
WILLOWBROOK DR
100 PHME 93041 552-F6
WILLOWBROOK LN
1400 SIMI 93065 497-H3
WILLOW CANYON ST
- THO 91362 527-C2
WILLOW CREEK CT
2200 OXN 93036 522-D1
WILLOW CREEK LN
3900 MRPK 93021 496-G3
WILLOW FOREST DR
12300 MRPK 93021 496-C3
WILLOW GLEN CIR
23600 SIMI 93065 527-F1
WILLOW GLEN CT
- CMRL 93012 524-G5
WILLOW GLEN ST
4300 CALB 91302 558-H7
WILLOWGREEN CT
1900 THO 91361 557-A5
WILLOW GROVE CT
12400 MRPK 93021 496-D3
WILLOW HAVEN CT
- THO 91362 527-C2
WILLOW HILL DR
12200 MRPK 93021 496-C3
WILLOWICK DR
3500 VEN 93003 491-H2
WILLOW OAK ST
- SIMI 93063 498-J3
WILLOWOOD CT
11500 MRPK 93021 496-B2
WILLOWPARK CT
2200 THO 91362 527-A4
WILLOW SPRINGS DR
12200 MRPK 93021 496-C3
WILLOW TREE CT
1900 THO 91362 526-J4
1900 THO 91362 527-A4
WILLOWTREE DR
5700 AGRH 91301 557-H4
WILLOW VIEW DR
5300 CMRL 93012 525-A2
WILLSBROOK CT
1200 THO 91361 556-J5
1200 THO 91361 557-A5
E WILMOT ST
3200 SIMI 93063 498-D2
WILSHIRE PL
400 THO 91320 555-H3
WILSON AV
100 OXN 93030 522-H6
WILSON DR
800 VeCo 93015 455-D5
1000 SIMI 93065 498-C4
WILSON ST
2500 VeCo 93015 465-E1
23600 VEN 93003 492-E2
WILTON ST
1600 SIMI 93065 497-J2
WIMBLEDON CIR
1300 THO 91361 557-A5
WINCHESTER DR
300 OXN 93036 522-G1
6200 VeCo 93021 475-J6
WINCHESTER WY
5400 CMRL 93012 525-A1
WINDBREEZE AV
23600 THO 91362 527-B2
WINDBROOK CT
1900 THO 91361 557-A7
WINDCREST CT
2700 OXN 93036 492-F7
2700 OXN 93036 522-F1
WINDFLOWER CIR
3200 THO 91360 526-H2
WINDHARP LN
23600 SIMI 93065 497-A2
WINDHAVEN DR
4800 THO 91362 557-E2
WINDING LN
3000 THO 91361 557-C5
WINDINGWAY DR
800 VEN 93001 491-D1
WINDMILL LN
1000 VeCo 91377 528-B7
1000 VeCo 91377 558-A1
WINDMILL WY
- SIMI 93065 497-H3
WINDMIST AV
23600 THO 91362 527-B2
WINDOM ST
22800 CanP 91307 529-G4
23200 LA 91304 529-F4
WINDOVER RD
8400 VeCo 93021 476-D3
WINDRIDGE AV
- THO 91362 527-C2
WINDRIFT CT
3000 THO 91360 526-F2
WIND RIVER CIR
400 THO 91362 557-B2

WINDROSE CT
23600 THO 91320 556-C1
WINDROSE DR
100 THO 91320 556-C1
WINDSHORE WY
- OXN 93035 522-B7
- OXN 93035 552-B1
WINDSONG LN
29600 AGRH 91301 557-J5
WINDSONG ST
2900 THO 91360 526-F2
WINDSOR CT
2200 CMRL 93010 494-D7
WINDSOR DR
1000 THO 91360 526-G6
WINDSWEPT PL
500 SIMI 93065 497-D7
500 SIMI 93065 527-D1
WINDTREE AV
100 THO 91320 556-C1
WINDWARD CIR
2300 THO 91361 557-B6
WINDWARD WY
1000 OXN 93035 522-D7
WINDWILLOW WY
1500 SIMI 93065 497-D6
WINDY MOUNTAIN AV
5000 THO 91362 527-F7
WINFIELD ST
900 THO 91320 555-E4
WINFORD AV
1100 VEN 93004 492-G3
WING RD
200 Chat 91311 499-F6
WINGED FOOT CT
2200 OXN 93036 522-D2
WINIFRED ST
2000 SIMI 93063 498-G2
WINNCASTLE ST
500 SIMI 93065 527-D2
WINONA CT
6400 VeCo 91377 558-A1
WINROCK WY
23600 SIMI 93065 497-A1
WINSIDE ST
4800 THO 91362 557-G2
WINSTON CT
1000 THO 91361 557-B5
WINTER AV
12600 MRPK 93021 496-E4
WINTERBERRY AV
5200 SIMI 93063 498-J2
WINTERBROOK CT
3100 THO 91360 526-F2
WINTERDEW AV
23600 SIMI 93065 497-D2
WINTERGREEN LN
13200 MRPK 93021 496-E4
WINTERSET PL
1800 SIMI 93065 497-D2
WINTERWOOD CT
4000 MRPK 93021 496-C3
WINTHROP CT
2500 SIMI 93065 497-J1
WINTHROP LN
1000 VEN 93001 491-E4
WINTON CT
- SIMI 93065 497-E2
WISCASSET DR
- CanP 91307 529-C4
- LA 91304 529-D4
WISDOM CT
3200 SIMI 93063 478-D6
WISHARD AV
600 SIMI 93065 497-J5
WISTERIA LN
900 SPLA 93060 473-J1
WISTERIA ST
2000 SIMI 93065 498-B2
WISTERIA WY
- VEN 93004 473-C7
WITHERSPOON DR
900 THO 91360 526-G2
WOLF CREEK CT
3300 SIMI 93063 479-A6
WOLFF RD
100 VeCo 93030 523-E7
500 VeCo 93033 523-E7
500 VeCo 93033 553-E1
WOLFF ST
100 OXN 93033 522-F7
WOLSEY CT
4500 WLKV 91361 557-C5
WOLVERINE ST
7000 VEN 93003 492-E5
WOLVERTON AV
1300 CMRL 93010 524-F1
1700 CMRL 93010 494-F7
WOLVERTON ST
9000 VEN 93004 492-H3
WOOD PL
1900 VEN 93003 492-A5
WOOD RD
- CMRL 93010 523-H3
400 VeCo 93010 523-H5
1000 VeCo 93012 523-H5
1100 VeCo 93012 553-H3
1100 VeCo 93033 523-H7
1100 VeCo 93033 553-H3
6400 VeCo 93033 583-G1
6800 VeCo 93041 583-G1
WOODBINE CT
3000 THO 91360 526-D3
WOODBLUFF CT
23600 THO 91362 527-A2
WOODBRIAR PL
30100 AGRH 91301 557-H4
WOODBRIDGE LN
- SIMI 93063 498-H1
WOODBROOK DR
29500 AGRH 91301 557-J4
WOODBURN AV
2000 THO 91361 557-A7
2600 WLKV 91361 557-A7
WOODBURY ST
5300 VEN 93003 492-B3
WOODCREEK CT
29000 AGRH 91301 558-A3
WOODCREEK RD
600 CMRL 93012 525-A1
1700 CMRL 93012 495-A7
N WOODCREEK RD
- CMRL 93012 495-A7
WOODCREST PL
6500 VeCo 91377 558-B2
WOODCUTTER LN
1900 THO 91320 525-J7
1900 THO 91320 526-A7
WOODED VISTA
24600 CanP 91307 529-C7

WOODFERN CIR
3100 THO 91360 526-H2
WOODFLOWER ST
- THO 91362 527-B2
WOODGATE CT
1000 CMRL 93010 524-C2
WOODGLADE LN
24500 CanP 91307 529-C5
WOODGLEN DR
4300 MRPK 93021 496-E3
5800 AGRH 91301 557-H4
WOODGLEN ST
1800 SIMI 93065 478-A7
WOODGREEN CT
2900 THO 91362 527-B2
WOODGROVE RD
800 FILM 93015 456-A5
WOODHALL AV
7600 LA 91304 529-F3
WOODHAVEN ST
3500 SIMI 93063 498-D1
N WOODHAVEN ST
2400 SIMI 93063 498-E1
WOODHILL DR
11200 MRPK 93021 496-B3
WOODLAKE AV
6100 WdHI 91367 529-G7
6400 CanP 91307 529-G5
7500 LA 91304 529-G2
WOODLAKE MNR
3900 MRPK 93021 496-F4
WOODLAND AV
700 VeCo 93023 451-B3
WOODLAND DR
1000 SPLA 93060 464-B3
WOODLAND RD
23600 SIMI 93065 497-G7
WOODLAND ST
1400 OXN 93035 552-E1
5900 VEN 93003 492-C2
6200 VeCo 93003 492-C2
WOODLAND GROVE CT
1300 THO 91362 527-E7
WOODLAND OAK PL
- THO 91320 555-F3
WOODLAND VIEW DR
6000 WdHI 91367 529-C7
WOODLANE CT
4100 THO 91362 527-C6
WOODLAWN DR
500 THO 91360 526-D7
WOODLET WY
- THO 91361 556-F2
WOODLEY AV
- THO 91362 527-C2
WOODLOCH LN
23600 SIMI 93065 497-A2
WOODLOW CT
1300 THO 91361 557-A6
WOOD OPAL WY
2400 OXN 93030 522-D3
WOODPECKER AV
2300 VEN 93003 492-E5
N WOOD RANCH PKWY
300 SIMI 93065 497-D5
S WOOD RANCH PKWY
- SIMI 93065 527-E1
200 SIMI 93065 497-E7
WOODRIDGE AV
1100 THO 91362 527-A6
WOODROW AV
2300 SIMI 93065 498-B1
2600 SIMI 93065 478-C7
WOODROW CT
2600 SIMI 93065 498-B1
WOODSCENT LN
23600 SIMI 93065 497-A2
WOODSIDE DR
1600 THO 91362 526-J3
WOODSIDE PL
1100 OXN 93036 522-F1
WOODSTEAD WY
100 SIMI 93065 497-F3
WOODSTOCK LN
900 VEN 93001 491-E4
WOODSTONE CT
3100 THO 91360 526-C2
WOODSTONE PL
7100 CanP 91307 529-C5
WOODVALE CT
7000 CanP 91307 529-F5
WOODVIEW CT
3200 THO 91362 527-C3
WOODWIND CT
2000 SIMI 93063 498-J2
WOODWORTH AV
- THO 91362 527-C2
WOOLEY RD
100 OXN 93030 522-C7
100 OXN 93033 522-C7
1000 OXN 93035 521-J7
1600 OXN 93035 522-C7
1800 VeCo 93030 522-C7
1800 VeCo 93030 523-A7
1800 VeCo 93033 522-C7
1800 VeCo 93033 523-A7
3800 VeCo 93035 522-A7
E WOOLEY RD
- OXN 93030 522-H7
- OXN 93033 522-G7
WOOLSEY CANYON RD
23700 LA 91304 499-D7
23900 WHil 91304 499-D7
24900 VeCo 93063 499-B7
WOOSTER ST
4300 VEN 93003 491-J2
4300 VEN 93003 492-A2
WORDSWORTH CT
2600 THO 91362 527-B3
WORDSWORTH WY
6500 VEN 93003 492-D3
WORKMAN AV
2100 SIMI 93063 498-G2
WORMWOOD ST
- VeCo 93023 451-B4
WORTH WY
5200 CMRL 93012 495-A7
5200 VeCo 93012 495-B5
N WRANGLER LN
- VeCo 91307 529-B3
WRANGLER RD
- SIMI 93065 497-J7
WREN CT
6900 VEN 93003 492-E4
WRIGHT RD
200 VeCo 93036 522-H1
2500 VeCo 93066 493-F6
3200 VeCo 93010 493-F6
WYANDOTTE ST
22000 CanP 91303 529-J5

WYANDOTTE ST
22700 CanP 91307 529-G5
WYCHOFF AV
1600 SIMI 93063 499-A3
WYETH LN
500 VEN 93003 492-D1
WYNN CT
300 THO 91362 557-A1
WYNNEFIELD AV
1300 THO 91362 527-C6
WYSTERIA DR
6100 VeCo 93063 499-B4

X

XANADU WY
- OXN 93036 492-H5
300 SIMI 93065 527-D1
XAVIER AV
100 VEN 93003 492-B2

Y

YACHT WY
- OXN 93035 522-D7
YAGER WY
3300 WLKV 91361 557-B7
YALE AV
100 VEN 93003 492-B3
N YALE AV
6400 MRPK 93021 476-H6
YALE CT
100 SPLA 93060 464-A6
400 OXN 93036 522-H2
YALE PL
500 OXN 93033 552-H4
YALE ST
200 SPLA 93060 464-A6
1100 OXN 93033 552-J4
YANA CT
5900 SIMI 93063 479-B7
YANKEE DR
4000 AGRH 91301 558-E7
YARDARM AV
2500 PHME 93041 552-B2
YARDLEY PL
3200 SIMI 93063 478-D6
YARNELL AV
3200 SIMI 93063 478-F6
YARNELL PL
800 OXN 93033 552-H1
YARNTON CT
23600 VeCo 91361 556-F6
YARROW DR
- SIMI 93065 527-E1
YEARLING CT
800 CMRL 93010 524-C2
YEARLING PL
2600 OXN 93036 492-F7
2600 OXN 93036 522-F1
YEATS LN
600 VEN 93003 492-D1
YELLOW HILL RD
12000 VeCo 90265 625-G1
YELLOWSTONE AV
200 THO 91320 556-D2
YELLOWSTONE DR
100 OXN 93033 553-C3
YELLOW THROAT PL
- THO 91320 525-J5
- THO 91320 526-A5
YELLOWWOOD DR
2600 WLKV 91361 557-A7
YERBA BUENA RD
8400 VeCo 90265 586-A3
9800 VeCo 90265 585-H4
12600 VeCo 90265 625-F2
YERBA SECA AV
6200 AGRH 91301 558-B3
YEW DR
2300 THO 91320 555-J1
YOKUTS CT
2700 SIMI 93063 479-A7
YOLANDA ST
1900 CMRL 93010 524-D2
YOLO ST
10600 VEN 93004 472-H7
YORBA LINDA PL
400 CMRL 93012 524-G3
YORK PL
1000 THO 91362 527-A7
YORK ST
1100 OXN 93033 552-J4
YORKFIELD CT
4400 WLKV 91361 557-D6
YORKSHIRE AV
800 THO 91360 526-G7
YOSEMITE
100 OXN 93033 553-C3
YOSEMITE AV
- SIMI 93063 478-J6
1500 SIMI 93063 499-A2
2600 SIMI 93063 479-A6
YOSEMITE CT
- VEN 93003 492-C2
YOSEMITE DR
100 OXN 93033 553-B5
YOUMANS DR
200 VEN 93003 492-B3
YOUNAN DR
- Chat 91311 479-H7
- Chat 91311 499-H1
YOUNG AV
1900 THO 91360 526-E4
YOUNG RD
2100 VeCo 93015 455-D5
YOUNG WOLF DR
- SIMI 93065 478-A5
YSRELLA AV
1500 SIMI 93065 498-A3
YUBA CT
8100 VEN 93004 492-F1
YUBA DR
2800 SIMI 93063 479-A7
YUCCA CT
3700 OXN 93033 552-H4
YUCCA DR
500 FILM 93015 455-J5
1800 VeCo 93012 495-J7
1800 VeCo 93012 525-J1
YUCCA LN
- THO 91362 557-A3
YUCCA ST
- OXN 93033 552-H4
800 PHME 93041 552-H4
W YUCCA ST
100 OXN 93033 552-G3
YUCCA WY
2300 VeCo 93012 495-J7

YUKON AV
4200 SIMI 93063
YUKON TR
8400 LA 91304
YUKONITE PL
1000 OXN 93030
YUMA CT
2400 VEN 93001
YUMA ST
4100 SIMI 93063
YUROK CT
2800 SIMI 93063

Z

ZACHARY ST
300 MRPK 93021
ZAHARIAS CT
- MRPK 93021
ZALTANA ST
22500 Chat 91311
N ZANJA LN
- VeCo 91307
ZAPATA CT
2800 SIMI 93063
ZELDA WY
9200 Chat 91311
ZELZAH AV
6800 VeCo 93001
ZENITH AV
3600 THO 91360
ZENO DR
400 VeCo 91377
ZEPHYR CT
2300 VEN 93001
ZIEGLER DR
- SIMI 93063
ZIMMAN LN
2600 SIMI 93063
2600 SIMI 93063
ZINNIA CT
600 THO 91360
ZINNIA WY
- VEN 93004
ZION AV
400 OXN 93033
ZION WY
1300 VEN 93003
ZIRCON AV
1600 OXN 93030
ZIRON AV
- SIMI 93065
ZOCALO CIR
4400 THO 91360
ZOLA AV
500 VEN 93003
ZUNI CT
2400 VEN 93001
ZUNIGA RIDGE PL
1700 THO 91362

#

1ST AV
- PHME 93043
1ST ST
- MRPK 93021
100 SIMI 93065
200 THO 91320
300 FILM 93015
700 FILM 93015
E 1ST ST
200 OXN 93030
W 1ST ST
100 OXN 93030
2ND ST
- MRPK 93021
100 FILM 93015
100 PHME 93041
200 THO 91320
700 FILM 93015
1400 SIMI 93065
E 2ND ST
200 OXN 93030
W 2ND ST
100 OXN 93030
3RD ST
- VeCo 93042
- MRPK 93021
100 FILM 93015
100 OXN 93030
100 PHME 93041
200 THO 91320
700 FILM 93015
1400 SIMI 93065
23600 VeCo 93063
E 3RD ST
100 OXN 93030
W 3RD ST
100 OXN 93030
4TH AV
- PHME 93043
4TH PL
400 PHME 93041
4TH ST
- VeCo 93042
- FILM 93015
- OXN 93030
600 FILM 93015
1000 SIMI 93065
N 4TH ST
100 SPLA 93060
S 4TH ST
100 SPLA 93060
5TH PL
1000 PHME 93041
5TH ST
- VeCo 93042
100 PHME 93041
700 FILM 93015
1600 SIMI 93065
1700 VeCo 93015
5TH ST Rt#-34
100 OXN 93030
1800 VeCo 93030
1800 VeCo 93030
1800 OXN 93030
2600 OXN 93033
2600 VeCo 93033
E 5TH ST Rt#-34
- VeCo 93012
- VeCo 93012
N 5TH ST
200 SPLA 93060
S 5TH ST
300 SPLA 93060
W 5TH ST
100 OXN 93030
3800 OXN 93030
3800 OXN 93035

City ZIP Pg-Grid
T
VeCo 93030 522-A6
PHME 93041 552-F4
VeCo 93042 583-G2
OXN 93030 522-F6
FILM 93015 455-J4
FILM 93015 456-A4
VeCo 93015 456-A4
PHME 93041 552-F4
T
OXN 93030 522-G6
T
SPLA 93060 464-A5
PHME 93041 552-F4
VeCo 93042 583-F2
OXN 93030 522-F6
FILM 93015 455-J4
FILM 93015 456-A4
PHME 93041 552-F4
OXN 93035 522-E6
VeCo 93015 455-F6
T
SPLA 93060 464-B5
T
SPLA 93060 464-B6
PHME 93043 552-D2
PHME 93041 552-F3
PHME 93041 552-F4
OXN 93035 522-E6
VeCo 93042 583-G3
OXN 93030 522-G7
PHME 93041 552-F4
VEN 93003 492-C5
VeCo 93003 492-C5
T
SPLA 93060 464-B5
T
SPLA 93060 464-B6
NW
VeCo 93023 451-C2
VeCo 93042 583-G2
OXN 93030 522-G7
SPLA 93060 464-B5
OXN 93035 522-E7
V
PHME 93043 552-D3
T
VeCo 93042 583-F3
VeCo 93063 498-G7
VeCo 93063 528-G1
ST
SPLA 93060 464-B4
ST Rt#-150
SPLA 93060 464-B5
ST Rt#-150
SPLA 93060 464-C6
V
PHME 93043 552-D3
T
VeCo 93042 583-F3
VeCo 93041 583-F3
VeCo 93063 528-G1
ST
SPLA 93060 464-C5
ST
SPLA 93060 464-C5
T
VeCo 93042 583-G4
VeCo 93063 528-G1
ST
SPLA 93060 464-C4
ST
SPLA 93060 464-C5
T
VeCo 93042 583-F4
ST
SPLA 93060 464-C4
ST
SPLA 93060 464-C5
T
VeCo 93042 583-E3
SPLA 93060 464-C4
V
PHME 93043 552-E3
T
VeCo 93042 583-E4
EPTIEMBRE
VEN 93004 492-J3
VEN 93004 493-A3
T
VeCo 93042 583-D4
T
VeCo 93042 583-D4
VeCo 93063 528-F1
T
VeCo 93042 583-D5
VeCo 93063 528-G1
V
PHME 93043 552-E3
T
VeCo 93042 583-E6
V
PHME 93043 552-E3
T
VeCo 93042 583-F6
VeCo 93063 528-F1
V
PHME 93043 552-D3
T
VeCo 93063 528-F1
V
PHME 93043 552-E3
T
VeCo 93063 528-F1
V
PHME 93043 552-E3
V
PHME 93043 552-E3
V
PHME 93043 552-D3
V
PHME 93043 552-E4
AV
PHME 93041 552-D4
PHME 93043 552-C4
AV
PHME 93041 552-E4
V
PHME 93041 552-D4
V
PHME 93043 552-D4

STREET Block City ZIP Pg-Grid

36TH AV
- PHME 93041 552-E4

41ST ST
- PHME 93041 552-E5
- PHME 93043 552-E5

NW 144TH ST
400 OJAI 93023 451-G1

NW 171ST ST
1300 VeCo 93023 451-D2

N 188TH ST
700 OJAI 93023 451-H1

N 201ST ST
2000 VeCo 93023 451-C3

Rt#-N1 LAS VIRGENES RD
3700 CALB 91302 558-H7
4800 LACo 91302 558-H7

Rt#-N9 KANAN RD
4100 Ago 91301 558-A7
4100 AGRH 91301 558-A7

Rt#-1 OLD RINCON HWY
2900 VeCo 93001 470-F6
4200 VeCo 93001 366-G9
4200 VeCo 93001 459-F7
4200 VeCo 93001 469-H1
23600 VeCo 93001 490-G1

Rt#-1 OXNARD BLVD
- OXN 93033 553-A2
- VeCo 93033 553-B3
100 OXN 93030 522-G7
1200 OXN 93030 552-H1
1200 OXN 93033 522-G7
1200 OXN 93033 552-H1
1500 OXN 93036 522-G1
19200 OXN 93036 492-G7

Rt#-1 PACIFIC COAST FRWY
- OXN - 553-C4
- VeCo - 553-C4
- VeCo - 583-H1

Rt#-1 PACIFIC COAST HWY
2900 VeCo 93001 470-B3
4200 VeCo 93001 366-G9
4200 VeCo 93001 459-F6
4200 VeCo 93001 469-H1
9000 VeCo 90265 387-F4
9000 VeCo 90265 625-A3
9400 VeCo - 584-A6
12300 LACo 90265 625-F5
19900 VeCo 93033 583-J5
19900 VeCo 93033 584-A6
23600 VeCo 93001 490-G1
34100 MAL 90265 625-F5

Rt#-23 A ST
- FILM 93015 456-A6
- FILM 93015 466-A1

Rt#-23 BELLEVUE AV
700 VeCo 93015 465-J3
700 VeCo 93015 466-A3

Rt#-23 BROADWAY
14900 VeCo 93021 476-D4

Rt#-23 CHAMBERSBURG RD
300 FILM 93015 466-A2
300 VeCo 93015 466-A2

Rt#-23 DECKER CANYON RD
1400 LACo 90265 586-F7

Rt#-23 FRWY
- MRPK - 496-G1
- THO - 496-J7
- THO - 497-A7
- THO - 526-J1
- THO - 556-H1
- VeCo - 496-H3
- VeCo - 497-A4

Rt#-23 GRIMES CANYON RD
1300 VeCo 93015 465-J4
4800 VeCo 93015 466-A5
4800 VeCo 93021 466-A5
8000 VeCo 93021 476-B2

Rt#-23 MOORPARK AV
- MRPK 93021 476-E7
500 MRPK 93021 496-E1

Rt#-23 N MOORPARK AV
- MRPK 93021 496-E1

Rt#-23 MULHOLLAND HWY
33000 LACo 90265 586-G6

Rt#-23 WALNUT CANYON RD
800 MRPK 93021 476-E7
1100 VeCo 93021 476-E4

Rt#-23 WESTLAKE BLVD
100 LACo 90265 586-H4
400 WLKV 90265 586-H4
400 WLKV 91361 586-H4
800 LACo 91361 586-H4
800 THO 91361 586-H4

Rt#-23 S WESTLAKE BLVD
100 THO 91362 557-C4
100 THO 91361 557-C4
600 THO 91361 556-J7
800 THO 91361 586-H1

Rt#-27 TOPANGA CANYON BLVD
9500 Chat 91311 499-J6

Rt#-33 HIGHWAY
- VeCo 93023 366-J6
- VeCo 93252 366-G1

Rt#-33 MARICOPA HWY
1000 OJAI 93023 441-E6
1000 OJAI 93023 451-F1
1700 VeCo 93023 441-B2
10000 VeCo 93023 366-J6

Rt#-33 OJAI FRWY
- VeCo - 461-B6
- VeCo - 471-C3
- VEN - 471-B7
- VEN - 491-A1

Rt#-33 VENTURA AV
- VeCo 93022 451-B5
4400 VeCo 93001 461-A2
4400 VeCo 93022 461-A2
11200 VeCo 93023 451-D2
11800 OJAI 93023 451-F1

Rt#-34 5TH ST
100 OXN 93030 522-H6
1800 VeCo 93030 522-H6
1800 VeCo 93030 523-A6
1800 OXN 93030 523-A6
2600 OXN 93033 523-A6
2600 VeCo 93033 523-D6

Rt#-34 E 5TH ST
- VeCo 93012 523-H6
- VeCo 93012 524-C6

Rt#-34 N LEWIS RD
- CMRL 93010 524-G2
1700 CMRL 93010 494-H7

Rt#-34 S LEWIS RD
- CMRL 93010 524-F4
200 CMRL 93012 524-F4

Rt#-34 PLEASANT VALLEY RD
2200 VeCo 93012 524-F5
2200 CMRL 93012 524-F5

Rt#-34 SOMIS RD
2400 CMRL 93010 494-J6
2400 VeCo 93010 494-J6
2400 VeCo 93066 494-J6
2600 VeCo 93066 495-A5

Rt#-118 LOS ANGELES AV
- MRPK 93021 496-F1
900 VeCo 93066 493-H4
900 VeCo 93066 494-A4
1200 VeCo 93004 493-B2
2000 VeCo 93036 493-B2
4500 VeCo 93066 495-A4
8000 VeCo 93021 495-H3
10700 VeCo 93021 496-A2

Rt#-118 RONALD REAGAN FRWY
- Chat - 499-E2
- MRPK - 476-H7
- MRPK - 477-B6
- MRPK - 496-G1
- SIMI - 477-B6
- SIMI - 497-G1
- SIMI - 498-F1
- SIMI - 499-E2
- VeCo - 477-B6

Rt#-118 S WELLS RD
300 VEN 93004 472-J7
700 VEN 93004 473-A7
800 VEN 93004 493-A1
900 VeCo 93004 493-A1

Rt#-126 HENRY MAYO DR
31100 Cstc 91384 458-H5
31800 VeCo 93040 458-H5

Rt#-126 KOREAN WAR VET MEM HY
2500 VeCo 93015 455-E7
2700 VeCo 93015 465-B2
17900 VeCo 93060 464-F3
18400 SPLA 93060 464-F3
20100 VeCo 93060 465-B2

Rt#-126 OLD TELEGRAPH RD
2500 VeCo 93015 455-E7
2700 VeCo 93015 465-E1

Rt#-126 SANTA PAULA FRWY
- SPLA - 463-J7
- SPLA - 464-D5
- SPLA - 473-F4
- VeCo - 473-B6
- VeCo - 492-D3
- VEN - 472-J7
- VEN - 473-B6
- VEN - 491-J4
- VEN - 492-D3

Rt#-126 TELEGRAPH RD
- FILM 93015 456-E6
- VeCo 93015 456-E6
900 VeCo 93015 457-E5
1400 VeCo 93040 457-G4
2200 VeCo 93040 458-B5
2700 VeCo 93015 465-C1
17900 VeCo 93060 464-F3
18400 SPLA 93060 464-F3
20100 VeCo 93060 465-A2

Rt#-126 E TELEGRAPH RD
100 FILM 93015 456-C6
300 VeCo 93015 456-C6

Rt#-126 VENTURA ST
100 FILM 93015 456-A6
400 FILM 93015 455-F7
800 VeCo 93015 455-F7

Rt#-126 E VENTURA ST
- FILM 93015 456-B6

Rt#-150 N 10TH ST
100 SPLA 93060 464-B5

Rt#-150 S 10TH ST
100 SPLA 93060 464-C6

Rt#-150 BALDWIN RD
- VeCo 93001 450-H3
- VeCo 93023 450-H3
600 VeCo 93023 451-A3

Rt#-150 CASITAS PASS RD
2000 VeCo 93001 450-D5
3500 VeCo 93001 460-B1
4000 VeCo 93001 366-G8
4000 VeCo 93001 459-G1
7100 StBC 93013 459-G1

Rt#-150 E OJAI AV
200 OJAI 93023 441-H7
1100 OJAI 93023 442-B7
1600 VeCo 93023 442-B7

Rt#-150 N OJAI RD
100 SPLA 93060 464-B3
300 VeCo 93060 464-B3

Rt#-150 W OJAI AV
100 OJAI 93023 441-G7
1000 OJAI 93023 451-G1

Rt#-150 OJAI SANTA PAULA RD
3100 VeCo 93023 442-D7
7000 VeCo 93023 452-E1
11900 VeCo 93023 453-A1

Rt#-150 RINCON RD
6600 StBC 93013 459-A1
23600 VeCo 93001 366-G9
23600 VeCo 93001 459-A1

Rt#-150 SANTA PAULA OJAI RD
4300 VeCo 93060 464-A1
4400 VeCo 93060 454-A7
4600 VeCo 93060 453-H4
12400 VeCo 93023 453-H4

Rt#-192 CASITAS PASS RD
6800 StBC 93013 459-A1

Rt#-232 E VINEYARD AV
500 OXN 93036 522-G2
2600 VeCo 93036 522-G2
2800 OXN 93036 492-H7
2800 VeCo 93036 492-H7
4100 VeCo 93036 493-A4
5100 VeCo 93066 493-A4

U.S.-101 EL CAMINO REAL
- VeCo - 366-E8
- VeCo - 459-C5
- VeCo - 469-H1
- VeCo - 470-E5
- VeCo - 490-H1
- VEN - 490-H1
- VEN - 491-G4

U.S.-101 VENTURA FRWY
- Ago - 558-D6
- AGRH - 557-G6
- AGRH - 558-D6
- CALB - 558-D6
- CMRL - 523-A3
- CMRL - 524-A3
- CMRL - 525-C5
- LACo - 558-D6
- OXN - 492-F7
- OXN - 522-H2
- OXN - 523-A3
- THO - 525-C5
- THO - 526-D7
- THO - 555-J1
- THO - 556-E1
- THO - 557-B4
- VeCo - 366-F9
- VeCo - 459-A3
- VeCo - 469-J1
- VeCo - 470-B3
- VeCo - 490-H1
- VeCo - 492-F7
- VeCo - 523-A3
- VeCo - 525-C5
- VEN - 490-H1
- VEN - 491-A2
- VEN - 492-F7
- WLKV - 557-B4

VENTURA COUNTY POINTS OF INTEREST

AIRPORTS

FEATURE NAME Address City, ZIP Code	PAGE-GRID
CAMARILLO, CMRL	523 - G4
HELIPORT, VEN	491 - F7
OXNARD, OXN	522 - D5
SANTA PAULA, SPLA	464 - B6

BEACHES, HARBORS & WATER REC

FEATURE NAME Address City, ZIP Code	PAGE-GRID
CARRILLO, LEO ST BCH, VeCo	625 - G5
CHANNEL ISLANDS BEACH PK, OXN	552 - B4
COUNTY LINE BEACH, VeCo	625 - E5
HOLLYWOOD BEACH, VeCo	552 - A4
WESTLAKE YACHT CLUB, WLKV	557 - C7
MANDALAY STATE BEACH, OXN	521 - G4
MARINA COVE BEACH, VEN	491 - F7
MCGRATH STATE BEACH, OXN	521 - G2
MUSSEL SHOAL BEACH, VeCo	459 - D6
NICHOLAS CANYON CO BEACH, MAL	625 - J6
OIL PIERS BEACH, VeCo	459 - E6
OXNARD BEACH PK, OXN	551 - J1
SAN BUENAVENTURA STATE BEACH, VEN	491 - D3
SILVER STRAND BEACH, VeCo	552 - C6
VENTURA YACHT CLUB, VEN	491 - F7
WOOD, EMMA STATE BEACH, VeCo	470 - G7

BUILDINGS

FEATURE NAME Address City, ZIP Code	PAGE-GRID
FOR DOWNTOWN BLDGS SEE PAGE F	-
ASSOC FOR RETARDED CITIZENS-VENTURA-CO 1183 CL SUERTE, CMRL, 93012	524 - H1
BOY SCOUTS COUNTY HEADQUARTERS 509 E DAILY DR, CMRL, 93010	524 - B3

BUILDINGS - GOVERNMENTAL

FEATURE NAME Address City, ZIP Code	PAGE-GRID
AGOURA HILLS CITY HALL 30001 LADYFACE CT, AGRH, 91301	557 - H6
BRANDEIS-BARDIN INSTITUTE 1101 PEPPERTREE LN, VeCo, 93064	498 - F4
CALABASAS CITY HALL 26135 MUREAU RD, CALB, 91302	558 - H5
CAMARILLO CITY HALL 601 CARMEN DR, CMRL, 93010	524 - D2
COUNTY ADMIN BLDG 800 S VICTORIA AV, VEN, 93009	492 - C3
CRIMINAL JUSTICE COMPLEX 800 S VICTORIA AV, VEN, 93009	492 - C3
EAST COUNTY COURTHOUSE 3855 ALAMO ST, SIMI, 93063	478 - E7
FILLMORE CITY HALL 250 CENTRAL AV, FILM, 93015	456 - A6
JUVENILE COURTHOUSE 4353 E VINEYARD AV, VeCo, 93036	492 - J5
MOORPARK CITY HALL 799 MOORPARK AV, MRPK, 93021	476 - E7
OJAI CITY HALL 401 S VENTURA ST, OJAI, 93023	441 - H7
OXNARD CITY HALL 300 W 3RD ST, OXN, 93030	522 - G6
PORT HUENEME CITY HALL 250 N VENTURA RD, PHME, 93041	552 - E6
SANTA PAULA CITY HALL 970 VENTURA ST, SPLA, 93060	464 - C6
SIMI VALLEY CITY HALL 2929 TAPO CANYON RD, SIMI, 93063	478 - F7
THOUSAND OAKS CITY HALL 2100 E THOUSAND OAKS BLVD, THO, 91362	556 - J2
VENTURA CITY HALL 501 POLI ST, VEN, 93001	491 - C1
VENTURA COUNTY COURTHOUSE 800 S VICTORIA AV, VEN, 93009	492 - C3
VENTURA COUNTY HONOR FARM 370 BALDWIN RD, VeCo, 93023	451 - B3
VENTURA COUNTY JAIL 600 TODD RD, VeCo, 93060	473 - F5
VENTURA CALIFORNIA YOUTH AUTHORITY 3100 WRIGHT RD, VeCo, 93010	493 - F7
WESTLAKE VILLAGE CITY HALL 31200 OAK CREST DR, WLKV, 91361	557 - F6

CEMETERIES

FEATURE NAME Address City, ZIP Code	PAGE-GRID
ASSUMPTION CEM, SIMI	497 - H4
BARDSDALE CEM, VeCo	465 - G4
CONEJO MTN MEM PK, VeCo	554 - J1
F & AM CEM, OXN	553 - B4
IVY LAWN CEM, VEN	492 - C6
JAPANESE CEM, OXN	553 - A4
MOUNT SINAI MEM PK, SIMI	479 - B7
NORDHOFF CEM, OJAI	441 - F7
OAKWOOD MEM PK, Chat	499 - H5
PIRU CEM, VeCo	457 - D4
SANTA CLARA CEM, OXN	522 - F2
SANTA PAULA CEM, SPLA	463 - J5
SIMI CEM, SIMI	497 - J3
VALLEY OAKS MEM PK, WLKV	557 - F5

COLLEGES & UNIVERSITIES

FEATURE NAME Address City, ZIP Code	PAGE-GRID
AQUINAS, THOMAS COLLEGE 10000 N SANTA PAULA OJAI RD, VeCo, 93060	453 - H2
CALIFORNIA LUTHERAN UNIV 60 W OLSEN RD, THO, 91360	526 - E2
CSU CHANNEL ISLANDS 1 UNIVERSITY DR, VeCo, 93012	554 - E3
ITT TECHNICAL INSTITUTE 2051 SOLAR DR, OXN, 93036	523 - B3
MOORPARK COLLEGE 7075 CAMPUS RD, MRPK, 93021	476 - J6
OXNARD COLLEGE 4000 ROSE AV, OXN, 93033	552 - J3
SAINT JOHNS SEMINARY COLLEGE 5012 SEMINARY RD, CMRL, 93012	494 - J7
VENTURA COLLEGE 4667 TELEGRAPH RD, VEN, 93003	491 - J2
VENTURA COLLEGE EAST CAMPUS 115 DEAN DR, SPLA, 93060	464 - A6

ENTERTAINMENT & SPORTS

FEATURE NAME Address City, ZIP Code	PAGE-GRID
CAMARILLO SKATEPARK 1030 TEMPLE AV, CMRL, 93010	524 - F1
CIVIC ARTS PLAZA 2100 E THOUSAND OAKS BLVD, THO, 91362	556 - J2
KAVLI, FRED THEATRE FOR THE PERF ARTS 2100 E THOUSAND OAKS BLVD, THO, 91362	556 - J2
NEWBURY PARK SKATEPARK 190 N REINO RD, THO, 91320	555 - F1
OJAI SKATEPARK 414 E OJAI AV, OJAI, 93023	441 - H7
OXNARD SKATEPARK 3250 S ROSE AV, OXN, 93033	552 - J3
PERF ARTS & CONV CTR 800 HOBSON WY, OXN, 93030	522 - F7
SANTA PAULA SKATEPARK S 10TH ST & VENTURA ST, SPLA, 93060	464 - C6
SEASIDE PARK & VENTURA CO FAIRGROUND 610 W HARBOR BLVD, VEN, 93001	491 - B2
SIMI VALLEY CULTURAL ARTS CTR 3050 LOS ANGELES AV, SIMI, 93065	498 - C2
SKATELAB SKATEPARK 4226 VALLEY FAIR ST, SIMI, 93063	498 - F2

GOLF COURSES

FEATURE NAME Address City, ZIP Code	PAGE-GRID
BUENAVENTURA GC, VEN	492 - C7
CAMARILLO SPRINGS GC, CMRL	525 - A5
CLARK, JOHN E GC, VeCo	583 - G2
ELKINS RANCH GC, VeCo	466 - A3
LAKE LINDERO CC, AGRH	557 - G4
LAS POSAS CC, VeCo	493 - J6
LOS ROBLES GREENS GC, THO	556 - D1
LOST CANYONS GC, SIMI	478 - D3
MALIBU CC, LACo	586 - J6
MOORPARK CC, MRPK	476 - C5
MOUNTAIN VIEW GC, VeCo	474 - B1
NORTH RANCH CC, THO	527 - D7
OJAI VALLEY INN AND SPA, OJAI	441 - G7
OLIVAS PK GC, VEN	491 - H7
RIVER RIDGE GC, OXN	522 - D1
RUSTIC CANYON GC, VeCo	476 - G4
SATICOY CC, VeCo	493 - F3
SATICOY REGL GC, VEN	492 - J1
SEABEE GC, PHME	552 - D2
SHERWOOD CC, VeCo	556 - F7
SHERWOOD CC, VeCo	586 - E1
SIMI HILLS GC, SIMI	478 - H6
SINALOA GC, SIMI	497 - F4
SOULE PK GC, OJAI	442 - A7
SPANISH HILLS GOLF & CC, CMRL	523 - H1
STERLING HILLS GC, CMRL	493 - H6
SUNSET HILLS CC, THO	496 - J7
TIERRA REJADA GC, VeCo	496 - J2
WESTLAKE VILLAGE GC, THO	557 - D5
WOOD RANCH GC, SIMI	497 - D6

HISTORIC SITES

FEATURE NAME Address City, ZIP Code	PAGE-GRID
CAMARILLO RANCH 201 CAMARILLO RANCH RD, CMRL, 93012	524 - H3
FATHER SERRA CROSS GRANT PARK, VEN, 93001	491 - B1
MISSION SAN BUENAVENTURA 211 E MAIN ST, VEN, 93001	491 - B1
OLIVAS ADOBE 4200 OLIVAS PARK DR, VEN, 93001	491 - J7
ORTEGA ADOBE 215 W MAIN ST, VEN, 93001	491 - B2
REYES ADOBE HIST SITE 5464 REYES ADOBE RD, AGRH, 91301	557 - H5
SANTA SUSANA PASS STATE HIST PK DEVONSHIRE ST, Chat, 91311	499 - G3
STAGECOACH INN MUS 51 S VENTU PARK RD, THO, 91320	556 - B2
STRATHEARN, ROBERT P HIST PK & MUS 137 STRATHEARN PL, SIMI, 93065	497 - E2
VENTURA COUNTY COURTHOUSE 501 POLI ST, VEN, 93001	491 - C1

HOSPITALS

FEATURE NAME Address City, ZIP Code	PAGE-GRID
COMMUNITY MEM HOSP 147 N BRENT ST, VEN, 93003	491 - G2
LOS ROBLES REGL MED CTR 215 W JANSS RD, THO, 91360	526 - E4
OJAI VALLEY COMM HOSP 1306 MARICOPA HWY, OJAI, 93023	441 - F7
SAINT JOHNS PLEASANT VALLEY HOSP 2309 ANTONIO AV, CMRL, 93010	494 - G7
SAINT JOHNS REGL MED CTR 1600 N ROSE AV, OXN, 93030	523 - A3
SANTA PAULA HOSP 825 N 10TH ST, SPLA, 93060	464 - B4
SIMI VALLEY HOSP & HEALTH CARE SERV 2975 SYCAMORE DR, SIMI, 93065	478 - B7
VENTURA COUNTY MED CTR 3291 LOMA VISTA RD, VEN, 93003	491 - H2
WEST HILLS HOSP & MED CTR 7300 MEDICAL CENTER DR, CanP, 91307	529 - G4

HOTELS

FEATURE NAME Address City, ZIP Code	PAGE-GRID
CASA SIRENA MARINA RESORT 3605 PENINSULA RD, OXN, 93035	552 - B3
CLOCKTOWER INN, THE 181 E SANTA CLARA ST, VEN, 93001	491 - B2
COUNTRY INN & SUITES BY CARLSON 298 CHESTNUT ST, VEN, 93001	491 - C1
COUNTRY INN AT PORT HUENEME 350 E PORT HUENEME RD, PHME, 93041	552 - E6
COURTYARD BY MARRIOTT 600 ESPLANADE DR, OXN, 93036	522 - H2
COURTYARD MARRIOTT 4994 VERDUGO WY, CMRL, 93012	524 - J3
CROWNE PLAZA VENTURA BEACH 450 E HARBOR BLVD, VEN, 93001	491 - C2
EMBASSY SUITES MANDALAY BEACH RESORT 2101 MANDALAY BEACH RD, OXN, 93035	552 - A2
FOUR POINTS VEN HARBORTOWN BY-SHERATON 1050 SCHOONER DR, VEN, 93001	491 - G6
GRAND VISTA HOTEL 999 ENCHANTED WY, SIMI, 93065	497 - G1
HAMPTON INN 30255 AGOURA RD, AGRH, 91301	557 - G6
HOLIDAY INN SIMI VALLEY 2550 ERRINGER RD, SIMI, 93065	498 - A1
HYATT WESTLAKE PLAZA 880 S WESTLAKE BLVD, THO, 91361	557 - C4
LA QUINTA INN 5818 VALENTINE RD, VEN, 93003	492 - C6
LA QUINTA INN & SUITES 1320 NEWBURY RD, THO, 91320	556 - B1
MARRIOTT VENTURA BEACH 2055 E HARBOR BLVD, VEN, 93001	491 - E3
OJAI VALLEY INN 905 COUNTRY CLUB RD, OJAI, 93023	451 - G1
PALM GARDEN HOTEL 495 N VENTU PARK RD, THO, 91320	556 - A1
POSADA ROYALE HOTEL 1775 MADERA RD, SIMI, 93065	497 - E3
RENAISSANCE AGOURA HILLS HOTEL 30100 AGOURA RD, AGRH, 91301	557 - H6
RESIDENCE INN BY MARRIOTT 2101 W VINEYARD AV, OXN, 93036	522 - E1

LAW ENFORCEMENT

FEATURE NAME Address City, ZIP Code	PAGE-GRID
CALIFORNIA HIGHWAY PATROL-VENTURA 4656 VALENTINE RD, VEN, 93003	492 - A4
CAMARILLO POLICE STA 3701 LAS POSAS RD, CMRL, 93010	494 - G7
FILLMORE POLICE STA 524 SESPE AV, FILM, 93015	456 - A6
MALIBU/LOST HILLS POLICE STA 27050 AGOURA RD, CALB, 91301	558 - F7
MOORPARK POLICE DEPARTMENT 610 SPRING RD, MRPK, 93021	
OJAI POLICE DEPARTMENT 402 S VENTURA ST, OJAI, 93023	
OXNARD POLICE DEPARTMENT 251 C ST, OXN, 93030	5
PORT HUENEME POLICE DEPARTMENT 250 N VENTURA RD, PHME, 93041	
SANTA PAULA POLICE DEPARTMENT 214 S 10TH ST, SPLA, 93060	
SHERIFFS STA 2101 OLSEN RD, THO, 91360	
SIMI VALLEY POLICE STA 3901 ALAMO ST, SIMI, 93063	
VENTURA POLICE STA 1425 DOWELL DR, VEN, 93003	

LIBRARIES

FEATURE NAME Address City, ZIP Code	PAGE-GRID
AGOURA HILLS 29901 LADYFACE CT, AGRH, 91301	5
AVENUE 606 N VENTURA AV, VEN, 93001	4
BLANCHARD 119 N 8TH ST, SPLA, 93060	4
CAMARILLO 3100 PONDEROSA DR, CMRL, 93010	5
CAMARILLO 4101 LAS POSAS RD, CMRL, 93010	4
COLONIA CTR 1500 CM DL SOL, OXN, 93030	5
DOHENY, CARRIE ESTELLE MEM 5118 SEMINARY RD, CMRL, 93012	4
DOHENY, EDWARD LAURENCE MEM 5012 SEMINARY RD, CMRL, 93012	4
FILLMORE 502 2ND ST, FILM, 93015	4
FOSTER, E P 651 E MAIN ST, VEN, 93001	4
MEINERS OAKS 114 N PADRE JUAN AV, VeCo, 93023	4
MOORPARK 699 MOORPARK AV, MRPK, 93021	4
NEWBURY PARK 2331 BORCHARD RD, THO, 91320	5
OAK PARK 899 KANAN RD, VeCo, 91377	5
OAK VIEW 555 MAHONEY AV, VeCo, 93022	4
OJAI 111 E OJAI AV, OJAI, 93023	4
OXNARD 251 S A ST, OXN, 93030	5
PIRU 3811 CENTER ST, VeCo, 93040	4
PLATT BRANCH 23600 VICTORY BLVD, WdHl, 91367	5
PRUETER, RAY D 510 PARK AV, PHME, 93041	5
SATICOY 11426 VIOLETA ST, VeCo, 93004	4
SIMI VALLEY 2969 TAPO CANYON RD, SIMI, 93063	4
SOLIZ, ALBERT H 2820 JOURDAN ST, VeCo, 93036	5
SOUTH OXNARD 200 E BARD RD, OXN, 93033	5
THOUSAND OAKS 1401 E JANSS RD, THO, 91362	5
VENTURA CO MUS HIST RESEARCH 100 E MAIN ST, VEN, 93001	4
WESTLAKE VILLAGE 31220 OAK CREST DR, WLKV, 91361	5
WRIGHT, H P 57 DAY RD, VEN, 93003	4

MILITARY INSTALLATIONS

FEATURE NAME Address City, ZIP Code	PAGE-GRID
CALIFORNIA AIR NATL GUARD 4146 NAVAL AIR RD, VeCo, 93033	55
NATL GUARD ARMORY 1270 ARUNDELL AV, VEN, 93003	49
NAVAL BASE VENTURA COUNTY 311 MAIN RD, VeCo, 93033	58
US COAST GUARD STA 4201 VICTORIA AV, OXN, 93035	55
US NAVAL CONSTRUCTION BATTALION CTR N VENTURA RD & PLEASANT VLY RD, PHME, 93043	55

MUSEUMS

FEATURE NAME Address City, ZIP Code	PAGE-GRID
ALBINGER ARCHAEOLOGICAL MUS 113 E MAIN ST, VEN, 93001	49
CALIFORNIA OIL MUS 1001 E MAIN ST, SPLA, 93060	46
CARNEGIE ART MUS 424 S C ST, OXN, 93030	52
CBC SEABEE MUS CUTTING RD & DODSON ST, PHME, 93043	55
COMSTOCK, A J FIRE MUS FIGUEROA ST & E SANTA CLARA ST, VEN, 93001	49
FILLMORE HIST MUS 350 MAIN ST, FILM, 93015	45
GULL WINGS CHILDRENS MUS 418 W 4TH ST, OXN, 93030	52
MUSEUM OF VENTURA COUNTY 100 E MAIN ST, VEN, 93001	49
OJAI VALLEY HIST SOCIETY AND MUS 130 W OJAI AV, OJAI, 93023	44
SAN BUENAVENTURA MISSION MUS 225 E MAIN ST, VEN, 93001	49
SANTA MONICA MTNS NRA MUS 401 W HILLCREST DR, THO, 91360	52
STRATHEARN MUS 137 STRATHEARN PL, SIMI, 93065	49
VENTURA COUNTY MARITIME MUS 2731 S VICTORIA AV, OXN, 93035	55

OPEN SPACE

FEATURE NAME Address City, ZIP Code	PAGE-GRID
BELL CANYON OPEN SPACE, LA	52
CHATSWORTH RESERVOIR NATURE PRESERVE, LA	49
CONEJO OPEN SPACE, THO	52
MCCREA, JOEL WILDLIFE PRESERVE, THO	49
POINT MUGU GAME RESERVE, VeCo	58
POTRERO OPEN SPACE, THO	55
SANTA CLARA RIV ESTUARY NATURAL RESRV, - OXN	52
SESPE CONDOR PRESERVE, VeCo	36
VENTURA COUNTY GAME RESERVE, VeCo	58

OTHER

FEATURE NAME Address City, ZIP Code	PAGE-GRID
CABRILLO RACQUET CLUB 3945 N CLUBHOUSE DR, VeCo, 93066	493
CAMP BLOOMFIELD MULHOLLAND HWY, LACo, 90265	625
CHANNEL ISLANDS NATL PK HDQTRS 1901 SPINNAKER DR, VEN, 93001	491

NAME City, ZIP Code	PAGE-GRID
H INDIAN INTERPRETIVE CTR NG RANCH PKWY, THO, 91362	527 - D4
VALLEY BOTANIC GARDEN AINSBOROUGH RD, THO, 91360	526 - E6
CH RANCH ELLOW HILL RD, VeCo, 90265	625 - G1
USE E RD, PHME, 93043	552 - D6
HOT SPRINGS A RD S, VeCo, 93023	441 - A2
RONALD PRESIDENTIAL LIBRARY DENTIAL DR, VeCo, 93065	497 - C4
SH HATCHERY APH & FISH HATCHERY RD, VeCo, 93015	456 - D7
IDS EQUESTRIAN CTR LYNN RD, VeCo, 91320	555 - C5
GROVE EQUESTRIAN CTR IEL CT, THO, 91320	556 - C1

PARK & RIDE

NAME	PAGE-GRID
ATL GUARD, VEN	491 - J4
LO METROLINK, CMRL	524 - F3
N ST, SIMI	498 - D1
R, SIMI	498 - A1
& SPRING RD, MRPK	496 - E1
THO	526 - H5
RD (NW LOT), AGRH	558 - A5
RD (SE LOT), AGRH	558 - A6
RD (SW LOT), AGRH	558 - A6
SPLA	473 - J1
AS RD, CMRL	524 - B3
VO METROLINK, VEN	492 - D6
RK, MRPK	476 - J6
ALL, THE, THO	526 - E7
W COMM CTR, VeCo	451 - B6
AI	441 - J7
METROLINK, OXN	522 - G6
THE, OXN	523 - B3
T VALLEY RD, CMRL	524 - J4
CONEJO BLVD, THO	525 - J7
RD, THO	556 - H2
18, SIMI	498 - C1
ETER CLAVER, SIMI	499 - A1
LLEY, SIMI	498 - J1
LLEY METROLINK, SIMI	498 - H2
ANYON, SIMI	498 - F1

PARKS & RECREATION

NAME	PAGE-GRID
PK, CMRL	524 - G1
VICH, MICHAEL D REGL PK - LACo, -	479 - G3
RANCH PK, CMRL	524 - E1
PK, SIMI	497 - F2
SEQUIT, LACo	586 - D7
SIMI EQUESTRIAN CTR, SIMI	498 - E3
STOW PK, SIMI	499 - A3
VERDE PK, VEN	472 - A7
VISTA COMM PK, MRPK	496 - D2
LL LINEAR PK, VEN	491 - H4
OOD PK, SIMI	478 - B7
PK, THO	555 - F4
ICHARD BUBBLING SPRINGS PK, PHME	552 - F4
CA VISTA PK, VEN	492 - E4
, OXN	552 - G2
LINEAR PK, VEN	492 - H3
NYON PK, CanP	529 - C5
T, BERNIECE PK, WLKV	557 - D6
OOD PK, SIMI	498 - B2
K, THO	557 - A1
PK, SIMI	478 - B4
IEW PK, CMRL	525 - A2
AUNCH RAMP & PK, OXN	552 - B2
PK, PHME	552 - D2
ARD OAK PK, OXN	522 - H3
ARD PK, THO	555 - F1
MAE REC CTR, CanP	529 - E6
MAE PK, VeCo	558 - A2
L BAY LINEAR PK, VEN	492 - E6
LINEAR PK, VEN	471 - D6
NG SPRINGS LINEAR PK, PHME	552 - F6
LO PK, OXN	522 - D4
SAS PK LAND, CALB	558 - F7
UAS CREEK PK, CMRL	524 - H2
LLO GROVE PK, VeCo	525 - D5
REAL PK, VEN	491 - J3
OMFORT PK, VeCo	451 - G3
S CANYON PK, MRPK	476 - J5
S PK, MRPK	476 - H6
S PK, OXN	522 - F6
A PK, THO	496 - J7
N, MARION PK, VEN	492 - B4
N OAKS PK, WLKV	557 - F3
NITA PK, CMRL	524 - D4
LO, LEO STATE PK, LACo	625 - J4
PK, OXN	552 - G4
C LAKE STATE REC AREA, LACo	367 - F5
PEAK PK, LA	529 - D4
AL PK, FILM	456 - A6
NGER PK, SIMI	497 - H7
EL ISLANDS NATL PK, VeCo	386 - F6
EL VIEW PK, OXN	552 - B4
RRAL PK, VeCo	558 - A2
ER OAK PK, CMRL	494 - E7
PK, LA	529 - H2
WORTH OAKS PK, Chat	499 - G6
WORTH PK NORTH, Chat	499 - J3
BORO CANYON, VeCo	528 - D5
ASH PK, AGRH	558 - B5
ASH PK, SIMI	479 - B7
ASH PK, VEN	492 - G2
X RANCH, VeCo	585 - H3
GROVE PK, SIMI	498 - A2
SET MELBA PK, CanP	529 - F4
GE ESTATES PK, OXN	552 - J3
GE PK, OXN	552 - J3
GE VIEW PK, MRPK	477 - A6
IA PK, OXN	522 - H5
CTR PK, CMRL	524 - D2
CTR PK EAST, OXN	522 - F6
CTR PK WEST, OXN	522 - F6
O CANYONS PK, THO	525 - H3
O COMM PK, THO	526 - E6
O CREEK EQUESTRIAN PK, THO	526 - H5
O CREEK PK, THO	526 - H6
ELLY PK, OXN	522 - E2
ITUTION PK, CMRL	524 - C3
GANVILLE PK, SIMI	499 - E3
RY TRAIL PK, MRPK	496 - B4
Y OWNED LAND, Chat	499 - J2
Y SQUARE LINEAR PK, VEN	492 - C3
E HILLS PK, SIMI	497 - F6
VIEW PK, CMRL	524 - A2
SS PK, THO	555 - E3
PK, OJAI	441 - J5
AH VOLUNTEER PK, SIMI	498 - E3
ILL PK, VeCo	528 - A7
RIDGE PK, THO	555 - G4
ES PK, FILM	455 - J5

FEATURE NAME Address City, ZIP Code	PAGE-GRID
DEL SOL PK, OXN	522 - J5
DENNISON PK, VeCo	452 - E1
DEWAR PK, PHME	552 - E6
DIZDAR PK, CMRL	524 - E3
DOS CAMINOS PK, CMRL	494 - G7
DOS VIENTOS COMM PK, THO	555 - C2
DOS VIENTOS NEIGHBORHOOD PK, THO	555 - C4
DURLEY PK, OXN	552 - F1
EAGLE VIEW PK, VeCo	527 - H6
EASTWOOD MEM PK, OXN	522 - F4
EASTWOOD PK, VEN	491 - B2
EBELL PK, SPLA	464 - B6
EL ESCORPION PK, CanP	529 - C5
EL PARQUE DE LA PAZ, THO	557 - A2
ENCANTO PK, CMRL	525 - A3
ESTELLA PK, THO	556 - J1
EVENSTAR PK, THO	557 - A5
FARIA COUNTY PK, VeCo	469 - J3
FIORE, ALEX PLAYFIELD, THO	526 - J4
FOOTHILL PK, SIMI	499 - D2
FOOTHILL PK, CMRL	494 - D7
FOREST COVE PK, AGRH	557 - H5
FORT WILDWOOD PK, THO	526 - D3
FOSTER PK, VeCo	460 - J6
FOXFIELD PK, WLKV	557 - C7
FREEDOM PK, CMRL	523 - J5
FREMONT PK, OXN	522 - F4
FRONTIER PK, SIMI	498 - A3
GATES CANYON PK, LACo	558 - J3
GLEN WOOD PK, THO	526 - G6
GLENWOOD PK, MRPK	496 - C2
GRANT PK, VEN	471 - C7
GRAPE ARBOR PK, CALB	558 - G6
HAPPY CAMP CANYON REGL PK, VeCo	466 - H7
HARDING PK, SPLA	464 - D5
HERITAGE PK, CMRL	525 - B1
HERTEL LINEAR PK, VEN	492 - F3
HICKORY PK, THO	555 - E4
HOBERT PK, VEN	492 - G1
HOBSON COUNTY PK, VeCo	469 - G1
HUNGRY VALLEY STATE VEH REC AREA, LACo	367 - C1
HUNTSINGER, FRITZ YOUTH SPORTS, VEN	492 - J1
INDIAN SPRINGS PK, VeCo	557 - H1
JOHNSON CREEK PK, OXN	552 - H4
JUANAMARIA PK, VEN	492 - E1
KENNEY GROVE PK, VeCo	455 - F5
KIMBER PK, THO	555 - G2
KNAPP RANCH PK, CanP	529 - C7
KNOLL PK, THO	525 - F7
KNOLLS PK, VeCo	499 - B3
LA JANELLE PK, PHME	552 - C6
LAKE CACHUMA REC AREA, StBC	366 - A5
LAKE CASITAS REC AREA, VeCo	450 - E5
LANG RANCH PK, THO	527 - C3
LAS PIEDRAS PK, SPLA	464 - C4
LAS POSAS EQUESTRIAN PK, VeCo	494 - A7
LAS VIRGENES CANYON, VeCo	528 - F5
LATHROP PK, OXN	552 - H1
LAURELWOOD PK, CMRL	524 - E2
LAZY J RANCH PK, LA	529 - E3
LEMONWOOD PK, OXN	553 - A2
LIBBEY PK, OJAI	441 - H7
LINCOLN PK, SIMI	497 - H4
LINEAR PK, VEN	492 - J3
LINEAR PK, VEN	492 - H2
LINEAR PK, VEN	492 - E1
LOKKER, ELDRED PK, CMRL	494 - C7
LOS PADRES NATL FOREST, VeCo	441 - D2
LYNN OAKS PK, THO	556 - C2
LYON, HARRY PK, VEN	471 - C6
MAHOOD SENIOR CTR, WLA	387 - J4
MALIBU CREEK STATE PK, LACo	387 - E3
MARINA PK, VEN	491 - F5
MARINA WEST PK, OXN	552 - D1
MASONIC PK, FILM	456 - A6
MAYFAIR PK, SIMI	497 - J1
MEDEA CREEK PK, VeCo	528 - A7
MEM PK, VEN	491 - D2
MILLER PK, MRPK	496 - G2
MILL PK, SPLA	464 - B4
MISSION OAKS COMM PK, CMRL	525 - B1
MISSION PK, VEN	491 - B2
MISSION VERDE PK, CMRL	525 - A1
MONTALVO NEIGHBORHOOD PK, VEN	492 - D4
MONTE VISTA NATURE PK, MRPK	496 - G3
MORANDA, WALTER B PK, PHME	552 - F6
MORRISON PK, AGRH	557 - J4
MOUNTAIN MEADOWS PK, MRPK	496 - D3
NEPTUNE SQUARE PK, OXN	551 - J1
NEWBURY PK, THO	555 - J1
NORTHBANK LINEAR PK, VEN	492 - J4
NORTH RANCH PK, THO	527 - C6
NORTH RANCH PLAYFIELD, THO	557 - G1
OAKBROOK NEIGHBORHOOD PK, THO	526 - J3
OAKBROOK PK, THO	527 - B4
OAKBROOK REGL PK, THO	527 - E4
OAK CANYON COMM PK, VeCo	527 - J7
OAK PK, SIMI	477 - C7
OBREGON PK, SPLA	463 - J6
OCEAN AVENUE PK, VEN	491 - E2
OLD AGOURA PK, AGRH	558 - D5
OLD MEADOWS PK, THO	526 - J5
OLD WINDMILL PK, SIMI	497 - F7
ORCHARD PK, OXN	522 - G2
ORCUTT RANCH HORTICULTURAL CTR PK, LA	529 - F2
PALO COMADO CANYON, VeCo	527 - J5
PARK AT WESTPORT, OXN	522 - A7
PEACH HILL PK, MRPK	496 - E3
PENINSULA PK, OXN	552 - B3
PEPPER TREE PLAYFIELD, THO	525 - E7
PITTS RANCH PK, CMRL	524 - H1
PLAZA PK, VEN	491 - C2
PLAZA PK, OXN	522 - G6
PLEASANT VALLEY PK, CMRL	524 - F2
PLEASANT VALLEY PK, OXN	552 - H4
POINDEXTER PK, MRPK	496 - D1
POINT MUGU STATE PK, VeCo	554 - G7
PORT HUENEME BEACH PK, PHME	552 - E7
PROMENADE PK, VEN	491 - B2
QUITO PK, CMRL	495 - D7
RALSTON VILLAGE LINEAR PK, VEN	492 - C4
RANCHO CONEJO PLAY FIELD, THO	526 - B6
RANCHO MADERA COMM PK, SIMI	497 - D6
RANCHO SANTA SUSANA COMM PK, SIMI	498 - H2
RANCHO SIERRA VISTA / SATWIWA PK, VeCo	555 - F5
RANCHO SIMI COMM PK, SIMI	497 - J3
RANCHO SIMI REC AREA, SIMI	497 - F7
RANCHO SIMI REC AREA, VeCo	528 - B7
RANCHO TAPO COMM CTR & VETERANS, SIMI	478 - E7
RANCHO VENTURA LINEAR PK, VEN	492 - E4
REYES ADOBE PK, AGRH	557 - H5
REYNOLDS, BLANCHE PK, VEN	491 - G4
RIO LINDO PK, OXN	522 - H2
RIVERVIEW LINEAR PK, VEN	492 - G4
ROCKY PEAK PK, VeCo	479 - D4
ROCKY POINTE NATURAL PK, SIMI	499 - C3
ROSCOE-VALLEY CIRCLE PK, LA	529 - D3
ROTARY COMM PK, OJAI	441 - G7
RUSSELL PK, THO	557 - B2
RUSSELL RANCH PK, WLKV	557 - F5

FEATURE NAME Address City, ZIP Code	PAGE-GRID
SAGE RANCH PK, VeCo	499 - A6
SANTA SUSANA PK, VeCo	499 - C4
SARZOTTI PK, OJAI	441 - J6
SATICOY PK, VeCo	493 - B1
SCHREIBER, HOUGHTON PK, SIMI	478 - F6
SEA AIR PK, OXN	522 - D7
SEASIDE WILDERNESS PK, VEN	490 - J2
SEAVIEW PK, OXN	522 - C7
SEQUOIA PK, SIMI	498 - E2
SERRA, JUNIPERO PK, VEN	492 - H4
SHADOW RANCH PK, CanP	529 - H6
SHIELLS PK, FILM	455 - H5
SIERRA LINDA PK, OXN	522 - F2
SIMI HILLS NEIGHBORHOOD PK, SIMI	478 - H7
SOULE PK, OJAI	442 - A7
SOUTHBANK PK, OXN	522 - F1
SOUTH SHORE HILLS PK, THO	557 - A6
SOUTHWEST COMM PK, OXN	522 - D6
SOUTH WINDS PK, OXN	552 - G6
SPRING MEADOW PK, THO	526 - F2
SPRINGVILLE PK, CMRL	523 - H2
STAGECOACH INN PK, THO	556 - B1
STARGAZE PK, SIMI	497 - D2
STECKEL PK, VeCo	453 - J5
STRAUSS, PETER RANCH, Ago	387 - D3
SUBURBIA PK, THO	526 - E3
SUMAC PK, AGRH	558 - B4
SUNSET HILLS PK, THO	526 - J2
SYCAMORE CANYON PK, SIMI	527 - D1
SYCAMORE DRIVE COMM CTR, SIMI	498 - C3
SYCAMORE PK, SIMI	498 - B5
TAPO CANYON PK, VeCo	478 - F2
TAXCO TRAILS PK, LA	529 - F3
TEAGUE PK, SPLA	463 - J7
THILLE PK, VEN	492 - B4
THOMPSON PK, OXN	523 - A5
THOUSAND OAKS COMM PK, THO	526 - F3
THREE SPRINGS PK, WLKV	557 - B7
TIERRA REJADA PK, SIMI	497 - D1
TIERRA REJADA PK, MRPK	496 - C3
TOLAND PK, VeCo	454 - J7
TOPANGA STATE PK, PacP	387 - G3
TRAILSIDE PK, CMRL	525 - A2
TRIUNFO COMM PK, THO	556 - J4
VALLE LINDO PK, CMRL	524 - C2
VALLEY VIEW PK, VeCo	557 - H1
VENTU PK, THO	556 - A2
VENTURA COMM PK, VEN	492 - E3
VERDE PK, SIMI	499 - B2
VETERANS MEM PK, SPLA	464 - B6
VIA MARINA PK, OXN	552 - C1
VIRGINIA COLONY PK, MRPK	476 - H7
VISTA DEL ARROYO PK, SIMI	498 - D3
WALNUT GROVE PK, THO	556 - C1
WARRING PK, VeCo	457 - F3
WAVERLY PK, THO	526 - H5
WENDY PK, THO	555 - G4
WEST HILLS REC CTR, CanP	529 - D5
WEST PK, VEN	491 - B1
WEST VILLAGE PK, OXN	522 - J4
WILDFLOWER PLAYFIELD, THO	526 - C3
WILDWOOD REGL PK, THO	496 - D7
WILLOWBROOK PK, SIMI	497 - H3
WILSON PK, OXN	522 - G5
WOOD CREEK PK, CMRL	525 - A1
WOODSIDE LINEAR PK, VEN	472 - J7
WOODSIDE PK, CMRL	524 - H4
ZUMA TRANCAS CANYONS, LACo	387 - D4

POST OFFICES

NAME Address City, ZIP Code	PAGE-GRID
AGOURA HILLS 5158 CLARETON DR, AGRH, 91301	558 - B5
CAMARILLO 2150 PICKWICK DR, CMRL, 93010	524 - E3
CONEJO VALLEY 235 N MOORPARK RD, THO, 91360	556 - F1
EAST VENTURA 41 S WAKE FOREST AV, VEN, 93003	492 - B2
FEDERAL BLDG 350 S A ST, OXN, 93030	522 - G6
FILLMORE 333 CENTRAL AV, FILM, 93015	456 - A6
LAS POSAS 528 LAS POSAS RD, CMRL, 93010	524 - B2
MONTALVO 2481 GRAND AV, VEN, 93003	492 - D6
MOORPARK 215 W LOS ANGELES AV, MRPK, 93021	496 - E1
MOUNT MCCOY STA 225 SIMI VILLAGE DR, SIMI, 93065	497 - F2
NEWBURY PARK 1602 NEWBURY RD, THO, 91320	556 - A1
OAK VIEW 360 VENTURA AV, VeCo, 93022	451 - B7
OJAI 201 E OJAI AV, OJAI, 93023	441 - H7
OXNARD MAIN 1961 N C ST, OXN, 93036	522 - G3
PIRU 652 N MAIN ST, VeCo, 93040	457 - F4
PORT HUENEME 560 E PLEASANT VALLEY RD, PHME, 93041	552 - F5
SANTA PAULA 111 S MILL ST, SPLA, 93060	464 - B5
SATICOY 11043 CITRUS DR, VEN, 93004	473 - A7
SAVIERS 2532 SAVIERS RD, OXN, 93033	552 - G2
SIMI VALLEY 2551 GALENA AV, SIMI, 93065	498 - D1
SOMIS 3349 SOMIS RD, VeCo, 93066	495 - A5
THOUSAND OAKS 3435 E THOUSAND OAKS BLVD, THO, 91362	557 - B3
VENTURA MAIN 675 E SANTA CLARA ST, VEN, 93001	491 - C2
WEST HILLS 23055 SHERMAN WY, CanP, 91307	529 - G5

SCHOOLS

NAME Address City, ZIP Code	PAGE-GRID
ACACIA ELEM 55 W NORMAN AV, THO, 91360	526 - F6
AGOURA HIGH 28545 W DRIVER AV, AGRH, 91301	558 - B5
ANACAPA MID 100 S MILLS RD, VEN, 93003	491 - H3
APOLLO HIGH 3150 SCHOOL ST, SIMI, 93065	498 - D2
ARROYO ELEM 225 ULYSSES ST, SIMI, 93065	497 - F2
ARROYO MONTESSORI ELEM 9 W BONITA DR, SIMI, 93065	497 - F3
ARROYO WEST ELEM 4117 COUNTRY HILL RD, MRPK, 93021	496 - B3
ASCENSION LUTHERAN ELEM 1600 E HILLCREST DR, THO, 91362	556 - J1
ASPEN ELEM 1870 OBERLIN AV, THO, 91360	526 - E5

FEATURE NAME Address City, ZIP Code	PAGE-GRID
ATHERWOOD ELEM 2350 GREENSWARD ST, SIMI, 93065	498 - B1
BALBOA MID 247 S HILL RD, VEN, 93003	492 - D2
BANYAN ELEM 1120 KNOLLWOOD DR, THO, 91320	555 - F4
BARD, RICHARD ELEM 622 PLEASANT VALLEY RD, PHME, 93041	552 - F5
BEDELL, THELMA B ELEM 1305 LAUREL RD, SPLA, 93060	464 - B2
BERYLWOOD ELEM 2300 HEYWOOD ST, SIMI, 93065	498 - B3
BETHANY CHRISTIAN ELEM 200 BETHANY CT, THO, 91360	526 - E5
BIG SPRINGS ELEM 3401 BIG SPRINGS AV, SIMI, 93063	478 - G5
BLACKSTOCK, CHARLES JR HIGH 701 E BARD RD, OXN, 93033	552 - H4
BLANCHARD ELEM 115 N PECK RD, SPLA, 93060	463 - J7
BREKKE ELEM 1400 MARTIN LUTHER KING JR DR, OXN, 93030	522 - J4
BRIGGS ELEM 14438 W TELEGRAPH RD, VeCo, 93060	473 - F2
BROOKSIDE ELEM 165 SATINWOOD AV, VeCo, 91377	558 - B2
BUENA HIGH 5670 TELEGRAPH RD, VEN, 93003	492 - C2
CABRILLO MID 1426 E SANTA CLARA ST, VEN, 93001	491 - E2
CAMARILLO, ADOLFO HIGH 4660 MISSION OAKS BLVD, CMRL, 93012	524 - H3
CAMARILLO CHRISTIAN 579 ANACAPA DR, VeCo, 93010	494 - D7
CAMARILLO HEIGHTS ELEM 35 W CATALINA DR, VeCo, 93010	494 - D7
CAMPUS CANYON ELEM 15300 MONROE AV, MRPK, 93021	476 - J5
CAPISTRANO AVENUE ELEM 8118 CAPISTRANO AV, LA, 91304	529 - J3
CARDEN CONEJO 975 EVENSTAR AV, THO, 91361	557 - B5
CARDEN OF CAMARILLO 1915 LAS POSAS RD, CMRL, 93010	524 - D1
CHAMINADE COLLEGE PREP HIGH 7500 CHAMINADE AV, LA, 91304	529 - F4
CHANNEL ISLANDS HIGH 1400 RAIDERS WY, OXN, 93033	552 - J3
CHAPARRAL MID 280 POINDEXTER AV, MRPK, 93021	496 - D1
CHATSWORTH PK ELEM 22005 DEVONSHIRE ST, Chat, 91311	499 - J4
CHAVEZ, CESAR ELEM 301 N MARQUITA ST, OXN, 93030	522 - H5
CHIME CHARTER MID 22280 DEVONSHIRE ST, Chat, 91311	499 - J4
CITRUS GLEN ELEM 9655 DARLING RD, VEN, 93004	492 - H2
COLINA MID 1500 E HILLCREST DR, THO, 91362	556 - J1
COLLEGE HEIGHTS CHRISTIAN 6360 TELEPHONE RD, VEN, 93003	492 - D4
COLUMBUS MID 22250 ELKWOOD ST, LA, 91304	529 - J3
COMM HIGH 5700 CONDOR DR, MRPK, 93021	476 - H7
CONEJO ADVENTIST ELEM 2645 W HILLCREST DR, THO, 91320	525 - J7
CONEJO ELEM 280 CONEJO SCHOOL RD, THO, 91362	557 - A1
CONEJO VALLEY HIGH 1872 NEWBURY RD, THO, 91320	556 - A1
CORNERSTONE CHRISTIAN HIGH 1777 ARNEILL RD, CMRL, 93010	524 - E1
CORNERSTONE CHRISTIAN 1777 ARNEILL RD, CMRL, 93010	524 - E1
CRESTVIEW ELEM 900 CROSBY AV, SIMI, 93065	498 - B5
CURREN, BERNICE ELEM 1101 N F ST, OXN, 93030	522 - F4
CYPRESS ELEM 4200 W KIMBER DR, THO, 91320	555 - E3
DE ANZA MID 2060 CAMERON ST, VEN, 93001	471 - C6
DOS CAMINOS ELEM 3635 APPIAN WY, CMRL, 93010	494 - G7
DRIFFILL ELEM 910 S E ST, OXN, 93030	522 - G7
EL CAMINO HIGH 3777 DEAN DR, VEN, 93003	491 - J3
EL DESCANSO ELEM 1099 BEDFORD DR, CMRL, 93010	524 - D2
ELMHURST ELEM 5080 ELMHURST ST, VEN, 93003	492 - B3
ELM STREET ELEM 450 E ELM ST, OXN, 93033	552 - H1
EL RIO ELEM 2714 E VINEYARD AV, VeCo, 93036	522 - H1
FAITH BAPTIST 7644 FARRALONE AV, LA, 91304	529 - J4
FILLMORE HIGH 555 CENTRAL AV, FILM, 93015	456 - A5
FILLMORE MID 543 A ST, FILM, 93015	456 - A6
FIRST BAPTIST ACADEMY 1250 ERBES RD, THO, 91362	527 - A6
FLORY ELEM 240 FLORY AV, MRPK, 93021	496 - E1
FOOTHILL TECHNOLOGY HIGH 100 DAY RD, VEN, 93003	492 - B2
FOSTER, E P ELEM 20 PLEASANT PL, VEN, 93001	471 - B7
FRANK, ROBERT J INTERMED 701 N JUANITA AV, OXN, 93030	522 - H4
FREMONT, JOHN CHARLES INTERMED 1130 N M ST, OXN, 93030	522 - F4
FRIENDS ELEM 3503 ARUNDELL CIR, VEN, 93003	491 - H5
FRONTIER HIGH 545 AIRPORT WY, CMRL, 93010	524 - A5
GARDEN GROVE ELEM 2250 N TRACY AV, SIMI, 93063	498 - E2
GLEN CITY ELEM 141 S STECKEL DR, SPLA, 93060	463 - J6
GLENWOOD ELEM 1135 WINDSOR DR, THO, 91360	526 - G6
GOOD SHEPHERD LUTHERAN ELEM 2949 ALAMO ST, SIMI, 93063	478 - C7
GRACE BRETHREN ELEM 1717 ARCANE ST, SIMI, 93065	497 - J4
GRACE BRETHREN JR/SR HIGH 1350 CHERRY AV, SIMI, 93065	498 - B3
GRACE LUTHERAN CHRISTIAN DAY 6190 TELEPHONE RD, VEN, 93003	492 - D4
GREEN, E O JR HIGH 3739 C ST, OXN, 93033	552 - G4
HAMLIN STREET ELEM 22627 HAMLIN ST, CanP, 91307	529 - H6
HARRINGTON, NORMA ELEM 2501 GISLER AV, OXN, 93033	552 - H2

FEATURE NAME Address City, ZIP Code	PAGE-GRID
HATHAWAY, JULIEN ELEM 405 DOLLIE ST, OXN, 93033	552 - H5
HAYCOX, ART ELEM 5400 PERKINS RD, OXN, 93033	552 - G6
HAYDOCK, RICHARD B INTERMED 647 HILL ST, OXN, 93033	522 - F7
HAYNES ELEM 6624 LOCKHURST DR, CanP, 91307	529 - E6
HERCHEL DAY WEST 27400 CANWOOD ST, Ago, 91301	558 - F6
HILLCREST CHRISTIAN ELEM 384 ERBES RD, THO, 91362	556 - J1
HILLCREST CHRISTIAN HIGH 384 ERBES RD, THO, 91362	556 - J1
HILLSIDE MID 2222 FITZGERALD RD, SIMI, 93065	498 - A4
HOLLOW HILLS ELEM 828 GIBSON AV, SIMI, 93065	497 - J5
HOLLYWOOD BEACH ELEM 4000 SUNSET LN, VeCo, 93035	552 - A2
HOLY CROSS ELEM 211 E MAIN ST, VEN, 93001	491 - B2
HUENEME CHRISTIAN ELEM 312 N VENTURA RD, PHME, 93041	552 - E5
HUENEME ELEM 354 3RD ST, PHME, 93041	552 - E6
HUENEME HIGH 500 W BARD RD, OXN, 93033	552 - G4
INDIAN HILLS HIGH 4345 N LAS VIRGENES RD, CALB, 91302	558 - H7
ISBELL MID 221 S 4TH ST, SPLA, 93060	464 - B6
IVY ACADEMIA CHARTER 6221 FALLBROOK AV, WdHl, 91367	529 - H7
JORDAN, JAMES CHARTER MID 22250 ELKWOOD ST, LA, 91304	529 - J3
JUANAMARIA ELEM 100 S CROCKER AV, VEN, 93004	492 - F2
JUSTICE STREET ELEM 23350 JUSTICE ST, LA, 91304	529 - F3
JUSTIN ELEM 2245 N JUSTIN AV, SIMI, 93065	498 - A2
KAMALA ELEM 634 W KAMALA ST, OXN, 93033	552 - F2
KATHERINE ELEM 5455 KATHERINE ST, SIMI, 93063	499 - A3
KNOLLS ELEM 6334 KATHERINE RD, SIMI, 93063	499 - C3
LADERA ELEM 1211 CL ALMENDRO, THO, 91360	526 - H3
LAGUNA VISTA ELEM 5084 ETTING RD, VeCo, 93012	553 - H4
LA MARIPOSA ELEM 4800 CTE OLIVAS, CMRL, 93012	524 - J1
LANG RANCH ELEM 2450 WHITECHAPEL PL, THO, 91362	527 - B3
LA REINA HIGH 106 W JANSS RD, THO, 91360	526 - F5
LARSEN, ANSGAR ELEM 550 THOMAS AV, OXN, 93033	552 - H3
LAS COLINAS MID 5750 FIELDCREST DR, CMRL, 93012	525 - B1
LAS POSAS ELEM 75 E CL LA GUERRA, CMRL, 93010	524 - B2
LAUREL SPRINGS ELEM 302 EL PASEO RD, OJAI, 93023	441 - H7
LAUREL SPRINGS HIGH 302 EL PASEO RD, OJAI, 93023	441 - H7
LAW, MARY PRIVATE ELEM 2929 ALBANY DR, OXN, 93033	552 - H3
LEMONWOOD ELEM 2200 CARNEGIE CT, OXN, 93033	553 - A2
LINCOLN ELEM 1107 E SANTA CLARA ST, VEN, 93001	491 - D2
LINCOLN, ABRAHAM ELEM 1220 4TH ST, SIMI, 93065	497 - G4
LINDA VISTA JR ACADEMY 5050 PERRY WY, VeCo, 93036	493 - B4
LINDERO CANYON MID 5844 LARBOARD LN, AGRH, 91301	557 - G4
LOCKHURST DRIVE ELEM 6170 LOCKHURST DR, WdHl, 91367	529 - E7
LOMA VISTA ELEM 300 LYNN DR, VEN, 93003	491 - H2
LOS ALTOS MID 700 TEMPLE AV, CMRL, 93010	524 - F2
LOS CERRITOS MID 2100 AVD DE LAS FLORES, THO, 91362	527 - A4
LOS PRIMEROS STRUCTURED ELEM 2222 E VENTURA BLVD, CMRL, 93010	524 - E3
LOS SENDEROS ELEM 1555 KENDALL AV, CMRL, 93010	524 - F1
LUPIN HILL ELEM 26210 ADAMOR RD, CALB, 91302	558 - H3
MADERA ELEM 250 ROYAL AV, SIMI, 93065	497 - F4
MADRONA ELEM 612 CM MANZANAS, VeCo, 91360	526 - D6
MANZANITA ELEM 2626 MICHAEL DR, THO, 91320	555 - H1
MAPLE ELEM 3501 KIMBER DR, THO, 91320	555 - F2
MARINA WEST ELEM 2501 CAROB ST, OXN, 93035	552 - D1
MARSHALL, THURGOOD 2900 THURGOOD MARSHALL DR, OXN, 93036	522 - D3
MAR VISTA ELEM 2382 ETTING RD, OXN, 93033	553 - B4
MATILIJA JR HIGH 703 EL PASEO RD, OJAI, 93023	441 - G7
MCAULIFFE, CHRISTA ELEM 3300 W VIA MARINA AV, OXN, 93035	522 - C7
MCKEVETT ELEM 955 PLEASANT ST, SPLA, 93060	464 - B5
MCKINNA, DENNIS ELEM 1611 J ST, OXN, 93033	552 - F1
MEADOWS ELEM 2000 LA GRANADA DR, THO, 91362	527 - A6
MEDEA CREEK MID 1002 DOUBLETREE RD, VeCo, 91377	558 - A1
MEINERS OAKS ELEM 400 S LOMITA AV, VeCo, 93023	441 - E7
MESA ELEM 3901 MESA SCHOOL RD, VeCo, 93066	493 - H4
MESA VERDE MID 14000 PEACH HILL RD, MRPK, 93021	496 - G3
MIRA MONTE ELEM 1216 LOMA DR, VeCo, 93023	451 - D2
MONICA ROS ELEM 783 MCNELL RD, VeCo, 93023	442 - E5
MONTALVO ELEM 2050 GRAND AV, VEN, 93003	492 - D5
MONTESSORI OF OJAI, THE 806 BALDWIN RD, VeCo, 93001	451 - A3
MONTE VISTA HIGH 1755 BLACKSTOCK AV, SIMI, 93065	498 - D3
MONTE VISTA MID 888 LANTANA ST, CMRL, 93010	524 - C2
MOORPARK HIGH 4500 TIERRA REJADA RD, MRPK, 93021	496 - C3

FEATURE NAME Address City, ZIP Code	PA
MORGAN CREEK CHRISTIAN ELEM 723 S D ST, OXN, 93030	
MOUND ELEM 455 S HILL RD, VEN, 93003	
MOUNTAIN MEADOWS ELEM 4200 MOUNTAIN MEADOW DR, MRPK, 93021	
MOUNTAIN VIEW ELEM 2925 FLETCHER ST, SIMI, 93065	
MUPU ELEM 4410 SANTA PAULA-OJAI RD, VeCo, 93060	
NEVADA AVENUE ELEM 22120 CHASE ST, LA, 91304	
NEWBURY PARK ADVENTIST ACADEMY HIGH 180 ACADEMY DR, THO, 91320	
NEWBURY PARK HIGH 456 N REINO RD, THO, 91320	
NEW COMM JEWISH HIGH 7353 VALLEY CIRCLE BLVD, CanP, 91307	5
NORDHOFF HIGH 1401 MARICOPA HWY, OJAI, 93023	4
OAK GROVE-KRISHNAMURTI ELEM 220 W LOMITA AV, VeCo, 93023	4
OAK GROVE-KRISHNAMURTI HIGH 220 W LOMITA AV, VeCo, 93023	4
OAK HILLS ELEM 1010 KANAN RD, VeCo, 91377	5
OAK PARK HIGH 899 KANAN RD, VeCo, 91377	5
OAKS CHRISTIAN HIGH 31749 LA TIENDA RD, WLKV, 91362	5
OAKS CHRISTIAN MID 31749 LE TIENDA RD, WLKV, 91362	5
OAK VIEW HIGH 5701 CONIFER ST, VeCo, 91377	5
OCEAN VIEW JR HIGH 4300 OLDS RD, OXN, 93033	5
OJAI VALLEY ELEM 723 EL PASEO RD, OJAI, 93023	4
OJAI VALLEY HIGH 723 EL PASEO RD, OJAI, 93023	4
OLIVELANDS ELEM 12465 FOOTHILL RD, VeCo, 93060	4
OUR LADY OF GUADALUPE ELEM 530 N JUANITA AV, OXN, 93030	5
OUR LADY OF THE ASSUMPTION ELEM 3169 TELEGRAPH RD, VEN, 93003	4
OXNARD HIGH 3400 GONZALES RD, VeCo, 93030	5
PACIFIC HIGH 501 COLLEGE DR, VEN, 93003	4
PACIFIC VIEW HIGH 1701 GARY DR, OXN, 93033	5
PACIFICA HIGH 600 E GONZALES RD, OXN, 93030	5
PARK OAKS ELEM 1335 CL BOUGANVILLA, THO, 91360	5
PARKVIEW ELEM 1416 6TH PL, PHME, 93041	5
PARK VIEW ELEM 1500 ALEXANDER ST, SIMI, 93065	4
PEACH HILL ELEM 13400 CHRISTIAN BARRETT DR, MRPK, 93021	4
PHOENIX RANCH 1845 OAK RD, SIMI, 93063	4
PIERPONT ELEM 1254 MARTHAS VINEYARD CT, VEN, 93001	4
PINECREST ELEM 449 WILBUR RD, THO, 91360	5
PINECREST ELEM 4974 COCHRAN ST, SIMI, 93063	4
PINECREST - MOORPARK PRIVATE ELEM 14100 PEACH HILL RD, MRPK, 93021	4
PIRU ELEM 3811 E CENTER ST, VeCo, 93040	4
PLEASANT VALLEY CHRISTIAN 1101 PONDEROSA DR, CMRL, 93010	5
POINSETTIA ELEM 350 N VICTORIA AV, VEN, 93003	4
POMELO DRIVE ELEM 7633 MARCH AV, LA, 91304	5
PORTOLA ELEM 6700 EAGLE ST, VEN, 93003	4
PUENTE HIGH 545 CENTRAL AV, VeCo, 93036	4
RAMONA ELEM 804 COOPER RD, OXN, 93030	5
RED OAK ELEM 4857 ROCKFIELD ST, VeCo, 91377	5
REDWOOD MID 233 W GAINSBOROUGH RD, THO, 91360	5
RENAISSANCE HIGH 325 N PALM AV, SPLA, 93060	4
REYNOLDS, BLANCHE ELEM 450 VALMORE AV, VEN, 93003	4
RIO DEL NORTE ELEM 2500 LOBELIA DR, OXN, 93036	5
RIO DEL VALLE JR HIGH 3100 ROSE AV, VeCo, 93036	5
RIO LINDO ELEM 2131 SNOW AV, OXN, 93036	5
RIO MESA HIGH 545 CENTRAL AV, VeCo, 93036	4
RIO PLAZA ELEM 600 SIMON WY, VeCo, 93036	4
RIO REAL ELEM 1140 KENNY ST, VeCo, 93036	5
RIO ROSALES ELEM 2001 JACINTO DR, OXN, 93030	5
RITCHEN, EMILIE ELEM 2200 CABRILLO WY, OXN, 93030	5
ROGERS, WILL ELEM 316 HOWARD ST, VEN, 93003	4
ROSE AVENUE ELEM 220 DRISKILL ST, OXN, 93030	5
ROYAL HIGH 1402 ROYAL AV, SIMI, 93065	4
SACRED HEART ELEM 10770 HENDERSON RD, VEN, 93004	4
SAINT ANTHONY ELEM 2421 C ST, OXN, 93033	55
SAINT BERNARDINE OF SIENA ELEM 6061 VALLEY CIRCLE BLVD, WdHl, 91367	52
SAINT BONAVENTURE HIGH 3167 TELEGRAPH RD, VEN, 93003	49
SAINT JOHNS LUTHERAN ELEM 1500 N C ST, OXN, 93030	52
SAINT JUDE THE APOSTLE 32036 W LINDERO CANYON RD, WLKV, 91361	55
SAINT MARY MAGDALEN ELEM 2534 VENTURA BLVD, CMRL, 93010	52
SAINT PASCHAL BAYLON ELEM 154 E JANSS RD, THO, 91360	52
SAINT PATRICKS ELEM 1 CHURCH RD, THO, 91362	52
SAINT PAULS ELEM 3290 LOMA VISTA RD, VEN, 93003	49
SAINT ROSE OF LIMA ELEM 1325 ROYAL AV, SIMI, 93065	49
SAINT SEBASTIAN ELEM 325 E SANTA BARBARA ST, SPLA, 93060	46

NAME City, ZIP Code	PAGE-GRID
ONIO ELEM NE RD, VeCo, 93023	442 - D6
ETANO ELEM UNTAIN VIEW ST, FILM, 93015	456 - B5
LARA ELEM ELEGRAPH RD, VeCo, 93060	464 - J2
LARA ELEM ST, OXN, 93030	522 - F6
LARA HIGH VIERS RD, OXN, 93033	552 - G2
AULA HIGH TH ST, SPLA, 93060	464 - A5
OSA ELEM ANTA ROSA RD, VeCo, 93012	496 - F6
USANA ELEM RICOT RD, SIMI, 93063	498 - G1
USANA HIGH COCHRAN ST, SIMI, 93063	498 - E1
ELEM MIN AV, VEN, 93004	492 - J1
MID RCHARD RD, THO, 91320	555 - H1
UNIPERO ELEM ALIFAX ST, VEN, 93004	492 - H3
EM HARD ST, FILM, 93015	456 - A6
D OF THE VALLEY LUTHERAN ELEM ITTRIDGE ST, CanP, 91307	529 - E6
N WAY ELEM RIDAN WY, VEN, 93001	491 - B1
INDA ELEM SMINE ST, OXN, 93036	522 - F2
M HOOL ST, SIMI, 93065	498 - C3
LLEY HIGH OCHRAN ST, SIMI, 93063	499 - A1
MID YAL AV, SIMI, 93065	497 - G3
LEM ORTH ST, VeCo, 93066	495 - A5
ELEM ALMFIELD AV, AGRH, 91301	558 - B3
ELEM SANTA PAULA OJAI RD, VeCo, 93023	453 - C1
ELEM AKWOOD ST, PHME, 93041	552 - E3
ELEM NSET AV, VeCo, 93022	461 - A1
RE ELEM AVENNA ST, SIMI, 93065	498 - C2
RE CANYON ELEM A RIO, THO, 91320	555 - D2
CHRISTIAN ELEM ALSTON ST, VEN, 93003	492 - C4
R HIGH HACHER RD, VeCo, 93023	442 - F4
GRACE S ELEM ENTURA ST, SPLA, 93060	464 - C6
ND OAKS BAPTIST ABEDUL, THO, 91360	526 - G3
ND OAKS HIGH OORPARK RD, THO, 91360	526 - F4
LINDA ELEM OODCREEK RD, CMRL, 93012	525 - A1
VISTA ELEM ANFORD ST, OXN, 93033	553 - A5
PA ELEM UNTAIN VIEW AV, OJAI, 93023	441 - J5
HIP ELEM OWNSHIP AV, SIMI, 93063	478 - F6
SITY ELEM TLAS AV, THO, 91360	526 - F3
SITY PREP MPLE AV, CMRL, 93010	524 - F2
VIEW MID APO ST, SIMI, 93063	478 - G6
A COUNTY CHRISTIAN ELEM CMILLAN AV, VEN, 93001	491 - E2
A COUNTY CHRISTIAN HIGH CMILLAN AV, VEN, 93001	491 - E2
A HIGH TALINA ST, VEN, 93001	491 - F2
A MISSIONARY CHRISTIAN ELEM GH POINT DR, VEN, 93003	472 - E7
OVA PREP HIGH VENTURA AV, VeCo, 93023	451 - F2
UNDAMENTAL ELEM VISTERIA ST, SIMI, 93065	498 - B2
T ELEM NA DR, VeCo, 91320	555 - G1
CANYON ELEM ASEY RD, MRPK, 93021	476 - D7
ERSFIELD ELEM ARLINGTON DR, THO, 91360	526 - G2
R, BARBARA ELEM ATICOY ST, SPLA, 93060	464 - C5
WAY ELEM WELBY WY, CanP, 91307	529 - F6
AKE ELEM OTRERO RD, THO, 91361	556 - J6
AKE HIGH LAKEVIEW CANYON RD, THO, 91362	557 - D3
AKE HILLS ELEM MEDICINE BOW CT, THO, 91362	557 - B3
ALLEY CHRISTIAN SHERMAN WY, CanP, 91307	529 - J5
OAK ELEM ALSCOT AV, SIMI, 93063	499 - C2
OAK ELEM W VILLAGE SCHOOL RD, WLKV, 91361	557 - D6
OOD ELEM ELARDE DR, THO, 91360	526 - D3
MS, FRED ELEM ANCHORAGE ST, OXN, 93033	552 - J4
V ELEM LARO DR, AGRH, 91301	558 - A4
RANCH ELEM RCLE KNOLL DR, SIMI, 93065	527 - D1
, ARTHUR E MID N LAS VIRGENES RD, CALB, 91302	558 - H7
BUENA ELEM ARBOARD LN, AGRH, 91301	557 - G4

SHOPPING CENTERS

NAME City, ZIP Code	PAGE-GRID
RILLO PREMIUM OUTLETS VENTURA BLVD, CMRL, 93010	524 - C3
RPOINT MALL SAVIERS RD, OXN, 93033	552 - G2
NADE, THE SPLANADE DR, OXN, 93036	492 - G7
ROOK MALL FALLBROOK AV, CanP, 91307	529 - G6
MARKETPLACE MOORPARK RD, THO, 91360	526 - E7
N OAKS VILLAGE LCREST DR & WILBUR RD, THO, 91360	556 - E1
THE HILLCREST DR, THO, 91360	526 - D7

FEATURE NAME Address City, ZIP Code	PAGE-GRID
PACIFIC VIEW MALL 3301 E MAIN ST, VEN, 93003	491 - H4
SHOPPING AT THE ROSE ROSE AVE & VENTURA FRWY, OXN, 93036	522 - J3
SIMI VALLEY TOWN CTR 1555 SIMI TOWN CENTER WY, SIMI, 93065	497 - J1
SYCAMORE SQUARE 2845 COCHRAN ST, SIMI, 93065	498 - C1
TELEPHONE ROAD PLAZA TELEPHONE RD & VALENTINE RD, VEN, 93003	492 - A4

TRANSPORTATION

FEATURE NAME	PAGE-GRID
AMTRAK/METROLINK STA, SIMI	498 - H2
AMTRAK STA-VENTURA, VEN	491 - B2
GREYHOUND BUS TERMINAL, OXN	522 - G6
GREYHOUND STA-VENTURA, VEN	491 - C2
METROLINK CAMARILLO STA, CMRL	524 - F3
METROLINK MONTALVO STA, VEN	492 - D6
METROLINK-MOORPARK STA, MRPK	496 - F1
METROLINK OXNARD STA, OXN	522 - G6

VISITOR INFORMATION

FEATURE NAME Address City, ZIP Code	PAGE-GRID
SANTA MONICA MTNS NRA PK VISTOR CTR 401 W HILLCREST DR, THO, 91360	526 - E7
VENTURA VISITORS BUREAU 89 S CALIFORNIA ST, VEN, 93001	491 - C2

FEATURE NAME Address City, ZIP Code	PAGE-GRID

Note Page

Note Page

CUT ALONG DOTTED LINE

The Thomas Guide®

Thank you for purchasing this Rand McNally Thomas Guide! We value your comments and suggestions.

Please help us serve you better by completing this postage-paid reply card.
This information is for internal use ONLY and will not be distributed or sold to any external third party.

Missing pages? Maybe not... Please refer to the "Using Your Street Guide" page for further explanation

Thomas Guide Title: Easy-to-Read Ventura County **ISBN-13# 978-0-5288-6851-1** **MKT: L**

Today's Date: ______ Gender: ☐M ☐F Age Group: ☐18-24 ☐25-31 ☐32-40 ☐41-50 ☐51-64 ☐6

1. What type of industry do you work in?
   ☐Real Estate ☐Trucking ☐Delivery ☐Construction ☐Utilities ☐Governm
   ☐Retail ☐Sales ☐Transportation ☐Landscape ☐Service & Repair
   ☐Courier ☐Automotive ☐Insurance ☐Medical ☐Police/Fire/First Response
   ☐Other, please specify: ______
2. What type of job do you have in this industry? ______
3. Where did you purchase this Thomas Guide? (store name & city) ______
4. Why did you purchase this Thomas Guide? ______
5. How often do you purchase an updated Thomas Guide? ☐Annually ☐2 yrs. ☐3-5 yrs. ☐Other: ______
6. Where do you use it? ☐Primarily in the car ☐Primarily in the office ☐Primarily at home ☐Other: ______
7. How do you use it? ☐Exclusively for business ☐Primarily for business but also for personal or leisure use
   ☐Both work and personal evenly ☐Primarily for personal use ☐Exclusively for personal use
8. What do you use your Thomas Guide for?
   ☐Find Addresses ☐In-route navigation ☐Planning routes ☐Other: ______
   Find points of interest: ☐Schools ☐Parks ☐Buildings ☐Shopping Centers ☐Other: ______
9. How often do you use it? ☐Daily ☐Weekly ☐Monthly ☐Other: ______
10. Do you use the internet for maps and/or directions? ☐Yes ☐No
11. How often do you use the internet for directions? ☐Daily ☐Weekly ☐Monthly ☐Other: ______
12. Do you use any of the following mapping products in addition to your Thomas Guide?
    ☐Folded paper maps ☐Folded laminated maps ☐Wall maps ☐GPS ☐PDA ☐In-car navigation ☐Phone maps
13. What features, if any, would you like to see added to your Thomas Guide? ______
14. What features or information do you find most useful in your Rand McNally Thomas Guide? (please specify) ______
15. Please provide any additional comments or suggestions you have. ______

We strive to provide you with the most current updated information available if you know a map correction, please notify us here.

Where is the correction? Map Page #: ______ Grid #: ______ Index Page #: ______

Nature of the correction: ☐Street name missing ☐Street name misspelled ☐Street information incorrect
☐Incorrect location for point of interest ☐Index error ☐Other: ______

Detail: ______

CUT ALONG DOTTED LINE

I would like to receive information about updated editions and special offers from Rand McNally
☐via e-mail E-mail address: ______
☐via postal mail
Your Name: ______ Company (if used for work): ______
Address: ______ City/State/ZIP: ______

Thank you for your time and help. We are working to serve you better.
This information is for internal use ONLY and will not be distributed or sold to any external third party.

TAPE SHUT

TAPE

get directions at

randmcnally.com

CUT ALONG DOTTED LINE

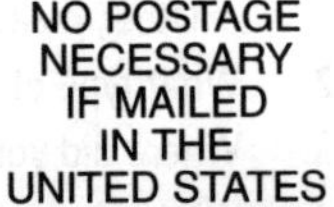
NO POSTAGE
NECESSARY
IF MAILED
IN THE
UNITED STATES

BUSINESS REPLY MAIL

FIRST-CLASS MAIL PERMIT NO. 388 CHICAGO IL

POSTAGE WILL BE PAID BY ADDRESSEE

RAND MCNALLY
CONSUMER AFFAIRS
PO BOX 7600
CHICAGO IL 60680-9915

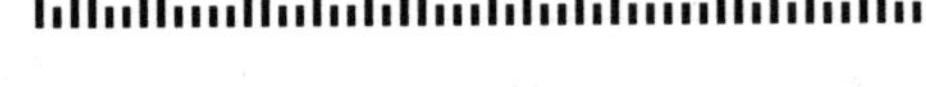

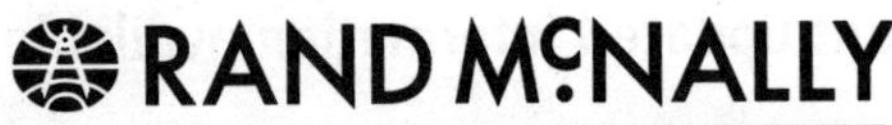
RAND McNALLY

The most trusted name on the map.

You'll never need to ask for directions again with these Rand McNally products!

- EasyFinder® Laminated Maps
- Folded Maps
- Street Guides
- Wall Maps
- CustomView Wall Maps
- Road Atlases
- Motor Carriers' Road Atlases

CUT ALONG DOTTED LINE

SGTG_07

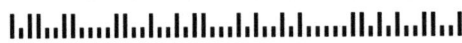

"Precise and Professional"

A Workbook of
Heirloom and Couture Techniques to
Perfect Everyday Sewing

with Lyn Weeks

Illustrations by
Peggy Falk, Rockford, MI

Artwork on Front and Back Covers by
Christine Thompson, Naperville, IL

Photography by
Brian Weeks

Published by Lyn Weeks, 2005

Printed in the United States of America by

FXWB Reprographics
50 Lakeview Pkwy., Ste 112
Vernon Hills, Illinois 60061

Weeks, Lyn.
Precise and Professional – A Workbook of Heirloom & Couture Techniques to Perfect Everyday Sewing

ISBN 1-59975-158-5

"Precise and Professional"

A Workbook of Heirloom and Couture Techniques to Perfect Everyday Sewing

Table of Contents

Introduction and Acknowledgements....................................7

Heirloom Sewing Glossary..10
Lace Terms, **10**
Trims and Stitches, **11**
Fabrics, **11**
Embroidery and Lace Identification, **13**
Interfacing, **15**

Let's talk 'Precise and Professional'......................................18

Lets talk 'Couture'..20

Finished Measurement Chart..22

General Information..24

Heirloom Sewing Techniques..25
Fine Rolled Hem (Roll and Whip), **25**
Fine Rolled Hem with Gathers, **26**
Rolled Hem with Lace, **28**
Attaching Lace to Fabric (creating a Rolled Edge), **30**
Attaching Gathered Lace to Fabric (creating a Rolled Edge), **32**
Working with Entredeux, **33**
Attaching Entredeux to Fabric, **34**
Rolled Hem with Entredeux, **36**
Attaching Entredeux to Gathered Fabric, **37**
Joining Entredeux to Lace Insertion or Straight Edge of Lace, **39**
Joining Entredeux to Gathered Lace, **40**
Joining Lace Insertion to another Straight Lace Edge, **42**
Applying Lace Insertion (or Straight Edge of Lace) to Fabric, **43**
Inserting Lace into Gathered Fabric, **45**
Applying Lace with a Mitered Corner to a Design within the Fabric, **47**
Applying Lace with a Mitered Corner to a Fabric Edge, **49**
Applying Entredeux and Gathered Lace to a Mitered Lace Corner, **53**
Applying Entredeux to a Corner, **56**
Applying Entredeux into a Lined Corner, **57**
Applying Lace with a gathered corner to Entredeux, **58**
Rolling and Whipping a Bias or Curved Edge, **60**
Applying Entredeux to a Curved Edge (Concave Curve), **61**
Applying Entredeux to a Curved Edge (Convex Curve), **62**
Corded Edge Trim, **63**

Creating with Tucks...65
*Adding Pleats and Tucks, **67***
*Basic Tucks, **68***
*Whipped Tucks, **70***
*Shell Edged Tucks, **72***
*Twin Needle Tucks, **74***
*Corded Pintucks, **76***
*Straightening Tucks, **78***
*Release Tucks, **79***
*Reverse Threading for Tucks, **80***
*Single-thread Dart, **82***
*Decorative Tucked Hem, **84***
*Tucked Hem with Embroidered Edge, **86***

Using the Bias...89
*Making Corded Piping, **91***
*Double Corded Piping, **93***
*Piping a Pointed Corner, **94***
*Applying Cording to a Seam, **94***
*Binding a Collar (or outer curve), **96***
*Binding the Neckline (Double Binding or French Binding), **98***
*Folded Bias Piping, **100***
*Rouleau (or 'Shoe-String') Tubes, **102***

Seams and Seam Finishes...103
*Seams, **103***
*Seams with Gathers, **105***
*French Seam, **107***
*French Seam incorporating Gathered Fabric, **109***
*Flat-Fell (Run-and-Fell) Seam, **111***
*Hong Kong Seam Finish, **112***
*The Self Bound Seam, **114***
*A Decorative Seam, **115***
*Making a Narrow Hem, **116***

Plackets and Closures..118
*Chart for Placket Lengths, **118***
*Continuous Lapped Placket, **119***
*Extension Placket, **121***
*Antique Tab or Flat Placket, **123***
*Buttons and Buttonholes, **127***
*Lapped Zipper, **131***

Basic Yoke Dress Alterations..133

Bibliography...136

About the Author..137

Introduction and Acknowledgements

I have been asked on many occasions if I intend to write a book. One of the advantages of teaching heirloom and couture machine techniques is that you meet so many sewers – from basic beginners to highly proficient seamstresses. And as much assistance as I am able to provide in class, I receive equally as much to help me understand just what type of information is necessary when preparing for these classes.

It was never my intention to write a book, as there seemed to be several books of this type already on the market. However, from years of gathering together information and refining the techniques that I teach, it became apparent that, whether I wanted it or not, a book was well underway with the amassing paperwork for class workbooks.

There is almost never an absolute right or wrong way to execute any sewing technique. There are certain rules that are meant to 'never be broken', and those that fall within the realm of 'design changes'. It is by using guidelines, such as I have provided in this book, and developing them to your own personal style, that we all become more accomplished sewers.

This book is written, printed and bound in the form of a Work Book. Keep it close by when you need reassurance with a certain technique, make your own notes within the text and know that it is just another sewing tool – it is not a coffee table book and, I suspect, will never appreciate in value for your retirement fund; however, the basic learnings in this book will not go out of date.

Of course, while all techniques have been written just as I would stitch them myself, they are not original thoughts that simply pop into my head. Please refer to the Bibliography at the end of this book for further reading on the topics covered, and discover for yourself the many ways there are to stitch one simple technique.

Apart from the referenced books and magazines in the Bibliography that I used for assistance, there are certainly many other people who assisted with this book. I guess I shouldn't even try and put them in any sort of order, just start writing the list.

Nothing would have been started or completed without the dozens and dozens of sewers who have been class participants, many of whom have become friends. These people willingly give feedback during and after class, help proof samples, notes, patterns and email regularly with their thoughts that may help my endeavor. Many have even trusted me with their vintage garments. There are too many to name and I hope I remember to personally acknowledge each and every one when next we meet.

Finding time to work on the many aspects of putting my class notes in order for this book was difficult. It seems that class preparation, managing web orders, drafting and testing patterns is always more pressing (and exciting) than sitting at the computer. Nancy Stuebe, a close friend and local chapter member, is always available to help with the mundane parts of my job. We cut fabric, lace, piping cord etc. into little pieces and pack them into plastic bags; we then coordinate these bags with handouts into class kits. And all throughout this process and many other labor-intensive jobs, Nancy tells me just how much she loves working in this business. Nancy definitely affords me the luxury of doing the work I love, and I treasure her for her friendship and support.

I would like to thank my friend Carol Harris. Although not directly involved with this book, Carol always graciously and selflessly shares her prized collection of vintage and antique garments. I am able to study these treasures, analyze various old techniques and gain enough inspiration for patterns and books for the next fifty years. I thank her for this contribution and for the opportunity to teach on so many occasions in her beautiful heirloom and fine sewing store in Tennessee. It is such a joy to know Carol.

Just when I thought I had my class notes in order, reworked sufficiently to stand alone, along came two sewing friends who, when asked would they mind proof-reading my notes, agreed with such enthusiasm that I should have realized I was not quite at the end of this adventure. My friends Cathy Hall and Kris Curtis, both extremely talented hand and machine sewers, not only read my notes, they made samples of the techniques, wrote copious suggestions on every page of text and generally created more work than I care to admit. I could not believe things were in such disarray, but now cannot begin to thank both Cathy and Kris for such an extraordinary amount of dedication and work. I believe they should be listed as 'The Editors' of this book.

Many hours of work were undertaken by Peggy Falk who drew illustrations even when she didn't have a clue what they represented, but still proceeded to fine tune in order to achieve meaningful drawings that clearly enhance the text. We worked so long and hard on some parts, lost other illustrations somewhere in the computer, faxed, emailed and slow mailed so often that I believe there will be withdrawal symptoms until we start a new series of techniques.

To my friend Angela Pfaff, I am indebted for the countless hours of computer assistance, proof reading, editing and technical content support – this sounds delightfully vague but, believe me, I would not have progressed to the printing stage without such electronic help, and with Angela to willingly visit me at a moments notice when needed.

And to the newest artistic person to come into my life, I thank Christine Thompson for her excitement in recreating my fabrics and techniques into original artwork for the book covers, and doing so with such flair. Christine provided a professional focus on the book's marketability as well as my, all too close, deadlines. I believe the covers look wonderful.

To my sewing friends, too numerous to name, who simply stitch with me from time to time to provide some R&R (both in Australia and the US), fellow teachers who are always willing to share and the various shops and needlework groups for whom I have taught, I say 'thank you'.

It is also extremely important for me to recognize the vital role that the Smocking Arts Guild of America has played in my life. They offered classes with excellent teachers when I was hungry for information, they invited me to teach when no-one was aware of Lyn Weeks and they have continued to support and push me to always offer the best I can, stretching me to think outside the box, not only with class offerings, but trying to master it all electronically.

*There are many reasons why we do what we do, and whether we do it "**Precisely and Professionally**" or are much more relaxed in our attitude, I believe sewing is in my blood. I can remember sitting with my mother as a child, pinning nothing in particular while she sewed, receiving doll dresses from 'Santa Clause' that had been made by one of my aunts, collecting award-winning artist bears made by yet another aunt and working with my grandmother when my sewing business first began. These are all very important people in my life and I am grateful they shared and passed on their talents.*

*It seems strange to end this introduction with what was really the catalyst for my total indulgence with sewing. Like most mothers, the birth of your children gives the perfect excuse to be involved in a world of designing, stitching and creating heirlooms for the next generation. Gregory and Melanie have accommodated my passion since they were too little to know. I remember on one Saturday-morning-shopping-trip as we walked down the street from our car, the voice of one (remaining nameless) child cried painfully "**not the Fabric Shop again**"! It seems, on reflection, I punished them with this trip all too often. But I now thank them sincerely for their love and support all these years, and for providing the reason for this book.*

I could not finalize this book without acknowledging the lifetime of love and support from my best friend – my husband Brian. For over 30 years he has supported every sewing endeavor, funded more sewing classes than I can remember, purchased fabric and lace for my 'stash' even when the stash has overtaken many rooms of the house, cooked, cleaned, babysat, proof-read, offered inspiration and on, and on, and on. He has always been totally involved in this love of mine and I love him for always being there.

As a postscript to this Introduction, Brian and I proudly announce that we are soon to become 'first-time grandparents'. Our son Greg and his wife Rachael are due to have their baby in October and thus will commence the next generation of babies in our family – and just one more reason to sew. Of course we are thrilled about the new baby, but I am particularly excited at the prospect of being allowed to sew for him or her.

Enjoy your sewing and enjoy the reason you sew, Lyn

Heirloom Sewing Glossary

Lace Terms

Alençon Lace: A light hexagonal mesh net ground developed in the French region of Alençon during the mid 18th century – a slow and difficult lace to make, continuing to sell to the upper end of the market.

Baby Lace: A light, narrow lace edging or insertion not more than ⅜" (1 cm) wide – generally Valenciennes or Cluny.

Beading: A lace or embroidered insertion, edging, or galloon having small holes through which ribbon may be laced.

Binche Lace: A very fine cotton straight-edge lace characterized by a spotted design. Originally hand made in Flanders; reproductions machine made in England, France and the United States.

Bobbin Lace: General term describing hand-made lace made with bobbins on a special lace making pillow or bolster. Following a pricked pattern, pins are inserted into the lace while it is being made to keep all the thread crossings in place until that lace portion is secure. Handmade Valenciennes, Binche, Mechin, Chantilly, and Honiton are some examples of Bobbin Lace.

Broderie Anglaise: A form or white embroidery which is characterized by eyelet holes surrounded by buttonhole stitches.

Cluny Lace: A course, strong cotton lace with a geometric design. It was formerly made by hand in France and Belgium of linen thread.

Cordonnet: A distinct, heavier thread that outlines the design in a lace. Cordonnet can also refer to a type of needlework thread as in DMC's Cordonnet special.

Filet Lace: A needle made lace formed with square meshes partially filled in to create a design – also the name given to Crochet Lace of similar design.

Irish Crochet Lace: A cotton lace made by crocheting to form characteristic designs of layered rose petals and shamrocks with picoted brides.

Limerick Lace: A delicate lace made by hand by embroidering a variety of stitches on to a fine cotton net. This lace is well suited for collars, cuffs, and medallions. May be French hand or machine sewn.

Maline: Originally made by hand in Maline, Belgium, now made by machine in France and England. An open textured diamond-shaped fine mesh with small, pretty floral designs. Motifs on the mesh background are hand trimmed.

Mechlin: A bobbin lace mesh of very fine thread. Early Mechlin lace had a six-sided mesh ground. However, present day Mechlin lace is often found with diamond shaped ground. It is usually characterized by floral motifs with a fine cordonnet. It is lighter in weight than Alencon, not as strong as Valenciennes.

Picot Lace: An edging with narrow, triangular or rounded loops along the outer edge.

Tatting: A kind of lace made by looping and knotting a thread that is wound on a hand shuttle.

Valenciennes Lace (Val): A fine cotton bobbin lace with usually a hexagonal or diamond shaped mesh background, originally made by hand and later by machine in Valenciennes, France. French Val lace is the most widely used lace in fine hand sewing.

Vraile: French for 'real' or 'handmade'.

Trims

Entredeux: a ⅛" to ½" (3mm – 12mm) embroidered veining stitched on Swiss batiste to create a ladder effect. Entredeux is used to strengthen the seam or join – loosely translated, the French word entredeux means "between two".

Galloon: A trim, lace or embroidery finished on both sides, which can range from ½" to 10" (12mm – 25 cm) in width.

Hand Loom: Fabrics or trims which are woven on either the hand or hand-and-foot power loom. These are now scarcely made and hard to find.

Insertion: A band of lace, eyelet or embroidery with two straight edges set into fabric. Refer to '*Beading*' as another example.

Lace: A fine netting or open work fabric of linen, cotton or silk produced by stitching interlacing or twisting threads in several directions to produce a porous trim or lace.

Medallion: An oval or circular design resembling a medal in shape, made of lace or embroidery, and used as decoration on a garment.

Rick Rack Trim: A firmly woven cotton trim that forms a zigzag effect. Available in several widths and a variety of colors – can be used to trim collars, yoke and hem lines and shaped for decorative designs.

Stitches

Bullion Knot: Similar to a French knot but covering a length of stitches – formed by wrapping the thread around the needle and passing the needle through the cloth to anchor it.

Faggoting: An open, decorative stitch to join two finished edges – embroidering over the space between the two. The stitches may be either plain or knotted.

Feather Stitch: A tiny decorative surface embroidery stitch loosely resembling a vine, often found on infant garments – may also be done as double or triple feather stitch.

French Knot: A small knot on the surface of a piece of work, formed by wrapping the thread around the point of the needle to form a knot on the surface of the fabric and then carrying the thread back to the wrong side.

Hemstitch: A decorative hand stitch made by drawing out (withdrawing) threads running parallel to the hem and fastening the cross threads by stitches, leaving an open work effect. This work my be used as insertion or hem finish and includes many variations – can also be adapted with variations for machine.

Pinstitch (or Pointe de Paris): A decorative stitch characterized by tiny pierced holes, used to apply edging, curved lace, Madeira appliqué, to finish a flat-felled seam and as a decorative method of sewing a hem.

Satin Stitch: A straight stitch solidly covering a given motif – can be lightly padded, or more so for high relief.

Shadow Work: Embroidery worked on a transparent fabric so that the threads on the back show through with a delicate shadow effect. It may be worked from the right side using double back stitch, or from the wrong side using closed herringbone.

Shell Stitch: A decorative scalloped stitch formed by folding a narrow hem and working a blanket stitch at intervals over the folded edge.

Fabrics

Batiste: A sheer, fine woven fabric with a plain weave of either cotton, cotton blends, wool, silk, rayon or other fibers.

Broadcloth: A fine, closely woven fabric with very fine crosswise ribs, made from cotton or a cotton/polyester blend. Filling yarns in this plain weave are heavier and have less twist than the lengthwise warp yarns. The best grades are made with combed ply yarns of Pima cotton.

Cambric: A soft, white, closely woven cotton fabric calendared to give a luster on the right side;. originally made in Cambrai, France, of linen.

Challis: One of the softest fabrics made, usually with a plain weave; originally made of wool, but now of cotton, rayon, and a wide variety of blends.

Chambray: A soft fabric made with a plain weave, colored warp (lengthwise) yarns and white fillings. The flat, smooth fabric may be all cotton or a cotton/polyester blend. Chambray gets its name from Cambrai, France, where it was first made.

Dimity: From the Greek word meaning "double thread", Dimity is a cotton lightweight woven fabric (similar to lawn). It is made by weaving two or more yarns as one, and separating them by areas of plain weave, giving a checked or barred effect.

Dotted Swiss: A lightweight cotton or cotton blend fabric woven of fine yarns embellished with woven or flocked small dots.

Flannel: Downy soft, warm fabric that is brushed on one or both sides to raise the nap. Flannel is usually cotton or a cotton blend, woven with a twill or plain weave.

Handkerchief Linen: A lightweight fabric with a plain weave made from the flax plant. Handkerchief linen is similar in luster to batiste but the yarns are more uneven than cotton yarns.

Lawn: A lightweight cotton fabric with a plain weave – crisper than batiste, but not as crisp as organdy.

Nainsook: A soft finished cotton fabric similar to batiste but less transparent and slightly heavier and coarser than lawn.

Organza: A very light, sheer, stiff fabric similar to organdy but made of silk or man-made fiber yarns.

Organdy (Organdie): A very light, sheer, cotton fabric with a plain weave and a finish added to give it a characteristic crispness.

Ramie: A natural fiber fabric made from a nettle plant. Similar in character to handkerchief linen, Ramie has more luster than linen and can be woven into fabric as fine as imported Swiss batiste.

Swiss Batiste: A sheer, transparent fabric with a high luster which is achieved by a special finish and the use of special grades of long staple cotton and Swiss mercerization

Combed Cotton: The finest quality of batiste is made with very thin yarns of combed cotton. All cotton fibers are carded, but only the finest cotton is combed. The combing process removes shorter fibers and impurities from the longer, choice, more desirable fibers. Combed yarns are finer, cleaner, more compact and more even than carded yarns. Fabrics made from combed yarns are tightly woven and more expensive than ordinary cotton cloths.

Mercerized Cotton: Mercerized cotton is stronger, more lustrous, easier to dye and more resistant to mildew. Tension is applied to the fabric, which is then saturated with a cold, caustic soda solution that is later neutralized. The fiber swells permanently, increasing the luster and making it easier to apply other finishes. The process was discovered by accident and patented by John Mercer in England in 1844.

Pima Cotton: is used to make fine knitted goods and expensive woven fabrics. It flourishes in the irrigated fields of Arizona, New Mexico, Texas and California. The best Pima cottons are Egyptian, Sea Island and the US Southwest high-grade cotton.

Piqué: A light to heavyweight cotton fabric with a raised woven design. Piqué has more body than flat fabrics.

Voile: A semi-sheer, dainty fabric made with tightly twisted yarns and a loose plain weave, usually with the same number of yarns in both directions.

Lace and Embroidery Identification

French Galloon

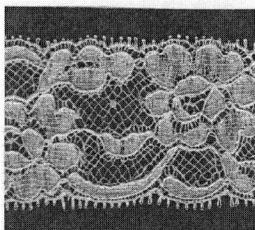

Valenciennes Lace Edgings

French Maline Lace Family

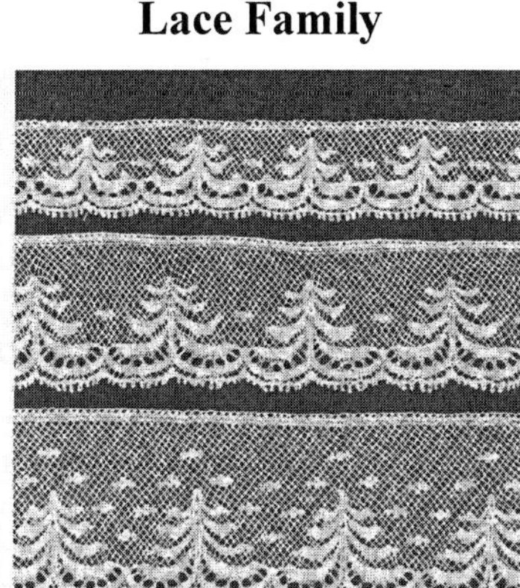

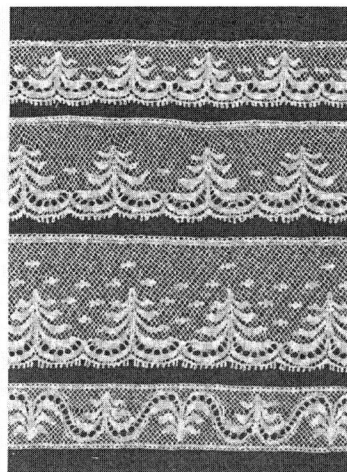

Lace Beading Galloon

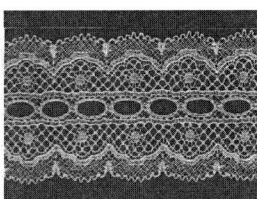

French Lace Beading

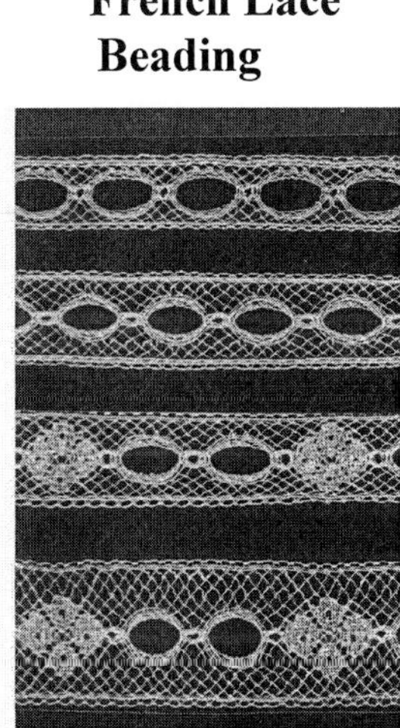

Valenciennes Lace Insertions

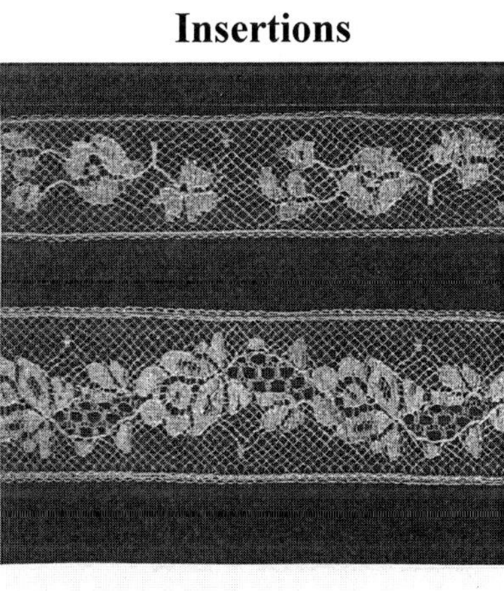

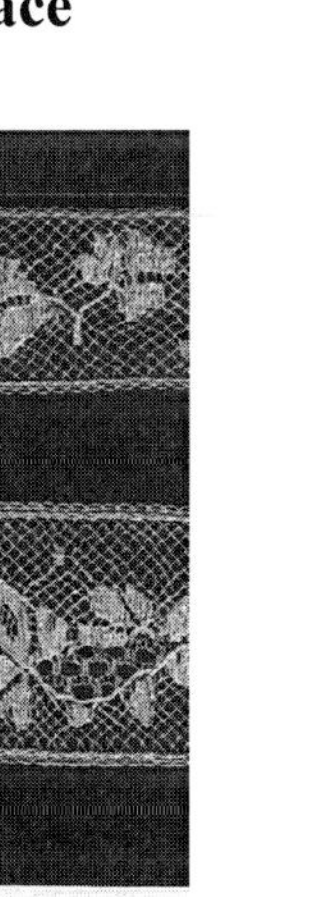

Maline Lace Edgings

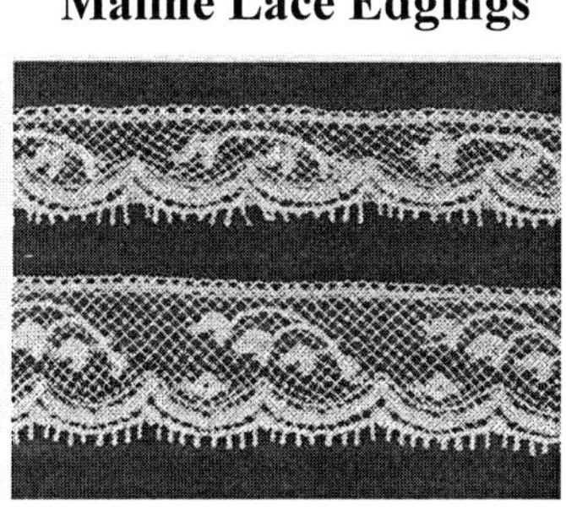

Narrow French Edging

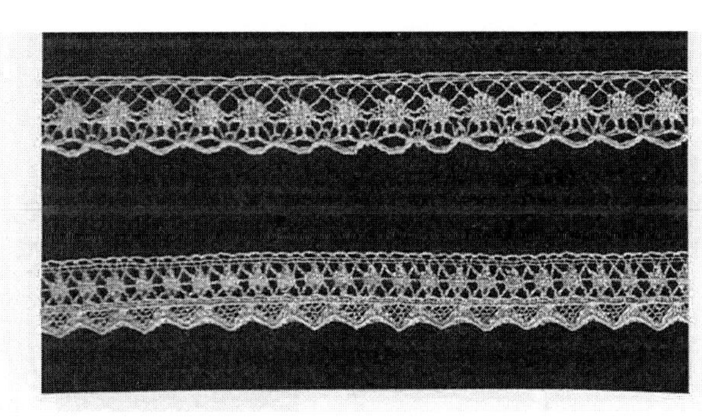

Maline Lace Insertions

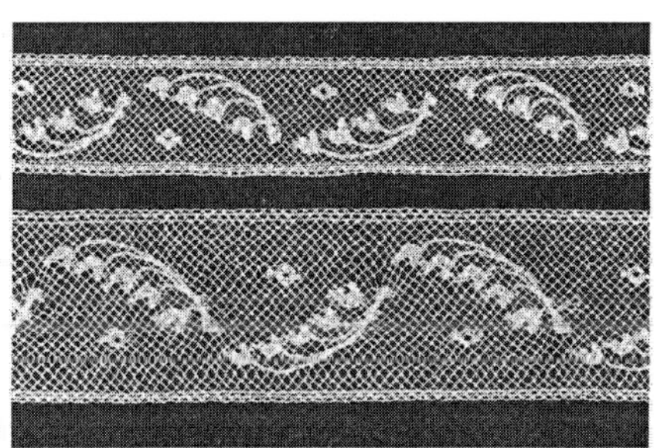

All Embroidery and Lace samples depicted in these two pages are courtesy of **Capitol Imports Inc**. These, and many other families, can be purchased from **www.lynweeks.com** or your favorite needlework store.

Baby Entredeux, Entredeux
Double Entredeux

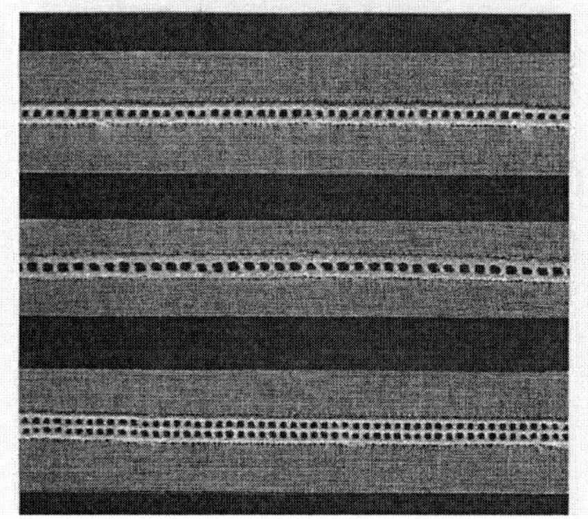

Entredeux, Swiss Beading

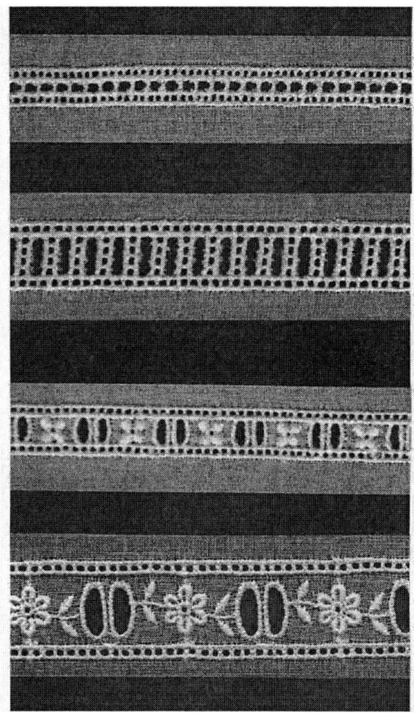

Swiss Insertion; Edging with Entredeux

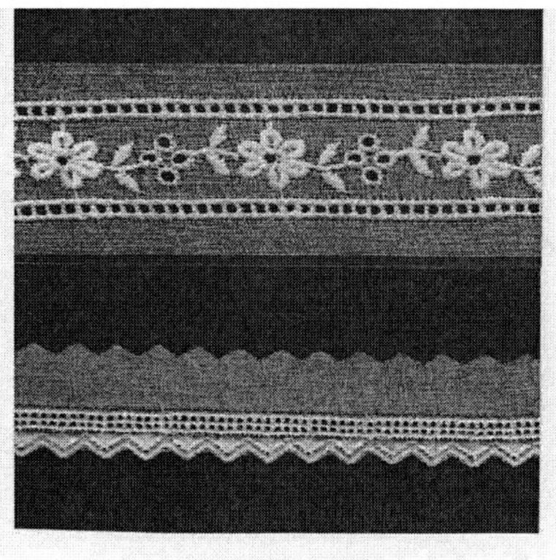

Matching Swiss Insertion and Edging

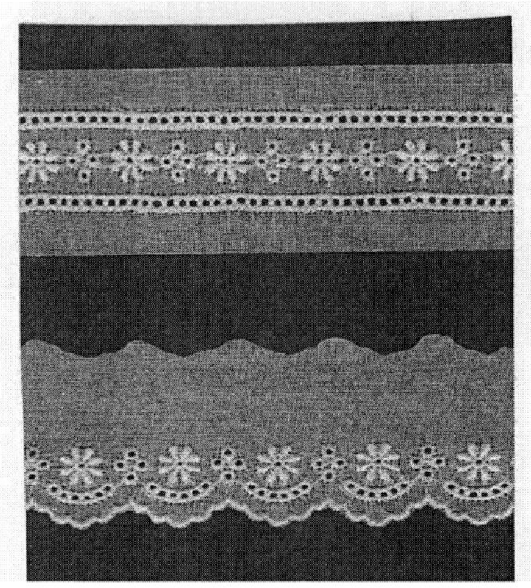

Swiss Embroideries

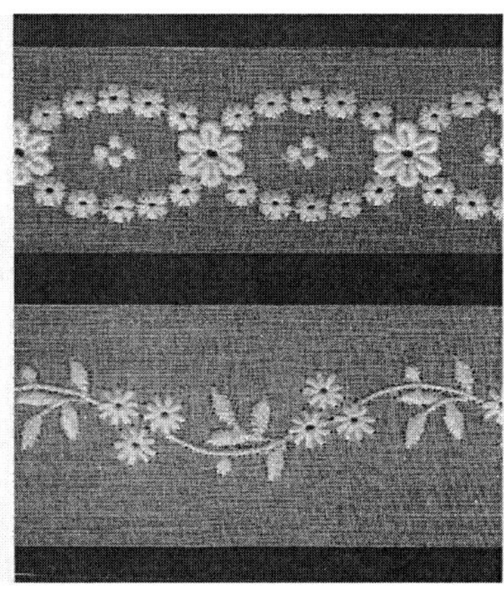

Swiss Edging without Entredeux

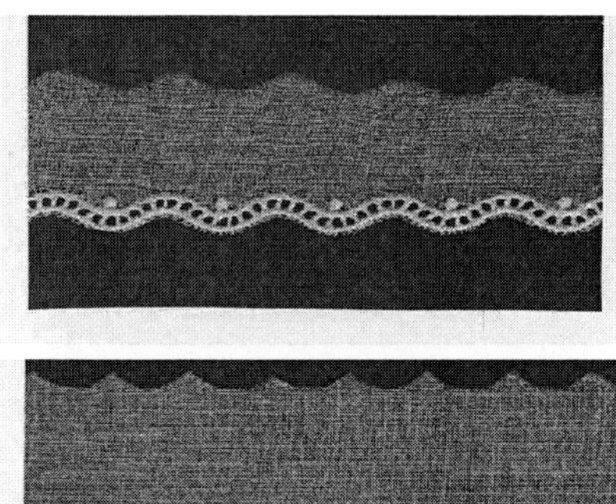

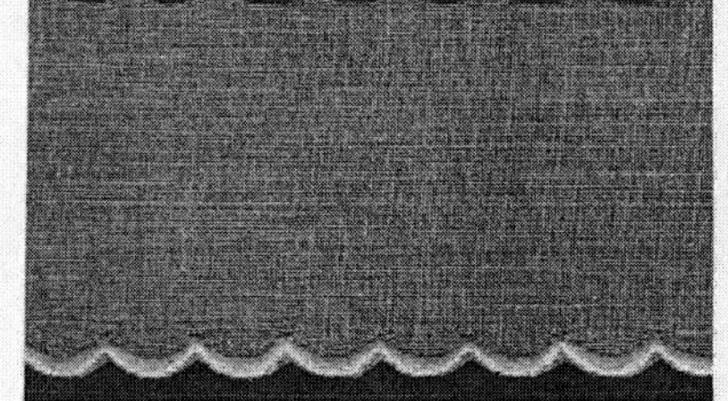

Interfacing

Almost every garment needs the support of interfacing in one area or another. And there are tests and debates on every aspect of interfacing – '***Sew-in or Fusible***', '***Woven, knit or non-woven***', '***Light or heavy weight***'.

Despite the myriad of choices, there is one simple route to more consistent success: **TESTING!**

We could devote several pages of information to the various interfacings for such garments as draped evening gowns, tailored jackets, and couture suits, and provide an in-depth reference tool. However, the content of this book deals primarily with Heirloom and Couture Techniques (for *Everyday Sewing* – babies, children, blouses, nightgowns etc.). It is important that we cover the relevant aspects associated with this type of sewing.

Sew-in or Fusible?

Except when the heat or pressure of fusing would harm the fabric or when the fusing agent shows through sheer fabric, you can almost always choose either fusible or sew-in interfacing for your garment.

Sew-in interfacings provide the widest range from minimal ultralight to very firm and they are easy to test, compared with fusibles which have to be bonded to a sample to be evaluated.

Some of the best sew-in interfacings come from using an additional layer of your garment fabric or such other fabrics as cotton batiste and high quality cotton organdy, or silk organza.

Fusible interfacings that are sold today are not only much more reliable and easier to apply than those of a few years ago; they can also be used on a wider range of fabrics than ever.

I have always been comfortable with the precision process of using sew-in interfacings, but my first choice of interfacing is usually a fusible. Once fused, the fabric and interfacing become one layer, which has multiple benefits:

- one layer is much easier to handle than two layers of fabric that have been basted together
- the finished garment is usually easier to press
- a fusible interfacing can more effectively limit the stretch and ease characteristics of the fashion fabric than can a separate, unattached interfacing layer.

Preshrink before Testing

Shrinkage after construction of either the fabric or the interfacing, or both, is the single most common cause of problems. As a result, the most fundamental issue in selecting iron-on interfacings is that the care requirements for fabric and iron-on interfacing are the same.

Preshrink both the fashion fabric and the interfacing (sew-in or iron-on) to be sure of the results. The feeling and drape of either or both may be changed by pre-shrinking. Make sure you know the care requirements of your interfacing, either from reading the label or from asking when you purchase it.

Your success rate with interfacings will depend on your familiarity with the types of fabric you sew most often, the techniques you use when applying interfacing, how often the garment is laundered or dry-cleaned, and even your pressing equipment.

Preshrinking Sew-ins
If possible, preshrink sew-in interfacings in the same way as you will care for the finished garment. A washable sew-in such as silk organza can be steam-shrunk by holding a steaming iron 2 inches (5 cm) above the interfacing if you want to preserve its unwashed crispness and if the fashion fabric will be dry-cleaned only.

Preshrinking Fusibles
Shrinkage rates vary with how the interfacing is constructed. Both the fabric and the fusible interfacing should be preshrunk. Preshrink washable woven or knit interfacings by placing them folded (to reduce wrinkling) into a sink of warm to hot water for 15 minutes, or until the water cools to room-temperature. Then the water is poured off and the excess is gently squeezed out.

Take care not to wring out or otherwise wrinkle the interfacing, since it can not be pressed out before you use it. Allow woven interfacings to air dry over a shower rod; knit interfacings should be laid out horizontally on a towel to air dry, to avoid stretching out of shape.

Testing the Interfacing

Hold the *sew-in interfacing* in your hand and drape the fashion fabric over it. The garment fabric should be a little heavier than the interfacing and should not show any undesirable change in color or texture.

Draping won't tell you much with *fusible interfacings* because the interfacing always feels crisper when fused to fabric. Make a fused sample at least 6 in. (15 cm) square by following the manufacturer's fusing instructions, and thus avoid bubbling and puckering in the finished garment.

Effective fusing of interfacing requires using a specific amount of **heat**, **moisture**, **pressure**, and **time**. Times may vary from 10 to 15 seconds, specified temperature settings may be silk, wool or cotton, and you may be advised to use either a damp press cloth or a shot of steam – follow the manufacturer's instructions!

Evaluate your Sample

Fold the square in half and evaluate as follows:

- Check for a nice rounded fold. If the interfaced square won't stay folded, it is likely that the interfacing is too heavy. If the fold is too flat, the fusible is probably too light.
- Check the right side of the fused section to ensure there are no undesirable color changes or shading and you have a pleasing result with regard to the weight of the fused fabric.
- Check for any changes in texture on the fabric caused by the bonding agent. This could indicate either a poor fuse or residual shrinkage of fabric or interfacing during fusing.
- The ultimate test is to launder and press the sample just as the garment will be laundered.

Label your test samples and keep them together after your project is finished so you continue to build a library of test swatches for future reference.

Don't be afraid to experiment with cutting the interfacing on the crossgrain or bias to achieve favorable results, or interface a biased area with interfacing on the straight grain to stabilize.

Hints and Tips from my own experience with Iron-on Interfacing

So, after all this basic information and the recommendation to spend precious time 'testing', my interfacing choices are limited to just one or two. I will use a sew-in interfacing (or third fabric layer) on extremely light or sheer fabrics, but for the most part I like to use the lightweight '***German woven cotton, iron-on interfacing***'* that I have tested and used for more than twenty years.

This interfacing is produced in Germany specifically for the high end ready-to-wear shirt manufacturers and does not have a commercial brand name. It is a lightweight, woven interfacing with a very firm bond once it has been fused. From experience it gives body to fine machine sewing projects, without making them stiff, and because it is cotton (not rayon or a blend) will stay permanently fused after repeated laundering.

If you've lost the directions that came with your fusible, try the method summarized below as a good default technique.

1. Set your iron for wool (or the hottest temperature your fabric will stand) and for steam.
2. Place the fabric, wrong side up, on the ironing board and remove all specs of thread or hair. Press the fabric to eliminate wrinkles and to warm it in preparation for fusing.
3. Remove any threads from the interfacing by shaking. Place the interfacing fusible side down, smoothing it into position without stretching it. To ensure that the interfacing is completely preshrunk before fusing steam-shrink it by holding the steaming iron above all surfaces of the interfacing for five seconds. Then lightly fuse a few spots to hold it in position.
4. Cover the interfacing with a dry, see-through press cloth and press firmly on all surfaces for 10 – 12 seconds, without moving the iron (thicker fabrics may require more time). Then lift, overlap the iron placement, and repeat until the entire surface is fused. Allow the garment pieces to cool.
5. Turn the fused fabric to the right side, cover with a dry press cloth, and repeat, pressing each section for 10 – 12 seconds. Allow the fused garment pieces to cool before lifting.

What parts of a garment would I interface?

- The outer layer of a collar, cuffs, pocket flap or romper crotch facing/extension.
- The buttonhole width for extra stability and to maintain a professional look. Cut strips of woven interfacing just large enough to cover the buttonhole area, along the lengthwise grain to prevent stretching; position them between the outer and lining layers, and fuse.
- The outer layer of the front and back yoke of a garment made from fine cotton floral fabric. This adds stability to the yoke, support for smocking (if included) and prevents the floral print from bleeding from the lining through to the outer layer.
- The wrong side of a piece of Swiss embroidery where extra stability is required. Be sure to trim any whiskers from the wrong side of the embroidery before fusing the interfacing.
- Interface the outer layer of a bias cut yoke with interfacing cut on the straight grain.
- I have even interfaced a 2" (5 cm) piece of flat bias with a bias cut interfacing where I needed more body in the fabric being used to bind a baby blanket.

Take time now to experiment with various interfacings to get a feel for how they behave with different fabrics. Although interfacing should be an invisible factor in the finished project, your interfacing know-how will show in the '*Precise and Professional*' garments you produce.

Much of the information on **Interfacing** has been sourced from ***Threads*** magazine, February/March 1998

* To purchase interfacing check my website – **www.lynweeks.com**

Let's talk 'Precise and Professional'

Heirloom sewing was once done only by hand. Many long and loving hours were invested in Christening gowns, trousseaux, dresses, blouses and undergarments.

Heirloom sewing is fun and very forgiving. In effect, you will be 'making fabric' with lots of little bits and pieces – combining fabrics, embroidered insertions, laces, entredeux and tucked panels to make confections of which dreams are made.

Just as it is imperative you understand the balance between fabric, needle size and thread weight, it is also important that you know your machine and that it is set correctly for the task at hand. All sewing machines will have different width and length settings and these settings may need to be very slightly adjusted for the same task with a different lace, or entredeux.

With attention to detail we can duplicate "French Hand Sewing" (as it was known) on our machines and bring back the more genteel times, as well as provide "***Precise and Professional***" heirlooms for the future.

Here are some of the guidelines that should always be a priority in your work.

Pattern Testing – After removing the pattern from the envelope, always check the pattern measurements against those of the child for whom the garment is being made, or against a garment that you know is the correct fit.

- If the pattern is not long enough, or is too long, it must be altered on the *'Lengthen or Shorten'* line. If this is not stated, then assume it can be adjusted at the bottom hemline.
- Check the waist length, if appropriate, and again either lengthen or shorten at the bottom of the waistline.
- Check the shoulder length and either add or subtract at the armhole.
- Remember, that once you start getting into more than simple '*lengthen or shorten*' adjustments, there are usually counter-adjustments to be made. These, then, fall into another category of Pattern Alterations.

Tip*: One of the rules when working with a pattern is to try never to make major changes in any one area – it may be that you simply need a different size pattern.*

Fabrics – There are three kinds of fabrics:
Natural (cotton, linen, wool and silk)
Synthetic (man-made fibers)
Blends (a combination of natural and synthetic)

- It is always recommended that you analyze your fabric requirements and purchase the best quality fabric you can afford. When putting so much time and effort into making beautiful garments that definitely are not "off the rack", you will achieve a better looking and longer lasting garment that truly is an heirloom.
- Better quality fabric will stay looking new after many washings, whereas cheaper fabrics will lose their sheen and body almost immediately. This is because cheap fabrics are presented from the manufacturer with large amounts of sizing, or starch, to make them appear crisp.
- It is always recommended that you preshrink fabrics. If using good quality fabrics and laces for *Heirloom* sewing it is not imperative that you preshrink these pieces; however, you will definitely need to preshrink cheaper cotton and linen fabrics to remove the sizing.
- Before commencing to sew I would recommend that you mist the laces, insertion, embroideries etc. with water and press with steam. This will ensure that they hold their shape once stitched.

Preparation Hints

Fabric has <u>three</u> grainlines: The ***warp*** grain (lengthwise or strongest grain)
The ***weft*** grain (cross grain or weakest grain – selvage to selvage)
The ***bias*** grain (the grain with the most memory) –
*Refer to **Using the Bias***

- The woven edge on the lengthwise grain is called the selvage. This is woven more tightly than the body of the fabric and should be removed before the pattern pieces are laid out for cutting. Be sure, however, to mark and maintain the lengthwise grain.
- It is imperative that you cut your garment in the direction indicated by the grainline arrows on each pattern piece. A garment will not hang correctly and could, quite possibly, be ruined by neglecting to get the warp and weft grains in the correct position.
- Be sure to square your fabric before positioning pattern pieces. The best way to commence is to pull a weft thread at each end and cut on this pulled thread. Fabric that has been torn is quite often out of square and must be pulled on the short, opposite diagonal ends to straighten. Square the fabric on a large pressing surface and steam well.
- Pay particular attention to the nap or pile and/or one-way design of your fabric so that your pattern pieces are all laid in the same direction if necessary. Always match designs and plaids before cutting.

Machine Maintenance – clean and oil your machine on a regular basis. Mechanical machines should be oiled according to your machine instruction manual. Electronic and computer sewing machines should be serviced regularly by a professional.

Threads – for best results use 100% Cotton thread on all natural fiber fabrics
Mettler 60/2 or DMC 50 for embroidery/zigzag stitching and construction of fine fabrics
Mettler 50/3, DMC 30 or Cotona 50 for seams of medium-weight fabrics OR
Coats and Clark's Dual Duty Extra Fine thread for garment construction
Tanne 80 for hemstitching (Venetian stitch, Parisian stitch etc.)

***Tip**: For correct tension, always use the same thread on both the top spool and the bobbin.*

Needles – Change the needle after approximately 8-12 hours of sewing time
Universal System 130/705H
No. 60/8, 65/9 or 70/10 for fine fabrics
No. 70/10 or 80/12 for slightly heavier cottons, soft winter fabrics
Twin Needles 1.6/70; 2.0/75 for fine fabrics
2.0/80; 2.5/80 for slightly heavier cottons and soft winter fabrics
*Refer to **Creating with Tucks,** Twin Needle Tucks*
Wing Needles used for decorative stitching such as pinstitching. I use and recommend a #110 Jeans needle for this type of sewing as it does not damage the fibers of fabric or lace.

***Tip**: You will need to change the needle more often when sewing with tear-away or stabilizer backing as the paper dulls the needle more rapidly.*

The techniques I use are those I have found to be the neatest and strongest. Depending on the fabric and trims used, you may need to change techniques from one project to the next, and I have included more than one method wherever possible.

Always sew a sample first and make note of all settings and adjustments. Machine settings vary from one machine to another, even if they are identical models, therefore making samples is even more important.

As you go through the pages of this book, I suggest you tape or staple your sample piece to the appropriate page, making note of the fabric type, presser foot, stitch settings, thread etc. Remember, by experimenting with your own inspirations, you will open a whole new world of sewing.

Let's talk 'Couture'

Couture Sewing can be thought of in many ways – from the Couture houses of Paris to the catwalks in Milan. It conjures up visions of the most expensive fabrics being used in the most elaborate ways and being worn by the most perfect figures.

But "Couture" is best described as simply the **ultimate** in quality sewing. There are no rules for how something should *always* be done, but the recognition that there are alternative techniques.

Couture is almost a way of life: it means attention to detail, from selection of pattern and fabric to the final stitch taken. "Couture, for the home sewer, requires time, patience and refinement of basic skills, and the commitment to make a garment to the best of your ability".

Here are some guidelines that should always be a priority in your work:

- **Maintain Accuracy in cutting, pressing and stitching**
- **Reduce Bulk**
- **Know when (and when not) to stabilize and clip seams**
- **Accept the fact that pressing goes hand-in-hand with quality sewing**
- **Believe that the final garment will give 'reward for effort'**
- **Above all – enjoy the process as well as the result**

Preshrinking

Everything involved in the construction of a garment should be preshrunk. The development of a couture garment relies totally on pressing, shaping, shrinking and stretching to permanently shape the finished garment..

If the garment is going to be washed, wash the fabric in the washing machine with detergent to remove any surface-finish.

Have the drycleaner steam press the fabric if the finished garment is to be dry-cleaned.

Grain

Grain direction is paramount in your preparations, whether it is the lengthwise, crosswise or bias grain that plays the key to the particular garment. You cannot expect the final garment to hang perfectly if the grain of the fabric has not been established at the beginning.

To prepare fabric, pull a thread until it breaks, then begin cutting across the width of fabric on this pulled thread. At the 'break-point' pick up another thread and continue with the *pull-and-cut* method for cutting a straight line.

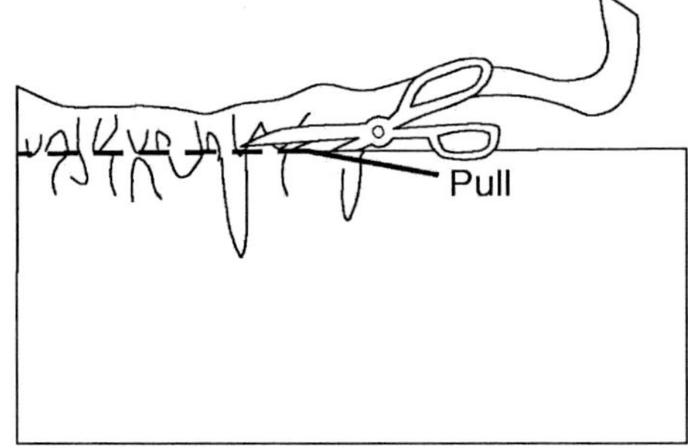
Pull

To square the fabric, lay the fabric out so that the crosswise and lengthwise grains are at **perfect** right angles. A grid cutting board or a T-square is helpful for this.

Marking
Just as important as the grain is the marking of all notches, seam intersections, darts, pleats, grainlines, center front, center back, and buttonhole and pocket placement from the pattern to the fabric.

Choose from the following marking tools and methods:

- Tailors chalk or chalk marking pencil for temporary marks
- Dressmakers carbon that comes in a variety of colors – use on the wrong side of the fabric only and apply by way of a tracing wheel
- Chalk or blue-lead mechanical pencils, water-soluble markers or air erase markers – always test these on your fabric before commencing
- Thread tracing by taking a long stitch, then short, then another long stitch.

Couture Seams
There are two rules for seams that sit inconspicuously and without puckering:

- Do not backstitch! Start and stop each seam by commencing with a stitch length of approximately 0.5 to 0.75 (20 stitches per inch/8 stitches per centimeter) for the distance of the seam allowance. This method allows for a single, yet secure, row of stitches at the beginning and end of each seam.

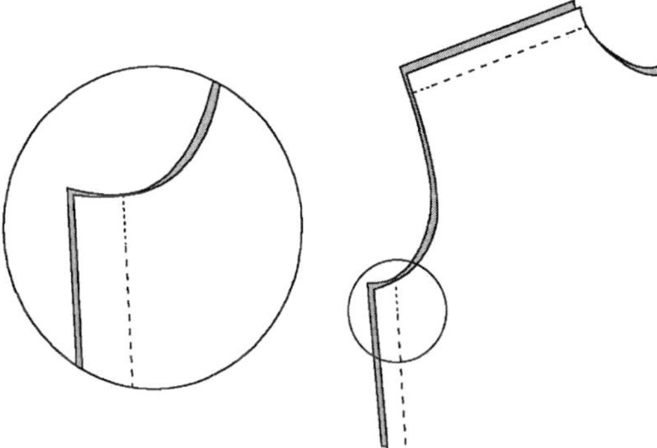

*Tip: It is important for accurate seams that you hold both top and bobbin threads as you commence stitching, to avoid the fabric being pulled into the bobbin casing. This rule is **absolutely essential** when working with laces, entredeux and embroideries for heirloom projects.*

- Always hold your work taut from in front of the presser foot as well as from behind. You are not pulling the seam through, but rather keeping tension on it to eliminate any puckers.

Gathering
More gathering rows are better than less! Once you have inserted the <u>three</u> rows of gathering threads, isolate the <u>bobbin threads</u> at each end, or the threads with more tension (taut), and tie them together in a simple overhand knot. This is a good habit to ensure you always *hold* the knotted group and *draw up* the bobbin threads in one single movement, thus avoiding locking the upper and bobbin threads by not consistently gathering with the same set of threads.

*Tip: The golden rule for gathering is **"The finer the fabric, the shorter the stitch length"**. To gather fine batiste I use a stitch length of not more than 3.0.*

Flexibility
Don't be afraid to change thread type and machine feet often. For example, I use polyester and/or colored thread for gathering but <u>never</u> for construction of fine fabrics. You will also find that many feet are named, but have a more beneficial use for a different purpose. Experiment and make note of which feet you have used to give the more professional result.

From accurate preparation and accurate construction comes the final "***couture***" garment.

Finished Measurement Chart

These suggested measurements are recommended as a guide ONLY. There is no industry standard for children, and those below represent a balance from such text books as *Patternmaking for Fashion Design* and *Childrenswear Design* – refer to the ***Bibliography***.

Size Inches (cm)	**6 Mo.**	**1 year**	**2**	**3**	**4**
Front Yoke across armscye center	8½ (21.5)	9 (23)	9 (23)	9½ (24)	9½ (24)
Back Yoke across armscye center	8¾ (22)	9¼ (23.5)	9½ (24)	9¾ (25)	9¾ (25)
Natural Shoulder neck to shoulder bone	2⅝ (6.75)	2¾ (7)	3 (7.75)	3⅛ (8)	3¼ (8.25)
Neck Jewel neckline	10 (25.5)	10½ (27)	11 (28)	11¼ (28.5)	11½ (29)
Length to Waist measured from neck	7½ (19)	8 (20.5)	8½ (21.5)	9 (23)	9½ (24)
Dress Length measured from neck	14½ (37)	16 (40.5)	18½ (47)	21 (53)	24 (61)
Long Sleeve Length shoulder to wrist with a bent elbow	11 (28)	11½ (29)	12½ (32)	13½ (34)	14½ (37)
Wrist loose for a cuff	5⅜ (13.75)	5½ (14)	5¾ (14.5)	6 (15.25)	6¼ (16)
Short Sleeve Band loose for a cuff	6¾ Girl 7¼ Boy	7½ (19) 8 (20.5)	7¾ (19.75) 8¼ (21)	8¼ (21) 8¾ (22.25)	8¾ (22.25) 9¼ (23.5)
Waist circumference at natural waistline	19 Girl 19½ Boy	19¼(49) 19¾ (50)	20 (51) 20½ (52)	20½ (52) 21 (53.5)	21 (53.5) 21½ (54.5)

Size Inches (cm)	**5**	**6**	**7**	**8**
Front Yoke across armscye center	9¾ (24.75)	10¼ (26)	11 (28)	11½ (29)
Back Yoke across armscye center	10 (25.5)	10½ (27)	11½ (29)	11¾ (30)
Natural Shoulder neck to shoulder bone	3⅜ (8.5)	3½ (9)	3⅝ (9.25)	3¾ (9.5)
Neck jewel neckline	11¾ (30)	12 (30.5)	13 (33)	13 (33)
Length to Waist measured from neck	9¾ (24.75)	10½ (26.75)	11¼ (28.5)	11¾ (30)
Dress Length measured from neck	25½ (65)	27 (68.5)	28½ (72.5)	30 (76)
Long Sleeve Length shoulder to wrist with a bent elbow	15 (38)	16¼ (41)	16¾ (42.5)	17½ (44.5)
Wrist loose for a cuff	6¼ (16)	6¼ (16)	6¾ (17)	6¾ (17)
Short Sleeve Band loose for a cuff	9¼ (23.5)	9½ (24)	9½ (24)	9¾ (25)
Waist circumference at natural waistline	21½ (55)	22 (56)	22½ (57)	23 (58.5)

Finished Measurement Chart

This page may be photocopied as needed for personal use only. Insert the child's name and measurements for easy reference.

Name:

Size **Inches (cm)**	**6 Mo.**	**1 year**	**2**	**3**	**4**
Front Yoke across armscye center					
Back Yoke across armscye center					
Natural Shoulder neck to shoulder bone					
Neck jewel neckline					
Length to Waist measured from neck					
Dress Length measured from neck					
Long Sleeve Length shoulder to wrist with a bent elbow					
Wrist loose for a cuff					
Short Sleeve Band loose for a cuff					
Waist circumference at natural waistline					

Size **Inches (cm)**	**5**	**6**	**7**	**8**
Front Yoke across armscye center				
Back Yoke across armscye center				
Natural Shoulder neck to shoulder bone				
Neck jewel neckline				
Length to Waist measured from neck				
Dress Length measured from neck				
Long Sleeve Length shoulder to wrist with a bent elbow				
Wrist loose for a cuff				
Short Sleeve Band loose for a cuff				
Waist circumference at natural waistline				

General Information

MELD
Press the stitching line with steam to settle the machine stitches into the fibers of the fabric. Always meld, or press, each seam before pressing the seam open or attaching another part of the garment.

STAYSTITCH
Stitch a scant ⅛″ (3mm) from seam line within the seam allowance with a stitch length of 2.0.

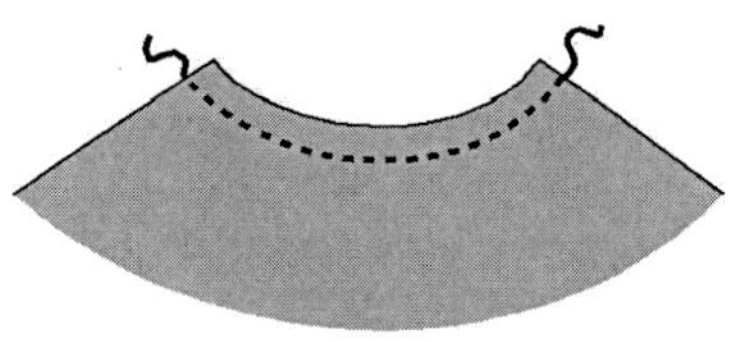

GRADING
Trim the seam allowance and interfacing in layers close to the stitching. The seam allowance closest to the outside of the garment will be the one with the widest allowance.

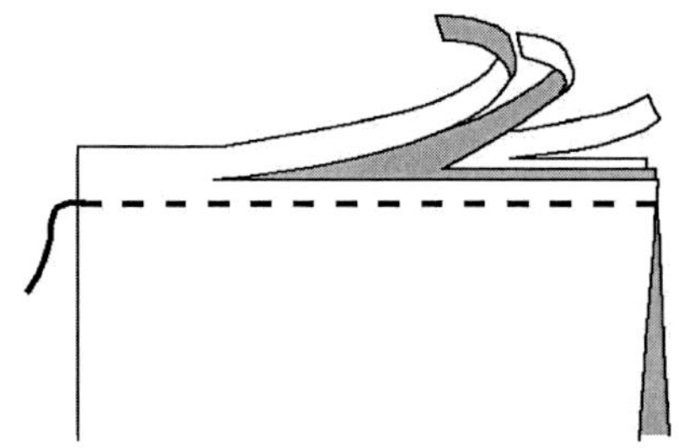

UNDERSTITCH
After grading and clipping the seam allowance, press the facing away from garment, onto the seam allowance. With facing uppermost, stitch close to the seam through the facing and the seam allowance.

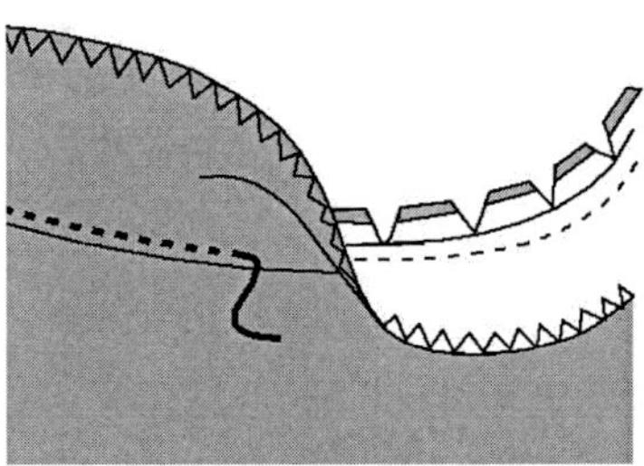

***Tip**: When understitching a curved line, always pull the seam against the curve to avoid re-stitching the allowance and thus eliminating any flexibility.*

TOPSTITCH
With right side uppermost, stitch ¼″ (6mm), or desired amount, from the seam line or finished edge, using the presser foot or an edge-joining foot as a guide.

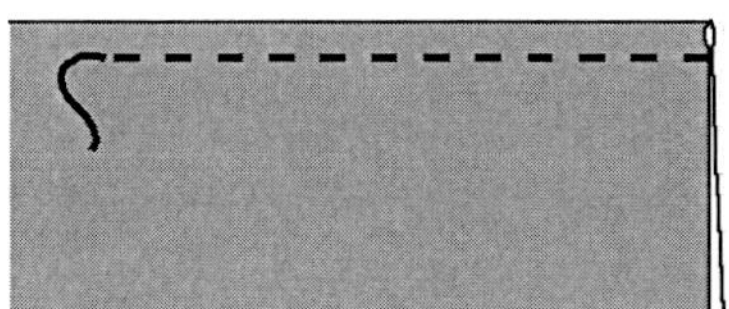

***Tip**: Don't be afraid to use a heavier and/or contrasting thread to highlight this design feature. You could also try a longer stitch length or topstitching stitch on embroidery machines.*

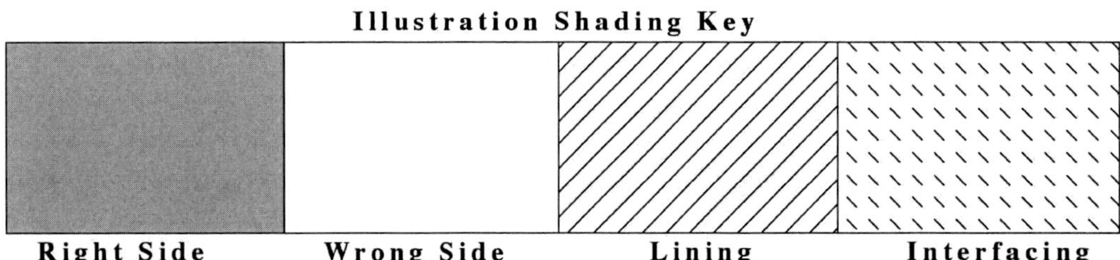
Illustration Shading Key
Right Side
Wrong Side
Lining
Interfacing

FINE ROLLED HEM
(Roll and Whip)

The 'Roll and Whip' technique is used for best results on fine fabrics such as batiste, voile, lawn etc. It is used to add strength and a neat finish to the raw edge of fabric and trimmings.

Before commencing to stitch a fine rolled hem always neaten the straight fabric edge by pulling a thread and cutting off the excess threads.

To ensure a fine, even roll, the left needle swing will need to stitch approximately 3/16" (5mm) onto the fabric and the right needle swing will completely clear the edge of the fabric. You will need to test your machine to determine a position, stitch setting and machine foot that gives a nice roll.

Place the edge of the fabric under the presser foot slightly to the right of center.

Holding the machine threads firmly, the first stitch should go down into the fabric on the left.

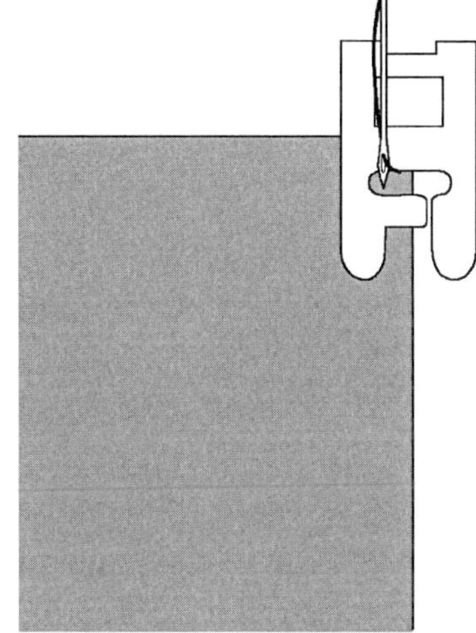

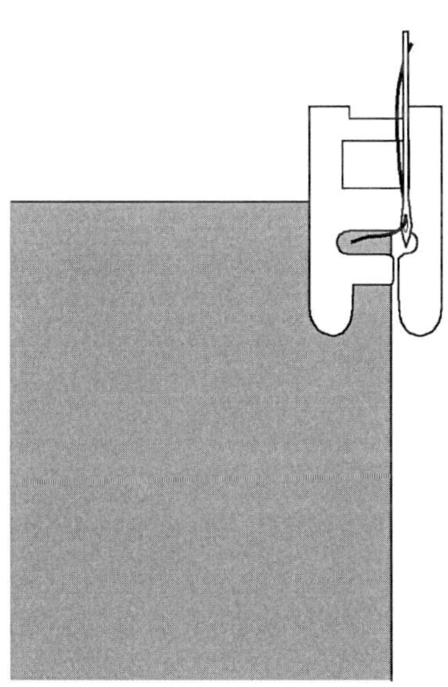

As the needle stitches to the right it will clear the fabric edge, causing the fabric to roll.

As you experiment with varying fabric samples you will note that different weights of fabric require different width and length settings.

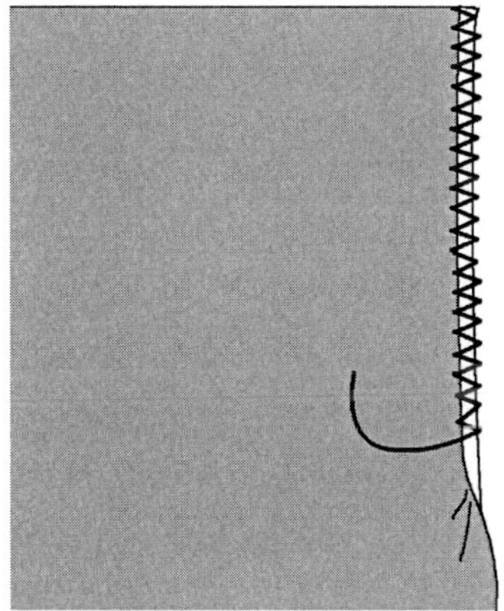

SUGGESTED MACHINE SETTING
Zigzag Stitch:
W: 2.5 to 3.0
L: 0.75 to 1.0
Needle Position: Center
Foot: Buttonhole (not automatic)

For a fluted effect, place very fine clear fishing line or nylon thread to the left of the presser foot center and the fabric edge to the right of center - the fishing line will be encased as the fabric folds over it. Slightly pull the fishing line while sewing. Be careful not to use a slightly colored line as this will show through the fabric – 20lb. breaking strain gives the best result.

FINE ROLLED HEM WITH GATHERS

Apart from the traditional method of sewing rows of long machine stitches, there are three accepted methods for gathering fabric using heirloom techniques. The basic 'Roll and Whip' settings that you have just established will be used for each of these methods.

Before commencing to stitch a fine rolled hem always neaten the straight fabric edge by pulling a thread and cutting off the excess threads.

TECHNIQUE #1

Insert a row of straight basting stitches ⅛" (3mm) from the edge of the fabric. Do not remove the tails from the basting stitches. You may want to use a stronger thread for this step.

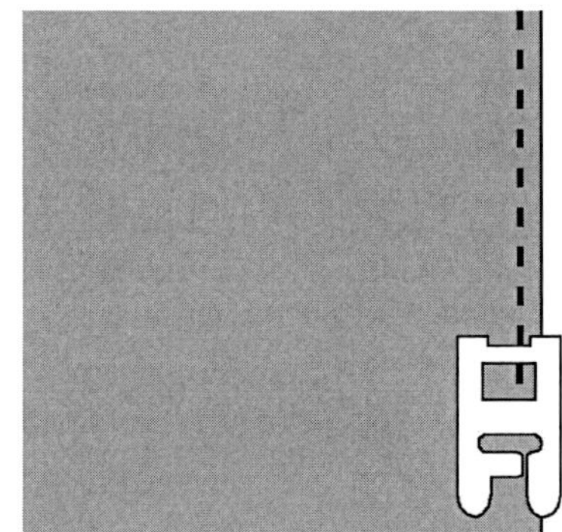

SUGGESTED MACHINE SETTING
Straight Stitch:
L: 2.5 to 3.0
Needle Position: Center
Foot: Basic Sewing

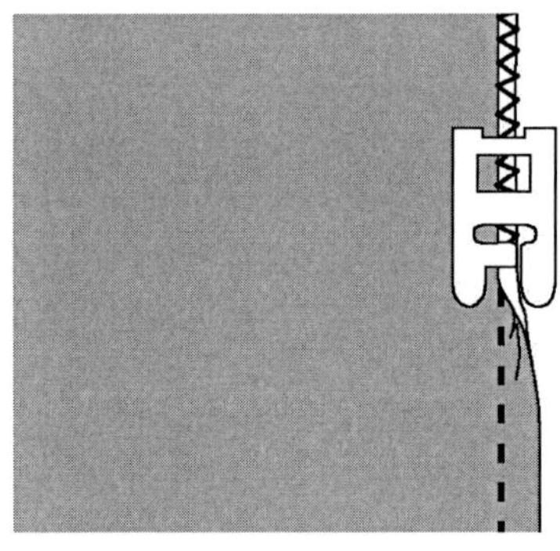

Change to a fine machine embroidery thread and carefully zigzag over this row of stitches so that the left swing of the needle clears the basting line and the right swing is off the edge of the fabric. The basting stitches will be encased in the roll.

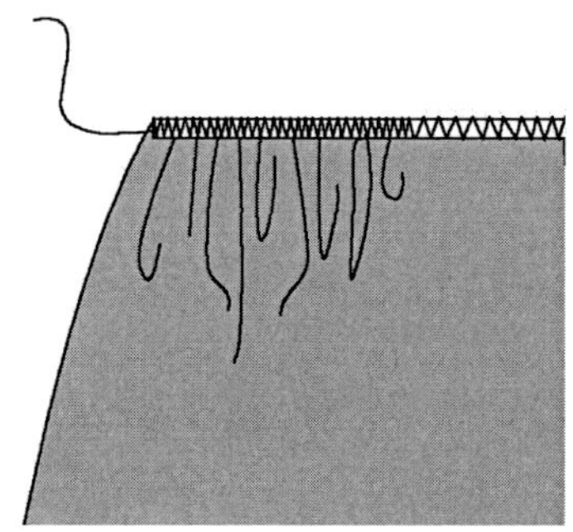

Pull the <u>bobbin thread only</u> to gather the fabric to the required measurement.

***Tip**: On long lengths of fabric to be gathered, gather from both ends, thus causing less strain on the thread encased in the zigzag.*

SUGGESTED MACHINE SETTING
Zigzag Setting:
W: 2.5 to 3.0
L: .75 to 1.0
Needle Position: Center
Foot: Buttonhole (not automatic) or Pintuck

TECHNIQUE #2

Replace the row of machine basting stitches (as in Technique #1) with a length of quilting thread that matches the color of the fabric. Be sure to work with a length that is slightly longer than the length of fabric to be gathered.

***Tip**: There is no need to cut the thread off the spool unless you only need a short length.*

Tie a large knot in one end. Hold the quilting thread next to the fabric edge as you place the fabric and thread under the presser foot.

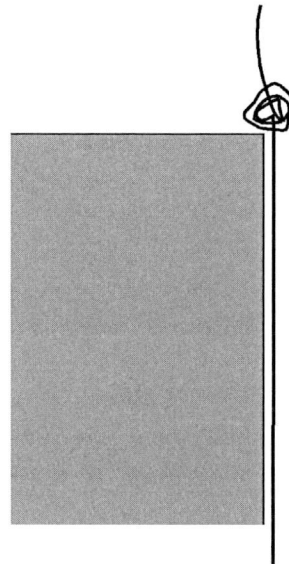

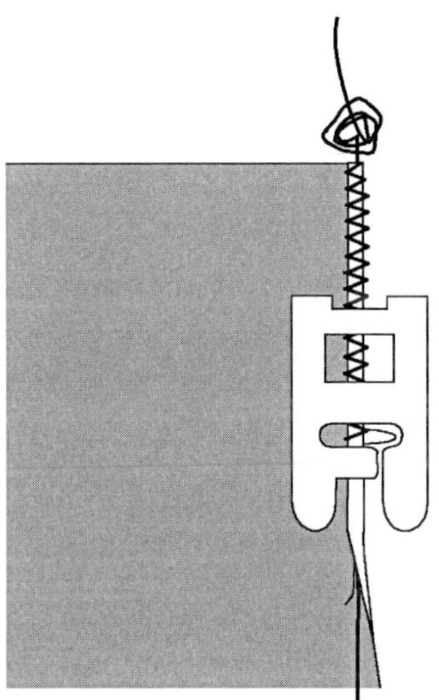

Continue to hold the thread along the raw edge of the fabric, keeping both taut with your left hand.

Zigzag over the thread causing the raw edge of fabric to roll over the thread encasing it in a roll.

Refer to the techniques for a ***Fine Rolled Hem.***

Using this method, you can pull the quilting thread and gather from both ends, without the worry of breaking the gathering thread.

This is an quick and very reliable method when gathering long pieces for ruffles, etc.

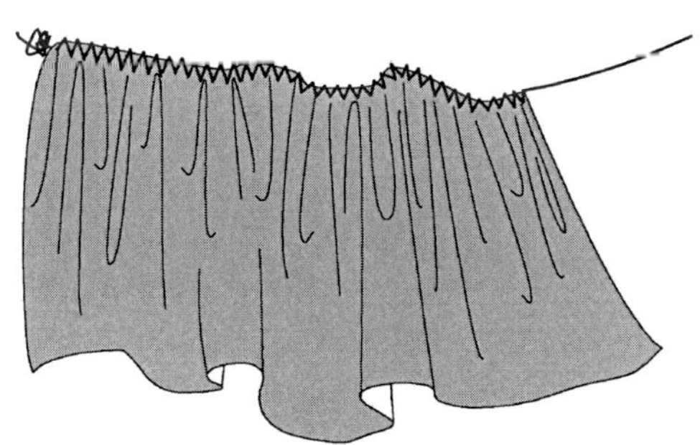

SUGGESTED MACHINE SETTING
Zigzag Setting:
W: 2.5 to 3.0
L: 0.75 to 1.0
Needle Position: Center
Foot: Buttonhole (not automatic) or Pintuck

TECHNIQUE #3

While the sewing machine is still threaded, pull a length of both the top thread and the bobbin thread toward you for the full length of the fabric to be rolled, whipped and gathered.

Hold the two threads close to the edge of the fabric as you place the fabric under the presser foot.

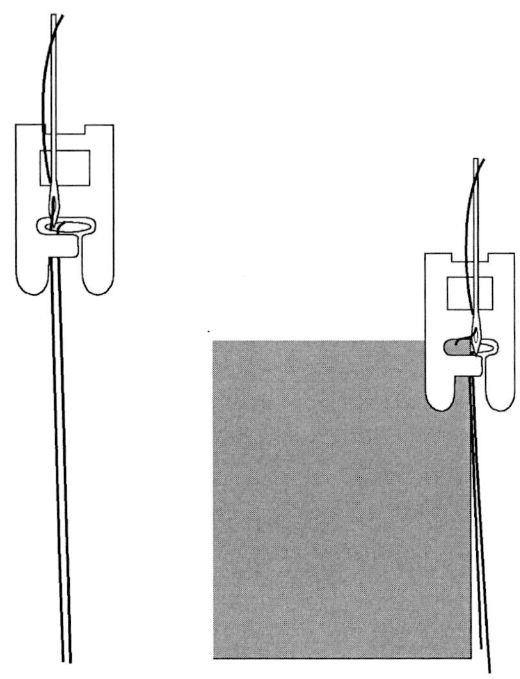

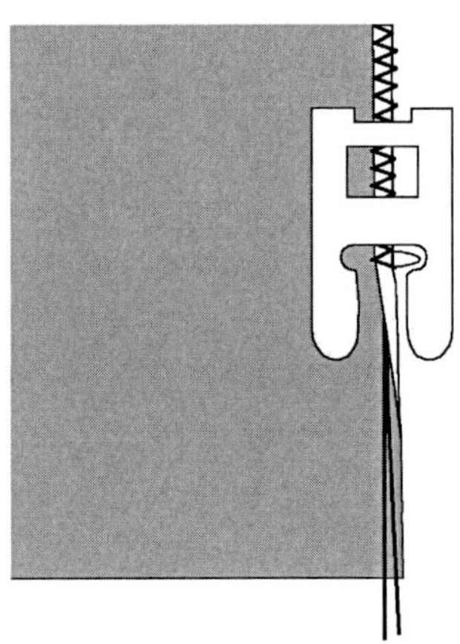

Make a fine rolled hem by zigzagging over both threads so that the left swing is approximately 3/16" (5mm) onto the fabric and the right needle swing will completely clear the edge of the fabric.

Pull both threads and gently gather the fabric to the required measurement. Distribute the gathers evenly.

This method works best for shorter lengths of fabric as you will be putting the strain of gathering onto fine cotton thread, and are only able to gather from one end.

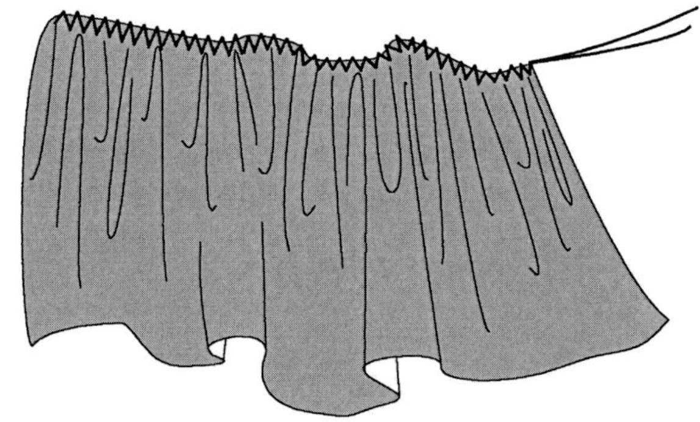

SUGGESTED MACHINE SETTING

Zigzag Setting:
W: 2.5 to 3.0
L: 0.75 to 1.0
Needle Position: Center
Foot: Buttonhole (not automatic) or Pintuck

ROLLED HEM WITH LACE

This method for attaching lace to fabric can be used when extra strength is required and when it is not desired to have visible stitches on the front of your work. The best presentation is obtained when this technique is worked on the straight grain.

Roll and whip the straight edge of fabric.
*Refer to technique for a **Fine Rolled Hem***

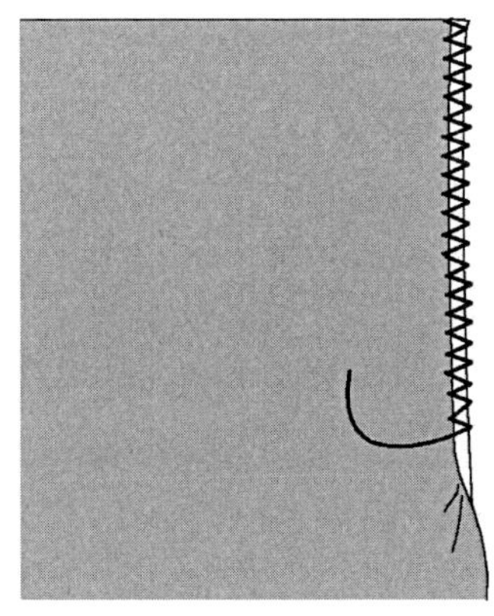

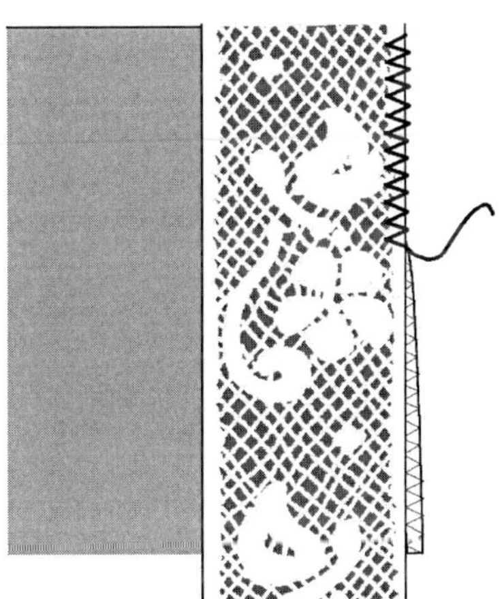

With right sides together and the lace on top, butt the lace heading up to, but <u>not on top of</u>, the rolled and whipped edge.

Zigzag with the left needle swing going just over the lace heading and the right needle swing off the edge of the rolled fabric.

Note: *The zigzag will pull the rolled edge and lace together as you stitch.*

SUGGESTED MACHINE SETTING
Zigzag Setting:
W: 2.5 to 3.0
L: 0.75 to 1.0
Needle Position: Center
Foot: Buttonhole (not automatic) or Pintuck

ATTACHING LACE TO FABRIC
(creating a Rolled Edge)

This method for attaching lace to fabric is very quick and best used for decorative purposes, or where there will not be a lot of strain on the project.

Before commencing to stitch a fine rolled hem always neaten the straight fabric edge by pulling a thread and trimming off the excess threads. Mist the fabric and the lace with water and press with steam.

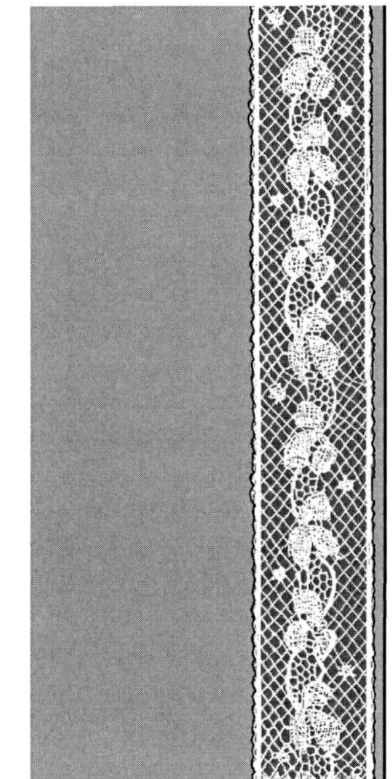

With the right side of the fabric facing up place the edge of fabric to the right of center under the foot.

Position the edge of the lace, wrong side facing up (right side facing the fabric), under the center line of the foot.

> ***Tip**: There should be approximately ⅛" (3mm) of the fabric edge showing.*

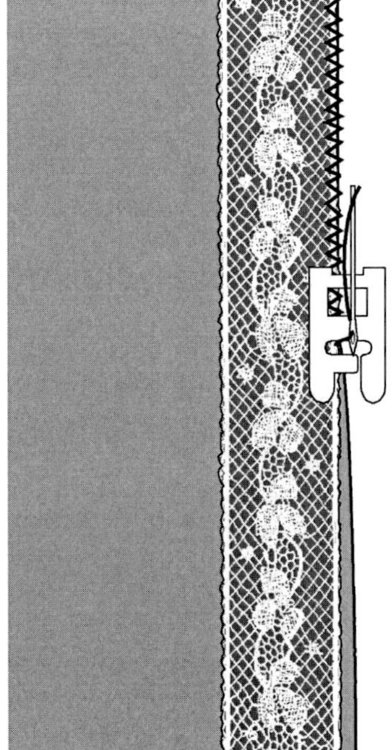

Zigzag with the left needle swing going just over the lace heading and the right swing off the edge of the fabric.

Hold the fabric taut from behind and in front of the foot as you sew.

Meld the stitches and press the rolled seam away from the lace.

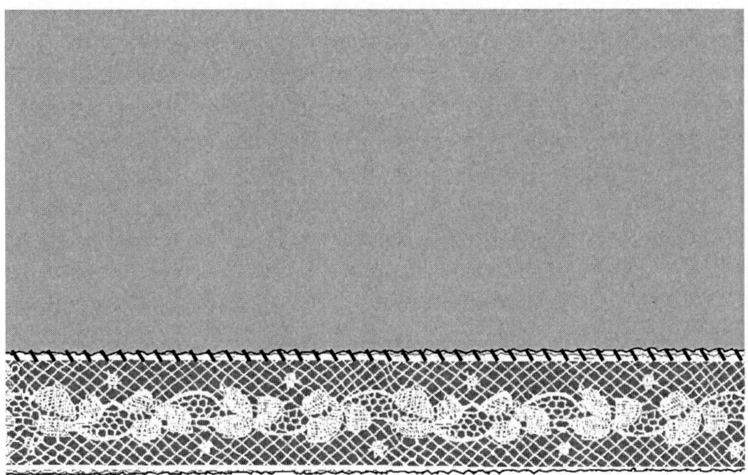

This method may show tiny stitches on the front of the work once the seam is pressed behind the fabric.

Notes

ATTACHING GATHERED LACE TO FABRIC
(creating a Rolled Edge)

The strongest method for attaching *Gathered Lace to Fabric* is to join the two with entredeux. However, there are times when it may be necessary to attach the lace directly onto the fabric.

Gather the lace by pulling the heading threads, <u>one at a time</u>. I start with the top 'loopy' thread (usually the strongest thread) and pull this thread taut until the lace gathers and is approximately the length required.

Then very carefully pull all remaining threads, one at a time, distributing the gathers evenly.

***Tip**: It is always a good idea to gather from both ends toward the middle wherever possible.*

This method for gathering lace takes longer than just pulling one thread, but it creates a firm 'ribbon' of threads which will lay very flat on the fabric.

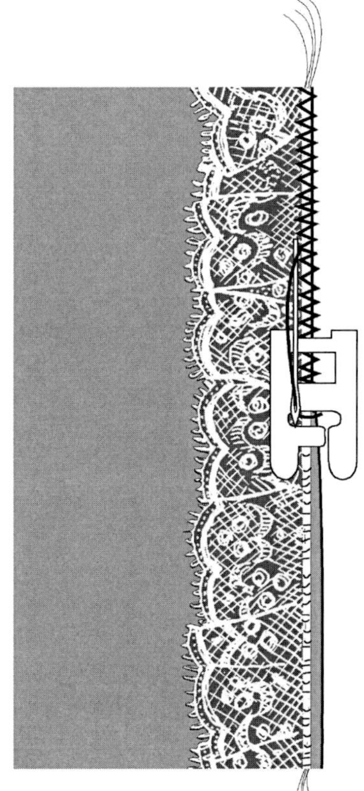

Place the edge of the gathered lace approximately ⅛" (3mm) from the neatened raw edge of the fabric, right sides together.

Set the width of the zigzag so that it goes off the edge of the fabric on the right and just over the lace heading on the left.

*Refer to technique for **Attaching Lace to Fabric***

The edge of the fabric will roll up and over the heading of the lace.

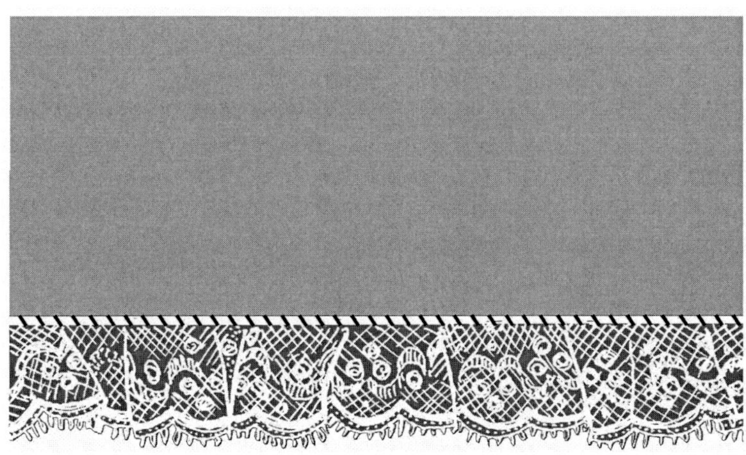

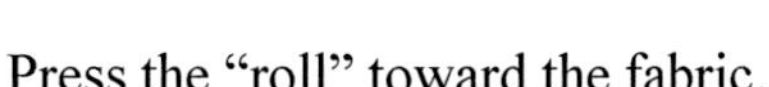

Press the "roll" toward the fabric.

WORKING WITH ENTREDEUX

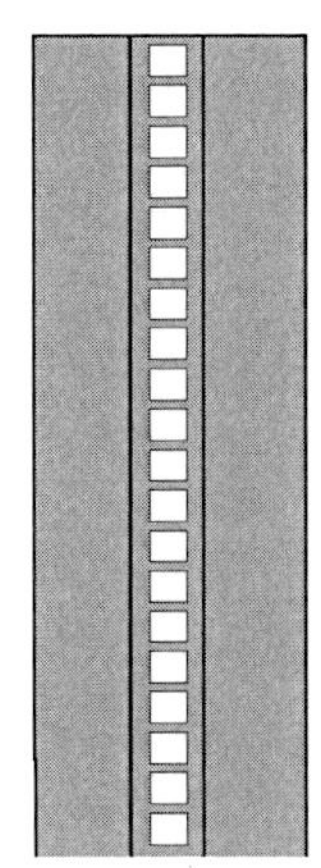

Before beginning a project incorporating entredeux it is important to test your machine settings. Cut a piece of entredeux approximately 4" (10 cm) long. Do not cut the batiste off either side while testing your stitch width and length settings.

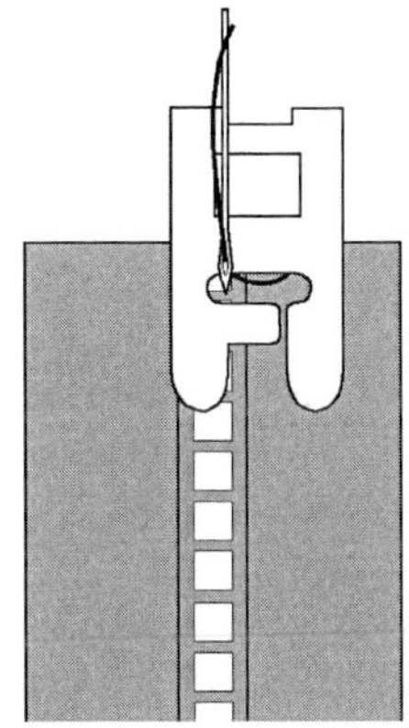

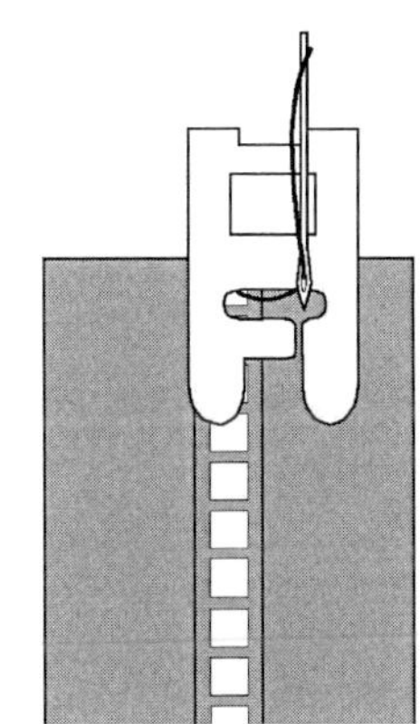

Holding the entredeux taut from in front and behind the presser foot, and with a zigzag setting on your machine, begin with the needle in one of the entredeux holes and make your first stitch into the batiste fabric

Stitch very slowly; paying particular attention to ensure the needle goes into a new hole with each left swing. The right needle swing will be positioned on the batiste.

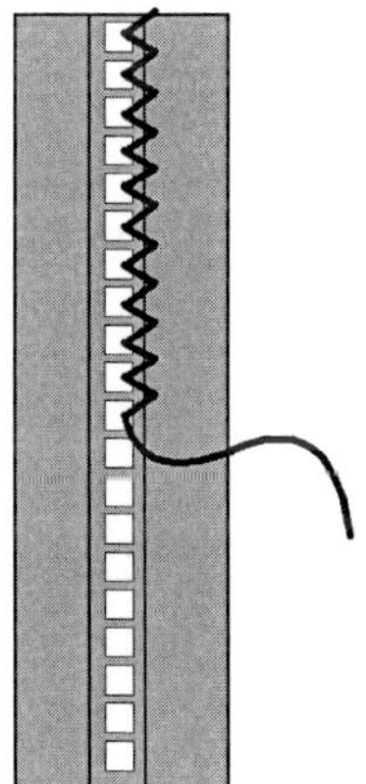

SUGGESTED MACHINE SETTING
Zigzag Stitch: (for basic-size entredeux)
W: Approximately 2.5
L: .Approximately 1.0

Watch carefully as the needle zigzags back and forth into the hole and onto the batiste. No matter how much you are able to fine tune your machine, there will come a time when the entredeux holes have worked themselves out of synchronization with your machine setting. When you notice this occurring, stop stitching, lift the presser foot and reposition the needle to continue with the correct zigzag sequence.

***Tip**: I like to hold the entredeux taut with my thumb positioned in front of the presser foot and third finger behind the foot – don't stretch or pull; just keep it taut! Imagine it feeding under the foot like a piece of cardboard – if (and when) the zigzag misses a hole, fabric and thread will not be dragged into the bobbin casing if you are holding it firm.*

ATTACHING ENTREDEUX TO FABRIC

This method for attaching entredeux to fabric creates the strongest and most stable join.

Do not trim the batiste from the entredeux. Lightly spray the entredeux piece with water and press with steam.

***Tip**: Trim the seam allowance of the garment to the same measurement as the batiste fabric beside the entredeux holes. It may be necessary to trim both the batiste <u>and</u> the garment fabric, as different entredeux have differing widths of batiste – sometimes even on the same piece.*

This trimming will allow you to match the raw edges so you do not have to accommodate varying seam allowances.

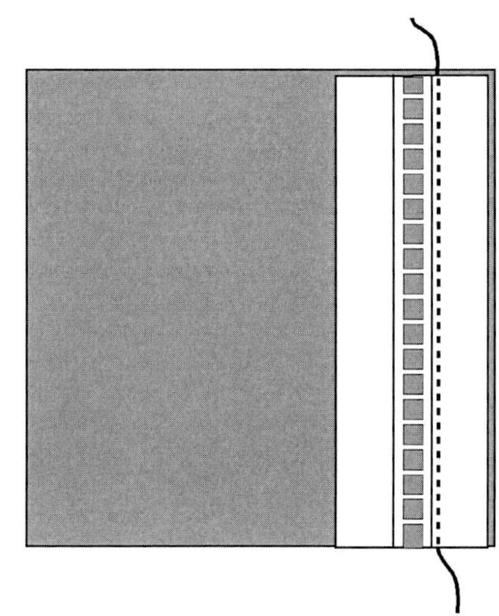

Place the edge of the fabric and the untrimmed entredeux with right sides together – the raw edges will be even.

Stitch with short straight machine stitches along the right hand side of the entredeux, or *'in the ditch'*, next to the entredeux holes.

***Tip**: Use an Edge-joining Foot with center flange positioned next to the entredeux holes.*

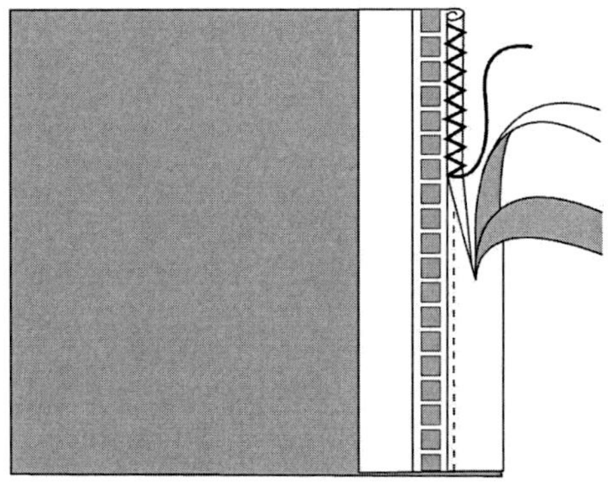

Trim the edges of the fabric and entredeux leaving a seam of <u>not less than</u> 1/8" (3mm).

Roll and whip the trimmed edges together with a tight zigzag stitch. The left needle swing will go into the ditch beside the entredeux (<u>not</u> into the holes) and the right swing will go all the way off the edge of the fabric.

This zigzag will completely encase the fabric and cause a tight roll.

*Refer to the technique for a **Fine Rolled Hem** (Roll and Whip)*

***Tip**: When using a heavier weight fabric such as course linen or broadcloth, it may be necessary to trim the garment fabric to <u>less than</u> 1/8" (3mm) but <u>not less than</u> 1/16". This will allow the 1/8" batiste allowance to roll over the garment fabric and secure the raw edge.*

Open out the fabric with the right side facing down on the ironing board. Using the side of the iron and gently pulling the fabric away from the iron, press the rolled seam toward the fabric. The holes of the entredeux should be clearly visible, with the seam pressed towards the garment.

Turn the garment with the right side facing up on the ironing board and press again to set the fabric roll away from the entredeux holes.

SUGGESTED MACHINE SETTING
Straight Stitch Setting:
Length: 2.0
Foot: Edge-joining
Needle Position: Center

Zigzag Setting:
W: 2.5 to 3.0
L: 0.75 to 1.0
Foot: Edge-joining
Needle Position: Far right (wherever possible to move the needle position while in a zigzag setting)

Note: when it is not possible to move the needle position with the machine set for a zigzag stitch, use the embroidery or regular foot and the needle position in the center. Be sure to position the fabric under the foot so that the left swing of the needle touches the row of straight stitches and the right swing goes off the edge of the fabric.

Notes

ROLLED HEM WITH ENTREDEUX

This method is another variation for attaching entredeux to fabric. It can be used when extra strength is required and it is desirable not to have visible stitches on the front of your work.

The best presentation is obtained when this technique is worked on the straight grain.

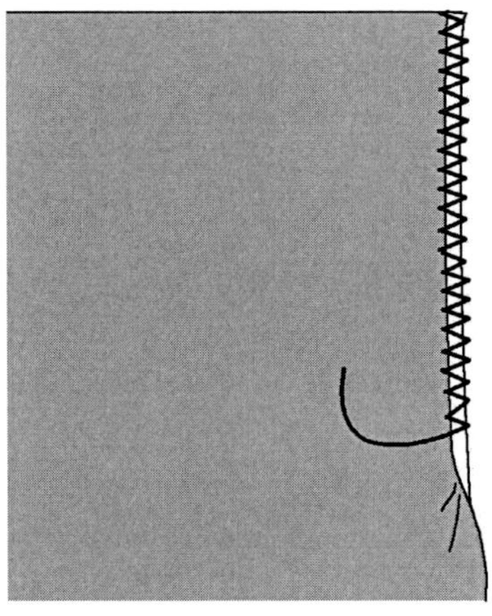

Roll and whip the straight edge of fabric.
Refer to the technique for a ***Fine Rolled Hem***
(Roll and Whip)

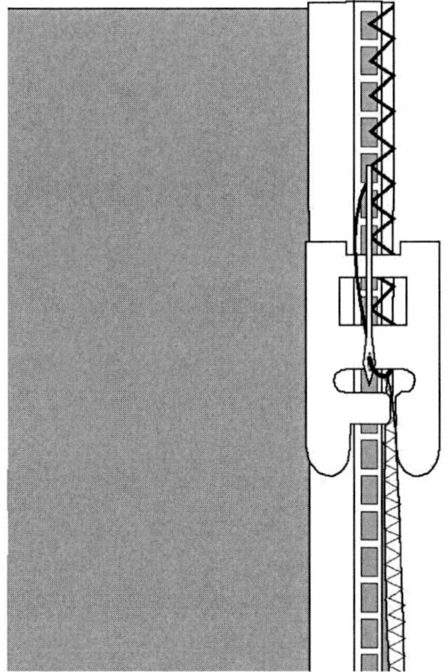

Trim the batiste from one side of the entredeux. With right sides together and the entredeux on top, butt the entredeux up to, but not on top of, the rolled and whipped edge.

Zigzag with the left needle swing going into each hole of the entredeux and the right needle swing off the edge of the rolled fabric edge.

Adjust the machine length so the needle does not hit the bars. All entredeux holes should be clean and visible.

Steam and press from the wrong side, and then the front of work. The edge of the fabric will roll up and over the heading of the lace.

ATTACHING ENTREDEUX TO GATHERED FABRIC

This is a very strong method for attaching the entredeux to fabric, particularly for areas of stress such as joining the yoke to a gathered skirt.

Note: *These guidelines are written for a 3/8" (1 cm) seam allowance on both the garment and the entredeux batiste. The position of the gathering threads will need to be adjusted for a narrower or wider seam allowance.*

Mark the halfway points on both the entredeux and the fabric to be gathered.

Stitch the first row of machine gathering just below the seam line and **NOT** within the seam allowance.

Tip: *position the edge of the fabric on the ⅜" (1cm) line on the machine sole plate, and move the needle position one or two notches to the left for this first row.*

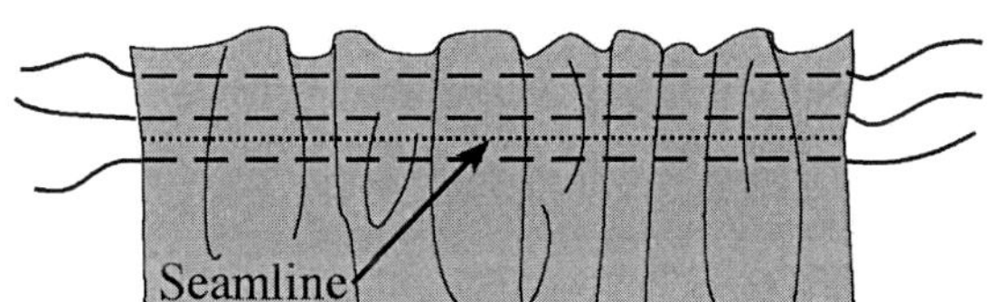
Seamline

Stitch the 2nd row of machine gathering ⅛" (3mm) from the seam line and a third row ⅛" from the 2nd row of gathering stitches (or ⅛" from the raw edge).

Tip: *More gathering rows are better than less! Once you have inserted the three rows of gathering threads, isolate the bobbin threads and knot them together. This way you will always hold the knotted group and gather with the bobbin threads, thus avoiding locking the upper and bobbin threads by not consistently gathering with the same set of threads.*

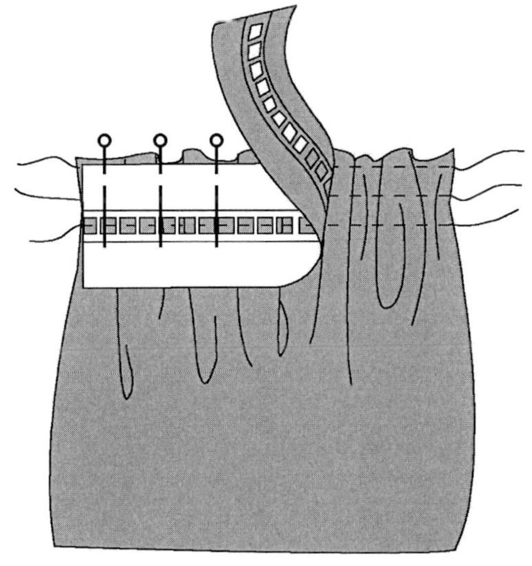

Gently pull the bobbin threads and gather the fabric to the correct measurement.

Tip: *Gather from each end towards the center of the piece wherever possible as this helps keep the fullness even.*

Place the **right side** of the untrimmed entredeux to the **right side** of the gathered fabric, matching the center points.

Commencing at the center, pin in place to secure. On projects where there are lots of gathers, it is recommended that you hand baste before stitching.

Hints:

- Two rows of gathering threads will be within the seam allowance and the other barely outside the seam line.
- Stitch the gathering row that is furthest from the edge of the fabric (just below the seam line) first. Use a colored thread, as this will be visible through the holes in the entredeux and will assist with keeping the fabric and entredeux pieces lined up.
- Do not make the stitch length for the gathering rows too long as this will cause fine fabric to 'pleat' rather than gently gather.

***Tip**: The golden rule for gathering is **"The finer the fabric, the shorter the stitch length"**. To gather fine batiste I use a stitch length of not more than 3.*

The right side of the untrimmed entredeux is now positioned to the right side of the gathered fabric with the center points matching. The raw edges should be even.

Straight-stitch close to the entredeux holes (or "*in the ditch*") with a short straight stitch. **DO NOT** stitch into the holes.

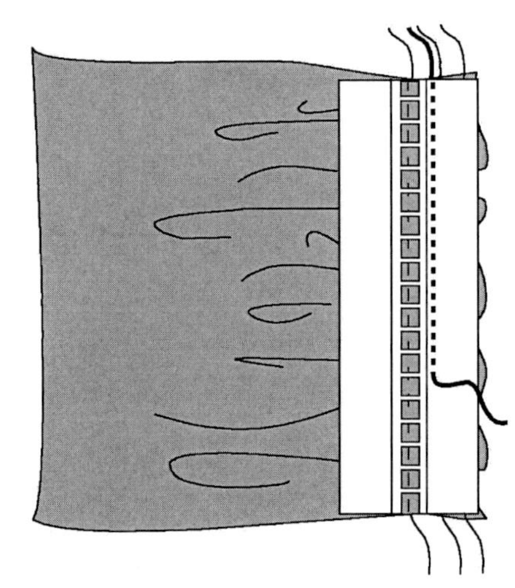

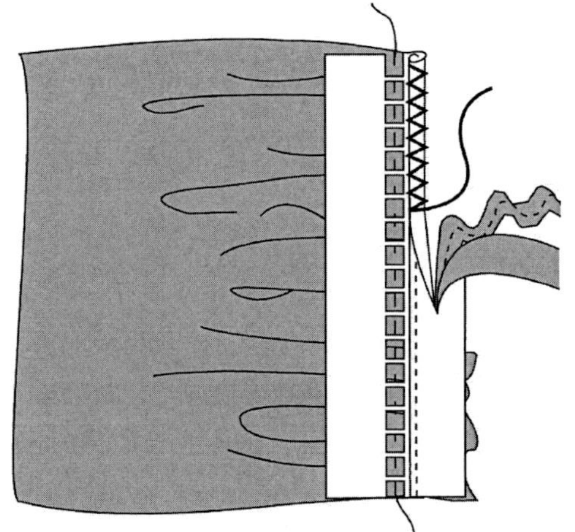

Trim the seam allowance of both the fabric and entredeux to approximately ⅛″ (3mm).

Roll and whip with a zigzag stitch up to the entredeux holes and over the edge of the fabric.

Refer to the technique for ***Attaching Entredeux to Fabric***

Note:
It will most likely be necessary to grade the seam allowance when applying *Entredeux to Gathered Fabric*, to reduce the bulk. The gathered fabric is trimmed to approximately (and not less than) 1/16-inch (1.5mm) and the batiste a little longer to ⅛″ (3mm), so that it wraps around the gathered bulk.

JOINING ENTREDEUX TO LACE INSERTION OR STRAIGHT EDGE OF LACE

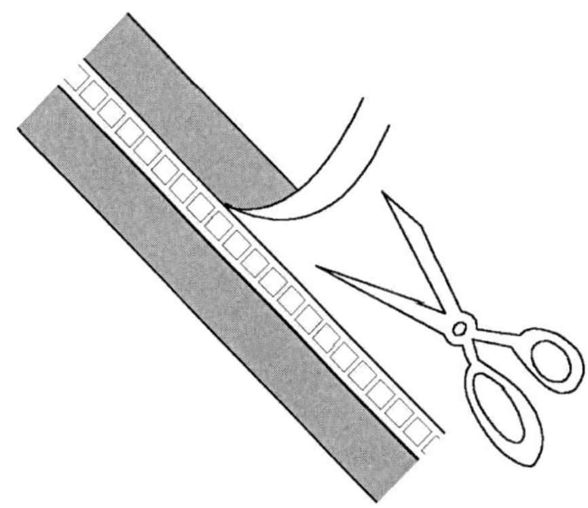

Lightly mist the lace and entredeux pieces with water and press with steam.

Trim one of the batiste fabric edges from the entredeux.

> ***Tip**: The entredeux is always more stable if you remove the batiste only as you are about to stitch. Removing both sides at once leaves very little to hold taut and maintain tension.*

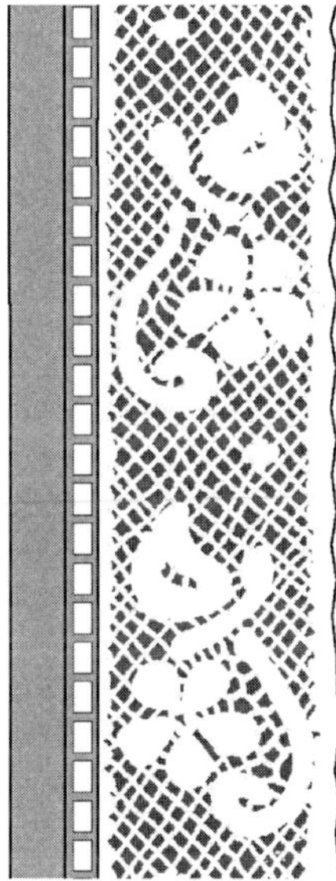

With right sides facing up, butt the trimmed edge of the entredeux against the lace heading – they should not overlap.

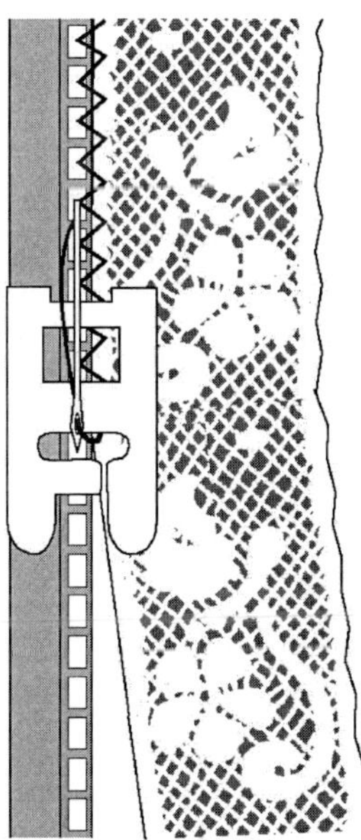

Sew together using a zigzag stitch, with the left swing going into each of the entredeux holes and the right swing just over the lace heading.

DO NOT have the width setting so wide that it takes up more than just the heading threads of the lace. If the zigzag is too wide it will bit into the lace design and not look as pretty

Experiment with the machine settings, as they will vary according to the size of the holes in the entredeux.

***Tip**: Be careful not to pull or put any pressure on the lace while stitching as this creates "ripples" or "ruffles" in the lace. Hold the entredeux taut (Refer to the techniques for **Working with Entredeux**) and allow the lace to feed itself.*

JOINING ENTREDEUX TO GATHERED LACE

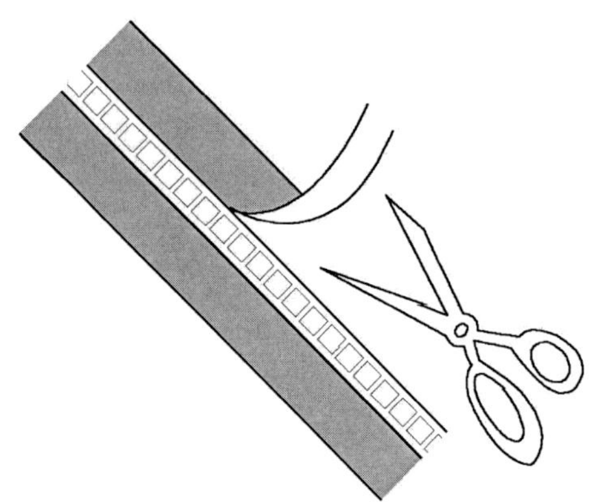

Lightly mist the lace and entredeux pieces with water and press with steam.

Trim one of the batiste fabric edges from the entredeux.

***Tip**: The entredeux is always more stable if you remove the batiste only as you are about to stitch. Removing both sides at once leaves very little to hold taut and maintain tension.*

Gather the lace by pulling the heading threads, one at a time. I start with the top 'loopy' thread (usually the strongest thread) and pull this thread taut until the lace gathers and is approximately the length required. Wherever possible pull the threads from both ends.

Then very carefully pull all remaining threads, one at a time, distributing the gathers evenly.

This method for gathering lace takes longer than just pulling one thread, but it creates a firm 'ribbon' of threads which will lay very flat next to the entredeux.

Be mindful of the fullness of the gathers in your project. Too many gathers are not necessarily better, as they tend to eliminate the pattern in the lace. And too few gathers can give the appearance that you did not have sufficient yardage of lace. I like to gather with a ratio of between 1.5:1 or 2:1.

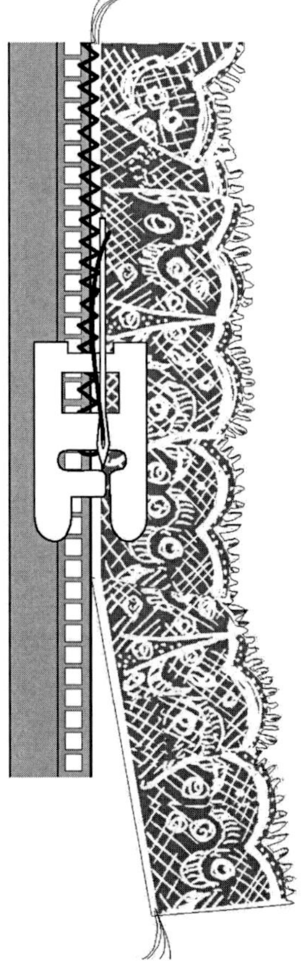

With right sides facing up, butt the trimmed edge of the entredeux against the edge of the lace – they should not overlap.

Sew together using a zigzag stitch, with the left swing going into each of the entredeux holes and the right swing just over the lace heading.

***Tip**: Use a firm, sharp-pointed tool such as an awl or stiletto to "push" the gathers toward the foot. And Remember – hold the entredeux taut as you assist the gathered lace to feed evenly!*

DO NOT make the width setting so wide that it takes up more than just the heading threads of the lace.

Meld the stitches with the tip of the iron, being careful not to flatten the gathers of the lace.

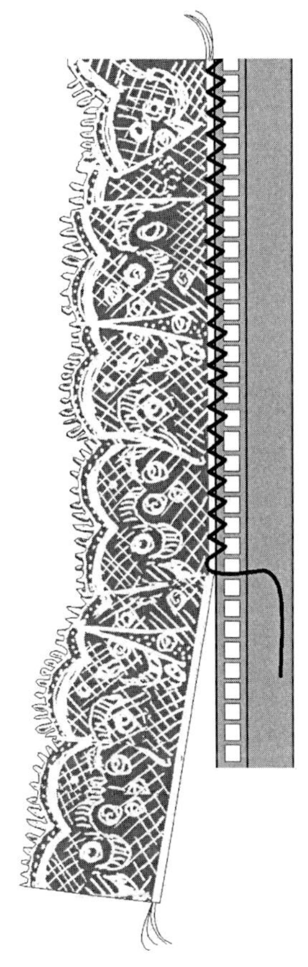

Note: The above instructions work well for right-handed sewers because they can hold the entredeux taut between the thumb and third finger of the left hand, while controlling and adjusting the gathers in the lace with the right hand. Don't be afraid to attach the lace from the other side if this is more comfortable for you. Remember – good results are achieved when you are relaxed and confident with your stitching.

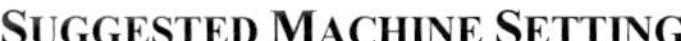

SUGGESTED MACHINE SETTING

Zigzag Setting:
W: 2.0 to 2.5
L: Approximately 1.0
Needle Position: Center
Foot: Buttonhole (not automatic) or Basic
Experiment with the edge-joining foot as this foot is the preference for many heirloom sewers.

Notes

JOINING LACE INSERTION TO ANOTHER STRAIGHT LACE EDGE

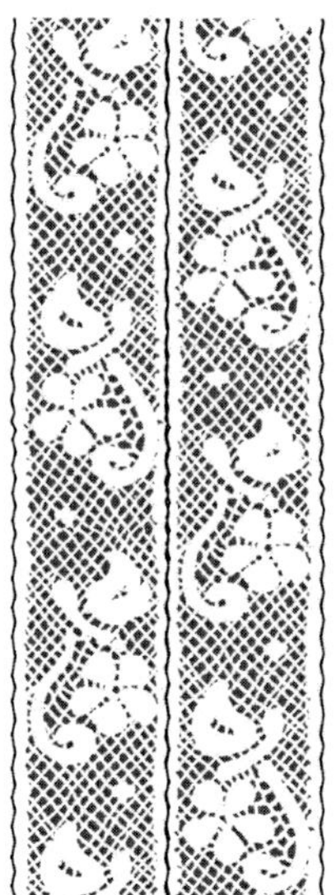

Lightly spray the two lace lengths with water and press (not iron) with steam.

Attach the appropriate machine foot for zigzag stitching, and adjust the stitch length and width settings.

Place the two lace pieces side by side with right sides facing up and matching the pattern in the lace, as you prefer. Do not overlap the laces.

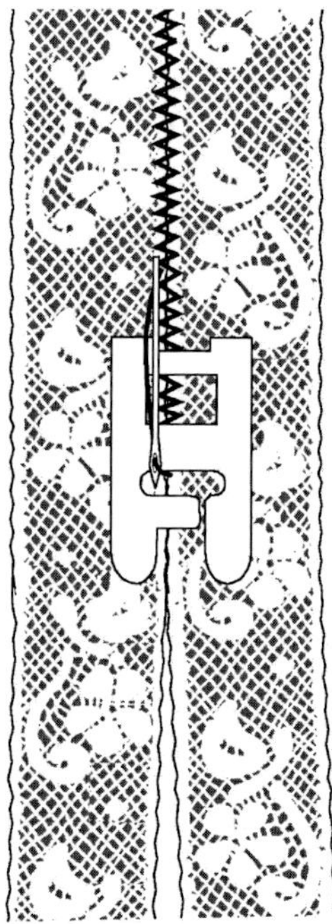

With the butted lace underneath the center of the foot, zigzag over both lace headings. Aim for a discreet stitch: do not take in more than the heading of the adjoining lace, yet be sure to secure both pieces firmly.

Tip: *Use the very finest thread available for an almost-invisible join – suggest Tanne or Cotona 80, Lacis 120*

SUGGESTED MACHINE SETTING
Zigzag Stitch:
W: 2.0 to 2.5
L: .Approximately 1.0
Needle Position: Center
Foot: Basic or Edge-joining
Experiment with the edge-joining foot as this foot is the preference for many heirloom sewers.

Be careful NOT to stretch or hold back either piece of lace.

To repair a section where laces do not meet, stitch over this area again, reducing the stitch width a little.

Note: After zigzagging the laces together, you may find "ripples" in the panel. These can easily be straightened by lightly applying spray starch and using a steam iron to press.

Tip: *For a very fine join on laces with a small band of heading threads, try overlapping the lace headers only and joining with a small zigzag stitch (not more than W-1.5; L-0.7) using the Jeans or Quilting foot. Be careful, as these feet have been designed for straight stitching only. Try it for a wonderful result, but tread carefully!*

APPLYING LACE INSERTION (OR STRAIGHT EDGE OF LACE EDGING) TO FABRIC

For applying lace insertion in a straight line, or on the grain of fabric, commence by drawing a line in the center of the lace placement or by removing two or three fabric threads to highlight the straight grain of the fabric and to highlight the position of the lace being inserted.

Note: If you wish to apply the lace to the edge only of a piece of fabric, follow these directions working on one side (heading) of the lace only.

Center the lace insertion or edging over these pulled threads and baste in position through the center of the lace (not the heading), with the right side of the lace and the fabric facing upwards.

Align the center of the foot over the lace heading. Using a small straight machine stitch and matching fine machine embroidery thread, stitch in the center of the lace heading.

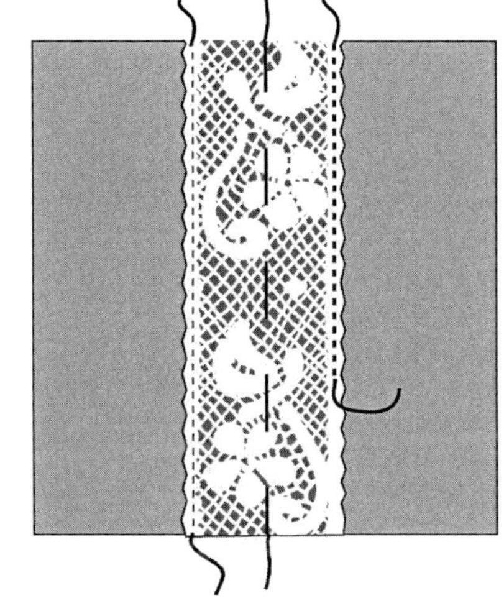

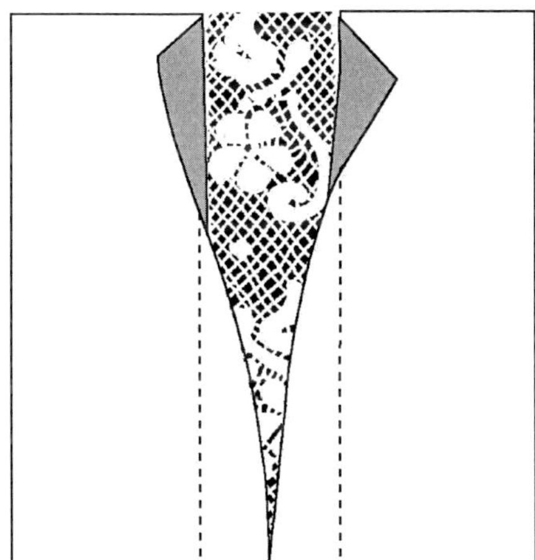

Remove the basting thread.

Turn the work to the wrong side and, with small, sharp scissors, cut the fabric behind the lace using the pulled threads as a guide. Be careful not to cut the lace.

Tip: *my preference is to use 3½" (9 cm) or 4" (10 cm) mini-appliqué (or duck-bill) scissors, however, you may also want to try round nose scissors. Both these help reduce the risk of accidentally cutting the lace.*

Press the cut edges of the fabric away from the lace insertion pushing with the side of the iron.

Baste if necessary to hold the small seam allowance in place.

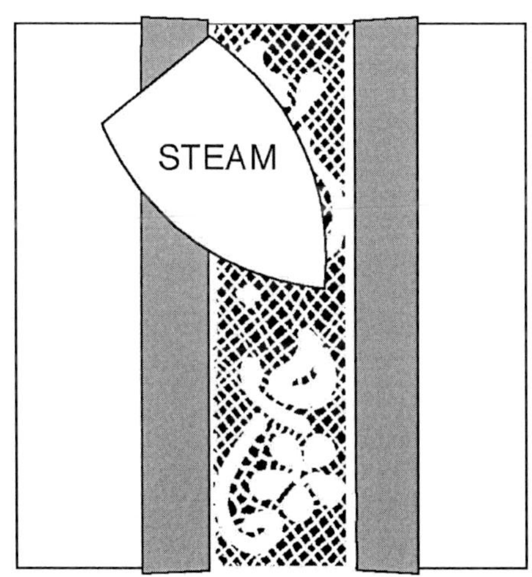
STEAM

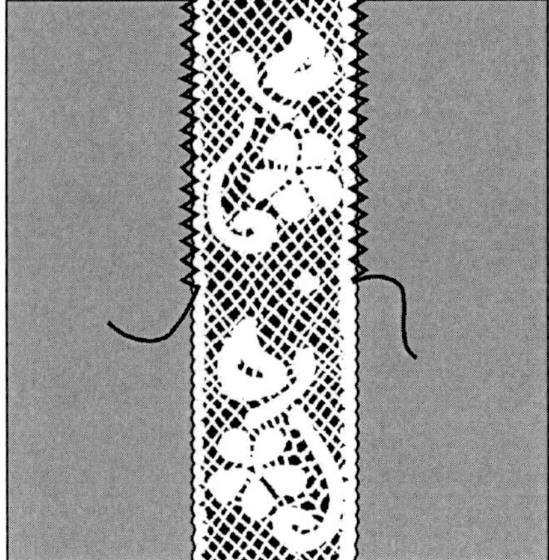

Working from the right side, secure the insertion with a tiny zigzag stitch, a pin stitch (Parisian Stitch) or hemstitch (Venetian Stitch).

***Tip**: It is important that you meld the stitches so they settle into the fabric and allow you to trim close in the next step.*

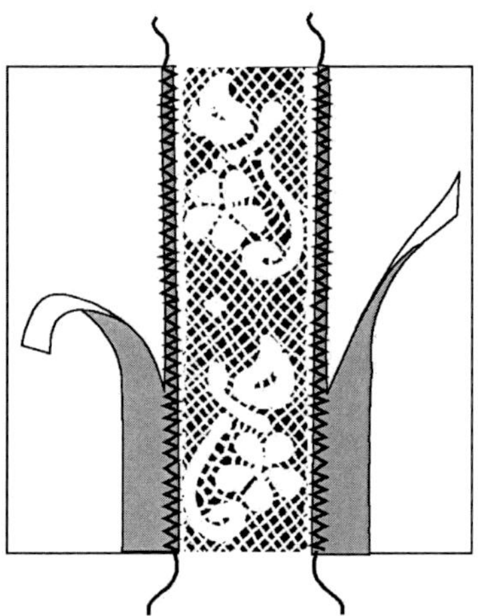

Turn to the wrong side and trim the remaining seam allowance right up to this second row of stitching.

***Tip**: Hold the scissors flat, with the fabric being cut resting over the tips of your fingers.*

Although the illustrations for this technique directly relate to lace insertion being applied to a design line within the fabric, exactly the same steps will be taken for ***Applying a Lace Edging to Fabric***.

If you are using this technique to apply an edging lace to fabric, first pull a thread (wherever possible) to straighten the fabric edge. Position the lace on at least ¼" (6mm) of fabric for the turn-back allowance and follow the above guidelines, working on the lace heading (or one side of the lace) only.

SUGGESTED MACHINE SETTINGS
Straight Stitch:
L: 2.0
Needle Position: Center
Foot: Straight Stitch or ¼"

Zigzag Stitch:
W: 1.0 to 1.5 (2.0 on some laces)
L: Approximately 0.75
Needle Position: Center
Foot: Straight Stitch or ¼"

***Note**: If using the straight stitch or ¼" foot for the zigzag step, be very careful to hand test the width first – needles could be broken on the sides of the foot if the width setting is too wide!*

INSERTING LACE INTO GATHERED FABRIC

This technique can be used to best advantage for such purposes as:

- applying a beading lace at the bottom edge of a sleeve. The fabric can be cut away from behind the beading, but it does not have to be.
- drawing up fabric to secure with a lace or folded fabric casing.

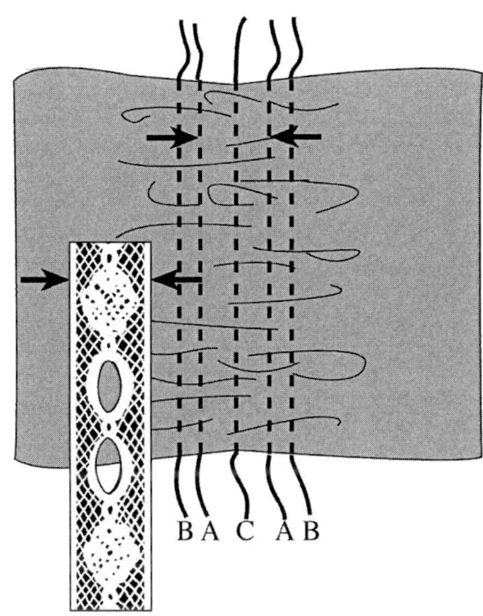
B A C A B

Stitch two rows of machine gathering just a little closer together than the distance between the headings on the beading or lace insertion (shown by the arrows and labeled **A**).

Stitch two more rows of machine gathering just a little further apart than the distance between the headings on the beading or lace insertion (on the outer sides of the first gathering rows, labeled **B**).

Stitch a final row of machine gathering at **C** in the center of the space created by the previous rows.

Pull the bobbin threads to gather the fabric to the correct measurement for the length of the beading or insertion being applied.

***Tip**: I like to isolate all (five) bobbin threads at both ends and knot them together so I am always sure to gather with the bobbin threads only.*

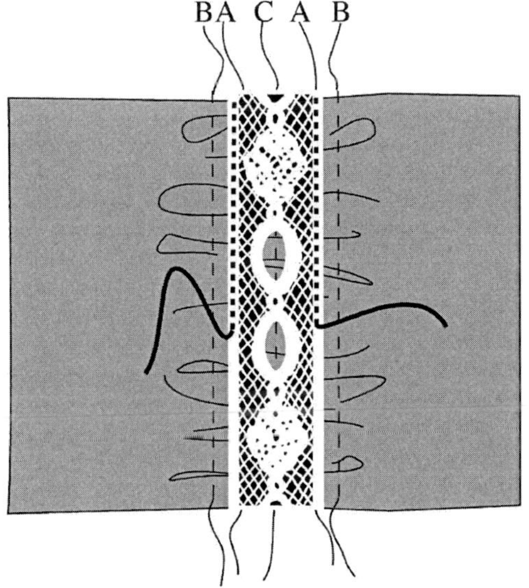
BA C A B

With the right side of the fabric facing upward and the right side of the insertion facing upward and on top, match the center points and pin at intervals to secure.

Stitch through the heading on both sides of the lace (or fabric casing) with a short straight stitch.

Meld the stitches with the tip of the iron being careful not to flatten the gathers.

***Note**: The center of the beading or lace insertion will lie on the center row of the gathering stitches.*

Remove the <u>center gathering thread only</u> and, using a pair of mini-appliqué scissors or round nose scissors, carefully cut up the center of the fabric behind the lace.

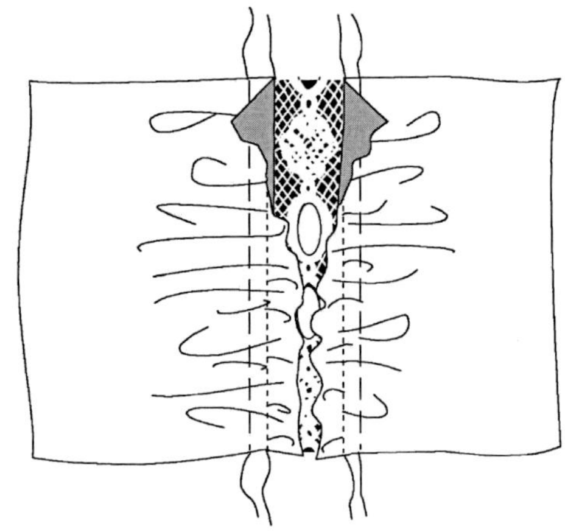

Finger press the cut edges back from behind the lace and baste to hold in place – it is important to baste on this occasion, so don't skip this step!

*Refer to the techniques for **Applying Lace Insertion into Fabric***

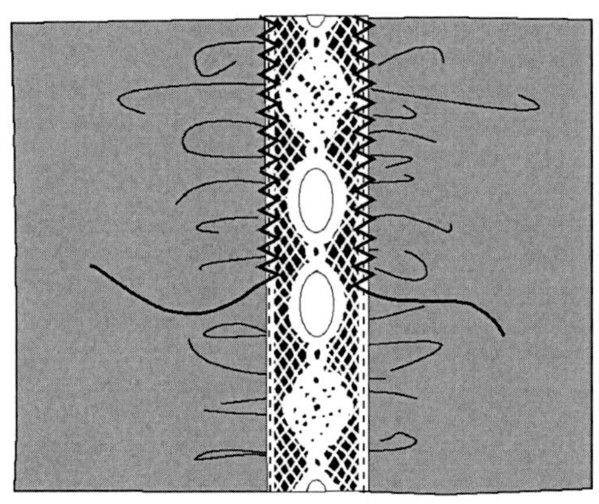

Working from the right side, secure the insertion with a tiny zigzag stitch, a pin stitch (Parisian Stitch) or hemstitch (Venetian Stitch).

Remove the remaining machine basting threads.

From the wrong side, hold the scissors flat and trim the fabric up to this row of zigzag stitching, to neaten the finished application.

***Tip**: It is not imperative that you remove the fabric from behind the lace, especially if you are working on a heavier fabric or are threading ribbon through a beading. In these instances, work the steps on the previous page and neaten the lace heading with a zigzag or pin stitch as per the final step.*

SUGGESTED MACHINE SETTINGS

Straight Stitch:
L: 2.0
Needle Position: Center
Foot: Straight Stitch or ¼"

Zigzag Stitch:
W: 1.5 to 2.0
L: 0.75 to 1.0
Needle Position: Center
Foot: 5 or 7 groove pintuck foot

APPLYING LACE WITH A MITERED CORNER TO A DESIGN WITHIN THE FABRIC

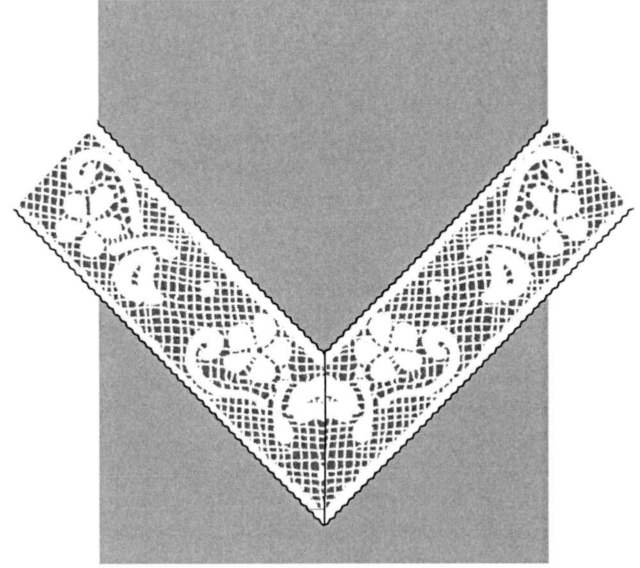

To miter the corner of the lace, refer to the instructions for ***Applying Lace with a Mitered Corner to a Fabric Edge*** (METHOD 1), up to the point of positioning the lace onto the fabric edge.

At this point you will center the mitered lace in position over the mitered design line on your project.

Hand-baste the insertion onto the fabric through the center of the lace.

Using a short straight stitch, (approximately L -1.5) machine stitch through the heading on **both sides** of the lace, pivoting at each corner. Meld these stitches.

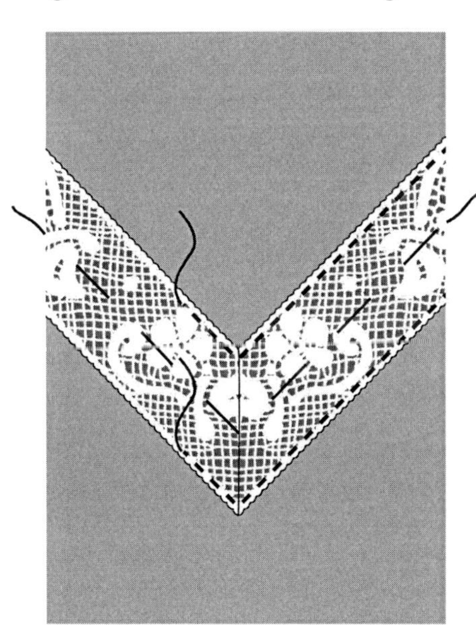

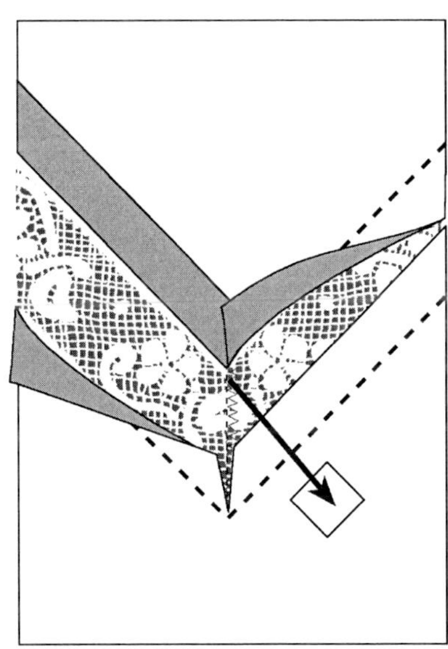

From the wrong side, clip up to the stitching line and into the corners at each angle. Remove the box that will be created at the top when you clip into the corner as shown – this will allow the seam allowance to lay flat without too much overlap in the top corner.

Working from the wrong side, press the fabric away from behind the lace, using steam to make a sharp crease, and allowing no tiny tucks to extend beyond the stitching line.

Hand baste these small seams in place to keep them away from the next row of stitching.

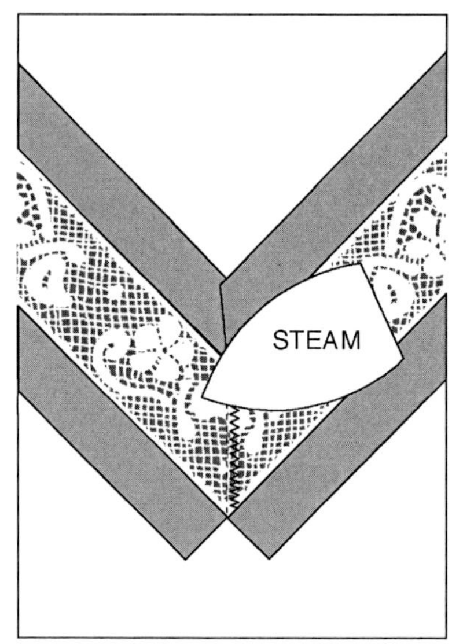
STEAM

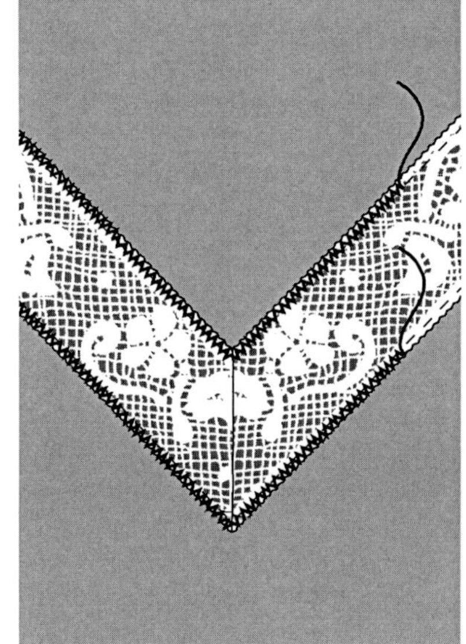

On the right side, zigzag (or pinstitch) over the lace headings to secure both sides of the lace.

Use a stitch width that will just encompass the lace heading and a length that is a little longer than a satin stitch. Press well.

***Tip**: I like to use the very finest cotton thread for this type of decorative stitching, as it makes the stitching almost invisible and does not detract from the lace itself.*

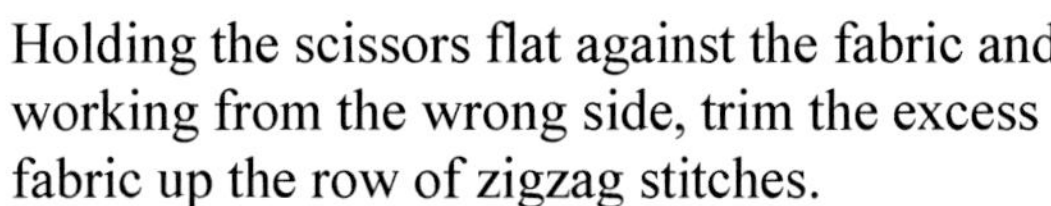

Holding the scissors flat against the fabric and working from the wrong side, trim the excess fabric up the row of zigzag stitches.

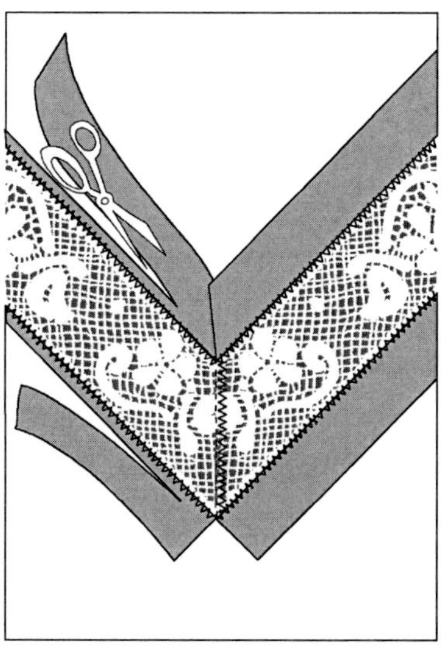

*Refer to the techniques for **Applying Lace Insertion (or Straight Edge of Lace) into Fabric***

APPLYING LACE WITH A MITERED CORNER TO A FABRIC EDGE

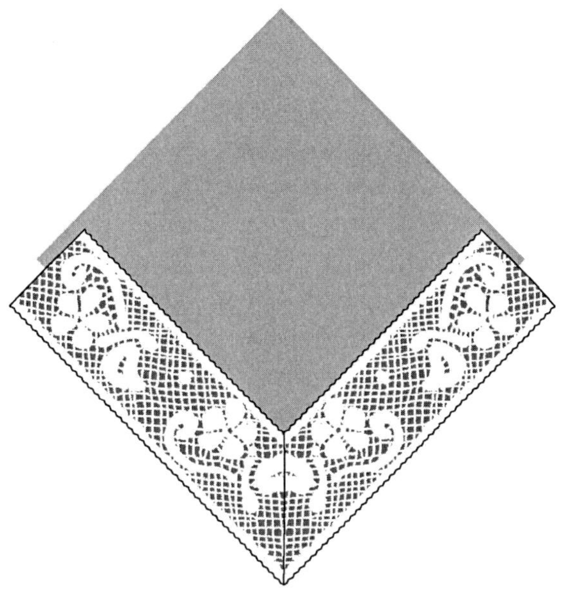

METHOD 1

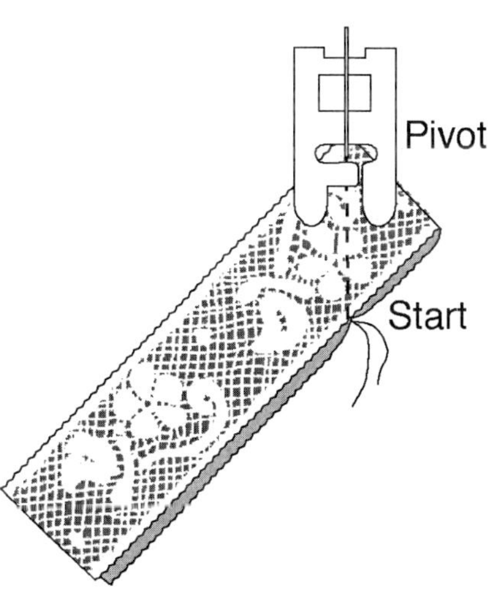
Pivot
Start

With right sides together, fold the lace insertion, matching the pattern within the lace if desired, and mark a 45° angle. Commencing at the widest point, stitch across the angle to the fold (just above the heading) with a short straight stitch– be careful **NOT** to stitch through the top heading thread at the end of the stitching (pivot point).

Stop with the needle in the '**down**' position, lift the presser foot and pivot the lace.

Pull the starting tails back under the presser foot (over the original row of straight stitches) and stitch again with a short zigzag stitch that comes up to the first row of stitches or <u>just barely</u> over theses stitches <u>and</u> the thread tails. I use a machine zigzag setting of approximately W-1.0; L-0.5.

Meld the stitches.

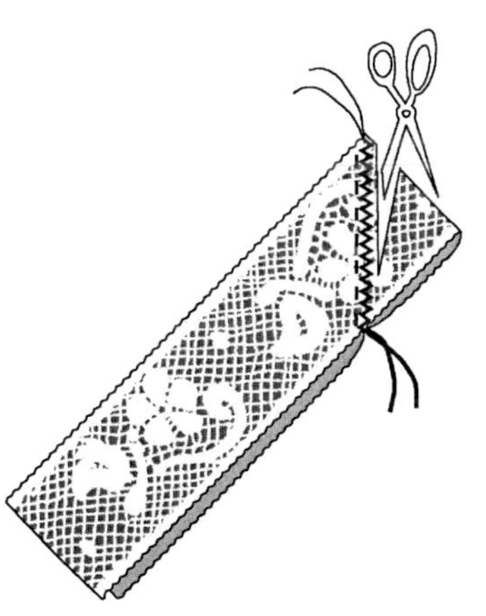

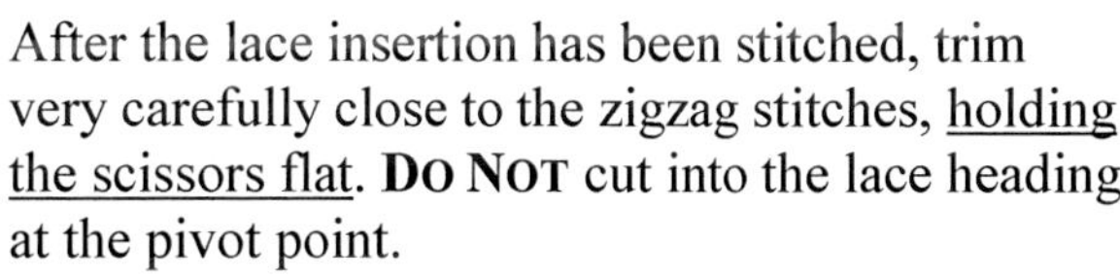

After the lace insertion has been stitched, trim very carefully close to the zigzag stitches, <u>holding the scissors flat</u>. **DO NOT** cut into the lace heading at the pivot point.

Lightly mist the mitered lace with water and press to ensure that the finished lace angle matches the angle on the pattern piece.

Position the lace on the fabric corner with at least ¼" (6mm) of fabric for the seam allowance, and baste the insertion to secure.

Refer to the techniques for ***Applying Lace Insertion (or Straight Edge of Lace) into Fabric***

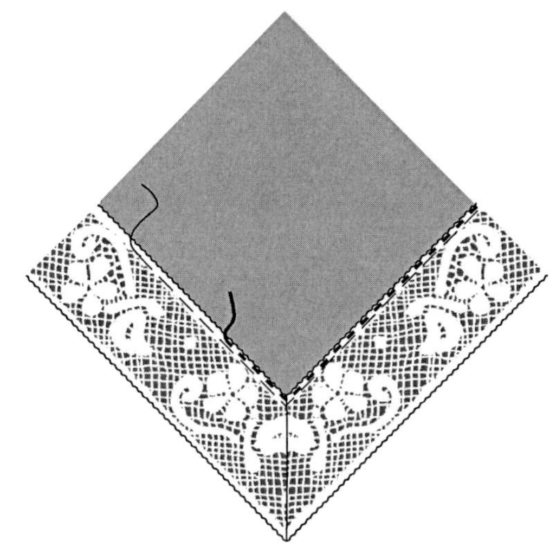

Straight stitch through the top lace heading only. Meld the stitches, and lightly spray starch only if necessary.

Clip up to the corner stitching, removing the small box of fabric and complete this lace application.

Refer to the techniques for ***Applying Lace with a Mitered Corner to a Design within the Fabric***

Lightly spray starch the mitered lace corner and press, being careful to maintain the correct angle of this piece.

METHOD 2

This second method can be used to miter a corner in a lace insertion or edging, where the fabric is left behind the lace without being cut away, and the lace remains folded at the corner.

Note: these illustrations show lace being applied to the edge of the fabric; however, this method is also appropriate for lace being applied as an insertion within the fabric.

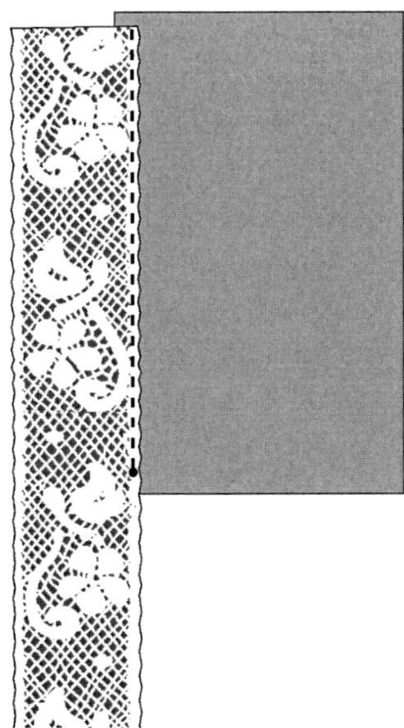

Position the lace on the outside edge of the fabric. Stitch through the lace heading to the corner. Leave the needle inserted in the lace at this corner point and raise the presser foot of the machine ready to pivot and miter the lace.

With right sides together fold the lace so that it extends beyond the corner point by the exact width of the lace.

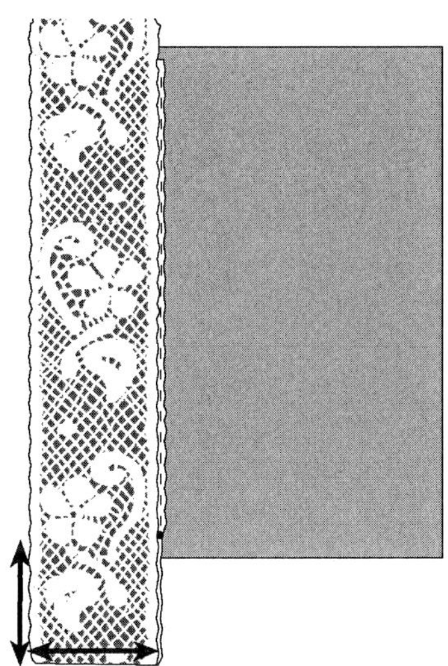

Pivot

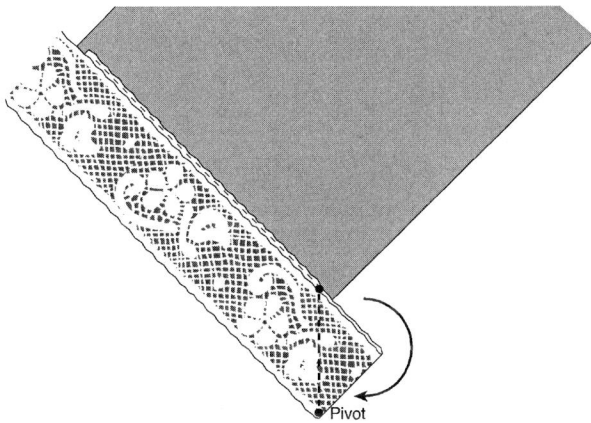

Continue stitching from the fabric to the point of the lace that is diagonally opposite. This stitching will be through the two layers of the folded lace and stop just short of the outside heading thread.

Stitch back to corner of fabric

Open lace to lay along this edge

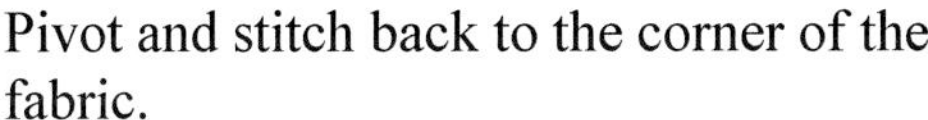

Pivot and stitch back to the corner of the fabric.

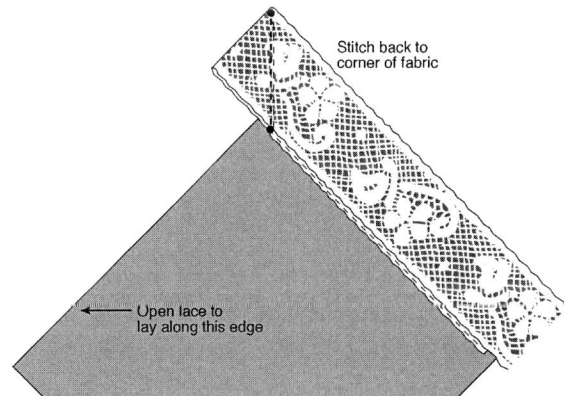

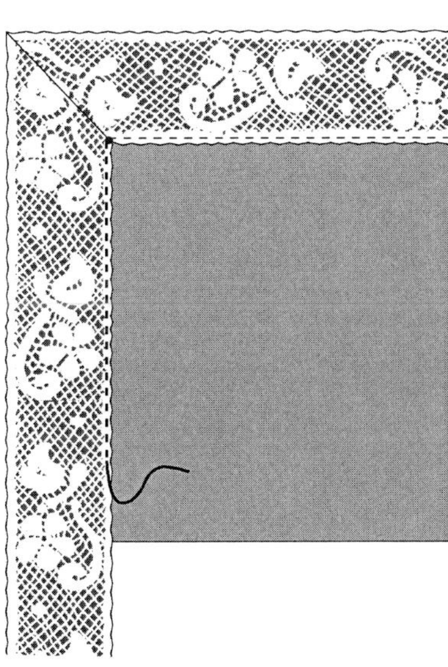

Open the mitered lace to expose the corner. At this point you will need to lift the needle and reposition – then stitch along the heading of the lace for the remainder of the lace attachment.

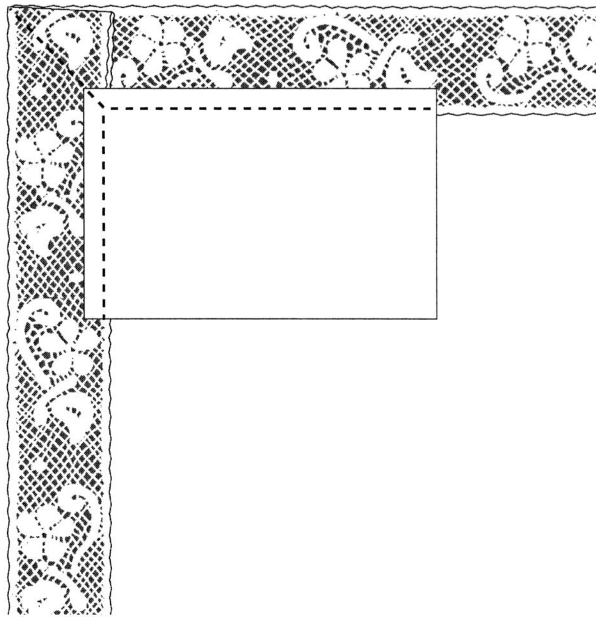

The lace has now been mitered, as above shown from the wrong side, with the fold of lace remaining in each corner.

At this point the lace needs to be secured from the right side by one of the following methods:

- Stitch with a narrow zigzag (W-1.5, L-0.7) or pin stitch over the heading of the lace, and then trim the seam allowance from behind **OR**
- From the wrong side clip the fabric close to each side of the miter stitch line and fold the seam allowance back behind the fabric. Hand baste the seam allowance in place and secure from the right side with a tiny zigzag or pinstitch.

Refer to the techniques for Applying ***Lace with a Mitered Corner to a Design within the Fabric***

Notes

APPLYING ENTREDEUX AND GATHERED LACE TO A MITERED LACE CORNER

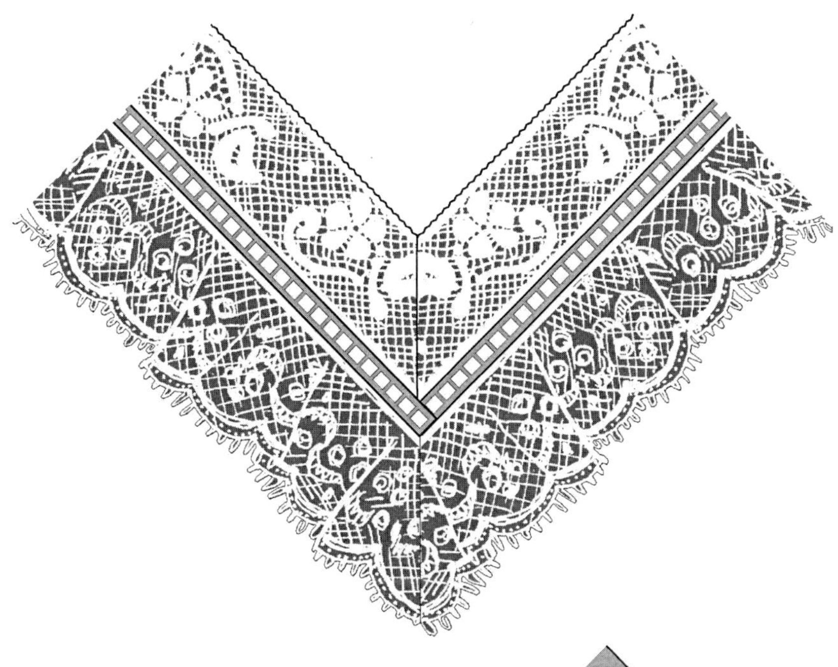

Cut a length of entredeux that is approximately ½" (12mm) longer than the fabric/lace edge. Trim the batiste from one side of the entredeux.

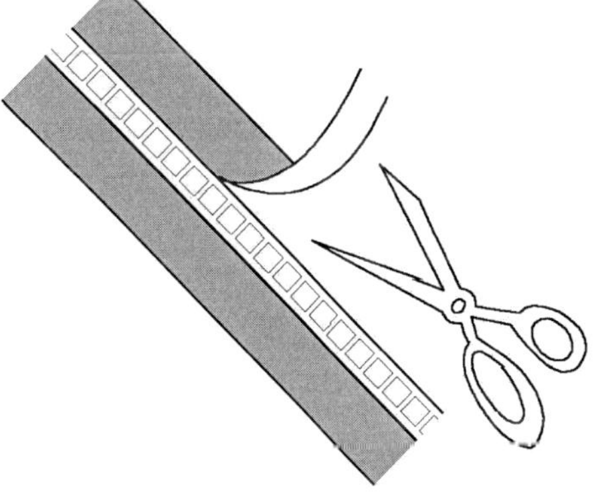

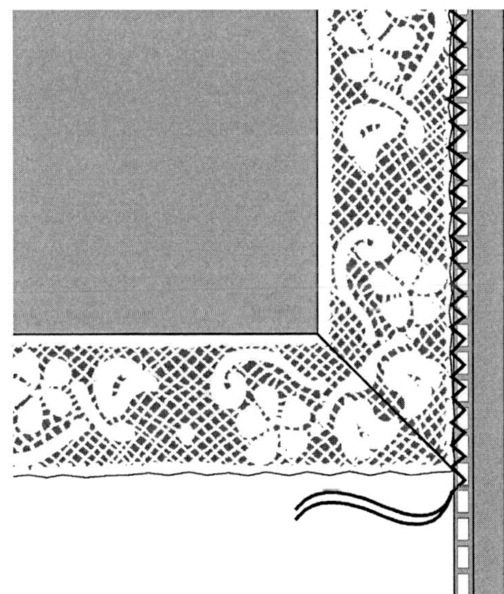

Zigzag with the right needle swing going into each hole of the entredeux and the left swing going over the heading of the lace.

***Tip**: Be sure to hold the lace taut between the thumb and third finger of your left hand, butting the entredeux up the lace with your right hand.*

Stitch up to the corner point and cut the machine threads, leaving a tail on each that is long enough to tie a knot.

Remove the remaining batiste from the other side of the entredeux.

Leaving ½" (12mm) of entredeux extending, butt the second piece of entredeux, with one side of the batiste removed, up to the edge of the lace and on top of the entredeux which has already been stitched,.

Zigzag this piece into position from the corner point to the end of the lace as above. Be sure to leave machine thread tails to secure.

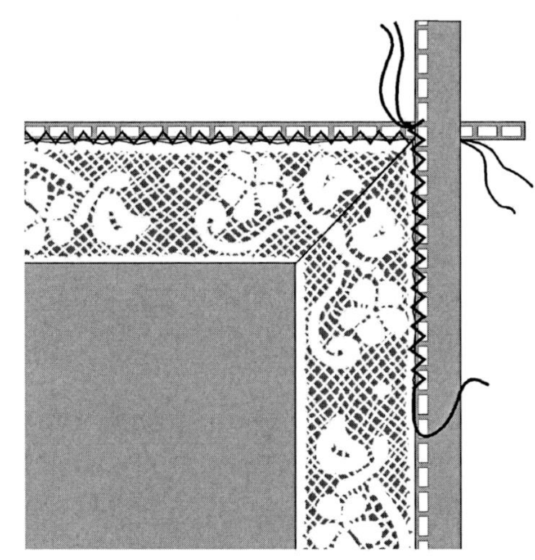

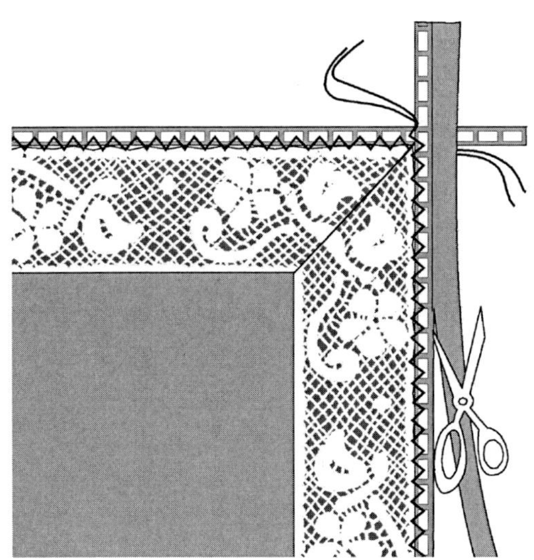

Trim the remaining side of batiste from the entredeux.

Pull both sets of thread tails to the wrong side of your work and tie together with a small, firm square knot.

***Tip**: The thread tails can be clipped, leaving about ½" (12mm) remaining. These tails will be much more secure if they are caught within the zigzag stitches when the lace edging is attached, rather than cutting them off at the knot.*

Each corner should be squared by removing the extending ½" (12mm) of entredeux just prior to the lace edging being attached.

SUGGESTED MACHINE SETTINGS

Zigzag Stitch:
W: Approximately 2.0
L: Approximately 1.0
Needle Position: Center
Foot: Basic, Buttonhole or Edge-joining foot

***Tip**: Using a clear plastic, or open-toe, boot will allow you to see your work and align the stitch in the holes of the entredeux – especially at the corners.*

For the gathered lace edging you will first need to determine the fullness desired for each side. Multiply this by the amount of fullness and cut as one length of lace only.

***Tip**: My preference is to have less gathers for two reasons: the edging is easier to apply with less fullness and the lace pattern remains more visible. I gather the lace with just a little more than 1½ times the amount of fullness.*

With right sides together, fold the lace edging over and mark a 45° angle. Straight-stitch across this angle from the widest point (on the heading) to the lace edge.

***Tip**: be careful to stop at the foldline just above the edge of the lace – this will allow the lace to turn and maintain a continuous scalloped edge.*

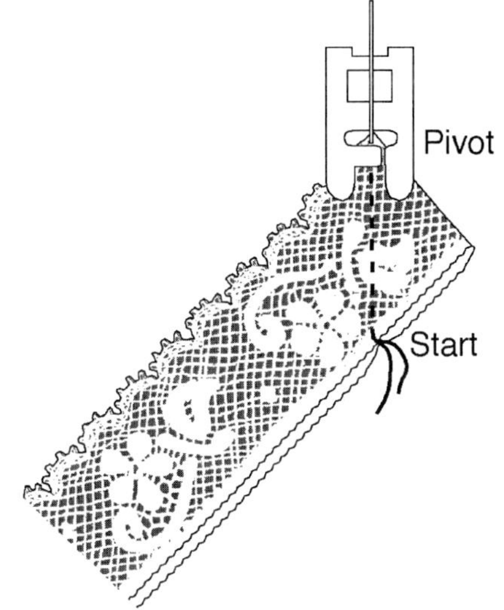
Pivot
Start

Stop with the needle in the '**down**' position, lift the presser foot and pivot the lace.

Pull the starting tails back over this first row of stitching so they are now lying on top of the straight stitches and extending behind the presser foot.

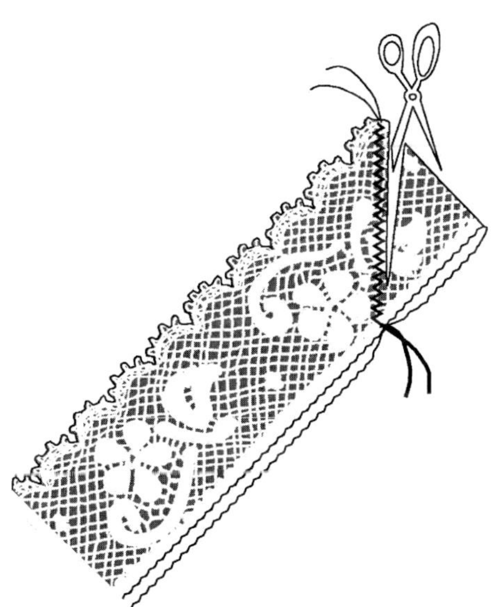

Hold the starting tails and stitch again with a short zigzag stitch that comes up to the first row of stitches, or just barely over these stitches. I use a machine setting W-1.0; L-0.5.

Meld the stitches.

After the lace edging has been stitched, trim very carefully close to the zigzag stitches, holding the scissors flat against your fingers. **DO NOT** cut into the scalloped edge of the lace.

Lightly mist the mitered lace with water and press to ensure that the finished lace angle matches the angle of the lace/entredeux.

Pull the lace heading threads (**NOT** the stitching threads) and gather each side of the lace separately and from both ends.

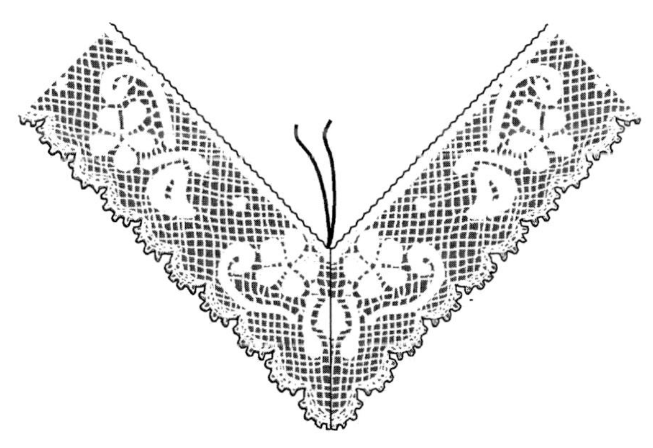

Refer to the techniques for
Attaching Gathered Lace to Fabric

APPLYING ENTREDEUX TO A CORNER

(on a single thickness of fabric)

Consider this method for applying entredeux or Swiss beading to the edge of a single fabric thickness:

- collar or handkerchief
- mitered hemline of a skirt

Cut the entredeux approximately ½" (12mm) longer than the fabric and trim the batiste off one side of the entredeux. Trim the remaining seam allowance to ¼" (6mm), or to match the seam allowance of the garment piece.

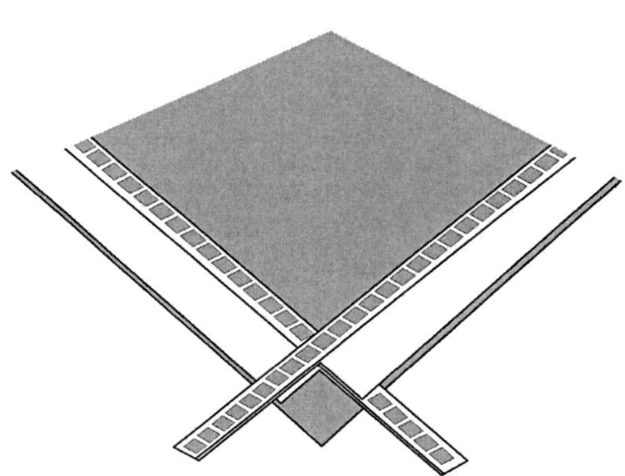

With raw edges even position the entredeux on the seam line of the project and pin in place.

Where the two lengths of entredeux overlap, trim the batiste from the other side, by the same amount as the overlap.

Allow the entredeux to extend approximately ½" (12mm) beyond the end of the fabric.

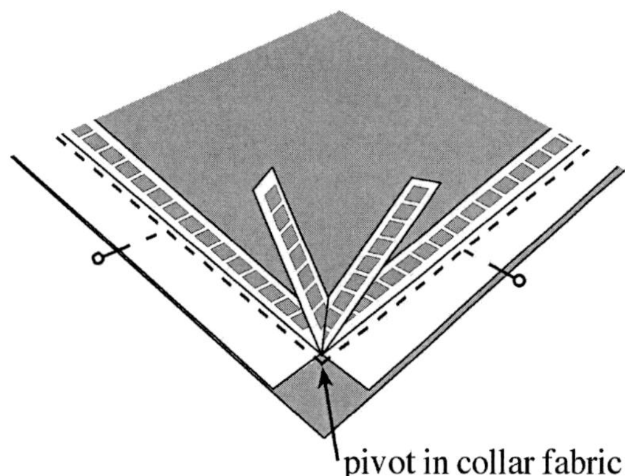
pivot in collar fabric

With right sides together and raw edges matching, straight stitch '*in the ditch'* beside the embroidered holes of the entredeux. Use a short machine stitch length and stitch all the way around the project.

At the points where the entredeux overlaps, fold it back so as not to catch it in the stitching. The pivot of the machine stitch will be in the **<u>collar</u>** <u>fabric</u> **<u>only</u>**.

Trim the seam allowance of the garment and the batiste to approximately 1/8" (3mm). With the tails of the overlapping entredeux pinned away from the stitching line, roll and whip each side of the project, using a short zigzag stitch. Roll and whip one side and stop. Roll and whip the remaining side – **DO NOT** try to round the corner.

Refer to the techniques for ***Attaching Entredeux to Fabric.***

Press the Rolled and Whipped Seam away from behind the entredeux holes. Working from the right side, align the two corner holes and hand catch these together using very small stitches and fine thread. Trim the entredeux to form a neat corner – the corner is now ready for attaching lace or applying a decorative hand embellishment.

APPLYING ENTREDEUX INTO A LINED CORNER

(between two layers of fabric)

Consider this method for applying entredeux or Swiss beading to the edge of

- a square collar
- a baby pillow, quilt or cot cover

Apply interfacing to the wrong side of the outer collar, if desired. Follow the steps for ***Applying Entredeux to a Corner*** *(on a single thickness of fabric)*. ***DO NOT*** complete this technique with the Rolled and Whipped edge.

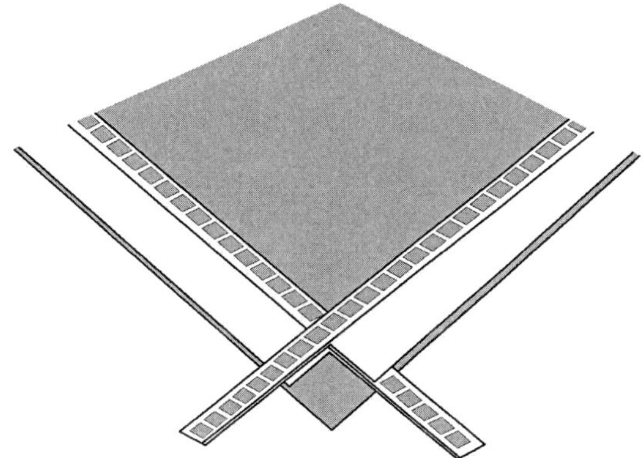

At the points where the entredeux overlaps, fold the entredeux back so as not to catch it in the stitching. Pin to secure.

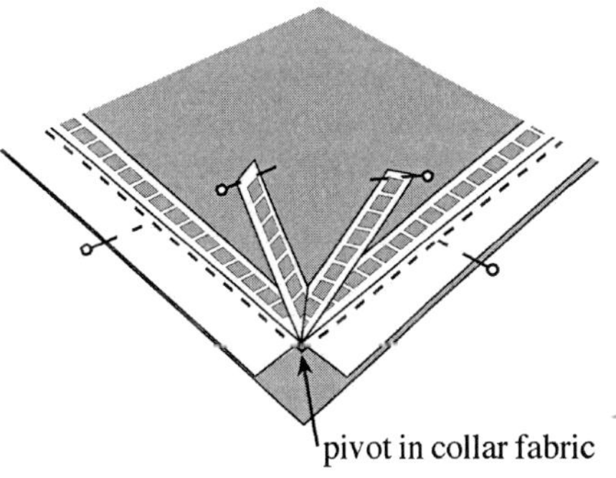
pivot in collar fabric

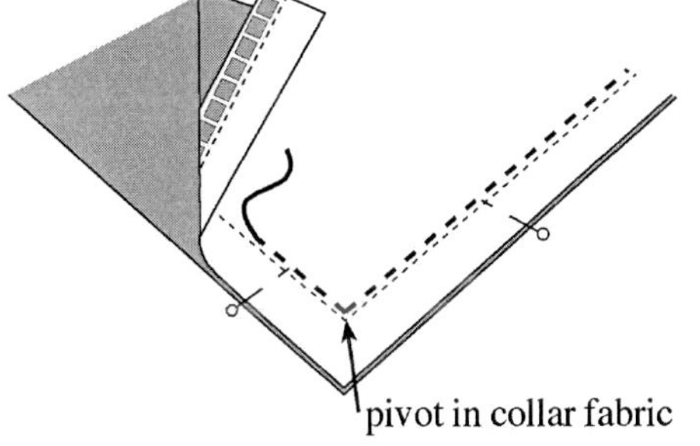
pivot in collar fabric

With right sides together and interfaced (outer) collar on top, join the outer collar and lining being careful to stitch just a little bit closer to the entredeux. Pivot exactly on the previous pivot point.

Meld this stitching line with a steam iron.

Grade the seam allowance so that the widest seam allowance is on the outer (interfaced) layer of the collar, and turn the corners right sides out.

Tack overlapping corner holes of the entredeux together by hand.

APPLYING LACE WITH A GATHERED CORNER TO ENTREDEUX

For many applications a prettier effect can be achieved by gathering the lace at the corners, rather than mitering it. Suggested examples would be:

- around a delicate pillow
- the corners of a baby bonnet
- a square collar or handkerchief.

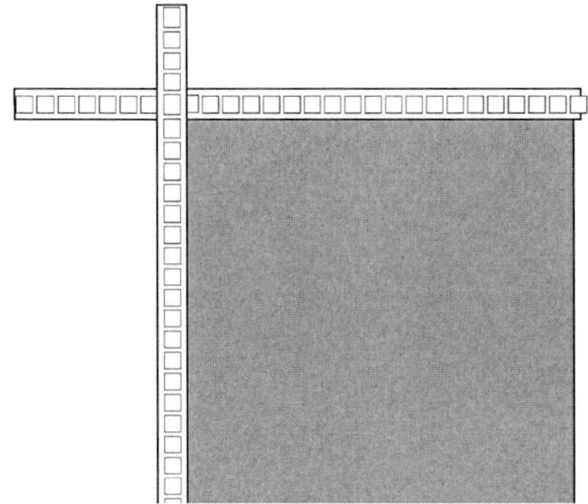

Attach the entredeux to all edges of your project and neaten the corners.

Tip**: Refer to the techniques for **Applying Entredeux to a Corner

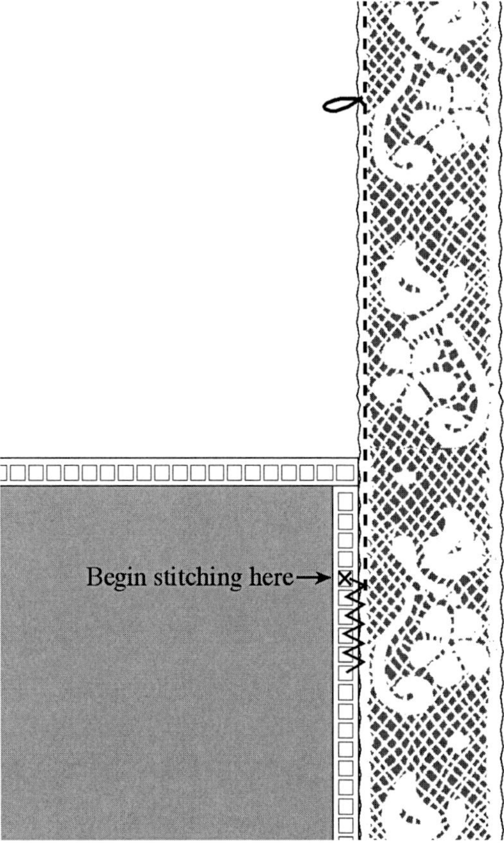
Begin stitching here

Lay out the lace edging next to the entredeux but do not gather it at this point. Be sure to leave a tail of about 3" – 4" (7-10 cm) before you begin stitching.

Using the method for *Attaching Lace to Entredeux*, begin about five holes from the corner and attach the lace with the left swing of the needle going into each entredeux hole and the right swing going over the heading of the lace.

Stop stitching about five entredeux holes from the next corner. Leave your machine needle in the down position in the entredeux hole.

Pull a thread in the lace heading, about 5" (12 cm) from where you stopped stitching, to form the gathers for rounding the corner. Maintaining tension on the pulled thread with your left hand, use a small stiletto or awl to gently push the gathers into the corner. Zigzag the lace into position, with the excess thread from the lace being sewn into the zigzag stitches.

Continue applying the lace to each corner in the same way until you reach the last corner. Gather the lace as if you intend to turn the corner, but stop stitching about five entredeux holes from the corner.

Remove the work from your sewing machine and cut the lace leaving a 3" – 4" (7-10 cm) tail.

Join the two lace ends at the corner with a small zigzag join or a French seam.

Refer to the techniques for ***Applying Lace with a Mitered Corner****.*

Pull up the heading threads on this last corner until the lace fits. Zigzag the gathered lace into position as before. Press well.

This method of finishing the last corner will hide the lace join in the gathers.

Notes

ROLLING AND WHIPPING A BIAS OR CURVED EDGE

This technique will be used to firmly hold any edge that may stretch. Examples include:

- the neckline or armhole of a petticoat or dress.
- the scallops at the hemline of a petticoat or dress.

Make a row of straight stitching a scant 1/16″ (1.5mm) from the seam line, within the seam allowance. This will help stabilize the neckline and secure the grainline. Use a short stitch length (L-1.5) and Cotton Embroidery thread (60/2 or 50/3).

***Tip**: Be aware of the neckline seam allowance before you begin as patterns vary from ¼" - ⅝" (6mm – 15mm).*

Lightly spray starch the curved edge and press.

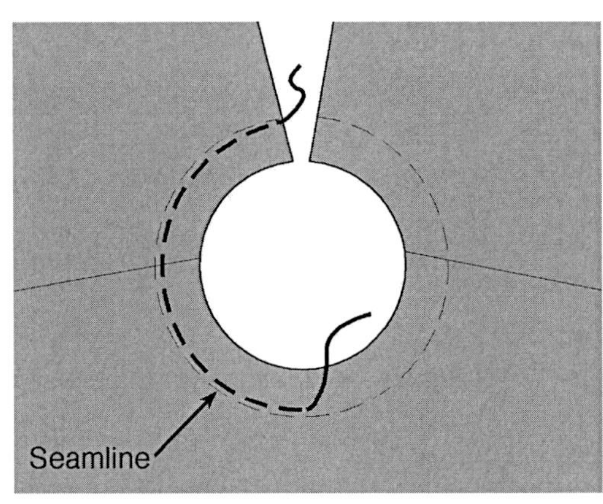
Seamline

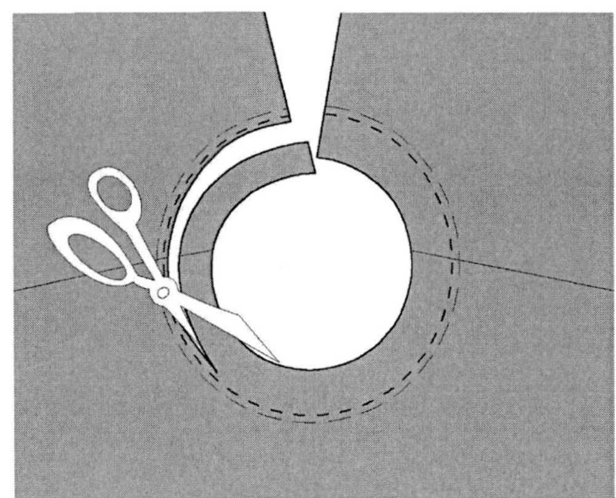

Trim **close** to the stitching line, and not more than 1/16″ (1.5mm) away. There should now be approximately ⅛″ (3mm) to roll and whip.

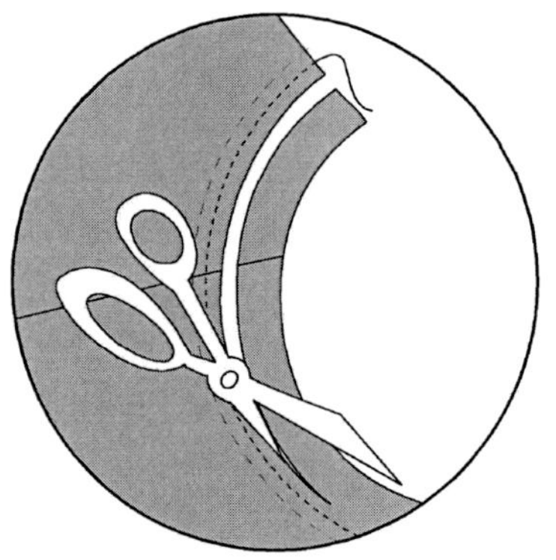

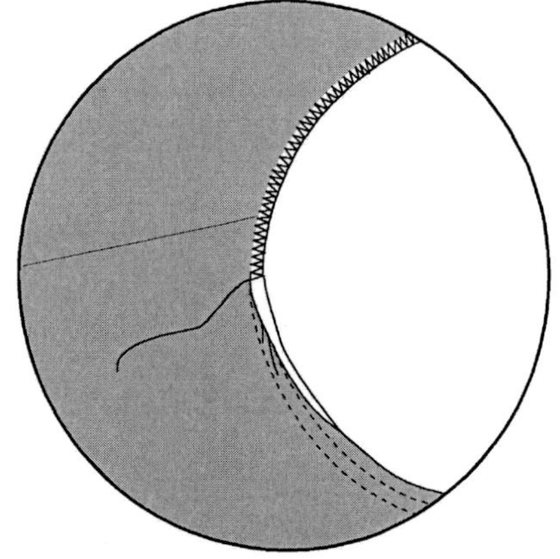

Roll and whip the curved edge with a zigzag stitch so that the fabric rolls over the original line of straight stitches. I use my buttonhole foot (not the automatic buttonhole foot), centered over the straight stitches – L-0.75; W-2.0.

*Refer to the techniques for making a **Fine Rolled Hem**.*

APPLYING ENTREDEUX TO A CURVED EDGE
(Rolled and Whipped Concave Curve)

One method for applying entredeux to a curved edge (e.g. neckline or armhole) is to start with a rolled and whipped edge.

Refer to the techniques for ***Rolling and Whipping a Bias or Curved Edge***

Remove the batiste from one side of the entredeux by trimming up to the row of embroidered holes.

Clip the batiste on the remaining side of the entredeux at approximately ¼″ (6mm) intervals.

Press the entredeux into a curve, following the same line as the edge to which it will be attached. Lightly mist with spray starch and press again using steam. Repeat the pressing process until the entredeux is stable, but not too stiff.

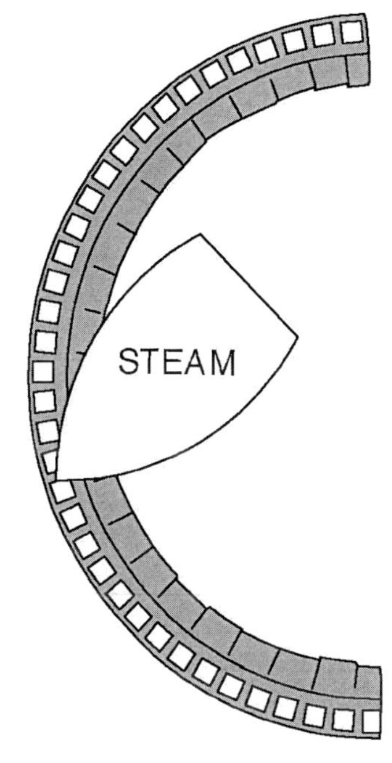
STEAM

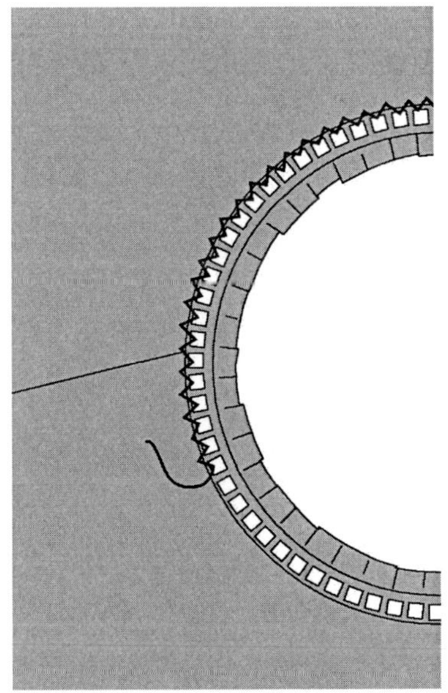

Attach the entredeux to the rolled and whipped edge by butting the edges together and zigzagging into each hole of the entredeux and over the roll of fabric.

Tip: *This technique is very similar to* ***Attaching Entredeux to a Straight Edge of Lace****. The stitching will be over a rolled edge instead of a lace heading, with the rolled edge to the left of the entredeux for ease in working.*

SUGGESTED MACHINE SETTINGS
Zigzag Stitch:
W: Approximately 2.0
L: Approximately 1.0
Needle Position: Center
Foot: Basic or Buttonhole foot

Tip: *Experiment with an open-toe or clear presser foot as this allows for greater visibility*

APPLYING ENTREDEUX TO A CURVED EDGE

(Rolled and Whipped Convex Curve)

One method for applying entredeux to a curved edge (e.g. scallops at the hemline, or a round yoke or collar) is to start with a rolled and whipped edge.

Tip*: refer to the techniques for* ***Rolling and Whipping a Bias or Curved Edge***

Remove the batiste from one side of the entredeux by trimming up to the row of embroidered holes.

Clip the batiste on the remaining side of the entredeux at approximately ¼″ (6mm) intervals.

Press the entredeux into a curve, following the same line as the edge to which it will be attached. Lightly mist with spray starch and press again using steam. Repeat the pressing process until the entredeux is stable, but not too stiff.

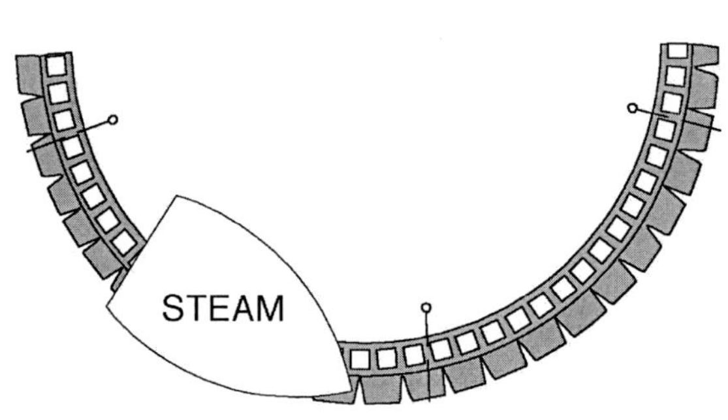
STEAM

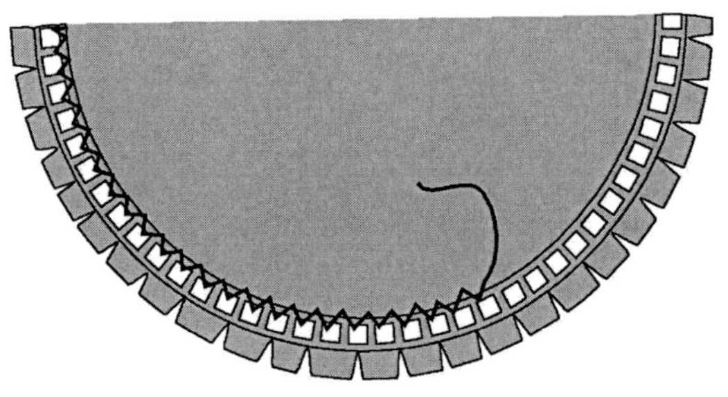

Attach the entredeux to the rolled and whipped edge by butting the edges together and zigzagging into each hole of the entredeux and over the roll of fabric.

Tip: *This technique is very similar to* ***Attaching Entredeux to a Straight Edge of Lace****. The stitching will be over a rolled edge instead of a lace heading, and the rolled edge will be to the left of the entredeux.*

It is important that you apply ample ease to the entredeux when you attach it to the outside curve of fabric, as even the slightest stretch on the entredeux will cause the fabric within the scallop or curve to pucker.

SUGGESTED MACHINE SETTINGS

Zigzag Stitch:
W: Approximately 2.0
L: Approximately 1.0
Needle Position: Center
Foot: Basic or Buttonhole foot

CORDED EDGE TRIM

This application is an excellent treatment on which to apply lace or a hand embellishment for:

- Collars or cuffs on a single or double thickness of fabric. Collars and cuffs must be cut as a pair
- Single top layer of a decorative bib attached over a soaker pad

Make all necessary adjustments to the pattern piece to allow for the addition of a trim or hand embellishment. For example, if the pattern does not allow for a trim, but you wish to add a ¼" (6mm) lace edging, then you must reduce the outer edge (NOT the neck edge) by ¼" (6mm).

The pattern can be traced onto the fabric block following the seam line (NOT the cutting line) or, if using more than one layer of fabric that is too dense to trace, a pattern template that finishes on the seam line of the outer collar edge can be produced for tracing around. In either case the seam allowance of the neck edge must remain on the template.

Cut a block of fabric that is larger than the pattern piece. If using a double layer of fabric, place the *wrong* sides together and baste across the fabric in two or three places. Lightly spray starch and press the fabric block.

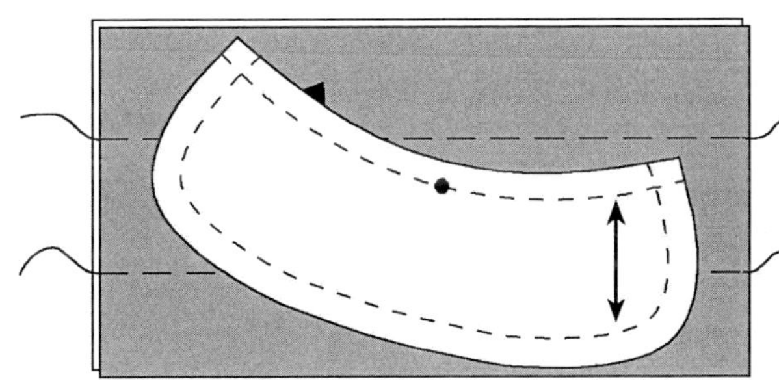

Position the template on the fabric block, or the pattern piece underneath for tracing. Be careful to match the grain lines.

Using a water-soluble marker, trace the seam line of the pair of collars or cuffs and transfer all notches from the pattern.

***Note**: The diagrams show the pattern with seam allowances maintained all round – you may prefer to make a new master pattern with the seam allowances removed from the outer edge and the neck edge seam allowance in tact.*

***Tip**: Machine stitch, using a short stitch length, on the **cutting line of the neck edge**. Include all notches and the shoulder position, as this will be the only reference you have for cutting out once the Corded Edge is applied and the collars are rinsed.*

Thread **Perle 8 cotton** or **gimp cord** through the tunnel in the center front of the foot. With the **right side** facing up, stitch around the outer edge of the collar (not the neckline) on the **seam line**. The zigzag stitch should be just wide enough to pass over the filler cord.

Stitch with an even, steady speed, very slightly pivoting at regular intervals on the outside edge of the curve. This will make a smooth and rounded stitching line. Keep the fabric taut from in front and behind the presser foot.

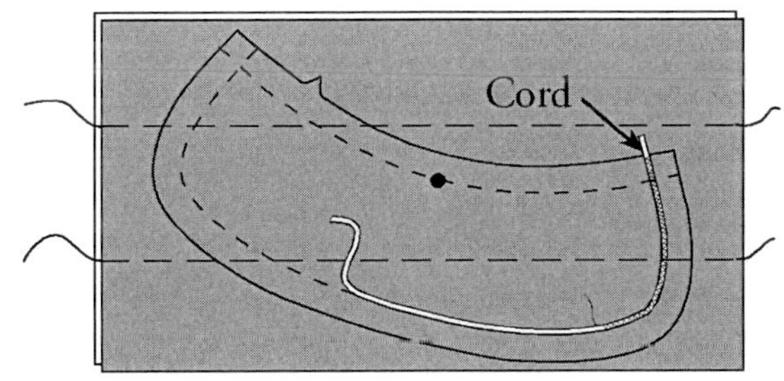
Cord

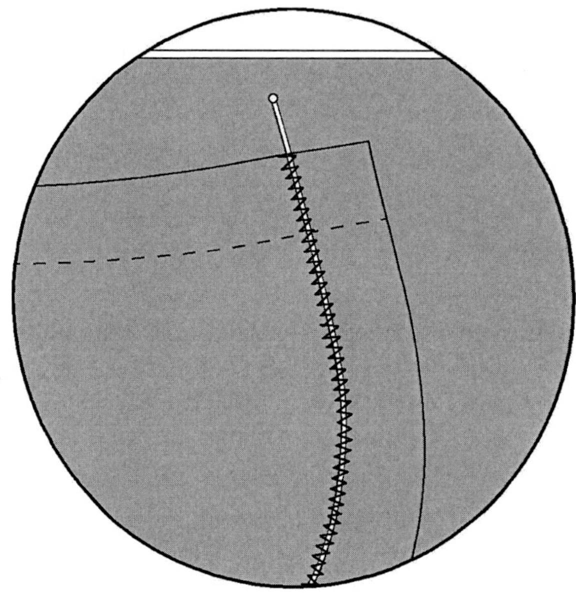

The fabric must be washed at this point to remove all tracing lines. First remove the basting threads and gently agitate in lukewarm water until all blue markings have disappeared; dry flat. When dry, press well from the wrong side, being careful to square up the block of fabric again. Lightly spray starch and press again to meld the stitches and remove any wrinkles.

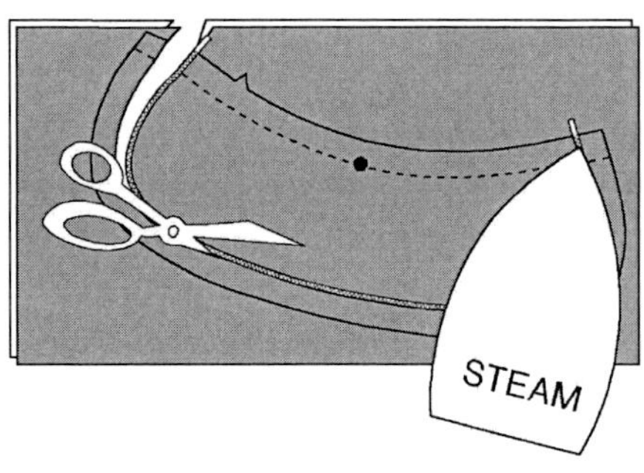
STEAM

Use a very fine, sharp pair of scissors and trim the seam allowance close to the zigzag stitches. Work from the right side and be careful not to cut any of the threads.

***Tip**: I find it easier to trim close when using a pair of micro-serrated scissors, as the blades on these scissors maintain their grip on fine fabric, especially on the bias grain. My preference is the 4″ or 6″ size.*

The collar is now complete and ready to be trimmed or attached untrimmed to the neckline of the garment. Experiment with this technique as it can produce exciting results. For example, the cording and zigzag stitching could be of a contrast color creating a highlighted edge; or the collar trimmed with lace, tatting, rick-rack trim or a hand embroidered finish.

SUGGESTED MACHINE SETTINGS

Zigzag Stitch:

Width	*Approximately 1.0 – 1.25*
Length	*Approximately 0.75 – 1.0 (not as tight as satin stitch, but not too open so as to allow whiskers)*
Tension:	*Tighten the bobbin tension as for working buttonholes*
Needle Position:	*Center*
Foot:	*A single cording foot, or the center hole in a multi-cord foot*
Thread:	*Fine cotton embroidery thread (Tanne 80 or Cotona 80), Lacis #120, Mettler 60/2 or DMC 50)*

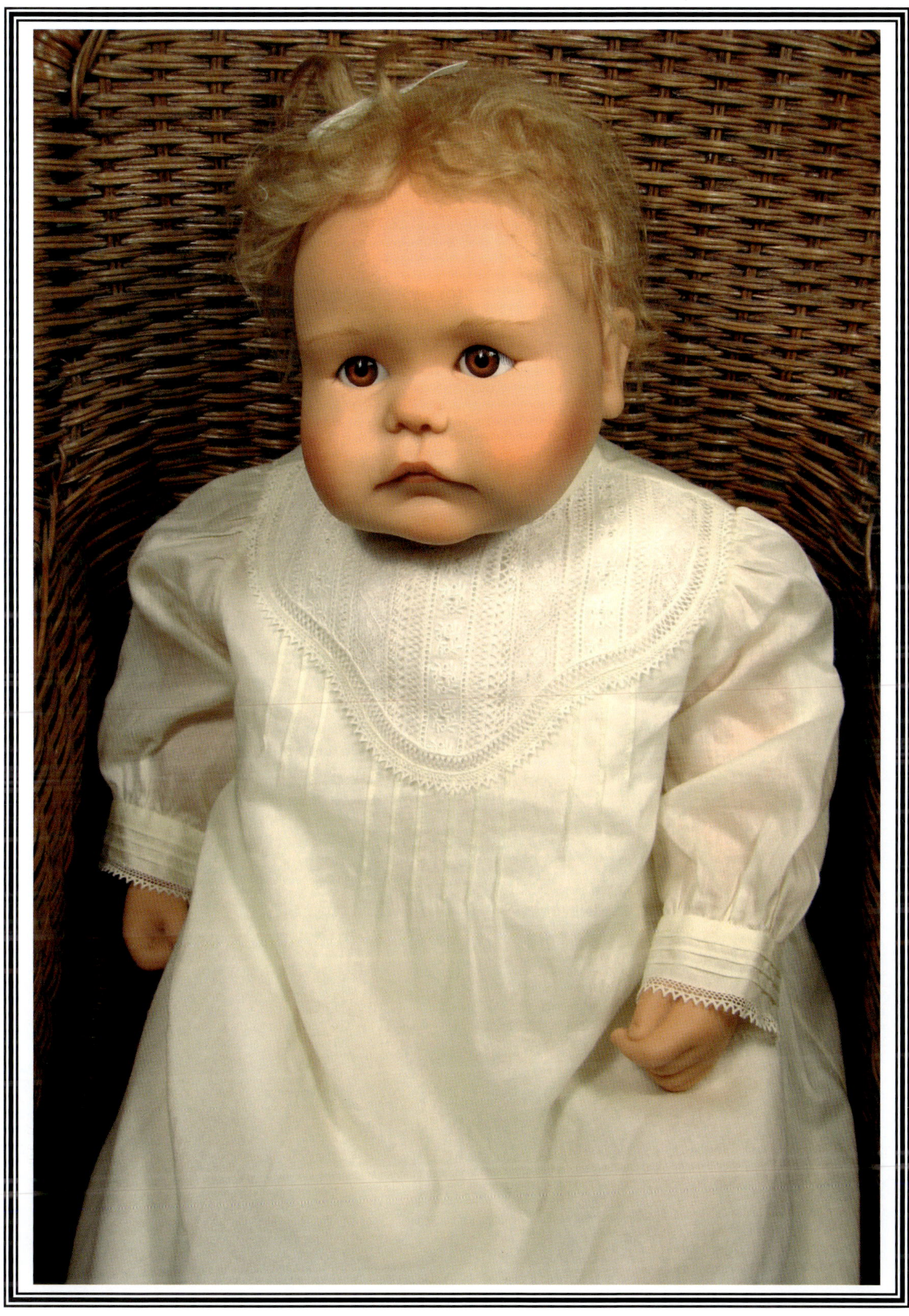

'Delicate Daydreams' with Release Tucks

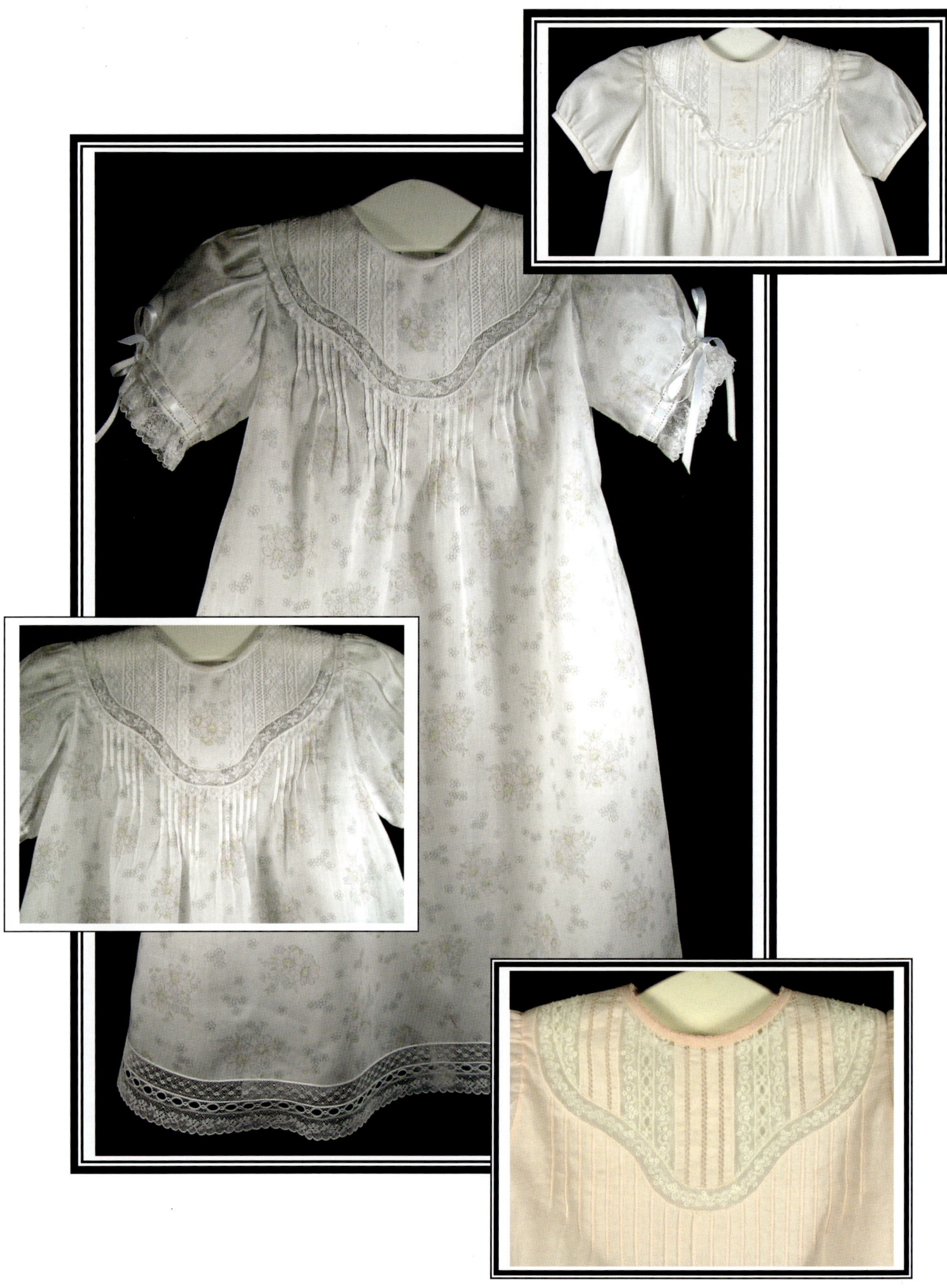

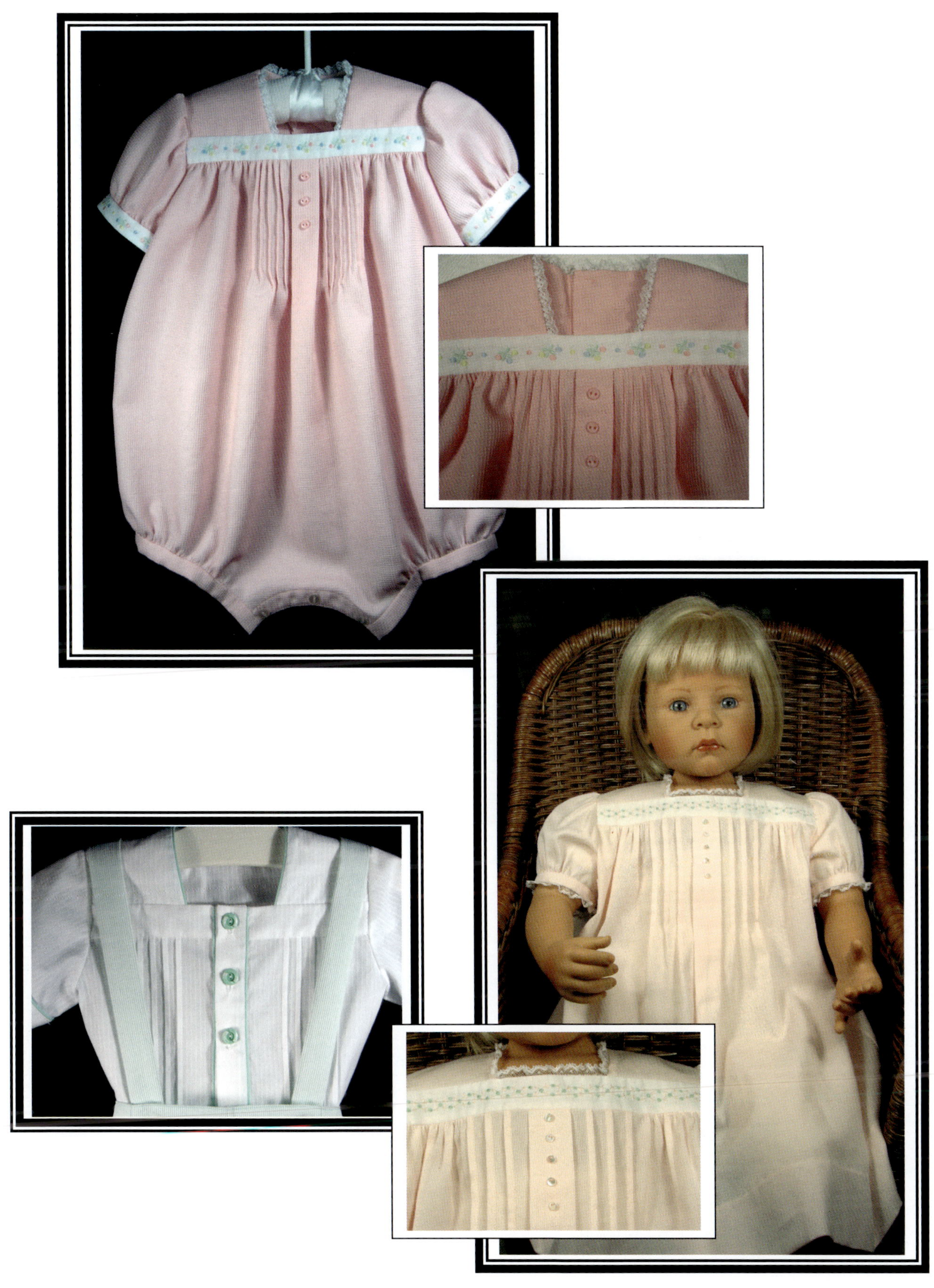

'Carol & Christopher' with Release Tucks

'The Edwardian Baby' showing Lace-to-Fabric

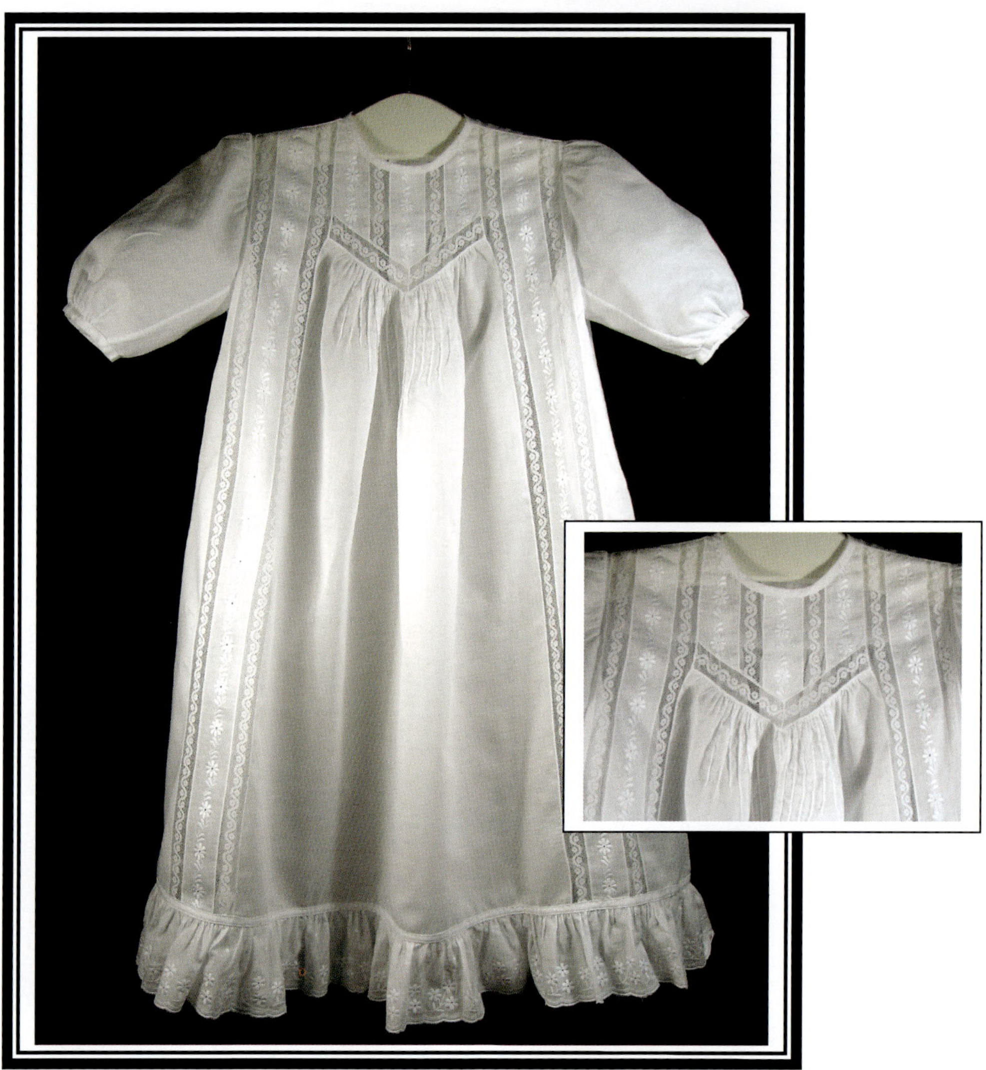

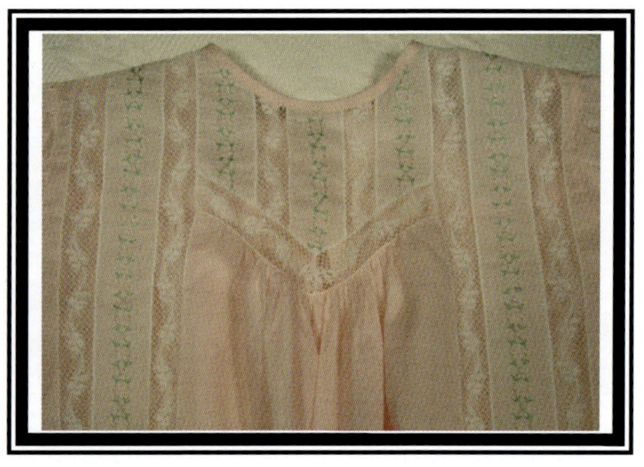

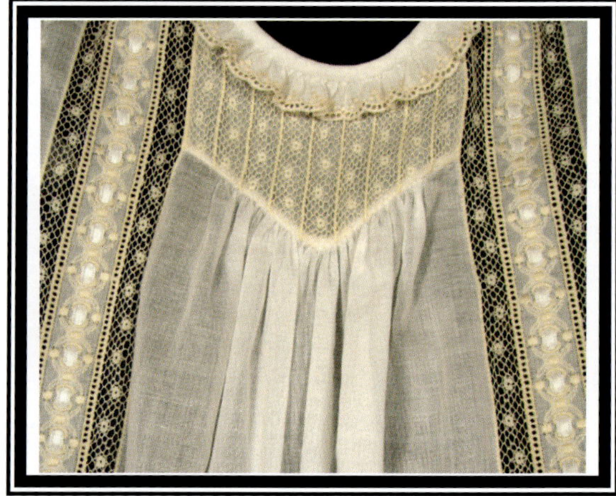

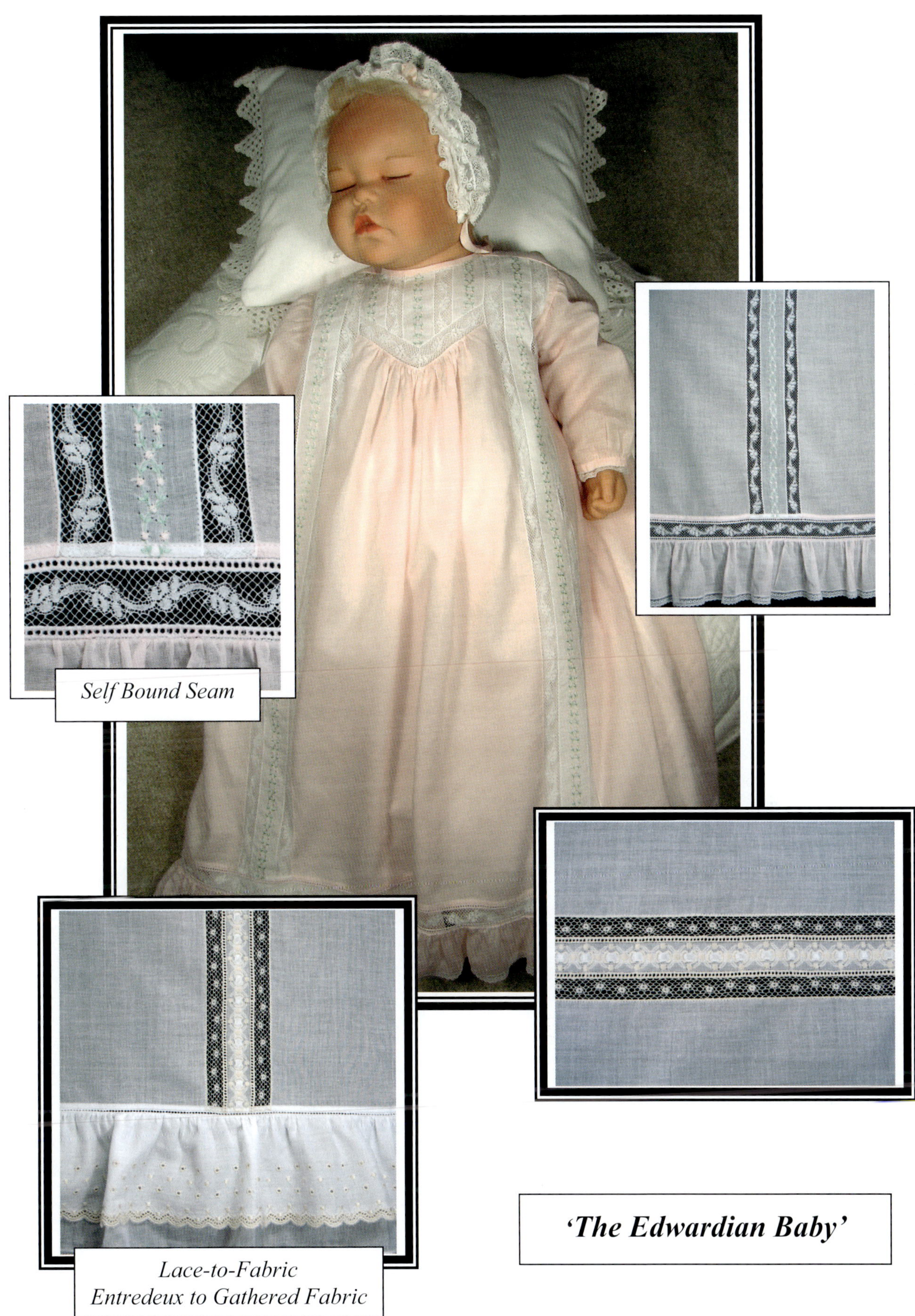

Self Bound Seam

Lace-to-Fabric
Entredeux to Gathered Fabric

'The Edwardian Baby'

'Frannie'

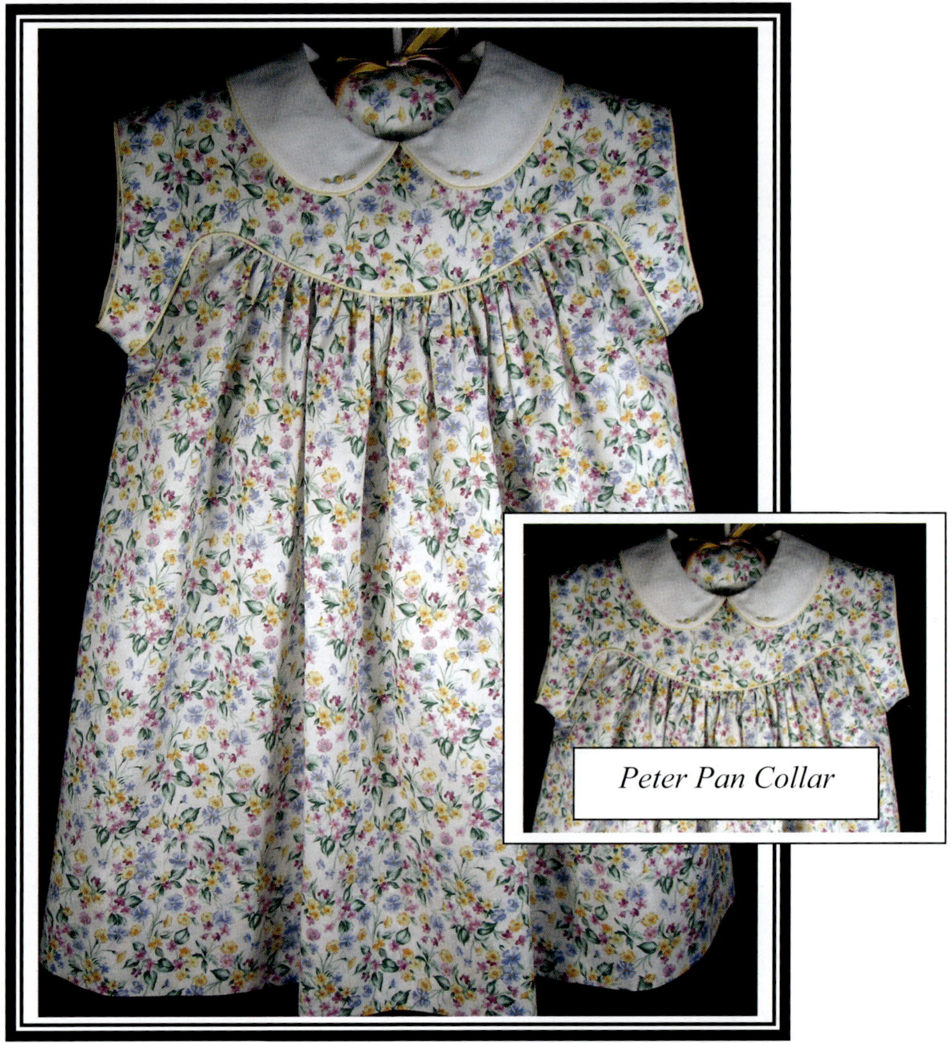

Peter Pan Collar

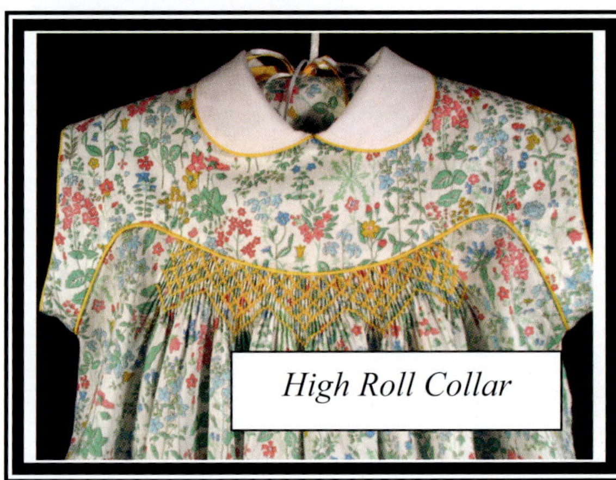

High Roll Collar

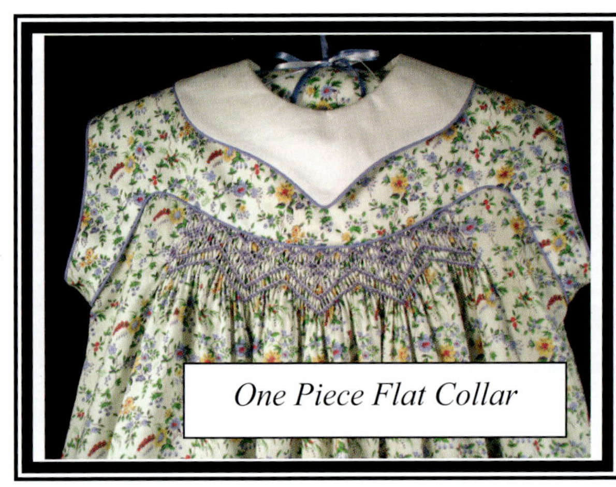

One Piece Flat Collar

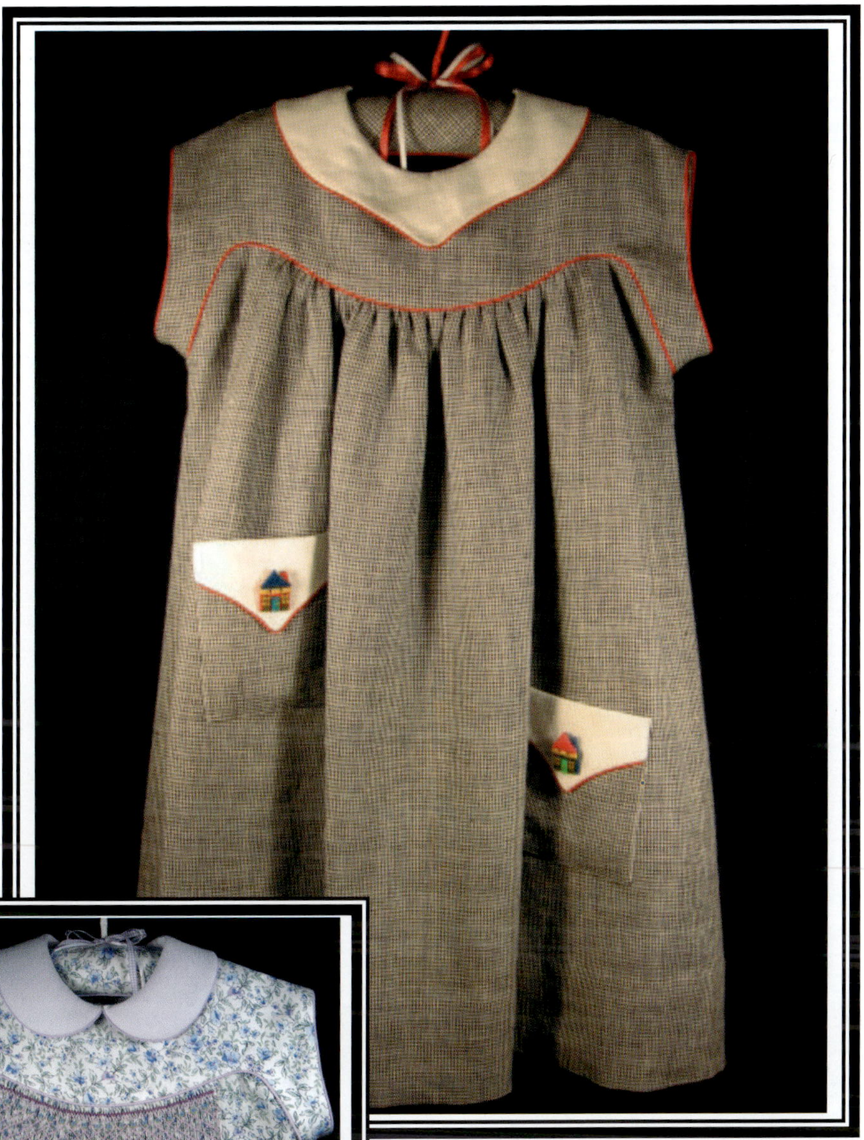

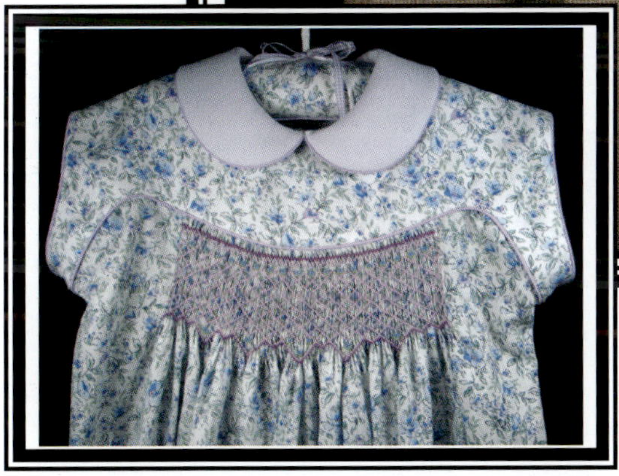

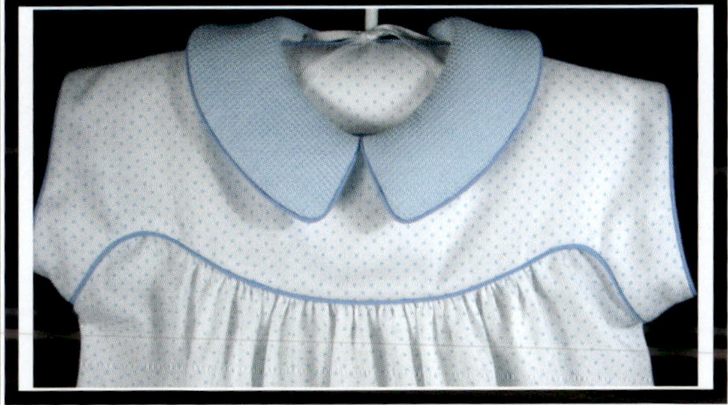

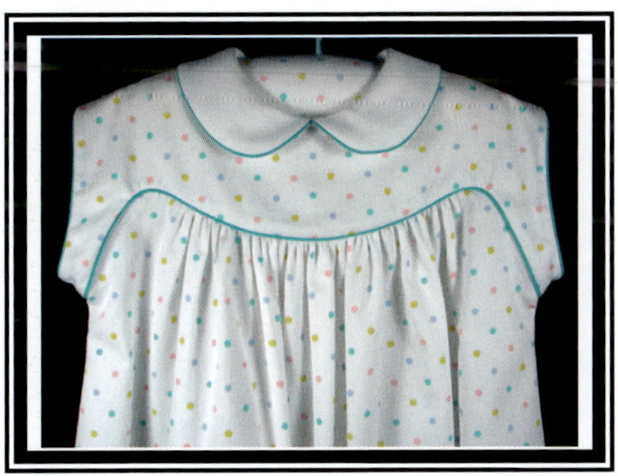

'Frannie'-with Piping Detail

'Gabrielle'-Daygown & Jacket

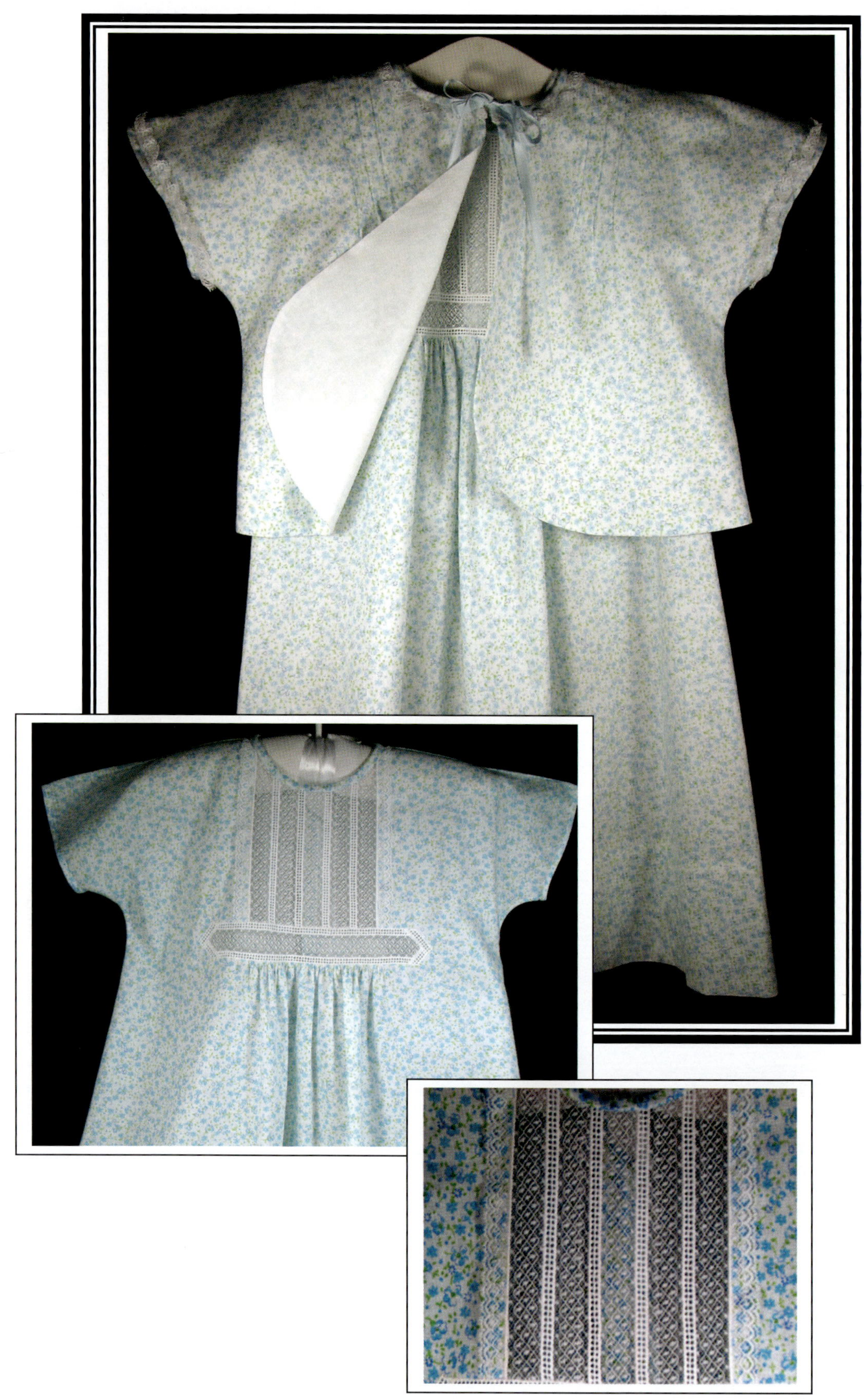

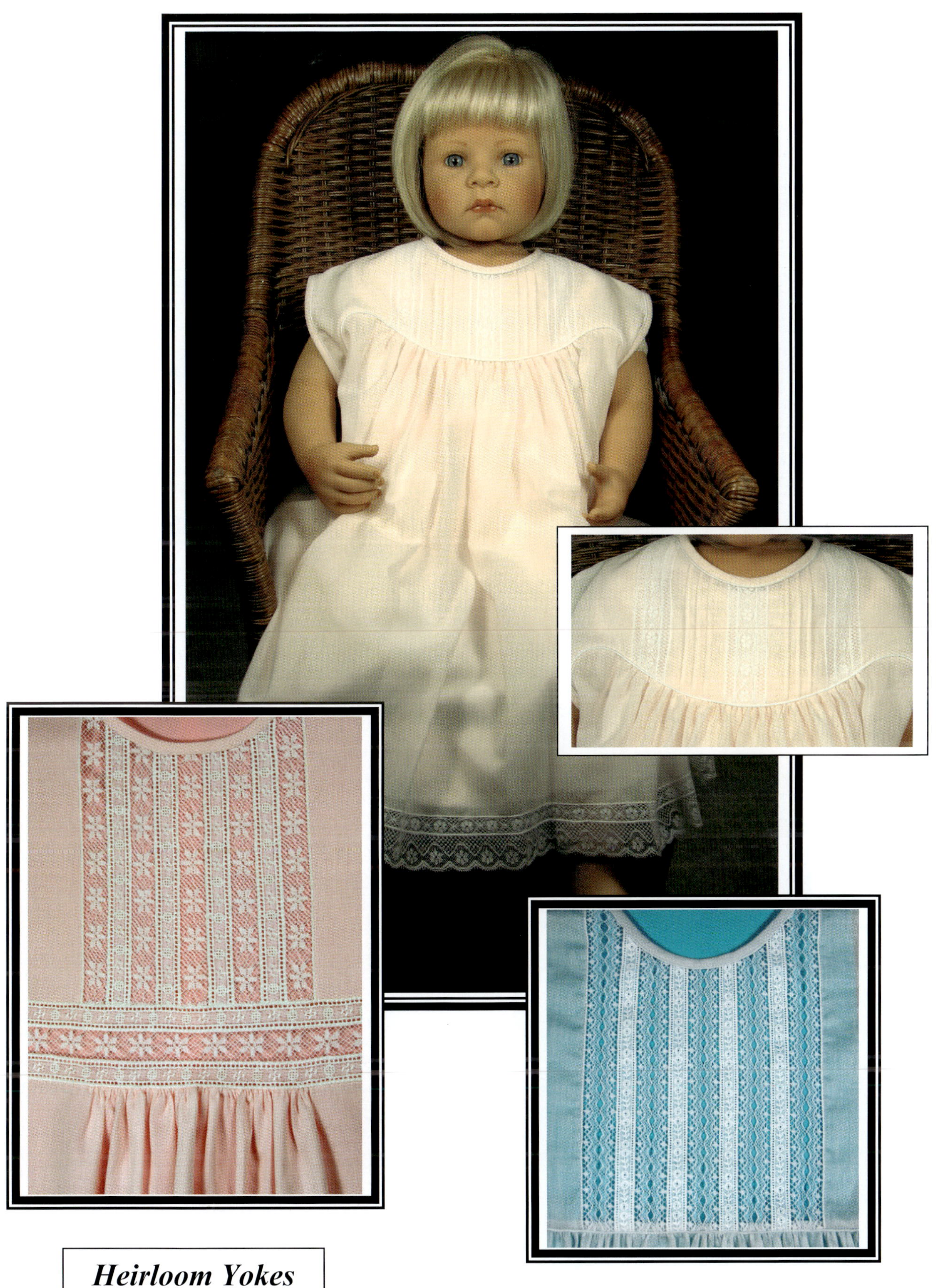

Heirloom Yokes

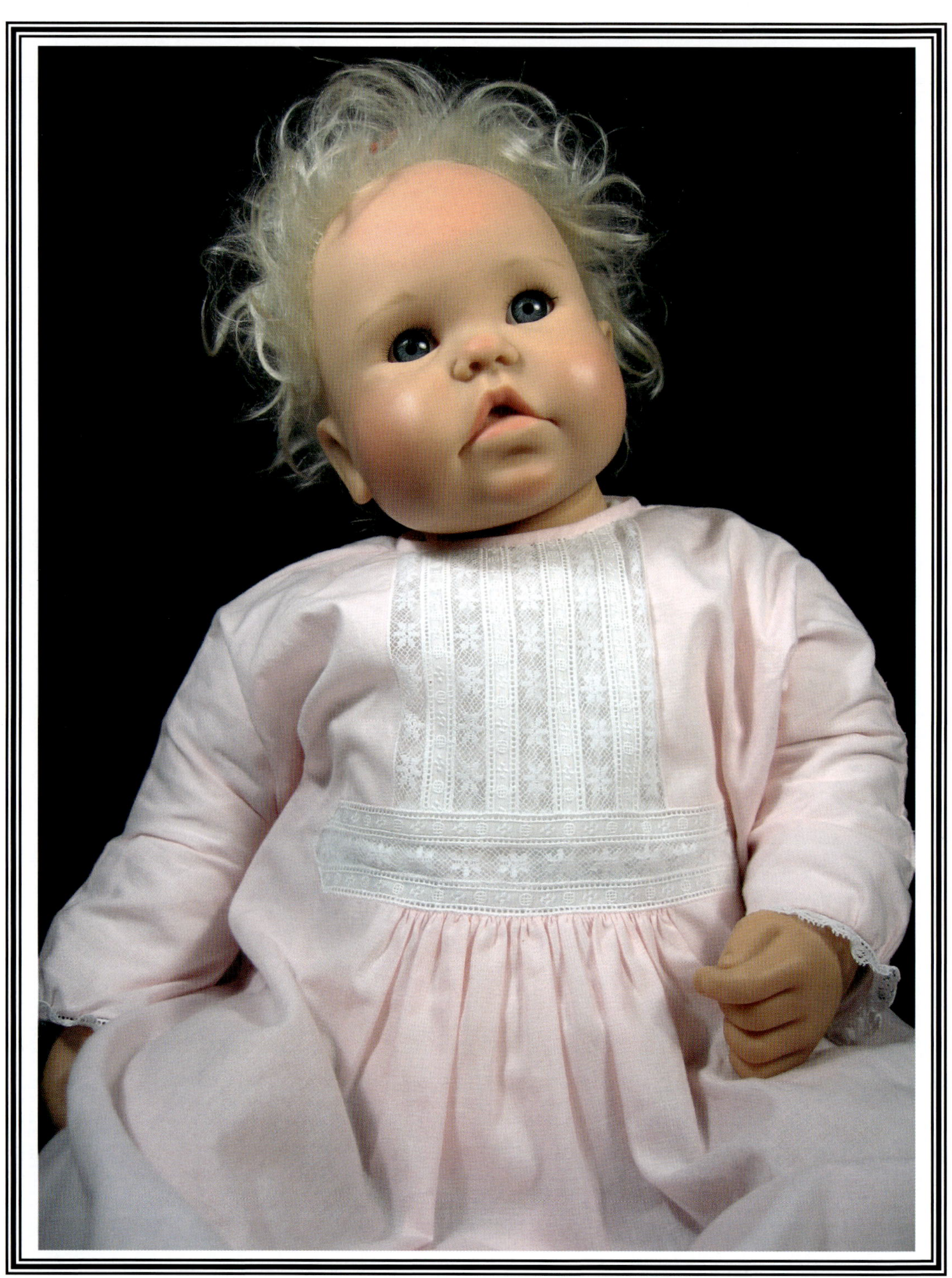

CREATING WITH TUCKS

Tucks create a wonderful opportunity to add texture and interest to any project, without any additional expense. They are beautiful, versatile and combine well with other heirloom or basic sewing techniques. Despite the simplicity of executing tucks, they are also a rich addition to everything from a sweet and dainty baby's layette to a sophisticated, elegant linen blouse. There is only one main point to remember and that is:

Tucks can enhance any project if they are perfectly even and stitched well; poorly worked tucks can ruin the project.

Tucks fall into two basic categories:

- Traditional Pintucks
  - Narrow Pintucks
  - Blind Tucks
  - Growth Tucks
  - Grouped Tucks
  - Whipped Pintucks
  - Shell Edge Tucks
  - Released Pintucks

- Twin Needle Tucks
  - Corded Twin-needle Tucks
  - Scalloped or Shaped Tucks
  - Cross-over Tucks

Other Types of tucks fall into the category of:

- Fabric Manipulation
  - Sharks Teeth or Prairie Point Tucks
  - Mexican or back-folded tucks

BASIC TUCKS

These are the traditional tucks stitched along the fold of the fabric with a single needle, and one top and one bobbin thread.

Measure accurately, or pull a thread to mark the fold of the tuck and stitch the desired distance from the fold.

Select a foot that makes accuracy achievable (e.g. an edge-joining foot for tucks of less than ⅛" (3mm)) and don't be afraid to play with the needle position on your machine.

Hold the fabric taut from in front of and behind the presser foot, and stitch with a steady even pace.

Tucks that lie horizontal are always pressed down. Vertical tucks are usually pressed away from the center.

TWIN NEEDLE TUCKS

Twin Needle tucks are created by using the combination of a twin needle, a special grooved foot that complements the needle size and a spool of thread for each of the two needles.

Measure and mark the placement of the first tuck only. Stitch this first tuck on the marked line – it will then automatically “ride” in one of the grooves underneath the foot to evenly space the next tuck being stitched.

The stitch length is determined by the weight of the fabric. The finer the fabric, the shorter the stitch should be.

Because we want the fabric to create a tuck or ridge, stabilizer should not be used. You may, however, choose to lightly spray starch and press the fabric before commencing.

Notes

ADDING PLEATS OR TUCKS

A pleat or tuck is a stitched fold of fabric which is most often decorative, and can either be added to the pattern pieces or stitched into the fabric before the fabric is cut. The following directions would add a box pleat or inverted pleat to the garment. For a single tuck follow the directions working on one side only of the center line.

The ratio of fabric to pleat is 3:1. It takes 3" (7.5 cm) to make a 1" (2.5 cm) pleat.

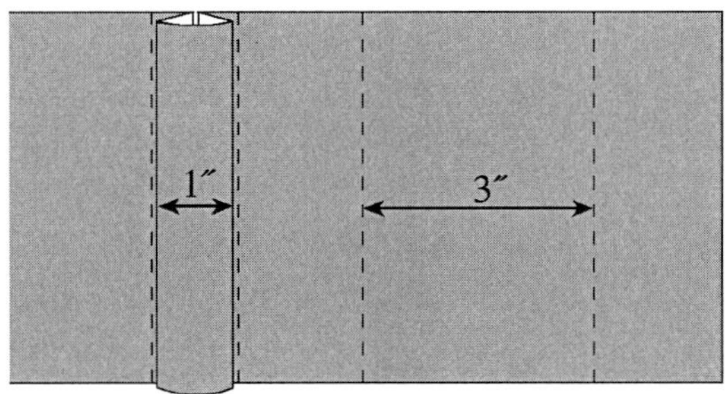
1″
3″

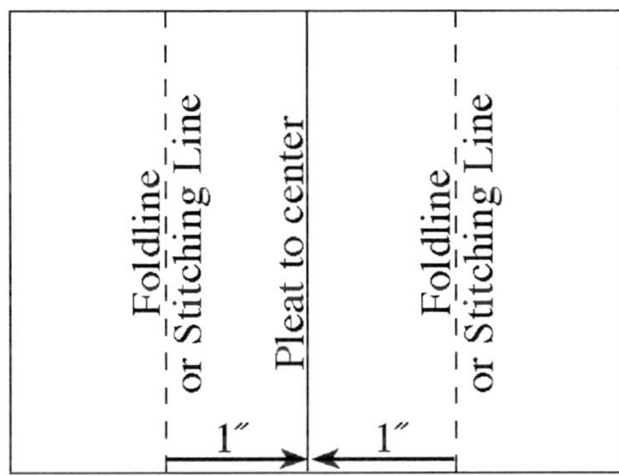
Foldline or Stitching Line
Pleat to center
Foldline or Stitching Line
1″
1″

To add pleats to a pattern:
Locate the desired position of the pleat and draw a vertical line at that point.

Draw a parallel line on either side equal to the finished pleat width. These parallel lines will be the fold lines for the pleat

Crease the pattern along these two parallel foldlines.

Bring these lines together to meet at the original pleat position line. Crease the pattern piece well on both sides.

Repeat the above steps for any remaining pleats being careful to allow for the distance between each pleat.

***Tip**: Start with the center pleat and work toward the sides. This will help maintain symmetry.*

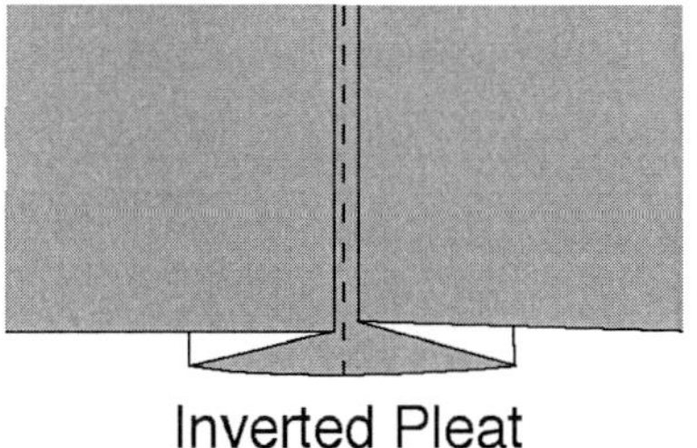
Inverted Pleat

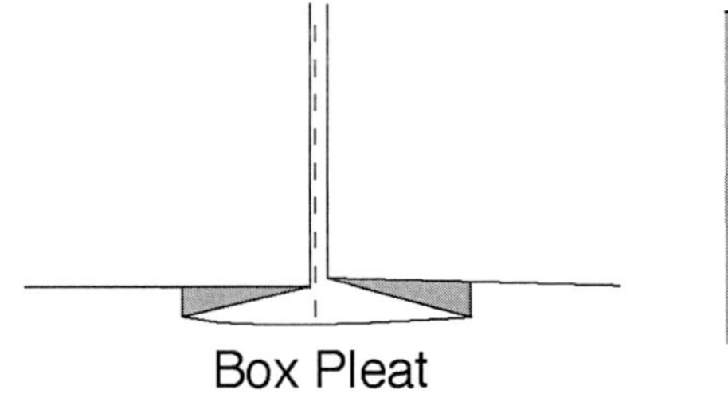
Box Pleat

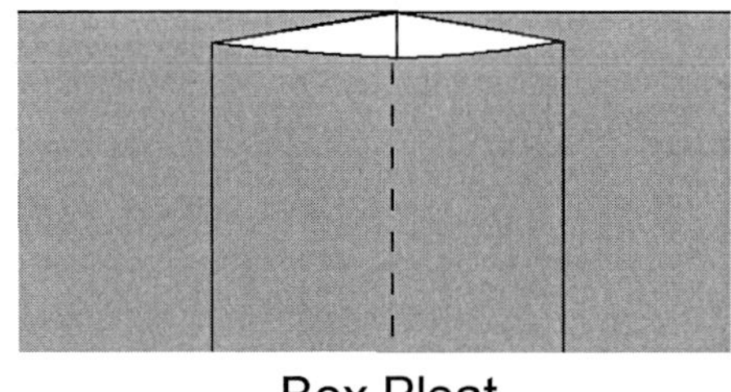
Box Pleat

BASIC TUCKS

A tuck is nothing more than a stitched fold of fabric that is most often decorative in purpose. Tucks may vary in width from very narrow pintucks to much wider tucks of up to 1"-1¼" in width. Using an edge joining (or edge stitching) foot as a guide makes creating traditional delicate pintucks almost effortless. Despite how simple these tucks are to make, they are a beautiful addition to any project.

Tucks may be all the same length, or they may be of graduated lengths; they may be held at each end as decorative embellishment or stitched to a certain point and released for added fullness. If the tuck is made on the wrong side of the garment it is used to create fullness only and not for decorative purposes.

A tucks width is the distance from the fold of fabric to the stitching line. The width can vary, as can the space between the tucks. You may choose *'Blind Tucks'* where each tuck touches or overlaps the next tuck, or those with a space between them called *'Spaced Tucks'*. A very narrow tuck is called a *'Pintuck'*.

Because traditional tucks, or basic pintucks, are stitched along the fold of the fabric, the fold lines need to be marked. There are several ways to mark the foldline:

- Pull a thread on the straight grain for each tuck – this works best when making lots of very long, narrow tucks on fine fabric and not as well when working on linen where the slubs can cause gaps on the foldline.
- Use the '*Measure, Pin and Press'* method, executing only one tuck at a time for complete accuracy – the most versatile method, especially for working with linen.
- Mark the foldline with a water-soluble marker – usually a 'last resort' as the fabric MUST be washed before the tucks can be pressed.

Traditional tucks have a depth of approximately ⅛″ so each tuck takes up a full ¼″ of fabric. This involves some preparation so plan ahead. Always make a series of test tucks to gauge the amount of fabric needed, the most appropriate distance between each tuck, the foot that will make the job easiest and the needle position. There is no magical answer to these questions – just practice. It is advisable to write every detail directly onto the stitched sample for future reference.

To embellish a project without so much measuring, tuck a large area of fabric and then cut the stitched pieces to the correct size – i.e. you will be *making fabric* by piecing panels together. This new fabric could comprise tucks that are joined to Swiss embroidery (or plain fabric) and then joined to more tucks.

PRESSING

Always press tucks firmly from the wrong side of the fabric first, to eliminate any pleats that might form behind the tuck. Use the side of the iron and steam to create a smooth, sharp line.

Alone, or in groups, tucks can be used to add fullness or to incorporate a decorative touch to a garment.

BASIC TUCKS

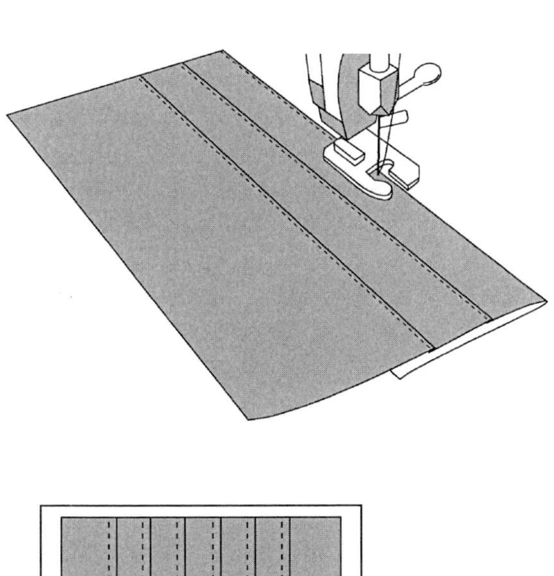

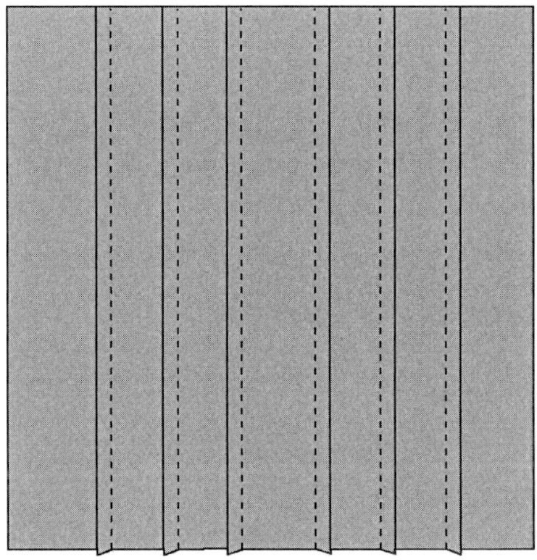

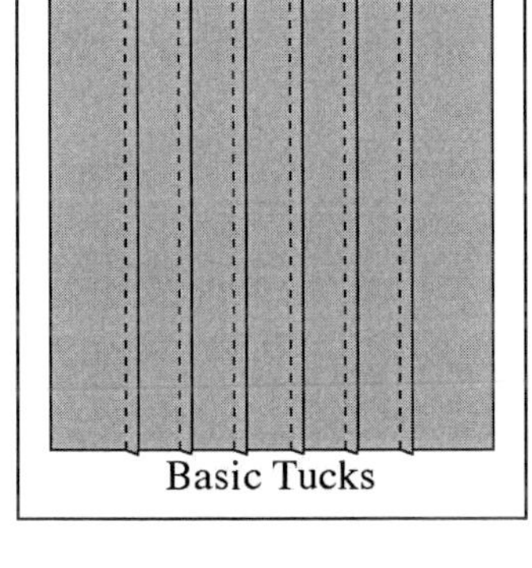

Basic Tucks

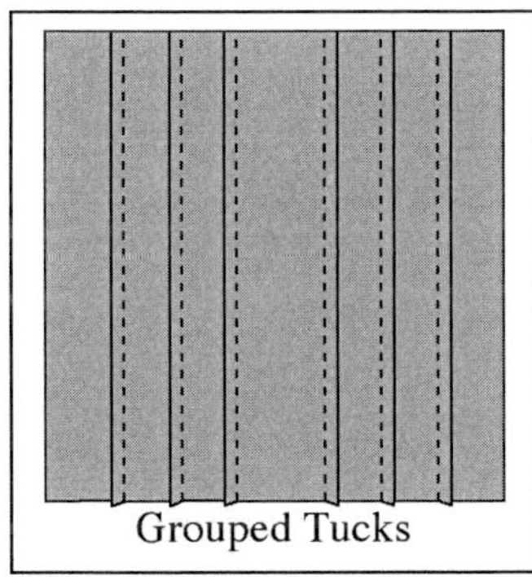

Grouped Tucks

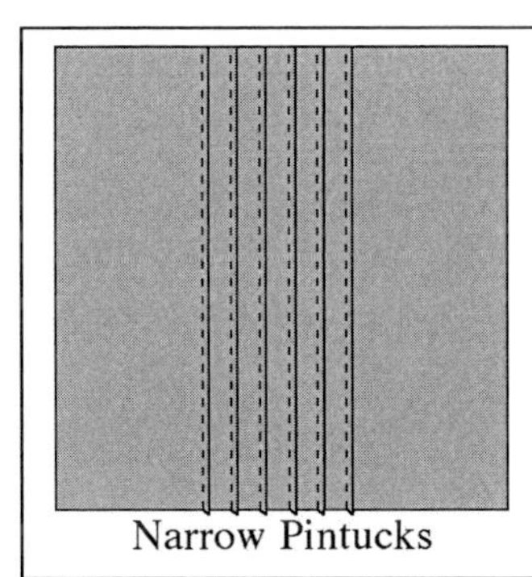

Narrow Pintucks

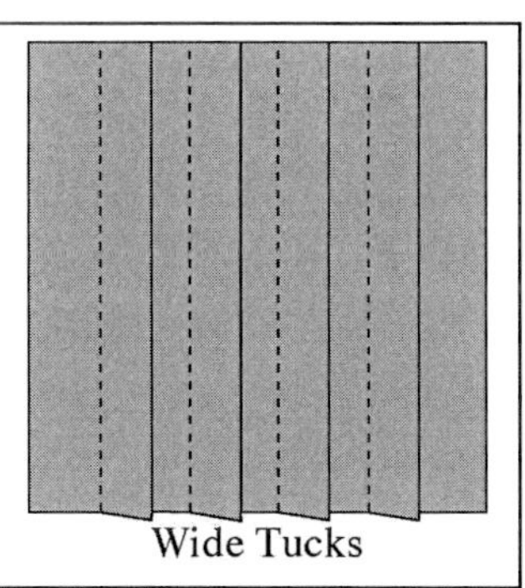

Wide Tucks

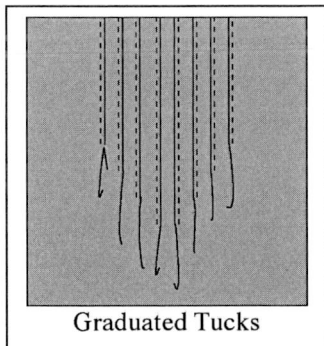

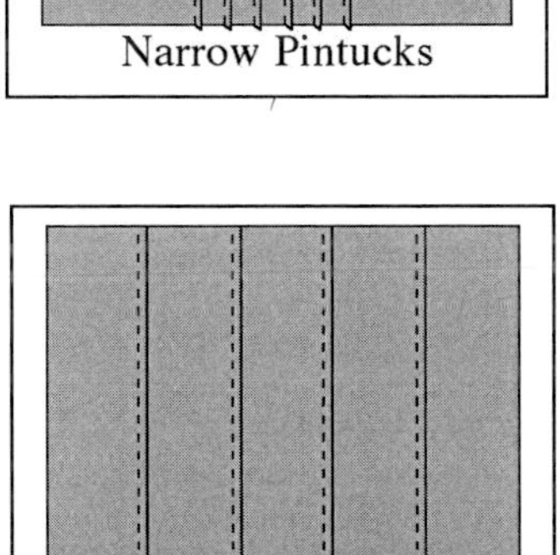

Graduated Tucks

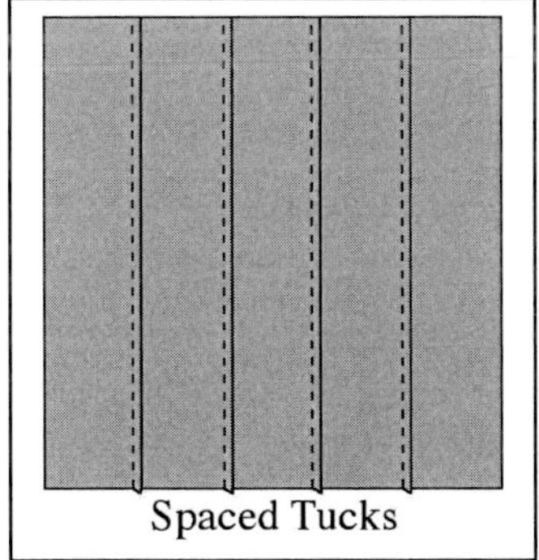

Spaced Tucks

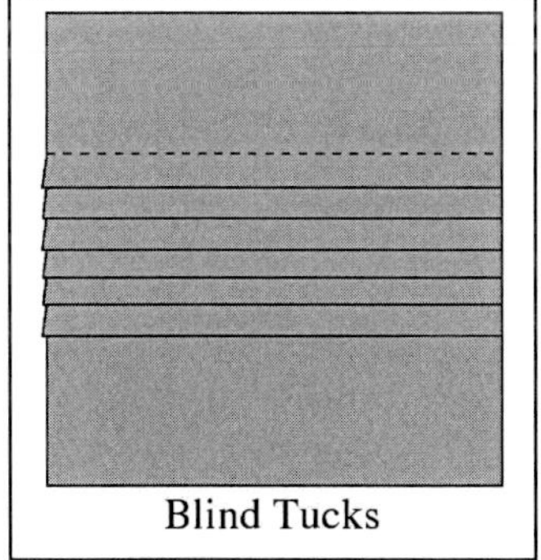

Blind Tucks

WHIPPED TUCKS

Whipped tucks are made using a very small zigzag stitch and are perfect for lingerie and baby clothing. The thread in the top spool can be fine and the same color as the fabric so as to blend when melded, or it can be of contrasting color and thickness.

Whipped tucks are purely decorative, and although they make a special statement when used as released tucks, they do not add any great amount of fullness to the garment. Whipped Release Tucks can be made using the technique for Reverse Threading.

***Tip**: Tucks should be made with the stitching from the top spool of thread on the front, or top, of the tuck. This will ensure that the decorative thread will be on top when the tucks are pressed away from center. For Release Tucks you will need to pull the two threads to the back at the release point and tie off using a square knot.*

Mark the placement for the Whipped Tucks and fold the fabric on this line. Press in a sharp crease.

Place the folded edge of the fabric under the presser foot and stitch with a small zigzag stitch.

*Refer to the techniques for **Reverse-threading** if making Release Tucks.*

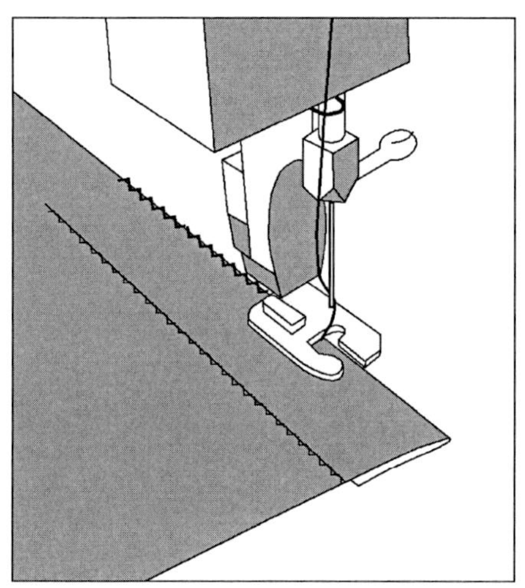

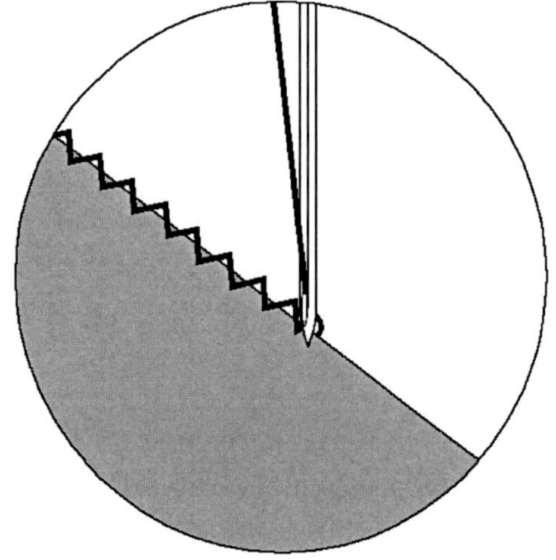

The left swing of the needle should pierce two to three threads on the edge of the tuck and then just barely clear the fabric with the right swing.

SUGGESTED MACHINE SETTINGS
Zigzag Stitch:
W: Approximately 0.5 –0.75
L: 1.0 to 1.5
Needle Position: center
Foot: edge-joining or basic sewing

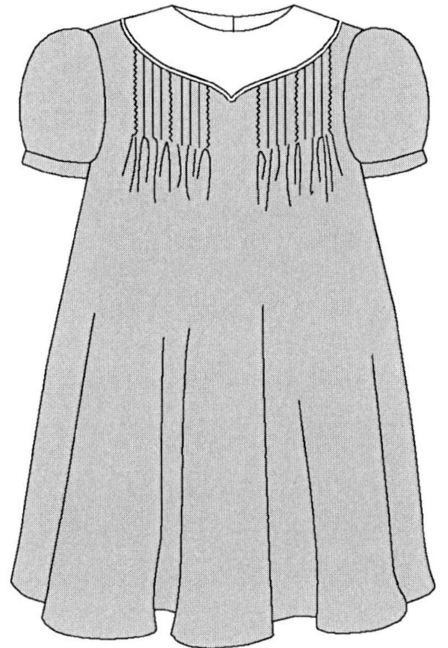

Notes

SHELL EDGE TUCKS

Shell Edge tucks form a decorative feature when used on lingerie, nightwear and delicate baby and children's clothing. They are formed by sewing over a fold of fabric with the stitch being sewn off the edge of the fold. They can be worked on the straight grain, bias grain or around a tiny curved neckline – in fact, the Shell Edge is even prettier when made on a curved edge rather than on the straight grain. The most suitable fabric is soft, lightweight woven cotton or cotton blend.

The principle for making a shell edge hem or neckline finish as shown by the hand-stitch illustrations, is to turn (or roll) a very narrow double turning of ⅛" (3mm) to ¼" (6mm). Fasten the thread in the hem and secure the hem with one or two small running stitches, then one or two whip stitches at right angles over the edge of the fabric. Continue as follows either by making one or two small running stitches, or taking a tiny stitch in the garment, then slipping the needle to the next shell and repeat.

***Tip**: Always make a test hem so you can determine how wide you want the hem and how far apart each shell should be – sometimes wider shells are prettier than the smaller ones.*

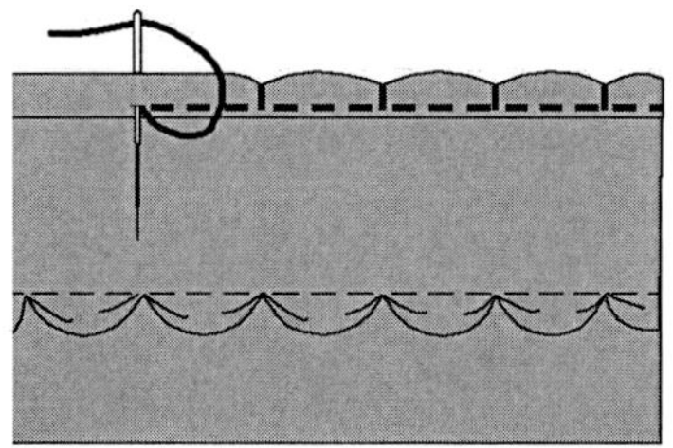

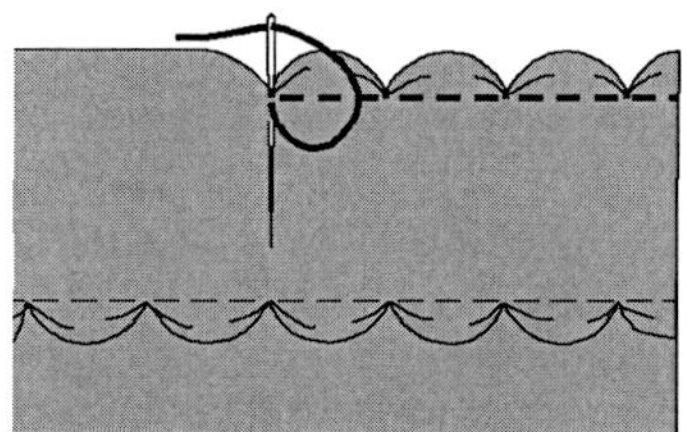

When working with only one stitch over the fold, stitch four or five scallops and then carefully pull the thread until the fabric puckers into gentle folds.

***Tip**: Keep the running stitches small and even and the scallops will be even. Use a stronger thread when working by hand so the thread doesn't break when you pull up the scallops.*

When making Shell Edge tucks by machine, mark the placement line on the fabric and fold on this line.

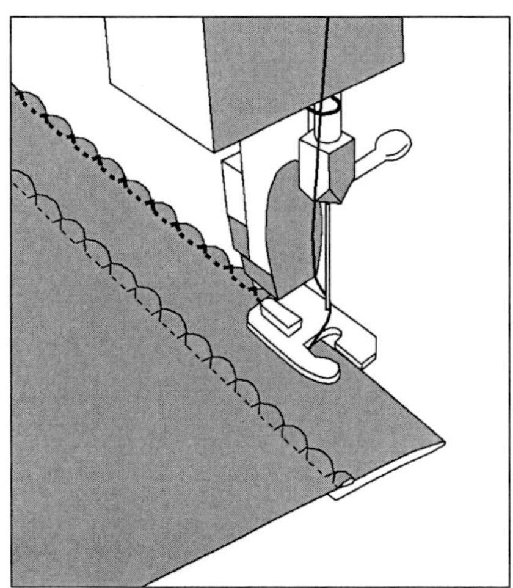

The machine stitch used to make a Shell Edge tuck could be a simple zigzag stitch, a blind hem stitch or single-swing hemstitch.

***Tip**: Be careful that the right hand needle swing in any of these stitch sequences just barely clears the fold of the fabric, thus causing the fabric to pinch in and form a scalloped edge.*

It will look like this on the stitch panel board:

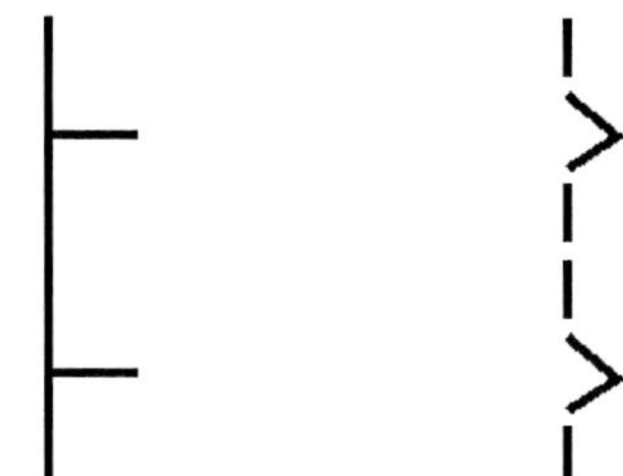

SUGGESTED MACHINE SETTINGS
Blind Hem Stitch ***or*** *as shown above:*
W: Depends on the placement of fabric and the width of the tuck
L: Each scallop should be no longer than 3/16" (5mm)
Needle Position: center
Foot: basic sewing or edge-joining foot
Thread: Fine Cotton – Mettler 60/2 or DMC 50
Tension: Upper tension will need to be slightly tightened

Notes

TWIN NEEDLE TUCKS

Twin Needle tucks are created by using the combination of a twin needle, two spools of thread and a special grooved (Pintucking) foot. Thread the machine, treating both threads as one, through all guides except at the tension where they will be separated (one thread onto each side of the center tension disc), and at the needles.

The two needle threads work with the bobbin thread, which forms a small zigzag on the wrong side of the work. It is the bobbin thread that actually pulls the two rows of the needle threads together to form the tuck. The smaller the stitch length, the more likely the tucks will sit up and form a ridge.

FEET

Pintuck feet have additional grooves under the foot that serve as spacing guides for stitching multiple rows of tucks. The groove or space in the foot allows the tuck room to form and doesn't flatten it after it is stitched. The first tuck is stitched in the center and can then "ride" in a different groove under the foot. This is an automatic guide to evenly space the next tuck while it is being stitched.

The number (or size) of grooves in the foot help determine the size of the tuck being formed. Pintuck feet are generally available with 3, 5, 7 or 9 grooves. Feet with fewer grooves have wider, deeper channels and form larger tucks.

NEEDLE SIZE

The needle size on twin needle packages is given in two sets of numbers with a slash in between – example 2.0/80. The first number designates the distance between the needles and the second number is the needle size. Thus, 2.0 means that the distance between the needles is 2mm, and the size of the needle is an 80.

The spacing between the needles helps determine the size of the pintuck. The needle size is selected to complement the type of fabric and the thread being used. It is important to understand this relationship between the fabric, the needle spacing and the size of the grooves under the foot. All these factors work together to make unique and varied combinations

SPACING

Remember, making tucks for texture or fullness creates a form of wearable art. The best advice is to always test your tucks, or doodle a little, before stitching on your project. This is how you determine the spacing you like, and time spent in preparation is never wasted.

SUGGESTED GUIDE

- Very Fine fabric such as Swiss voile, batiste, cotton lawn
  No. 1.6/70 needle 9 groove pintuck foot Cotton Embroidery thread (60/2)

- Medium weight fabric such as cotton sateen, dress-weight batiste, handkerchief linen
  No. 2.0/80 needle 7 or 5 groove pintuck foot Cotton Embroidery thread (60/2)

- Heavier weight fabric such as tightly woven cotton and cotton sateen, linen
  No. 2.5/80 needle 5 or 3 groove pintuck foot Cotton Silk Finish thread (50/3)

PRESSING

Always press twin needle tucks from the wrong side of the fabric first.

TWIN NEEDLE TUCKS

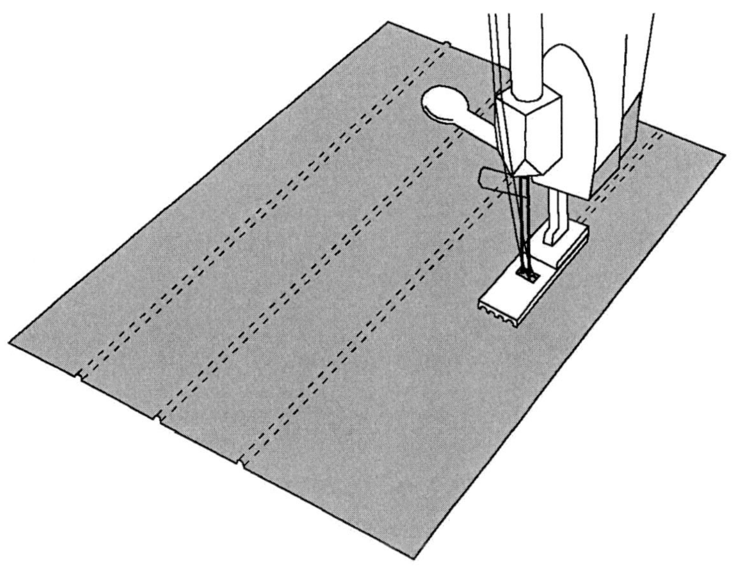

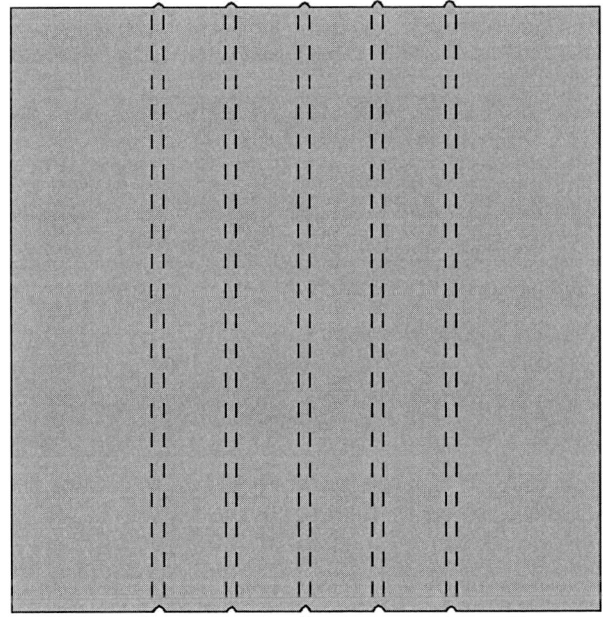

CORDED PINTUCKS

Different sewing machines have different methods for incorporating a fine cord underneath the fabric being drawn up into the twin-needle tuck. The most appropriate weights of cord to be used are Perle 8, Cordonnet or gimp cord to name a few. This cord will give the tuck a full, rounded look and create tucks that are resilient and will not flatten with continued laundering.

***Tip**: Experiment with various weights of thread for the fabric you intend to tuck, and don't be afraid to try a colored cord for a more pronounced or decorative tuck. For example, you could use pink cord and pink stitching thread on white voile for a very pretty tucked feature.*

Thread the cord from underneath the sole-plate on your machine, through the hole that sits directly below the needle.

Alternatively, for sewing machines without the above feature, pass the cord through the guide that will be attached on top of the sole plate, directly in front of the needle, and thread the cord between the two needles, as follows. Refer to your Sewing Machine Manual to find out which method to use.

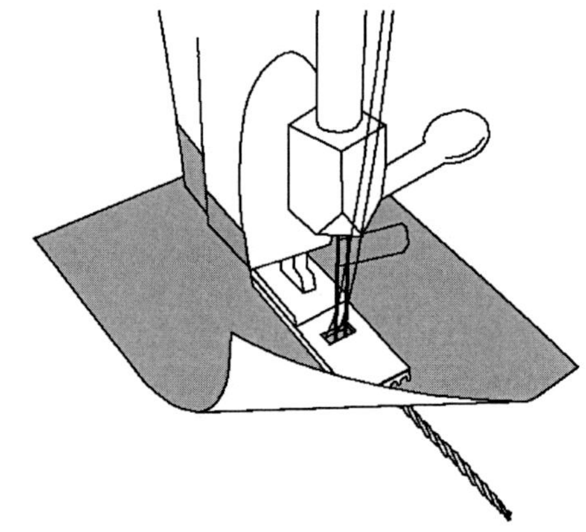

With the twin needle installed and the machine threaded correctly, take a few stitches and stop with the needle in the down position.

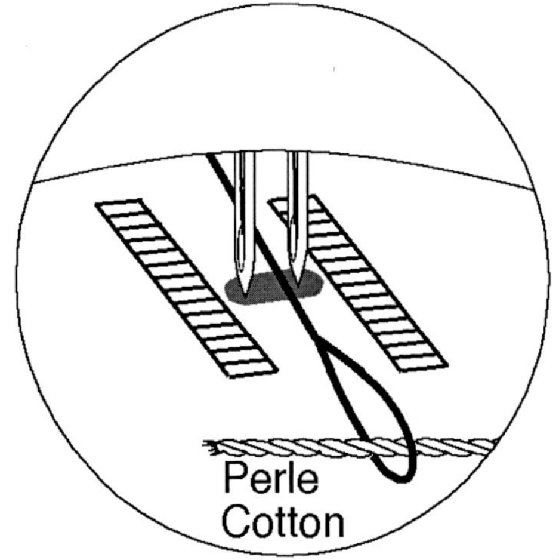
Perle
Cotton

Raise the presser foot and lift the fabric so that you can see the twin needle underneath the fabric.

Thread the cord between the two needles using a dental floss or loop-style threader. Place the threader between the needles, thread the cord through the loop and pull the threader through the needles bringing the cord with it.

***Tip**: Be sure the cord is under the center groove of the pintuck foot.*

Lower the presser foot, gently pull the cord upwards in front of the presser foot to be sure it will stay in the groove of the foot.

Straight stitch using the same settings as for uncorded twin needle tucks.

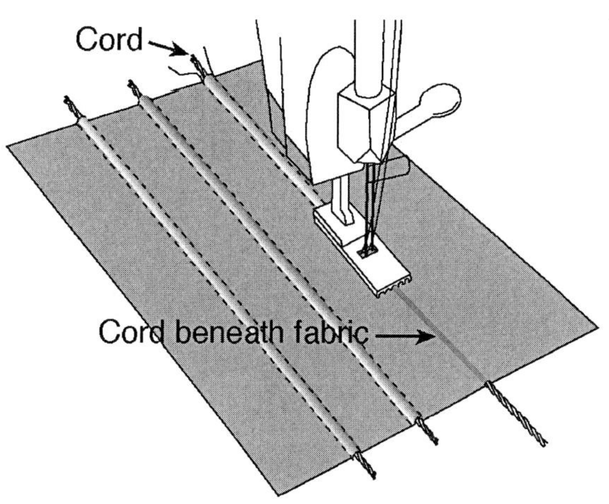
Cord
Cord beneath fabric

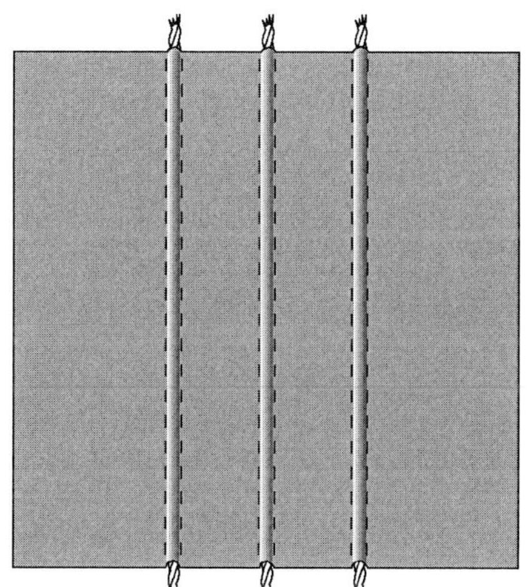

Suggested Machine Settings
Straight Stitch:
L: approximately 2.0
Needle Position: center
Foot: Pintuck foot that directly corresponds to the size of the needle and the thickness of fabric

Refer to the techniques for
Twin Needle tucks

Notes

STRAIGHTENING TUCKS

Sometimes when stitching multiple rows of pintucks, the fabric looks out of shape, or the pintucks look as if they are almost on the bias. This is more obvious when stitching a large block of tucks all in the same direction.

Before straightening, press the tucks from the wrong side using steam and the side of the iron to firmly push against the stitching line of each tuck. Be sure that the tucks are being pressed in the correct direction and no pleats are being formed between the tucks.

To straighten a block of pintucks:

- Lightly mist the pin tucked fabric with water or spray starch.
- Work on a board into which the pins will go easily.

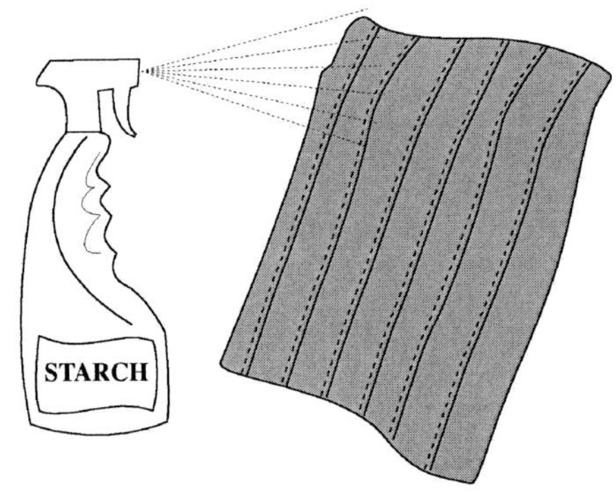
STARCH

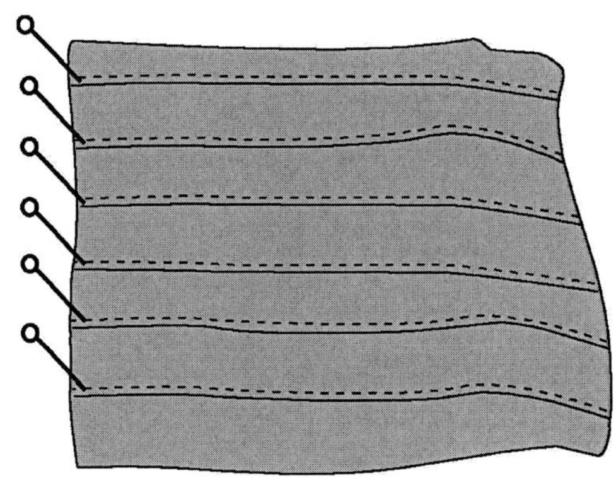

Pin one end of the tucked fabric onto the blocking board and pull the other end so that the tucks are straight.

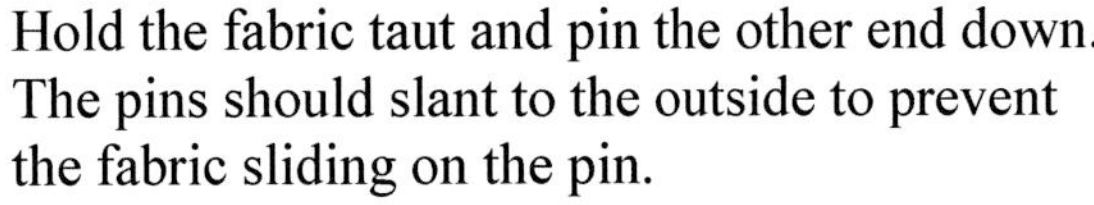

Hold the fabric taut and pin the other end down. The pins should slant to the outside to prevent the fabric sliding on the pin.

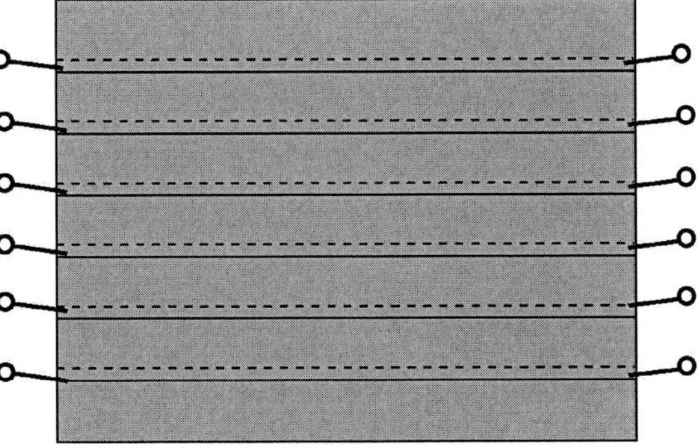

Allow the piece of fabric to dry. When you remove the fabric from the board, the tucks and the fabric will be straight and even.

RELEASE TUCKS

Release tucks are stitched in the same way as any other tuck – i.e. using the most suitable foot, needle position and with the fabric held taut. However, release tucks are not stitched from the top to bottom of the fabric, but stop somewhere in between to create fullness.

Release tucks can be any width and may be a single needle pin tuck, twin needle tuck or a whipped tuck.

The threads of the tuck ends will need to be pulled to the back and tied off to make the release point inconspicuous.

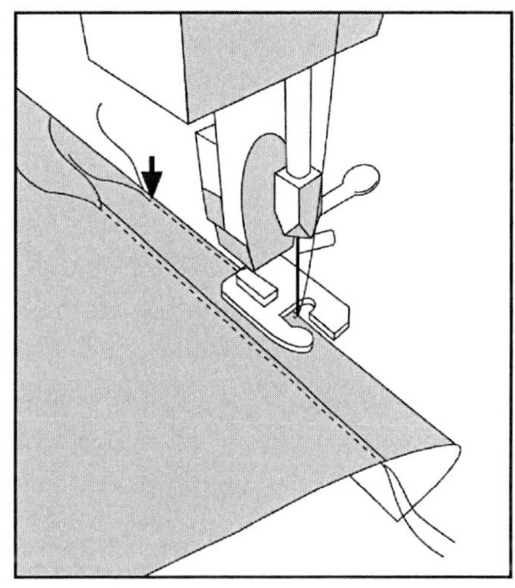

To avoid having to tie off the threads of each and every tuck, or backstitching the end of each tuck, you can make released pintucks using the ***Reverse Threading Technique***.

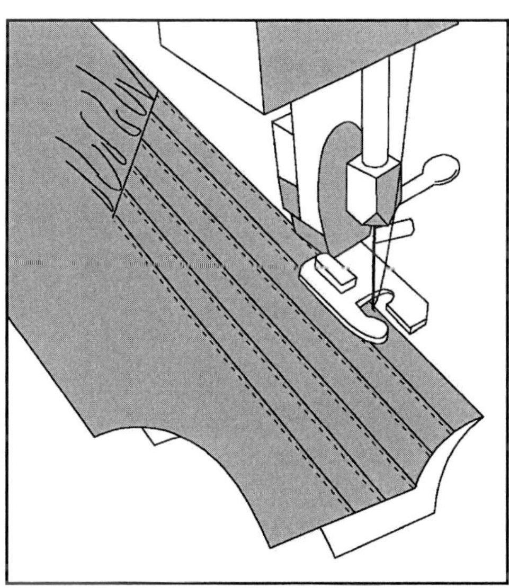

Always begin stitching the release pintuck where the fullness is to be released.

In this case you will stitch from the marked line at the bottom (or release point), to the top edge of the fabric.

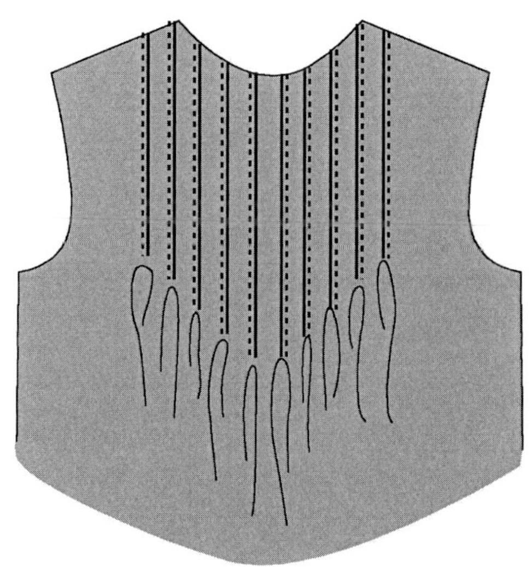

REVERSE THREADING FOR TUCKS

The following method for executing **Reverse Threaded** tucks works well for very narrow pintucks or release tucks, and is even more impressive on wider tucks.

Remove the top thread from the machine and pull the bobbin thread up.

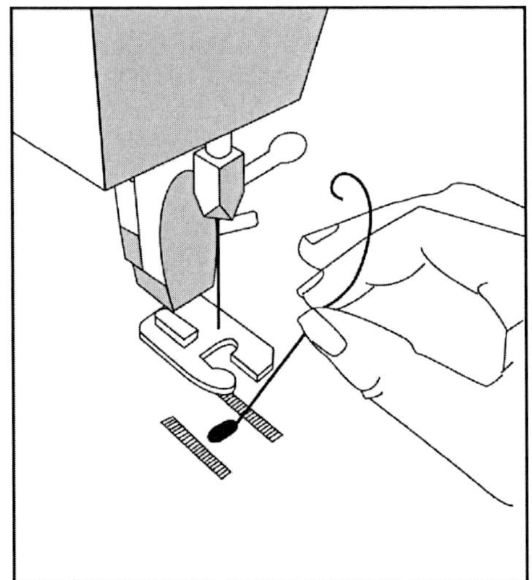

Using a needle threader, thread the needle from the **back to the front**. Although the following diagrams show a loop-style needle threader, you may find a hook-style needle threader easiest to use for this step. The needle threader is inserted into the eye of the needle. The end of the bobbin thread is then passed through the loop of the needle threader and pulled to the front.

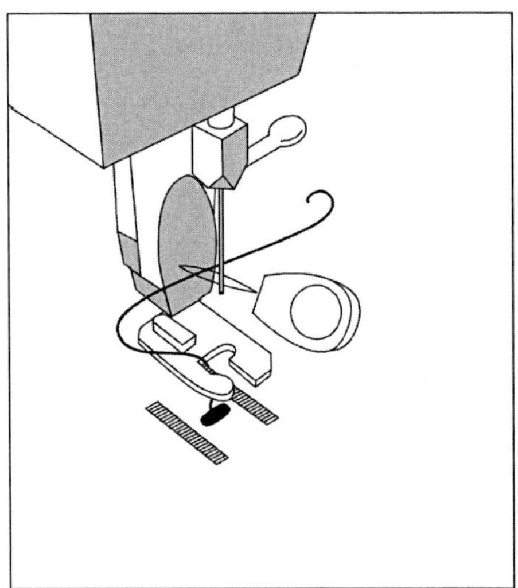

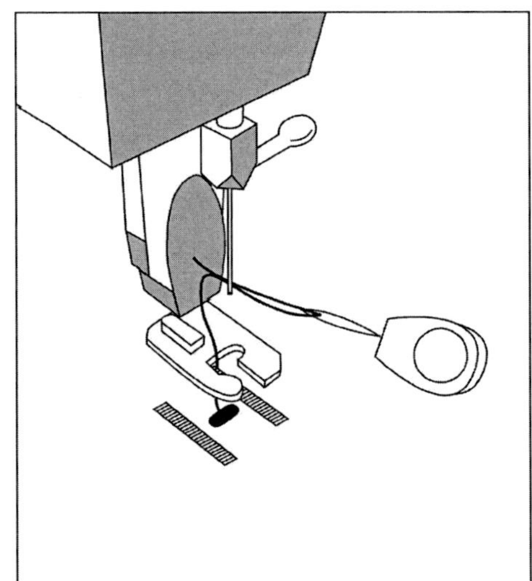

Alternatively, if you are using the hook-style needle threader, this is pushed from front to back through the eye of the needle. Hold the bobbin thread directly behind the needle eye and rotate the needle threader vertically until it picks up the thread. Always pull the threader straight towards you, **NOT** deviating to the left or right, or the wire could break from the handle.

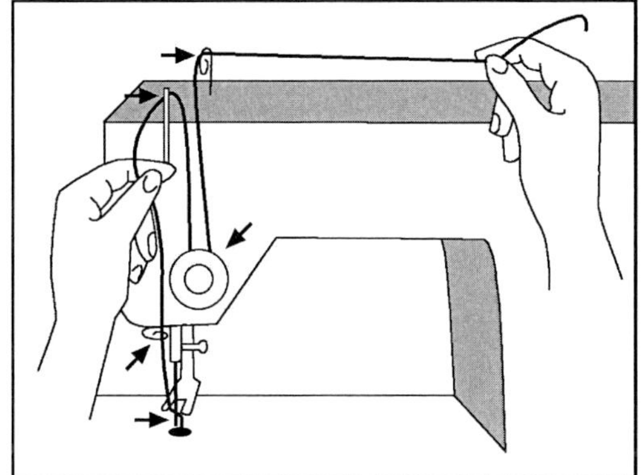

Continue threading the machine in reverse.

***Tip**: hold the thread on top of the machine in the same position as if the spool of thread was in place, and thread the machine as you would normally.*

The end of the bobbin thread is now located at the top of the sewing machine where the spool of thread would be positioned.

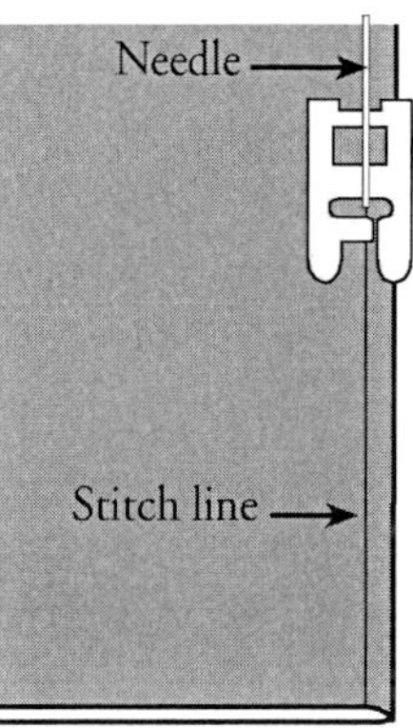
Needle
Stitch line

Place the fabric under the needle so the first stitch is **exactly** on the fabric at the marked starting point, and lower the needle. This may be the point of a dart or the 'release line' for a tuck.

Before making the first stitch, gently pull backwards on the thread to tighten any slack that will have been created when lowering the needle. Hold the thread firm, but not tight, as you make the first few stitches, sewing at a steady pace.

For tucks that are ⅛″ or wider, you will need to pull the bobbin thread through the fabric at the exact starting point for each tuck. The first tuck will be made with the bobbin thread being pulled through the fabric using the spool of thread already in place on the top of the machine. All consecutive tucks will be made with the bobbin thread being pulled through the fabric before the top thread that remains from the previous tuck is removed.

Do this by lowering the presser foot and then the needle into the exact starting position of the tuck. Hand wheel the needle (down and then up) until the take-up lever is at its highest position. Lift the presser foot and pull the bobbin thread through to the top of the fabric by holding the two threads that are lying across the top of the fabric and gently easing the bobbin thread up.

Once the bobbin thread has been passed through the two layers of fabric, remove the top thread left from previous tuck and continue ***Reverse Threading*** as above.

***Note:** This method for making tucks uses more thread than normal sewing techniques, and can **ONLY** be perfected by practice, practice, practice. The result, however, is well worth the effort and the threads that have been cut off before commencing each successive tuck can be kept for all the hand-basting that should be done to accomplish professional results in your Couture and Heirloom sewing projects.*

SINGLE-THREAD DART
(Reverse-thread Release Tuck)

A single thread dart has no thread tail at the point – it is made using the '**Reverse-Threading**' technique. It is a little more time consuming than making the dart, tying the ends to secure and then weaving them through the double fabric thickness of the dart. However, it is well worth the effort for a perfectly finished dart.

A single-thread (or reversed-thread) dart can be used to best advantage:

- on light weight or sheer fabrics where the tail ends may show through
- on short darts (4″ [10 cm] or less) as in the cap of a sleeve
- on tailored garments

Once you make a single-thread dart (or tuck) with its smooth point, and experience the ease of pressing it, I am confident you will much prefer this method. It just takes a little practice and patience to perfect this "couture" technique.

Reverse Threading

Thread the machine as you normally would, stopping just before threading the needle.

Using a needle threader, thread the bobbin thread through the needle eye, from the ***back*** to the ***front***.

Tip*: A hook-style works well for this technique*

Tie the bobbin thread to the top machine thread with a tiny square knot.

Note*: this is an alternate method for Reverse Threading to the one described previously*

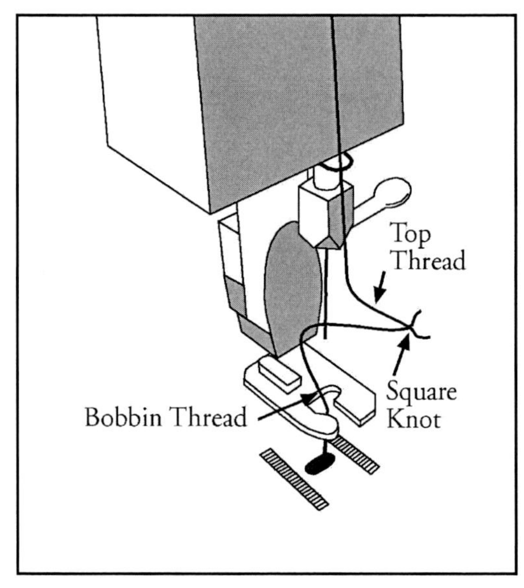
Top
Thread
Square
Knot
Bobbin Thread

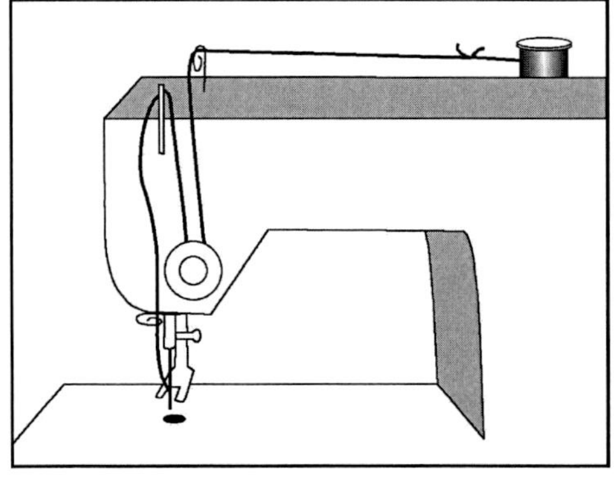

Gently rewind the needle thread until the bobbin thread comes up to the spool and wraps around two or three times.

You will need enough thread to sew only one dart (or tuck).

Place the dart point under the needle so the first stitch is **exactly** on the fabric fold and lower the needle.

You will sew the dart from the ***point*** to the **seam edge**, the opposite direction from the traditional dart stitching method.

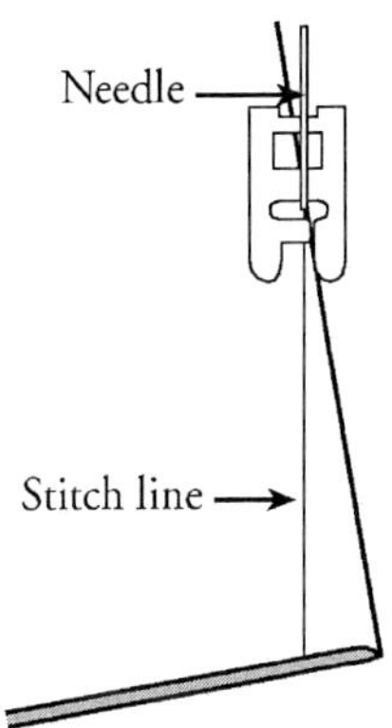
Needle
Stitch line

Before making the first stitch, gently pull the thread backwards through the machine to tighten any slack that will have been created when lowering the needle.

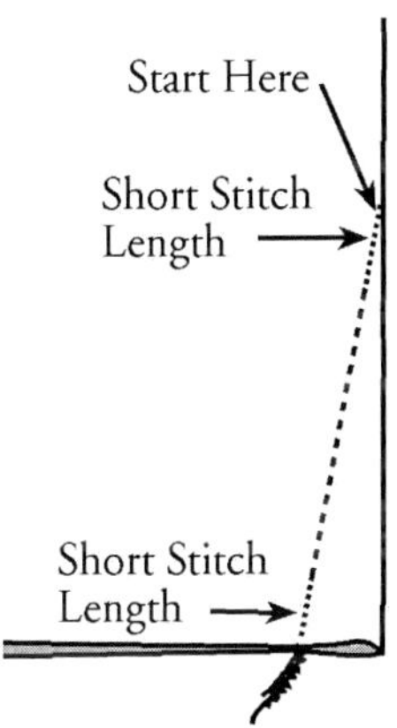
Start Here
Short Stitch Length
Short Stitch Length

Stitch the first ¼″ (6mm) with a very short stitch length, say 0.50 – 0.75 (20 stitches to the inch/8 stitches per centimeter) then change to a regular stitch length of not more than 2. Finish stitching the last ¼″ (6mm) of the dart with the shortened stitch length. Cut the threads.

***Tip**: Shortening the stitch length at the beginning and end of every seam eliminates the need to backstitch (thus, eliminates thread bulk and fabric stress)*

To sew the next dart (or tuck), re-thread the machine in the same manner as previously described using your preferred method for ***Reverse-threading***.

Notes

DECORATIVE TUCKED HEM

This hem treatment is among the most versatile, suitable for light to medium weight fabrics. It is executed in two quick steps and requires only a minor adjustment to the skirt length.

First, determine the finished length of the skirt and to this measurement add the hem depth and three times the tuck size.

For example: Add 7" (18 cm) to allow for a 4" (10 cm) hem with a 1" (2.5 cm) tuck. Cut the skirt to this measurement.

Turn the garment to be hemmed inside out. With wrong sides together, press under the hem allowance plus the tuck depth and baste in place.
For our example: 4" hem, 1" tuck

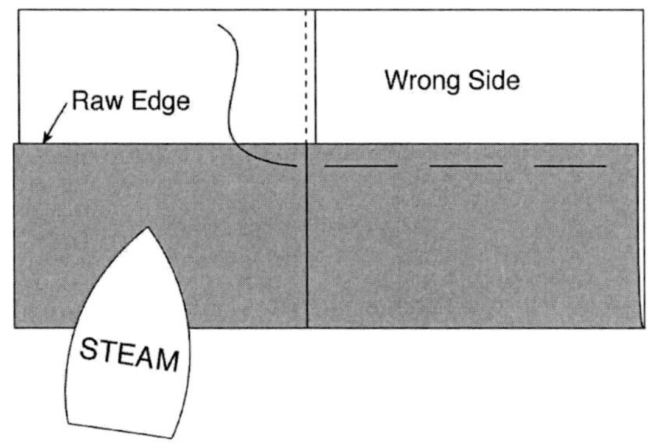
Raw Edge
Wrong Side
STEAM

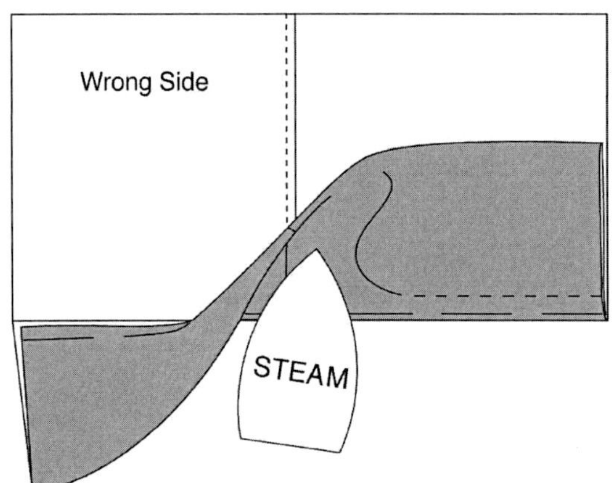
Wrong Side
STEAM

Press under the same size hem allowance once more to the inside of the garment (example 5"). Straighten the edges carefully and press the bottom edge.

Pin or baste in place.

Stitch the tuck from the fold at the lower edge of the garment, enclosing the raw edge.

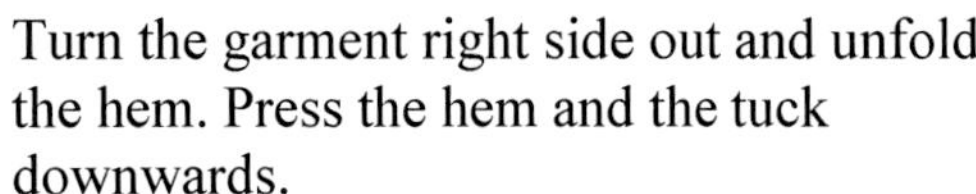

Turn the garment right side out and unfold the hem. Press the hem and the tuck downwards.

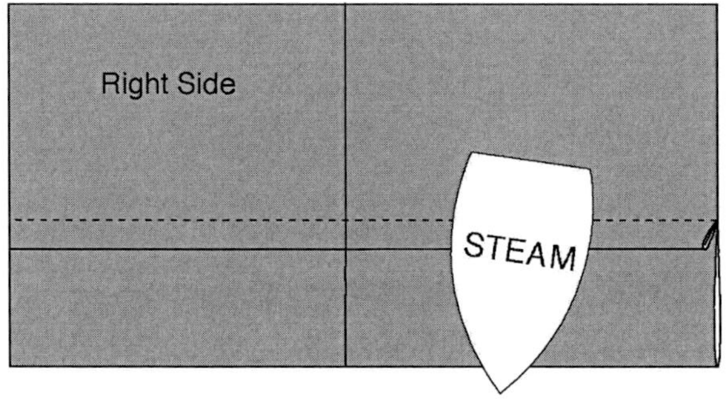
Right Side
STEAM

You will have a neat hem with a decorative tuck that looks like a cuff. The size of the hem or tuck can be adjusted by varying the size of the folds you make.

These particular tucks work well if they are added above the hem tuck, and overlapped slightly so the stitching lines do not show.

To add extra tucks, increase the finished garment for each tuck. Measure twice the tuck size, minus ¼" (6mm) for the tuck overlap, and fold the fabric again to the wrong side.

Stitch the tuck in place with a short stitch length. Meld the stitches and fold the tuck downward. Press from the wrong side, using the side of the iron to push against the tuck stitching line.

Repeat for each successive tuck.

For added variety, trims such as lace, Swiss edging, rick rack trim, picot trim or a decorative machine scallop stitch may be added to the tuck. These trims are simply zigzagged to the edge of the tuck.

Notes

TUCKED HEM WITH EMBROIDERED EDGE

This is a wonderful hem treatment when you need to lengthen a dress and are able to incorporate a Swiss edging on an heirloom-style dress. It also gives a nice finish to baby dresses and Christening gowns that don't need to be let down, but can be enhanced by the addition of a fancy hemline.

This hem band is completed after both side seams have been joined. You will need to measure the circumference of the skirt, add approximately ¾" (2 cm) for ease and a seam allowance to each end of the Swiss embroidered edging.

Join the edging into a circle with a small French seam. Mark the half and quarter points on the skirt and the embroidered eyelet/edging.

Refer to the techniques for making a ***French Seam***

METHOD 1 – for use with a narrow embroidered edge or eyelet
Determine the finished length of the garment and do not add a hem allowance.

Measure the width of the eyelet or edging being used and subtract the width of this embroidered edging from the finished length.

Add 1" (2.5 cm) to allow for the seam and the tuck.

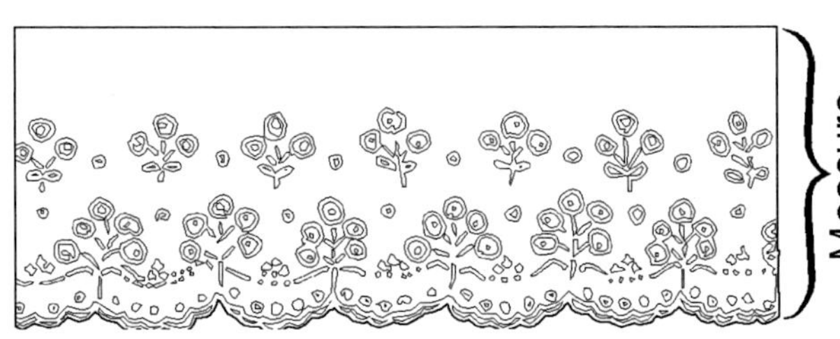
Measure

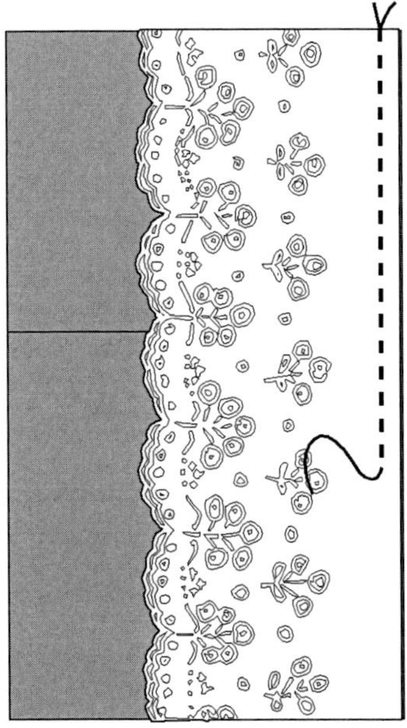

With right sides together, place the eyelet or edging onto the skirt and stitch a ¼" (6mm) seam. Meld the stitches, trim the seam allowances to ⅛" (3mm) and roll and whip the seam.

Open out the edging and press the seam allowances away from the edging – i.e. towards the garment.

To determine the foldline of the tuck, measure up ¾" (2 cm) from the seamline and press in a crease with wrong sides together.

Pin or baste the tuck in place to keep it from twisting. Stitch a ⅜" (1 cm) seam.

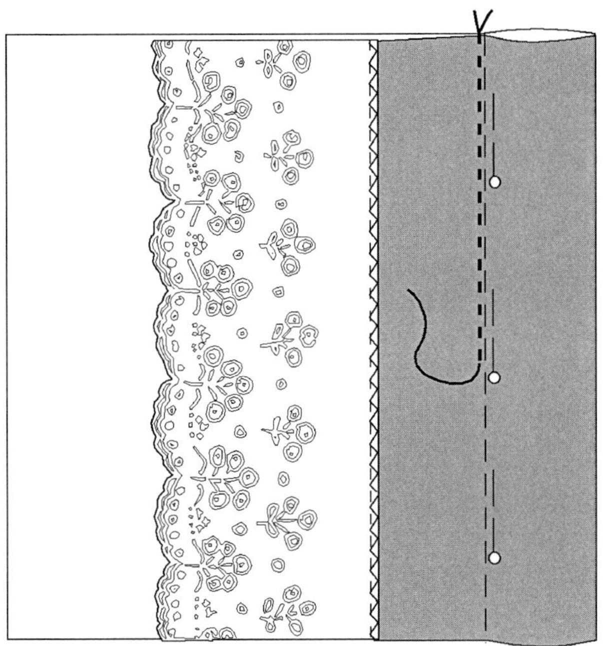

***Tip**: Make a test hemline tuck to be sure the tuck is positioned over the first seam (where the edging and garment have been joined) and this seamline cannot be seen. It may be necessary to move the needle position slightly to the left to ensure a hidden seam.*

METHOD 2 – when making a wider tuck

An alternative to this narrow embroidered edging and small tuck is to choose an edging with more plain batiste above the embroidery and a deeper tuck. Measure the depth of plain batiste fabric above the embroidery and this will be the depth of the tuck.

Determine the finished length of the garment and do not add a hem allowance. To the finished length add twice the tuck depth and a ¼" (6mm) seam allowance.

With right sides together and raw edge even, place the eyelet or edging onto the skirt and stitch a ¼" (6mm) seam. Meld the stitches and grade the seam allowance with the smaller allowance being on the garment.

Open out the edging and press the seam allowances away from the edging – i.e. towards the garment.

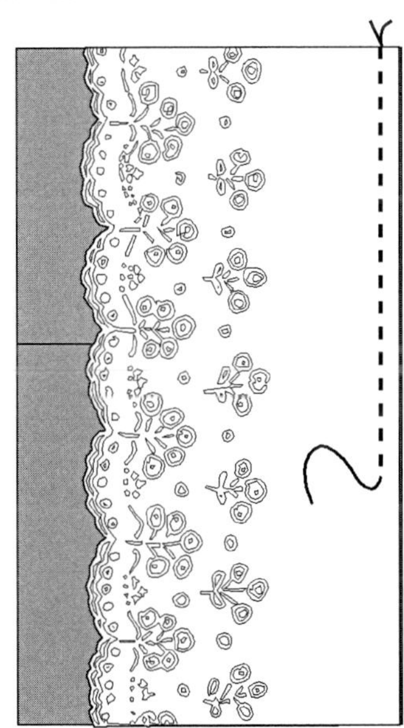

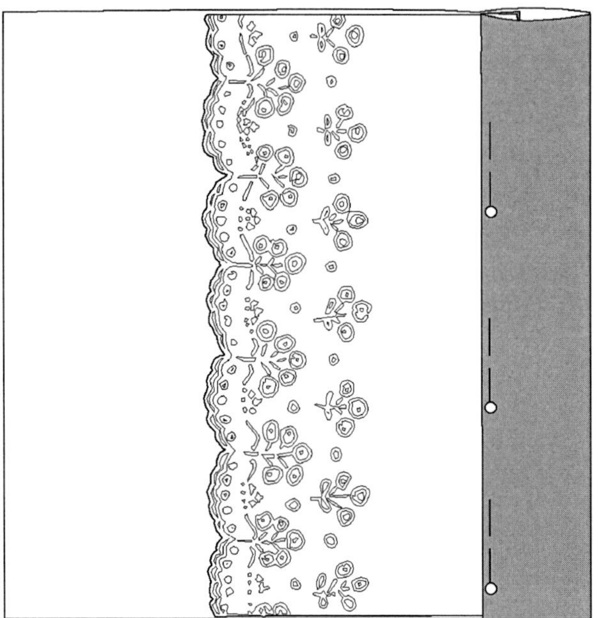

On the right side of the garment measure from the seamline to the fold for the tuck depth.

With wrong sides together, press in a crease for the foldline of the tuck.

Pin or baste the tuck in place to keep it from twisting.

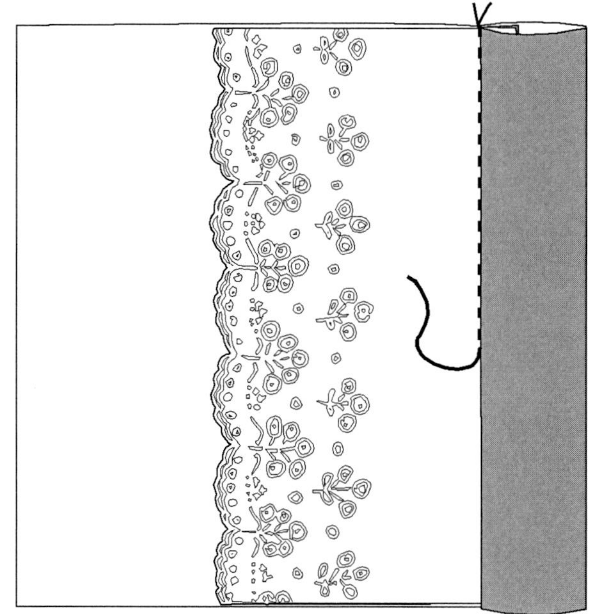

Using the edge-joining foot, stitch in the ditch between the fabric of the tuck and the embroidered edging. The seam should now be enclosed within the tuck.

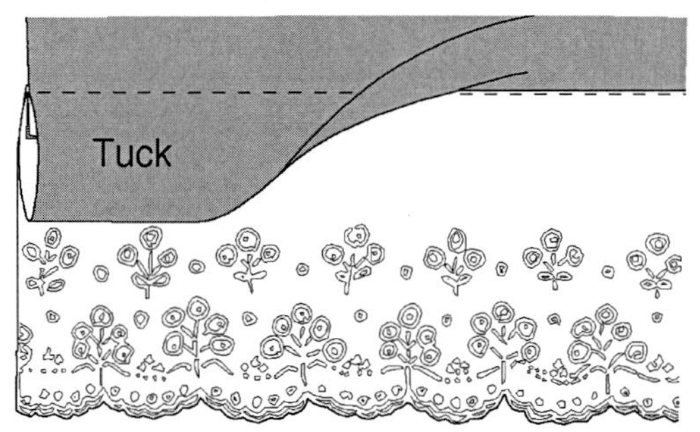
Tuck

USING THE BIAS

Making use of the ***Bias*** grain will surely show your skills as a 'Couture' seamstress. The bias does have a mind of its own, but understanding how to work with this **grain** of the cloth will produce remarkable results.

The bias grain can be both decorative and functional. It can be used in two ways:

- Bias cut fabric strips can be used to bind both concave and convex curves, create piping, or to make rouleau (tiny bias tubes).

- Garment sections or entire garments can be cut on the bias grain to create interesting effects in the fit, drape and visual design of the garment.

The following guidelines for cutting and joining bias fabric will ensure a professional finish to your garments.

When working on the bias, the fabric must be perfectly grained up and the bias line established. Always cut strips of fabric at a 45° angle to the lengthwise and crosswise grains, or on the **true bias.**

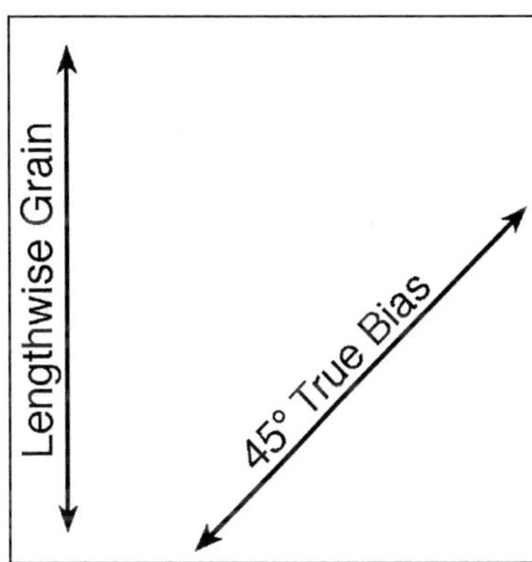
Lengthwise Grain
45° True Bias

For self-stripe or twilled fabric, cut the bias so that the self-stripe will be perpendicular to the bias edge.

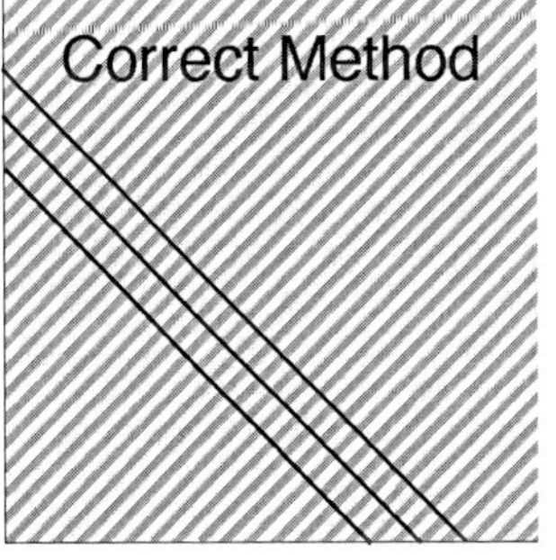
Correct Method

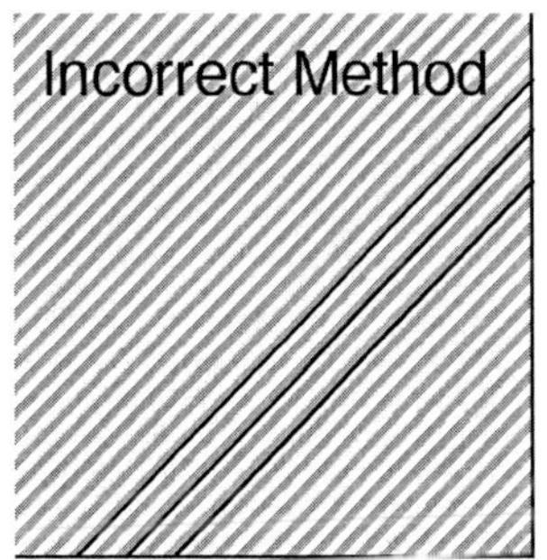
Incorrect Method

The less piecing the better, but sometimes it is necessary to join the bias strips in order to obtain the required length.

Cut the ends square and place strips, right sides together, at right angles.

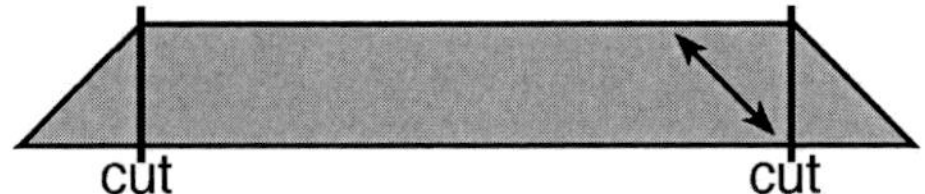
cut
cut

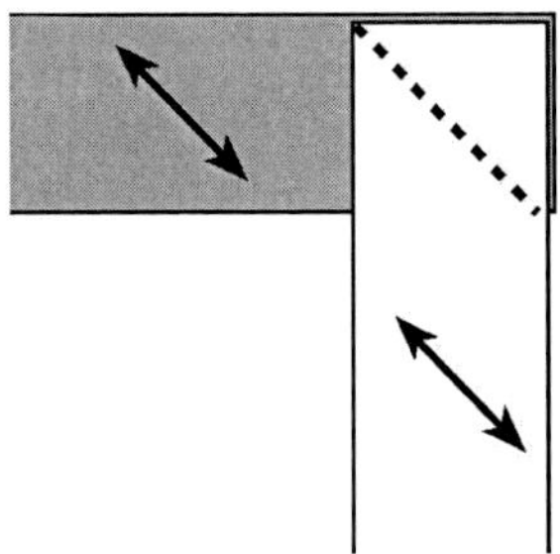

Stitch corner to corner as marked on the **lengthwise**, or straight of grain, only.

The bias grain is perfect for ruffles because:

- it can be gathered more fully than any other grain, and
- bias ruffles have a soft, rounded edge

Bias ruffles do use substantially more fabric so be sure to buy extra if you are incorporating them into a design.

Bias ruffles can be cut double width, and then folded in half lengthwise, gathered and inserted into a seam, around a collar, or to a hemline.

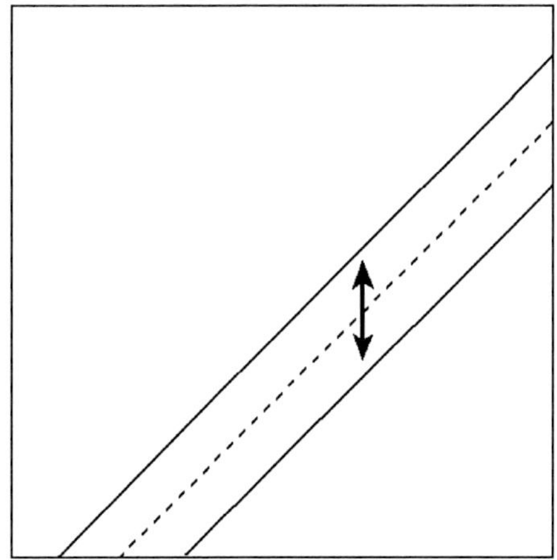

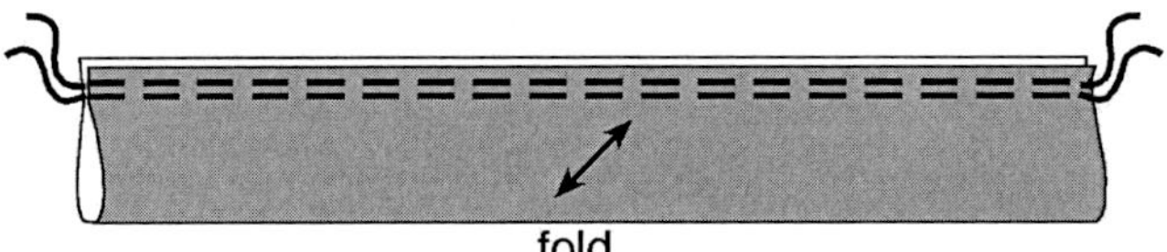
fold

MAKING CORDED PIPING

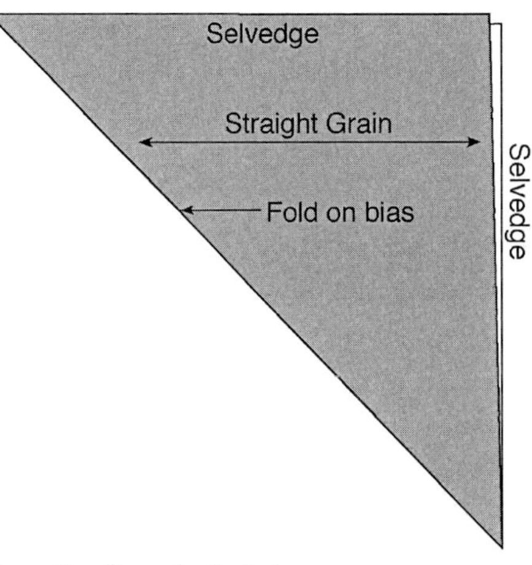
Selvedge
Straight Grain
Fold on bias
Selvedge

Bias Strips

Cut fabric to the required length at 45° to the selvage, or on the "true bias".

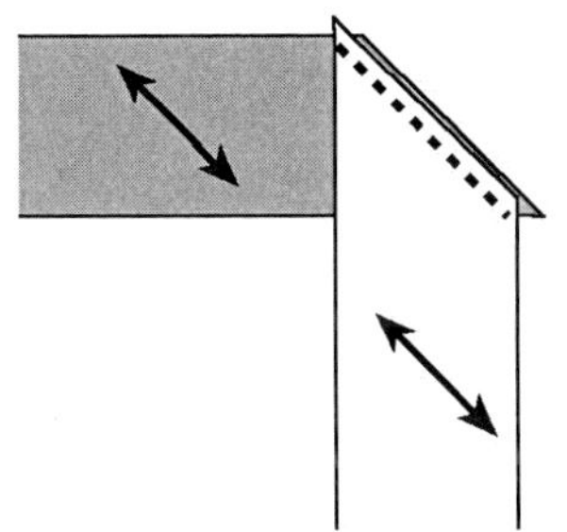

To piece bias strips to make a length of corded piping, always sew the ends of the strips together along the ***straight grain*** of the fabric. The resulting small diagonal seam will be strong, relatively invisible and will allow the bias strip to stretch. Attach the remaining strips in the same manner to form one long piece of bias fabric.
*Refer to **Using the Bias** for an alternative bias joining method.*

Meld the seam and press open. Trim away the small protruding triangles then proceed to add the cording.

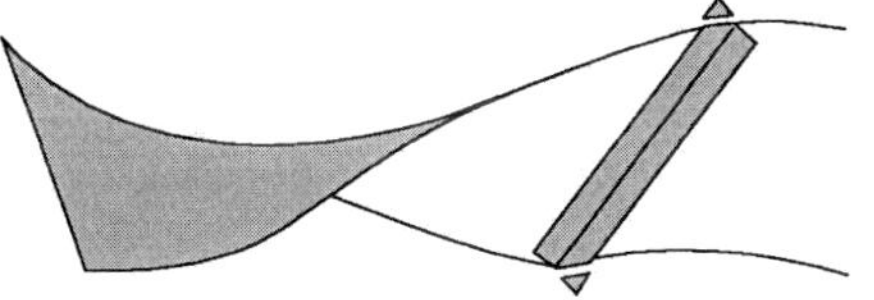

Choose a fine cord suitable for use with fine fabrics. Mini piping can be made from:

- Size 000 cotton cord – difficult to find
- 4 or 6-ply knitting cotton – very soft and flexible
- Size 00 piping cord – use as is, or with one strand removed

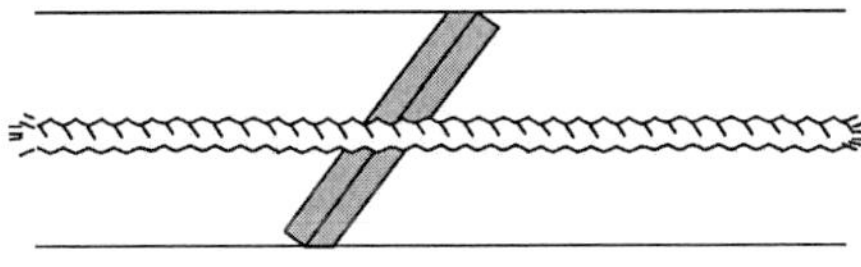

Lay the piping cord along the center of the *wrong side* of the bias strip.

Fold the fabric over the filler cord with the raw edges together and pin firmly in place.

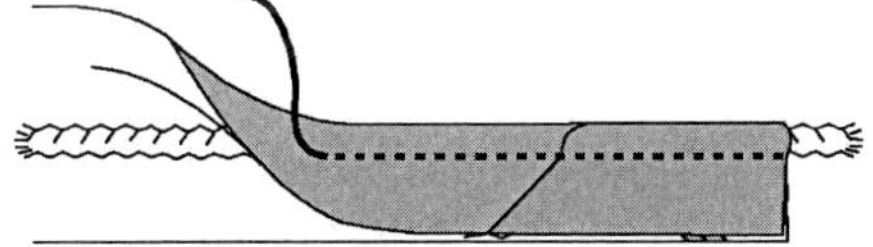

Attach a machine presser foot to the sewing machine that allows the cord to be contained within the groove underneath the foot (e.g. buttonhole, pintucking or cording foot). On some machines the best results can be obtained by using the zipper foot.

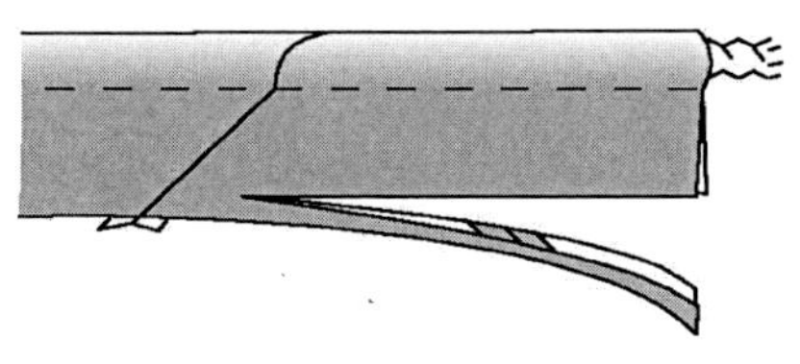

Using a slightly longer-than-normal straight stitch, sew through both layers of fabric close to the cord, leaving a little "air space" between cord and stitching.

The cord will be firmly enclosed within the fabric roll when the piping is stitched again onto the garment.

If necessary, trim the raw edges so that the finished piping is the same width as the seam allowance.

Do not stretch the bias. After removing the corded piping from the sewing machine, run your thumb and forefingers along the cord to remove any tightness the machine may have caused.

It is often recommended to pre-wash the cord to avoid shrinkage. I prefer not to pre-wash, as the soaking tends to make the cord 'swell' or 'puff' a little and the idea of mini-piping is to have a very fine cord for use on collars, cuffs, smocking etc.

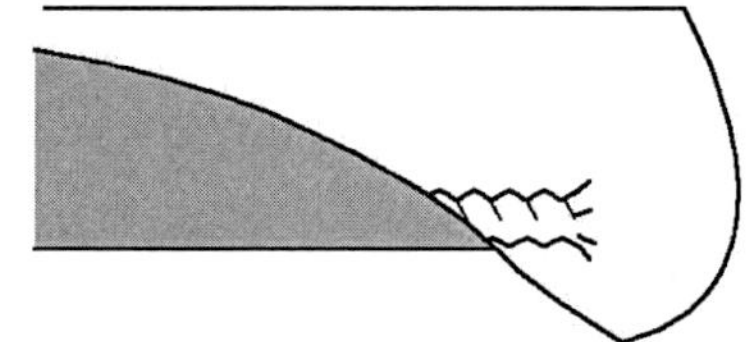

The alternative to pre-washing the piping cord is to remove the cord from within the seam allowance at each end. In this way the small amount of shrinkage will not affect the garment's professional finish.

***Tip**: Remove the cord from the beginning end before commencing to attach the piping, and remove cord from the other end once the piping has been attached.*

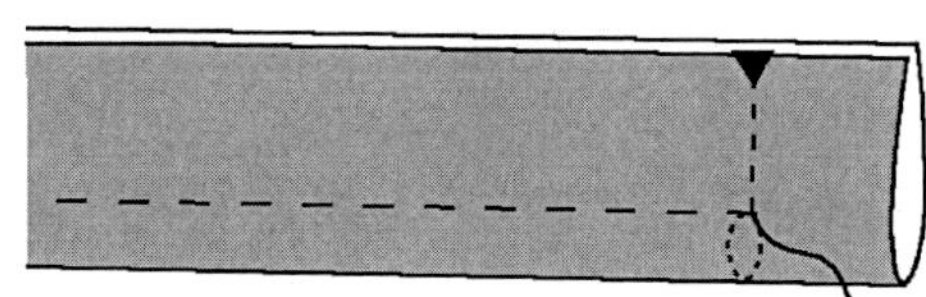

DOUBLE CORDED PIPING

Double piping adds design detail and can be used as follows:

- it is ideal on a lined edge where there is no facing (on necklines and hems) hand stitching the lining in place to the piping
- as a feature detail on patch pockets or where you need a contrasting decorative line
- applied between the lining and facing of a tailored jacket or coat

MAKING THE DOUBLE PIPING

Using a machine presser foot that allows the cord to be contained within the groove underneath the foot, make two separate pieces of piping.

For the piece that will be nearer to the garment (the top color), cut the bias to equal the circumference of the piping cord, plus ½″ (13mm) to allow for two ¼″ (6mm) seam allowances.

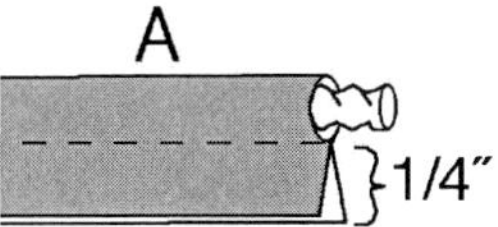
A
1/4″

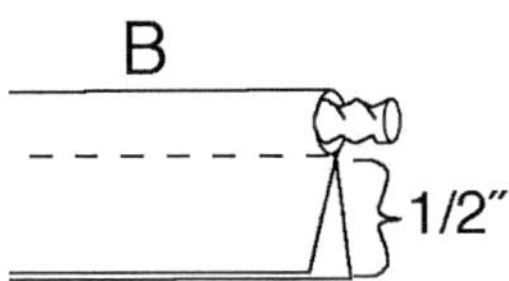
B
1/2″

For the piece that will be at the outer edge (the underneath color) cut the bias strip to equal the circumference of the piping cord, plus 1″ (2.5 cm) to allow for two ½″ (13mm) seam allowances.

***Tip**: Use a longer-than-normal stitch length so it can be removed if necessary.*

Place the top color **A** on top of **B** and stitch, following the stitching line of **A**.

***Tip**: Use a zipper foot and thread to match the color of the underneath fabric.*

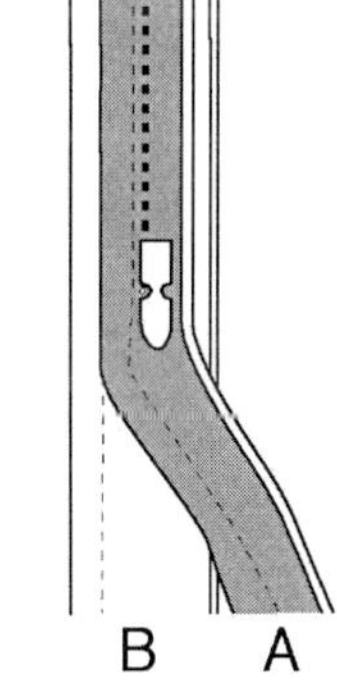
B
A

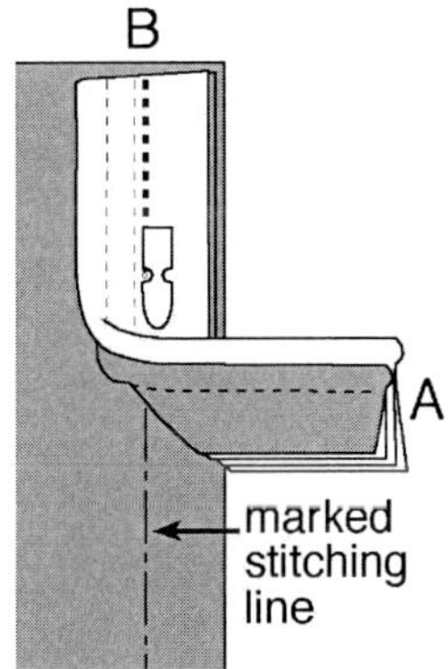
B
A
marked
stitching
line

With right sides together, position the double piping on the garment with **A** nearer the edge of the garment. Use the stitching line of **A** as a guide, matching it to the marked stitching line on the garment. Attach using a zipper foot.

Double piping makes an attractive burst of complementary or contrasting color to many garment applications. It does, however, take practice to accurately incorporate it into curved and pointed areas.

PIPING A POINTED CORNER

Using a regular stitch length, sew piping to within ½″ (13mm) of the corner. Shorten the stitches to ½ - ¾ (20 stitches per inch/8 stitches per centimeter) and stop stitching one stitch short of the turning point.

Once the needle reaches this point, with the needle in the fabric, lift the presser foot. Clip the piping seam allowance only up to the point directly in front of the needle to allow the piping to turn. Take one stitch at 45° across the corner.

Pivot the work again, lower the presser foot and continue stitching, using the shortened stitch length for ½″ (13mm). When making the turn it will be necessary to guide the cord from being caught underneath the needle by pushing it away from the needle with a stiletto or pointed laying tool.

> ***Tip**: You may also find it easier to make one additional clip 1/8″ (3mm) on each side of the corner (or pivot) clip, thus allowing more flex in the bias at the turn.*

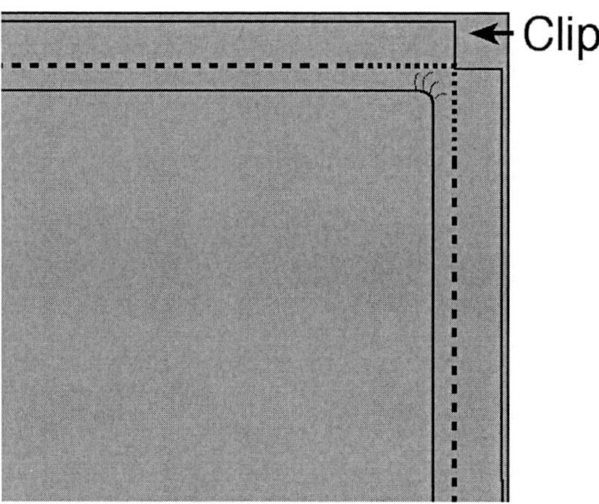
Clip

APPLYING CORDING TO A SEAM

The corded seam is a decorative seam or edge and can be used as a design feature on your garment. Many vintage garments included the tiniest cording (or piping) to add detail around the armhole and at the yoke or waistline. Baby and children's clothing can be brought to life with the addition of piped seams in contrasting fabric.

The size of the cord being used should be directly proportional to the weight of the fabric and the size of the garment or project. Try using soft knitting cotton for baby piping.

For precise and consistent application of piping, use a presser foot with one or more grooves (such as the standard buttonhole foot, or pintuck foot) to guide small piping cord. For stitching close to large cord, use a zipper foot.

When making the piping, set the needle to stitch one position away from directly beside the cord. Then, when sewing the piping into the project, use the needle position closest to the piping. This prevents the common problem of having the first row of stitching visible.
Place the outer layer of fabric on the sewing table with the right side facing up.

Place the raw edge of the piping even with the raw edge of the fabric. Stitch the two together with a slightly longer stitch length and the needle de-centered from the cord.

***Tip**: Trim the size of the seam allowance beside the piping cord to equal that of the seam allowance on the garment (or vice versa) to help achieve perfectly even seams.*

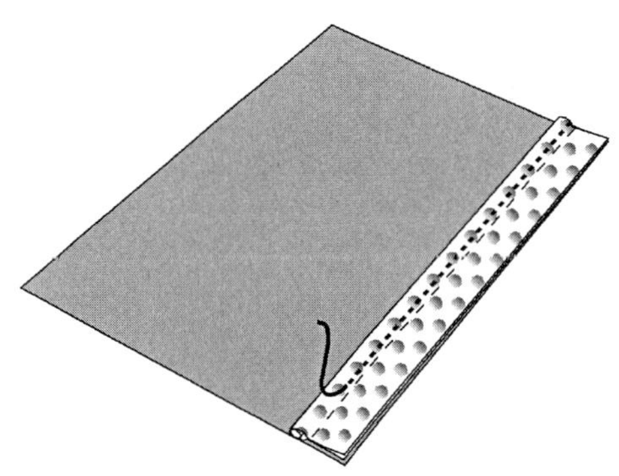

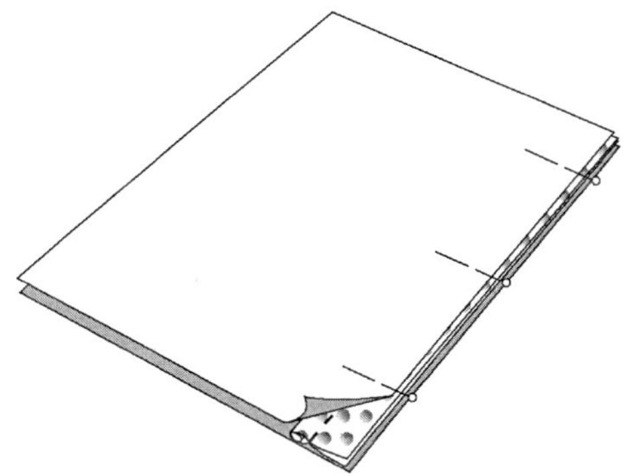

With right sides together and raw edges even, place the lining or underneath garment piece to the piped fabric.

Pin these together and baste if necessary.

Using the buttonhole, piping or zipper foot, stitch along the edge of the cording, just a little closer to the cord than the first row of stitches. You should be stitching on the seamline.

Meld the stitches and grade the seam allowance.

***Tip**: I like to grade the underneath and one layer of piping fabric to ⅛" (3mm) and the outer layer and piping fabric just a little wider – 3/16" (5mm).*

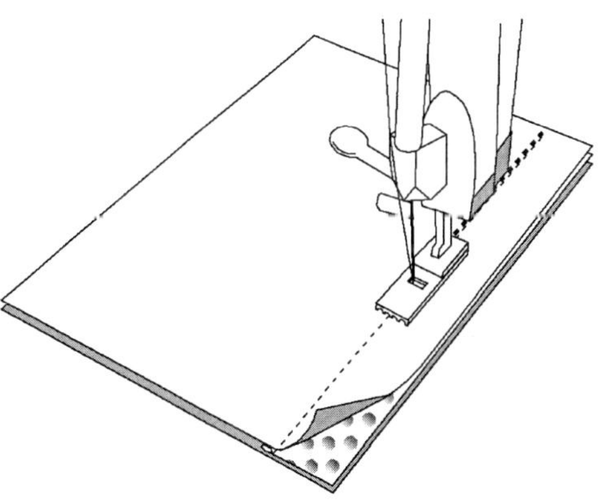

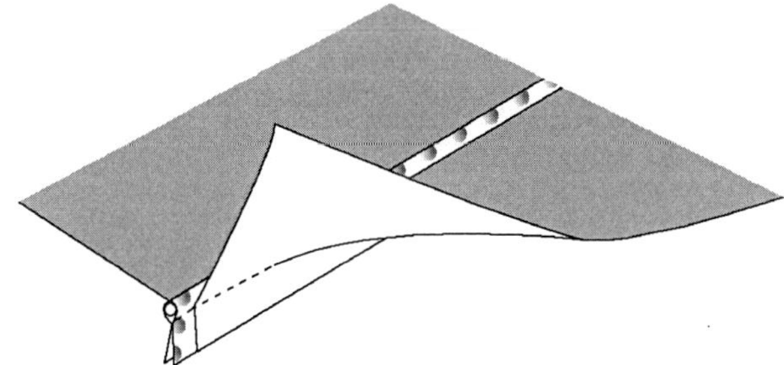

BINDING A COLLAR
(or outer curve)

This trim technique makes use of contrasting fabric to highlight the collar, cuffs, pocket or even a bound scalloped hemline.

If the collar pattern is NOT designed for a bound finish, you will need to trim away the seam allowance from the ***outer edge*** only (**NOT** the neck edge). This permits the edge of the finished collar to fall along the original seamline.

The pattern can be traced onto the fabric block following the seam line (NOT the cutting line) or, if using more than one layer of fabric that is too dense to trace, a pattern template that finishes on the seam line of the outer collar edge can be produced for tracing around. In either case the seam allowance of the neck edge must remain on the template

With *wrong* sides together, baste the upper and underneath collar and/or cuff fabric pieces together. **DO NOT** cut out the collar at this stage.

Position the pattern on the fabric (matching the grain lines) and trace the seamline of the pattern.

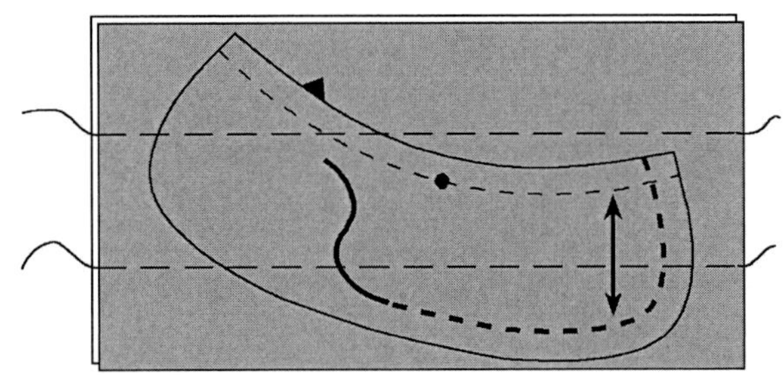

***Note**: The diagrams show the pattern with seam allowances maintained all round – you may prefer to work with a new master pattern that has the seam allowances removed from the outer edge and the neck edge seam allowance in tact.*

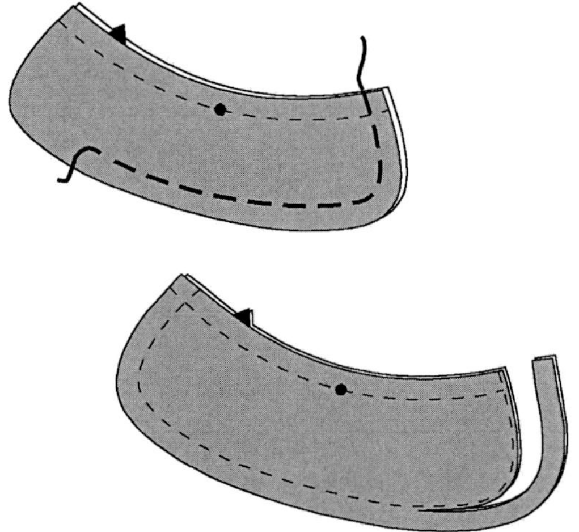

Staystitch on the seamline – this will be within the collar shape, NOT on the original cutting line. Cut away the excess fabric up to this stitching line.

Cut bias strips four times the desired finished width plus ⅛" (3mm) to ¼" (6mm) depending on the thickness of the fabric. The additional fabric allows for folding the binding.

Fold the strip in half, wrong sides together, and press lightly. Open the fold, turn both raw edges in toward the center fold and press again. Refold along the center so that the bias now equals the finished width.

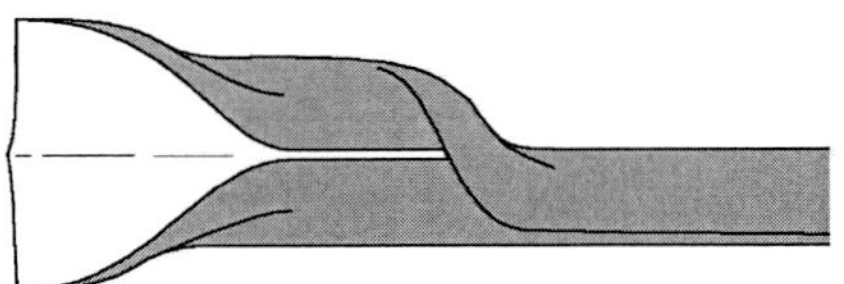

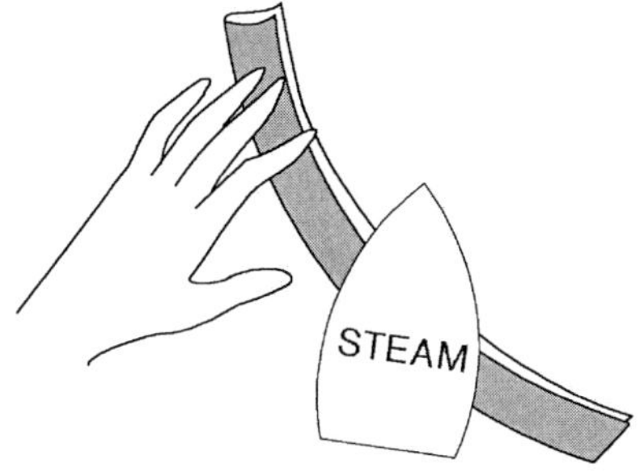
STEAM

Pre-shape the bias strip by steaming to match the curve of the garment edge, gently easing in any fullness, and being careful not to stretch the bias.

Note: *Illustration is designed to show the direction in which to shape the bias for an outer curve, but does not show all four layers of the binding.*

If using joined bias strips, place the seam lines at inconspicuous locations wherever possible.

Open out one folded edge of the binding strip. With right sides together and raw edges even, pin and hand baste the binding to the garment at a distance from the edge that is slightly less than the width of the finished binding. **Be very careful NOT to stretch the bias.**

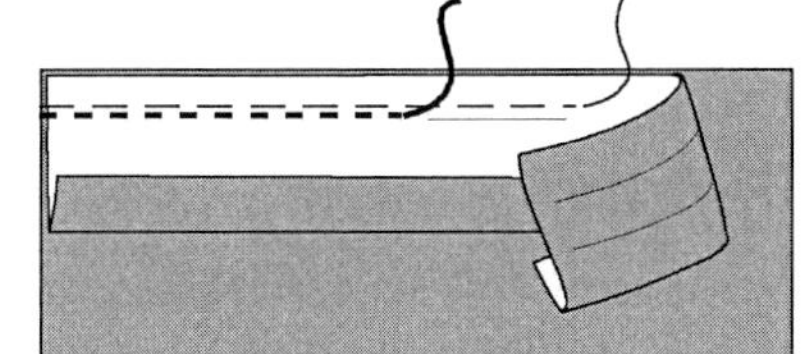

Stitch on the fold line (or finished binding width measurement).

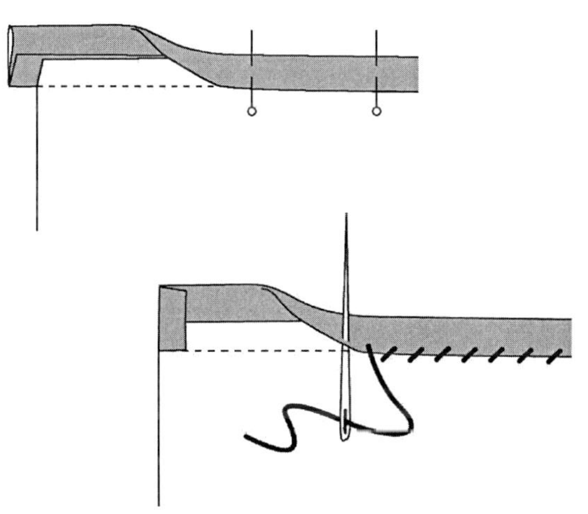

Turn the binding over the seam allowance.

Commencing at the center, pin in place by pinning through all layers <u>except</u> the outer binding layer.

Secure with tiny slipstitches, catching the fold of the binding and passing the needle under one of the machine stitches made when attaching the binding – pull stitches firm, but not tight. This will ensure that no stitches appear on the front.

Note: Always be sure the garment completely fills the binding roll. It may be necessary, therefore, to trim the bias <u>slightly</u> to ensure a firm, non-roll binding.

The above instructions for working with bias on a convex curve would be applied to *Neatening an attached Collar with a Bias Facing*. The following are some general guidelines:

- Wherever possible the bias strip should be the same color as the collar.
- Trim the neckline seam allowance to not more than ¼" (6mm) and clip around the curves.
- Cut the bias ¾" (2 cm) wide, fold in half and steam to shape.
- Sandwich the collar(s) between the garment and the pre-shaped bias, with the bias on top.
- After stitching, neaten the seam by trimming the whiskers so the seam is 3/16" (5mm).
- For preference, whip the folded edge of the bias by hand to secure.

BINDING THE NECKLINE
(Double Binding or French Binding)

If your pattern is NOT designed to incorporate a bound neckline finish, staystitch on the seam line and trim away the seam allowance very close to the row of staystitching. This permits the top edge of the finished binding to fall along the original seamline.

Refer to the techniques for ***Binding a Collar***

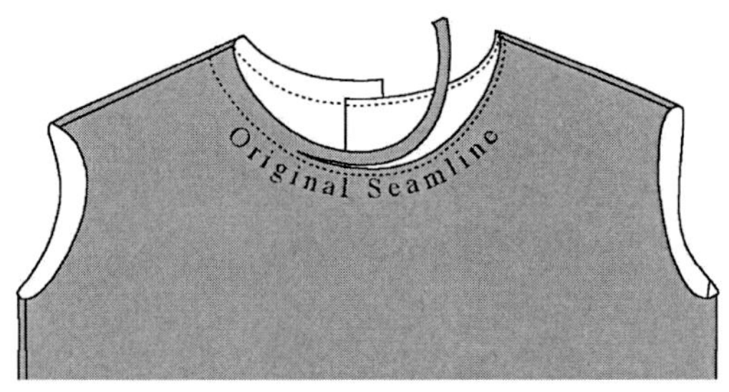
Original Seamline

The length of the binding strip equals the length of the garment seamline plus 1" (2.5 cm) for ease and finishing the ends. The width of the bias strip should be six times the desired finished width plus ⅛" – ¼" (3mm – 6mm), depending on the thickness of the fabric.

These instructions allow for a finished binding of not more than ¼" (6mm).

Cut out the neckline binding on the true bias, 1⅝" (4.2mm) wide x the length on the pattern or the neck measurement, plus 1" (2.5 cm). This measurement is reached by adding six times the finished binding width (6 x ¼") plus ⅛" for 'the turn of the cloth'.

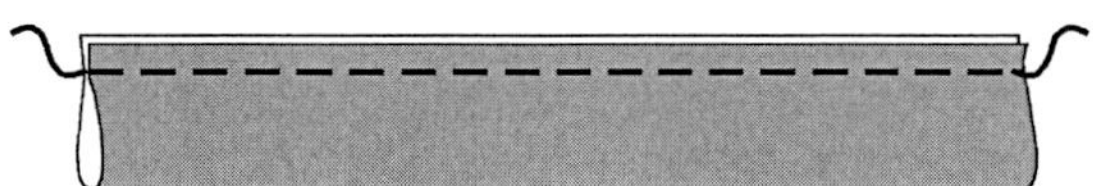

With wrong sides together, fold the bias strip in half lengthwise, baste and press.

Steam the bias to the shape of the curve, gently and very slightly stretching the bias – be sure to keep the raw edges even. Do NOT flatten the bias strip when pressing.

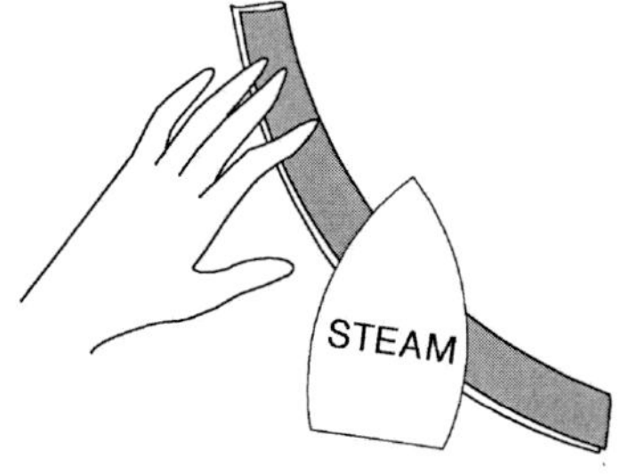
STEAM

***Tip**: Be sure to keep the folded edge on the inside of the curve as shown in the illustration, and thus avoid wrinkles in the finished binding.*

Place any seamline joins in the bias at inconspicuous locations wherever possible.

With raw edges even, pin the binding to the right side of the garment. **Commencing at the center**, hand baste (or glue baste) the folded bias in position at a distance from the edge that is slightly less than the width of the finished binding. In this example the basting would be slightly less than ¼" (6mm) from the edge or, say, 3/16" (5mm).

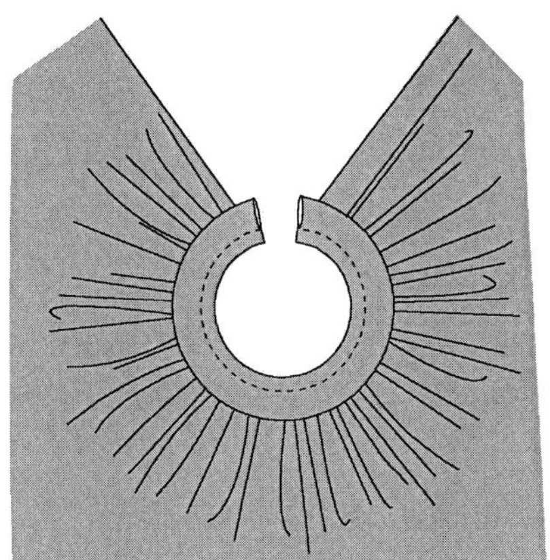

Leave at least ⅜" (1 cm) of binding free beyond the beginning and ending of any application, for finishing.

Stitch next to (not on) the basting. The stitching should be ¼" (6mm) from the edge for a finished binding width of ¼" (6mm).

Note*: the basting stitches will remain within the seam allowance.*

Check and correct any unevenness or tiny pleats in the binding at this stage.

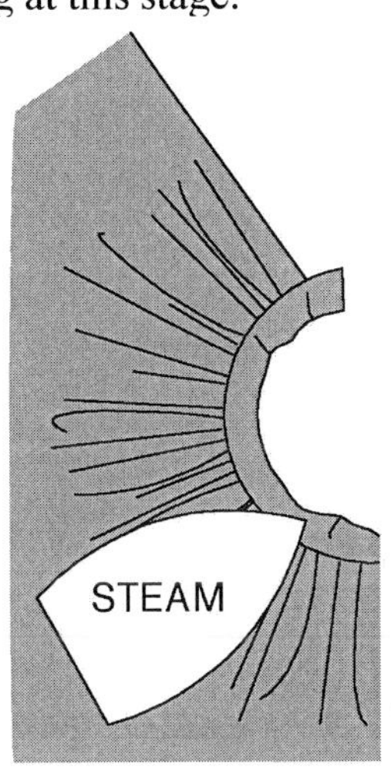
STEAM

With the tip of the iron press the bias strip towards the seam allowance, shaping it into a curve. Do not allow the iron to flatten the bias. From the right side baste this strip down to the seam allowance through all layers of the garment and the binding fabric.

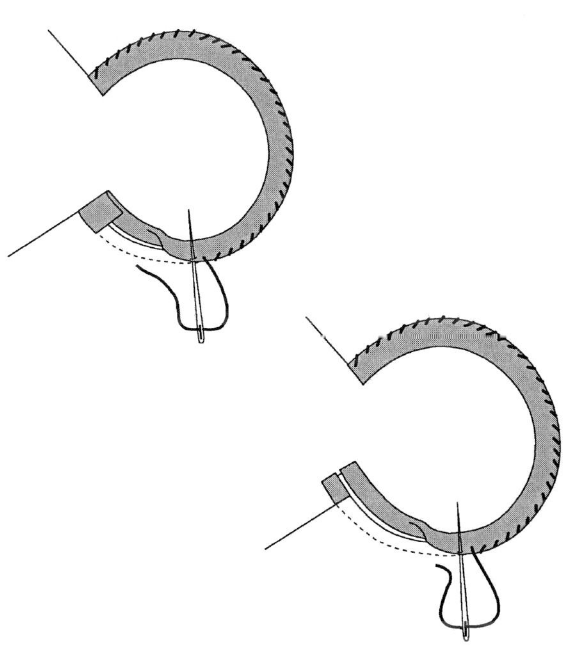

Roll the binding over the seam allowance so that the binding is completely filled with the garment fabric. Pin in place, working from the center out to each end.

Check for puckers on the top side. Trim the excess at each end to ¼" (6mm) and fold in before hand stitching the folded edge to the stitching line on the wrong side of the garment.

Tip*: Some reasons that bias bindings pucker are:*

- *The bias band was not cut accurately on the true bias grain*
- *The bias band was stretched during steaming, pinning or stitching*
- *The bias band was not stitched from the <u>center out</u> and with an exact seam allowance*

Note*: This method for* ***Binding a Neckline*** *can be used as a replacement for a collar on a basic garment, or executed in the same way on a gathered or smocked neckline. You will note that the drawings reflect both types of garment.*

FOLDED BIAS PIPING

As we continue to learn, from books, teachers and one another, it will become very clear that the bias, the strongest grain of the fabric, is a most useful couture tool.

Folded Bias Piping has the same finished appearance as you would see on a piped collar or cuff. This technique is yet another example of the versatility of using bias to make an easy, but very tailored, edge treatment. By working with a double fold of bias fabric you will be able to add piping trim and face the garment edge in just one step.

This technique could be used for:

- Piping and binding the neckline and armholes of a dress, petticoat, diaper shirt or nightgown
- Making a two-layer reversible baby blanket that features piping on one side and binding on the other

Cut a length of bias fabric not more than 1¾" (4.5 cm) wide and long enough to bind the edge of the garment. Fold the bias in half lengthwise and press.

Lay a length of piping cord on the center of the double layer of bias cut fabric and fold the bias again, wrapping it around the piping cord. Bring the folded edge and the raw edges together.

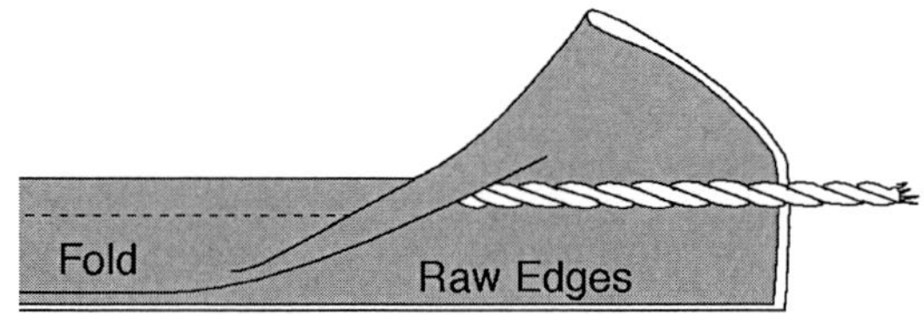
Fold
Raw Edges

***Tip**: Because it will not be possible to reduce the width of the 'seam allowance' beside the cord, it is imperative that you are accurate with the bias measurement and the placement of the cord when folding the fabric.*

Place the folded bias under the piping foot (or buttonhole foot) so it rides in the groove on the underside of the foot.

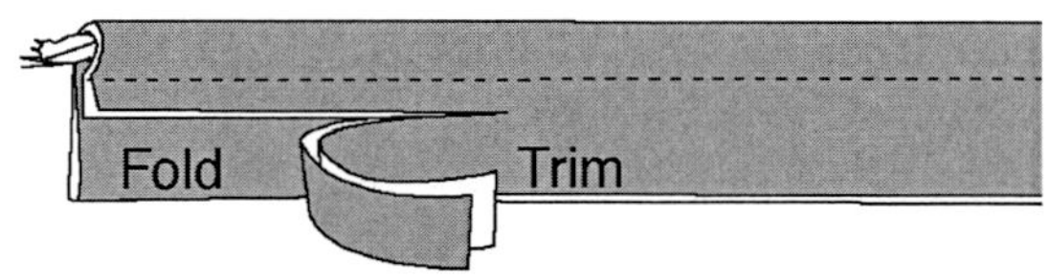
Fold
Trim

Straight stitch to hold the cord in place, but not right up next to it – leave a little 'breathing room' around the cord!

Trim the <u>raw edges</u> of the fabric close to the stitching line – <u>**DO NOT trim the folded edge**</u>.

Place the piping on the right side of the garment edge with the trimmed edge of the bias against the right side of the garment. Be sure that the bias fold and the raw edge of the garment are even.

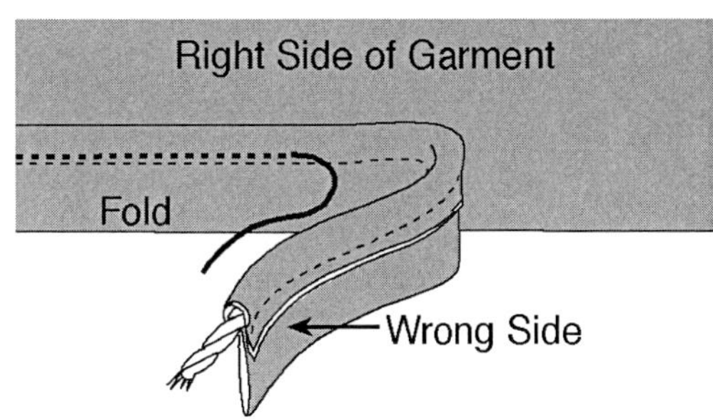
Right Side of Garment
Fold
Wrong Side

Place the piping in the groove of the foot and straight stitch again, just a little closer to the cord. Meld the stitches.

***Tip**: Before attaching the piping, be sure to steam and shape the double folded bias using exactly the same techniques as you would for single bias. Trim and clip the garment if necessary, but **DO NOT** trim the folded edge of the bias fabric.*

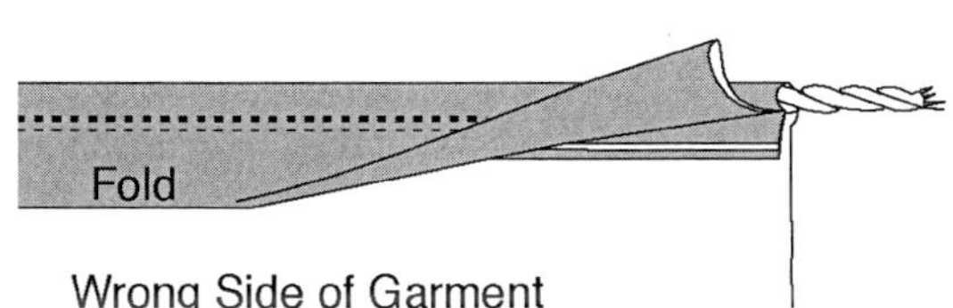
Fold
Wrong Side of Garment

Press the seam to the wrong side, revealing the piped edge.

Topstitch from the right side to secure the folded edge to the wrong side. Alternately, the folded allowance can be hand caught on the inside of the garment.

Notes

ROULEAU (OR SHOE-STRING) TUBES

Rouleau, or fabric tubing, is made by stitching the raw edges of a bias strip together then turning right side out. Rouleau tubes make pretty trims when used as:

- A neckline bow between two collars – tie a knot at each end and pull hard to make it tight
- Ties on an opening of a baby jacket, ties for a baby bonnet and bootees, straps on a camisole or nightgown
- or even shaped and stitched to a garment as a decorative feature

Avoid using fabrics, which fray easily or are difficult to turn. Thick fabrics are necessarily more bulky and the dimensions given should be treated as a guide only. Always make samples from your garment fabric to be sure the loops or tubes are correctly sized.

Begin with a 1″ (2.5 cm) wide bias strip, folded lengthwise with right sides together.

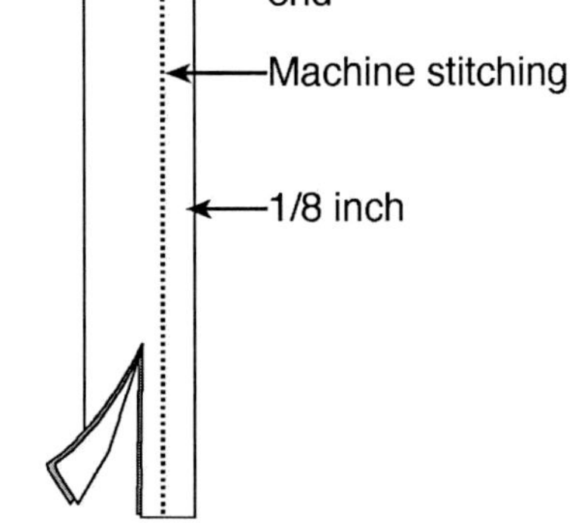
Funnel-shaped end
Machine stitching
1/8 inch

Baste together 1/8″ from the <u>folded</u> edge, increasing slightly at one end of the tube to make a funnel shape.

Shorten the machine stitch length to 0.5 – 0.75 (20 stitches per inch) and stitch on the basted line, stretching the strip as much as possible. This will narrow the tube. Leave long threads at the 'funnel' end.

Trim the seam allowance to slightly less than the tube's width and remove the bastings.

Thread a tapestry needle with the two long machine threads. Pass the needle inside the tube, pull it out the other end and turn the tube right side out. If the tube turns easily, it's probably too wide!

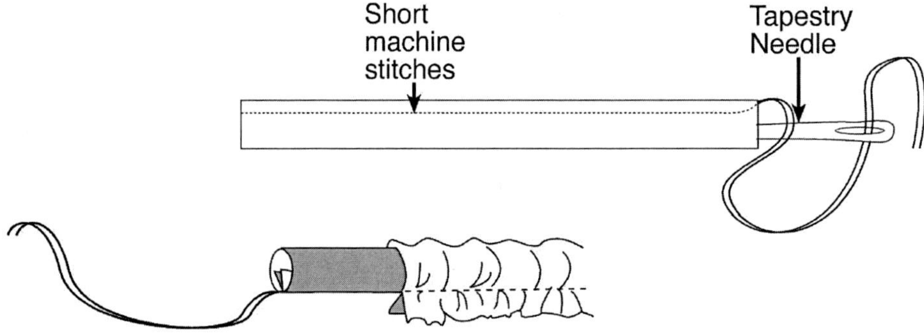
Short machine stitches
Tapestry Needle

After turning the tubing, wet it and squeeze it dry in a towel. Pin one end securely to the pressing board. Straighten the tubing so the seam is not twisted and stretch it as much as possible. Pin the other end securely and leave it to dry.

An alternative method of turning the bias tube right side out is to double stitch across one end of the bias and, using the flat end of a bodkin, gently push against the stitches.

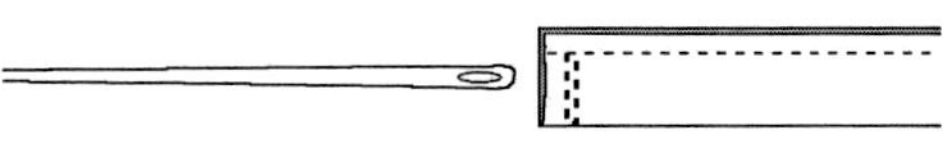

SEAMS AND SEAM FINISHES

SEAMS

The distinguishing feature of a neat, professional looking garment is in the preparation and precision with which you begin. Perfect seams are a critical point – they should not pucker, or appear stretched in any way.

There are several points that I like to recommend and emphasize over and over again, that will help maintain even and consistent stitching, and seams that sit perfectly smooth.

- Work with a stitch length that is suitable for the fabric. Fine fabric should be stitched with a short stitch length – I suggest not more than L-2.0.
- Always use thread that will not add bulk to fine heirloom and couture sewing – I like to use the Mettler 60/2 or DMC 50 for construction on nearly all my projects where the fabrics are lawn, batiste, voile, soft cotton flannel etc.

***Remember**, the strength of your seams comes from the size of the stitch length,* NOT *the weight of thread being used. A short stitch length gives a secure seam, even when using fine cotton thread.*

- Never clip a seam unless it is the only option – narrow French seams are an excellent alternative.
- Always apply even pressure to the fabric when sewing, both in front of and behind the presser foot. Keeping the fabric taut will prevent puckers from spoiling the look of your seams.

- Stitch seams in the direction of the fabric grain to prevent stretching – usually from the widest to the narrowest part of each piece.

Sew the shoulder seams from the neck to the armhole, and side seams from the armhole to the hem.

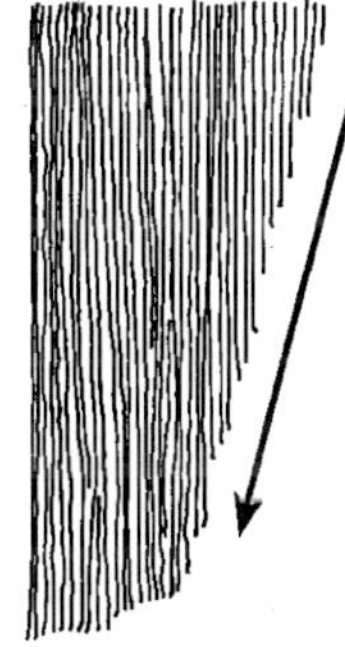
With Grain

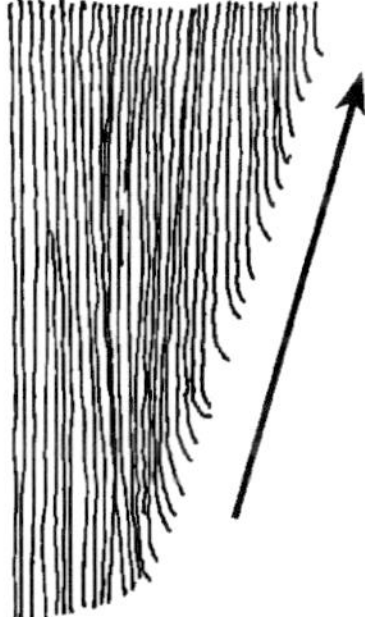
Against Grain

- Start and end the stitching of seams by making very small locking stitches, approximately ¼" to ⅜" (6mm to 1 cm) from the end (or for the distance of the seam allowance).
- To help make edges flat and help prevent seam allowances from making a ridge on the garment during pressing, trim and grade seam allowances when they are to be turned in one direction, or enclosed.

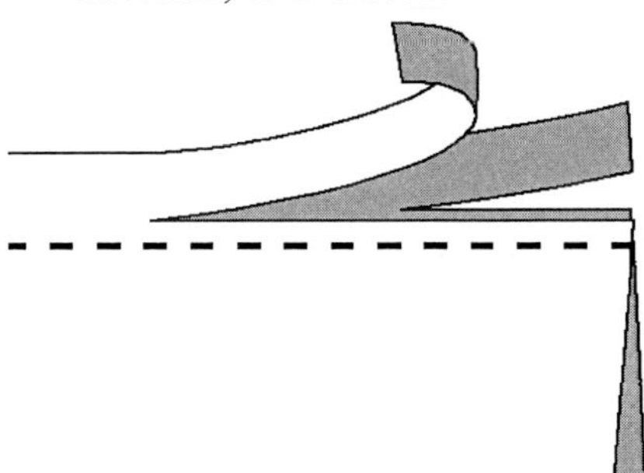

Trim enclosed seams (inside collars, cuffs, etc.) to ¼" (6mm) and **grade** them to cut down the bulk.

***Tip**: I like to first trim the underneath seam allowance to ⅛" (3mm) and the outer layer a little longer – say 3/16" (5mm).*

- Cut diagonal corners from the ends of seams and trim the enclosed seam allowances diagonally at points and corners.

  This step is not mandatory when working with a right angle corner – simply grade the seams and fold the corner seam allowances firmly on the stitching line.

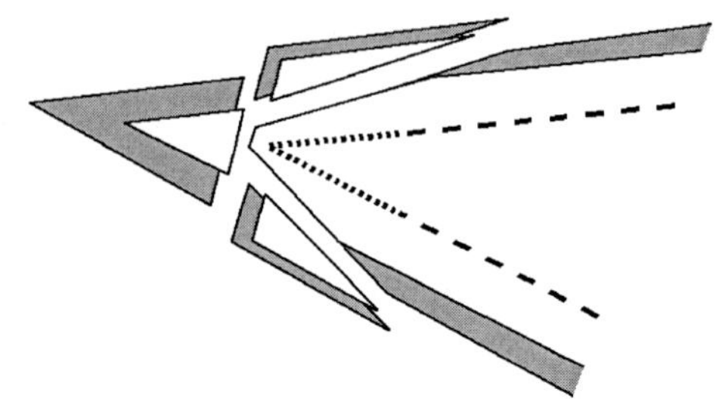

__Tip__: Never turn and poke into the corner with a skewer – this will create a ball of fabric in the corner. Never pull with a needle at the corner threads to help turn from the right side of the point – you will risk drawing threads out of the fabric at the corner (or point).

Instead, carefully fold on the seam line and turn the point, then lever the point into the correct angle by lifting the seam allowance from the outside with a large needle – insert the needle straight down into the fold of the seam, approximately ⅜" (1 cm) from the corner and with the tip of the needle facing the point, gently lift the tip of the needle, forcing the seam line to create a firm angle. Repeat on the other seam.

- Press seams flat or over a seam roll or tailors ham if necessary, in the direction specified by the pattern.
- When joining a bias edge to a straight edge, pin and baste the bias edge to the straight edge, and stitch with the bias edge on top, or facing upwards, in order to control the stretch of the bias and prevent puckers.
- If you are stitching two bias edges together, stretch the fabric **slightly** and stitch over tissue paper. Once the tissue paper has been removed, meld the stitches and steam press the seam to shape, removing all wrinkles or stretch marks.

In order to make a garment look as neat on the inside as it does on the outside, the seams should be secured – not left with raw edges showing. A garment with finished seams will last through many launderings. Remember, the seam and seam finish must be appropriate for particular garment area and the fabric being used.

- A Plain Seam is usually the beginning point for most seams. Place right sides together and, with raw edges even, join the two layers of fabric together.

  Should one of the seams have more fullness than the other keep the full edge facing upwards (on top) when stitching. Pin at close intervals and baste to hold. Stitch carefully, being sure to prevent tiny pleats from forming.

  If the seam is on a curve it must be clipped after melding and before pressing in order to prevent puckering

SEAMS WITH GATHERS

Gathering is the process of drawing a given amount of fabric into a pre-determined, smaller area, along one or several stitching lines, to create soft, even folds. Fabric is usually gathered to one-half or one-third the original width. Gathering most often occurs in a garment at the waistline, cuffs or yoke, or as ruffles.

These instructions have been written for working with a ⅜" (1 cm) seam allowance.

Stitch the first row of machine gathering just below the seam line, **NOT** within the seam allowance.

***Tip**: position the edge of the fabric on the ⅜" (1 cm) line on the machine sole plate, and move the needle position one (or two) notch(es) to the left.*

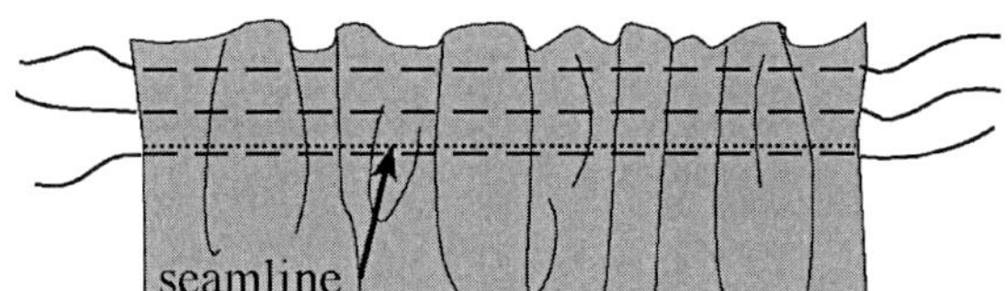
seamline

Stitch the 2nd row of machine gathering ⅛" (3mm) from the seam line, within the seam allowance, and a third row ⅛" (3mm) from the 2nd row of gathering stitches (or ⅛" (3mm) from the raw edge where the seam allowance is ⅜" (1 cm).

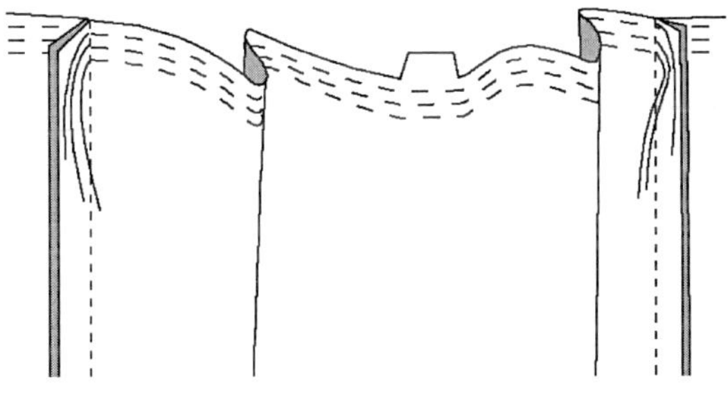

Leave long thread ends. Break stitching at the seams, as illustrated, as it is difficult to gather through two thicknesses and maintain even gathers in this area.

With right sides together, pin the stitched edge to the corresponding straight edge, matching the notches, center lines and seams.

Anchor the bobbin threads (now facing you) at one end by twisting in a figure 8 around pins. Excess material is now ready to gather.

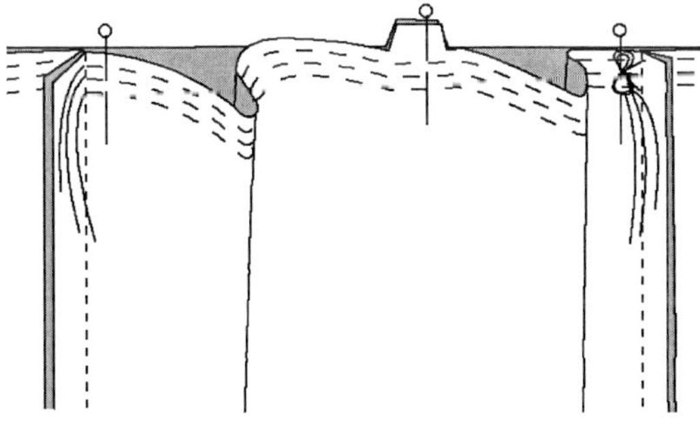

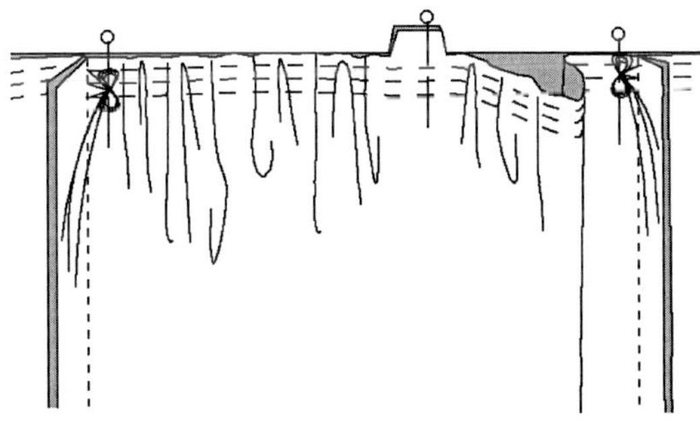

Gently pull on the bobbin threads while, with the other hand, you slide the fabric along the thread to create uniform gathers. When this first gathered section fits the adjoining edge secure the thread ends by winding them in a tight figure 8 around a pin.

To draw up the ungathered portion, untie the bobbin threads and repeat the process from the other end. When the entire gathered edge matches the straight edge fasten the thread end. Adjust the gathers uniformly and pin at frequent intervals to hold the folds in place. Repeat for each section.

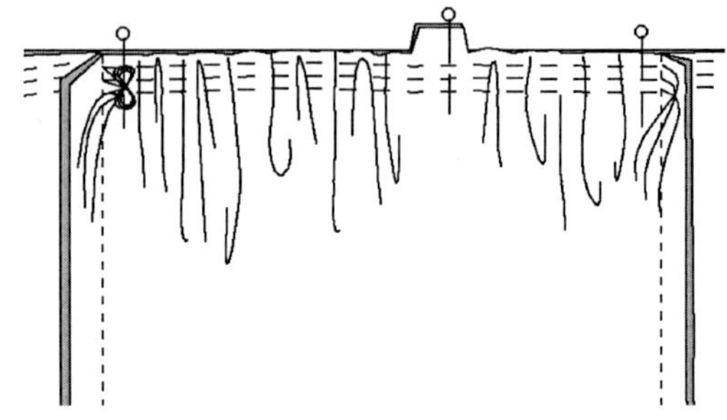

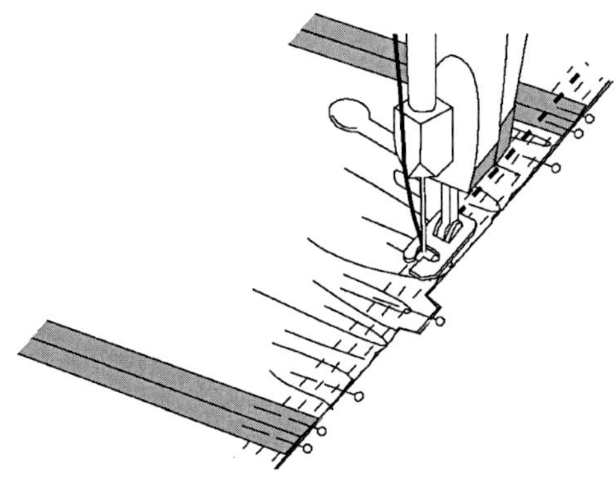

Before seaming the gathered sections, be sure the sewing machine is set to a short stitch length suitable to the fabric. With the gathered side facing up, stitch on the seamline, holding fabric on both sides of the needle so that the gathers will not be stitched into little pleats.

Trim any seam allowances, such as side seams, which are caught into the gathered seam. Once stitched, press the seam allowances only using just the tip of the iron.

The raw edges are now ready to be finished as appropriate to the garment – zigzag or overcast.

Refer to the techniques for a ***Self-Bound Seam*** *and a* ***Hong Kong Seam Finish****.*

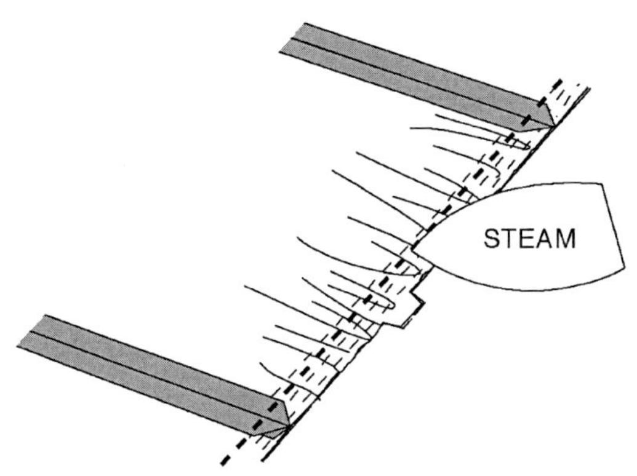
STEAM

Open the garment section out flat and press the seam in the direction it will be in the finished garment – toward the bodice if a waistline seam, toward the shoulder if a yoke seam, toward the wrist if a cuff.

Again work with just the tip of the iron, pressing flat the seam gathers only, taking care not to crease folds.

Press the gathers by working the point of the iron into the gathers toward the seam. Press from the wrong side of the fabric, lifting the iron as you reach the seam. Do not press across the gathers as this will flatten and cause them to go limp.

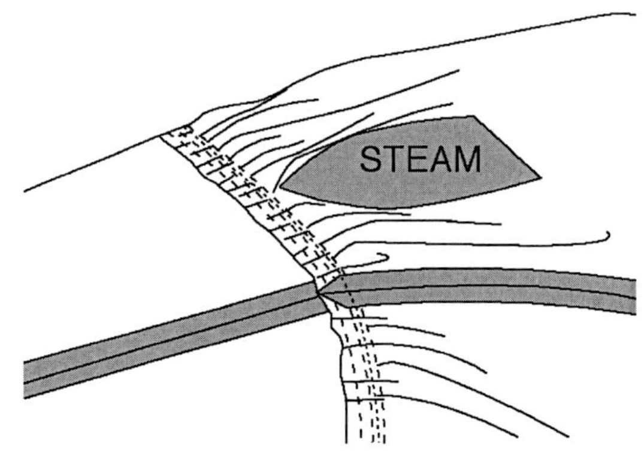
STEAM

FRENCH SEAM

It is almost impossible to execute a neat French seam where the seam allowance is less than ⅜″ (1 cm). Adjust the seam allowances to ⅜″ (1 cm) minimum to accommodate the French seam.

For seams on sheer or lightweight fabrics make a French seam – a neat, narrow seam of not more than 3/16" (5mm) which encloses the raw edges.

Tips:

- *When making a French Seam always stitch the first row (wrong sides together) and the second row (right sides together) in the same direction, otherwise it will surely wrinkle.*
- *If making the French Seam on very fine and/or fabric not cut on the grain (e.g. flared side seam or sleeve seam), stabilize the fabric before making the first row of zigzag stitches. Lightly spray starch the fabric two or three times until firm, or work with a fine tissue paper underneath. Meld the zigzag stitches and carefully remove the tissue paper before trimming the seam allowance for the next step.*

With ***wrong sides together*** and raw edges even, mark the seam allowance with a basting thread or water-soluble marker. Mark a second line ⅛" (3mm), but not more than 3/16" (5mm), from the seam line, within the seam allowance.

***Tip**: Always marking the seam allowance until this technique is perfected will help maintain a precise seam. This is especially important on sheer fabrics – no "eyeballing" allowed!*

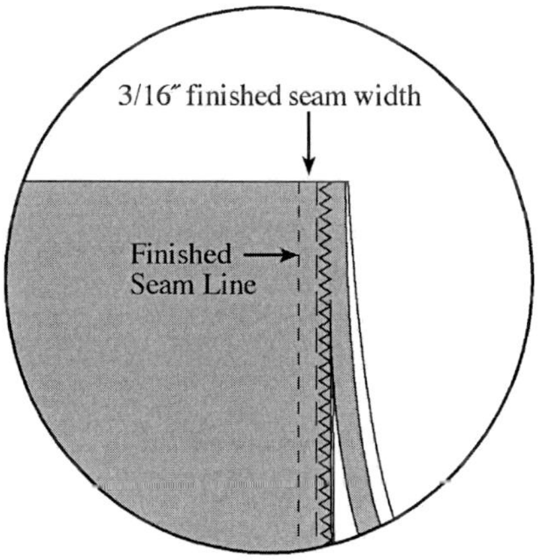

3/16″ finished seam width
Finished Seam Line

Stitch the first row with a small zigzag stitch (W: 2.0; L: 1.2 - 1.5 approx.) with the left swing almost on the 'seam width' line (see cameo).

Meld the row of zigzag stitches – very important!

Trim the seam allowance very close to the zigzag stitches, being careful not to cut the stitches.

With the wrong side facing upward on the ironing board, press the seam flat from both sides of the zigzag stitching, using the side of the sole plate to push firmly against the row of stitches. This will eliminate any tiny tucks in the French seam.

Finger-roll ***right sides together***, with the seam forming the fold line at the edge. It may be necessary to baste the fabric together at this point, especially if you are making the seam on a curved line.

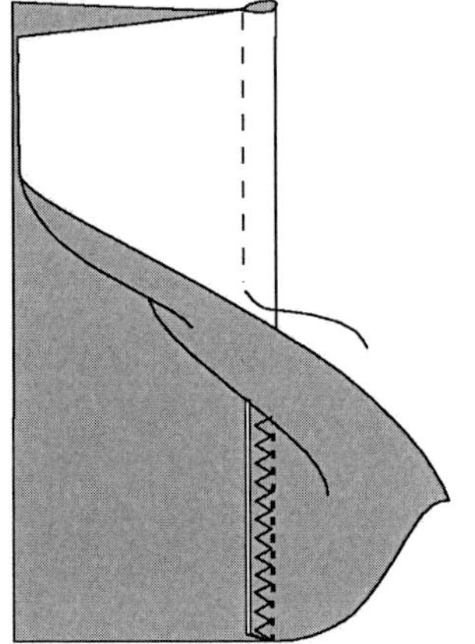

Pin and straight stitch along the *Finished Seam Line*. This should be ⅛" (3mm), but <u>not more than</u> 3/16" (5mm) from the edge. The raw edges and the previous row of stitching have now been enclosed within the seam.

Meld the stitches, and press the seam flat and to one side.

Notes

FRENCH SEAM INCORPORATING GATHERED FABRIC

For seams on sheer or lightweight fabrics make a French seam – a neat, narrow seam of not more than 3/16″ (5mm) finished width, which encloses the raw edges

Suggested applications for this technique would include:

- Attaching the sleeve in lingerie or a baby gown.
- Attaching a ruffle to lingerie or a Christening gown
- Joining the skirt to the bodice of a garment constructed from fine fabric.

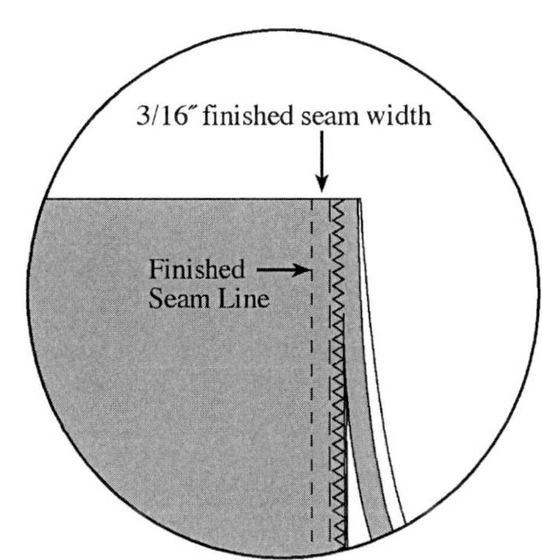
3/16″ finished seam width
Finished
Seam Line

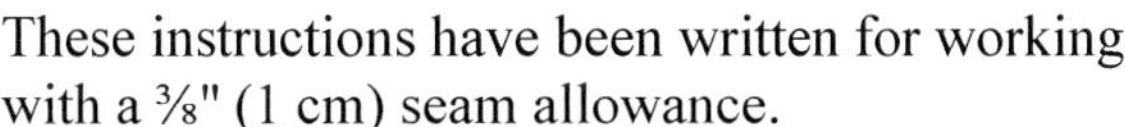

These instructions have been written for working with a ⅜" (1 cm) seam allowance.

Stitch the first row of machine gathering just below the seam line and **NOT** within the seam allowance.

Tip*: position the raw edge of the fabric on the ⅜″ (1 cm) line on the machine sole plate, and move the needle position one or two notches to the left.*

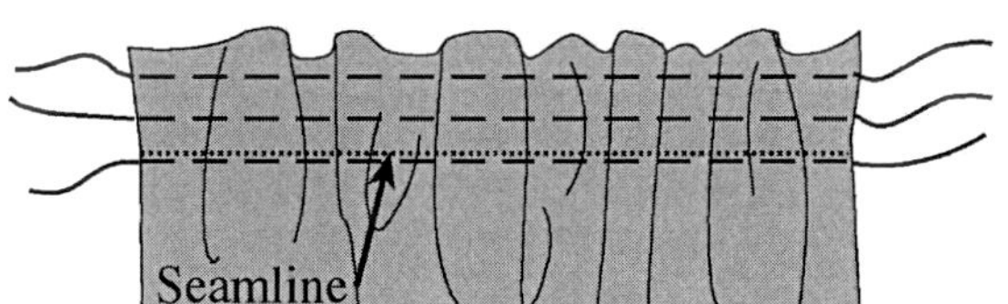
Seamline

Stitch the 2nd row of machine gathering ⅛″ (3mm) from the seam line and a third row ⅛″ (3mm) from the 2nd row of gathering stitches (or ⅛″ [3mm] from the raw edge where the seam allowance is ⅜″ [1 cm]).

Gently pull the bobbin threads and gather the fabric to the correct measurement.

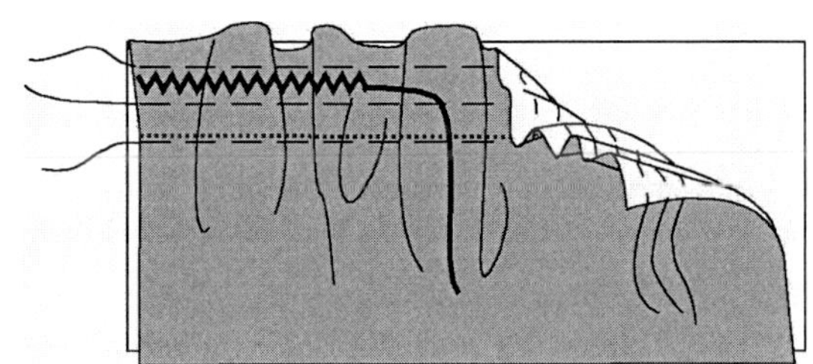

Tip*: Be sure to mark the center points (or shoulder/underarm positions) on both pieces of fabric. If adding a long ruffle mark at least the half and quarter points on both pieces.*

With **wrong** sides together, raw edges even, and the gathered fabric on top, use a small zigzag stitch to join the two pieces together. This should be between the 2nd and 3rd gathering lines.

Refer to the techniques for a ***French Seam***

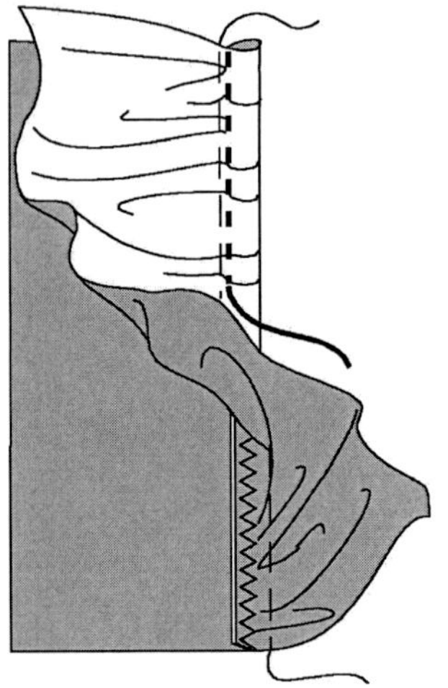

Meld the stitches with the tip of the iron and trim away the excess seam allowance, trimming as close as possible to the zigzag stitches. Finger-roll **right** sides together and hand baste.

Straight stitch on the seam line, not more than 3/16″ (5mm) from the folded edge. The raw edges and zigzag stitches are now enclosed within the seam.

***Tip**: Be sure to maintain the first row of machine gathering in the fabric until the technique is complete. You will be able to pull on the bobbin thread as you straight stitch and thus ensure the gathers remain perpendicular to the folded edge.*

Suggested Machine Settings

Zigzag Stitch:
W: Approximately 2.0
L: 1.0 to 1.5
Needle Position: center
Foot: basic sewing foot

***Tip**: If you are able to use your zigzag setting with the needle de-centered, use the basic 7mm sewing foot with the right hand edge of the foot aligned with the raw edges of the fabric and the needle position far right.*

Straight Stitch:
L: 2.0
Needle Position: center
Foot: basic sewing foot or a foot with a ⅛" guide

Notes

FLAT-FELL (or Run and Fell) SEAM

The Flat-Fell seam is an excellent choice of seam finish for sportswear, shirts and blouses or heavier fabrics, as it is very sturdy as well as being decorative. It would be the best seam to use when joining two pieces of fabric that may have tucks and heirloom sewing details incorporated in them.

Care must be taken to keep the seam widths uniform. These instructions have been written for working with a ⅜" (1 cm) seam allowance – width measurements will need to be adjusted for seam allowances that vary from this measurement.

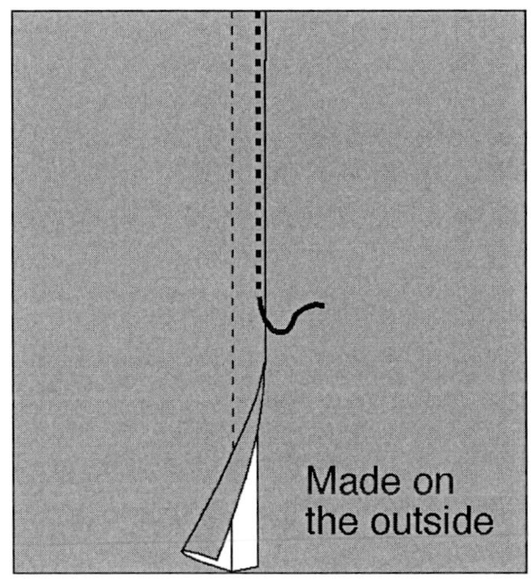
Made on
the outside

With the ***wrong*** sides of fabric together and raw edges even, stitch on the seamline. Press the seam open, then to one side and in the direction in which it will be stitched.

Trim the inner seam allowance (seam allowance closest to the right side of the garment) leaving either 3/16" (5mm) or ¼" (6mm).

If you have trimmed to an accurate 3/16" (5mm), press under the edge of the outer seam allowance until it barely meets the stitching line. The inner seam allowance is now encased by the outer seam allowance.

> ***Note:*** *With these measurements the inside seam allowance will be exactly half of the outer allowance that wraps around it.*

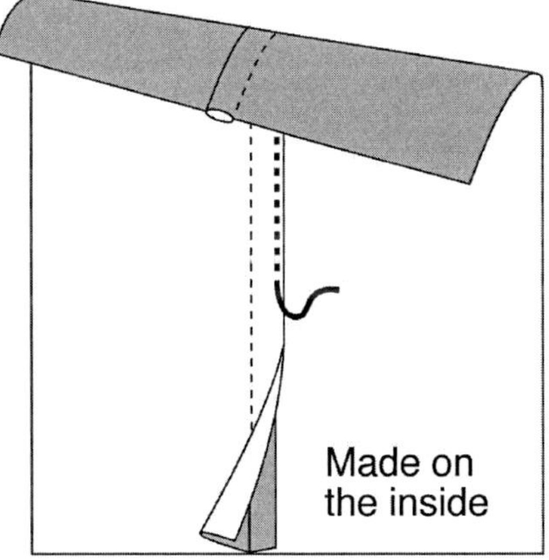
Made on
the inside

If you trimmed the inside seam allowance to ¼" (6mm) the outer seam allowance will be folded ¼" from the original stitching, leaving only ⅛" (3mm) pressed under to wrap around the inner seam allowance.

This seam finish is usually formed on the right side as per the above directions. However the final row of stitching can be made on either the inside **or** the outside of the fabric. Make a test sample of both and decide which one you prefer for the garment being constructed.

Baste the seam allowance into position and edgestitch this pressed edge to the garment, using the *edge-joining* foot for preference, and with the needle de-centered. Be careful to trim and press like seams in the same direction – e.g., both shoulder seams to the front, side seams to the back.

HONG KONG SEAM FINISH

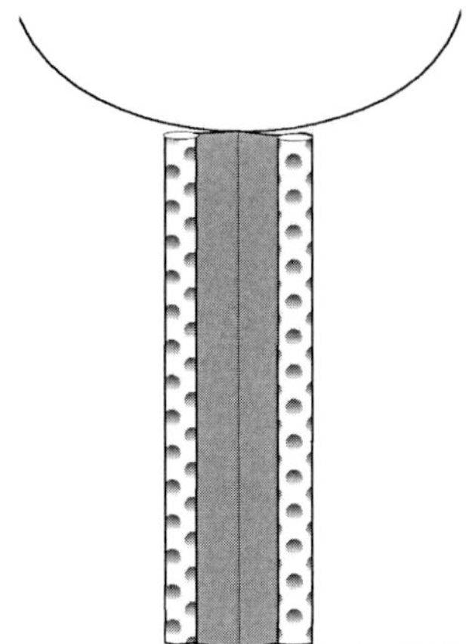

The Hong Kong finish is an elegant detail created by binding the hem, facing or seam allowance with a piece of bias fabric. It is a smooth finish that eliminates all possibility of raveling and is used when a couture finish is required.

The Hong Kong seam finish is particularly effective for seams in an unlined jacket, heavy fabric or where bulk needs to be enclosed. For most effective use, seam allowances should be not less than ⅝" (1.5 cm).

Fabrics suitable for use as the binding include silk organza, silk crepe de Chine, cotton organdy or batiste, or any extremely lightweight fabric – natural fibers work best. You might also like to try a product called 'Seams Great' – a lightweight knit fabric available in varying widths and colors.

For a binding of not more than 3/16" (5mm), cut the bias strips 1" (2.5 cm) wide; or refer to the instructions with your bias binding maker before cutting.

Run the bias fabric through the small (or ¼") bias maker and press the fold on one edge only.

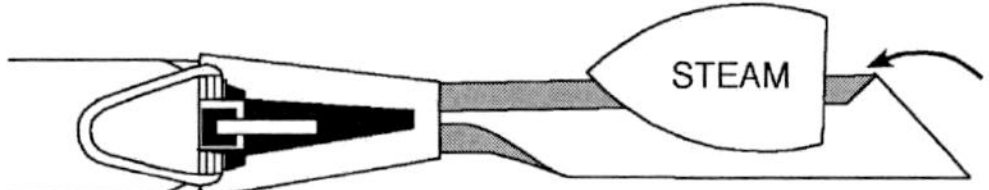
STEAM

Open out the fold after the crease has been pressed. This fold should be ¼" (6mm) and you will use it as the stitching guide in the next step.

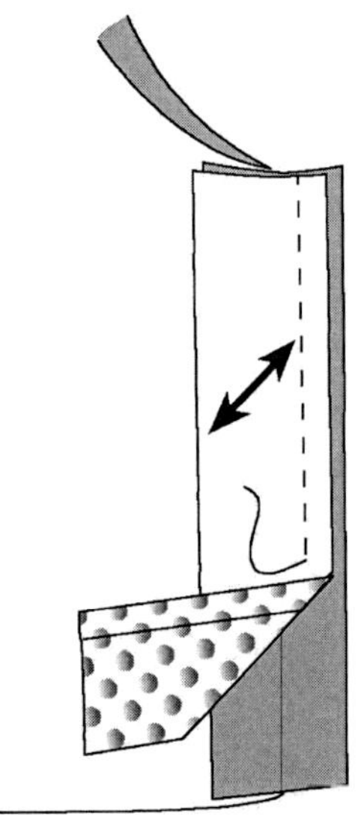

Using the edge of the bias which has been creased, place the ***right*** side of the bias to the right side of the seam allowance with raw edges even.

Stitch the bias strip to the seam allowance ¼" (6mm) from the edge, or on the pressed crease.

Meld the stitches.

Trim all layers (seam allowance and bias trim) to approximately ⅛" – 3/16" (3mm - 5mm).

Finger-roll the bias over the raw edges to the wrong side of the seam. Pin, with pins at right angles to the stitching line. The bias fabric on the back of the seam must be flat and not twisted.

From the right side, stitch in the ditch using an edge-joining foot with a center bar.

Trim the raw edge of the bias strip <u>close</u> to the stitching line on the wrong side, or underneath side, of the seam allowance.

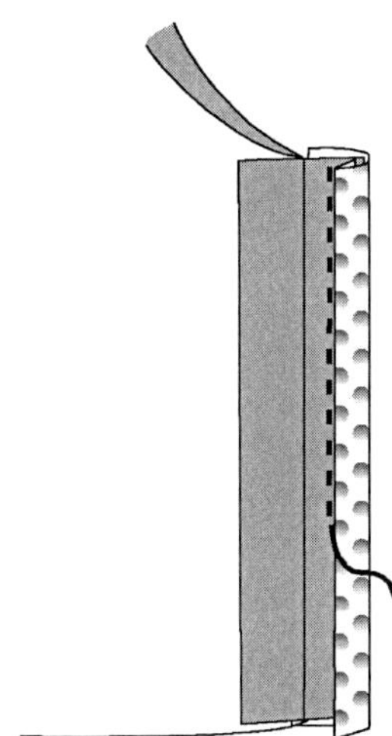

Using the Hong Kong Seam Finish to neaten the seam allowance of a seam with gathered fabric:

One way to neaten the seam allowance of a seam that includes gathered fabric is to encase the seam allowance in a bias strip.

- Prepare the bias strip as above, pressing under only one edge.

- With right sides together and raw edges even, stitch a bias strip of lightweight fabric on top of the original seam line (or <u>barely</u> within the seam allowance). Stitch with the flat fabric against the feed teeth and the bias strip against the presser foot so that the gathered fabric is sandwiched between the flat fabric and the bias.

  This placement will ensure that, when completed, the bias finish does not interfere with the fall of the gathers.

- Meld the stitching line with the tip of the iron, being careful not to flatten the gathers.

- Neaten the raw edges and finger-roll the bias binding over the seam allowance so that the binding is completely filled. Pin or baste the rolled bias in place. The unstitched edge of the bias strip will not be folded under, but will lay flat and extend beyond the seam allowance.

- With the seam allowance facing upwards and the gathered fabric on top (the bias will be folded to the underside), stitch in the ditch. On the underside trim the edge of the bias strip close to this stitching line

  OR

  Do not machine stitch in the ditch, but turn the remaining allowance of the bias strip under and hand catch to the stitching line.

Refer to the techniques for ***Binding a Neckline*** *or*
Binding a Collar *for hand stitching closure*

THE SELF-BOUND SEAM

The self-bound seam is so named because one seam allowance wraps around and binds the other. It works best on loosely woven fabrics or lightweight fabrics that do not fray easily. However, it is also a seam treatment that was used before the invention of the zigzag stitch on the sewing machine where, for example, a gathered skirt seam could be enclosed by using the seam allowance from the yoke to form a binding. This seam treatment looks similar to a French seam but is not as durable.

On fine, single thickness fabrics accurate results can be achieved with a ⅜" seam allowance, but you would be wise to consider using a ⅝" (1.5 cm) seam allowance where one layer of fabric has been gathered.

With ***right*** sides of fabric together and raw edges even, stitch on the seam line.

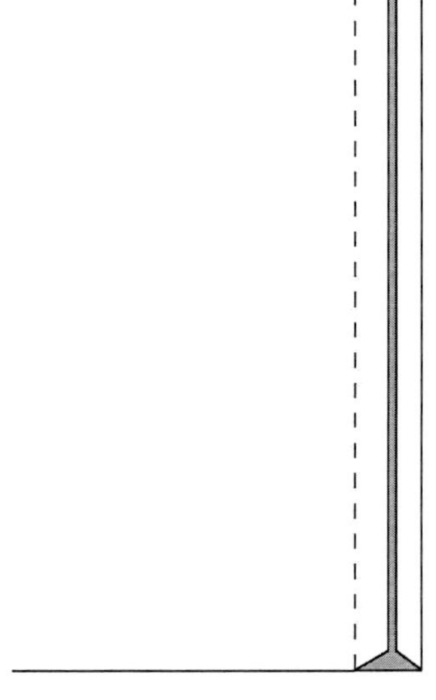

Trim one seam allowance to ⅛" (3 mm), or ¼" (6mm) narrower than the other.

Turn under the edge of the longer, uncut, seam allowance ⅛" (3 mm) and press.

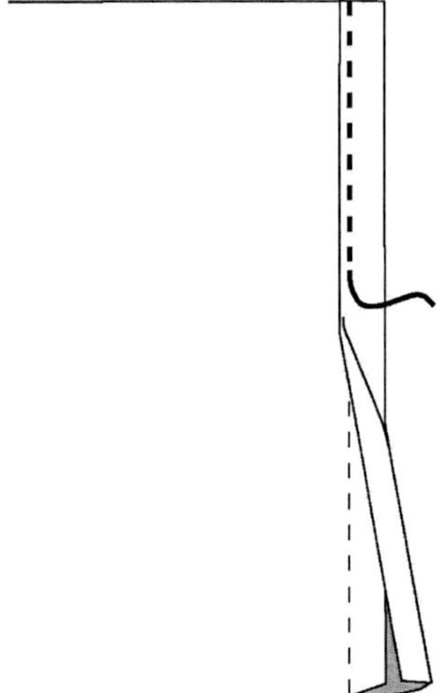

Turn and press again, bringing the folded edge up to, but not over, the seamline, so that the trimmed edge is now enclosed.

***Tip**: When working with a ⅜" (1 cm) seam, I like to trim to 3/16" (5mm) and fold to 3/16" (5mm) so that the bound seam is completely filled.*

Stitch close to the fold and as near as possible to the first line of stitching (within the seam allowance).

***Tip**: use an edge joining foot with the center bar positioned beside the binding and the needle position offset just barely to the right of center.*

This final row of stitching can also be worked by hand.

Prepare the seam binding as above, trimming the seam allowance and folding the longer edge over to meet the row of machine stitches.

Press and baste the seam into position.

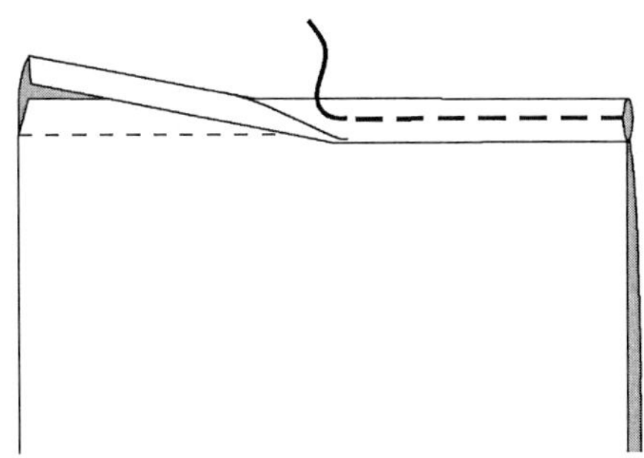

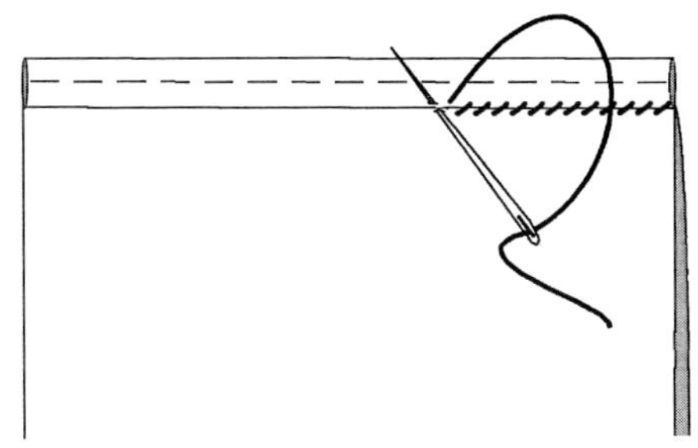

Secure the binding by whip-stitching the edge of the fold to the first row of stitching.
Refer to this step in the techniques for ***Binding a Collar***.

Be careful to trim and press like seams so they fall in a consistent direction – both shoulder and side seams towards the back.

A DECORATIVE SEAM

In some garments a seam can be turned into a design feature without the need for neatening the seam allowances. A decorative ribbon, tape or Swiss beading is placed over the seam in such areas as joining a yoke to a skirt, a ruffle to the bottom of a daygown or an eyelet edge to a sleeve.

Construct a plain seam with the seam allowance on the right side of the garment (**wrong sides together**). Meld the stitches.

Trim or grade the seam allowances so they are less than the width of the trim, and press the seam in the direction it will lay once the trim has been added (away from the gathered fabric):

- the seam on a hemline ruffle of a skirt will be pressed up towards the garment
- the seam on a waistline (or high waist) will be pressed up towards the bodice

Position the trim over the seam so that any embroidery or design in the trim is centered (from right to left on a yoke) and the trim completely encloses the seam allowances. Baste to hold.

Edgestitch the trim on the top and bottom. This finishes the seam on the inside of the garment as well as on the outside.

MAKING A NARROW HEM

In fine sewing, it is sometimes desirable to finish an edge without a traditional hem.

Opportunities to use this very narrow hem are:

- the hem of a full or sheer garment
- the edges of a ruffle
- the hem of a garment lining
- the curved edge of a garment where it would be impossible to turn a large hem (e.g. the lower or curved edge of a shirt or blouse)

The narrow hem provides couture detail in such instances. It is stitched twice to keep it smooth and without wrinkles.

Add ⅝″ (1.5 cm) to the finished length. Stitch through a single layer 3/8″ (1 cm) from the edge. Fold the hem up following this stitching line, with machine stitches to the underneath side. Press perpendicular to the hem and steam the excess fabric into place.

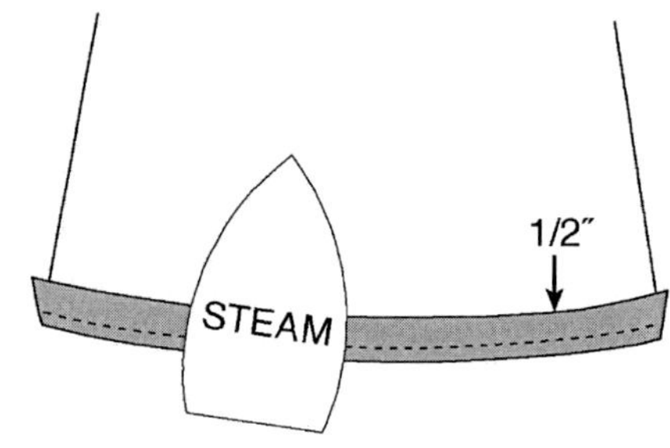
1/2″
STEAM

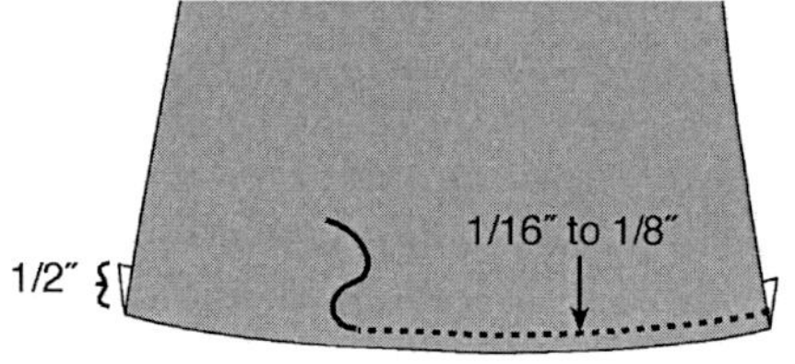
1/2″
1/16″ to 1/8″

From the **right side** machine stitch 1/16″ (1.5mm) – 1/8″ (3 mm) from the edge.

Meld the stitches. Press the stitched edge – the original stitches should be centered in the hem you have turned up

***Tip**: Always press at right angles to the stitching line – this is especially true on a rounded hemline.*

Working from the wrong side and with very sharp scissors (mini appliqué or duckbill scissors work well), cut away the seam allowance as close to the stitches as possible.

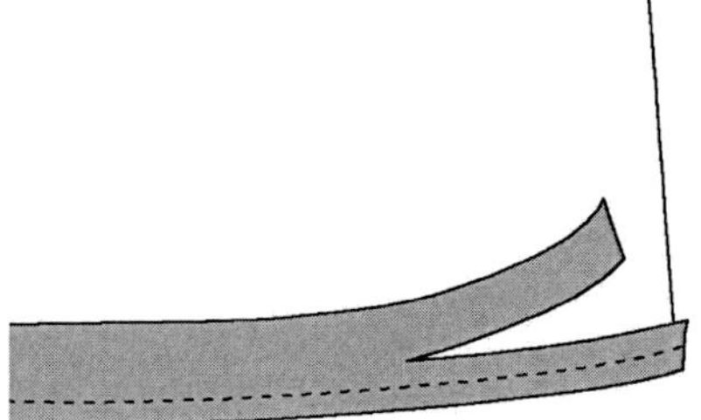

.

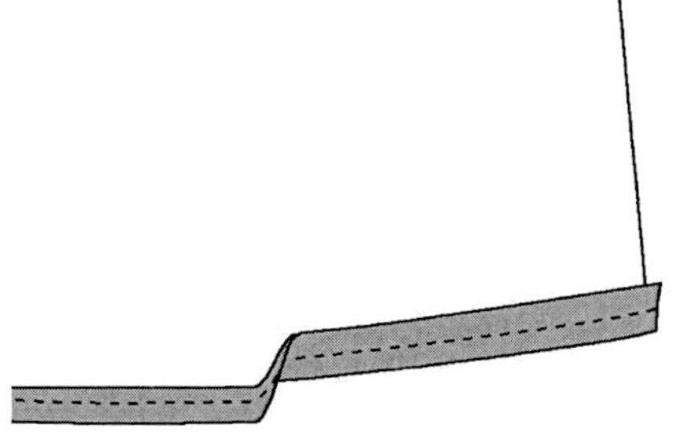

Turn the hem a second time to enclose the raw edges. From the wrong side, slowly machine stitch directly over the first stitches holding the fabric taut.

Press again to meld the stitches and to ensure the hem sits flat.

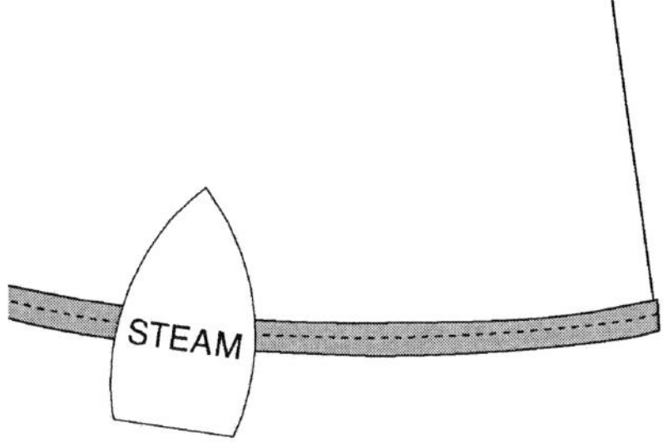
STEAM

QUICK STEPS TO COMPLETE A CURVED EDGE

A thinly rolled hem which curves gently must sit smooth and flat.

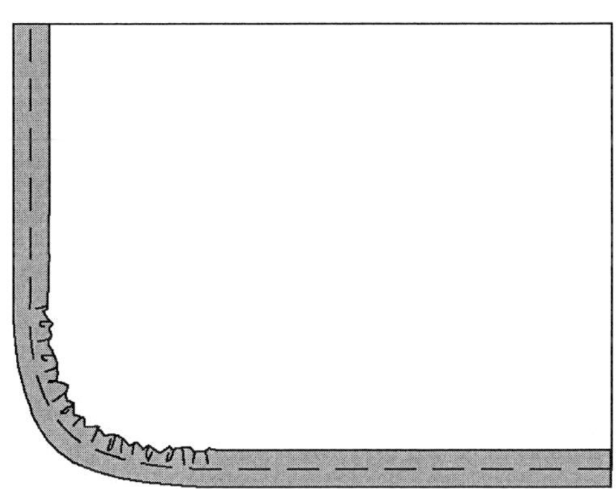

Sew an ease line 3/16" (5mm) from the raw edge around the curve. Use a stitch length of about 2.5 so as to gather gently and not create pleats.

Pull the bobbin threads at the curves until the raw edge fits the garment shape without puckering, and the edge turns under ⅜" (1 cm).

Fold the raw edge in 3/16" (5mm) at the ease line to meet the pressed crease. Press lightly.

Stitch the rolled hem by hand or machine.

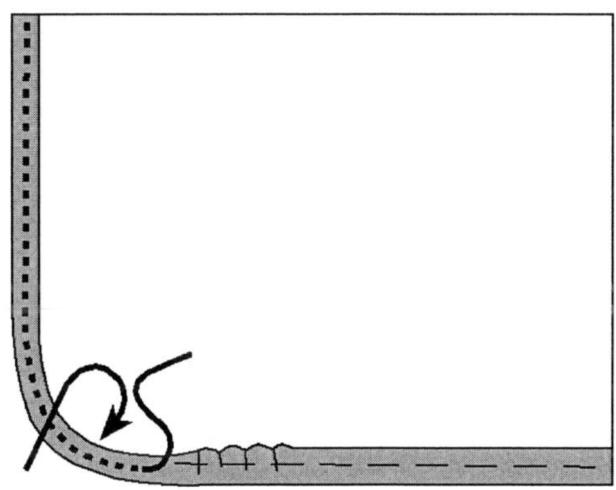

PLACKETS AND CLOSURES

Very few garments have a large enough neckline to slip over the head, so most garments will need an opening in one form or another. These openings can be creative and form the feature of the garment –

- Create an extension to the front and back shoulder seams in order to use feature buttons
- Open the garment from the neckline to the hem by adding a button lap (see *Buttons and Buttonholes*) and facing, and incorporating decorative buttons
- Insert a Keyhole or Slot Seam opening at the neckline

However, when a feature is not being made of the opening and the placket is either an *Antique Tab Placket* or a placket being incorporated within the width of fabric (*Continuous Lapped Placket*) or into a seam (*Extension Placket*) of a skirt, this opening must be adequate to serve the purpose.

Note: When a garment does not have a waistline the placket does not need to be as long as it would for a garment with a waistline. A waistline on a garment creates a tighter fit.

The easiest method of determining a placket length is to use the measurement from a garment that already fits. However, if working without such luxury, the following chart for approximate placket lengths should be of some assistance.

Chart for Placket Lengths

Size	**Garment with no Waistline (Bishop, A-line Dress or Daygown)**	**Garment with a Waistline (Placket in Skirt only)**
6 months	7½" (19 cm)	4" (10 cm)
1	8¼" (21 cm)	4" (10 cm)
2	8⅝" (22 cm)	4½" (11.5 cm)
3	9" (23 cm)	4½" (11.5 cm)
4	9½" (24 cm)	5" (12.5 cm)
5	10" (25.5 cm)	5" (12.5 cm)
6	11"(28 cm)	5¼" (13.5 cm)
7	11⅝" (29.5 cm)	5½" (14 cm)
8	12¼" (31 cm)	6" (15 cm)

CONTINUOUS LAPPED PLACKET

This is the most widely used of all plackets. It is incorporated into sleeves, skirts and dresses where the placket is intended to be as inconspicuous as possible. The Continuous Lapped Placket is the most appropriate for use within a width of fabric (on the fold) and NOT where a seam is involved.

The length of the placket is optional and primarily determined from the pattern recommendation. It is important to make continuous lapped plackets in baby garments equally as long as for child size garments, not shorter as we would be inclined. This allows for easier dressing of a baby.

Cut the placket binding to measure 1½" (4 cm) wide by twice the length of the opening plus ½" (12mm). Draw a line lengthwise on the binding fabric, 3/16" (5mm) from one long edge.

***Tip**: This is an important step, as it will allow you to sew a precise seam without having to guess where you should stitch.*

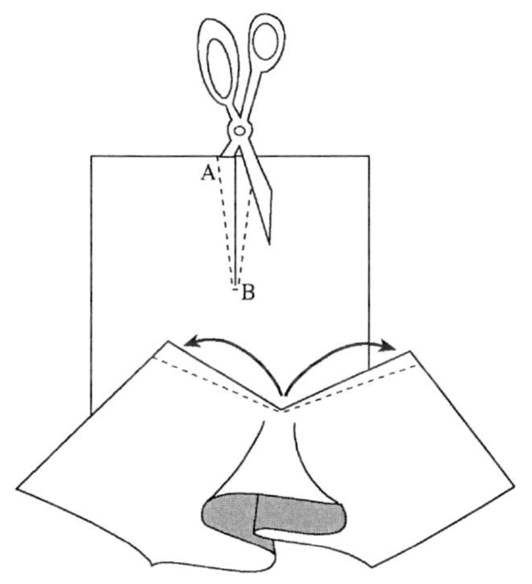
A
B

Mark the placket placement on the skirt back with a straight line A-B.

Reinforce the placket stitching line with small machine stitches, commencing 3/16" (5mm) from one side of placement line at the top tapering toward the bottom (point B) and making one stitch across the point. Use smaller stitches on each side of the pivoting point.

Continue stitching up the other side, finishing 3/16" (5mm) from the placement line at the top.

Slash through the garment fabric on the placket placement line (solid line A-B), from the top to the pivot-point as shown.

With right sides together pin the garment and binding together, matching the machined reinforcement line to the ruled line on the placket fabric.

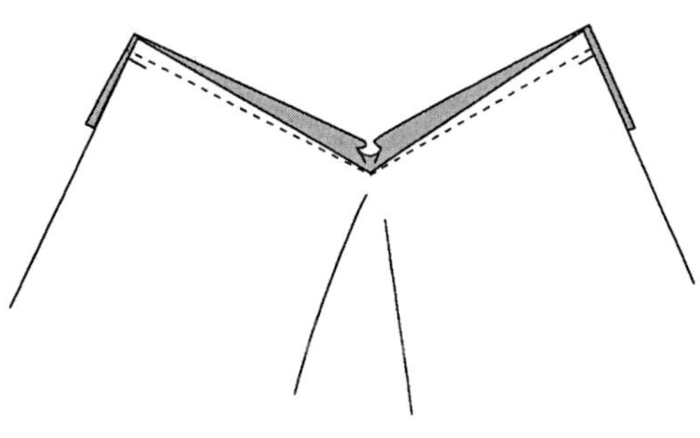

Machine stitch just outside the original line of reinforcing stitches. Sew with the slit on top and the placket fabric on the bottom in order that the end of the opening is visible and not to cause puckering (The placket strip will be straight – the garment fabric will form a slight 'V').

***Tip**: Stitching very slowly at the pivot point and lifting the presser foot while keeping the need down will allow you to adjust the extra fabric at the point. Use a sharp stylus or stiletto to assist.*

Meld the stitches.

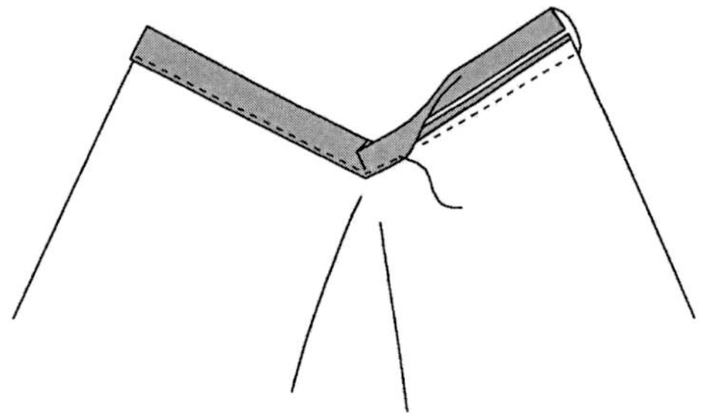

Extend the binding and press the seam toward the placket strip. Press again from the right side with the tip of the iron making a sharp crease at the seam line.

Measure the binding fabric in thirds and fold to the wrong side, encasing the raw edges. Pin in place and secure by hand whipping or machine stitching.

For extra strength at the point, pull the placket to the inside of the garment and fold the placket in half, allowing the top edges of the garment to meet. Machine stitch a dart diagonally across the folded edge of the placket only.

Tip*: Stitch from the widest point (placket edge) towards the garment, and back again – do* NOT *take a stitch into the garment fabric or you will create a slight tuck on the front of your work.*

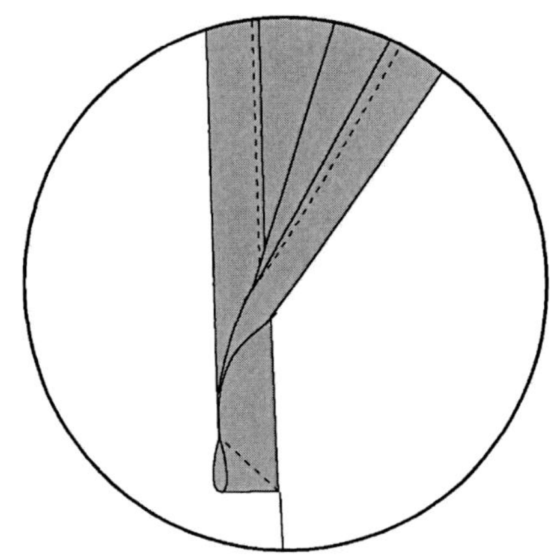

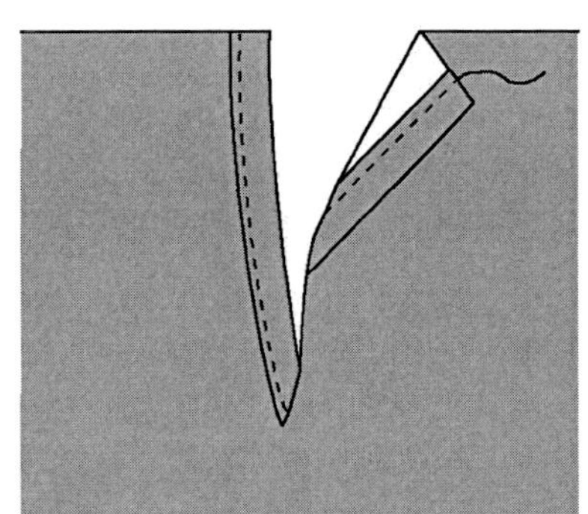

Turn back the side of the placket that will be on top when overlapped and press. The underneath side extends as shown.

Notes

EXTENSION PLACKET

This type of placket is perfect for any opening where a seam is involved.

If you are working with a pattern that has a ⅜" (1cm) seam allowance you will need to increase this allowance to at least ¾" (18mm) on the seam where the placket will be added.

In the case of a smocked bishop dress, when pleating leave approximately ¾"(18mm) – 1" (2.5 cm) from each back edge unpleated. This forms the foundation of the placket.

Neaten the seam edges. Stitch the seam with the bottom of the placket opening at the top of seam to the hemline, leaving open the desired portion for the placket. Meld the stitches and press the seam open and flat along the full length of the garment.

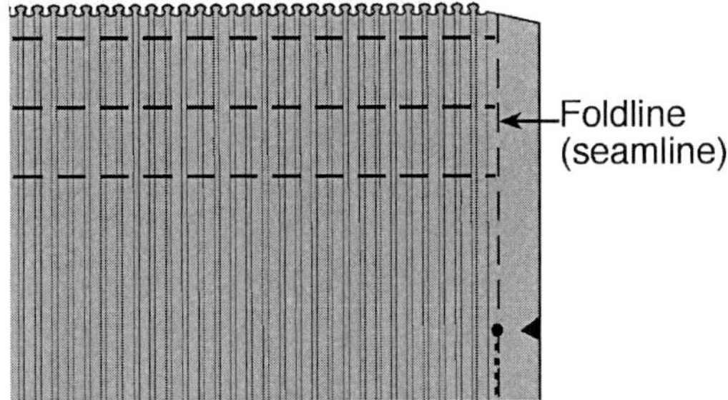
Foldline
(seamline)

Tip*: For a more accurate pressing line for the placket, stitch the seam from the raw edge to the top of the seam with a long basting stitch. Lock the stitches at the placket depth line and continue stitching to the hemline with a short stitch length. The basting threads will be removed after the seam has been melded and pressed open.*

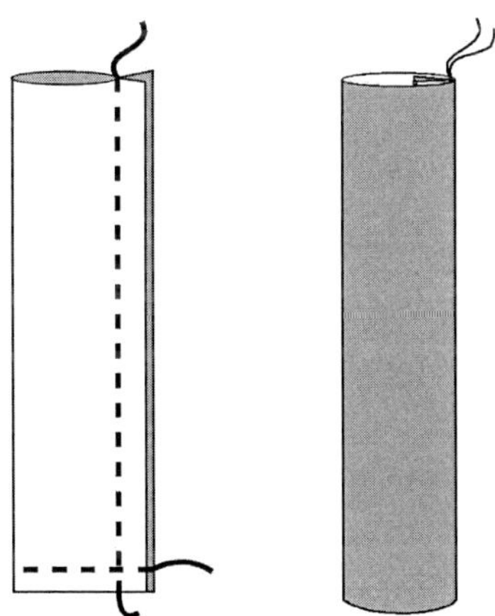

Cut a facing on the straight grain in the same fabric as the garment, approximately 2" (5 cm) wide and 1" (2.5 cm) longer than the opening.

Fold this strip of fabric in half lengthwise, with *right* sides together. Stitch down the length and across the bottom, using a ¼" (6 mm) seam allowance.

Turn right side out and press, ensuring that the point is turned out sharply.

The placket is positioned on the **left** side of the opening as you look at it. The right side is pressed back on the seam line into position for buttonholes or snaps, if required.

With the right side of the garment facing upwards and commencing at the neck edge, Match the **folded** edge of the placket to the seam line and pin in place. Continue pinning ¾" (2 cm) down beside the seam, past the placket opening point.

Work only on the single layer of seam allowance and do not attach this placket to any other part of the garment. Baste in place; check the finished result and then stitch on the very edge of the placket using a short straight stitch and an edge-joining foot with the needle de-centered one position.

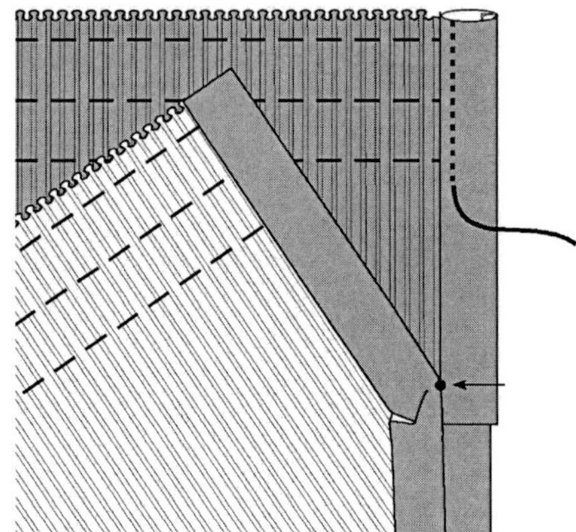

Meld the stitches and press with the side of the iron so that the seam allowance on which the placket tab is positioned is turned back against the garment. The placket only should extend and sit flat; the seam allowances will be turned back on the underside.

The result should be a neat, flat, invisible placket ready for your choice of closure Suggestions for closing this type of placket would be:

- Two or three snaps positioned on the placket extension and the seam allowance on the underneath side of the garment.
- Buttons positioned close to the seam line of the extension placket and buttonhole loops to correspond attached to the fold of the top fabric layer.
- Buttons and buttonholes (non-smocked garments only).

Notes

ANTIQUE TAB (OR FLAT) PLACKET

These instructions have been written for incorporation into a back-opening baby daygown – *('Gabrielle'*, or *'Delicate Daydreams' and 'Edwardian Baby'* with pattern modifications).

Note: If constructing this placket for the first time it is advisable to mark **ALL** guide lines on the placket and make a sample.

Position the pattern **facing upwards** on the **right** side of the fabric and cut out the placket from garment fabric (or contrasting fabric if desired).

- With ***right*** sides of the ***garment*** together, press the center crease into the daygown back. **DO NOT** cut the back opening.
- With ***wrong*** sides together press the center crease into the ***placket fabric***.

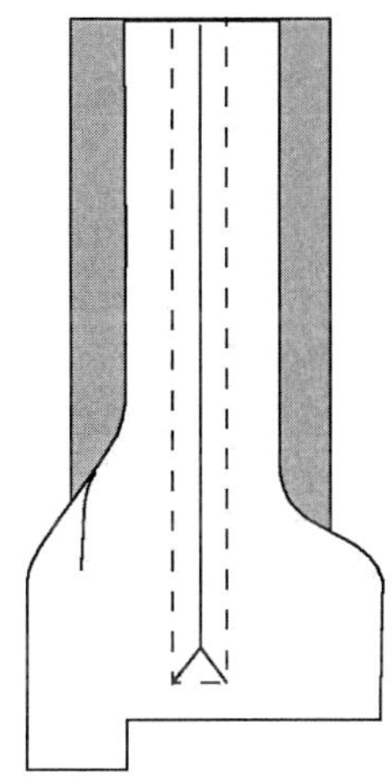

Turn and press ½" (12mm) to the wrong side on each side of the placket fabric.

With *right sides together*, position the placket on top of the fabric, nestling the two center creases together. Pin together and baste on the center line to keep both pieces on the straight of grain.

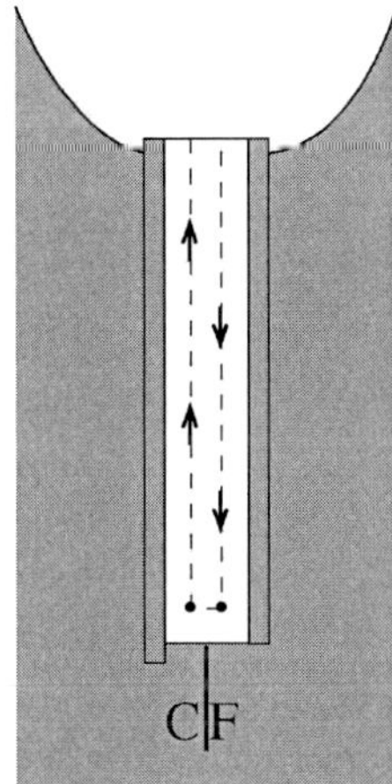
CF

Mark the center box stitching line with a water-soluble marker or tailor's chalk.

Tip*: Once you have made your sample placket you may not need to draw in this box every time. Instead, use the ¼" or quilting foot to stitch ¼" (6mm) from the center line.*

Stitch along the stitching lines in the direction marked by the ↓'s, pivoting at the '•'s at each corner, and reducing the stitch length around the bottom of the box.

Cut through the garment and the placket on the centerline between the lines of stitching, clipping diagonally to the corner '•'s. Meld and grade the long seam allowances and, from the wrong side, press them towards the placket.

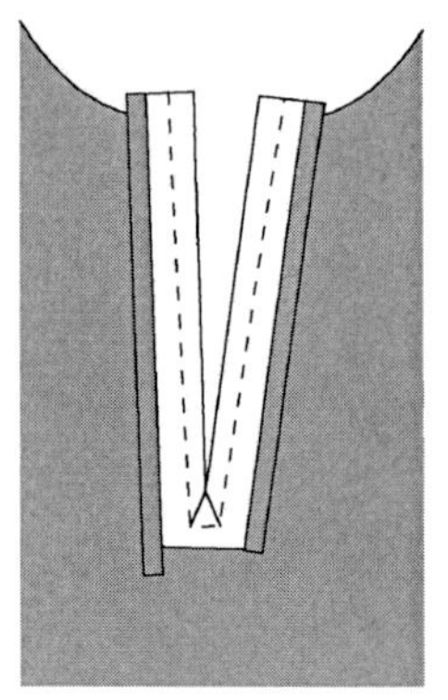

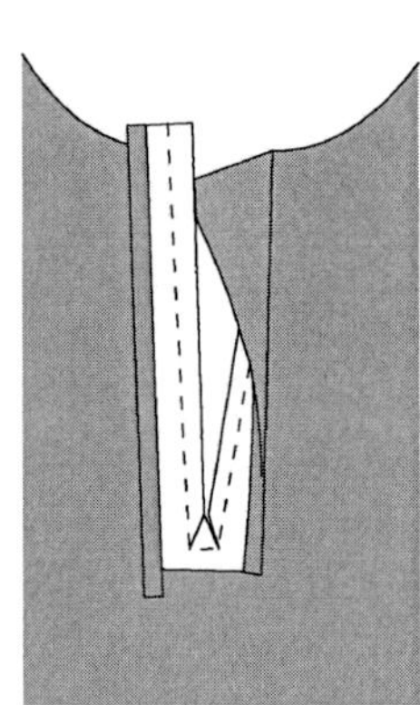

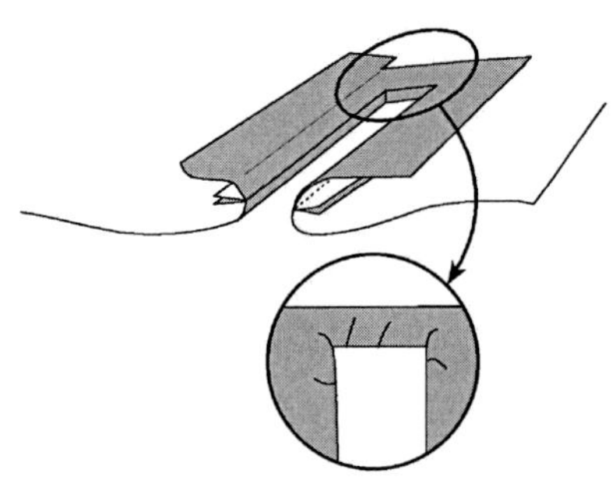

Pull the placket fabric through the opening to the wrong side of the garment. Press the bottom of the placket and the wedge away from the opening. There should be no pressed horizontal creases in the placket fabric.

Note: *The two sides of the placket fabric will now be positioned to fill in the box that has been created by pulling the placket fabric through to the wrong side of the garment.*

Finger press the shorter side of the placket along the fold line so that the first fold that was pressed with the iron, meets the stitching line of the 'box'. Pin in position and stitch the fold to the edge of the placket with tiny whipping stitches.

Finger press the longer side of the placket along the fold line so that the first fold meets the stitching line of the 'box'. Pin in position and stitch the fold to the edge of the placket with tiny stitches.

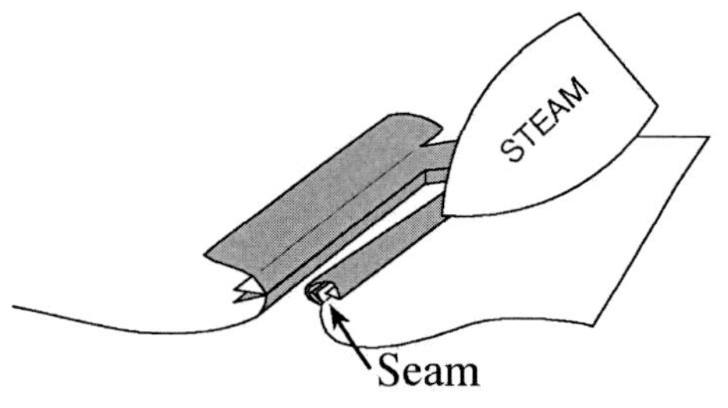
STEAM
Seam

The little tab at the bottom of the box is now positioned between the wrong side of the garment fabric and the folded placket. The placket now fills the opening that was created by stitching around the box.

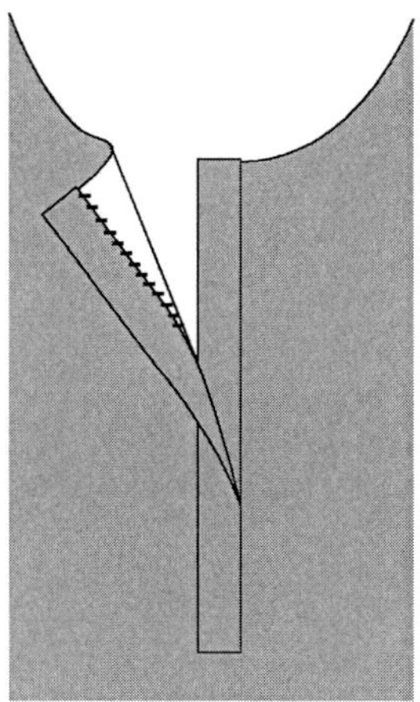

Make sure the placket bands are square and sitting exactly on top of one another. Pull the little tab and the placket bands free, and stitch across the top of the ▼ (wedge), on the original stitching line, to secure all layers.

Trim the shorter end of the placket extension to ¼″ (6mm) and finger press the extending end of the placket around it. Whip stitch to conceal the raw edges.

Alternately, zigzag across the bottom on the wrong side ¼″ (5mm) from the securing stitching row, and trim the excess fabric on both extensions close to this zigzag stitching.

Make buttonholes in the top placket band and sew buttons on the under placket band.

***Note**: Tradition is for button bands to lap*
***Right over left** for girls and **left over right** for boys.*

Antique garments were lapped right over left for all babies and small children.

Note: It is important to emphasize once again, the benefits of making at least one sample. By testing your placket placement on the fabric (right side of pattern up or down) you will be able to determine whether you want the placket lapped right over left or left over right, and make the necessary adjustments.

Notes

ANTIQUE TAB (OR FLAT) PLACKET

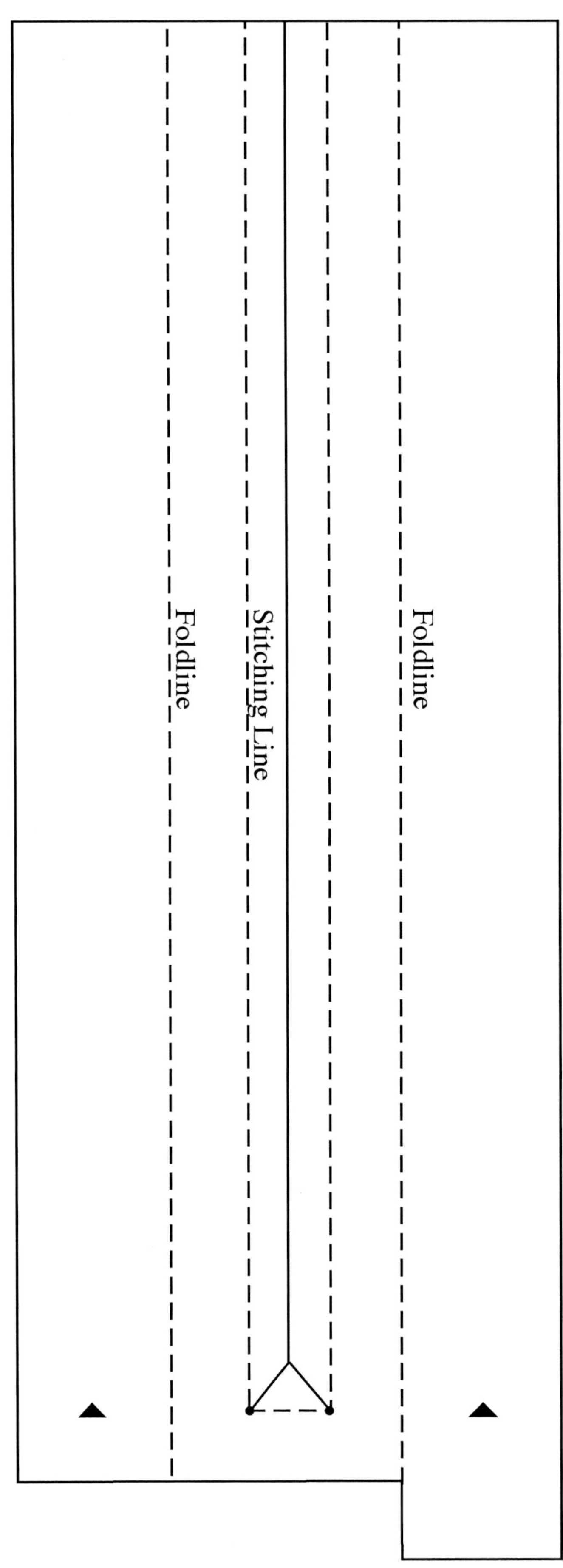
Foldline
Stitching Line
Foldline

BUTTONS AND BUTTONHOLES

When drafting and constructing garments with button closures it is paramount that you are aware of both center front and center back. These two points are critical to achieving professional results and they **never** vary – no matter how many fit and/or design changes are made to the garment, center front and center back remain constant.

It is the point at which the buttons/buttonholes come together and collars meet, and it is the grainline that is the determining factor for changes to the pattern. Any movement will alter the fit of the garment, therefore care must be taken when working buttonholes or altering the pattern (to accommodate larger buttons or a wider overlap), to be mindful of these two important reference points.

Chart for Button Sizes

Linge is the traditional European sizing of buttons.

Linge	Button Diameter (inches)	Button Diameter (metric)
100	2⅛"	64mm
75	1⅞"	51mm
60	1½"	38mm
45	1⅛"	29mm
40	1"	25mm
36	⅞"	22mm
30	¾"	19mm
24	⅝"	16mm
20	½"	13mm
18	7/16"	11mm
16	⅜"	10mm
14	a little less than ⅜"	9mm
12	5/16"	8mm
10	¼"	6mm

There are three types of buttonholes, and many variations of each:

- the worked buttonhole – by hand or machine
- the bound buttonhole – corded, patch, welt
- the in-seam buttonhole

The type of buttonhole you choose for a garment will depend on the design of that garment, the fabric being used and your level of sewing confidence. A buttonhole needs to be large enough to accommodate the button, but not so large that the button can slip through and become undone.

While I would recommend that you practice and perfect hand-worked buttonholes for fine garments such as Christening gowns and heirloom style baby clothes, in this chapter we will cover the principles of buttonholes and, more specifically, those worked by machine.

1. Never attach a button or make a buttonhole on a single thickness of fabric.
   There should always be at least two thicknesses of fabric, and for preference three. This means you could use three layers of the same fabric, or two layers of fabric, one having been interfaced with a fine cotton interfacing. The interfacing acts as a stay and prevents the buttonhole from stretching out of shape during use.

   ***Tip**: I like to use the lightweight German woven, cotton iron-on interfacing for all my heirloom and fine machine sewing projects – I have tested it over a long period an have had no problems.*

2. Refer to the pattern you are planning to use and check the size of the button.

   The distance between the center front or center back and the foldline for the facing (or lining) will be at least equal to the diameter of the button.

   If the button is too big for this "lap" area it will hang over the edge of the fold when the garment is fastened together. Conversely, if the button is too small the lap will appear to flap open beside the button.

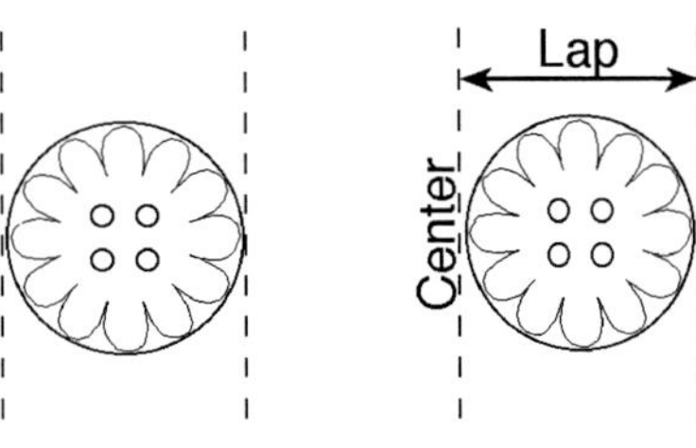
Lap
Center
Foldline

   If the button size is changed from the pattern specification, the space between the button position line and the finished edge of the garment must be changed accordingly. This space must always measure the diameter of the button, or <u>at least</u> three-quarters of that diameter.

   Note: Continue to be ever mindful of center front or center back as the case may be.

   If the button size is larger, add to the garment edge; if smaller, subtract.

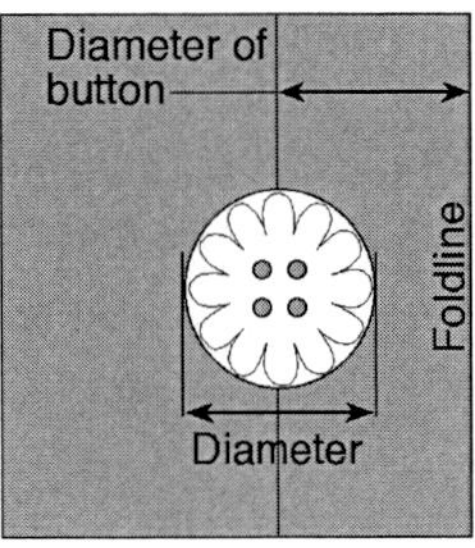
Diameter of
button
Foldline
Diameter

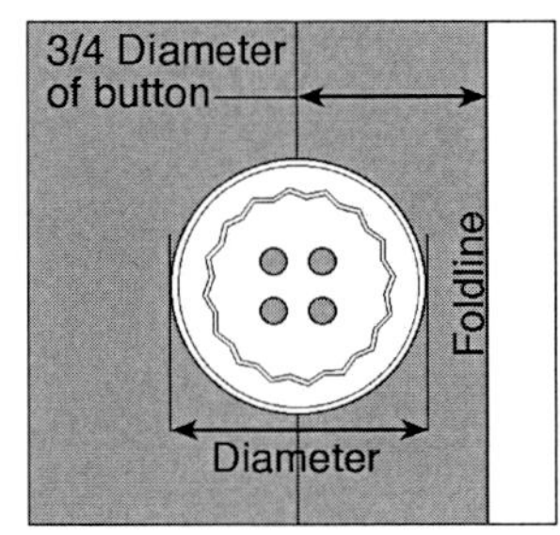
3/4 Diameter
of button
Foldline
Diameter

3. The placement of the buttonhole is the same whether it is made by hand or machine. For children's clothing in particular, always make the buttonholes in the direction of the greatest strain so the garment won't come unfastened too easily.

Horizontal buttonholes are the most secure, therefore used on most garments. When buttoned, the pull of the closure is absorbed by the end of the buttonhole, with very little distortion. These buttonholes are positioned to extend a scant ⅛" (3mm) beyond the button placement line.

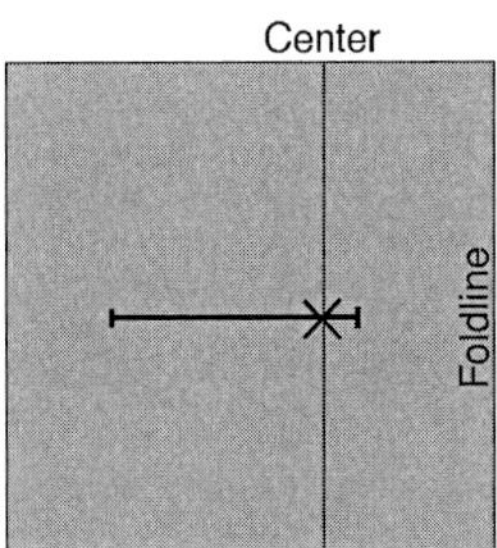
Center
Foldline

Vertical buttonholes are most often used with a placket or button band, such as on a shirt, or the shoulder buttons on a petticoat, pinafore or overalls. They are placed directly on the button placement line and the top of the buttonhole is ⅛" (3mm) above the mark for the center of the button.

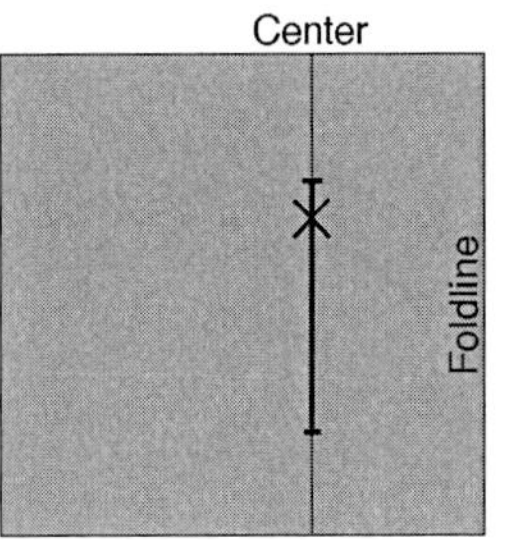
Center
Foldline

4. The direction of lap varies from girls to boys, and whether the garment is front or back buttoning. The guidelines below will help you determine the placement of the buttonholes; however, I believe that this is one of those rules that will not ruin the look of your garment if you inadvertently work your buttonholes on the incorrect side.

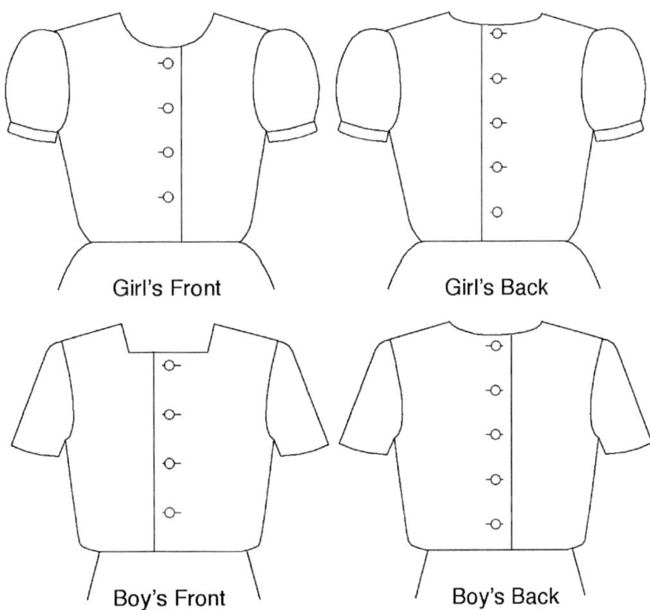
Girl's Front
Girl's Back
Boy's Front
Boy's Back

5. The size of the button has already been determined and the pattern adjusted accordingly, if necessary. It is important to make your buttonholes exactly the right length, so that they allow the button to pass through easily, yet hold the garment securely closed.

   The length of the buttonhole opening should equal the diameter of the button plus its height. Because of the bar tacks that are necessary at each end of a worked buttonhole, you should add a scant ⅛" (3mm) to the calculation for the actual length of the opening.

   An easy method for determining the length of the buttonhole for a flat button being worked on fine fabric is to place the button on a piece of paper and, with a sharp pencil, make a dot on each side of the button. Remove the button and measure the distance between the dots. Since the pencil marks are a little wider than the button, this a good starting point to which you will add the scant ⅛" (3mm) for buttonhole finishing.

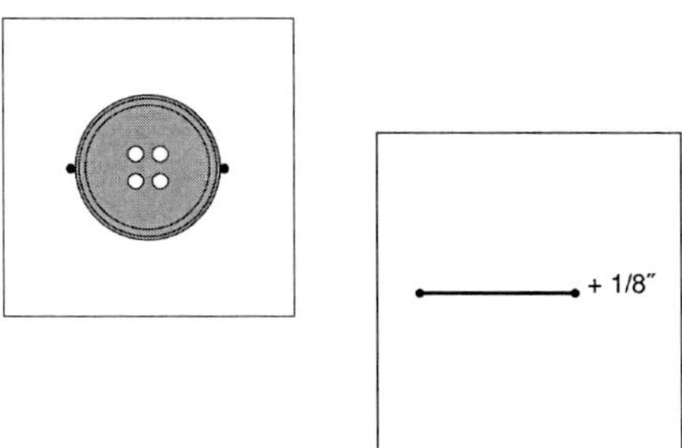
+ 1/8"

6. There are various ways in which a machine-worked buttonhole may be made. The best advice is to refer to your sewing machine manual and make a sample, and another, and another; 'playing' with the settings until you achieve the size and look you want. The following hints may help you reach the point where you are no longer afraid of buttonholes.

   - Determine whether you need a simple rectangular buttonhole, an elastic buttonhole made with the overedge stitch for stretch fabrics, a corded or reinforced buttonhole for extra durability or perhaps a keyhole buttonhole for thicker fabrics. Follow the steps in your machine manual to make a sample.
   - Always stitch your practice machine-worked buttonholes on the same fabric and number of layers as you have used for the garment.
   - Determine whether or not the buttonhole placement is suitable for using the automatic buttonhole attachment.

     ***Tip**: I find it almost impossible to use the automatic buttonhole attachment on areas where the foot will ride over two different thicknesses of fabric – e.g. at the neckline next to a binding or collar, and at the yoke or waistline where there are gathers on one side of the seam. Use the basic buttonhole foot in these instances.*

   - Although working the buttonhole on three layers of fabric, on fine fabrics it often helps to maintain stability and stop the fabric from puckering if you place a length of tracing paper (not heavier bond paper) underneath the fabric. This is easily pulled away from the buttonholes once you have completed the set.
   - Buttonholes are opened only after stitching of the full set is completed.

     Place pins at each end of the buttonhole opening to prevent cutting through the bar tacks. Slit the fabric down the center of the buttonhole. Use a seam ripper and not scissors to cut open a worked buttonhole.

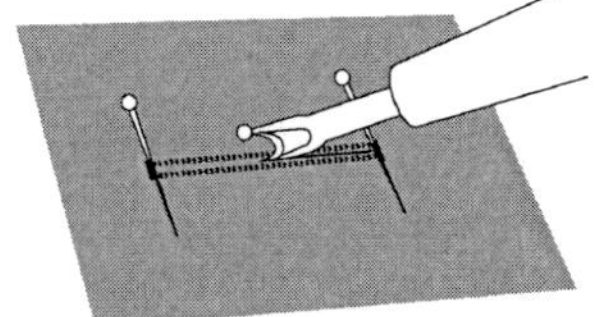

     Alternately, use a buttonhole chisel and a wooden block to cut the buttonholes. For buttonholes larger than ⅜" (1 cm) this is a one-step motion that makes a very clean cut.

7. Because of their odd shape or thickness, there are many 'fun' buttons that are better used as decoration. They are too hard to button and require an oversized buttonhole, and should be attached to the garment on top of a press stud (snap) or hook and eye.

LAPPED ZIPPER

The lapped zipper, although more time consuming than the centered zipper, gives a more professional closing and a truly hidden zipper.

A lapped zipper is applied the same way regardless of garment type; the only variable is in the placement of the zipper in relation to the garment edge. If there will be a facing finish, place the top stop *⅜" (1 cm) below* the seamline. If the garment will have a binding, waist band or standing collar, place the top stop *just below* the seamline.

Use the following guidelines to achieve correct results when putting in a zipper.

- Allow at least 7/8" (2.2 cm) seam allowance for the zipper when cutting out garment
- Work from the bottom to the top on all steps; this will ensure there are no bubbles at the end of the zipper
- Do all work on the inside of the garment, except topstitching

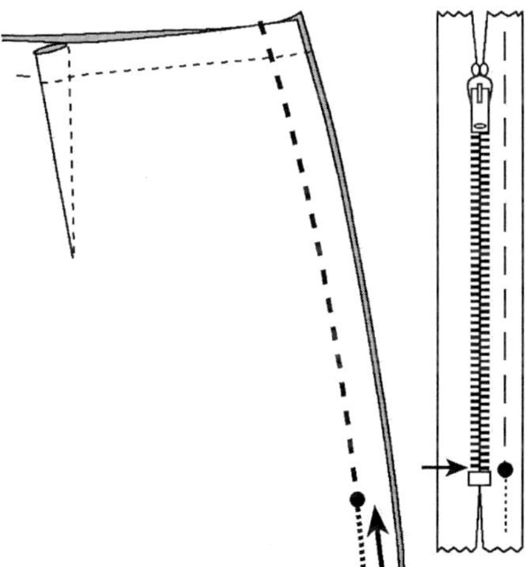

Measure the length of the zipper from the bottom of the zipper teeth to the top of the zipper tape and mark the bottom of the placket opening on the garment. Stitch the seam from the lower edge of the garment up to the bottom of the zipper placket, with a regular stitch length. Lock off the seam with tiny stitches – do not cut the threads.

Change to machine basting stitch length for the placket and continue stitching to the top of garment.

Meld the stitches and press the seam open.

To position the zipper, extend one of the seam allowances and place the zipper on it face down, with the top stop at the pre-determined position and the zipper teeth almost on the seamline. Pin the zipper, placing pins perpendicular to zipper teeth.

This extended seam is on the *right-hand* side for **boys** and *left-hand* side for **girls**.

Baste in the center of the zipper tape in the seam allowance only, keeping the garment free.

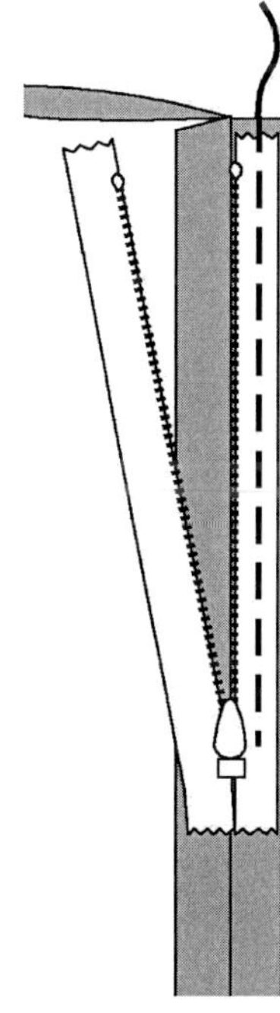

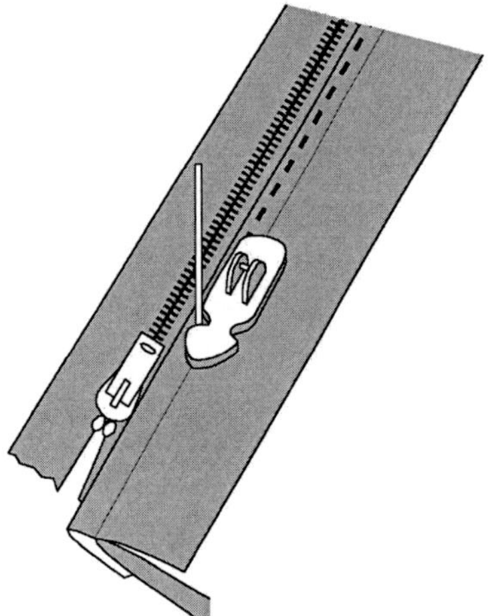

Close the zipper and turn the wrong side of the garment facing up, forming a fold in the seam allowance – the wrong side of the garment is facing up and the zipper is extended.

Bring the fold close to, but not over, the zipper teeth. Pin perpendicular to the zipper teeth if necessary. Stitch close to the fold through all thicknesses, to the top of the tape.

Turn the garment to the right side and spread the fabric as flat as possible over the unstitched zipper tape. Pin or baste into position about ⅜" (1 cm) from the seamline. This should place the basting close to the stitching guide line on the zipper tape.

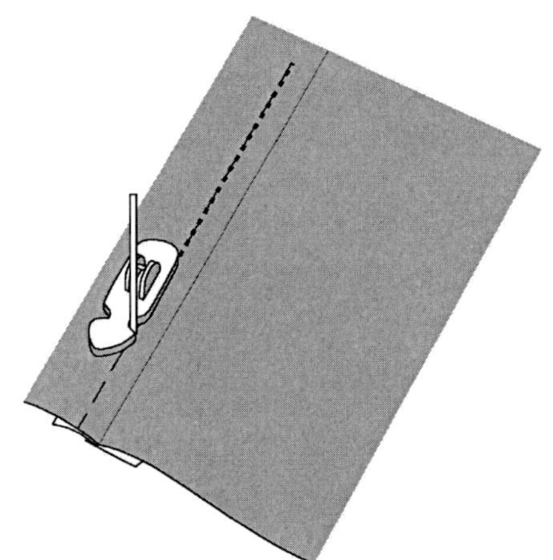

With the needle in the right-hand position and using the zipper foot, topstitch close to the basting, from the bottom to the top. Meld the stitches

Bring the thread ends to the underside and tie securely. Remove the basting stitches.

Open the zipper placket by clipping the original basting threads just above the locking stitches and removing the machine basting in the seam.

***Tip**: Tweezers are helpful for getting out any stubborn thread ends.*

Press the lapped zipper toward the fold. Do not press with up and down strokes or you will produce wrinkles.

Finish the top edge of the garment with an appropriate finish – facing, collar, or waistband – as the pattern directs.

BASIC YOKE DRESS ALTERATIONS

(for increased smocking fullness at front)

The following guidelines may be of assistance in maintaining ample fullness when working with fabric that is not wide enough to accommodate smocking pleats. In other words, the back yoke will be extended and redrawn to include the underneath and part of the front armhole.

From a visual point it is preferable not to remove large numbers of pleats at each end of the smocked panel to accommodate lack of fullness. Instead, smock the full width of fabric leaving a seam allowance at each end. The pattern will now be adapted to allow this smocked panel to be positioned between the armholes and the back yoke and skirt extended to meet the front smocked panel.

Using a basic square yoke pattern, alter the pattern as follows:

- Trace off the back bodice pattern piece and add the button/buttonhole facing extension to the back foldline. This will eliminate the need for double bodices.

  Tip*: The extension being added will need to be more than twice the diameter of the button (or center to fold line) – I would suggest three times the button diameter plus extra to turn a narrow hem. Refer to the techniques for* ***Making a Narrow Hem****.*

  Square across at right angles from the Facing Line to the Underarm Seam line. Square off from this point down to the waist, or finished smocking depth. This will add extra width to the waist but that fullness can be pulled in by the ties. The reason for squaring off at this point is to have the front of this extended bodice on the same straight of grain as the front smocked panel.

- Determine the finished back waist depth needed – e.g. short waisted or natural waistline. Square off again from the Back Facing line at the waistline (or bottom of dropped yoke depth) through to the front.

- Lap the front blocking guide seamline over the back yoke seamline at the underarm point.

- Square off again from the seamline on the front blocking guide (at the point where the yoke seam meets the armhole) down to the waistline. Add a seam allowance to this line and the waistline.

- Trace off the complete extended Back Yoke pattern piece.

- Pleat the number of rows required to the depth of this guide. Measure from seamline to seamline on the yoke edge of the guide. Allow for 5/8" (1.5 cm) seam allowances at each end and block the pleated fabric to this measurement.

1. Square off at underarm point down to waist
2. Lap the front blocking guide to the side seam on the stitching line, matching the underarm point
3. Square off a line from the seamline point 2 on the front. Add the seam allowance
4. Mark a notch at the underarm side seam for matching the sleeve seam
5. Your smocking then meets at the seamline of yoke and armhole
6. Measure across the top of blocking guide seamline to seamline. Block the pleated area to this width, leaving 2-3 pleats for seam allowance.

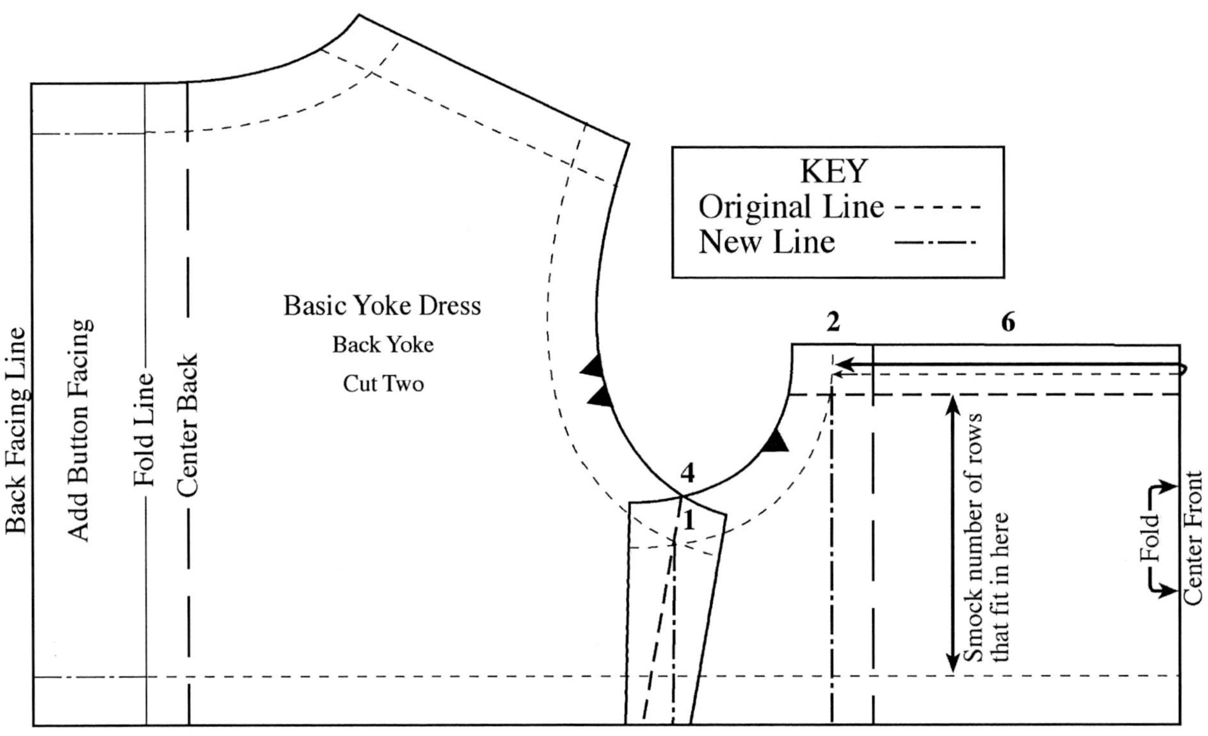

KEY
Original Line - - - - -
New Line —·—·
Basic Yoke Dress
Back Yoke
Cut Two
Back Facing Line
Add Button Facing
Fold Line
Center Back
2
6
4
1
Smock number of rows that fit in here
Fold
Center Front

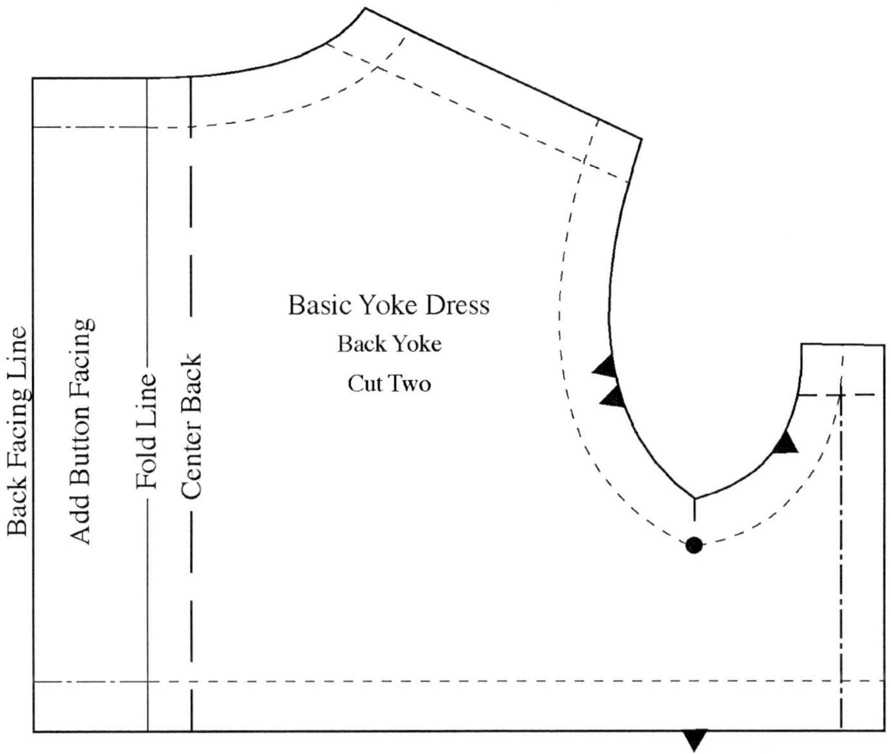
Basic Yoke Dress
Back Yoke
Cut Two
Back Facing Line
Add Button Facing
Fold Line
Center Back
Revised Extended Back Yoke

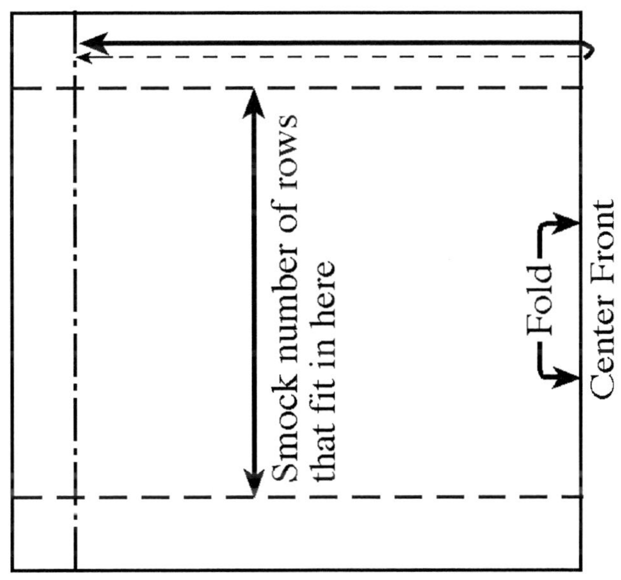
Smock number of rows
that fit in here
Fold
Center Front

Bibliography

All About Cotton – A Fabric Dictionary & Swatchbook, Julie Parker
Rain City Publishing, Seattle, WA, 1993

Antique Clothing – French Sewing by Machine, Martha Campbell Pullen, PH.D.
Published by Martha Pullen Company, Inc., Huntsville, AL, 1990

Childrenswear Design, Hilde Jaffe and Rosa Rosa
Published by Fairchild Publications, New York, NY, 1979

Couture – The Art of Fine Sewing, Roberta Carr
Published by Palmer/Pletsch Incorporated, Portland, OR, 1993

Couture Sewing Techniques, Claire B. Shaeffer,
Published by The Taunton Press, Newtown, CT, 1994

Creative Needle magazine
Published by Creative Needle, Lookout Mountain, GA

Exquisite Embroidery, Jennifer Newman
Published by Sally Milner Publishing Pty. Ltd., Australia, 1993

Fine Machine Sewing, Carol Laflin Ahles
Published by The Taunton Press, Inc., Newtown, CT, 2001

Mimi's Machine Heirloom Sewing, Mildred Turner
Published by Mimi's Smock Shoppe, Inc., Waynesville, NC, 1987

Patternmaking for Fashion Design, Helen Joseph Armstrong
Published by Harper Collins Publishers, New York, NY, 1995

Reader's Digest Complete Guide to Sewing
Published by The Reader's Digest Association (Canada) Ltd., 1995

Sew Beautiful magazine
Published by Martha Pullen Company, Huntsville, AL

The Complete Book of Sewing for Children, Elizabeth Travis Johnson
Albright & Company, Huntsville, AL 1990

The Vogue/Butterick Step-by-Step Guide to Sewing Techniques
Published by Simon & Schuster, New York, NY, 1989

Threads magazine
Published by The Taunton Press, Newtown, CT

About the Author

Lyn Weeks, was born in New South Wales, Australia and lived most of her life in Sydney. Lyn and her husband, Brian, have one son, Gregory, one daughter, Melanie, and a daughter-in-law, Rachael. Lyn and Brian have now resided in Illinois for the past ten years, following a business move in 1995.

In 1980 Lyn commenced her small business, *Melanie Jane*, designing and sewing for quality baby and children's boutiques around Australia. As the winner of Australia's first international smocking competition in 1989, the opportunity arose for Lyn to continue her passion for smocking and fine machine sewing by changing her business focus towards teaching. Although Lyn's business interests are still excited and fueled primarily by a classroom of fine needlework enthusiasts she has, once again, added another dimension to her activities. In 2000 Lyn produced her first pattern for commercial sale and, to date, successfully markets a range of ten patterns for baby, children and adult wear with the draft of "the next one" always on the drawing board.

In 1993 Lyn was instrumental in founding Australia's first Smocking Guild, joined the Smocking Arts Guild of America (SAGA) in 1994 and became a charter member and inaugural President of the *Midwest Heirloom Stitchers* SAGA chapter in the Chicagoland area in 1997. As well as being an active member of several other sewing related groups, Lyn's time is spent preparing and conducting workshops around the United States and focusing on presenting challenging and exciting classes at the SAGA National Convention each year – a continuous invitation since 1999.

Lyn has been published numerous times in *Australian Smocking and Embroidery*, *Inspirations*, *Sew Beautiful* and *Creative Needle* magazines. She has won awards in SAGA's *Design Show* and *Show and Share* competitions, including a *People's Choice* award for heirloom sewing.

Although excited at the prospect of a new pattern, enthusiastic about a forthcoming workshop or content in front of a sewing machine, Lyn will still always leap at the opportunity of becoming a student whenever possible and learning from someone else to help improve her own skills. With Lyn's admission of being "too much of a perfectionist", her most recent study focus has been five full days of concentrated *Fine Whitework Embroidery*, including *Ayrshire Embroidery*, at the Royal School of Needlework in 2003, 2004 and again in 2005. The exacting nature of this type of needlework excites new design thoughts, while at the same time, tests the eyesight.

Lyn Weeks
www.lynweeks.com

Notes

Notes

Notes

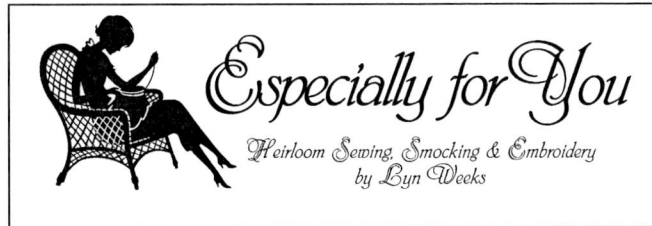

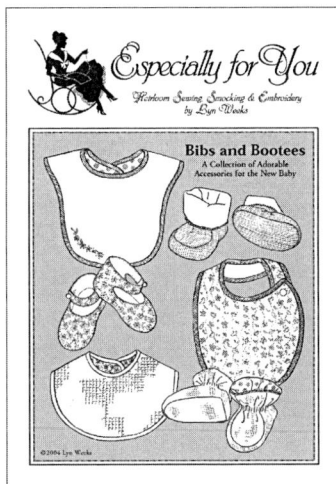

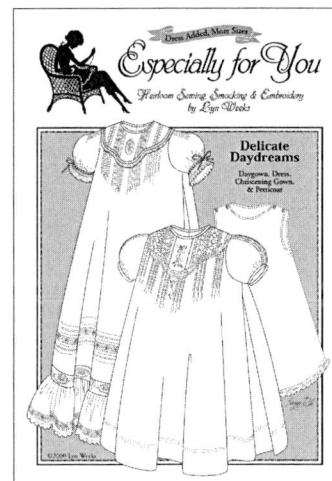

EDWARDIAN BABY
Daygown and Petticoat

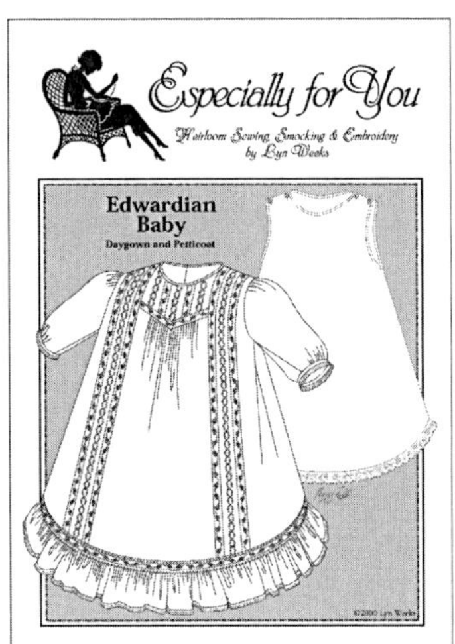

Especially for You
Edwardian
Baby
Daygown and Petticoat

There is nothing more exciting than finding an old garment and studying the detail to create something new. Using our needlework talents we provide a link to the past and an heirloom for the future.

The original Edwardian daygown was found dirty, wrinkled and in need of repair at a flea market in Illinois. It was clearly 'homemade' using inexpensive fabric, but it had a charm which reminds us of an era when mothers sewed for their children not only to save money, but for the love of creating something to be admired and passed on to the next generation.

The pattern for reproducing this garment incorporates an inverted underarm pleat that adds fullness to the garment and a long sleeve, the style of which dates back to the nineteenth century. The pattern also includes a short sleeve variation and a petticoat.

This Pattern includes sizes ***3 months, 6 months*** *and* ***12 months****.*

GABRIELLE
Dolman Sleeve Daygown, Dress, Jacket and Petticoat

'Gabrielle', is the result of inspiration from several vintage dolman-sleeve garments collected from flea markets, antique stores and estate sales. The simplicity of the pattern makes it perfect for a relatively quick project or allows capacity for a wide variety of design lines incorporating such heirloom techniques as pintucks and insertion of laces and embroidery.

The pattern incorporates a baby daygown, a front or back buttoning dress in two lengths with empire-line yoke and a dainty jacket to complete the ensemble. All garments can be made with either long or short sleeves. The matching A-line petticoat buttons on the shoulder.

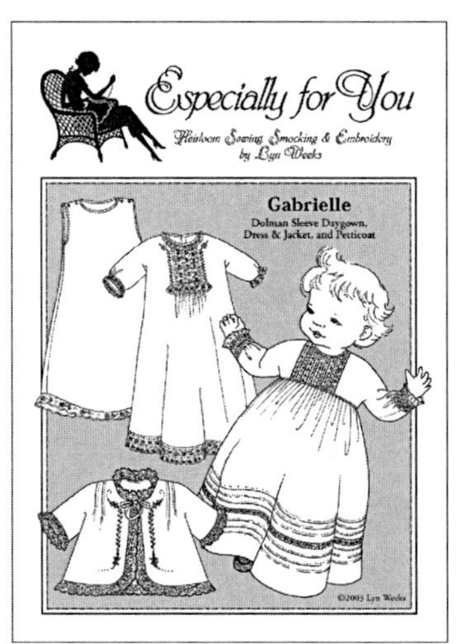

Especially for You
Gabrielle

This pattern includes sizes ***Preemie, 3 months, 6 months, 12 months*** *and* ***18 months****.*

FRANNIE
Toddler's Pocket Dress

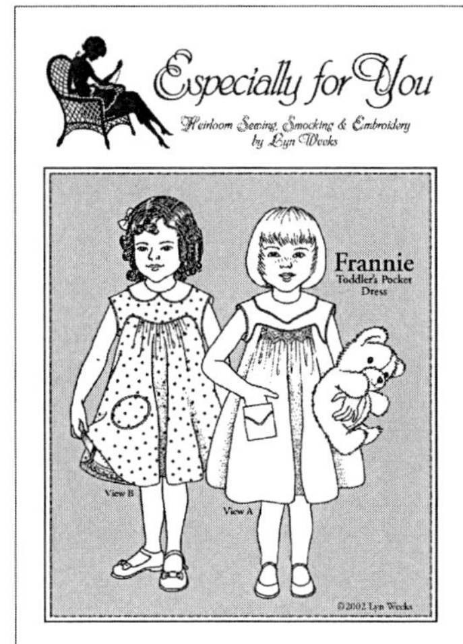

Especially for You
Heirloom Sewing, Smocking & Embroidery
by Lyn Weeks
Frannie
Toddler's Pocket Dress
View B
View A
©2002 Lyn Weeks

Children's garments from the early part of the twentieth century have a homemade and well-loved appeal, being creative in design but without the lavish use of expensive trim and embellishment.

***'Frannie'**, an adaptation of a 1930's garment, has been drafted to reflect this simplicity. The curved front yoke, which incorporates a small sleeve cap to protect delicate shoulders from the sun, buttons at the back and is piped to highlight the design line. The neckline can be embellished with a binding only or may include your choice of collar style. The skirt can be smocked or just gathered, with the added feature of one of the included pocket styles.*

There is also a pattern for a petticoat.

*This pattern includes sizes **6 months – 4 years**.*

FRANNIE'S BIG SISTER
Girls Cap Sleeve Dress

***'Frannie's Big Sister'** is drafted with the same cap-sleeve feature as the smaller-size 'Frannie' pattern. There is ample opportunity to embellish the curved yoke and hemline of this garment with heirloom techniques, and the garment can either be smocked or gathered-only for less fullness.*

There is also a pattern for a petticoat.

As an added bonus:
Drafted to the same design lines, the envelope also includes the pattern for a matching dress to fit an 18" Girl Doll (this pattern is also available separately).

*This pattern includes sizes **5 – 8 years.***

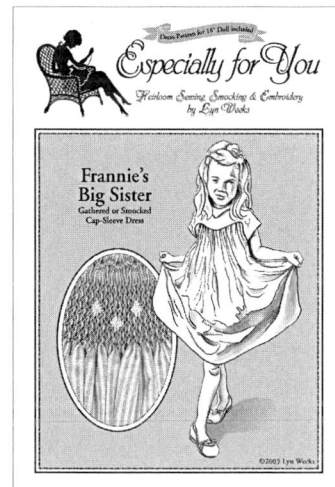

Especially for You
Heirloom Sewing, Smocking & Embroidery
by Lyn Weeks
Frannie's
Big Sister
Gathered or Smocked
Cap-Sleeve Dress
©2003 Lyn Weeks

All Patterns available at www.lynweeks.com

AMANDA

Tucked Heirloom Blouse

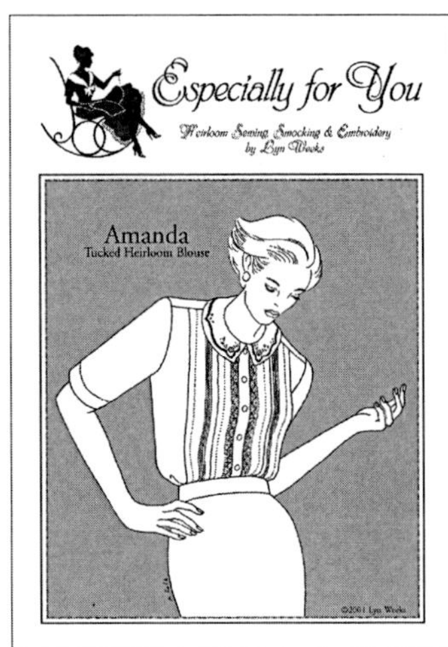
Especially for You
Heirloom Sewing Smocking & Embroidery
by Lyn Weeks
Amanda
Tucked Heirloom Blouse

Every woman's wardrobe should include a classic linen blouse with just enough "heirloom" detailing to make it feminine. This blouse is equally at home with a pair of denim jeans or a tailored straight skirt, which means it may spend more time out of your closet than in it.

The pattern for reproducing the 'Amanda' blouse features a yoke that comes forward of the shoulder and incorporates small pleats on the back bodice for added fullness. The collar, which can be embroidered or left plain, has a gentle roll and sits just below the collarbone. This pattern also includes a long or short sleeve version, plus guidelines for the heirloom sewing techniques used in the construction of the blouse.

*This pattern includes sizes **8 – 18.***

BRONWYN

Dolman Sleeve Blouse

There is nothing more exciting than having a pattern as versatile as this dolman sleeve blouse. The design detail on both the short and long sleeve versions is understated, yet sparks the imagination for a variety of other embellishments such as piping, entredeux, tucks and embroidery.

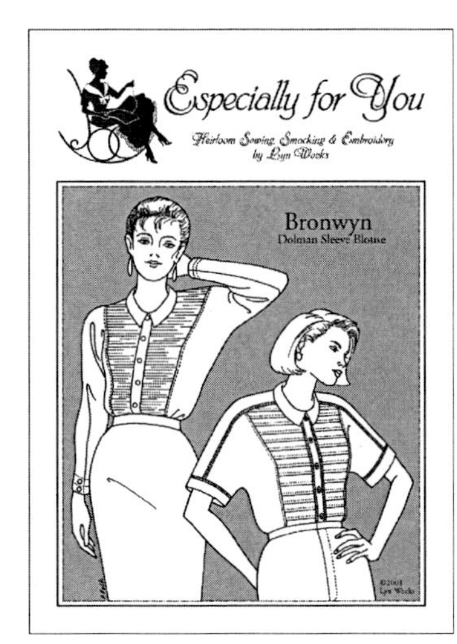
Especially for You
Heirloom Sewing Smocking & Embroidery
by Lyn Weeks
Bronwyn
Dolman Sleeve Blouse

A dolman sleeve blouse allows freedom of movement without the restrictions of a set-in sleeve, and is comfortable and simple to construct.

The long sleeve on this blouse is secured at the wrist with a mock cuff that is buttoned to fit, while the short sleeve version tapers to a cuff band. The collar has a full stand at the back neck, but sits fairly open at the front below the collarbone.

*This pattern includes sizes **8-18**.*

MELANIE
Round Yoke Heirloom Nightgown

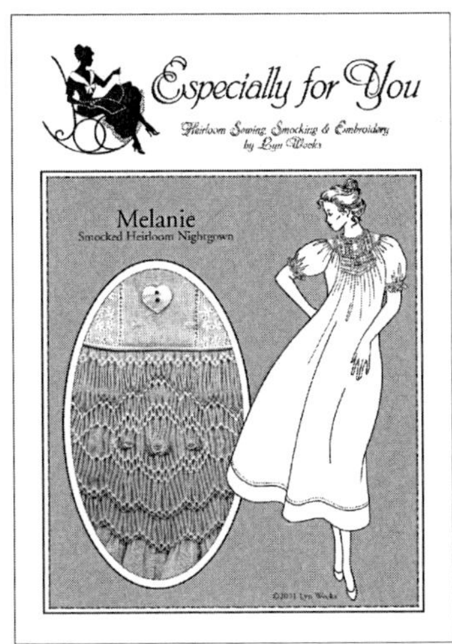
Especially for You
Melanie
Smocked Heirloom Nightgown

If pampering products like rose water, aromatherapy, and herbal tea are the pleasures that help you wind down after a hectic day, take these little indulgences a step further by slipping into something utterly elegant. An heirloom nightgown is the crowning comfort.

The round yoke works up beautifully in a selection of laces and embroideries, or perhaps with the inclusion of hand embroidery or tucks on inserted fabric. For a last-minute gift, this design would look just as pretty if made with gathers on both the front and back instead of the smocking.

There are also three sleeve variations, long, short or capped.

*This pattern includes sizes **Petite** (4-6) to **Ex. Large** (20-22).*

FRANNIE'S DOLL
Dress for 18" Girl Doll

Although included with the pattern for 'Frannie's Big Sister' the doll dress, which was inspired by Angela Pfaff, is also sold separately.

All Material Requirements, Cutting Layouts and Instructions are included in this one-size pattern that can either be smocked or gathered-only if you choose.

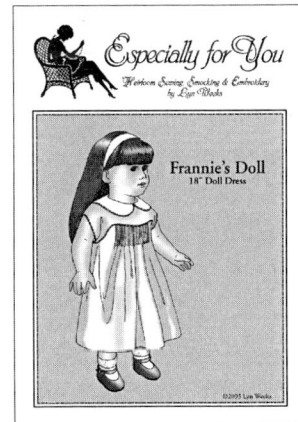
Especially for You
Frannie's Doll
18" Doll Dress

DELICATE DAYDREAMS SUPPLEMENT
Preemie Size Daygown, Dress and Christening Gown

This is a Supplement to the Delicate Daydreams pattern, drafted to the same design lines in one size only. This Preemie-size pattern will fit a baby weighing 3-7 pounds and a length of 18-20 inches.

The Preemie Supplement includes Material Requirements and the Cutting Layout but, as a supplement pattern, is designed to be used in conjunction with the Delicate Daydreams pattern containing the construction guidelines.

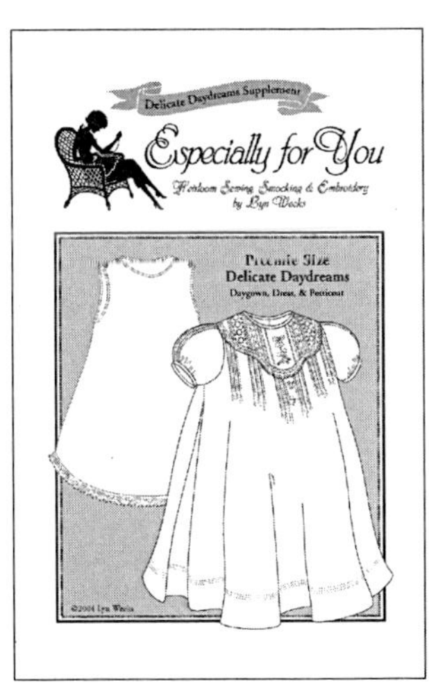
Delicate Daydreams Supplement
Especially for You
Preemie Size
Delicate Daydreams

Notes